MICROBIOLOGY

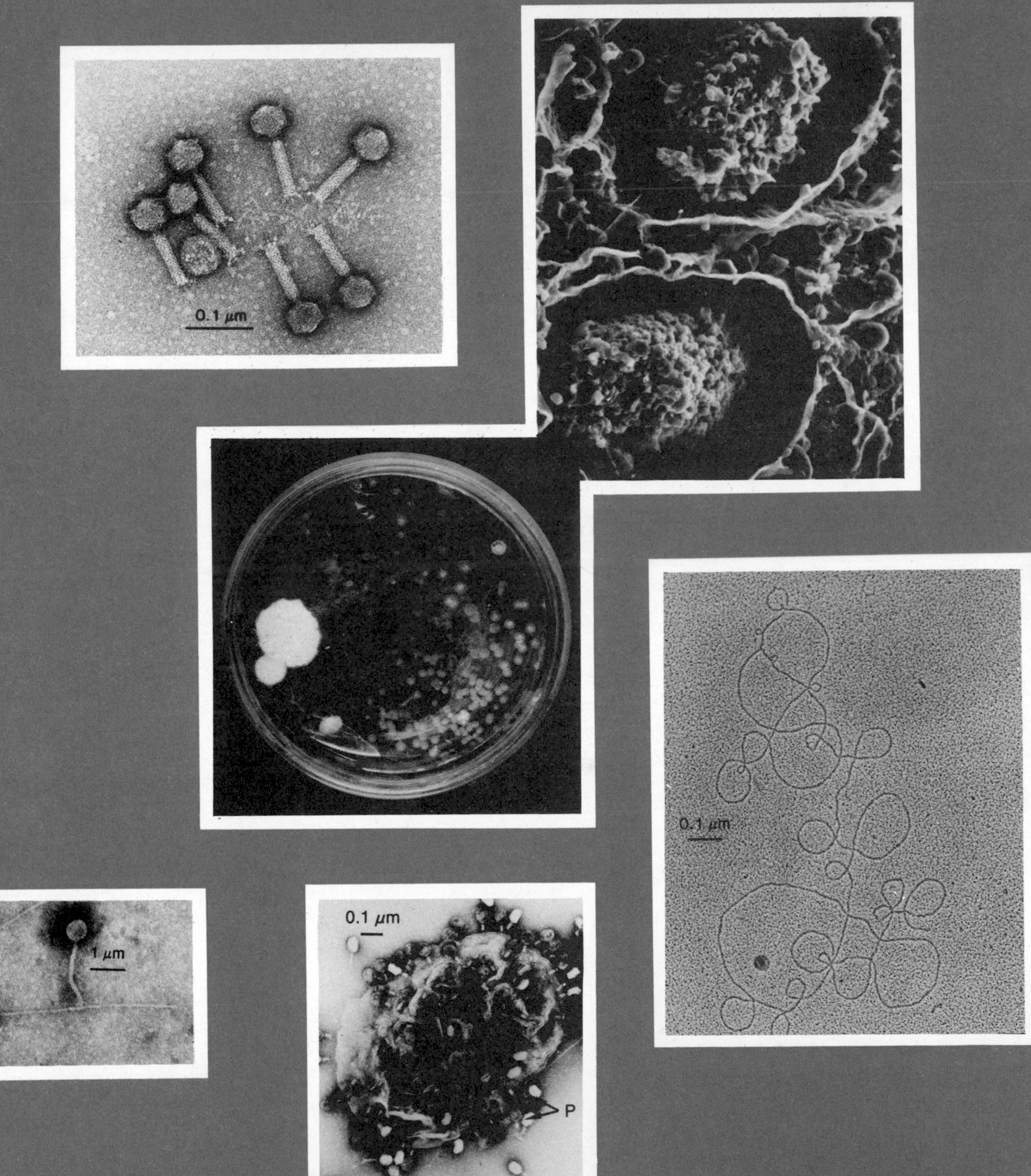
0.1 μm
0.1 μm
1 μm
0.1 μm
P

MICROBIOLOGY

THIRD EDITION

George A. Wistreich

EAST LOS ANGELES COLLEGE

Max D. Lechtman

GOLDEN WEST COLLEGE

Glencoe Publishing Co., Inc.
Encino, California
Collier Macmillan Publishers
London

To our families, whose encouragement, patience,
and sacrifices helped to make this book possible

Cover photo of *Mycobacterium phlei* courtesy of A. L. Vestal, Center for Disease Control, Atlanta, Georgia

Part-opening photos: Part 1, courtesy Chas. Pfizer & Co.; Part 2, from Paerl, H. W., *Microbial Ecology* 4:215–231 (1978); Part 3, courtesy of BioQuest, Division of Becton, Dickinson, and Company; Part 4, courtesy Dr. K. E. Muse, North Carolina State University; Part 5, from Tawara, J., et al., *Journal of Electron Microscopy* 25:37–38 (1976); Part 6, courtesy of The Taylor Wine Company.

Printed in the United States of America

Glencoe Publishing Co., Inc.
17337 Ventura Boulevard
Encino, California 91316
Collier Macmillan Canada, Ltd.

Library of Congress Catalog Card Number: 78-71751

1 2 3 4 5 6 7 8 9 10 83 82 81 80 79

ISBN 0-02-470910-7

Preface

Microbiology is designed for an introductory microbiology course. We assume that most students using this text will be somewhat like our students: they will have had some exposure to biology or chemistry, but not necessarily to both; they will not, however, be comfortable with sophisticated applications of either. They are also students who need a thorough grounding in the basic concepts and principles of microbiology and in some of the applications of these concepts to human disease, the environment, and industrial processes.

In a text intended for an introductory course, it is impractical, as well as inappropriate, to treat every facet of microbiology in detail. The intent of the fourth edition of *Microbiology* is to give beginning students a framework on which to build their knowledge. Basic principles and concepts are emphasized. We have also attempted to do justice to today's student by including some of the recent developments in microbiology, both theoretical and applied.

Organization of the Text

Microbiology is organized into six parts. The first three parts concentrate on basic principles, while the last three treat more sophisticated aspects of microbiology and its applications. The arrangement of the parts and of the chapters within the parts allows for flexibility in the use of the text, so that instructors are free to design a course that meets the particular needs of their students.

Part 1, "An Introduction to Microbiology," begins with an overview of microbiology as a discipline. This first chapter includes a discussion of the scientific method and of some of the challenges for microbiology in the near future. Chapter 2 gives the student a brief introduction to the historical development of microbiology, and Chapter 3 introduces the principles of classification and gives a brief survey of microorganisms. Chapter 4 discusses techniques for preparing specimens for most types of microscopy. For students whose background in biochemistry is limited, Chapter 5 provides a brief introduction to those biochemical principles needed to understand the chemical composition and life processes of microorganisms.

Part 2, "The World of Microorganisms," provides a comprehensive overview of the microbial world. The first chapter in this part reviews the cellular structure of higher-level animals and plants to provide students who have little or no background in cell biology with a frame of reference and basis for comparison.

Students who have fulfilled a biology prerequisite can usually skip this chapter. The next two chapters, 7 and 8, discuss and survey bacteria. This is followed by chapters 9 through 12, which focus on the structures, functions, and ecology of fungi, protozoa, algae, and viruses.

The basic principles and processes of microbial growth, metabolism, and genetics are discussed in chapters 13 through 15. Chapter 13 covers basic bacterial cultivation techniques, while chapter 14 includes some of the newer ideas about cellular regulation. Chapter 15, "Microbial Genetics," includes a section on genetic engineering and its implications. Part 2 concludes with chapters 16 and 17, which cover environmental microbiology, including the interrelationships among microbes in various environments and their involvement in the chemical cycles of life.

Part 3, "The Control of Microorganisms," discusses chemical and physical means of controlling microorganisms—topics of great practical significance. Both basic principles and particular techniques are presented. New developments are included—for example, chemotherapeutic control of fungi and viruses and techniques for determining the effectiveness of such chemotherapeutic agents.

Part 4, "Principles of Immunology," presents the concepts of immunology and some of their applications. Chapter 21 is devoted to the defense mechanisms of a host against disease agents. Chapter 22 discusses microbial virulence, and chapters 23 and 24 characterize antigens and antibodies and the techniques for their isolation, identification, and application. Chapter 25 discusses immunologic disorders, and Chapter 26 discusses immunizing materials, their preparation, administration, and side effects.

Part 5, "Microorganisms and Infectious Diseases," begins with chapters 27 and 28, which set the stage for the following chapters by giving the student a thorough introduction to the principles of disease transmission and the procedures used to identify microorganisms in the laboratory. Chapters 29 through 35 apply these basic ideas to a survey of microbial diseases of specific human tissues and organ systems. Chapter 36 discusses the relationship between microorganisms and cancer. Part 5 concludes with Chapter 37 on helminthic infections.

Part 6, "Microorganisms and Industrial Processes," begins with Chapter 38 on the role of microorganisms in the preparation of various industrial products. Chapter 39 discusses the role of microorganisms in food preparation, including wine and cheese making, and in food spoilage. The concluding chapter discusses the microbiology of soil and water and of waste treatment.

Features of the Third Edition

We have used the suggestions of many instructors as guidelines for a number of changes in the text. Foremost among these changes is the reorganization of the chapters on the structure, function, cultivation, and growth of microorganisms. These topics are now discussed according to the groups of microorganisms: bacteria, fungi, protozoa, algae, and viruses. Applied and environmental microbiology receive greatly expanded treatment, with two chapters on microbial ecology (chapters 16 and 17) and three on industrial microbiology (chapters 38, 39, and 40). Historical material has been deemphasized to make way for increased emphasis on basic concepts.

The review of biochemistry has been placed earlier in the text (Chapter 5), so students will be able to use this background in subsequent chapters. The material on metabolism, genetics, and immunology has been completely revised to reflect the latest thinking in these areas. Material on current research in immunology, virology, and cancer has been included.

In addition, the entire text has been updated and rewritten for greater clarity and readability. The physical layout of the text has also been completely reworked to accommodate the hundreds of two-color diagrams and black-and-white photographs that illustrate the text. Sixteen pages of full-color photographs show students the true appearance of microorganisms, disease states, and some important reactions. This is especially useful for students who do not have the benefits of a microbiology laboratory.

Learning Aids

The text includes a number of learning aids designed to help students absorb, review, and retain its content. Each chapter begins with a chapter overview which briefly describes the topics to be covered. This is followed by a list of learning objectives preceding the chapter text. Within the chapter, summarizing tables reinforce what the student has learned, and diagrams and photographs illustrate the ideas presented in the text. Key words printed in bold type help the student retain important vocabulary.

Each chapter concludes with a Summary in outline form and Questions for Review, including a photographic quiz. An annotated bibliography follows each chapter.

The Glossary at the end of the text contains definitions for all of the key words. The appendices contain classification schemes for bacteria, fungi, protozoa, algae, viruses, and helminths. The classification for bacteria follows that in *Bergey's Manual.*

Supplementary Materials

Study Guide to Accompany Microbiology, by George A. Wistreich and David W. Smith, contains vocabulary lists, review of important concepts, two self-tests for each chapter of the text, and enrichment sections.

Tests to Accompany Microbiology contains two equivalent objective tests of twenty-five questions each for each chapter of the text. Answers to all test questions are included. This package is available gratis to adopting instructors.

Instructor's Manual to Accompany Microbiology, also available gratis to adopting instructors, contains lists of current audiovisual materials with their sources, references for each chapter and general references, discussion questions for each chapter, and teaching suggestions.

Laboratory Exercises in Microbiology, Fourth Edition, contains fifty-two laboratory experiments that can be used either in conjunction with the text or independently. Specific laboratory procedures are explained by step-by-step diagrams, and concepts learned in the laboratory are reinforced by post-lab questions and photographic quizzes. Color photographs showing characteristic properties of microorganisms and experimental results are included in a separate section. An accompanying Instructor's Manual offers the instructor resources and suggestions for effective use of the Laboratory Manual.

Acknowledgments

This edition of *Microbiology* was greatly influenced by the many enthusiastic comments of students and by the wise guidance and counsel offered by many instructors and professionals—in particular, the comments of the reviewers whose names follow this preface. The authors are greatly indebted to these people, as well as to the many users of the Second Edition—too numerous to mention here—who contributed their suggestions for improving the text.

The authors would also like to thank the many others who contributed their time and efforts, especially Caroline Eastman and Janet Greenblatt, who advised us on many matters of wording and style, and Eileen Landrum, who researched many of the bibliographies. The authors would also like to thank Tanya Mink, development editor for Glencoe, who devoted a great deal of her patience, time, and editorial expertise to our text. We are also indebted to Francis Tsui and Janis Long for the care they exercised in typing portions of the manuscript, and to Tracy Moston, Eddie Wisztreich, Phillip Wisztreich, and Reneé Wisztreich for their assistance in preparing the manuscript.

Finally, we would like to thank the many contributors here and abroad who willingly provided us with photographs and diagrams. To these people we are especially indebted.

Reviewers

Theresa Arasim
Richland College

Anne Belovich
San Diego City College

Daniel Caylor
Palm Beach Junior College

Edward DeSchuytner
Northern Essex Community College

David Donaldson
Brigham Young University

Joan Handley
University of Kansas

Dennis Huff
California State University
at Sacramento

M. Ibanez
University of New Orleans

Russell Johnson
University of Minnesota

Phillip Loh
University of Hawaii

Richard C. Mellien
Grossmont College

Diane Michael
San Diego Mesa College

Richard Perras
Hudson Valley Community College

Joan Pontney
Orange Coast College

W. Stewart Riggsby
University of Tennessee

Geraldine Ross
Bellevue Community College

Charles San Clemente
Michigan State University

Maureen A. Shiflett
University of California at Los Angeles

David Smith
University of Delaware

Patricia Vary
Northern Illinois University

Carl E. Warnes
Ball State University

Brief Contents

PART 1: INTRODUCTION TO MICROBIOLOGY 1

1: The Scope of Microbiology 2
2: Early History of Microbiology 13
3: Principles of Classification and Survey of the Microbial World 30
4: Techniques Used in the Observation of Microorganisms 48
5: Introduction to Biochemistry 77

PART 2: THE WORLD OF MICROORGANISMS 99

6: The Structures of Typical Animal and Plant Cells 100
7: The Procaryotes, Their Structures and Organization 115
8: A Survey of Procaryotes 144
9: Fungi 160
10: Protozoa 180
11: Algae 194
12: Virus Structure, Organization, and Cultivation 211
13: Bacterial Growth and Cultivation Techniques 241
Color Atlas, Section One *following page 256*
14: Microbial Metabolism and Cellular Regulation 271
15: Microbial Genetics 297
16: Microbial Ecology 322
17: The Environmental Activities of Microorganisms 339

PART 3: THE CONTROL OF MICROORGANISMS 355

18: The Use of Chemicals in Disinfection and Sterilization 356
19: Physical Methods of Microbial Control 369
20: Antimicrobial Chemotherapy 386

PART 4: PRINCIPLES OF IMMUNOLOGY 409

21: Resistance in Host-parasite Interactions 410
22: Microbial Virulence 434
23: Antigens, Immunoglobulins, and States of Immunity 448
24: Diagnostic Immunologic and Related Reactions 468
25: Immunologic Disorders 492
26: Immunization and the Control of Infectious Diseases 510
Color Atlas, Section Two *following page 512*

PART 5: MICROORGANISMS AND INFECTIOUS DISEASES 525

27: Principles of Disease Transmission 526
28: The Identification of Disease Agents 546
29: Microbial Diseases of the Skin, Nails, and Hair 560
30: Oral Microbiology 582
31: Microbial Infections of the Respiratory Tract 596
32: Microbial Diseases of the Gastrointestinal Tract 621
33: Microbial Infections of the Circulatory System 644
34: Microbial Diseases of the Reproductive and Urinary Systems 660
35: Microbial Diseases of the Central Nervous System and the Eye 681
36: Microorganisms and Cancer 702
37: Helminths and Disease 717

PART 6: MICROORGANISMS AND INDUSTRIAL PROCESSES 735

38: Industrial Microbiology 736
39: Food and Dairy Microbiology 750
40: The Microbiology of Soil and Water and Waste Treatment 764

APPENDICES A1

A: Classification Outline of Division III, the Bacteria A2
B: Classification Outline of True Fungi A6
C: Classification Outline of Medically Important Protozoa A8
D: Classification Outline of the Algae A11
E: Classification Outline of the Pathogenic Helminths A11

GLOSSARY A13

INDEX A23

Contents

PART 1: INTRODUCTION TO MICROBIOLOGY 1

Chapter 1: The Scope of Microbiology 2

The Microbial World 3
Microbiology and Its Subdivisions 4
Taxonomic Arrangement 4 *Integrative Arrangement* 6
Applied Microbiology 8
Food and Dairy Microbiology 8 *Medical Microbiology* 9
Veterinary Microbiology 9
Microbiology and the Scientific Method 9
Resources in Microbiology 10
Some Challenges for Microbiology 11
Summary 11
Questions for Review 12
Suggested Readings 12

Chapter 2: Early History of Microbiology 13

Early Development of Microbiology 14
Leeuwenhoek 14 *Pasteur* 15
The Germ Theory of Fermentation 15
Nonvitalist versus Vitalist 15 *Pasteur's Contributions to Fermentation Research* 16
The Spontaneous Generation, or Abiogenesis, Controversy 17
The Macroscopic Level 17 *The Microscopic Level: The 'War of Infusions'* 18 *Filtration Approaches* 19 *A Word of Caution* 22
Antiseptic Surgery 22
The Germ Theory of Disease 22
Koch's Postulates 23 *Rivers' Postulates* 24
Early Technical Achievements 25
Microbial Cultivation 25 *Chemotherapy* 26
The Growth of Organized Microbiology 26
Summary 27
Questions for Review 28
Suggested Readings 29

Chapter 3: Principles of Classification and Survey of the Microbial World 30

The Importance of Biological Classification 31
Natural versus Artificial Classification 31

The Naming of Organisms: The Binomial System of Nomenclature 31
Groupings in the Linnaean System 32
The Position of Microorganisms in the Living World 33
Early Bacterial Classification Schemes 33
The Five-kingdom Approach 34
A Third Kingdom: The Protista 34 *Eucaryotic and Procaryotic Cellular Organization* 34 *The Components of the Five-kingdom System* 37
A Consideration of Viruses 39
Trends in Microbial Classification 40
Numerical Taxonomy 40 *Molecular Approaches to Taxonomy* 41
The Origin of Life 41
Oparin's Theory 41 *Oparin-Haldane Concept* 41 *Fossilized Evidence* 43 *Paleomicrobiology* 43 *Bacterial Evolution* 44 *A Third Form of Life* 44
Summary 45
Questions for Review 47
Suggested Readings 47

Chapter 4: Techniques Used in the Observation of Microorganisms 48

Microscopes and Microscopy 49
Units of Measurement 49 *Properties of Light* 51
Light Microscopes 54
Bright-field Microscopy 54 *Micrometry* 57 *Specimen Preparation for Bright-field Microscopy* 57 *Dark-field Microscopy* 63 *Fluorescence Microscopy* 63 *Phase Microscopy* 64
Electron Microscopes 65
The Transmission Electron Microscope 65 *Specimen Preparation for Electron Microscopy* 69 *High-voltage Electron Microscopy* 72 *The Scanning Electron Microscope* 73
Summary 74
Questions for Review 75
Suggested Readings 76

Chapter 5: Introduction to Biochemistry 77

Basic Chemistry Review 78
Atoms: The Particles of Matter 78 *Elements* 78 *Compounds, Molecules, and Macromolecules* 78

Functional Groups 79
Oxidation-reduction 80
pH and Buffers 81
The Organic Compounds 82
Lipids 82 *Carbohydrates* 84 *Nucleic Acids* 86
Proteins 90
Summary 96
Questions for Review 97
Suggested Readings 97

PART 2: THE WORLD OF MICROORGANISMS 99

Chapter 6: The Structures of Typical Animal and Plant Cells 100
The Cell's Role in Life 101
The Cell Theory 101
Types of Cellular Organization 102
The Anatomy of Animal Cells 103
The Cell Membrane and Cytoplasm 103 *The Nucleus and Nucleolus* 104 *Internal Membrane-associated Structures* 105
Microtubules 107
Plant Cells and Tissues 109
Cell Wall 109 *Plasma Membrane* 109 *Plastids* 109
Photosynthesis 111 *Vacuoles* 111 *Inclusions* 112

Chapter 7: The Procaryotes, Their Structures and Organization 115
Bacterial Size 116
Shapes and Patterns of Arrangement 116
Structures and Functions 119
The Bacterial Surface 119 *Structures Interior to the Cell Wall* 127
Specialized Cells 132
Bacterial Endospores 133
Dormancy, Sporulation, and Germination 134
Bacterial Cysts 137
Heat-susceptible Spores, Conidia 138
Heterocysts and Akinetes 138
Summary 140
Questions for Review 141
Suggested Readings 143

Chapter 8: A Survey of Procaryotes 144

Cultivation of Bacteria 145
Representative Procaryotes 145
Heterotrophic Bacteria 148
The Mycoplasma and Related Organisms 148 *Gliding Bacteria* 149 *Sheathed Bacteria* 150 *Stalked and Budding Procaryotes (The Prosthecate Bacteria)* 150 *Spiral and Curved Bacteria* 152 *The Obligate Intracellular Procaryotes* 152
Autotrophs 155
The Phototrophs 155
Summary 158
Questions for Review 159
Suggested Readings 159

Chapter 9: Fungi 160

Distribution and Activities 161
Structure and Function 162
Molds 162 *Yeasts* 162 *Dimorphism* 165
Reproduction and Spores 165
Asexual Spores 165 *Sexual Spores* 166
The Ultrastructure of Fungi 167
Cultivation of Fungi 168
Types of Media 168 *Distinctive Mycelia* 169
Classification 169
Ascomycetes 170 *Basidiomycetes* 171 *Deuteromycetes (Fungi Imperfecti)* 172 *Oomycetes* 174 *Zygomycetes* 174 *Myxomycetes, the Slime Molds* 175
Summary 177
Questions for Review 178
Suggested Readings 179

Chapter 10: Protozoa 180

Distribution and Activities 181
Structure and Function 181
Locomotion 181 *Feeding and Digestion* 182 *Excretion and Osmoregulation* 183 *Protective Structures* 183
Trophozoites and Cysts 185
Methods of Reproduction 186
Asexual Reproduction 186 *Sexual Reproduction* 186 *Regeneration* 187
Cultivation 187

Classification 187
Ciliata 187 *Suctoria* 188 *Opalinata* 188 *Sarcodina* 188 *Mastigophora* 189 *Sporozoa* 191
Summary 192
Questions for Review 193
Suggested Readings 193

Chapter 11: Algae 194
Algae: "The Grass of the Waters" 195
Structure and Organization 196
Means of Reproduction 196
Cultivation 196
Classification 196
The Green Algae (Chlorophycophyta) 197
Structure and Organization 197 *Reproduction* 197 *Economic and Ecological Importance* 197
The Golden-brown Algae and the Diatoms (Chrysophycophyta) 198
Structure and Organization 198 *Reproduction* 200 *Economic and Ecological Importance* 200
The Euglenoids (Euglenophycophyta) 201
The Brown Algae (Phaeophycophyta) 202
Structure and Organization 202 *Reproduction* 202 *Economic Value and Importance* 202
The Dinoflagellates (Pyrrophycophyta) 203
Structure and Organization 203 *Reproduction* 203 *Economic and Ecological Importance* 203
The Red Algae (Rhodophycophyta) 204
Lichens 205
Summary 209
Questions for Review 210
Suggested Readings 210

Chapter 12: Virus Structure, Organization, and Cultivation 211
What Is a Virus? 212
Basic Structure of Extracellular Viruses 212
The Nucleic Acid of the Mature Virion 212 *The Nucleocapsid* 213 *Enveloped Viruses* 215 *Shape and Size* 215
Classification 216
Bacteriophages (Bacterial Viruses) 218
The Basic Structure of Bacteriophages 218 *Filamentous Bacteriophages* 221 *The Cultivation of Bacteriophages* 221

Enumeration of Phages 222 *Phage Typing* 222
Replication Cycle of Bacteriophages 222
Lysogeny 223 *The Lytic Cycle* 223 *Growth Curve* 225
Cyanophages 226
Cyanophage Cultivation and Enumeration 227
Animal Viruses 227
Diseases 227 *Animal Virus Replication* 227 *Animal Virus Cultivation* 230 *Tissue Culture Cultivation of Viruses* 231
Plant Viruses 234
Plant Virus Structure and Shape 234 *Plant Virus Cultivation* 234 *Plant Virus Infections* 235
Viruses of Eucaryotic Microorganisms 235
Viroids 236
Summary 238
Questions for Review 239
Suggested Readings 240

Chapter 13: Bacterial Growth and Cultivation Techniques 241
An Introduction to Bacterial Cultivation 242
Nutrition and Other Conditions for Growth 243
Heterotrophy, Autotrophy, and Hypotrophy 243
Gaseous Requirements 243 *Thermal Conditions* 244
Acidity or Alkalinity (pH) 244
Properties of Bacteriological Media 245
Nitrogen Sources 246 *Carbon and Energy Sources* 246 *Vitamins and Growth Factors* 247 *Essential Mineral Salts* 247 *Water and Osmotic Pressure* 247
Preparation of Media 248
Media Usage and Categories 248
Differential Media 249 *Selective Media* 249 *Selective and Differential Media* 250 *Other Media* 250 *Media for the Cultivation of Anaerobes* 250 *Prereduced Anaerobically Sterilized Media* 251
Inoculation and Transfer Techniques 251
Techniques for the Isolation of Pure Bacterial Cultures 254
The Pour-plate Technique 254 *The Streak-plate Technique* 254
Anaerobic Transfer 255
Conditions of Incubation 256
Aerobic Incubation 256 *Anaerobic Incubation* 256
Color Atlas, Section One *following page 256*
Biological or "Sterility Test" Cabinets 259
Bacterial Growth 259
Bacterial Growth Curve 259 *Continuous Culture* 261 *Growth on Solid Media* 262

Measurement of Growth 262
Cell Mass Determination 262 *Viable Counts* 264 *Determining Total Counts of Microorganisms* 266
Summary 268
Questions for Review 269
Suggested Readings 270

Chapter 14: Microbial Metabolism and Cellular Regulation 271
General Metabolism 272
Processes Essential to Cellular Growth and Reproduction 272
Energy Metabolism 273 *Glycolysis* 274 *Krebs (Citric Acid) Cycle* 276 *Electron Transport System* 278 *A Summary of Energy Production During Glucose Catabolism* 279
Metabolic Interrelationship of Carboyhdrates, Fats, and Proteins 280
Autotrophic and Heterotrophic Metabolism 281
Autrotrophic Microorganisms 283 *Heterotrophic Microorganisms* 284
Protein Synthesis 285
Genetic Code 285
Control and Regulation of Metabolism 288
Feedback or End-product Inhibition 288 *Operons* 289
Measurement of Metabolism 290
Simple Fermentation Tests 290 *Manometry* 291 *Oxidation-Reduction Activity* 292 *Radioisotopes* 292 *Chromatography* 293
Summary 295
Questions for Review 296
Suggested Readings 296

Chapter 15: Microbial Genetics 297
Evolution and Inheritance 298
The Chemistry of Genetics 299
DNA and Chromosomes 299 *The Chemistry of Mutations* 300
Mutations in Microorganisms 301
Microbial Experiments and the Nature of Mutation 302 *The Lederbergs' Indirect Selection Procedure* 302
Recombination in Procaryotes 304
Transformation 304 *Bacterial Conjugation* 306 *Sexduction* 307 *Transduction* 309 *Lysogenic Conversion* 310 *Plasmids* 310 *Cytoplasmic Inheritance in Eucaryotes* 311
Mapping the Bacterial Genome 313
Applications of Microbial Genetics 314

Biological Assays 314 *Genetics and Taxonomy* 315
Gene Manipulation 316
Potential Benefits 316 *Potential Hazards* 316 *Techniques* 317
Summary 320
Questions for Review 320
Suggested Readings 321

Chapter 16: Microbial Ecology 322
Basic Ecological Principles 323
The Organization of the Biosphere 323
The Components of an Ecosystem 325
The Natural Habitats of Microorganisms 328
Terrestrial Habitats 328 *Aquatic Habitats* 328
Microhabitats 329 *Microbial Habitats* 329
Microbial Interactions 329
Syntrophism 330 *Competition* 330 *Predation* 330
Symbiosis 330
Summary 337
Questions for Review 338
Suggested Readings 338

Chapter 17: The Environmental Activities of Microorganisms 339
The Life-supporting Biogeochemical Cycles 340
The Carbon Cycle 340 *The Nitrogen Cycle* 342 *The Phosphorus Cycle* 345 *The Sulfur Cycle* 346 *The Oxygen Cycle* 346
Reactions of Ecological Concern 347
Bioconversion 348 *Bioconcentration* 352
Summary 353
Questions for Review 354
Suggested Readings 354

PART 3: THE CONTROL OF MICROORGANISMS 355

Chapter 18: The Use of Chemicals in Disinfection and Sterilization 356
Historical Background 357
Ignatz Semmelweis 358 *Surgical Antisepsis* 358

The Use of Antiseptics and Disinfectants 358
General Directions for Chemical Disinfection 358 *Chemical Antiseptics* 359 *Selected Disinfecting and Sterilizing Chemicals* 359
Testing Methods for Antiseptics and Disinfectants 365
Phenol Coefficient Test 365 *The Use-dilution Test* 366 *Bacteriostatic-bactericidal Test* 366 *Tissue Toxicity Test* 367
Virus Disinfection 367
Summary 367
Questions for Review 368
Suggested Readings 368

Chapter 19: Physical Methods of Microbial Control 369
Preparing Materials for Physical Sterilization 370
Danger of Hepatitis Infection 371
Heat Killing of Microorganisms 371
Terminology of Thermal Kill 371 *How Heat Works* 372 *Monitoring Sterilization* 372 *Moist Heat* 373 *Dry Heat* 376
Radiation 377
Ultraviolet Radiation 377 *Ionizing Radiation* 378
Filtration 379
Liquid Filtration 379 *Air Filtration* 381
Summary 384
Questions for Review 384
Suggested Readings 385

Chapter 20: Antimicrobial Chemotherapy 386
Historical Background 387
Chemotherapeutic Agents 387
Principles of Chemotherapy 388
Minimal Antibacterial (Active) Concentration (MAC) 389 *Properties of an Effective Antibiotic* 389 *Mechanisms of Action of Antimicrobial Agents* 389 *Specific Mechanisms of Action* 390
Some Commonly Used Antimicrobial Drugs 390
Sulfa Drugs 390 *Penicillins* 393 *Clindamycin: A Useful Alternative to Penicillin-cephalosporin Antibiotics* 395 *Chloramphenical and the Tetracyclines* 395 *Aminoglycosides (Streptomycins)* 395 *Polypeptides* 397 *Antimycobacterial Drugs* 397 *Rifampin* 398
Mechanisms of Drug Resistance 398
The Ominous Nature of Antibiotic 398 *Transferable Antibiotic Resistance* 399

Antibiotic Sensitivity Testing Methods 400
Minimum Inhibitory Concentration Determination 400
Drug Diffusion Methods 400
Blood Levels of Antimicrobial Agents 403
Antimycotic Agents 403
The Treatment of Protozoan Diseases 404
Antiviral Agents 404
Antiviral Agent Sensitivity Testing 405
Summary 407
Questions for Review 408
Suggested Readings 408

PART 4: PRINCIPLES OF IMMUNOLOGY 409

Chapter 21: Resistance in Host-parasite Interactions 410
Species or Racial Resistance 411
Mechanical and Chemical Barriers: The Body's First Line of Defense 411
Intact Skin 412 *Mucous Membranes* 412 *Genitourinary System* 412 *Eyes* 412 *Gastrointestinal System* 412
Indigenous or Normal Flora 413
Amphibiont Sites 413 *Development* 413 *Variety* 414 *Benefits* 414
The Immune System 415
The Components of Normal Blood and Their Roles in Health and Disease 416 *The Lymphatic System* 419
Phagocytosis 421
Phagocytic Cell Types 423 *Stages in Phagocytosis* 423
Inflammation 424
Signs 425 *Mechanism* 425 *Inflammatory Exudate* 425 *Fever* 425
Antimicrobial Substances 426
Complement 426 *Leukins* 427 *Lysozyme* 427 *Phagocytin* 427 *Properdin* 428 *Spermine* 428 *Interferon* 428
Conditions That Lower Host Resistance to Disease Agents 429
Summary 431
Questions for Review 432
Suggested Readings 432

Chapter 22: Microbial Virulence 434
Infectious Disease and Virulence 434

Invasiveness 436 *Relatively Nontoxic Bacterial Structures and Products Contributing to Invasiveness* 436
Microbial Toxin Production 437
Bacterial Toxins 437 *Bacterial Phytotoxins* 442 *Toxins of Blue-green Bacteria* 442 *Algal Toxins* 442 *Mycotoxins* 443
Viral Pathogenicity 443
The Pathological Effects of Viruses 444
Opportunists and True Pathogens 445
Summary 446
Questions for Review 447
Suggested Readings 447

Chapter 23: Antigens, Immunoglobulins, and States of Immunity 448
Antigens and Immunogens 449
Properties of Immunogens 449 *Factors That Determine Immunogenicity and Immune Responses* 450 *Classes of Antigens* 450
Antibodies 452
Immunoelectrophoresis (IEP) 452 *Immunoglobulins* 453 *Antibody Production* 456 *The Occurrence of Normal Immunoglobulins* 456
The Development of the Immunologic System 457
The Thymus Gland and Its Role 457 *The Immune Response in the Developing Individual* 458 *Mechanism of Antibody Formation* 460
Immunosuppression and Immunosuppressive Agents 461
States of Immunity 462
Acquired Immunity 462
Summary 465
Questions for Review 466
Suggested Readings 467

Chapter 24: Diagnostic Immunologic and Related Reactions 468
Production of Antisera 470
The Diagnostic Significance of Rising Antibody Titers 470
The Agglutination Reaction 470
Examples of Agglutination and Related Reactions 471
Hemagglutination Inhibition (HI) 472
The Precipitin Reaction 472
Ring or Interface Tests 473

In Vitro Hemolysis Tests 475
Complement Fixation 475 *Antistreptolysin Test* 477
In Vitro Immunologic Procedures Incorporating Differential Staining 478
Fluorescent Antibody Techniques 478
Diagnostic and Investigative Electron Microscopy 480
Immune Electron Microscopy 480 *Ferritin-conjugated Antibodies* 480
In Vivo Testing Procedures 481
Virus Neutralization 481 *Diagnostic Skin Tests* 481
Immunohematology 482
The ABO System 482 *The Rh System* 485
Blood Testing Techniques 487
Compatibility Testing or Cross Matching 487 *Coombs Tests* 488
Summary 488
Questions for Review 490
Suggested Readings 491

Chapter 25: Immunologic Disorders 492
Immunodeficiencies 493
Primary Immunodeficiencies 493 *Secondary Immunodeficiencies* 493
Hypersensitivity (Allergy) 494
Categories of Hypersensitivity 494
Type I (Classic Immediate) Hypersensitivity 496 *Representative Type I Allergic States* 496 *Type II (Cytotoxic) Hypersensitivity* 500 *Type III (Immune-complex-mediated) Hypersensitivity* 500 *Type IV (Cell-mediated, or Delayed), Hypersensitivity* 501 *Representative Type IV Allergic States* 502 *Autoallergy (Autoimmune) Diseases* 506
Summary 507
Questions for Review 508
Suggested Readings 508

Chapter 26: Immunization and the Control of Infectious Diseases 510
Immunization Preparation 511
The Preparation of Representative Vaccines 511
Color Atlas, Section Two *following page 512*
The Safety of Live versus Inactivated Preparations 514
Vaccine Safety 514
Vaccines Currently in Use 514

Combined Vaccines 515 *BCG and Tuberculosis Prevention* 515
Passive Immunization 516
Antitoxins 516
The Role of Allied Health Service Personnel 518
Administering Vaccines 518 *Complications Associated with Vaccinations* 520 *Immunization for International Travel* 521
Eradication Through Immunization 522
Summary 522
Questions for Review 523
Suggested Readings 523

PART 5: MICROORGANISMS AND INFECTIOUS DISEASES 525

Chapter 27: Principles of Disease Transmission 526

Morbidity and Mortality Rates 527
Reporting Communicable/Infectious Diseases 528
Sources and Resevoirs of Infection 528
Zoonoses 529
Principle Modes of Transfer for Infectious-disease Agents 531
Direct Contact 532 *Indirect Contact* 533 *Air- and Dustborne Infections* 533 *Fomites* 534 *Accidental Inoculation* 534 *Arthropods and Disease* 534
The Hospital Environment 539
Hospital Infections 539 *Principles of Control* 540 *Measures of Control* 541 *Institutional Policies for Control* 542
Diseases of Plants 543
Summary 543
Questions for Review 544
Suggested Readings 545

Chapter 28: The Identification of Disease Agents 546

Approaches to Identifying Pathogens 546
Protozoa and Helminths 547 *Fungi* 547 *Bacteria* 547
Collecting and Handling Specimens 548
Transporting Microbe-containing Specimens 549
Laboratory Procedures 550
Media 550 *The Blood Culture* 551
General Identification Procedures 552

Guidelines for the Identification of Selected Microorganisms 553
Gram-positive Aerobic Bacteria 553 *Gram-negative Aerobic Enteric Bacteria* 555 *Anaerobic Bacteria* 556 *Acid-fast Bacteria* 556
Quality-control Considerations 557
Summary 558
Questions for Review 559
Suggested Readings 559

Chapter 29: Microbial Diseases of the Skin, Nails, and Hair 560

The Organization of the Skin 561
Skin Lesions 562
Bacterial Diseases 562
Anthrax 562 *Gas Gangrene* 566 *Leprosy (Hansen's Disease)* 566 *Pseudomonas Infections* 568 *Staphylococcal Infections* 568 *Streptococcal Infections* 569 *Other Clostridial Infections* 571
Mycotic Infections 571
Classification of Mycotic Infections 572 *Diagnostic and Related Features of the Dermatophytes* 572 *Representative Dermatophycoses* 574 *Other Diseases Caused by Fungi* 575
Viral Infections 575
The Herpesvirus Group 576 *Warts (Papilloma Virus Infection)* 578 *The Paramyxoviruses* 578 *A Togavirus Representative* 579 *The Poxviruses* 579
Summary 580
Questions for Review 580
Suggested Readings 581

Chapter 30: Oral Microbiology 582

Structure of the Mouth 583
The Oral Flora 583
Nonspecific Infections of the Oral Region 584
Focal Infections 584
Diseases Related to Oral Foci of Infection 589
Bacterial Infections 590
Mycotic Infections 590
Viral Infections 593
Summary 595
Questions for Review 595
Suggested Readings 595

Chapter 31: Microbial Infections of the Respiratory Tract 596

Structures of the Respiratory System 597
The Pharynx 597 *The Trachea* 599 *The Lungs and the Primary Bronchi* 599
Normal Flora of the Respiratory Tract 599
Introduction to Microbial Infections of the Respiratory Tract 599
Control Measures 600
Representative Microbial Diseases 600
Diagnosis 600
Upper Respiratory Infections 600
Bacterial Diseases 602 *Virus Diseases* 605
Lower Respiratory Infections 606
Bacterial Pneumonias 606 *Fungus Diseases* 614 *Influenza Virus Infection* 616 *Pneumocystis Carinii* 618
Summary 618
Questions for Review 619
Suggested Readings 620

Chapter 32: Microbial Diseases of the Gastrointestinal Tract 621

Parts of the Gastrointestinal Tract 622
The Stomach 622 *The Small Intestine* 622 *The Large Intestine* 624 *The Liver* 624
Gastrointestinal Microbial Ecology 624
Bacterial Diseases 625
Asiatic Cholera 626 *Brucellosis* 629 *Leptospirosis* 629 *Salmonellosis: Food Infection* 630 *Shigellosis (Bacillary Dysentery)* 631 *Typhoid Fever* 632 *Two Bacterial Disease States of Increasing Frequency* 632 *Food Poisoning (Intoxications)* 633
Viral Infections 636
Picornavirus Infections 636 *Cytomegalovirus Inclusion Disease* 637 *Viral Hepatitis* 637 *Other Types of Viral Hepatitis* 639 *Prevention and Control* 639
Parasitic Protozoan Infections 640
Amebiasis (Amebic Dysentery) 640 *Balantidiasis* 641 *Giardia (Lamblia) Intestinalis* 642
Summary 642
Questions for Review 643
Suggested Readings 643

Chapter 33: Microbial Infections of the Circulatory System 644

Components of the Circulatory System 646
The Heart 646 *Arteries, Veins, and Capillaries* 646
Diseases of the Heart 647
Rheumatic Fever and Rheumatic Heart Disease 647 *Subacute Bacterial Vegetative Endocarditis (SBE)* 648
Other Microbial Diseases of the Circulatory System 648
Signs and Symptoms of Infections 648 *Bacterial Infections* 648 *Protozoan Infections* 654 *Infectious Mononucleosis* 656
Summary 658
Questions for Review 659
Suggested Readings 659

Chapter 34: Microbial Diseases of the Reproductive and Urinary Systems 660

Anatomy of the Urinary System 661
The Flora of the Normal Urinary Tract 661
Diseases of the Urinary Tract 663
An Introduction to Urinary Tract Infections 663 *Kidney (Renal) Diseases Caused by Bacteria* 665 *Diseases of the Urinary Bladder* 666 *Diseases of the Ureter* 666 *Urinary Tract Infections caused by Anaerobes* 667 *Immunological Kidney Injury* 666
The Functional Anatomy of the Reproductive System 667
The Female Reproductive System 667 *The Male Reproductive System* 669
Diseases of the Reproductive System 669
Anaerobic Infections of the Female Genital Tract 669 *Selected Diseases of the Male Reproductive System* 670 *The Venereal (Genitoinfectious) Diseases* 670
Summary 679
Questions for Review 680
Suggested Readings 680

Chapter 35: Microbial Diseases of the Central Nervous System and the Eye 681

Organization of the Central Nervous System 681
Diseases of the Central Nervous System 682
Selected Bacterial Diseases of the Nervous System 682 *Selected Viral Infections of the Nervous System* 686 *Protozoan Infections of the Central Nervous System* 690
The Eye 693

Flora of the Normal Conjunctiva 695
Selected Microbial Diseases of the Eye 695
Bacterial Diseases 695 *Eye Infections Caused by Viruses* 698
Summary 699
Questions for Review 700
Suggested Readings 700

Chapter 36: Microorganisms and Cancer 702

General Characteristics of Cancerous States 703
The Forms of Human Cancer 704
Carcinomas 705 *Leukemias* 705 *Lymphomas* 705
Sarcomas 705
Viral Transformation 705
Early Discoveries Relating Viruses and Cancer 706
Characteristics of Oncogenic RNA Viruses 706
Differences Among Oncogenic RNA Viruses 706
The Role of DNA Viruses in Carcinogenesis 707
Cancer Virus Hypotheses 709
Reverse Transcriptase 709 *Current RNA Cancer Hypotheses* 710
Microbial Carcinogens 712
Cancer Detection 712
Fetal Antigen 712 *Tumor-specific Antigens (TSAs)* 713
Microbial Detection of Carcinogens and Mutagens 713
The Use of Microorganisms in Cancer Treatment 714
A Future Outlook 714
Summary 715
Questions for Review 716
Suggested Readings 716

Chapter 37: Helminths and Disease 717

The Equipment of Parasitic Worms 718
Life Cycles and Control of Parasitic Helminths 718
Hosts Distribution and Transmission 720 *Symptoms and Pathology* 720 *Laboratory Diagnosis* 720 *Treatment of Parasitic Infections* 720
The Nematodes 721
Representative Animal Roundworm Infections 723 *Parasitic Nematodes of Plants* 726
The Platyhelminthes 726
The Cestodes 727 *The Trematodes* 727
Summary 733

Questions for Review 734
Suggested Readings 734

PART 6: MICROORGANISMS AND INDUSTRIAL PROCESSES 735

Chapter 38: Industrial Microbiology 736
An Introduction to Industrial Microbiology 737
Aerobic versus Anaerobic Processes 737
Alcoholic Beverages 737
Beer 738 *Wine* 738 *Sake* 739 *Distilled Beverages* 739
Antibiotics 739
Acids, Vitamins, and Alcohols 740
Vinegar 740 *Amino Acids* 741 *Vitamin Production* 742
Other Products of Fermentation 742
Microbial Enzymes 743
Immobilized Enzymes 744
Steroid Transformations 744
Microbial Insecticides 745
Automation for Microbiology 746
Summary 748
Questions for Review 748
Suggested Readings 748

Chapter 39: Food and Dairy Microbiology 750
Fermented Foods 751
Fermented Vegetables 751 *Dairy Products* 753
Single-cell Protein: Microorganisms as Food 755
Microbial Food Spoilage 757
Major Sources of Microorganisms 757 *How Microorganisms Affect Food* 759
Food Preservation 759
Drying 759 *Canning* 759 *Chemical Preservatives* 761
Summary 762
Questions for Review 762
Suggested Readings 763

Chapter 40: The Microbiology of Soil and Water and Waste Treatment 764
Soil and Its Formation 765
Steps in Soil Formation 765
The Aquatic Environment 767
The Water (Hydrologic) Cycle 767 *Aquatic Microorganisms* 768 *Properties of the Aquatic Environment* 768
Waste Treatment 773
Waste Water 773 *Environmental Effects* 774 *Waste Water Treatment* 778 *Solid Waste Disposal* 783 *Some Products and Problems of Waste Treatment* 784
Summary 784
Questions for Review 785
Suggested Readings 786

Appendices A1
Appendix A: Classification Outline of Division II, the Bacteria A2
Appendix B: Classification Outline of True Fungi A6
Appendix C: Classification Outline of Medically Important Protozoa A8
Appendix D: Classification Outline of the Algae A11
Appendix E: Classification Outline of the Pathogenic Helminths A11

Glossary A13

Index A23

PART ONE

Introduction to Microbiology

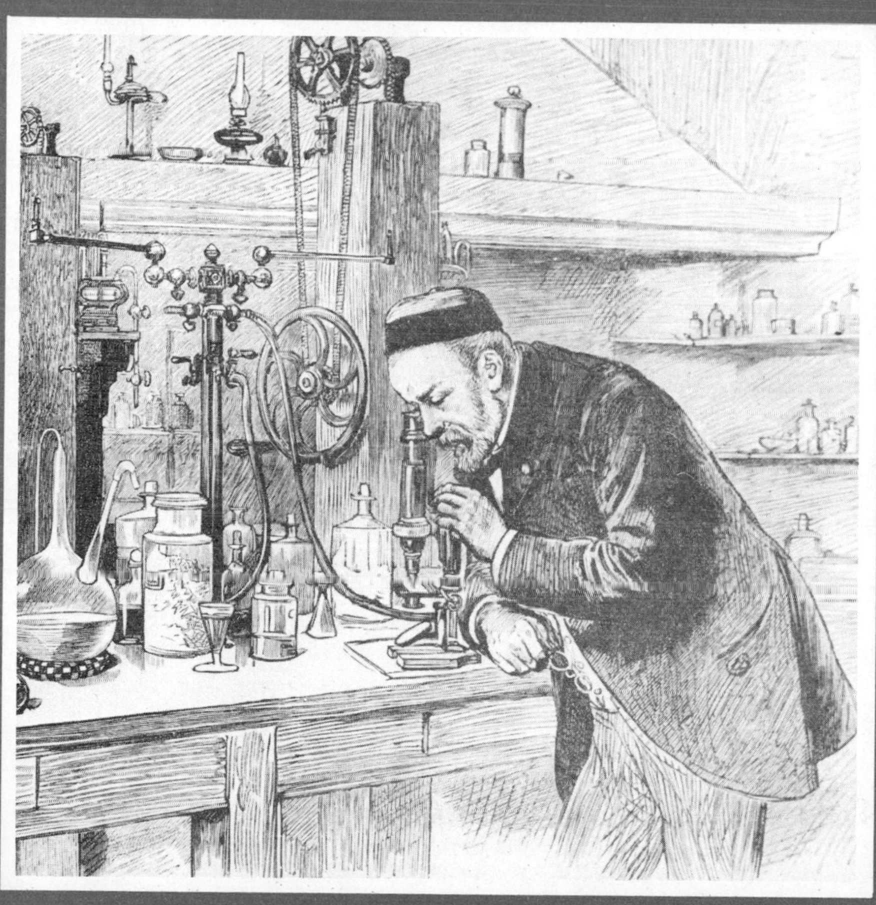

CHAPTER 1

The Scope of Microbiology

The first, simple forms of life appeared on earth more than three billion years ago. Their descendants have changed and developed into the several million types of animals, plants, and microorganisms recognized today. No doubt, thousands more remain to be discovered and officially described.

Throughout the centuries, humans have distinguished the living from the nonliving in different ways, have used various forms of life to meet their needs, and have been fascinated by the abundance and variety of life around them. This chapter introduces the reader to the world of microorganisms, their activities and their applications. Despite their small size, these microscopic forms of life play important roles in nature and in processes affecting the well-being of all other life forms.

After reading this chapter, you should be able to:

1. **List and explain the general properties common to microorganisms and other biological systems.**
2. **Describe the major divisions of microbiology and the type of microorganisms that each division involves.**
3. **Define immunology and describe its importance.**
4. **List and explain four subdivisions of microbiology.**
5. **Discuss the importance of microorganisms in everyday life.**
6. **Describe the scientific method.**
7. **Describe three areas of applied microbiology.**
8. **Discuss the need for scientific periodicals.**
9. **List three areas of study that pose particular challenges for microbiologists.**

The Microbial World

Microscopic forms of life are present in vast numbers in nearly every environment known. They are found in the soil, in bodies of water (Figure 1–1), in the food and water we consume, and even in the air we breathe. Since the conditions that favor the survival and growth of many microorganisms are the same as those under which people normally live, it is not unusual to also find these microscopic forms on the surfaces of our bodies and in the mouth (Figure 1–1), nose, portions of the digestion tract, and other body regions. Fortunately, the majority of such microorganisms are not harmful to humans or to the various other forms of life.

The microbial world, including both microscopic life forms and those too small to be seen with an ordinary microscope, displays a wide variety of forms and properties. Many microorganisms, or microbes, occur as single cells; others are multicellular; and still others, such as viruses, do not have a true cellular appearance. Certain organisms, called **anaerobes,** are capable of carrying out their vital functions in the absence of free oxygen. However, the majority of organisms, the **aerobes,** require free oxygen. Some microbes can manufacture the essential compounds for their physiological needs from atmospheric sources of nitrogen and carbon dioxide. Other microorganisms, such as viruses and certain bacteria, are totally dependent for their existence on the cells of higher forms of life. The branch of science known as *microbiology* embraces all of these properties of microorganisms and many more. For the most part, microorganisms exhibit the characteristic features common to biological systems, such features as reproduction, metabolism, and growth.

Reproduction. Living things have the ability to duplicate themselves, or multiply. Many microorganisms are capable of both asexual and sexual forms of this basic process. In **asexual reproduction** a single cell divides, resulting in the formation of two new cells. In **sexual reproduction** the nuclear material of two cells combines and unites, forming a genetically new individual. Variations of this process occur among different groups of microorganisms.

Metabolism. The ability to use a variety of substances as food and to obtain from them the energy needed for cellular activities is a necessary feature of most living systems. The sum total of the chemical reactions associated with such activities is known as *metabolism.* Metabolic reactions can be grouped into two categories. **Anabolism,** or constructive metabolism, includes all the reactions involved in the synthesis of cellular components needed for growth, reproduction, and repair. **Catabolism,** or destructive metabolism, includes the reactions of digestion and those by which harmful substances are broken down.

Growth. Most microorganisms, like other forms of life, increase in size as materials are produced inside the cell—a process of growth from within. This is in contrast to accretion, which is the accumulation of material from the external environment onto surfaces.

Irritability. Irritability is the ability to respond to environmental stimuli, including temperature, acidity, intense light, and toxic substances. Even the simplest microorganisms show some responses to their environment.

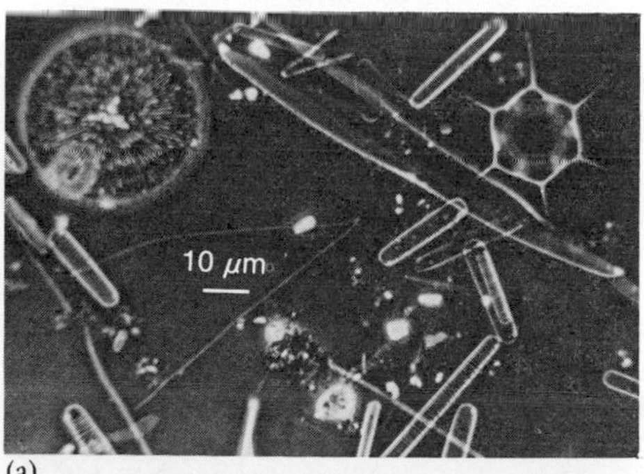

(a)

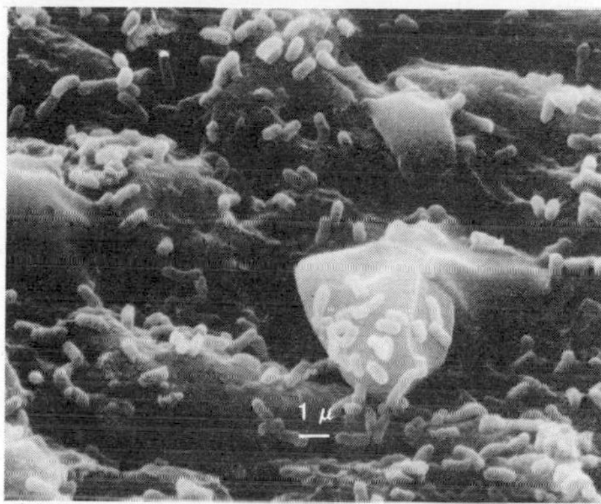

(b)

FIG. 1–1 Some environments of microorganisms. (a) A typical phytoplankton algal community from the antarctic pack ice area. The bar marker (short line) on this and later illustrations serves as a size reference. The length of marker represents the length of a metric unit at a particular magnification. The metric system is discussed in Chapter 4. *Courtesy of Dr. Paul E. Hargraves, Narragansett Marine Laboratory, Kingston, Rhode Island.* (b) Bacteria in the mouth. Short rodlike microorganisms can be seen on the tooth's surface. A few red blood cells are also present. *Allen, A. L., and J. B. Brady,* J. Peridontol. *49:415 (1978).*

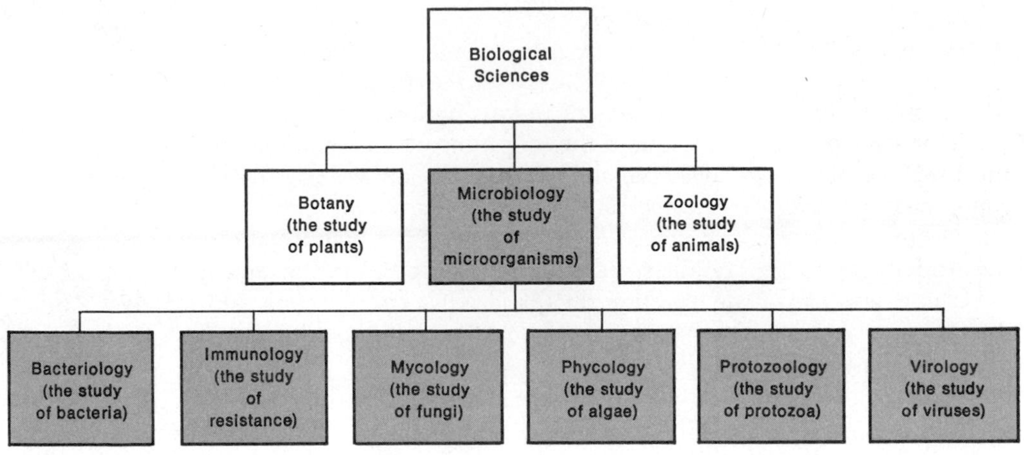

FIG. 1–2 The taxonomic approach to microbiology.

Adaptability. The ability to adjust to environmental stimuli is ***adaptability.*** Several microbial types survive unfavorable environments because they are capable of altering certain of their activities, for example, the direction of their movement (motility), or because they secrete substances to detoxify harmful substances in their environments.

Mutation. Mutation is genetic change. Certain environmental factors, either natural or experimentally produced, bring about changes in the genetic information of an organism. This changed gene is passed on to its offspring and to all future generations of the organism.

Organization. It is clear from the processes performed by microbial forms of life that they possess a certain level of organization and precision. Hence, it is quite appropriate to refer to microbes as small, organized units or ***microorganisms.***

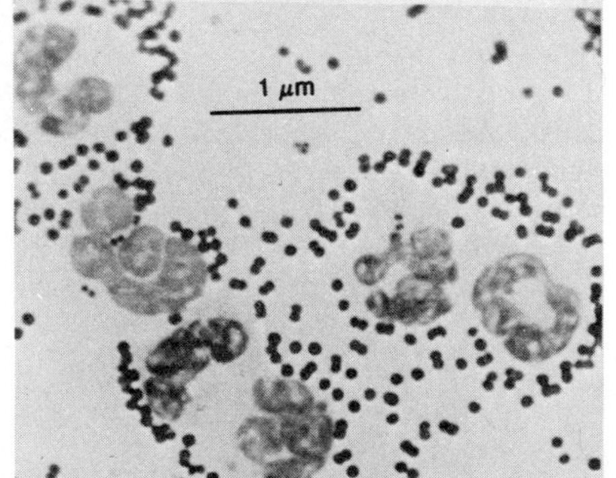

FIG. 1–3 Bacteriology. A photomicrograph of the bacterium ***Staphylococcus aureus*** in the presence of several white blood cells. This microorganism has a spherical shape. *S.* ***aureus*** is the cause of several infections, including boils, food poisoning, impetigo, and pneumonia. *Melly, M. A., L. J. Duke, D. F. Liau, and J. H. Hash,* Infect. Immun. *10:389 (1974).*

Microbiology and Its Subdivisions

Taxonomic Arrangement

The field of microbiology includes the study of algae, bacteria, fungi (molds and yeasts), protozoa, and viruses. As a matter of convenience, the branches of microbiology are frequently named according to which of these topics they focus on. This terminology, referred to as the taxonomic approach, is shown in Figure 1–2.

BACTERIOLOGY

Bacteria represent a large group of microscopic organisms in terms of both variety and numbers. They are found in numerous types of environments (Color Photograph 66), ranging from soil and bodies of water to the external and internal surfaces of humans, lower animals, and plants. The activities in which bacteria are involved include the causation of disease (Figure 1–3 and Color Photograph 2), the decomposition of decaying or dead organic matter, the digestion of food in humans and other organisms, and the production of various chemicals, foods, and other useful products.

IMMUNOLOGY

The study of a host's defense mechanisms against disease is called **immunology.** In general, studying an organism's resistance to disease involves determining the contributions made by certain body cells such as white blood cells, and by various chemical components of body fluids such as antibodies. Modern immunology is also concerned with the diagnosis (Figure 1–4) and prevention of disease. Immunological studies of the interaction between humans and disease agents are aimed at developing new methods of disease detection and prevention.

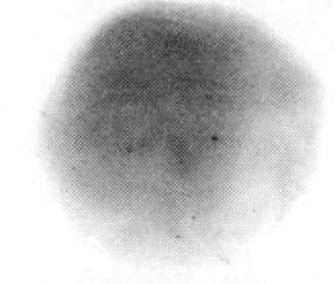
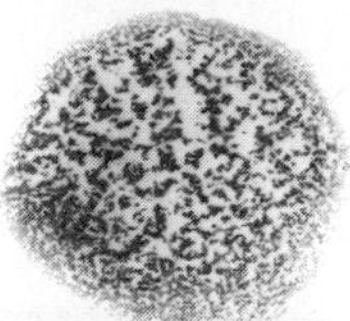

FIG. 1–4 Immunology. One example of immunological procedure, blood typing. The reaction on the left occurs when blood to be used in a transfusion is of the correct type; the clumping reaction on the right can result when blood of a group different from the recipient is used in a transfusion. *Courtesy of USDA.*

MYCOLOGY

Included in the fungi are molds, mushrooms, and yeasts (Figure 1–5). Fungi have a wide variety of sizes, colors, and shapes. Nonphotosynthetic, many fungi live in the soil and take an active part in the decomposition of organic matter (Color Photograph 3). In addition, fungi are involved in the production of several kinds of food and antibiotics and in the causation of disease in humans (Color Photograph 40), lower animals, and plants. All of these aspects of fungi are the subject matter of **mycology.**

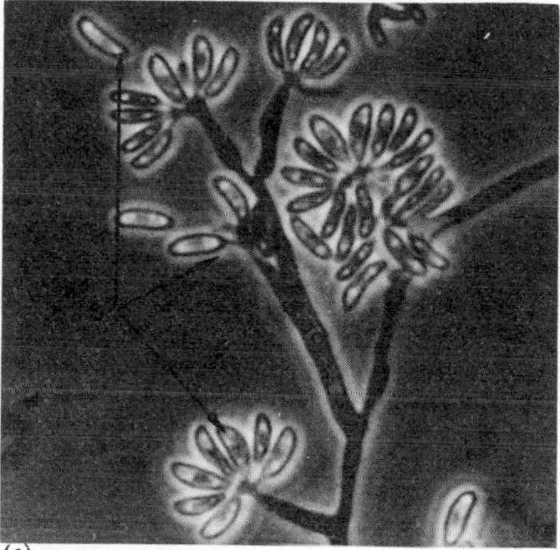

(a)

FIG. 1–5 Mycology. (a) The microscopic appearance of a mold that is found in many different environments. Its reproductive structures, spores (S), are in clusters. Molds of various types play a role in the production of antibiotics and in the decomposition of decaying matter. *Shearer, C. A., Mycologia* 56:16–24 (1974). (b) Brewer's yeast, *Saccharomyces cerevisiae,* is a fungus. This microorganism is frequently used in baking. *Courtesy of Standard Brands, Fleischmann Laboratories, Stamford, Connecticut.*

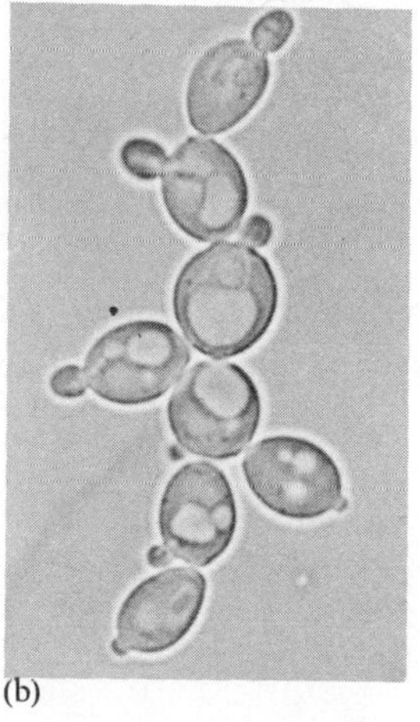

(b)

PHYCOLOGY

Phycology, the study of algae, is sometimes also called *algology.* These algae range in size from microscopic unicellular forms (Figure 1–6 and Color Photograph 4b) to the multicellular giant kelp (seaweed), which can reach lengths of 150 feet or more. The pigments in algae, which span the colors of brown, green, red, and yellow, give these organisms the ability to carry out photosynthesis. Algae are useful as decomposers of organic matter in sewage and as food sources for humans and livestock.

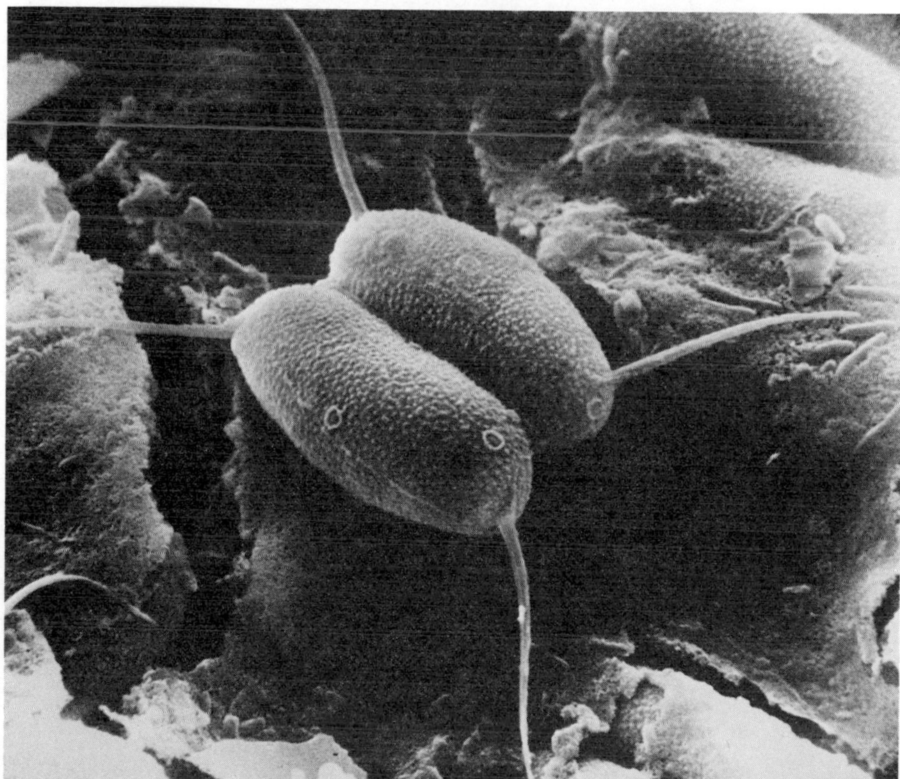

FIG. 1–6 Phycology. Microscopic algae are remarkable microorganisms, showing amazing variety in shape, surface appearance, and the way they group together. *Staehelen, L. A., and J. D. Pickett-Heaps,* J. Phycol. *11:163 (1975).*

Not all of the activities of algae are beneficial to higher life forms, however. For example, algae have recently caused water pollution problems ranging from formation of algal blooms (Color Photograph 4a) to vast fish kills.

PROTOZOOLOGY

Protozoa, the subject of **protozoology,** are larger than most other microorganisms and are complex in structure and activities. They are found in sewage, in various bodies of water (Figure 1-7), and in damp soil. Most protozoa live on rotting or dead organic matter and are harmless, but some types of protozoa are responsible for severe diseases of humans and other animals, such as African sleeping sickness (Color Photograph 5) and malaria.

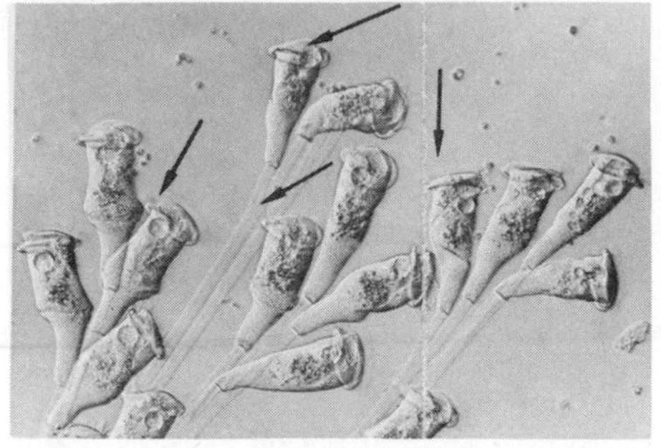

FIG. 1-7 Protozoology. A large number of protozoans such as the ones shown here are commonly found in marine and fresh waters. Note the stalked appearance of these microorganisms and the presence of short, hairlike structures called cilia (arrows), used to gather food. *Courtesy Carolina Biological Supply Company.*

VIROLOGY

The term *virus* comes from the Latin word for poison. **Virology** is concerned with these submicroscopic organisms, which have an organization (Figure 1-8) and patterns of growth and multiplication different from those of other microorganisms. Because viruses depend on the cells they invade (their hosts) for growth and reproduction, they are referred to as ***obligate intracellular parasites.*** Virtually every form of life, including microorganisms (Figure 1-8), can be parasitized by viruses.

Because viruses are smaller than other microorganisms, they could not until recently be viewed directly. They were surrounded by an aura of mystery because of their apparent invisibility and their disease-producing capabilities. Combating the effects of these invisible disease agents was for many years limited to prevention through vaccine development (Figure 1-9).

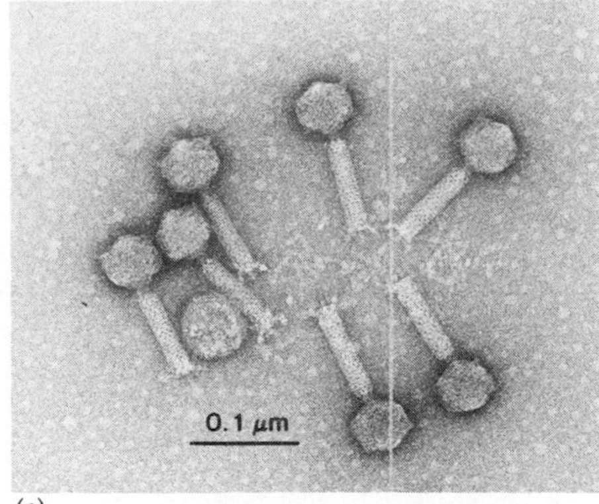

(a)

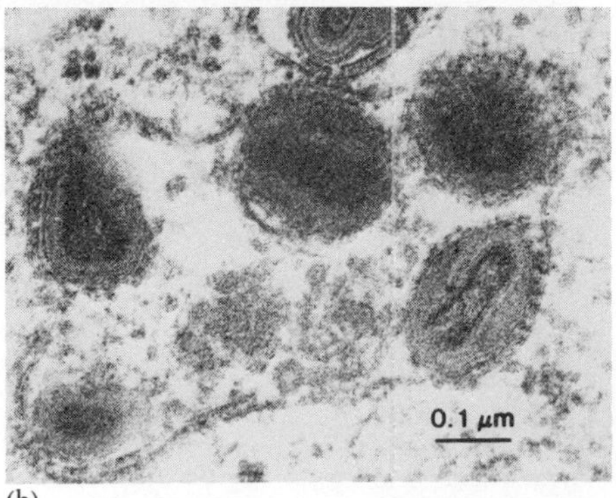

(b)

FIG. 1-8 Virology. The organization and appearance of viruses are different from those of other microbes. (a) Viruses that invade bacteria (bacteriophages) as seen through the electron microscope. Note the head and tail structures of the virus particles. *Gerdes, J. C. and E. R. Romig,* J. Virology 15:1231-1238 (1975). (b) An electron micrograph of vaccinia virus. This is the virus used for vaccination against smallpox, a disease that has been virtually eliminated by effective immunization. *Holowaczak, F. I., L. Flores, and V. Thomas, 61:376-396 (1975).*

The discovery of viruses, or at least the recognition of a nonbacterial infective agent, was made by Ivan Iwanowski in 1892. While working with diseased tobacco plants (Figure 1-10), he detected the infectious nature of the sap from these plants. As Iwanowski could neither observe any microscopic agent nor prevent its activity by passing infectious plant sap material through bacterial retaining filters, he concluded that here was a previously unknown form of life.

In 1898, Löffler and Frosch discovered the virus that causes foot-and-mouth disease (FMD), and two years later Walter Reed and his associates discovered the virus that causes yellow fever. With the discovery of several viruses responsible for diseases in animals, and with the subsequent demonstration of viruses capable of attacking and causing the destruction of bacteria in 1915, interest in these agents began to grow. Then in 1935, W. Stanley reported the crystallization of a pure virus, the tobacco mosaic virus, to the scientific world.

This discovery, in the words of W. Hayes, "gave birth to the romantic idea that viruses are a kind of missing link between living and nonliving material," a type of borderline of life. The debate as to whether viruses are alive continues today. Nevertheless, viruses have gained a prominent position in the scientific world, not only because of their obvious relationship to disease, but also because of their value as research tools in unlocking the intricate mechanisms of life's processes. Today, most scientists consider viruses a distinct category of living things.

Integrative Arrangement

Another approach to the study of microorganisms is the *integrative arrangement.* Here the boundaries between the subdivisions of microbiology are drawn in a way that emphasizes the common characteristics of microbes and their various interactions. These areas of study include the following:

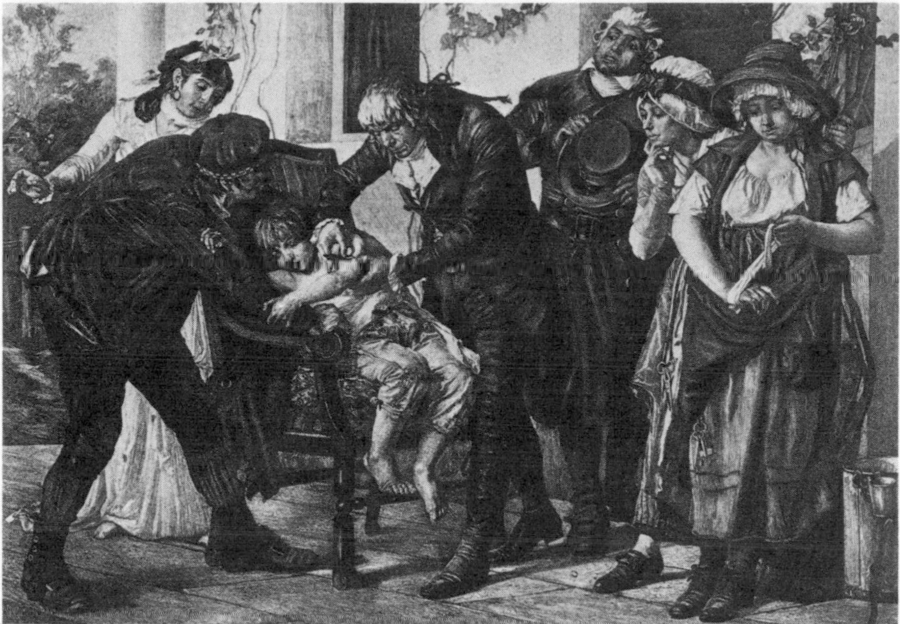

FIG. 1-9 The original vaccination procedure conducted by Edward Jenner (1749–1823). It was performed by removing some fluid from a lesion of cowpox on the hand of a dairymaid and injecting it into the arm of a small boy. The successful outcome of Jenner's vaccination against smallpox established a firm basis for the value of artificial immunization. *Courtesy of Fisher Scientific Co.*

Microbial cytology. Microbial cytology is the study of microscopic and submicroscopic details of microbial cells.

Microbial ecology. Microbial ecology is the study of the relationships between microorganisms and their environments. An investigation of the way microorganisms respond to unfavorable situations would be an example of this area of specialization.

Microbial genetics. Microbial genetics is the study of heredity. This area of investigation concerns the activities of the nuclear elements of microorganisms, how they regulate the growth and development of these forms of life and the effects of altering the nuclear material through mutation-causing agents.

Two important applications of microbial genetics are the use of microorganisms to screen chemicals in food and other materials for their cancer-causing abilities, and their use in producing hormones, such as insulin, through the transfer of genetic material from one type of organism to another. The latter application is only one aspect of *genetic engineering*. This somewhat controversial area holds great potential, if properly handled, for the control and possible elimination of certain genetic defects.

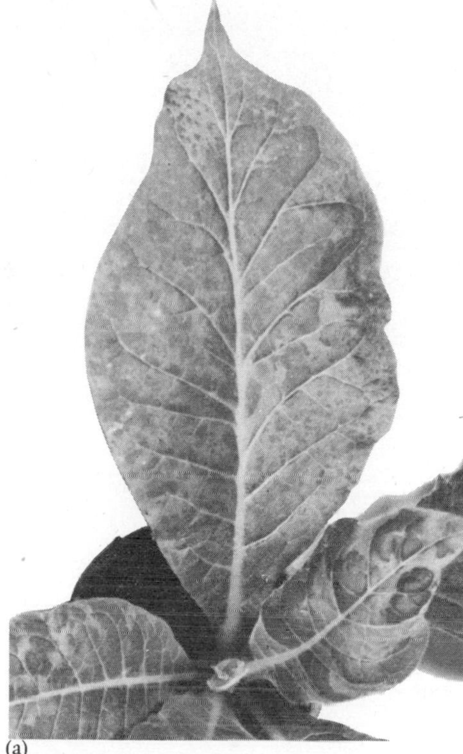

(a)

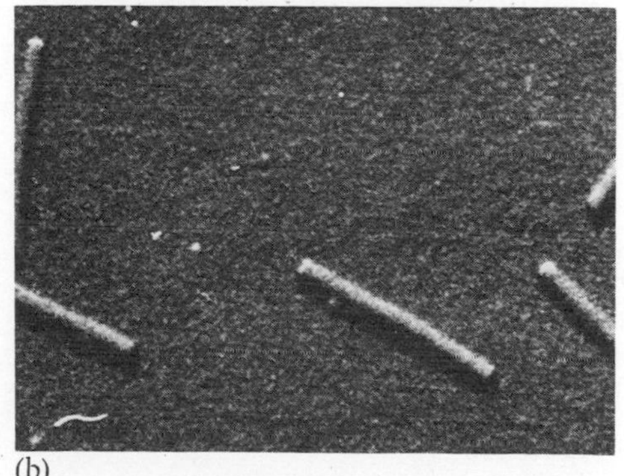

(b)

FIG. 1-10 (a) A leaf of a tobacco plant infected with tobacco mosaic virus. Note the variation in color shown on the infected leaf. Courtesy of the U.S. Department of Agriculture. (b) An electron micrograph of the cause of this plant disease, tobacco mosaic virus. *Courtesy of Dr. Robley C. Williams and the Virus Laboratory, University of California, Berkeley.*

Microbial physiology. Microbial physiology is the study of how microorganisms function. Metabolic activities, the effects of the environment on microbial synthetic pathways, and the nutritional requirements of different groups of microbes are a few of the subjects with which microbial physiology deals.

Molecular biology. Molecular biology is an extremely important and exciting area that has grown from the advances in knowledge and technology made in microbial genetics and physiology. The principal aim of molecular biology is to determine the relationship between the chemical structure and genetic makeup of microbial and higher forms. Microorganisms have played a central role in studies of the intracellular regulatory mechanisms and the expression of genetic information (Figure 1-11). Among the advances that contributed to this foundation were the discoveries relating to the structures and functions of deoxyribonucleic acid (DNA) and ribonucleic acid (RNA) and the mechanism by which genetic information in DNA controls the synthesis of proteins. In fact, how genetic information flows from DNA to RNA and finally results in the formation of a protein molecule is referred to as the "central dogma" of molecular biology.

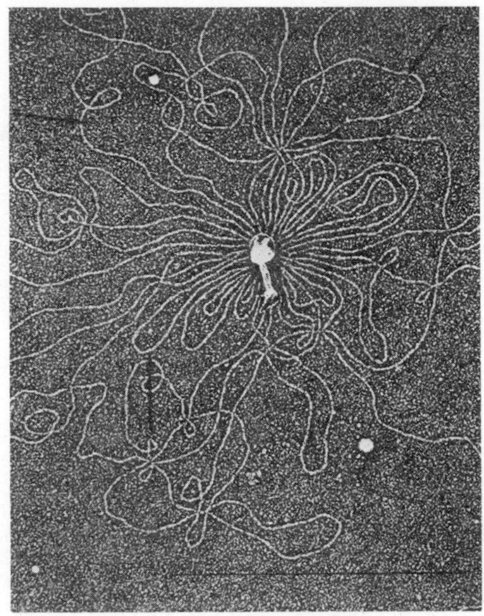

FIG. 1-11 A special preparation of a virus that infects bacteria (bacteriophage), showing its DNA (arrows), which contains the genetic information of the virus. The virus particle is located approximately within the center of the nucleic acid. The bar marker equals 1.0 micrometers. *Courtesy of Dr. A. K. Kleinschmidt; from Kleinschmidt, A. K., D. Lang, D. Jackerts, and R. K. Zahn,* Biochem. Biophys. Acta *61:857 (1962).*

Microbial taxonomy. Microbial taxonomy is the naming and classification of microorganisms. It involves determining the similarities and differences among microbial species and using these data to formulate a classification system that shows the relationship of microorganisms to one another.

Other specialties. Two other areas of investigation are ***biochemistry*** and ***biophysics.*** These specialized fields are "reductionist" sciences, analyzing basic processes in terms of electrons, atoms, and molecules. Biochemistry is concerned with the chemical basis of living matter and the reactions associated with it. Biophysics is devoted to the study of the principles of physics as they apply to all living matter.

Many of these branches overlap. Moreover, one specialty can include a number of narrower subdivisions. For example, microbial genetics may be further divided and restricted to bacteria or to viruses that infect bacteria.

The education of a microbiologist today includes a background of general information on the majority of subdivisions. Because of the tremendous accumulation of information in each specialization—which no single individual can hope to master—most microbiologists focus their advanced study and research on one or two of the branches of microbiology. The branches chosen for specialization depend upon the type of microbial work to be pursued.

Applied Microbiology

The many areas of applied microbiology use the principles, basic information, and techniques of the different subdivisions. These areas include the microbiology of dairy products and other foods, diseases of humans, lower animals, and plants; microbial production of commercially important products such as antibiotics; microbiology of soil and aquatic environments; and microbiology of outer space and the planets. Only some of these areas will be described.

Food and Dairy Microbiology

Many substances that we consume daily are products of microbial activity. Microbe-dependent activities such as brewing beer and making bread and cheese have been known since ancient times. Food and dairy microbiology involves the efforts of chemists, engineers, and microbiologists toward efficient control of **fermentation** or the conversion of raw materials into desirable end products by carefully selected microorganisms.

Food microbiology is also concerned with the prevention of spoilage and improvements in the nutritional value, aroma, flavor, and general quality of foods. Dairy microbiology deals with the manufacture of cheeses and other fermented milk products, such as yogurt. The production of foods free of disease-producing agents is the goal of both applied areas.

Medical Microbiology

Human welfare is affected by the activities of certain microbial species that interfere with the normal processes of the human body. Investigations concerned with the harmful effects of microorganisms (pathogens) are the basis of medical microbiology. The following types of studies are included in this area of specialization: determining the properties and disease capabilities of microorganisms; developing procedures to detect the presence of pathogens (diagnosis); seeking an antibiotic or antibiotics that will eliminate the disease agent or prevent it from exerting its harmful effects (antibiotic sensitivity testing); developing vaccines against pathogens; and incorporating both chemical and physical methods for the management and control of infectious diseases in the population as a whole. Today, individuals in the areas of public health and environmental microbiology are being trained in the principles of medical microbiology.

Veterinary Microbiology

Infectious diseases of various kinds are responsible for the death of our pets as well as for heavy economic losses of livestock and agriculturally important plants (Figure 1–12 and Color Photographs 3b and 6b). These diseases are caused by parasites, organisms that live on or within another form of life, the ***host***. The spread and control of diseases caused by such agents are the concern of veterinary microbiologists and others involved with public health and the livestock industry.

Since many animal parasites, such as hookworms and tapeworms, have microscopic stages in their life cycles, courses concerned with the medical aspects of microbiology may include the study of these forms (Color Photograph 6a). Ordinarily, however, these ***metazoan*** (multicellular) ***parasites*** are considered separately in the specialized branch of ***parasitology***. In this textbook the parasitic worms (helminths) will be considered in a separate chapter.

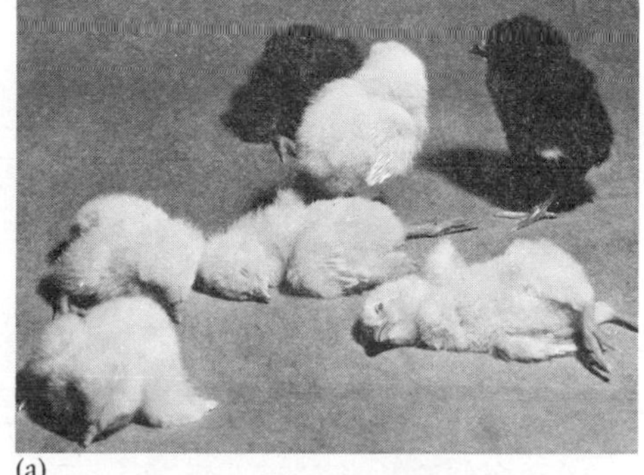

(a)

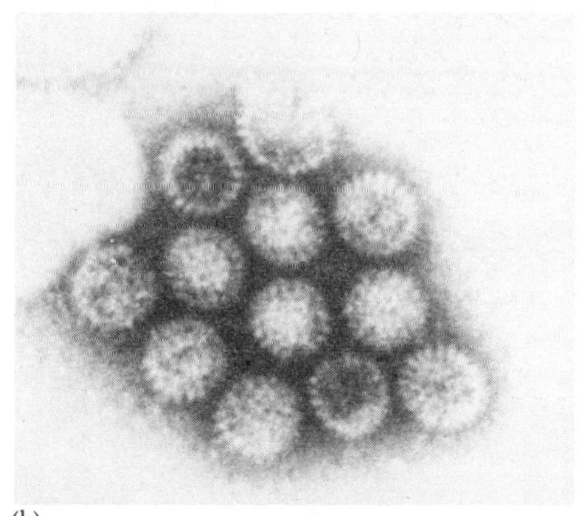

(b)

FIG. 1–12 Infectious diseases of poultry can spread quickly through a flock, causing significant economic losses. (a) Such losses are due not only to death, but also to reduced growth rate and decreased meat or egg production of the infected animals. (b) An electron micrograph of virus particles isolated from calves until gastrointestinal infections, the leading cause of death in newborn calves. *Courtesy of G. N. Woode, Institute for Research on Animal Diseases, Berkshire.*

Microbiology and the Scientific Method

One goal of microbiology and every other branch of the biological sciences is to find explanations for observed phenomena and to show interrelationships between them and related events. To achieve this aim, a type of organized common-sense approach, referred to as the "scientific method," is used in one form or another. While all of the steps of this procedure may not be applicable to every aspect of microbiology, the essence of the method does direct the investigator to pose pertinent questions and to look for testable answers (Figure 1–13).

The scientific method involves making ***careful observations*** of a particular event and then arranging them so that a generalization can be made to account for the observed phenomenon. This particular step is called a ***hypothesis***, or simply a "well-calculated guess." Once a hypothesis has been formulated, its validity must be tested. This phase of the scientific method is called ***experimentation***. The simplicity or complexity of the hypothesis will determine the type and number of experiments needed. Such experiments must be designed to test

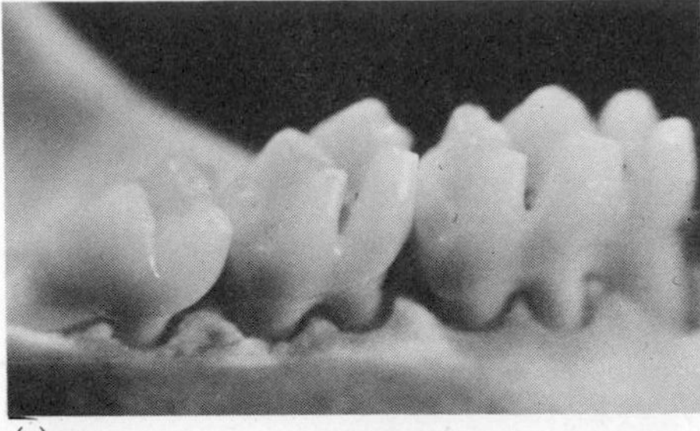
(a)

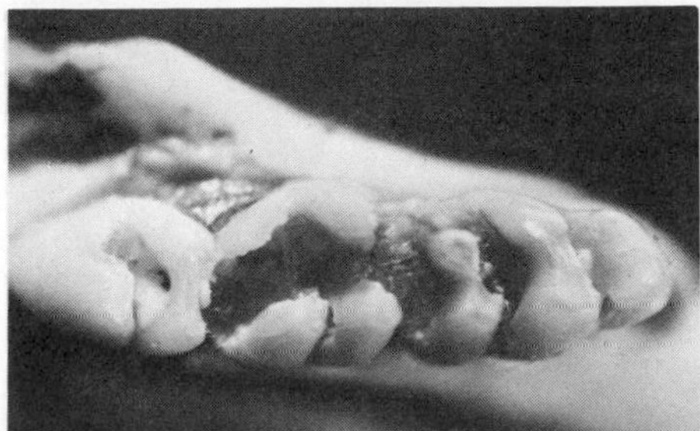
(b)

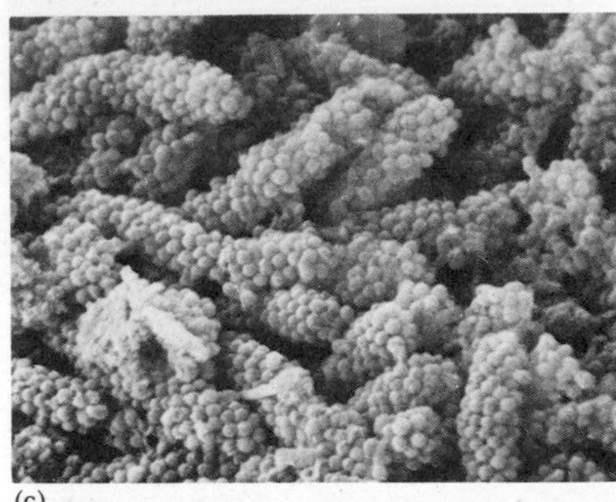
(c)

FIG. 1–13 The scientific method in action. Discovering the microbial cause of tooth decay demonstrates the formulation of a hypothesis and its testing by experimentation. For years hypotheses were formulated and attempts made to find the cause of tooth decay, or dental caries. It was shown that the bacterium *Streptococcus mutans* was a potent producer of caries in germ-free animals. This finding led to the isolation of these bacteria from humans and other animals and to attempts to reproduce tooth decay experimentally in laboratory animals. (a) The teeth of a control noninfected animal. (b) Here the caries producing effects of the suspected bacterium are quite obvious. *Hamada, S., T. Ooshima, M. Torii, H. I. Imanishi, N. Masuda, S. Sobue, and Kotanti,* Microbiol. Immunol. *22:301–314 (1978).* (c) Bacteria such as these *Streptococcus mutans* produce sugar substances that help them stick to the surfaces of teeth. Diets containing large amounts of the sugar sucrose support an increase in the number of bacteria. *Dr. Z. Skobe, Forsyth Dental Center.*

the pertinent point of the hypothesis, to include adequate controls for purposes of comparison, and to avoid the subjectivity, or bias, of the scientist. Experiments that cannot be repeated by other competent investigators are discarded.

The next stage of the scientific method is the ***theory***. This is an explanatory hypothesis that has been supported by various types of observations and experiments. A good theory can be used to predict new facts, to show relationships between phenomena, and to relate new information as it is uncovered. The term *law* is often used interchangeably with ***theory***. A distinction must be made, however, for a law is a theory that has attained universal acceptance. Many theories do not achieve this distinction.

There is no doubt that the scientific method is a functional tool for inquiry, but it is not without limitations and sources of frustration. The brief description given here cannot adequately depict the trials and errors experienced by investigators. Moreover, the individuals using the scientific method also have limitations. They are human, and being so, have feelings, failings, and even prejudices that may, from time to time, interfere with their reasoning and competence. Through the years, new techniques of observation, as well as refinements of older procedures, have caused scientists to reexamine scientific facts and, if considered valid, to make changes in hypotheses and conclusions.

While there is no one scientific method, the description presented here emphasizes some of the important elements associated with scientific inquiry. Discoveries of a scientific nature are made in a variety of ways, including intuition and imagination. Such discoveries involve diverse and challenging procedures and methods, and some of these will be presented in later chapters.

Resources in Microbiology

Within a relatively few years, an enormous body of experimental data has accumulated and been recorded in the journals for the various divisions of microbiology. Discussions and interpretations of these data are also published. Obviously, the need to communicate knowledge and ideas is vital to any phase of scientific endeavor. Knowledge of important developments constitutes a most powerful and necessary tool for scientific methodology.

In beginning the study of any new area of specialization, some understanding and information about the publications in the field is essential. Scientific periodicals are produced by scientific societies, individuals, institutions, private companies, and commercial publishing firms. They range in frequency from weeklies like *Science* to annuals such as *Annual Review of Microbiology*. The content of periodicals also may vary. Certain journals, such as *Applied Microbiology* and the *Journal of Phycology*, are devoted to providing reports of recent research developments in the pure and applied fields of microbiology. Other publications, such as *Advances in Immunology* and *Microbiological Reviews*, provide review articles that draw together information from many separate sources on a particular area. Such reviews are especially important to individuals approaching a new field of interest or a specialized topic for the first time. Still other periodicals, including *The American Scientist* and *The Sciences*, combine both these approaches and may include additional items such as book reviews, society developments, and announcements. Some periodicals contain advertisements of products useful to the microbiologist.

Most publications provide an annual index of subjects and authors, either in a separate issue or as part of the last issue of a volume. There are also reference publications devoted solely to providing brief summaries or article titles for specific subjects. *Biological Abstracts* and *Index Medicus* are two such publications. Others list the titles of all articles contained within selected periodicals *(Current Contents)*. Either type of publication helps the microbiologist keep abreast of publications in his or her particular specialization.

To list all of the available sources of information pertaining to microbiology would be impractical, not only because of space limitations, but also because new specialized publications appear each year. Science, medical, or related types of libraries should be consulted for further information.

Some Challenges for Microbiology

One of the attractive features of microbiology as well as other areas of science is the amount of investigation and work remaining to be done. Despite the years of intense study of microorganisms and their activities, key questions remain unanswered. Microbiology has assumed a position of great importance in modern society. Many decisions affecting the future of the world may depend upon and involve the activities of microorganisms in areas such as food production, pollution control, energy production, and the control and treatment of diseases not only of humans, but of domestic animals and plants.

SUMMARY

The Microbial World

1. Microscopic forms of life can be found in abundance in nearly every environment.
2. The majority of microorganisms are not harmful.
3. Most microorganisms are single cells and exhibit the characteristics common to all biological systems, including ***reproduction, metabolism, growth, irritability, adaptability, mutation,*** and ***organization.***
4. Viruses do not have a true cellular form.

Microbiology and Its Subdivisions

Taxonomic Arrangement

1. The general branches of microbiology include: ***bacteriology,*** the study of bacteria; ***immunology,*** the study of a host's resistance against disease, and the detection and prevention of disease; ***mycology,*** the study of fungi; ***phycology,*** the study of algae; ***protozoology,*** the study of protozoa; and ***virology,*** the study of viruses.
2. The first demonstration of the existence of a nonbacterial infective agent, the virus, was made by Iwanowski in 1892.
3. Demonstration that viral diseases infect plants, lower animals, and humans made viruses an important subject of study.

Integrative Arrangement

1. Specialty areas of microbiology are directed toward the study of common properties of microorganisms and their interactions.
2. Such areas of study include cellular features of microorganisms ***(microbial cytology),*** interactions between microorganisms and their environments ***(microbial ecology),*** hereditary mechanisms ***(microbial genetics),*** metabolic activities ***(microbial physiology),*** the relationship between chemical structure and genetic makeup ***(molecular biology)*** and naming and classification of microorganisms ***(microbial taxonomy).***

Applied Microbiology

1. Applied areas of microbiology utilize the basic principles, information, and techniques of microbiology in various ways.
2. Such applied areas deal with the microbiology of foods and other products formed by microorganisms and with the environments in which microorganisms may be found.

Microbiology and the Scientific Method

1. The scientific method is a common-sense approach to finding explanations for basic phenomena and showing their importance.
2. The steps of this approach include ***careful observation, hypothesis, experimentation,*** and ***theory.***

Resources in Microbiology

Scientific publications communicate knowledge and ideas. This means of communication is a powerful tool for scientific methodology.

Some Challenges for Microbiology

Microbiology has a position of importance in the modern world. Many decisions affecting the future of the world may depend on the activities of microorganisms.

QUESTIONS FOR REVIEW

1. a. What are the characteristic features of a *biological system?*
   b. Must all of these properties be present before a microorganism can be considered living? Explain.
2. Which of the properties of a biological system would you consider essential to the well-being of microorganisms in the following situations?
   a. pathogenic bacteria in the bloodstream
   b. a microorganism stranded on the surface of the moon
   c. bacteria in the human small intestine
3. a. List three ways in which viruses differ from other microorganisms.
   b. Give two examples of viral diseases.
4. Briefly describe the activities associated with the following areas of microbiology:
   a. food microbiology
   b. medical microbiology
   c. mycology
   d. phycology
   e. dairy microbiology
   f. microbial ecology
   g. microbial genetics
   h. biochemistry
5. a. Of what value is the scientific method?
   b. List the steps involved in this approach.
6. a. How important are scientific publications? What is their purpose?

SUGGESTED READINGS

Beveridge, W. I. B. *The Art of Scientific Investigation*. New York: Vintage Books, A Division of Random House, 1957. *A short, thought-provoking book dealing with the basis of scientific investigation, thought, and ethics.*

Dubos, R. J., and J. Dubos. *The White Plague: Tuberculosis, Man and Society*. Boston: Little, Brown and Co., 1952. *Many diseases caused by microorganisms continue to have an impact on society. This book presents a well-written account of the early history of one of these diseases, tuberculosis.*

Fuller, J. G. *Fever*. New York: Ballantine Books, A Division of Random House, 1974. *A true medical detective thriller about the events leading to the discovery of the viral cause of the deadly disease, Lassa fever.*

Porter, J. R. "The Scientific Journal—300th Anniversary." *Bact. Rev.* 28:211 (1964). *A short article emphasizing the importance and history of the scientific journal as a means of communication.*

Portugal, F. H., and J. S. Cohen. *A Century of DNA*. Cambridge, Mass.: The MIT Press, 1977. *A timely book describing the discovery of, and advances made with, the genetic substance deoxyribonucleic acid (DNA). The immediate and overwhelming impact of this genetic substance on the nature and basic properties of all forms of life, as well as the nature of scientific investigation, is presented in a readable and interesting manner.*

Postgate, J. *Microbes and Man*. Baltimore: Penguin, 1975. *An excellent, readable book that emphasizes the roles microorganisms play and their influence on our daily lives. Microbial applications are also included.*

Early History of Microbiology

CHAPTER 2

Chapter 2 surveys the ideas, discoveries, problems, and successes of early scientists in their approaches to studying microorganisms. Among the most important of these events were the discoveries of microorganisms and their roles in natural processes such as fermentation and disease, the disproof of the doctrine of spontaneous generation, and the development of measures for controlling microorganisms.

After reading this chapter, you should be able to:

1. **Describe the contributions of individual scientists and the events leading to the discovery of microorganisms, their activities, and their functions.**
2. **Show how early investigators applied the scientific method.**
3. **Define fermentation from the nonbiological and biological viewpoints.**
4. **Identify the problems and needs of early investigators attempting to study, grow, and control microorganisms.**
5. **Describe pasteurization and its applications.**
6. **Explain the doctrine of spontaneous generation and the experiments used to disprove it.**
7. **List both Koch's and Rivers' postulates and relate their importance to the germ theory of disease.**
8. **Define chemotherapy and explain its importance in the control of microorganisms.**

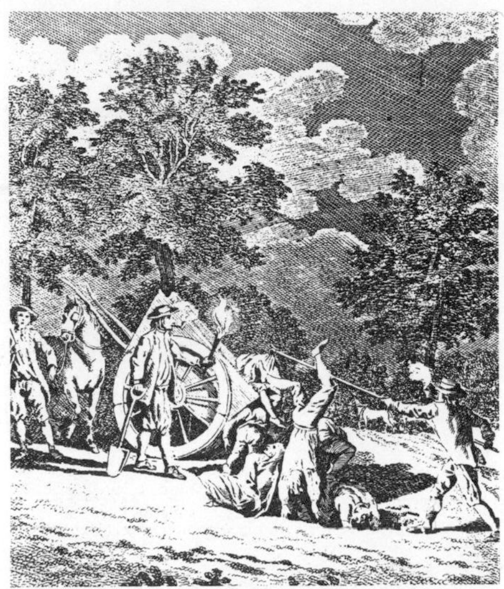

FIG. **2-1** Burying victims of the Plague of London of 1664 in mass graves. In the late seventeenth century, one physician estimated the annual number of deaths in London due to smallpox at 3,000—a number that was probably low. *The Bettmann Archive.*

Microbiology, like most other sciences, had its origin deeply rooted in curiosity. At first microorganisms were thought to be mysterious oddities of little practical importance. However, the work of many individuals, including Louis Pasteur, Robert Koch, and Joseph Lister, drastically changed this limited view of microbes during the late nineteenth century. For the first time, the world became aware of the desirable and undesirable effects of microorganisms on their environment—including spoilage, disease, and death (Figure 2-1). This realization unleashed a whole new era of research in microbiology.

This chapter will present many of the early historical landmarks in the growth of microbiology. The next chapter will introduce the major groups of microorganisms studied in this fascinating branch of the biological sciences.

Early Development of Microbiology

Leeuwenhoek

In 1673, in Delft, Holland, Anton van Leeuwenhoek, a successful linen merchant, was the first to observe the mysterious and exciting world of microorganisms (Figure 2-2a). For the next fifty years, until his death in 1723, Leeuwenhoek continued to watch microorganisms with the aid of small, ***simple (one-lens) microscopes*** (Figure 2-2b). Although the ***compound microscope*** had already been invented, Leeuwenhoek found his device more suitable for observing specimens with transmitted light. This was because his lenses provided greater detail, or ***resolving power.*** The magnifying power of his early instruments ranged from approximately 50 to 300 times the diameter of a particular specimen.

Leeuwenhoek's position in the development of microbiology has been firmly established because of his remarkable observations and descriptions of microscopic forms of life. His unending curiosity led him to spend hours upon hours examining specimens collected from lakes, rain barrels, and even from his own teeth and those of others. Among his first observtions were descriptions of protozoa and of the basic shapes of bacteria, yeasts, and algae.

Leeuwenhoek recognized the value of recording his observations (Figure 2-2c). He sent more than 200 handwritten, occasionally illustrated, letters to the Royal Society of London. Many of these were translated into English and published.

Leeuwenhoek's discoveries went beyond the world of microbes, for he made many other contributions of biological significance. For example, he provided confirming evidence for William Harvey's theory of blood circulation by constructing an aquatic microscope ("aalkijer"). This instrument enabled scientists to observe the flow of red blood cells through the capillaries of a fish's tail fin. Leeuwenhoek also observed muscle fiber striations (1682), nuclei of fish blood cells (1682), and the myelin sheath of nerve fibers (1717). No wonder such discoveries were provocative to investigators and inquisitive amateurs everywhere.

Because of his numerous observations and careful measurement and recording of specimens, Leeuwenhoek is considered the "father" of bacteriology, hematology, histology, protozoology, and other sciences for which the microscope is the main investigative tool. After Leeuwenhoek's death, the study of microorganisms was neglected for some time. This was because of the difficulty in constructing better microscopes and because many scientists still considered microorganisms to be nothing more than oddities—until the landmark work of Louis Pasteur.

Pasteur

Except for Leeuwenhoek, French and German scientists dominated early microbiology. One of the first scientists to recognize the true biological function of microbes was the chemist and physicist Louis Pasteur (Figure 2-3a). Pasteur was born on December 27, 1822, in the little French village of Dôle. A major figure in the development of biology and medicine, his discoveries brought to light dramatic new concepts as well as new approaches to age-old problems. Pasteur's contributions led to new, more effective measures for disease prevention (Figure 2-3b), to the improvement of health in general, and to the understanding of basic aspects of microbial life. Among the practical results of this understanding are the control of fermentation processes, pasteurization, and the development of vaccines against such dread diseases as rabies and anthrax.

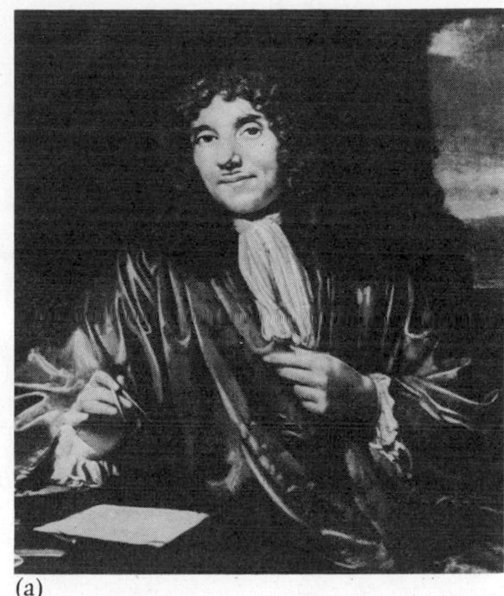

(a)

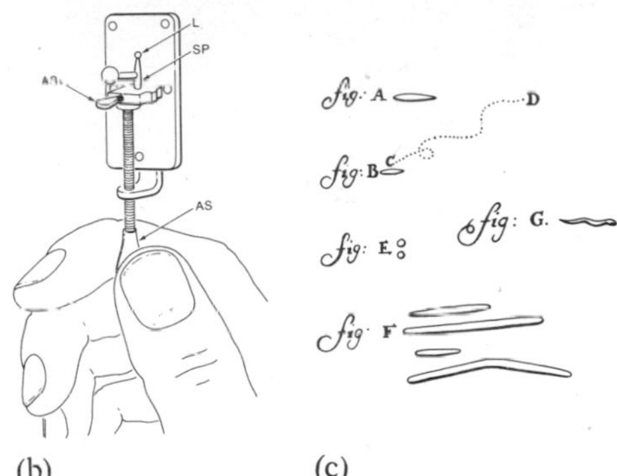

(b) (c)

FIG. 2-2 (a) Anton van Leeuwenhoek (1632–1723), the father of bacteriology and protozoology. ***Fisher Scientific Company, Chicago.*** (b) Leeuwenhoek's simple microscope (rear view). The small size of the instrument is apparent from its relationship to the fingers grasping it. A single magnifying lens (L) was held between two thin metal plates. Objects for examination were mounted on a specimen pin (SP) that could be moved by adjusting screws (AS). Specimens were viewed by holding the microscope close to the eye and placing a source of illumination in back of the lens. (c) Leeuwenhoek's drawings of bacteria. The recognizable forms include rodlike, spherical (coccus), and spiral forms. *Corliss, J. O., J. Protozool. 22:3–7 (1975).*

The Germ Theory of Fermentation

Nonvitalist versus Vitalist

Fermentation is a natural process in which alcohols and organic acids such as vinegar and lactic acid are formed from dissolved sugar, in the presence of microorganisms. The results of fermentation reactions, including the souring of milk and the preparation of alcoholic beverages, have been known and used all over the world throughout history. Yet, despite the recorded descriptions of microorganisms by Leeuwenhoek, the biological basis of fermentation was not formulated until well into the nineteenth century. Basically two viewpoints evolved to explain these processes—the *nonvital* (nonbiological) theory and the *vital* (biological) theory.

According to the nonvital view, yeasts seen in fermenting materials are by-products rather than causes of fermentation. During the period from approximately 1839 to 1869, supporters of the nonvital theory, including the three influential chemists Jöns Jakob Berzelius, Justus von Liebig, and Friedrich Wöhler, maintained that essential, unstable chemical entities called *ferments* produced the reactions by acting as **catalysts** or **enzymes,** simply activating the chemical reactions. These unstable ferments were formed by the action of air on sugar-containing fluids. The resulting ferments transmitted their instability to sugar molecules, which in turn decomposed to form the products of fermentation. Liebig used as support for the nonvital theory the absence of any yeasts in acetic and lactic acid fermentations. The nonvitalists neglected to consider the possibility that other microorganisms could produce these "essential ferments." Several years later these reactions were shown to be caused by bacteria.

The biological theory of fermentation was strengthened by the work of French and German scientists in the 1830s. German physiologist Theodor Schwann clearly demonstrated the role of yeasts in alcoholic fermentation. He showed that exposing these microorganisms to heat and chemical agents stopped all fermentation. In addition, Schwann described the **asexual** form of reproduction (budding) of yeasts, and showed that this "sugar fungus" *(Saccharomyces cerevisiae)* was needed in large numbers for fermentation to proceed. These observations were not readily accepted by the nonvitalists, and the stage was set for a bitter controversy that was not settled until Louis Pasteur provided experimental proof for the biological theory in 1857.

Pasteur's Contributions to Fermentation Research

Pasteur's fermentation studies occupied a major portion of his scientific career. They began as a search for the cause of souring and spoilage of beer and wines. In 1854 Pasteur was a professor at the University of Lille, France, and in that city the production of wine and beer was a very important industry. Pasteur found that the spoilage was caused by a different fermentation process, in which sugar is converted to lactic acid rather than to alcohol. The microscopic examination of sediments from wine vats in which this lactic acid fermentation occurred revealed microorganisms that were eventually recognized as bacteria and unwanted "wild" yeasts. The classification of such organisms was difficult, since no formal rules of identification had yet been developed.

On further experimentation, Pasteur found a way to destroy these microbes without altering the quality of the wine. He discovered that wine could be heated and held for a specific period of time at a temperature between 50° and 60°C. This procedure, which came to be known as **pasteurization,** prevented the wine from spoiling.

Pasteur also showed that the souring of milk is caused by microorganisms. Today, milk and certain other foods are routinely pasteurized by heating at 63°C for 30 minutes or at 71°C for 15 seconds. These temperatures are adequate to destroy, or to reduce in number, food spoilage organisms and many **pathogenic** (disease-producing) organisms.

In investigating many other fermentative processes, Pasteur discovered some interesting things:

1. Each type of fermentation, as defined by its particular end products, is caused by a specific microbial type.
2. Each microorganism requires specific conditions, such as a definite degree of **acidity** or **alkalinity,** in order for fermentation to occur.

FIG. 2-3 (a) Louis Pasteur (1822–1885), the Freelancer of Science. *National Library of Medicine, Bethesda, Maryland.* (b) Pasteur in his laboratory during work on the viral disease of rabies in 1884. Pasteur's idea for weakening the rabies virus led to an effective control measure against the disease. *The Bettmann Archive.*

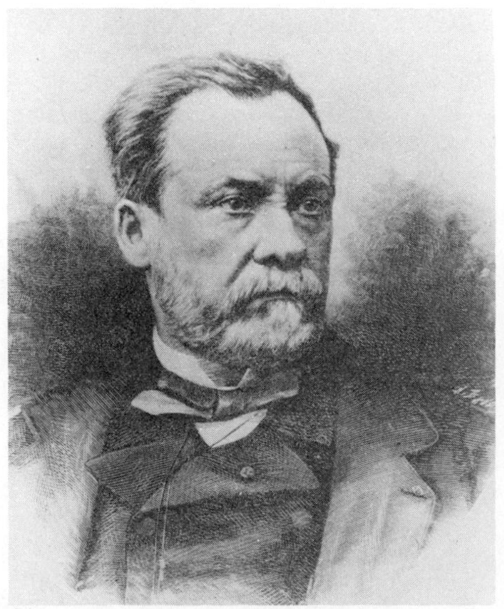

(a)

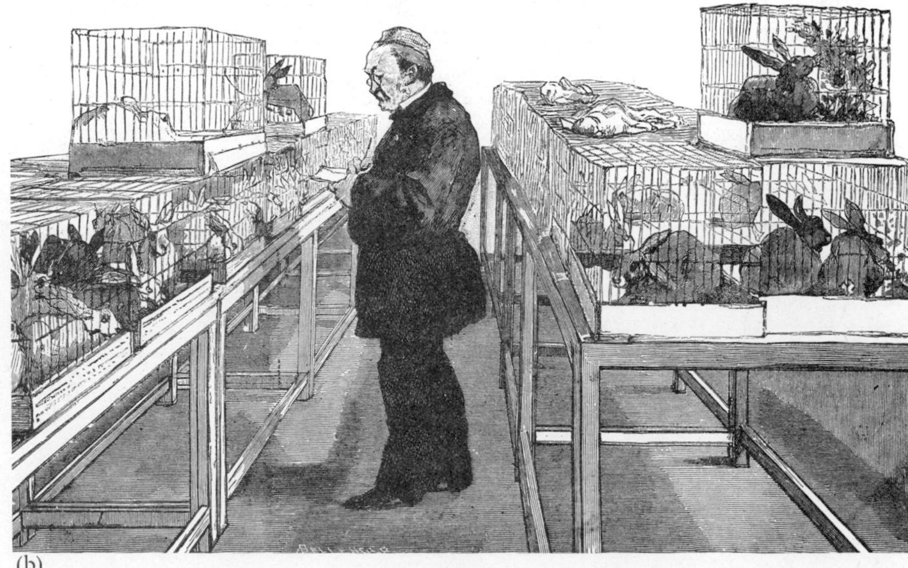

(b)

While studying the fermentation that produces butyric acid, a substance present in rancid butter, Pasteur discovered microorganisms that could live only in the absence of free oxygen. Normally these organisms are *motile*, but he noticed that those in close contact with air ceased to move. Pasteur quickly realized the possibility that air might inhibit these bacteria. He confirmed his suspicion by introducing a stream of air into fermentating systems. The effect was striking. The process either stopped totally or slowed down considerably. The terms **aerobic** and **anaerobic** were coined by Pasteur to distinguish between those microbes capable of living only in the presence of free oxygen and those capable of living only in the absence of free oxygen, or air.

Pasteur's discoveries contributed enormously to the control of microorganisms and demonstrated the relationship of numerous organisms to disease and to food spoilage.

The Spontaneous Generation, or Abiogenesis, Controversy

The theory of **spontaneous generation,** stated by Aristotle in 346 B.C., expressed a belief widely held as late as the nineteenth century—that life could and did appear spontaneously from nonliving or decomposing matter. People were constantly seeing what they thought were examples of this Aristotelian doctrine of spontaneous generation: snakes, frogs, and related forms of life developing from the mud of river banks, and maggots and flies appearing in decaying food. Aristotle taught that insects develop from morning dew and rotting manure and that tapeworms arise from animal wastes. These beliefs, held by all Greek scholars, were accepted and expanded throughout the Middle Ages and until comparatively recent times.

In the seventeenth century, the Belgian physician Jan Baptista van Helmont wrote a receipe for the generation of mice. According to his formula, a dirty shirt placed in a container with wheat grains for 21 days would form living mice. Although this result was not considered unusual by van Helmont, he was rather puzzled by the similarity between such spontaneously created mice and those born naturally.

Today the theory of spontaneous generation seems absurd. Certainly it was the product of inadequate observation and faulty deduction. Nevertheless, it figured importantly in scientific thought through the centuries—especially in the study of disease and of various natural processes such as fermentation. Before any relationship could be shown between microorganisms and disease, the concept of spontaneous generation had to be disproved.

The Macroscopic Level

FRANCESCO REDI

One of the first to refute the doctrine of spontaneous generation was Italian naturalist and physician Francesco Redi. Around 1665 he showed that maggots did not emerge spontaneously from putrefied (decayed) meat. Redi put meat in three separate containers. One of these was closed with a paper cover, another was left uncovered, and the third was covered with fine gauze (Figure 2–4). Naturally the meat readily putrefied and attracted flies. Redi made the following observations:

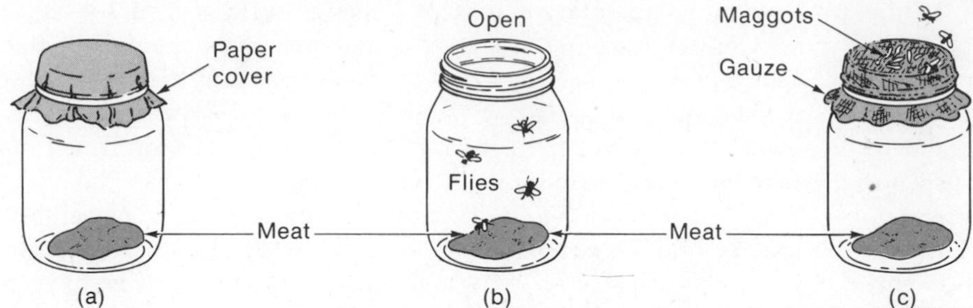

FIG. 2–4 Francesco Redi's experiment showing that flies were not spontaneously generated in meat.

1. The paper-covered container showed no evidence of any flies or maggots.
2. Flies laid their eggs on the meat in the uncovered container, and within a short period of time maggots and newly emerging adult flies appeared.
3. Although no maggots were present in the meat in the gauze-covered container, they did appear on the covering. Apparently the smell of putrefying meat attracted the flies. Unable to reach it, they laid their eggs on the gauze.

The conclusion seemed inescapable. Maggots, and the flies into which they develop, come not from the meat itself but from the eggs left on the meat by other flies. Thus Redi dealt a crushing blow to the myth that flies were spontaneously generated from meat. Even with his own evidence in hand, however, Redi himself continued to believe that insects in a type of plant tumor called *galls* arose spontaneously.

The Microscopic Level: The "War of Infusions"

Leeuwenhoek's later discovery of bacteria—*animalcules,* as they were called—revived the arguments over spontaneous generation on a microscopic level. Although he believed that his newly discovered forms came from the surounding air, Leeuwenhoek performed no systematic study to prove it. Another view shortly developed. Many individuals believed that nonliving material of animal or vegetable origin held a "vital," or life-generating, force that could give rise to animalcules. As proof, they cited the fact that microorganisms eventually appeared in boiled extracts *(infusions)* of hay and meat. In 1711 Louis Joblot found contradictory evidence when he observed that infusions stoppered tightly immediately after boiling remained free of microorganisms. However, if these stoppered preparations were later opened and exposed to the air, animalcules soon appeared. Joblot's findings were challenged, and thus the "war of infusions" began.

JOHN NEEDHAM

In 1749, John Needham, a Roman Catholic priest, reported the results of his experiments, which he believed proved that bacteria arose spontaneously where no such living forms existed before. Needham's studies consisted of tightly corking flasks of boiled mutton broth and observing them periodically for cloudiness as an indication of microbial growth. Some containers remained clear, but most eventually became turbid. Examining a few drops of these cloudy preparations with a microscope, Needham found them teeming with microorganisms. Since boiling was known to destroy microorganisms as well as any other living cells, Needham believed his experiments a clear demonstration of spontaneous generation. He postulated that the organic matter in his flasks possessed a "vital or vegetative force" that could confer the properties of life on the nonliving elements present.

LAZZARO SPALLANZANI

Sixteen years later, the Abbé Lazzaro Spallanzani, an Italian naturalist, reinvestigated Needham's findings and conclusions. He questioned the heating procedure used by his predecessor. Spallanzani found that flasks that were first sealed and then heated for one hour showed no cloudiness after a reasonable period. This experiment was repeated several times with the same results every time. Needham argued that the prolonged boiling procedure destroyed the life-rendering "vegetative force." Spallanzani responded by breaking the seal on his heated, closed flasks, allowing exposure to air. Within a short time, the contents of these flasks became turbid, showing that the long-heated organic matter was still capable of supporting life.

The effect of Spallanzani's experiments was short-lived. Soon after, the discovery of oxygen by Joseph Priestly, a Unitarian minister, and the demonstration of oxygen's importance to life by Antoine Laurent Lavoisier in 1775 rekindled arguments for spontaneous generation. Spallanzani's findings were criticized from the standpoint that sufficient oxygen was not present in his sealed flasks to support microbial growth.

Filtration Approaches

SCHWANN AND SCHULZE

It was now necessary to show that bacterial growth in nutrient-containing flasks was brought about by exposure to air containing these organisms and not by spontaneous generation. In 1836 Theodor Schwann set up two separate flasks, both of which held an infusion of some type. In one such experimental system (Figure 2–5), air passed through a red-hot tube before entering the flask containing the nutrient material. The other system, which received unheated air, served as the experimental control. Soon growth developed in the control, while the system receiving heated air remained **sterile** (free of any living organisms).

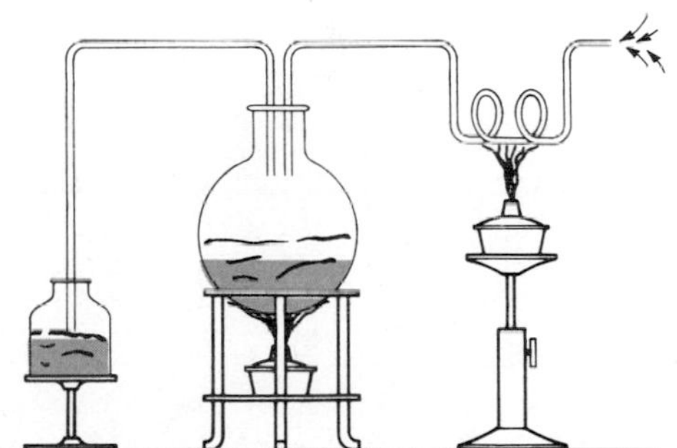

FIG. 2–5 Schwann's experimental system. When the center flask, containing an infusion or other nutrient material was exposed to heated air, growth did not occur in this system. Note the coiled glass tubing and the heating device on the right-hand side of the drawing.

Similar experiments were performed by Franz Schulze in the same year. However, his approach involved a different treatment of entering air. Air was allowed to enter nutrient flasks only after it had passed through solutions of such strong chemicals as sulfuric acid and sodium hydroxide. His results were the same as Schwann's. No growth developed in the flask receiving the treated air.

SCHRÖDER AND VON DUSCH

Upon learning of the experiments of Schwann and Schulze, the proponents of spontaneous generation insisted that the drastic treatments that the air systems were subjected to destroyed all possible "life-rendering power." This obviously would prevent life from being spontaneously generated. This objection was countered in 1854 by Heinrich Georg Friedrich Schröder and Theodor von Dusch, who introduced the use of cotton plugs for bacteriological culture flasks and tubes. Using a system similar to that of Schulze and Schwann, these scientists allowed air to enter untreated in any way except to filter it through cotton wool that had been previously heated in an oven (Figure 2–6).

The results of these experiments were the same as those observed by Schwann and Schulze. Flasks that received filtered air showed no signs of microorganisms, while those systems exposed to unfiltered air clearly contained microorganisms. These studies demonstrated that treatment of air with chemicals or with heat was unnecessary to prevent growth in nutrient-containing flasks and that the living forms in air could be removed from air by filtration through cotton wool. Pasteur later recovered some of the bacteria trapped in the cotton wool used for filtration, completing the proof of its filtering action.

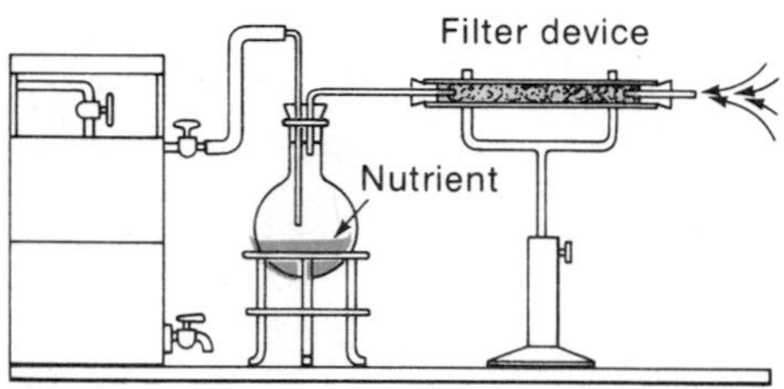

FIG. 2-6 The experimental system used by Schröder and von Dusch in 1854 to demonstrate the removal of living organisms from air by filtration. Draining liquid from the bottle on the left produced suction to draw air through the long tube containing cotton cool (at right). This air would then flow into the flask of nutrient material.

PASTEUR AND TYNDALL

Although these various experiments might seem conclusive, the issue was far from settled. In 1859, French naturalist Félix Pouchet claimed to have carried out experiments showing clearly that microbial growth could occur without contamination by air. About this time the studies of Pasteur were becoming known and several other scientists began to recognize the roles of microorganisms in fermentation and putrefaction processes. However, the acceptance of Pasteur's findings on the biological functions of microbes was threatened by the claims of Pouchet. Irritated by these arguments, Pasteur set out to disprove spontaneous generation once and for all.

Slightly altering the procedure of Schröder and von Dusch, Pasteur passed large volumes of air through a tube that held a plug of guncotton as a filter. A portion of the guncotton was then dissolved in an alcohol-ether mixture and the remaining sediment was examined under the microscope. Pasteur found small round and oval bodies that resembled the ***spores*** (reproductive structures) of plants. To show that the guncotton not only stopped the passage of microorganisms, but was heavily laden with these forms of life, Pasteur simply added a little of the used filter to sterile meat infusions. Soon microbial growth appeared. Thus Pasteur confirmed how microbes gained access to and how they could be prevented from reaching nutrients.

Despite his obvious success, Pasteur was not fully satisfied. He then performed what some regard as his most "elegant" experiment on the subject to show that microbe-free air did not create life in organic infusions. To special gooseneck flasks (Figure 2-7) liquid nutrient media were added after both flask and liquid had been boiled. No plugs of any type were used to prevent the passage of microorganisms into these systems. Although these systems were open to the environment, no growth occurred. Because of the length and the bend of the flask's gooseneck, microorganisms present in the air could not reach the flask proper. However, if the top of a system were broken off, or if a flask

FIG. 2-7 Pasteur's experiment disproving spontaneous generation.

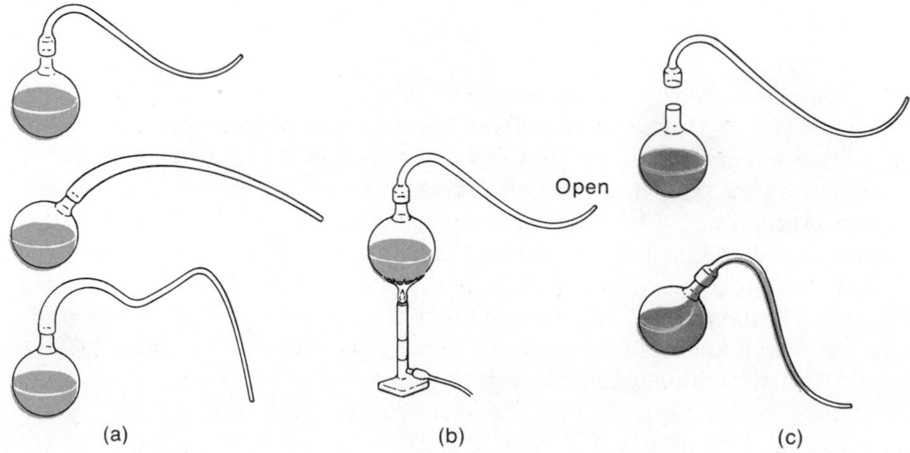

were tilted so that the sterile liquid nutrient ran into the exposed part of the neck and then returned, microbes soon appeared in the fluids.

Pasteur also demonstrated that the distribution of microorganisms is not uniform in the atmosphere. During a summer holiday, he took sealed flasks containing sterile nutrient fluids to many localities in France. A certain number of these flasks were opened at each location, exposed to the air, and then quickly resealed. Flasks exposed to the atmospheres of deep wine cellars or to mountain air in the Alps remained mostly free of microorganisms. However, the experiments carried out in the streets of Paris or on the road to Pasteur's home town, Dôle, produced several contaminated flasks. Thus Pasteur showed that microorganisms, although present in the atmosphere, are not evenly distributed.

Most authorities agree that the final blow to spontaneous generation was given by British physicist John Tyndall in 1877. In the course of his work on the optical properties of atmospheric dust, he observed that a beam of light passing through air without any dust particles was invisible. On the other hand, a light beam through a dust-laden environment was clearly visible. Moreover, the dust particles in such an atmosphere could also be seen. Aware of Pasteur's conclusions regarding the presence of microorganisms on dust and the greater likelihood of microbial contamination in a dusty environment, Tyndall devised a system (Figure 2–8) to determine if air lacking dust particles contained microorganisms. He built a chamber equipped with side windows and curved tubular vents through which bacteria could not enter. The inside surfaces of this box were coated with *glycerol* to trap the dust particles that sooner or later would come to settle on the surfaces. This chamber was fitted with a rack of test tubes. When the chamber was found to be optically empty of floating matter, as determined by shining a beam of light through its windows, the test tubes were filled with a broth, which was then sterilized by immersing the tubes in boiling brine. Tyndall observed that the broth remained sterile even though it was in direct contact with the air of the chamber. When dust-laden air was introduced, microbial growth appeared after a brief time. Thus, with his specialized chamber and techniques, Tyndall demonstrated that bacterial life occurred in sterile broth only after it was introduced from an outside source. His results also showed a correlation between the presence of particles in the air and the fermentation or putrefaction of the material exposed to it.

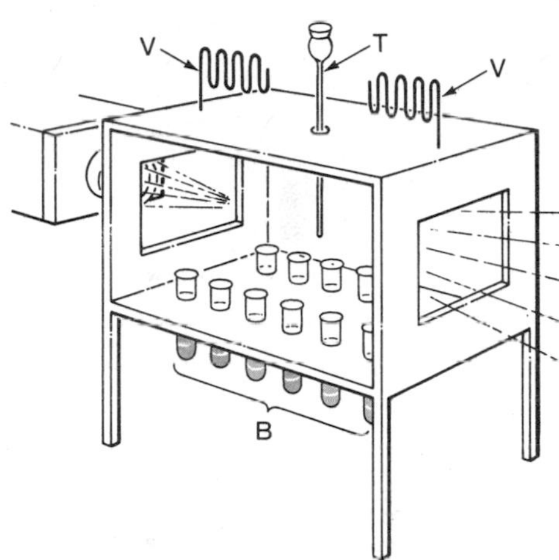

FIG. 2–8 The culture chamber designed by John Tyndall to investigate the relationship of bacteria and dust particles. Note the lateral windows, the specialized vent system (V) and the thistle tube (T) for the introduction of nutrient medium into the test tubes (B) located in the bottom of the chamber.

During the course of his studies, Tyndall concluded that bacteria existed in two forms. The *thermolabile* form was killed easily by a few minutes of exposure to boiling temperatures. However, the *thermostable* form was resistant to boiling for several hours. These incredibly heat-resistant bacterial structures, which are now known as *spores,* were independently found and named in 1877 by the German botanist-bacteriologist Ferdinand Cohn. While attempting to repeat his experiments with dust-laden environments, Tyndall was unable to obtain similar results after a bale of hay used in broth preparations was brought into his laboratory. The hay harbored too many spores and spore-forming bacteria. Only when tests were performed in different rooms could Tyndall duplicate his earlier results. In an effort to eliminate the spores, Tyndall developed an intermittent sterilization procedure, which subsequently became known as *tyndallization.* His procedure consisted of boiling the nutrient solutions for short periods of time on each of three successive days and incubating these preparations between heatings to allow microbial growth to occur. This was an effective procedure because growing bacteria are easily killed by boiling, and the time between heatings allowed the spores to germinate into growing bacteria, losing their heat resistance. Today, spores are destroyed in the laboratory by more rapid means, with the apparatus called the **autoclave** (Figure 19–2a). This device incorporates steam under pressure, usually at a temperature of 121.5°C, a higher temperature than Tyndall could attain without pressurized vessels.

A Word of Caution

We can safely conclude from the various studies reported here that microorganisms do not arise spontaneously from properly sterilized nutrient preparations. However, as a discussion in the next chapter will indicate, the possibility exists that the ***primary*** origin of life on earth did indeed involve a form of spontaneous generation. Moreover, these prehistoric events were quite different from those proposed by earlier investigators discussed in this chapter.

Antiseptic Surgery

When anesthetics were introduced into surgery and obstetrics during the 1840s, surgeons began performing longer, more complex procedures than ever before. Unfortunately, the number of surgical wound infections increased at the same time, often causing the death of patients. The young English surgeon Joseph Lister (Figure 2–9) undertook the task of preventing wound infection.

Impressed with Pasteur's studies showing the involvement of microorganisms in fermentation and putrefaction, Lister reasoned that surgical infection, *sepsis*, might actually be caused by microbes. He devised procedures designed to prevent access of microorganisms to wounds. Lister's system, which came to be known as ***antiseptic*** surgery, included the heat sterilization of instruments and the application of carbolic acid ***(phenol)*** to wounds by means of dressings. These procedures, critically received at first, ultimately proved to be effective in preventing surgical sepsis. Although Lister was not aware of the exact nature of the microorganisms involved, antiseptic surgery did provide an indirect source of evidence in support of the germ theory of disease.

The Germ Theory of Disease

In developed countries today, most major diseases, including cholera, plague, smallpox, typhoid, typhus, and yellow fever, are controlled by means of vaccination, sanitation, and the destruction of **arthropod** carriers such as fleas, lice, mosquitoes, and ticks, which serve to transmit specific infections. Unfortunately, in some parts of the world, many of these diseases still take a heavy toll. Because of the great suffering and disability caused by these diseases, humanity has benefited greatly from the contributions of Robert Koch (Figure 2–10), Louis Pasteur, and others who established the relationship between a specific disease agent and a disease, and who developed methods for the control of infections.

From earliest times, disease was associated with natural phenomena such as earthquakes and floods, mysterious and supernatural forces, and poisonous vapors called miasmas. Although ancient Greek and Roman physicians suspected that certain types of disease were caused by invisible, minute agents, no direct proof for this view was found until the nineteenth century. The concept of ***contagion***—the spread of infectious disease—preceded the proof of the existence of pathogenic agents by many centuries.

Fungi were the first microorganisms shown to be pathogenic. Agostino Bassi

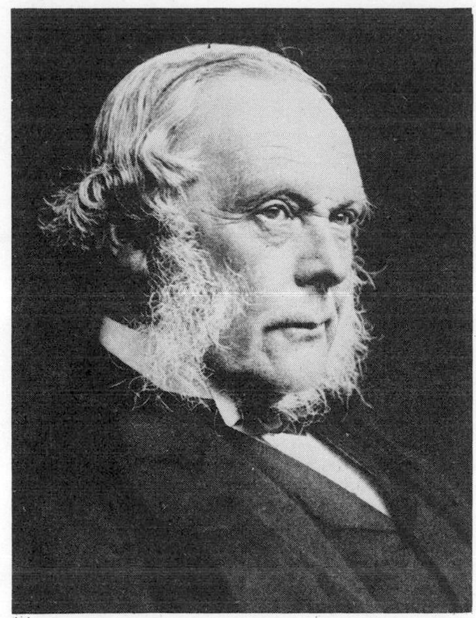
(a)

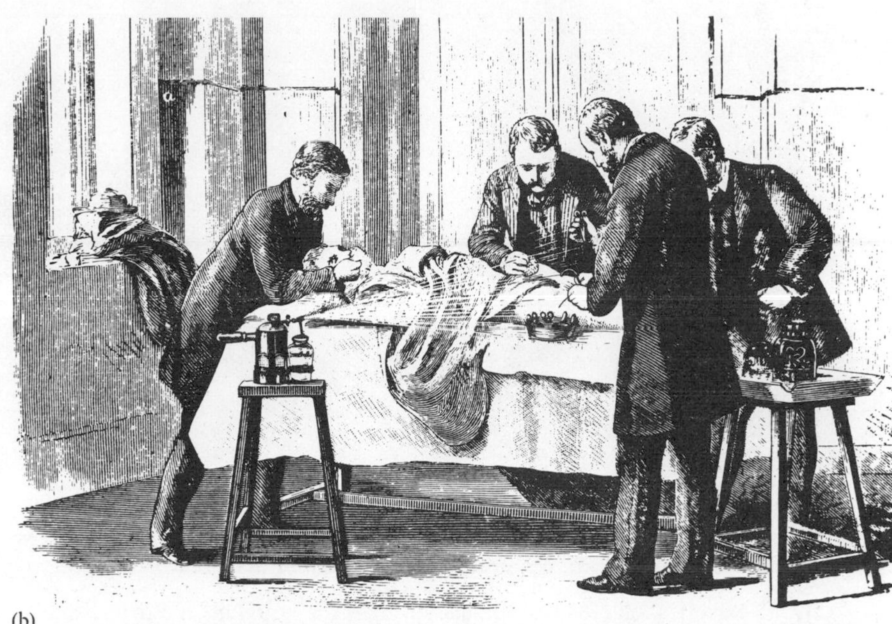
(b)

FIG. 2-9 (a) Dr. Joseph Lister (1827–1912). National Library of Medicine, Bethesda, Maryland. (b) A surgical operation in the early days of antiseptic surgery. Steam and the anesthetic, chloroform, are being administered to the patient. Lister's steam spray device is used here for the chloroform. *The Bettman Archive.*

proved experimentally that an agent of this type caused an infection in silkworms. This discovery was followed in 1839 by the first isolation of a fungus from a human skin disease by Johann Schönlein. As we will see in later chapters, many fungi are serious threats not only to humans, but to plants and other forms of animal life. Protozoa also were among the first micoorganisms shown to have an association with disease. This relationship is credited to Pasteur, who in 1865 discovered that an infection of silkworms, which were vital to the silk industry in Europe, was protozoan in nature. The disease was called pebrine.

Koch's Postulates

A direct demonstration of the role of bacteria as agents of disease was given by Koch in 1876 and confirmed by Pasteur and Jules Joubert. The organism used was *Bacillus anthracis* (Color Photograph 79), the cause of anthrax. Although rod-shaped structures had earlier been observed in the blood and organs of sheep dying of anthrax, there was no clear-cut proof at that time that these bodies caused anthrax.

Koch established a definite sequence of experimental steps by which the causal relationships between a specific organism and a disease could be proved beyond a doubt. Although this procedure is known as **Koch's postulates,** it is based upon the earlier theoretical work of the German scientist Jacob Henle. In showing the causal relationship of *B. anthracis* to anthrax, Koch first isolated the organism from an animal with the disease and ultimately completed the cycle by obtaining similar cultures from laboratory-inoculated animals with symptoms of anthrax. The steps of Koch's postulates are as follows:

1. The suspected causative agent must be found in every case of the disease.

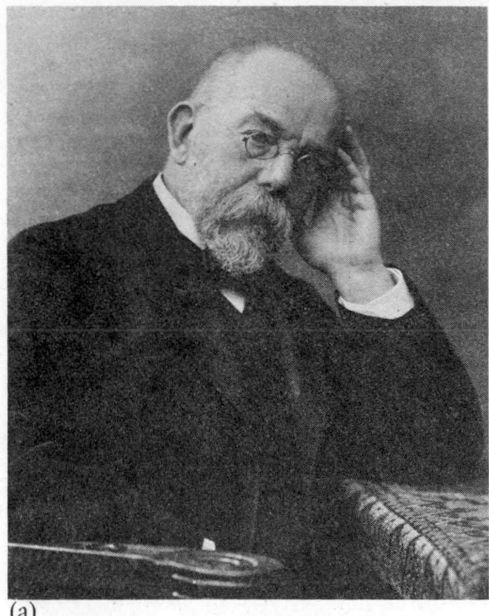

(a)

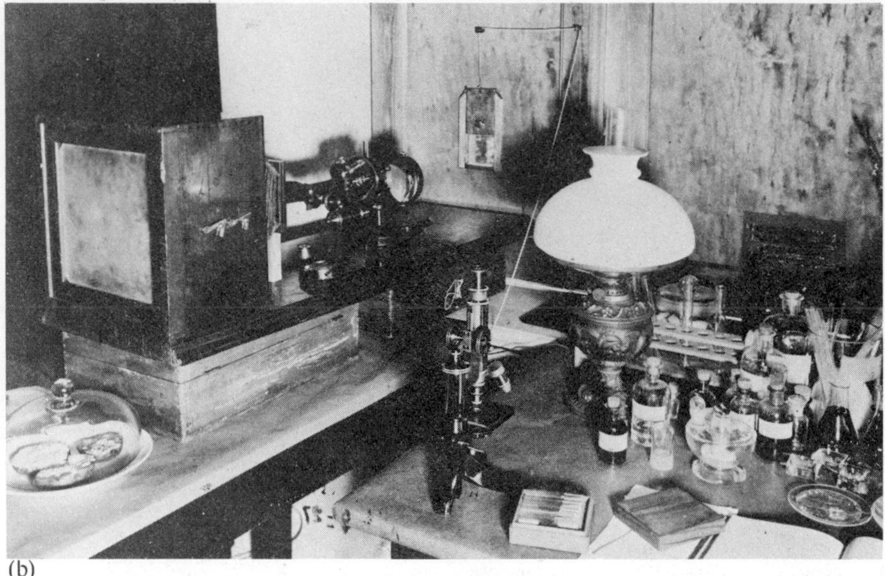

(b)

FIG. 2-10 (a) Robert Koch (1843–1910), one of the trailblazers of microbiology. This German-born bacteriologist identified human pathogens, developed bacteriological techniques, and discovered tuberculin, a tuberculosis skin-testing material. *National Library of Medicine, Bethesda, Maryland.*

(b) A view of Robert Koch's study. Note the various laboratory-related items: microscope, test tubes and rack, staining supplies, a bell jar under which microorganisms were incubated, and a photomicrographic camera (at left, horizontal position). *The Bettman Archive.*

2. This microorganism must be isolated from the infected individual and grown in a culture containing no other kinds of microorganism. (Koch utilized the fluid filling the eyeballs of cattle for this purpose.)
3. Upon inoculation into a normal, healthy, susceptible animal, a pure culture of the agent must reproduce the specific disease.
4. The same microorganism must be recovered again from the experimentally infected host.

With relatively few exceptions, the causal relationship between pathogenic bacteria and a particular disease has been shown according to the dictates of Koch's postulates. One notable exception is the causative agent of human leprosy, *Mycobacterium leprae,* for which the human body is the main natural host. Attempts to reproduce the disease under experimental conditions with organisms isolated from actual human infections have failed for the most part.

Rivers' Postulates

At the time Koch's postulates were formulated, true viral pathogens were unknown. In 1937, T. M. Rivers created a similar group of rules to establish the causal role of viruses in disease. *Rivers' postulates,* applicable to both animal and plant viruses, can be stated as follows:

1. The viral agent must be found either in the host's body fluids at the time of the disease or in the cells showing specific lesions.
2. The viral agent obtained from the infected host must produce the specific disease in a suitable healthy animal or plant or provide evidence of infection in the form of **antibodies** (substances produced in response to a virus) against the viral agent. It is important to note that all host material used for inoculation must be free of any bacteria or other microorganisms.
3. Similar material from such newly infected animals or plants must in turn be capable of transmitting the disease in question to other hosts.

Early Technical Achievements

Microbial Cultivation

With the growing interest in microorganisms, improved techniques for their handling and study developed rapidly. The advances included the preparation of several nutrient combinations, known as **media,** for the growth, or **culture,** of bacteria. Typical media included sources of carbon, nitrogen, vitamins, and trace chemical elements. All of these early preparations were in broth or liquid form. Although these media provided excellent growth conditions, they posed problems in the isolation and separation of bacteria from the mixed populations usually found in natural specimens. A general method of separating bacteria in mixtures was needed, especially in studies seeking the causative agents of infectious diseases.

The early approaches to isolating bacteria focused on the development of solid natural media. Freshly cut surfaces of potato were used to culture bacteria. After a suitable incubation period, distinctively colored bacterial growths, or *colonies,* formed (Color Photograph 21). Each isolated colony contained a single kind of organism. Other such media were carrot slices, freshly baked bread, meat, and coagulated egg white. Although each one proved satisfactory for bacterial culture, some were either difficult to work with or did not support the growth of all organisms of interest.

In 1881, Koch reported a relatively simple procedure for the surface isolation of bacteria from contaminated materials using a medium of coagulated blood plasma or gelatin-solidified broth. In the latter case, gelatin, a simple protein, would be added to a liquid medium that could support the growth of the desired organisms. While this preparation was still warm and liquid, it was poured on sterilized glass plates and allowed to harden. Organisms could then be introduced by spreading one drop of specimen solution across the surface of the gelatin. This process is known as *streaking* (Figure 13–8). The inoculated glass plate was covered by a bell jar and left to incubate. Some six years later, an assistant of Koch's, Richard J. Petri, introduced the **Petri dish** (Figure 13–1) as a more effective medium container than the glass plate.

Using his gelatin medium, Koch could obtain isolated colonies of bacteria that could not be grown on potato. However, the gelatin had several limitations, one of which was that it melted when warmed to more than 28°C. This made it impossible to obtain isolated colonies of human pathogenic bacteria, since the most favorable growing temperatures of these organisms range from 35° to 37°C. Other problems soon became apparent. Certain microorganisms were found to digest gelatin, leaving a liquified broth. Others would not grow well at low temperatures. Both limitations had to be overcome before pure cultures of human pathogens could be obtained.

Around this time, another associate of Koch's, Walter Hesse, learned of a far better solidifying agent than gelatin. The real credit for this new agent belongs to Hesse's wife. Upon learning of her husband's difficulty in finding a better way to grow pathogens, Frau Hesse told him of a substance used by her grandmother in the tropics to keep jams and jellies solid at warm temperatures. This material proved to be agar-agar (or simply **agar**), which is extracted from algae found along the coast of Ceylon, China, Japan, Malaya, and southern California. Agar is liquid at temperatures of nearly 100°C but settles into a firm gel at approximately 42°C. Most agar media now contain approximately 1.5 percent agar. As few bacteria are capable of digesting agar, it has proved to be indispensable in microbiology.

Chemotherapy

By 1900 the microbial causes of many important human diseases were known. These included cholera, diphtheria, leprosy, plague, tetanus, tuberculosis, and typhoid fever. During the ten years that followed, the bacterial agents of syphilis and whooping cough were added to the list. Despite the relative success in uncovering the cause of bacterial disease, advances in treatment were disappointing. Up to this time, infectious diseases were controlled mainly through the use of vaccines, such as the vaccine against smallpox. Furthermore, such approaches were largely preventative; little could be done to cure already infected individuals.

The modern era of control and treatment began with the use of chemicals that would kill or interfere with the growth of the disease agent without damaging the infected individual. This approach, known as **chemotherapy,** was introduced by Paul Ehrlich during his search for "magic bullets" to combat African sleeping sickness and syphilis (Figure 2–11 and Color Photograph 5). Ehrlich's efforts led to the discovery of an arsenic-containing compound that proved effective against syphilis (Color Photograph 87) and related diseases but produced undesirable side effects in patients.

Of all the advances made in the early part of this century, the one that is regarded as the major modern triumph of microbiology is the discovery and application of the wonder drugs known as **antibiotics.** In 1929, Alexander Fleming (Figure 2–12a) observed, as had many microbiologists before him, the presence of mold *(Penicillium)* in a Petri dish culture of the bacterium *Staphylococcus.* Strangely enough, the area in the immediate vicinity of the mold was free of bacteria (Figure 2–12b). On further study, Fleming isolated a mold-produced substance that inhibited bacteria but was nontoxic to laboratory animals. Fleming named his newly isolated antibacterial material *penicillin.* Years later, penicillin was purified sufficiently for human use. Today this antibiotic remains one of the most effective chemotherapeutic agents against bacterial disease.

Since Fleming's discovery, hundreds of new antibiotics have been developed for the control and treatment of infectious diseases. Almost all human bacterial infectious diseases that were once major causes of death have been brought under control through the use of these "miracle" drugs.

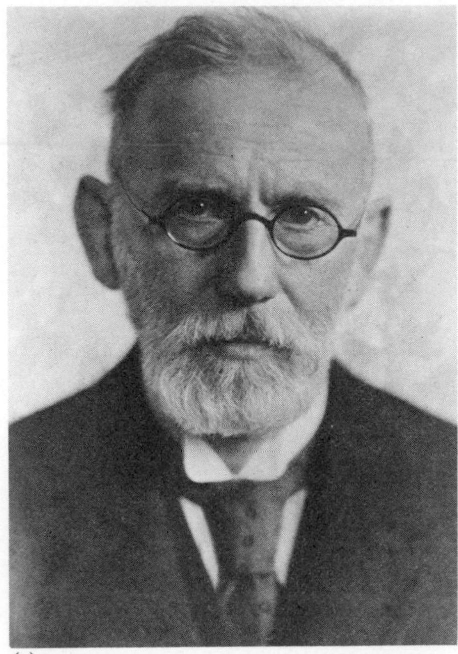
(a)

FIG. 2–11 (a) Dr. Paul Ehrlich (1845–1915), the famous physician-chemist who provided one of the first effective drugs to combat syphilis. In 1908 he and E. Metchnikoff were jointly awarded the Nobel Prize in immunology. *National Library of Medicine, Bethesda, Maryland.* (b) A microscopic view of the corkscrew-shaped bacteria that causes the venereal disease syphilis.

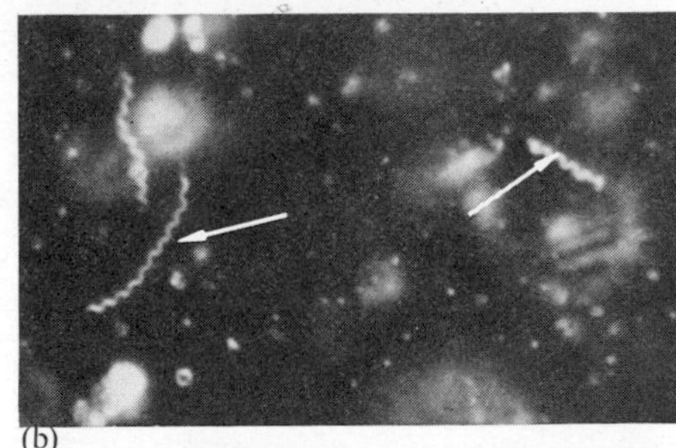
(b)

The Growth of Organized Microbiology

In approximately three quarters of a century, microbiology has become a significant influence in our society and one of the most dynamic and important branches of biology. Like any growing field, it requires a formal means of communication by which to exchange ideas and experimental findings. It is not surprising, therefore, to find that there are numerous journals, as well as several organizations, representing the specialties of microbiology. In the United States, for example, the American Society for Microbiology publishes several monographs, laboratory aids, and journals, including *Applied and Environmental Microbiology, Microbiological Reviews, Infection and Immunity, The Journal of Clinical Microbiology,* and *The International Journal of Systematic Bacteriology.* Comparable organizations are well established in other countries. Because these organizations are concerned with the advancement of

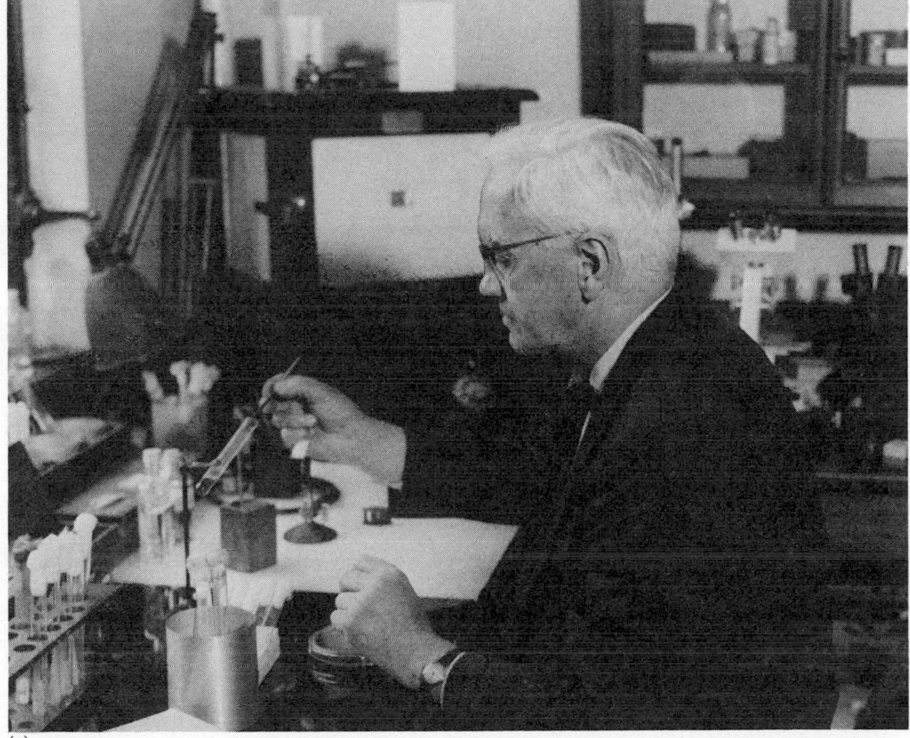

(a)

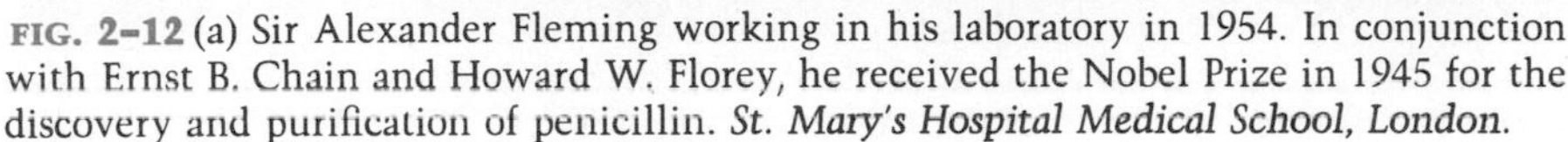

FIG. 2–12 (a) Sir Alexander Fleming working in his laboratory in 1954. In conjunction with Ernst B. Chain and Howard W. Florey, he received the Nobel Prize in 1945 for the discovery and purification of penicillin. *St. Mary's Hospital Medical School, London.*

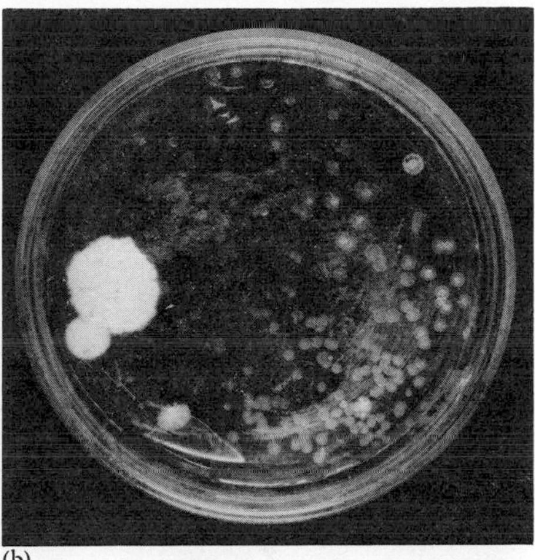

(b)

(b) The original culture plate on which Fleming observed the effect of penicillin on microorganisms. Note the limited number of bacterial colonies immediately around the fungus *Penicillium* (P). *St. Mary's Hospital Medical School, London.*

microbiology or one of its specialties, particular attention is given to maintaining the highest professional and ethical standards.

SUMMARY

Early Development of Microbiology

Leeuwenhoek

1. Leeuwenhoek designed and constructed simple microscopes with lenses that provided greater viewing detail *(resolving power)* than was previously possible.
2. He made the first accurate descriptions of most major types of single-celled microorganisms known today—*algae, bacteria, protozoa,* and *yeasts.*

Pasteur

1. Pasteur demonstrated the biological functions of microorganisms.
2. He developed effective vaccines against microbial diseases such as anthrax and rabies.

The Germ Theory of Fermentation

Nonvitalist versus Vitalist

1. *Fermentation* is a process in which alcohols and organic acids such as vinegar and lactic acid are formed from sugar-containing substances. Examples of the process include the souring of milk and the production of wine and beer.
2. According to the nonvital, or nonbiological, theory of fermentation, yeasts were by-products of fermentation. Supporters of this theory held that unstable chemicals called ferments caused fermentation.
3. The vital, or biological, theory of alcoholic fermentation, eventually proved true, held that yeasts were responsible for the reaction.

Pasteur's Contributions to Fermentation Research

1. Pasteur obtained experimental proof for the microbial nature of fermentation and for the specificity of fermentation reactions.
2. He developed the heating process, *pasteurization,* that kills or inactivates most disease- and spoilage-causing organisms.
3. He discovered *anaerobes,* microorganisms that can live only in the absence of free oxygen.

The Spontaneous Generation, or Abiogenesis, Controversy

According to the Aristotelian doctrine of *spontaneous generation,* lower forms of animal life arose spontaneously from inanimate or decomposing organic matter.

The Macroscopic Level

Francesco Redi demonstrated that spontaneous generation did not apply to animals by showing that flies did not develop spontaneously from putrefied meat.

The Microscopic Level: The "War of Infusions"

1. The eventual appearance of bacteria and protozoa in boiled hay or meat preparations *(infusions)* was offered as proof of spontaneous generation on a microscopic level.
2. Louis Joblot and Lazzaro Spallanzani independently showed that heating infusions under controlled conditions prevents the appearance of microscopic life.

Filtration Approaches

1. Various filtration methods were found to be effective in removing microorganisms from air.
2. Pasteur demonstrated that air free of microbes could not create life in organic infusions.
3. By means of a specially constructed chamber, John Tyndall showed that bacterial life occurred in sterile broth only after the broth was exposed to dust bearing bacteria from outside sources.
4. Tyndall and Ferdinand Cohn independently demonstrated the existence of heat-resistant bacterial bodies called *spores.*

Antiseptic Surgery

1. The introduction of anesthetics into surgery during the 1840s enabled surgeons to perform longer and more complex operations with a corresponding increase in the incidence of wound contamination and infection.
2. Joseph Lister developed methods to prevent the access of microorganisms to surgical wounds, instruments, and operating rooms.

The Germ Theory of Disease

1. From the earliest times, diseases were associated with natural phenomena, supernatural forces, and poisonous vapors.
2. Robert Koch, one of several individuals who established the causal relationship between a disease agent and a disease state, suggested a method of demonstrating this connection.

Koch's Postulates

Koch's postulates are a definite sequence of experimental steps by which to prove the causal relationship between a disease agent and a specific disease state:

1. Identification of the causative agent in all cases of the disease.
2. Isolation of the agent from the disease state and preparation of a pure culture.
3. Reproduction of the disease in a susceptible host by inoculation with the pure culture.
4. Recovery of the same microorganism from the experimentally infected host.

Rivers' Postulates

Rivers' postulates are a definite sequence of experimental steps similar to those developed by Koch, but applicable to both animal and plant viruses.

Early Technical Achievements

Microbial Cultivation

1. An important development in the study and handling of microorganisms was the development of nutrient combinations called *media.*
2. Richard J. Petri developed a foolproof medium container known as the *Petri dish.*
3. The introduction of the solidifying agent *agar-agar* into media made possible the study of microorganisms that grow over a wide temperature range.

Chemotherapy

1. Paul Ehrlich was the first to develop and apply chemicals for the treatment of disease and control of disease-causing microorganisms. This approach is known as *chemotherapy.*
2. Alexander Fleming is known for the discovery of *antibiotics.* The subsequent development and application of penicillin and other antibiotics have been important in the control of bacterial infectious disease agents.

The Growth of Organized Microbiology

1. Both national and international organizations exist that are directed toward the advancement of general microbiology and associated specialties. One such organization in the United States is the American Society for Microbiology.
2. Journals, laboratory aids, and special monographs are published by professional organizations as a formal means of communication for the scientific community.

QUESTIONS FOR REVIEW

1. Describe Leeuwenhoek's contributions to the development of microbiology. Did his discoveries go beyond the microbial world? Explain.
2. Why was the study of microbiology neglected after Leeuwenhoek's death?
3. Who first demonstrated the biological significance of microorganisms?
4. What were the major arguments used to support the nonvital and vital theories of fermentation? What are "ferments"? Describe the contribution of Schwann in demonstrating the role of yeasts in alcoholic fermentation.
5. What consistent patterns did Pasteur find in studying different fermentative processes? How did he show the microbial basis for fermentation?
6. What is pasteurization? What types of microorganisms are destroyed by this process?
7. What is the "doctrine of spontaneous generation"? How would you attempt to disprove it? Why did the discovery of oxygen in 1775 provide new support for the proponents of this concept?
8. Describe the experiments of Pasteur and Tyndall, and explain how they dealt the final blow to spontaneous generation.
9. Why was it important that the doctrine of spontaneous generation be disproved?
10. Describe the early concepts of the cause of diseases. What were some of the first indications of the role of microorganisms as a cause of disease?

11. What purpose do Koch's postulates serve? What significant contributions did Koch make to the germ theory of disease? What are Rivers' postulates?
12. What factors or situations made the early study of microorganisms difficult?
13. In what ways are the contributions of Paul Ehrlich and Alexander Fleming related? Describe their most important contributions.
14. Define or explain the following:
    a. antiseptic surgery
    b. pure culture
    c. spore
    d. agar
    e. fermentation
    f. antibiotic

SUGGESTED READINGS

Brock, T. D., *Milestones in Microbiology.* Reprint. Washington, D.C.: American Society for Microbiology, 1975. *An enjoyable publication containing the translated and edited papers of Koch, Pasteur, and many others involved in the history of microbiology.*

Burnet, M., and D. O. White, *Natural History of Infectious Disease.* Great Britain: University Press, 1972. *An interesting account of the discovery of various infectious disease agents and how diseases are spread and treated.*

Dobell, C., ed. and trans., *Antony van Leeuwenhoek and His 'Little Animals.'* Reprint. New York: Dover Publications, 1960. *A well-written introduction to the life and times of Anton van Leeuwenhoek.*

Dubos, R. J., *Louis Pasteur: Free Lancer of Science.* Boston: Little Brown and Co., 1950. *Pasteur's life and work are presented in an enjoyable and interesting manner.*

Lechavalier, H. A., and M. Solotorovsky, *Three Centuries of Microbiology.* New York: Dover Publications, 1974. *Traces the development of microbiology and includes descriptions of the works of individuals such as Pasteur and Koch, advances in immunology and chemotherapy, and the discovery of viruses. The importance of genetics to microbiology is also considered.*

CHAPTER **3**

Classification and Survey of the Microbial World

The world of living things appears to be made up of a bewildering number and variety of animals and plants. All of these forms of life are quite different, each going its own separate way at its own pace. But what about the portion of this biological world we don't see as easily? Where do algae, bacteria, fungi, protozoa, and even viruses fit in the scheme of life? To understand microorganisms—their functions and activities—and even to uncover the mysteries of how life originated requires a logical system by which to show differences, similarities, and relationships among organisms—a system of classification. In this chapter we shall see how a classification scheme developed. On an even more basic level, we shall consider differences in cellular organization and structure as criteria for classification. We will end the chapter with a survey of the theories of the origin of life.

After reading this chapter, you should be able to:

1. **State the importance of and need for classification.**
2. **List the taxonomic ranks.**
3. **Describe the early approaches to classification, and distinguish between natural and artificial systems.**
4. **Explain the arrangement of the five different kingdoms that make up the biological world.**
5. **Distinguish clearly between eucaryotic and procaryotic cellular organization.**
6. **Identify the positions of microbial groups in the biological world.**
7. **List the major characteristics of each kingdom in the biological world.**
8. **Describe how viruses differ from other microorganisms.**
9. **Describe modern concepts of the chemical origin of life and bacterial evolution.**
10. **Describe simulated prebiotic-environmental experiments and their limitations.**

The Importance of Biological Classification

Classification is an important aspect of most sciences, and similar classification principles and procedures have developed independently in many fields. The origin of classification dates back to the ancient Greeks, who first described the process of classification, the recognition of similarities, and the groupings of organisms.

There are several reasons for classifying organisms. The most obvious reasons are to establish the criteria for identifying organisms and to arrange similar organisms into groups. We shall also find that classification provides important information about how organisms evolved. And, above all, a good classification scheme is invaluable simply because it makes things less confusing.

Taxonomy, the study of classification, is the system used to make order out of chaos. Taxonomists name and identify different forms of life. They arrange the forms into a ranked series of categories that reflect their interrelationships. In this way the scientist is given the most probable explanation for the diversity of life, as well as insight into the evolution of different kinds of organisms.

Natural versus Artificial Classification

The classification of organisms is based on their similarities. Although there are several approaches to determining degrees of similarity, no agreement exists as to which one is best. The ideal goal is a *natural,* or *phylogenetic,* classification system, which identifies relationships between organisms on the basis of their probable origin. In such a system, organisms with a common origin are grouped more closely than those with dissimilar origins. The final outcome of a developed natural system resembles the structure of a tree, with the trunk representing the main course of evolution from its origin at the base, the branches and twigs representing later stages in evolutionary development, and the outermost leaves indicating biological forms now in existence.

The alternative to a natural classification system is an *artificial* one, based on easily recognizable properties of known organisms. This approach provides a practical and useful guide for the identification of unknown organisms.

The Naming of Organisms: The Binomial System of Nomenclature

For centuries, biologists have classified the forms of life visible to the naked eye as either animal or plant. This practice was eventually adopted as a scientific basis for separating the living world into the two kingdoms (groupings) **Animalia** and **Plantae.** In 1735, Swedish naturalist Carolus Linnaeus published *Systema Naturae,* which together with his later works served to organize much of the current knowledge about living things. Since Linnaeus knew nothing of

TABLE 3–1 Classification of the Human Species

Taxonomic Rank	*Designation*
Kingdom	Animalia (animals)
Phylum	Chordata (chordates)
Subphylum	Vertebrate (vertebrates)
Class	Mammalia (mammals)
Order	Order Primates (primates)
Family	Hominidae (humans and closely related forms)
Genus	*Homo* (the human and precursors)
Species	*sapiens* (modern human)

evolution, he based his classification system on structural and physiological properties of organisms.

Although the modern system of classification is based on evolutionary relationships, it makes use of one of Linnaeus' innovations, the **binomial system of nomenclature.** Under this system, all organisms have two-word names. For example, the name *Mycobacterium tuberculosis* first gives the genus *(Mycobacterium)* to which the organism belongs. The genus name always begins with a capital letter. The species name follows and begins with a lowercase letter. The **genus** is a group of related organisms; a simple definition of a species is more difficult to write. For higher animals and plants, a **species** is often defined as a group whose members have a limited geographic distribution and interbreed. Because this definition assumes sexual reproduction, it does not readily apply to microorganisms such as bacteria. For such biological forms, a species may be defined as a population of cells that are descended from a single cell and that therefore have the same genetic make-up. Such a population is called a *clone.*

Usually the genus and species names appear printed in either boldface or italics. They are Latin terms, or words from other languages to which Latin endings are added. The name of a microorganism frequently refers to a distinctive property of the organism, such as its color (*citreus,* yellow), the disease it causes *(pneumoniae)*, or its habitat (*coli,* colon). The name may also indicate its discoverer (*Escherichia,* by Escherich) or some other individual for whom it was named (*Yersinia,* for Yersin).

Groupings in the Linnaean System

In the Linnaean system, classification begins by dividing all life forms into **kingdoms.** Today five kingdoms are recognized. Each kingdom in turn is divided into general groupings, or taxonomic ranks, called **phyla** (plural of **phylum**) for animals, **divisions** for plants. For all kingdoms these ranks are subdivided into **classes,** classes into **orders,** orders into **families.** Families are subdivided into **genera** (plural of **genus**), and finally the genera are composed of **species.** Table 3–1 shows the classification of human beings according to the modern system.

The Position of Microorganisms in the Living World

In general, animals are characterized as lacking the typical structures of plants such as leaves, stems, and roots. In addition, they are noted as being actively motile, nonphotosynthetic, and quite complex. Plants are regarded as the opposite of animals in all of these respects.

Until about 1830, the taxonomic status of most forms of life remained fairly constant. However, the discovery of a great variety of microorganisms confronted biologists with several problems. While some microorganisms could be categorized as either plant or animal, many could not. Additional properties had to be considered. One of these was the presence of an outer structure called a **cell wall,** which would define a cell as a plant. Animal cells, such as protozoa, did not have this feature. Moreover, animal cells were able to capture and ingest solid foods, such as smaller protozoa and cell fragments, something plant cells could not do. Thus microscopic algae, bacteria, and fungi (molds and yeasts) were grouped into the Plantae while the protozoa were considered to be members of the Animalia.

Unfortunately, other problems soon became apparent. Microorganisms were discovered which had properties of both animals *and* plants. Biologists continued to assign these microscopic forms arbitrarily to one of the kingdoms. It was clear, however, that a suitable classification of microorganisms could not be based on the characteristics of larger animals and plants.

Early Bacterial Classification Schemes

Linnaeus himself studied bacteria and was quite detailed in his classification of these microorganisms. He, too, realized that microorganisms could not be easily grouped in terms of the established system. He therefore created a new category for them. Linnaeus classified all bacteria in a large group called *Vermes* and the genus *Chaos*. Later, bacteria were incorrectly shifted about into various other categories as a result of insufficient knowledge. In 1773, Otto F. Mueller placed all bacteria into the single species *Monas termo*, believing that these organisms were highly variable in shape *(pleomorphic)* but essentially the same in all other properties. Later, he decided that a second genus, *Vibrio*, was justified. The next step came in 1838, when the German biologist Christian Gottfried Ehrenberg proposed that all bacteria be placed into the class of Infusoria.

Up to the middle of the nineteenth century, bacteria were regarded as animal largely because of Leeuwenhoek's term "animalcule" for the microscopic forms he observed. The assumption that all such forms of life were of a similar type persisted until 1857, when the German botanist Carl Nägeli proposed that bacteria should have a class of their own in the plant kingdom. He designated this class Schizomycetes or "splitting fungi." Somewhat later Ferdinand Cohn published a new system of classification for bacteria, which was, as previous systems, based mainly on their **morphology** (form and structure).

The work of Pasteur and Koch, including the development of solid media and pure culture techniques, provided the tools with which to uncover a variety of characteristics for the classification and identification of bacteria. Thus, by the start of the twentieth century, an immense body of information on various organisms had been accumulated. In 1894, Walter Migula, a German botanist, described bacteria as belonging to two major divisions, the Eubacteria and Thiobacteria. The first group contained bacteria that were nonnucleated and colorless; the second group contained nonnucleated cells that had granules of sulfur or a bacterial pigment. Another notable contribution was made by Karl Lehmann and R. O. Neumann, who in 1903 established the beginnings of a formal manual for classification. For the first time, bacterial staining reactions and the ability of organisms to form the highly heat-resistant endospores were considered formal diagnostic features.

In the years that followed, a number of significant traits were incorporated into classification, including pathogenicity and metabolic activities. These and related developments led to the preparation in 1923 of the first edition of *Bergey's Manual of Determinative Bacteriology* by the Society of American Bacteriologists (now the American Society for Microbiology). Over the years, this most famous of modern texts on bacterial classification has incorporated all significant advances as they have been made. It records the discoveries of new species, new criteria of classification, and improved schemes for classification.

Unfortunately, no classification scheme entirely satisfactory to everyone has ever been developed, and several are in use. In this text we will use the most widely accepted terminology whenever possible.

The Five-kingdom Approach

The difficulties in applying the two-kingdom system to the classification of microorganisms are obvious. There is an enormous variety of microorganisms, differing widely in metabolic and structural properties. Some microorganisms are plantlike, others are animallike, and still others are totally different from all other forms of life.

A Third Kingdom: The Protista

In 1866, one of Charles Darwin's students, Ernst Haekel, proposed the establishment of a third kingdom to eliminate the existing confused status of microorganisms and to provide a logical position for them in the living world. This kingdom was to be called **Protista,** from the Greek word meaning "primitive" or "first." The new kingdom consisted of single-celled microbes, such as algae, bacteria, fungi, and protozoa, and multicellular organisms that were not differentiated (organized) into distinct tissues and organs as are higher animals and plants. The concept of protists gained in popularity over the years but was never universally accepted. In 1957, Roger Stanier and his associates gave new life to the term *protist*. They distinguished two subgroups based on cellular characteristics: the lower protists **(procaryotes),** microorganisms having a primitive nucleus, and the higher protists **(eucaryotes),** those having a well-defined nucleus.

Eucaryotic and Procaryotic Cellular Organization

Development of the electron microscope and of techniques for the preparation of biological specimens has clearly demonstrated the existence of two fundamental cellular organizations, namely, the **procaryotic** (with primitive nucleus) and **eucaryotic** (with true nucleus).

The more complex eucaryotic organization is found in fungi, protozoa, and certain algae (Figure 3–1a), as well as in typical animals and plants. Eucaryotic cells contain: (1) a nuclear membrane and structures within the nucleus that are called **nucleoli;** (2) organized structures in the **cytoplasm** outside the nucleus that are bound by membranes (for example, **endoplasmic reticulum, mitochondria, chloroplasts, golgi apparatus,** and **lysosomes**); (3) **flagella,** by which the cell moves; (4) a *mitotic spindle* during

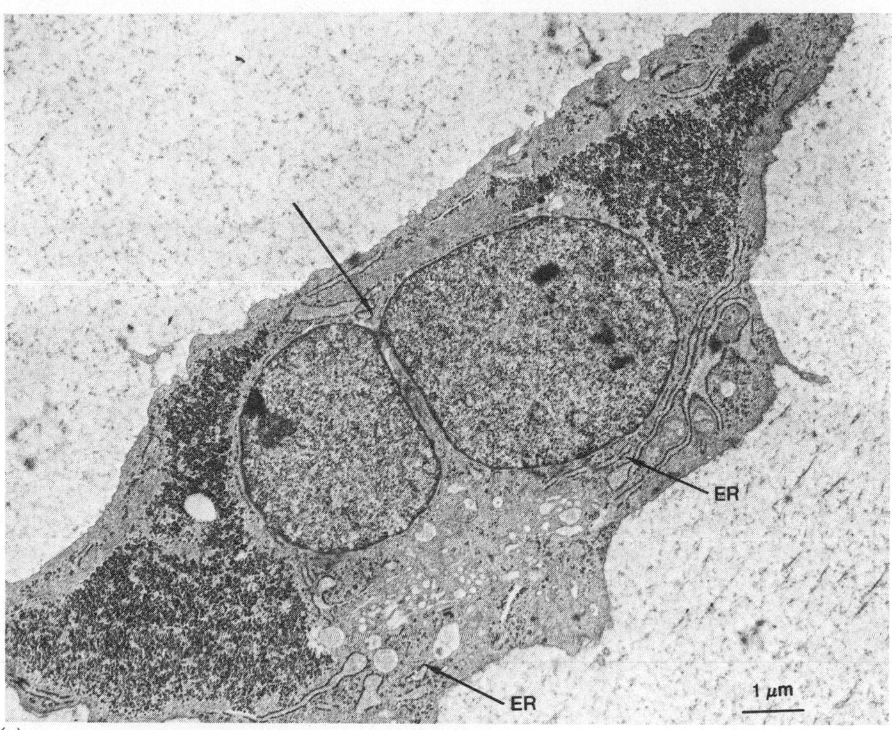

(a)

FIG. 3–1a Eucaryotic and procaryotic cells. A eucaryotic cell has a well-defined nucleus and nuclear membrane. The nucleus here is indented (arrow). The cytoplasm surrounding the nucleus contains the channels of the endoplasmic reticulum (ER), the major site for protein production in these cells. *Aparisi, T., B. Arborgh, J. L. E. Ericsson, G. Göthlin, and U. Nilsonne,* Act. Path. Microbiol. *Scand. Sect. A.* 86:*157–167 (1978).*

nuclear division; (5) ***chromosomes;*** and (6) the basic group of chromosomal proteins, called ***histones.***

Procaryotic organization is typical of bacteria (Figure 3–1b). Procaryotic cells lack most of the structures present in the cytoplasm of eucaryotic cells (Figure 3–1c). Because of this relative simplicity, the procaryotic cell is generally considered more primitive from an evolutionary standpoint than the eucaryotic cell. Procaryotic organisms, however, have some unique structural features. Among them are a nuclear region, or **nucleoid,** containing a single large

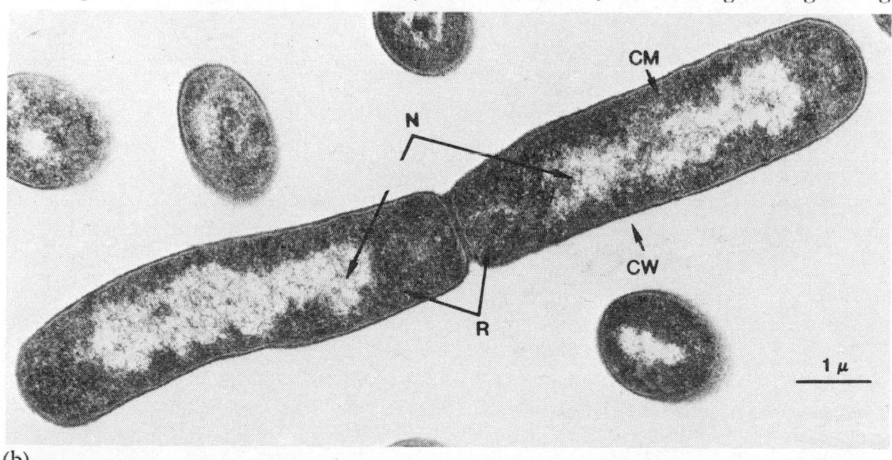

(b)

FIG. 3–1b A procaryotic cell lacks eucaryotic organelles such as a well-defined nucleus and an endoplasmic reticulum. The components present include cell wall (CW), cell membrane (CM), nuclear region (N), and ribosomes (R). *van Iterson, W., and J. A. Aten,* Antonie van Leeuwenhoek, 42:*365–386 (1976).*

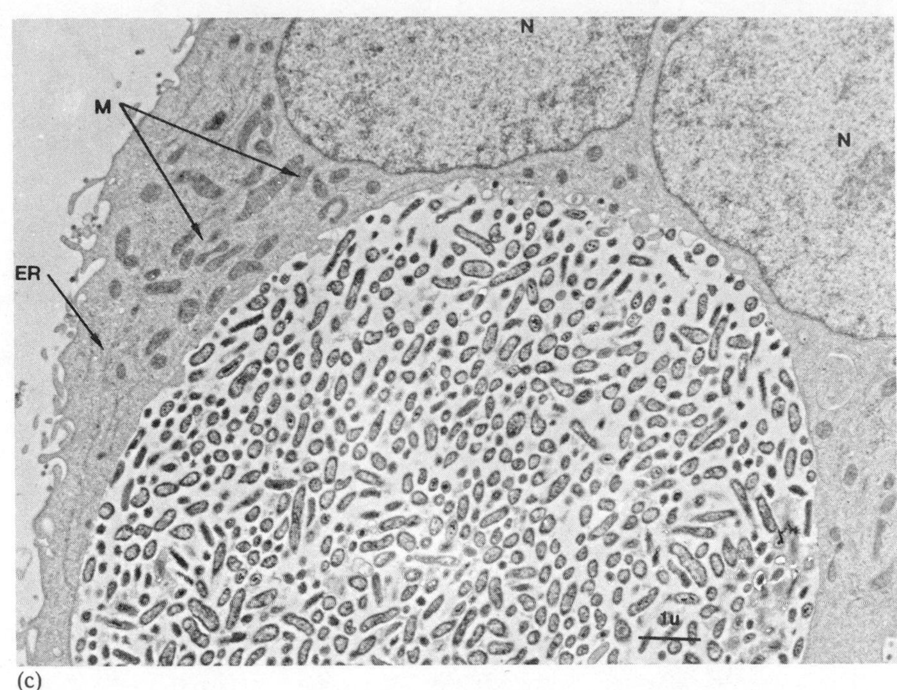

(c)

FIG. 3-1c Differences in procaryote and eucaryote cellular organization and size. Note the great number of bacteria (B) located within a white blood cell. It is obvious that none of these procaryotes have eucaryotic structures. Various components of eucaryotic cells are present, including endoplasmic reticulum (ER), mitochondria (M), and two nuclear segments (N). *Burton, P. R., J. Stueckemann, R. M. Welsh, and D. Paretsky,* Inf. Imm. 21*:556–566 (1978).*

deoxyribonucleic acid (DNA) molecule and a circular chromosome. All blue-greens, microorganisms formerly known as blue-green algae, and a few photosynthetic bacteria have layers of membrane, or *lamellae,* that are involved in photosynthesis utilizing bacterial chlorophyll. Table 3–2 compares these two types of cellular organization.

TABLE 3-2 A Comparison of Eucaryotic and Procaryotic Cells

Structure	*Eucaryotic Cell*	*Procaryotic Cell*
Nuclear membrane	Present	Absent
Nucleolus	Present	Absent
Chromosomes	Multiple and generally linear	Single and generally circular
Mitochondria	Present	Absent
Photosynthetic system	Chlorophyll, when present, and contained in chloroplasts	May contain chlorophyll, but not in chloroplasts
Golgi apparatus, endoplasmic reticulum, lysosomes, etc.	Present	Absent
Ribosomes	Large	Small
Mitotic apparatus	Present	Absent
Flagella	Present	Present but simpler structurally
Representative Microorganisms	Algae, fungi, and protozoa	Bacteria

The Components of the Five-kingdom System

Of all the classification schemes used in recent years, the one that now has gained widest acceptance is the **five-kingdom system** proposed by Robert H. Whittaker in 1969. According to this scheme, the living world is divided into the five kingdoms of **Plantae, Animalia, Protista, Fungi,** and **Monera** (Procaryotes). The relationships between the five kingdoms are shown in Figure 3–2, which suggests the descent of all organisms from a common ancestor, the first living cell. Whittaker's system is based on profound differences among eucaryotic and procaryotic forms of life, including their cellular organization—unicellular, unicellular-colonial, or multicellular—and their nutrition—absorptive, ingestive (Figure 3–3a), photosynthetic, or combinations of these. Brief descriptions of the kingdoms follow.

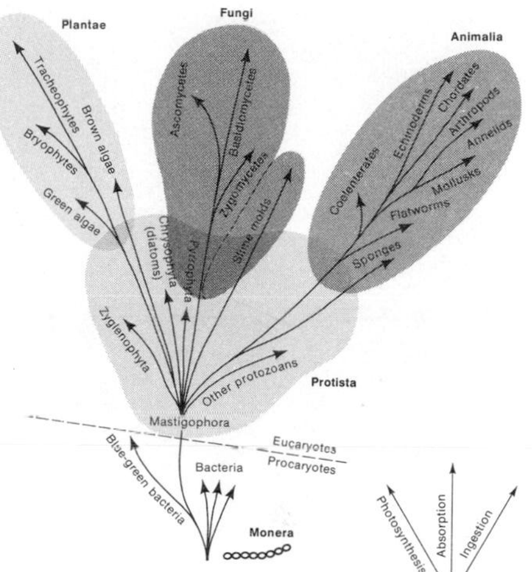

FIG. 3–2 The five-kingdom system of classification is based on three levels of cellular organization: procaryotic (Monera); eucaryotic, unicellular (Protista); and eucaryotic, multicellular and multinucleate (Fungi, Animalia, and Plantae). The divergence at each of these levels is based upon the three possible modes of nutrition: photosynthesis, absorption, and ingestion. The Monera lack an ingestive mode of nutrition, but at the highest level (multicellular-multinucleate), the nutritional modes distinguish the three higher kingdoms, Plantae, Fungi, and Animalia. *Modified from Whittaker, "New Concepts of Kingdoms of Organisms,"* Science *163:150–160 (1969).*

PLANTAE

Many of the species in this kingdom are well known and easily recognized green plants—garden vegetables, grasses, shrubs, mosses, and most algae. In general, plants are multicellular, eucaryotic, and have rigid cell walls. Most plants are photosynthetic, containing one or more types of chlorophyll, and, with few exceptions, they are nonmotile. Other properties of plant kingdom members include differentiation of their tissues (Color Photograph 7) into organized structures such as roots, stems, and leaves and complex life cycles, generally involving both asexual and sexual reproduction. Table 3–3 summarizes the characteristics of Plantae as well as the other kingdoms.

ANIMALIA

The animal life included in the kingdom Animalia ranges from organisms without backbones, such as sponges and worms, to highly developed forms with backbones, such as mammals. Animal cells are eucaryotic and enclosed only by a flexible membrane. They lack cell walls. Animals are multicellular, motile most of their lives, and they exhibit ingestive nutrition. Some show tissue differentiation. Animals may reproduce sexually and/or asexually.

PROTISTA

Various protozoa (Figure 3–3a and Color Photographs 5 and 43) and unicellular and colonial forms of algae (Figure 3–3b and Color Photographs 46 and 48) make up the Protista. Unlike typical animals and plants, protists are biologically and biochemically independent. There is no dependence upon other cells, such as exists in the tissues and organs making up higher plants and animals. The Protista is considered by some a transitional kingdom; in an evolutionary sense it falls between procaryotic organisms of the Monera kingdom and the more structurally sophisticated members of the animal and plant kingdoms. Others view Protista as a catchall kingdom for any organism that does not readily fit into another kingdom.

Protists are eucaryotic and obtain their nutrients in various ways, including absorption, ingestion, photosynthesis, and combinations of these modes. They exhibit both asexual and sexual reproduction.

FUNGI

This kingdom includes the familiar mushrooms (Color Photograph 3a), molds (Figure 3–3c and Color Photographs 34 and 41) and yeasts (Color Photograph

TABLE 3-3 Characteristics of the Five Kingdoms

Characteristics	Kingdoms: *Plantae*	*Animalia*	*Protista*	*Fungi*	*Monera*
Cellular organization	Eucaryotic and multicellular	Eucaryotic and multicellular	Eucaryotic, unicellular, and some colonial forms	Eucaryotic, multicellular, and unicellular	Procaryotic and unicellular
Cell wall	Present	Absent	Present with algae	Present	Present
Differentiation of tissues	Present	May be present or absent	Absent	Absent	Absent
Mode or type of nutrition	Primarily photosynthetic	Ingestive and some absorptive	Absorptive, ingestive, photosynthetic, and combinations	Absorptive	Absorptive
Reproduction	Generally both asexual and sexual	Generally both asexual and sexual	Asexual and sexual	Asexual and sexual with most	Asexual and rarely sexual
Motility (ability to move)	Mostly nonmotile	Motile	Both motile and nonmotile	Generally nonmotile	Both motile and nonmotile
Microbial representatives	None	None	Single-celled algae and protozoa	Molds and yeasts	Bacteria

35), as well as the less familiar slime molds, rusts, and smuts. An individual fungus organism may be microscopic or weigh several pounds (Color Photograph 37). Fungi are eucaryotic, possess cell walls, and may be unicellular or multicellular. Like animals, they are not photosynthetic. Fungi obtain their nutrition from the environment by absorption.

MONERA

The kingdom Monera consists of unicellular and colonial microorganisms with procaryotic cellular organization (Figure 3–1b). All of the functions and activities of life are carried out within the confines of these extremely small but far from simple cells. The monera includes a wide variety of bacteria (Figure 3–3d), such as the blue-greens and other photosynthetic organisms, agents of disease such as the rickettsia (Figure 3–4) and the chlamydia, and numerous beneficial and harmless forms. Most organisms in this group have absorptive nutrition, although some monerans are photosynthetic. Reproduction is mainly asexual, but a few species also reproduce sexually.

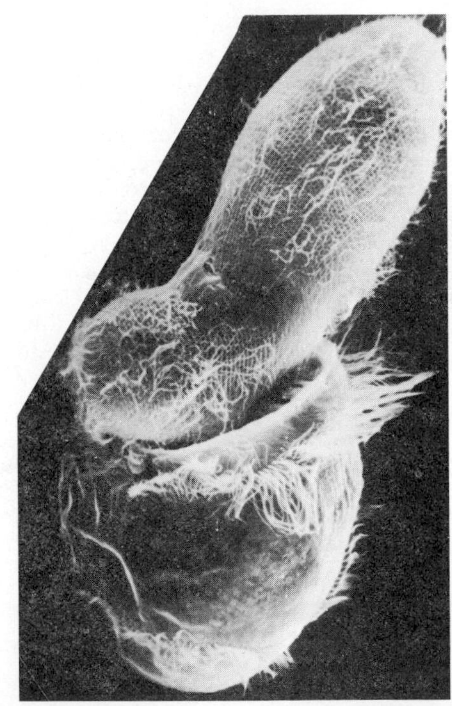

(a)

FIG. 3–3a Some members of the kingdoms of Protista, Fungi, and Monera. The carnivorous nature of certain protozoa is evident in this scanning micrograph. If the ciliate *Didinium* is hungry during a chance collision with the *Paramecium*, capture and ingestion of the larger protozoan almost always occurs. *Wessenberg, H., and G. Antipa,* J. Protozool. 17:*250–270 (1970).*

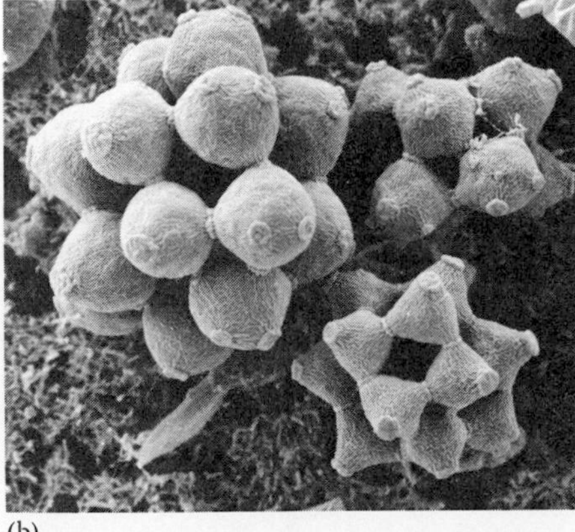

(b)

FIG. 3–3b A scanning micrograph of colony forming green algae *Coelastrum. Marchant, H. J.,* J. Phycol. 13:*102–110 (1977).*

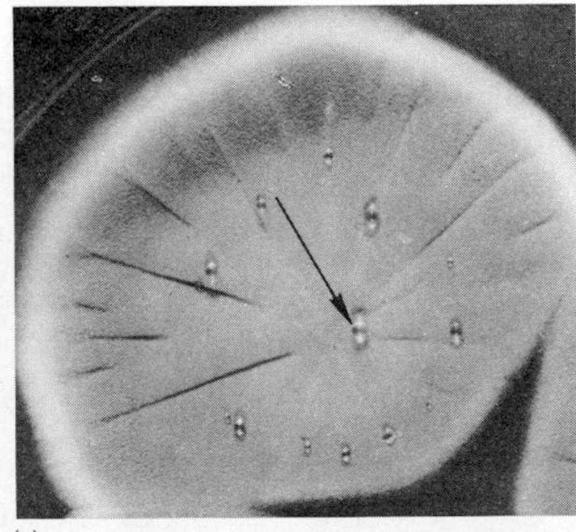

(c)

FIG. 3–3c The major sources of antibiotics are fungi. Here droplets of antibiotics (arrows) can be seen on the surface of the mold Penicillium. *Courtesy of Lederle Laboratories.*

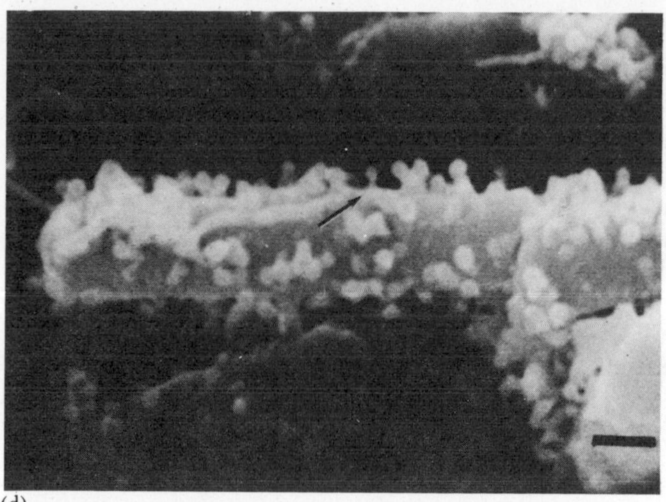

(d)

FIG. 3-3d A scanning micrograph showing the attachment of bacterial viruses to the cell wall of a susceptible procaryote. *Courtesy of Dr. K. Amako.*

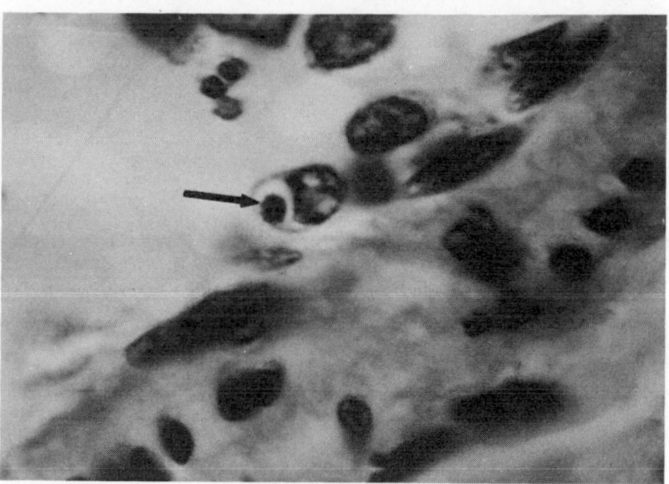

FIG. 3-4 Rickettsia, the bacterium causing ehrlichiosis in dogs. Its intracellular position (arrow) is evident. This microorganism is spread by ticks. *Hildebrandt, P. K., J. D. Conroy, A. E. McKee, M. B. A. Myindo, and D. L. Huxsoll,* Infect. Immun. 7*:265–271 (1973).*

A Consideration of Viruses

The classification of the submicroscopic microbes known as **viruses** has long been disputed by biologists. The debate has centered on whether these forms are living or not. Viruses are not cells (Figure 3–5). They do not possess the

FIG. 3-5 (a) Virus particles (arrows) inside a eucaryotic cell. Note the size of individual virus particles as compared to that of the nucleus (N), and other cellular components. *Grodums, E. I., and A. Zbitnew,* Inf. Imm. 14*:1322–1331 (1976). (b)* An electron micrograph of virus particles isolated from a case of human intestinal disorder. The absence of eucaryotic and procaryotic structures and organization is quite evident. The bar markers measure 1 micrometer (μm) or 1/25,000 of an inch. *Woode, G. N., J. C. Bridger, J. M. Jones, T. H. Flewett, A. S. Bryden, H. A. Davies, and G. B. B. White,* Inf. Imm. 14*:804–810 (1976).*

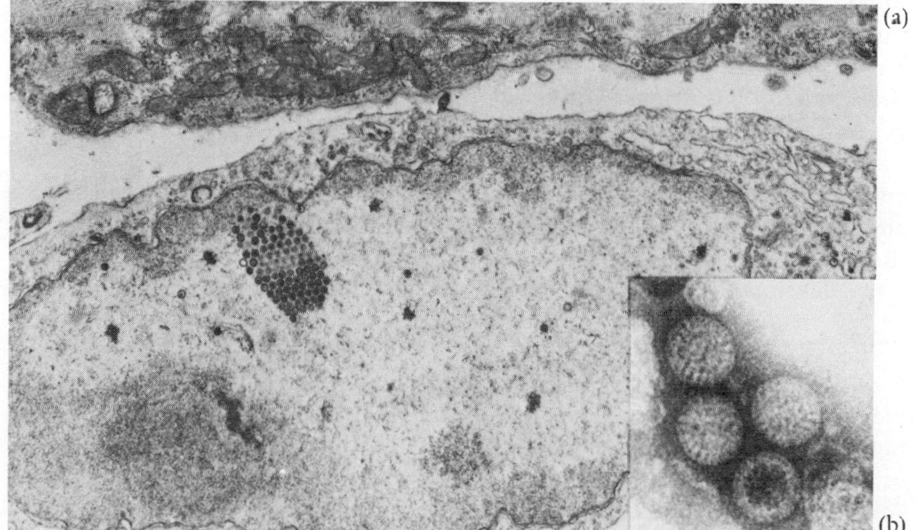

(a)

(b)

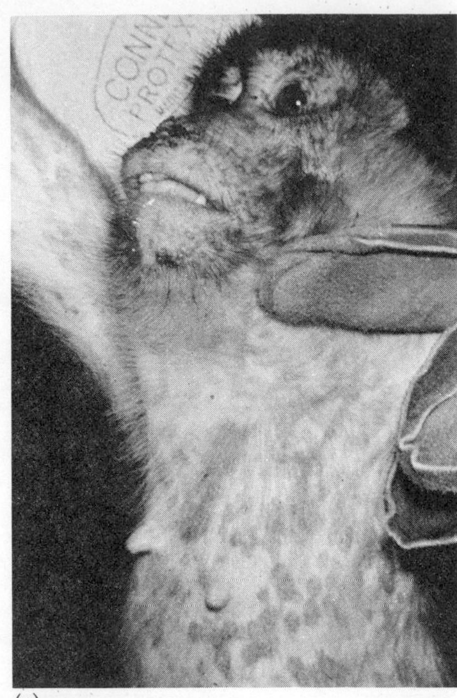

(a)

FIG. 3-6 Viruses have long been known to cause many human infections. They also cause infection of other forms of life, including lower animals. (a) A Macaque monkey with a chickenpoxlike skin disease. *Lourie, B., and A. F. Kaufmann,* J. Inf. Dis. *127:617-625 (1973).* (b) An acute case of foot-and-mouth disease, characterized by drooping and salivation. Foot-and-mouth disease is caused by one of the smallest viruses affecting animals. The disease is a continual potential threat to the beef and dairy industries of the world. *Courtesy of the U.S. Department of Agriculture.*

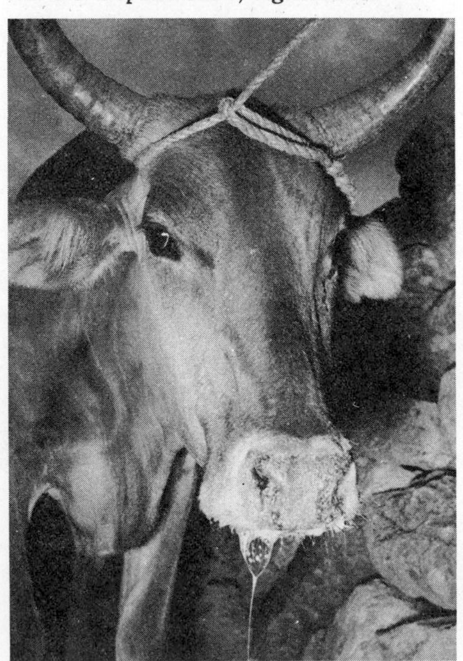

(b)

typical structures of procaryotic or eucaryotic cells, such as cell membrane, mitochondria, nucleus, and ribosomes. Most viruses consist of one type of nucleic acid, either deoxyribonucleic acid or ribonucleic acid, surrounded by a protein coat. Viruses invade living cells and use the metabolic and genetic machinery of the host cell to produce hundreds of new virus particles. Recent studies have also shown that some viruses can transform normal cells in laboratory animals into cancer cells. Viruses infect all types of life (Figure 3–6). Even microorganisms such as bacteria (Figure 3–3d), algae, protozoa, and fungi are not free from attack by these submicroscopic organisms.

Perhaps viruses exist at the boundary between living and nonliving matter. Although they resemble higher forms of life in that they undergo permanent genetic changes **(mutation)** and have a means of replicating and increasing their number, they do not readily lend themselves to classification by the type of rules and characteristics used in the classification of animals, plants, and other microorganisms. A further discussion of viruses is given in Chapter 12.

Trends in Microbial Classification

Some taxonomists consider certain properties of microorganisms to be more significant than other properties. For example, staining reactions or morphologic properties might be weighted more heavily than fermentative capability in assigning a microorganism to a group. Unfortunately, classification under such conditions tends to yield results that are biased.

Numerical Taxonomy

The purely mathematical method of **numerical taxonomy** eliminates the need to establish different weights for different characteristics. This method takes into account many properties, each with equal weight, in determining the similarity between microorganisms.

Using appropriately programmed computers, the properties of many organisms can be compared. This produces the information needed to arrange similar organisms in taxonomic groupings, or *clusters.* In this approach, each organism is classified as an *operational taxonomic unit,* or *OTU.* The computer determines the percentage of similarity between OTUs by finding the ratio of the number of characteristics they have in common to the total number of characteristics compared. This result is expressed as a percentage and is referred to as the *similarity coefficient.* Clusters of organisms are arranged according to the highest mutual similarity. Such similar clusters are called *phenons.*

The clusters showing the highest similarity are called *taxospecies,* to differentiate them from species that are shown to be related genetically, *genospecies,* and from species named according to the current method of binomial classification, *nomenspecies.* As more bacterial characteristics are analyzed, the possibility of developing a natural classification scheme of bacteria increases.

The amount of knowledge relating various organisms by numerical taxonomy will make a vast difference to microbial classification. In the field of medicine, the use of computers in classification offers greater potential for the identification of disease agents. It is possible that in the near future an instrument will be available that can obtain a pure culture, instantly perform 50 to 100 biochemical, morphological, and antibiotic sensitivity tests, and by consulting a computer, quickly identify a pathogen and suggest appropriate chemotherapy.

Molecular Approaches to Taxonomy

Genetic relatedness is an attractive addition to taxonomy, since it evaluates the relationship among organisms at a very fundamental level by comparing their genetic materials. Modern approaches to trace evolutionary relationships include (1) mating capabilities of organisms, (2) comparisons of the chemical composition of the DNA, which constitutes genetic material, and (3) comparisons of specific proteins or their components from different organisms.

The Origin of Life

Most theories of the origin of life suggest the guidance of a supernatural force to persons attuned to that philosophy. An opposite view can be taken by persons with an atheistic philosophy. This discussion takes a neutral viewpoint.

Before Pasteur's brilliant experiments refuting the spontaneous generation of life, it seemed obvious that the multitude of worms, snakes, and insects simply arose out of dirt, soil, water, decaying material, and so forth. When spontaneous generation was discredited, many looked to other planets for the origin of life. Such notable scientists as the German naturalist Hermann von Helmholtz and the Nobel Prize-winning physical chemist Svanti Arhennius proposed that life traveled to earth from outer space in the form of spores. Until and unless space missions find some proof of this hypothesis, the consensus is that we must look for the origins of life here on earth.

Oparin's Theory

At the beginning of the twentieth century, a new type of attack was launched on the problem of the nature and origin of life on earth. New concepts gradually arose that envisioned a long evolution of chemical substances before life actually appeared.

One of the first thorough presentations of a theory of the origin of life was published in 1936 by the Russian chemist A. I. Oparin. Oparin held that primitive earth had an atmosphere composed of simple hydrocarbons and superheated steam (steam above 100°C). As the earth cooled, steam condensed into large bodies of water forming a "hot dilute soup" of many organic compounds required by living organisms today. As proteins formed, several of them grouped together, thus creating ***colloidal*** (suspended) particles. This is an important aspect of Oparin's theory, since colloids have the ability to promote reactions much the way enzymes do. Colloidal particles tend to attract and attach other molecules to themselves. Thus they bring chemical compounds into intimate contact with one another. This contact, according to Oparin, favored new reactions forming new compounds. Ultimately, a droplet formed that was able to increase its stability, develop inheritable traits that were subject to mutation, and incorporate enzymatic activities. These activities included various metabolic pathways that allowed for rapid synthesis of compounds and production of the energy required for these reactions. At this point a living cell had formed.

Oparin-Haldane Concept

Working independently, the British-Indian biochemist B. A. Haldane applied the concept of spontaneous generation to the origin of life. He suggested that the primitive atmosphere contained carbon dioxide, ammonia, and water vapor. Upon exposure to ultraviolet light, these gases interacted to produce a variety of organic compounds. Both Oparin and Haldane believed that the evolution of matter was a slow process involving many levels of molecular and structural complexity. Neither scientist proposed the involvement of any mysterious mechanism.

SUPPORTIVE EVIDENCE

Although Haldane's concept could have been tested by simple experimentation in 1928, when he proposed it, it was not until 1953 that extensive study was begun (Figure 3–7). Stanley Miller and Harold Urey exposed a mixture of methane, ammonia, hydrogen, and steam, compounds believed present in the primitive atmosphere, to electrical discharges, simulating the lightning that must have existed then. Chemical analyses of the yellowish fluid that accumulated revealed a variety of amino acids, organic acids, and urea. With properly controlled experiments, Miller ruled out microbial contamination as a source of the organic compounds.

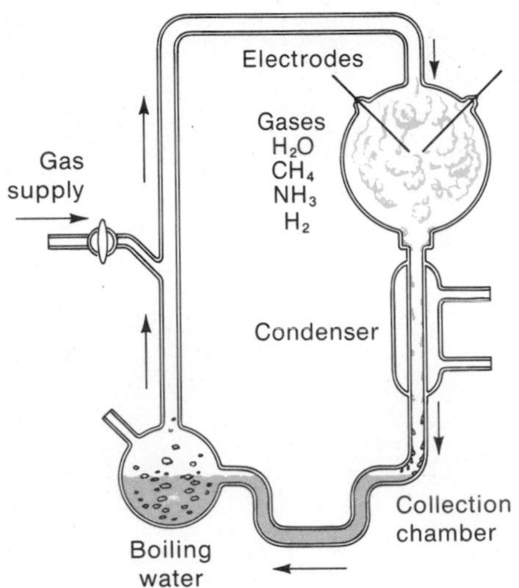

FIG. 3–7 Miller's apparatus, used to simulate the primitive atmosphere. Under these conditions, the gases of ammonia (NH_3), hydrogen (H_2), methane (CH_4), and water (H_2O) produced a variety of more complex organic molecules.

Miller's and Urey's findings stimulated other researchers. Using a wide range of reactants and energy sources and simulating a variety of different atmospheres, they identified several types of molecular products: amino acids; carbohydrates; numerous fatty acids and related compounds; biologically important purines, pyrimidines, and nucleotides, particularly adenosine triphosphate (ATP); and the components of chlorophyll and hemoglobin. Even evaluated cautiously, the results collectively indicate that a host of biochemically important compounds could have been formed in the primitive atmosphere of the earth. The "hot dilute soup" proposed by Haldane appears plausible.

THE NEXT EXPERIMENTAL STEP

The next step necessary in the series of events leading to the first living organisms would be the synthesis of macromolecules and ultimately their incorporation into a distinct system.

Probably the most significant experiments on macromolecular synthesis were performed by Sidney Fox and his colleagues, reported on from 1955 to 1963. These investigations undertook the synthesis of protein under primitive conditions. When amino acids are heated in a dry state at 150° to 200°C for 30 minutes to 3 hours, a linear ***polypeptide*** (several amino acids bonded together) is formed. This is called a ***proteinoid.***

One aspect of the behavior of these proteinoids is especially significant. When proteinoid material dissolved in hot water is allowed to cool for a few minutes, membranous structures appear (Figure 3–8). These ***microspheres*** are from 0.5 to 7.0 μm in diameter—roughly the size of some present-day bacteria. Some of the microspheres appear to form small extensions, or buds, and their membranes seem to be double-walled. These walls act as semipermeable membranes, that is, osmotic regulating structures. In addition, microspheres exhibit other properties found in contemporary cells, including catalytic activities, growth, motility, and a tendency to form junctions with one another.

LIMITATIONS OF THE SIMULATED PREBIOTIC-ENVIRONMENT EXPERIMENTS

On primitive (prebiotic) earth, with superheated steam preceding the formation of the oceans, amino acids forming on hot, dry rocks could possibly have yielded proteinoids. As temperatures dropped below 100°C, the oceans formed. The oceans could have transported proteinoid material into areas where conditions were favorable for microsphere formation. It is possible that Fox's microspheres in Oparin's "dilute soup" could have coexisted, and may have combined to yield double-walled membranes surrounding combinations of

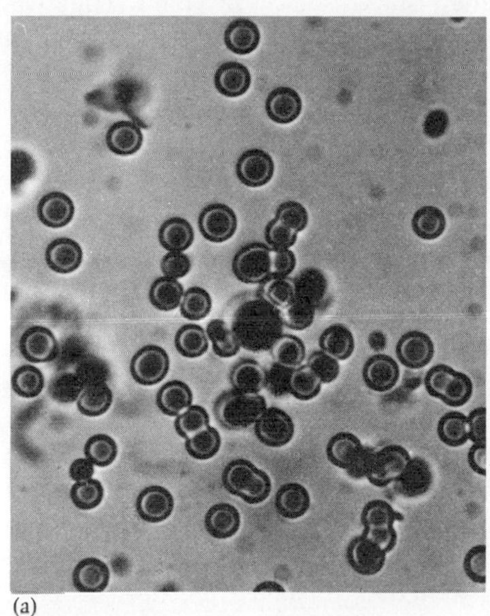
(a)

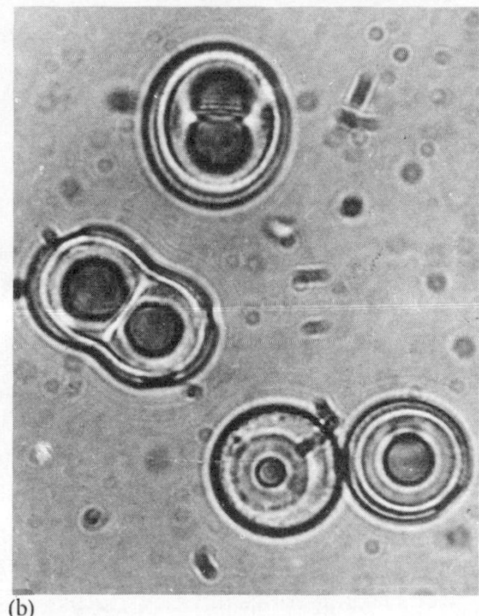
(b)

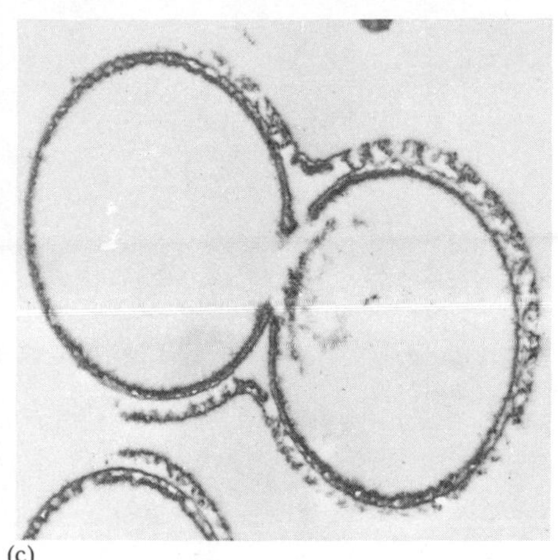
(c)

FIG. 3-8 Microspheres. Observed by S. W. Fox and associates, these microscopic spheres exhibit several properties common in contemporary cells, including osmotic properties, ultrastructure, and double-layered boundaries. Complex forms can be prepared by using additional types of molecular units. (a) Microspheres prepared by cooling hot, clear protenoid solutions. *Courtesy S. W. Fox, Institute of Molecular Evolution, Coral Gables, Fla.* (b) Protenoid micropheres in various stages of reproduction. *Courtesy S. W. Fox, Institute of Molecular Evolution, Coral Gables, Fla.* (c) Complex microspheres exhibiting substructure. *Courtesy S. W. Fox, Institute of Molecular Evolution, Coral Gables, Fla.*

organic molecules—proteins and carbohydrates, proteins and proteins or primitive cytoplasm. This arrangement would provide greater stability to the structure. If we assume that the membranes could rupture and reform, then Oparin's concept of coacervate mixing could function within the protection of membranes. If so, the first organisms could easily have been of microbial size and spherical shape.

The simulated prebiotic environment experiments have provided a number of provocative approaches to the question of the origin of life. Probably the most we can hope to achieve is to show how life *could* have originated—not how it actually *did* arise. The explorations of other planets hold great potential in this search. We may learn how similar or how different the processes of molecular and biological evolution are in various natural environments.

Fossilized Evidence

According to the present understanding of Darwin's theories of evolution and natural selection, life forms are constantly changing, usually very slowly, because of permanent genetic changes, or mutations. Such a change in a specific property of a particular species—for example, pigmentation, metabolism, or structure—might improve that species' chances for survival in a particular environment. The mutation serves as a selective advantage over other individuals. It favors the survival of the mutant to reproduce, passing along its new and favorable trait to its offspring. This condition would prevail until another change, either in the species or in the environment, upset the relative ability of the mutant to survive.

Paleomicrobiology

The evolution of various forms of life has been deduced largely from the study of ***fossils***, the remains of the past. A fossil may be in a petrified state, and therefore observed as a solid object, or it may be in the form of an imprint on a rock, left by a structure that has long since disappeared.

By studying fossils, we can observe changes in the body structure and appendages of animals and in the vascular systems of plants that have occurred since the time of fossil formation. Although it is easy to visualize the fossils of leaves, footprints, and bones, it is exceedingly difficult to imagine the appearance of

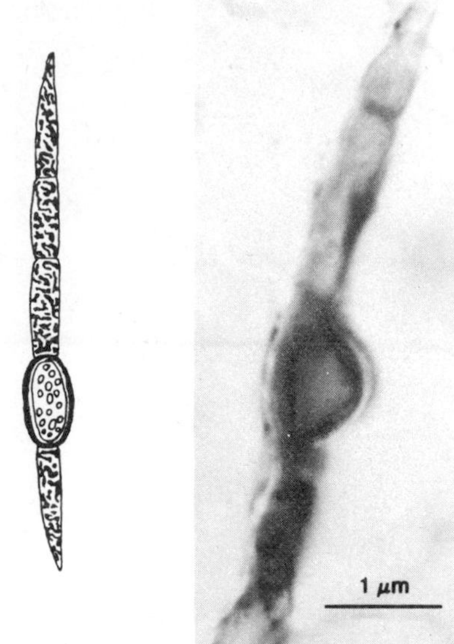

(a)

FIG. 3–9 (a) Microfossils. The microstructures shown are from the oldest known sediments on earth. These round or ellipsoidal microstructures appear to have double walls and are found individually or in chains or clusters. *Nagy, L. A.,* Science 138*:514 (1974).* (b) A photomicrograph of well-preserved microfossil filaments and spherical forms probably related to blue-green bacteria found in the late Pre-Cambrian Chuar Group from the eastern Grand Canyon. This area has long been considered a promising locale for the detection of early life. *Schopf, J. W., T. D. Fort, and W. J. Breed,* Science 170*:1319–1321 (1973).*

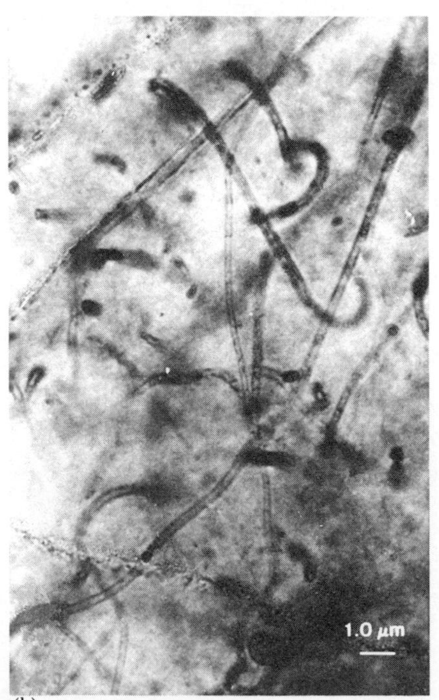

(b)

microfossils. Today's modern techniques, such as electron microscopy and microchemical analysis, are making it possible to study microbial genera that existed during Pre-Cambrian times, 2 to 3 billion years ago. With recent advances in this specialized area known as ***paleomicrobiology,*** microbial fossils have been discovered that indicate the existence of certain microorganisms 3 billion years ago.

Bacterial Evolution

Several hypotheses concerning the evolution of bacteria have been postulated. One of the first, and probably the most generally accepted, is a hypothesis proposed by A. J. Kluyver and C. B. Van Niel in 1936 but still unproved. According to them, the first or ***proto-bacterium,*** the ancestral source of bacteria, was spherical.

More recently, E. S. Barghoorn and his associates have uncovered direct evidence of the ancestors of modern blue-green, or photosynthetic, bacteria. During the examination of 3.5 billion-year-old rocks from South Africa's province of Transvaal, they discovered thousands of microfossils of individual and paired cells, some long and thin, others flat, wrinkled, or folded, but all similar to those found in much more recent rocks (Figure 3–9). If this fossil data is correct, oxygen-producing microorganisms were in existence 3.5 billion years ago. Presumably, the first organisms were anaerobic, since molecular oxygen did not accumulate until later.

In 1965, J. W. Schopf and his co-workers reported the presence of well-preserved rod-shaped and coccoid (spherical) "bacteria" in Pre-Cambrian iron formations. Their age was estimated to be 2 billion years old. By the use of surface replicas of ultrathin sections, rod-shaped "organisms" approximately 1.1 μm by 0.55 μm and coccoid "organisms" 0.35 μm in diameter were observed. Figure 3–10 shows the clumped and isolated rod-shaped "bacteria." The clumps of these "organisms" closely resemble the microcolonies of certain modern soil bacteria.

A Third Form of Life

In 1977, C. R. Woese and his co-workers found that the ribonucleic acid composition and genetic structure of specific bacteria known as the **methanogens** (methane-producing bacteria) (Figure 3–11) were distinctly different from those of other microorganisms or animals and plants. This discovery has far-reaching implications, since it suggests that there may be a third line of evolution. It has long been assumed that all terrestrial life evolved along two lines, one of which gave rise to animals and plants, the other to bacteria, fungi, and protists (Figure 3–2). On the basis of the genetic study of methanogens, it appears that a very ancient point of divergence occurred along these evolutionary lines.

Woese's findings also provide an important clue to the earth's early environment. Scientists have long believed that for about the first billion years after the formation of the earth, the planet was very warm and enveloped in clouds consisting largely of hydrogen, carbon dioxide, and other gases, but virtually no free oxygen. It was during this period that methanogens were to have evolved. In his studies of methanogens, Woese discovered the following properties: they thrive at high temperatures, between 65° and 70°C (Color Photograph 66), such as in the superheated springs at Yellowstone Park; they are anaerobic; and they utilize carbon dioxide and hydrogen and give off methane gas. These organisms may differ little from those single-celled methanogenic ancestors that evolved in the anaerobic primeval atmosphere.

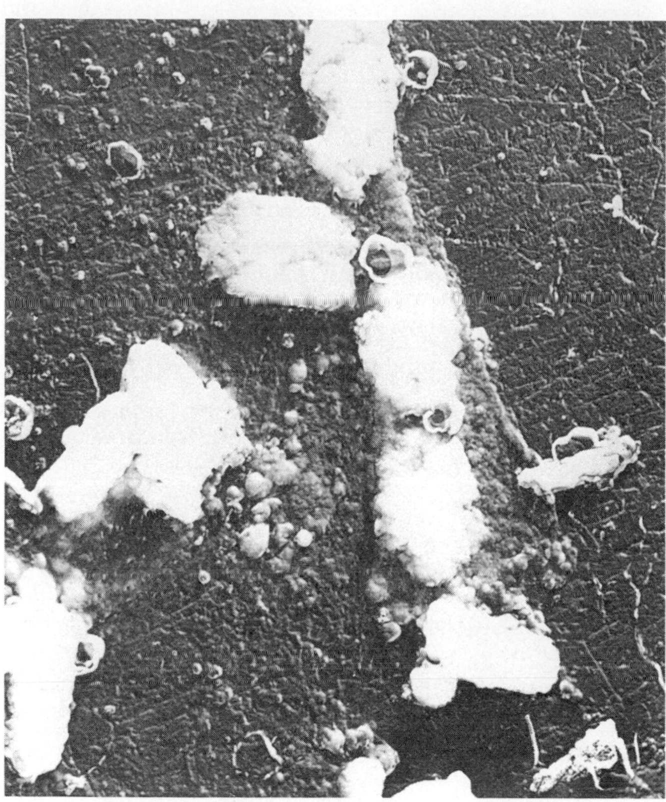

FIG. 3-10 Clumped and isolated fossil "bacteria" observed in Pre-Cambrian iron formations. *Schopf, J. W., E. S. Barghoorn, M. D. Maser, and R. O. Gordon,* Science 149:*1365–1366 (1965). Copyright 1965 by the American Association for the Advancement of Science.*

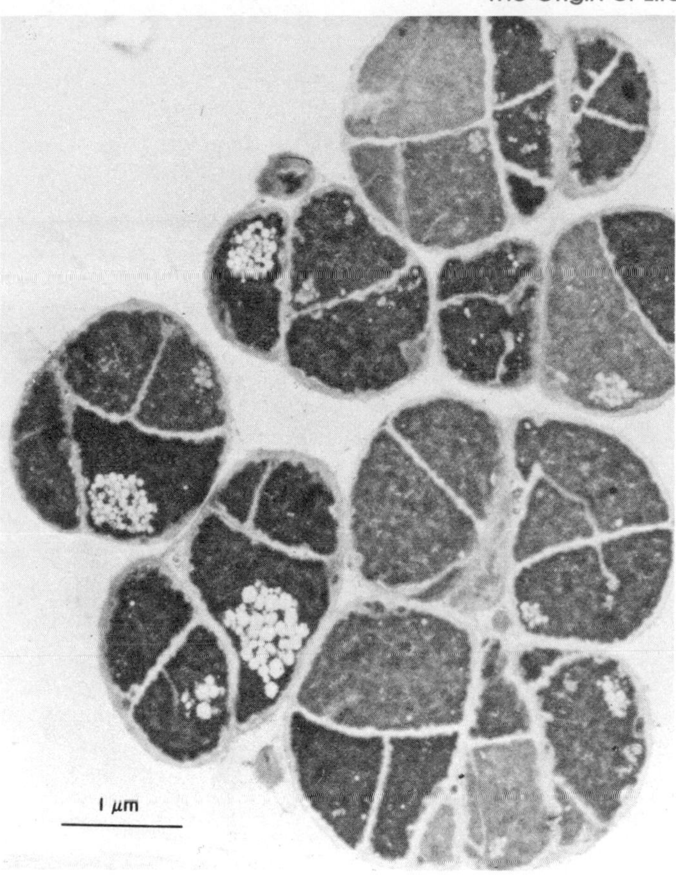

FIG. 3-11 An electron micrograph showing the methane-producing bacterium *Methanosarcina barkeri,* which has been identified as a descendant of a form of life that possibly dates back to the earth's first billion years. *Zeikus, J. G., and V. G. Bowen,* Can. J. Microbiol. 21:*121–129 (1975).*

SUMMARY

The Importance of Biological Classification

1. Classification of biological forms has several purposes: establishing the guidelines and properties necessary for identification; arranging organisms with similar properties into groups; determining evolutionary relationships; and lessening confusion.
2. Taxonomy is the study of classification.

Natural versus Artificial Classification

1. A *natural classification system* indicates relationships between organisms on the basis of their probable origin.
2. An *artificial classification system* is based on easily recognizable properties of known organisms. This approach is useful for the identification of unknown organisms.

The Naming of Organisms: The Binomial System of Nomenclature

1. All forms of life have two-word names, a system introduced by the Swedish naturalist Carolus Linnaeus.
2. The first name, the *genus* designation, always begins with a capital letter. The *species* name, which follows, is not capitalized. Both names are printed either in boldface or italic (italic in this text).
3. The scientific names of a microorganism frequently refer to a distinctive property or to its discoverer.
4. A species of higher animals or plants often is defined as a group of interbreeding organisms having a limited geographic distribution.

5. For microorganisms such as bacteria, a species may be defined in terms of a population of cells, or a *clone*, all descendents of a single cell and all genetically identical.

Groupings in the Linnaean System

1. All forms of life are classified in *kingdoms.*
2. Kingdoms are subdivided into smaller and more specific groupings or taxonomic ranks in the following sequence: *phyla* (singular, *phylum*) for animals, and *divisions* for plants; *classes, orders, families, genera* (singular, *genus*), and *species* (singular, *species*).

The Position of Microorganisms in the Living World

1. Until about 1830, all known forms of life, even microorganisms, were considered either animals or plants.
2. Newly discovered microorganisms with properties of both animals and plants presented taxonomic problems.

Early Bacterial Classification Schemes

1. Early systems were based on *morphological* (shape) properties.
2. Staining reactions, physiological reactions, and pathogenicity were incorporated into later classification schemes.
3. Since 1923, *Bergey's Manual of Determinative Bacteriology* has served as a significant text on bacterial classification.

The Five-Kingdom Approach

A Third Kingdom: The Protista

1. In 1866 Ernst Haekel proposed the establishment of the kingdom Protista for all single-celled microbes (such as algae, bacteria, fungi, and protozoa) and multicellular forms that were not organized into tissues and organs.
2. In 1957, Stanier and his associates suggested that two subgroups be established: the lower protists (procaryotes), or those with primitive nuclei, and the higher protists (eucaryotes), or those with well-defined nuclei.

Eucaryotic and Procaryotic Cellular Organization

1. Eucaryotic cells contain intracellular organized structures bounded by membranes internally, including nuclei, endoplasmic reticulum, mitochondria, mitotic spindle during nuclear division, linear chromosomes, and the basic group of chromosome proteins called histones.
2. Eucaryotic cellular organization is found in microorganisms such as fungi, protozoa, and certain algae, as well as in typical animals and plants.
3. Procaryotic cells lack most of the cytoplasmic structures of eucaryotic cells. However, procaryotic cells have unique properties that include single, circular chromosomes and bacterial chlorophyll associated with membrane layers.
4. Procaryotic organization is typical of bacteria.

The Components of the Five-Kingdom System

1. The living world is divided into the kingdoms of *Plantae, Animalia, Protista, Fungi,* and *Monera* (Procaryotes).
2. The system is based on the differences among eucaryotic and procaryotic forms, cellular organization, and modes of nutrition—absorptive, ingestive, photosynthetic, or combinations of these.

A Consideration of Viruses

1. *Viruses* are not cells. They do not have typical parts of procaryotic or eucaryotic cells.
2. Individual virus particles contain either DNA or RNA and require living cells to produce new viruses.

Trends in Microbial Classification

Numerical Taxonomy

1. This method utilizes a large number of equally weighted properties for microbial classification.
2. The degree of similarity between organisms is established by the ratio of number of characteristics they have in common to the total number of characteristics compared. This result, expressed as a percentage, is the *similarity coefficient.*

Molecular Approaches to Taxonomy

Modern approaches to finding the evolutionary relationships of microorganisms include the study of mating capabilities and comparisons of nucleic acids and specific proteins.

The Origin of Life

1. After the experimental results disproving spontaneous generation were accepted by the scientific world, other planets were considered as possible origins of life.
2. Spores from space seemed one possibility.

Oparin's Theory

1. Oparin held that the primitive earth had an atmosphere composed of simple hydrocarbons and superheated steam.
2. As the earth cooled, various organic compounds, such as proteins, and colloidal particles formed.
3. Ultimately, living cells were formed when these organic compounds came into contact with the colloidal particles.

Oparin-Haldane Concept

1. Haldane suggested that the primitive atmosphere contained carbon dioxide, ammonia, and water vapor. Upon exposure to ultraviolet light, these gases interacted to produce a variety of organic compounds.
2. Both Oparin and Haldane believed this process to be a gradual one.
3. Supportive experimental evidence was later provided by Miller and Urey in 1953.
4. Fox and his colleagues demonstrated the synthesis of protein-related compounds called *proteinoids.* These compounds possess the capacity to form microspheres with dimensions similar to contemporary bacterial cells.
5. The first organisms could easily have been of microbial size and spherical shape.

Fossilized Evidence

Paleomicrobiology

The specialized area of *paleomicrobiology* utilizes microfossils to study microbial forms that were in existence 2 to 3 billion years ago.

Bacterial Evolution

1. If current fossil data is correct, oxygen-producing microorganisms were in existence 3.5 billion years ago.
2. The first type of organisms were anaerobic, since molecular oxygen did not accumulate until later.

A Third Form of Life

Genetic studies of methane-producing bacteria suggest that there may be a third line of evolution. Currently existing *methanogens* may differ little from their ancestors that evolved in the anaerobic primeval atmosphere.

QUESTIONS FOR REVIEW

1. What is the significance of classification to the biological sciences?
2. What contribution(s) of Linnaeus are still used today?
3. Distinguish between natural and artificial classification systems.
4. What are taxonomic ranks?
5. Explain the binomial system of nomenclature.
6. Define *species*.
7. What are the advantages of the currently accepted five-kingdom system of classification?
8. Name at least five characteristics of each kingdom in the biological world.
9. What are the major differences between fungi and plants?
10. What important characteristics do the Monera and Protista have in common?
11. What is a virus?
12. Why is the classification of viruses in the biological world a problem?
13. Define, describe, or explain:
    a. paleomicrobiology
    b. genospecies, and nomenspecies
    c. clone
    d. proto-bacterium
    e. methanogen
14. What kinds of advances in microbiology have been critical to improvements in classification?
15. How were the following individuals involved in research concerning the origin of life, microbial classification, or evolution?
    a. Leeuwenhoek
    b. Fox
    c. Schopf
    d. Kluyver and Van Niel
    e. Oparin
    f. Miller
    g. Bergey
    h. Pasteur
    i. Koch
    j. F. Cohn
    k. Neumann and Lehmann
16. How does the fossil evidence for ancient microorganisms support the chemical theory of microbial evolution?

SUGGESTED READINGS

Dickerson, R. E., "Chemical Evolution and the Origin of Life," *Sci. Amer.* 238:70–86 (1978). *An easy-to-understand review of the various studies and speculations associated with biological evolution and the appearance of the first living organisms on earth.*

Holt, J. G., ed., *The Shorter Bergey's Manual of Determinative Bacteriology.* Baltimore: Williams and Wilkins, 1977. *As the title indicates, this book is a shorter version of a standard reference used for bacterial identification and classification. It contains descriptions of all genera, keys and tables for species identification, and an outline to bacterial identification.*

Lapage, S. P., P. H. A. Sneath, E. F. Lessel, V. D. D. Skerman, H. P. R. Seeliger, and W. A. Clark, eds., *International Code of Nomenclature of Bacteria.* Washington, D.C.: American Society for Microbiology, 1975. *Presents a glimpse into the future of naming microorganisms. It also outlines the rules under which such naming is to be based.*

Ponnamperuma, C., *The Origins of Life.* New York: E. P. Dutton & Co., 1972. *A clearly presented modern view of the origins of life on earth and the possibilities of life on other planets.*

Rossmoore, H. W., *The Microbes, Our Unseen Friends.* Detroit: Wayne State University Press, 1976. *A well-written and enjoyable book that emphasizes the beneficial importance of microorganisms, especially in food production. The author combines technical information with touches of humor.*

Schopf, J. W., "The Evolution of the Earliest Cell," *Sci. Amer.* 239:111–138 (1978). *An interesting account of the earliest of cells and of the events that led to the appearance of biochemical systems and the oxygen-enriched atmosphere on which life depends today.*

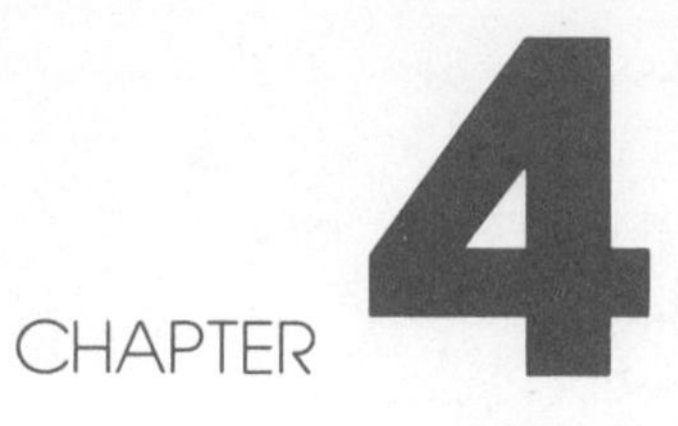

CHAPTER 4 Techniques Used in the Observation of Microorganisms

The microscope is the key investigative tool of microbiology. The microscopic observation of organisms involves staining procedures for identification and the use of the metric system to record the dimensions of organisms. These and the advantages and limitations of major types of microscopes are the subject of Chapter 4.

After reading this chapter, you should be able to:

1. **Apply the metric system of measurement to the structures of typical animal and plant cells and microorganisms.**
2. **Describe the general properties of light as it applies to microscopy.**
3. **Name and give the functions of the components of a bright-field microscope.**
4. **List the uses and relative advantages of microscope objectives in the examination of cells.**
5. **Describe the different types of microscopes, explaining associated techniques used in the study of microorganisms and other biological materials.**
6. **Outline the major differential staining techniques used in the identification of microorganisms and their parts.**
7. **List the advantages and limitations of staining procedures.**
8. **Describe how specimens and preparation techniques used with electron microscopes differ from those used with other microscopes.**
9. **Summarize the general advantages, limitations, and areas of application for different types of microscopy.**
10. **Define or explain the following terms: micrometer, resolving power, dyes, Gram-positive, acid-fast, freeze-fracture, sectioning, high-voltage electron microscopy.**

Microscopes and Microscopy

Microorganisms cannot be seen with the naked eye. Although several microbial forms—algae, bacteria, protozoa, and yeasts—had been observed by Anton van Leeuwenhoek as early as 1674, not until the development of modern compound microscopes did biologists the world over become aware of the tremendous number and variety of microorganisms.

The microscopes used today have evolved significantly from Leeuwenhoek's first simple microscopes (Figure 4–1). Depending upon the magnification principle involved, microscopes are known as either ***light microscopes*** or ***electron microscopes***. Light, or optical, microscopes may be bright-field, dark-field, fluorescence, or phase-contrast instruments. Electron microscopes are of two kinds—transmission and scanning electron microscopes. Before considering the various forms of microscopy, we shall review the units of measurement used in describing the morphologic characteristics of microorganisms and also review some fundamentals of optics.

Units of Measurement

For most of our everyday activities, we find it convenient to use familiar units of measurement, such as the inch, foot, yard, ounce, or pound. In addition, we usually use numbers that are neither very large nor very small to

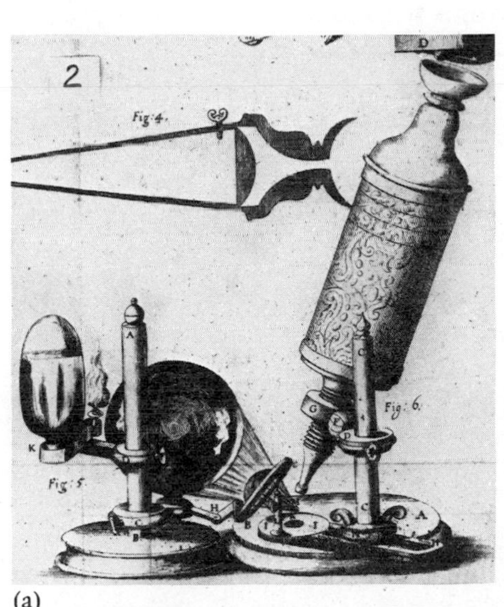

(a)

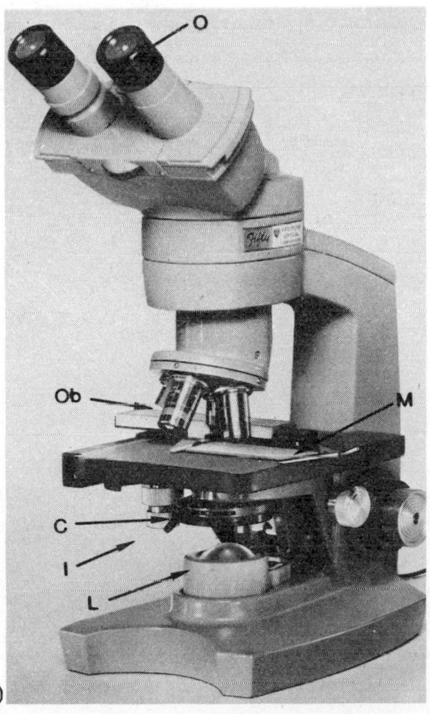

(b)

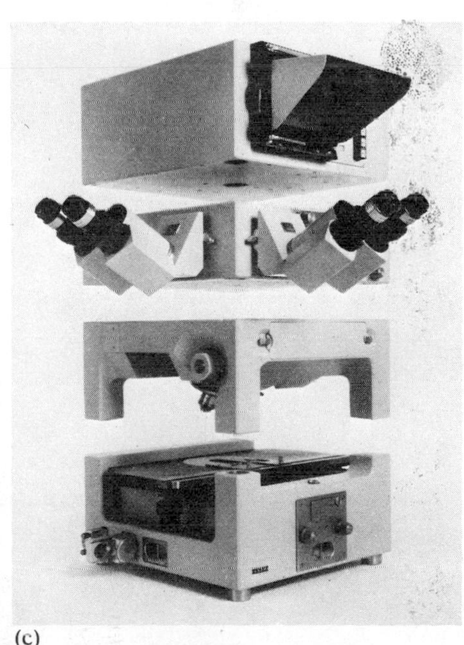

(c)

FIG. 4–1 Modification of light microscopes through the years. (a) An optical compound instrument designed and constructed by Robert Hooke in about 1650. The diagram in the upper left-hand corner shows a portion of the lens arrangement. Another lens at the far left is not shown. Note the lamp (source of illumination) at the lower left. *Courtesy of Rijksmuseum voor de Geschiedenis der Natuurwetenschappen, Steenstraat IA, Leiden, Holland.* (b) A modern-day laboratory compound microscope. Note the following components: ocular (O), objectives (Ob), mechanical stage (M), condenser (C), iris diaphragm (I), and source of illumination (L). *Courtesy of the American Optical Instrument Company, Buffalo.* (c) A special modification, the Axiomat, a microscope that incorporates a building block concept. Microscope modules (units) can be combined for different investigative needs, for example, metallurgy, biological sciences, medicine, and qualitative microscopy. *Courtesy Carl Zeiss, Inc.*

specify the quantities of these units. However, the exacting nature of science requires that experimenters must be able to repeat and verify results using the most precise measurements. Thus the quantitative nature of science has given rise to a variety of units of measurements and to procedures for writing both very small and very large numbers.

In the biological sciences, the two major systems of units used to express measurements are the *English system* (pounds, feet, and inches) and the **metric system.** The latter is by far the more widely used internationally and for scientific work. Since around 1960, an International System of Units based upon the metric system has quickly been gaining acceptance. It is referred to as the **SI system,** from the French *Système International d'Unités.*

The metric system has the great advantage of being simple, since using it requires remembering just a few basic terms. The basic unit of length is the *meter* (m); the basic unit of volume is the *liter* (l); the basic unit of mass (weight) is the *gram* (g); and the basic unit of temperature is the *Celsius degree* (°C). Converting to English units,

1 meter = 39.4 inches
1 liter = 1.06 quarts
1 gram = 0.0352 ounces

An additional feature of the metric system is that it involves decimal counting. Units are defined so that every unit is some power of 10 (10, 100, 0.01, and so on) times the basic unit. A meter, for example, consists of 100 centimeters (cm), or 1000 millimeters (mm); and one centimeter can then be seen to consist of 10 millimeters. Converting from one unit to another in the metric system merely involves shifting the decimal point.

Instead of having a number of different root words for length, as in the English system (league, mile, rod, yard, foot, inch, mil), the metric system has just one, the meter. With suitable prefixes, the meter can express a useful unit for even very small and very large distances (see Table 4–1). The same prefixes are applied to the measurement units of mass and volume as well.

TABLE 4-1 SI Units and Some Common Prefixes

Quantity	*SI base unit*	*Symbol*
length	meter	m
mass	kilogram	kg
time	second	s
temperature	kelvin	K
Prefix	*Means multiply by*	*Symbol*
giga	10^9 = 1,000,000,000	G
mega	10^6 = 1,000,000	M
kilo	10^3 = 1,000	k
hecto	10^2 = 100	h
deca	10^1 = 10	da
deci	10^{-1} = 0.1	d
centi	10^{-2} = 0.01	c
milli	10^{-3} = 0.001	m
micro	10^{-6} = 0.000,001	μ
nano	10^{-9} = 0.000,000,001	n
pico	10^{-12} = 0.000,000,000,001	p

For example:
1 millimeter = 10^{-3} meter, or 0.001 meter
1 nanometer = 10^{-9} meter, or 0.000,000.001 meter
1 kilogram = 10^3 grams, or 1,000 grams
In symbols, 1 mm = 10^{-3} m, 1 nm = 10^{-9} m, 1 kg = 10^3 g

TABLE 4-2 Some Metric Units and Useful Equivalents

Unit	*Symbol*	*Equivalents*[a]
meter	m	1 m = 39.37 in.
centimeter	cm	1 cm = 10^{-2} m = 0.39 in.
micrometer	μm	1 μm = 10^{-6} m = 0.39×10^{-4} in.
nanometer	nm	1 nm = 10^{-9} m = 0.39×10^{-7} in.
Angstrom	Å	1 Å = 10^{-10} m = 0.39×10^{-8} in.
liter	ℓ or L	1 ℓ = 1 dm^3 = 0.001 m^3 = 1.06 qt
milliliter	ml or mL	1 ml = 0.001 ℓ = 0.001 qt
degree Celsius	°C	1 °C = 1 K = 1.8°F
		0 °C = 273.15 K = 32°F

[a]English equivalents are approximate.

In the study of biological materials, the most commonly used measurements of length are the *centimeter* (cm = 10^{-2} m), the *millimeter* (mm = 10^{-3} m), the **micrometer** (**μm** = 10^{-6} m), the **nanometer** (**nm** = 10^{-9} m), and the **Angstrom unit** (**Å** = 10^{-10} m). Most animal, plant, and microbial cells are measured in micrometers, cellular parts and viruses in nanometers. Table 4–2 gives some common metric units and their equivalents.

To estimate distances from a map, one usually looks for a scale or bar marker as an aid. The same approach is used in the biological sciences to indicate the dimensions of cellular structures and associated components in a drawing or photograph. The *bar marker,* a short, straight line usually found at the bottom corner of each photograph, is placed there as a size reference. The length of the marker represents the length of a metric unit at that particular magnification. Typical units include 1 micrometer, 1 nanometer, and fractions or multiples of these units.

Each type of microscope has definite limitations. Each instrument can be used to observe cells or other objects that are at least a certain size and no smaller. For example, an ordinary light *(bright-field)* microscope can be used to observe objects with dimensions down to about 0.2 μm. An electron microscope can be used with specimens only one tenth that size—15 nm (or 0.015 μm). The limitations of these and other instruments are compared in Figure 4–2. The advantages, disadvantages, and special features of each form of microscopy are given in the sections that follow.

To understand microscopy, one must be aware of certain fundamental properties of light and optics. With this foundation, many of the problems encountered in using a microscope will be more readily understood.

Properties of Light

Light travels with a velocity of approximately 186,300 miles, or 3×10^{10} centimeters, per second. According to the wave theory, light is propagated through space as waves of varying electric and magnetic fields.

AMPLITUDE

Light waves are described in terms of their amplitude, frequency, and wavelength (Figure 4–3). An analogy can be made between a light wave and a jump rope. When two people pull on the rope and stretch it tight, a position of equilibrium is established. Now if the rope is swung, a wavelike effect is produced. The maximum displacement of the rope from the equilibrium position, as represented by the crests and troughs of the curves produced, is the amplitude of the wave.

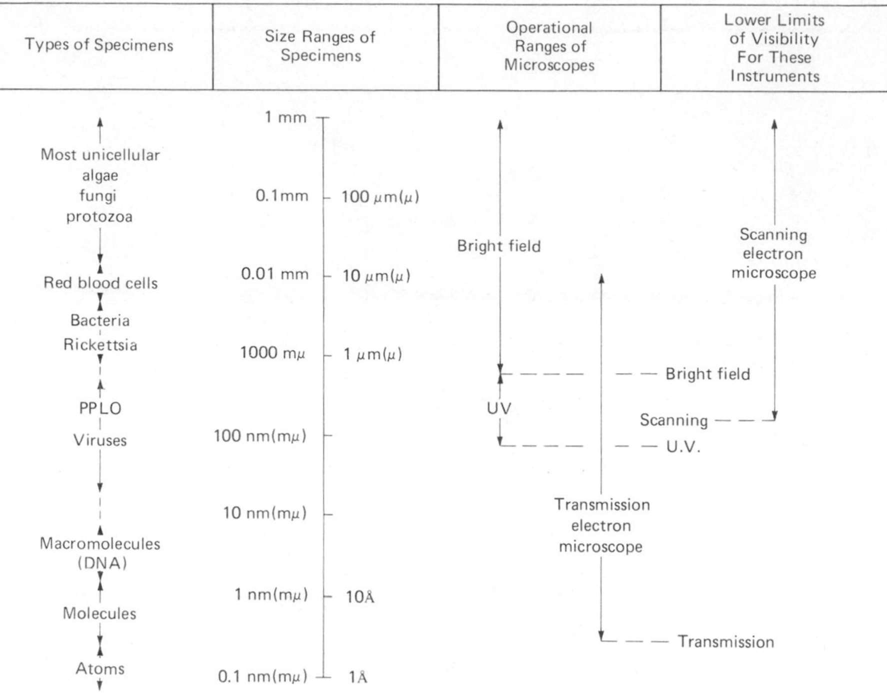

FIG. 4–2 A diagrammatic representation of the types of specimens that can be viewed by three different instruments commonly used in microbiology and related areas, and one microscope that is being used with increasing frequency, the scanning microscope. The operational ranges are also indicated. *Adapted in part from Rhodes, A. J., and C. E. Van Rooyen,* Textbook of Virology. *Baltimore: Williams & Wilkins Co., 1968.*

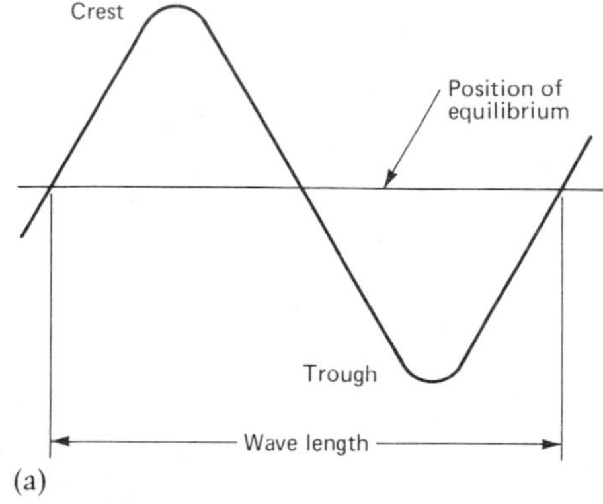

FIG. 4–3 Properties of light waves. (a) The anatomy of a wavelength. Note the position of equilibrium. (b) A representation of frequency.

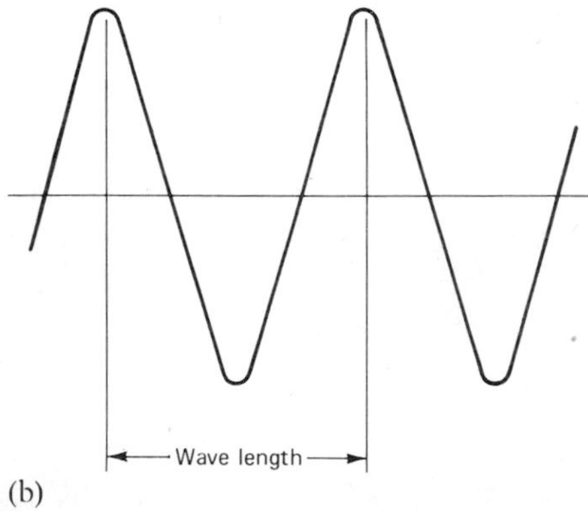

FREQUENCY

This property of a light wave refers to the number of vibrations that occur in one second. Specifically, ***frequency*** is the number of times a wave crest or trough passes a particular point per second (See Figure 4–3). If two people take a rope and shake it, the frequency of the wave can be regulated by the speed with which the rope is shaken.

WAVELENGTH AND FREQUENCY

A ***wavelength*** is the distance between two corresponding points on a wave, such as the distance between two successive peaks or crests (Figure 4–3a). Because the frequency of light is the number of wave crests or troughs that move past a point in one second, and because the speed of light in a medium is constant, frequency is inversely related to wavelength:

$$\text{Frequency} = \frac{\text{Velocity}}{\text{Wavelength}}$$

The wavelengths of light rays that make up the visible spectrum range from approximately 4000 to 7000 Å (400 to 700 nm) (Figure 4–4). The colors we see result from a combination of factors, including amplitude and wavelength. Wavelengths either less than or greater than the limits of the visible spectrum also exist. *Ultraviolet* light rays, for example, have wavelengths ranging from approximately 1000 to 3850 Å (100 to 385 nm). Infrared light has wavelengths greater than those of visible light.

The **resolving power** (RP) of a microscope—its ability to reveal the fine details of a specimen—depends on wavelength. As a general rule, the shorter

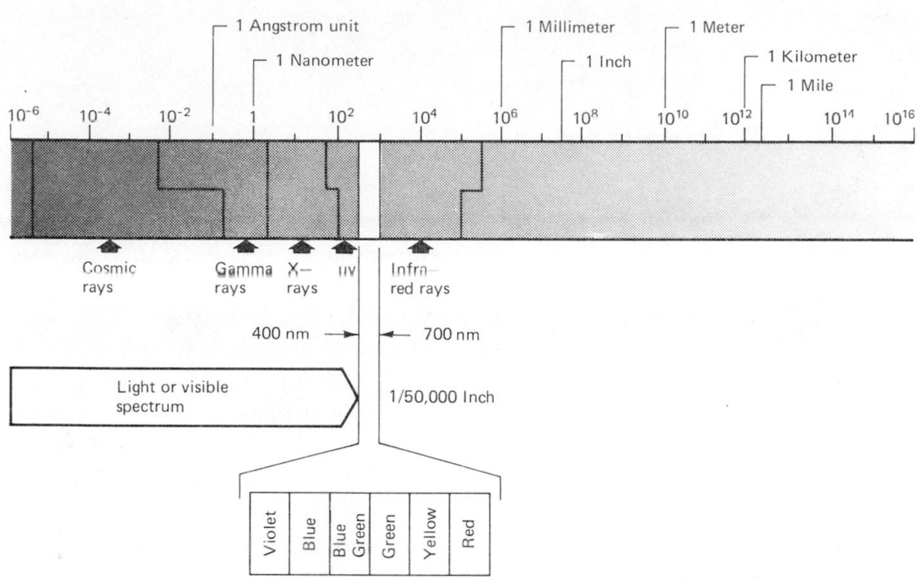

FIG. 4–4 Relative wavelengths of representative forms of radiation. Which of these are important in studying microorganisms? Would any type of radiation be harmful to these and other forms of life?

the wavelength of illuminating light, the greater the resolving power. Thus, with ultraviolet light as illumination, finer details can be seen than with visible light.

REFRACTIVE INDEX AND REFRACTION

The nature of the medium through which light passes during the operation of a microscope affects the image seen. The rate at which light moves is not the same for all transparent media. Denser materials exert a slowing effect on light rays. This difference in velocity is expressed in the form of a ***refractive index***, or index of refraction. The refractive index, represented by the Greek letter η (eta), is defined by the formula

$$\eta \text{ (refractive index)} = \frac{\text{Speed of light in a vacuum}}{\text{Speed of light in the medium being tested}}$$

In making determinations of light velocity, it is important to keep the temperature constant during the testing period. The indexes of some commonly used materials are 1.00003 for air, 1.33 for water, an average of 1.6 for various glasses, and 1.55 for immersion oil.

Light rays traveling in a single medium generally move along a straight path. However, if these rays pass at an oblique angle from one material into another material having a different refractive index, the light wave changes direction. This phenomenon, called ***refraction***, takes place at the boundary between the two media. The importance of refraction and the refractive indexes of materials is clearly demonstrated in the use of the oil-immersion objective and other forms of microscopy.

Successful operation of a microscope depends upon understanding the principles involved in its operation, the functions of the instrument's components, and the procedures for proper maintenance and use. We shall now review the most important types of optical microscopes and their uses in microbiology.

Light Microscopes

Bright-field Microscopy

Leeuwenhoek's early microscopes were simple in the sense that they used a single lens—rather like a magnifying glass. There are fundamental limitations to the magnifying power of a simple microscope, no matter how carefully it is constructed. For this reason, the development of the compound microscope was a welcome advance in microbiology. Credit for the invention and early development of the compound microscope is still debated, but most experts acknowledge the basic contributions of Hans and Zaccharias Janssen. Around 1590, the Janssens introduced a second lens to magnify the image formed by the primary lens. This is the principle upon which today's compound microscopes are based.

A ***compound microscope*** consists of at least two lens systems: the ***objective,*** which magnifies the specimen and is close to it, and the ***ocular,*** or ***eyepiece,*** which magnifies the image produced by the objective lens. The total magnification thus obtained is equal to the product of the magnifying powers of the two sets of lenses. Under optimal conditions, maximum magnifications can range from approximately 1000 to 2000 times (×) the diameter of a specimen being observed.

The compound microscopes used today consist of a series of optical lenses (systems), mechanical adjustment parts, and supportive structures for these components. The optical lenses include the ocular, the objectives (usually three with different magnifying powers), and the substage condenser. The coarse, fine, and condenser adjustment knobs, together with the iris diaphragm level, comprise the major mechanical parts. The various components of the scope are held in position by supportive structures such as the base, arm, pillar, body tube (barrel), and revolving nosepiece. Several of these microscope components are shown in Figure 4–5 and discussed in the following sections.

OCULAR (EYEPIECE)

A short tube generally containing two lenses, the ocular fits into the upper portion of the microscope's body tube. Several different types of eyepieces can be used to examine specimens. The specific type used generally depends upon the objective lenses on the instrument. The magnifying power of the ocular is usually engraved on it. Common magnifications for oculars include 1×, 2×, 5×, 10×, and 15×. Eyepieces are used to magnify the image of the specimen produced by the objective and to correct certain distortions produced by the objective. Commonly used oculars include compensating, Huygenian, and hyperplane eyepieces. The ***compensating*** type is designed to neutralize distortions introduced by some objectives because of different wavelengths of light. The ***Huygenian*** is used with low-power objectives. ***Hyperplane*** eyepieces are generally used with objectives of intermediate power.

OBJECTIVES

These are considered the most important of the microscope's optical parts, primarily because they affect the quality of the image seen by the observer. Most microscopes are equipped with three objectives with different magnifying powers: the low-power, high-power (or high-dry), and oil-immersion lenses.

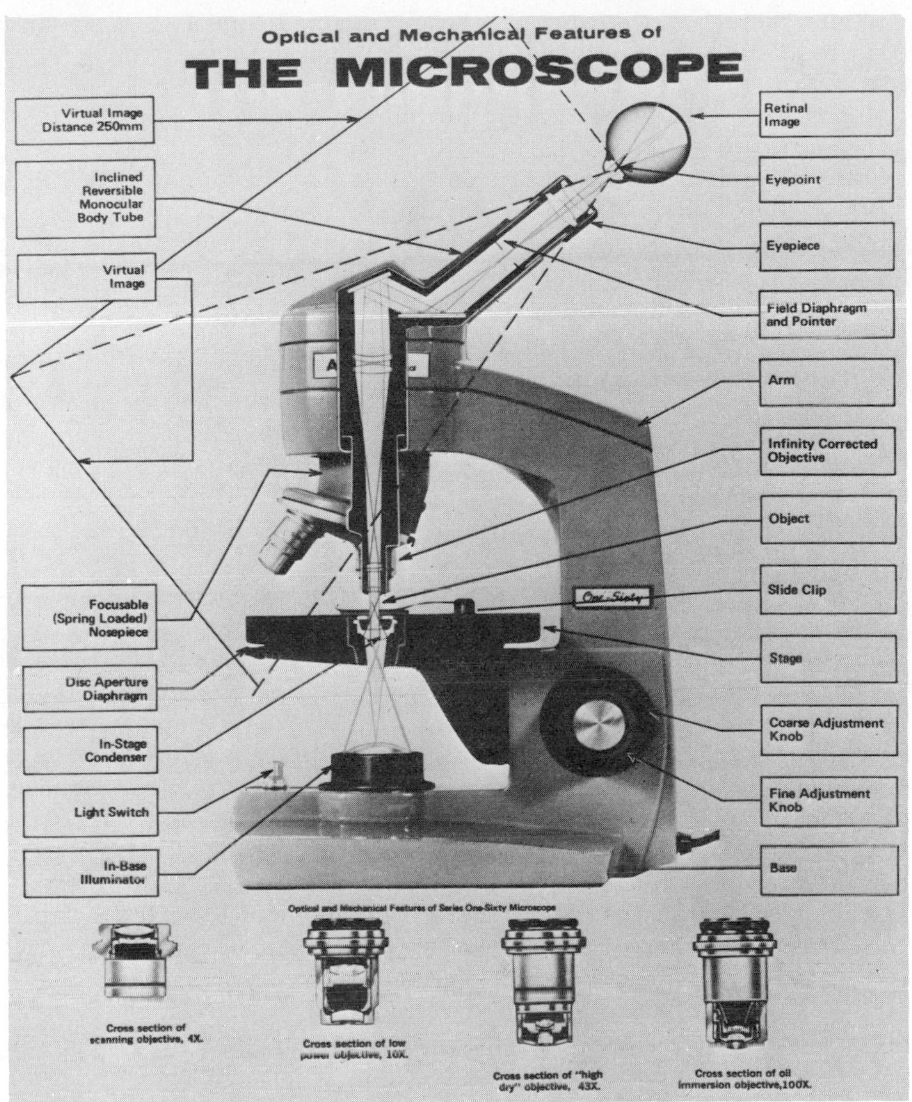

FIG. 4–5 A cutaway diagram of a representative compound monocular microscope. The various components of the instrument and the pathways followed by light waves through the microscope are shown. *Courtesy of the American Optical Instrument Company, Buffalo.*

Several microscope manufacturers differentiate the individual objectives by sets of differently colored rings—for example, green for low-power, yellow for high-dry, and red or black for oil-immersion. If not color-coded, the individual objectives commonly can be distinguished by their respective lengths (low-power is the shortest, oil-immersion the longest).

Objective lenses are used to gather, or concentrate, the light rays coming from the specimen being viewed, form the image of the specimen, and magnify this image. Several important properties of a microscope are directly associated with the objectives. One of these is resolving power, or resolution, which is specifically defined as the ability to distinguish clearly two points that are close together within the structure of the specimen. This feature is largely determined by the wavelength of the light source (with a shorter wavelength providing finer detail) and the angle formed by the outer edges of the lens and a point on the object. The resolution is also affected by the refractive index of the medium through which light passes before entering the microscope objective. The relationship of these factors is expressed in the combined formula

$$\text{Numerical aperture } (NA) = \eta \sin \theta$$

where η represents the refractive index of the medium through which light passes before entering the objective lens and θ (Greek theta) is the angle formed by light rays (in the shape of the cone) coming from the condenser and passing through the specimen. Light in this form frequently is referred to as "a pencil of rays." Sin θ is the trigonometric sine of this angle. Figure 4–6 depicts the explanation of numerical aperture. Values for NA are engraved on the barrels of objectives and indicate the maximum obtainable resolution.

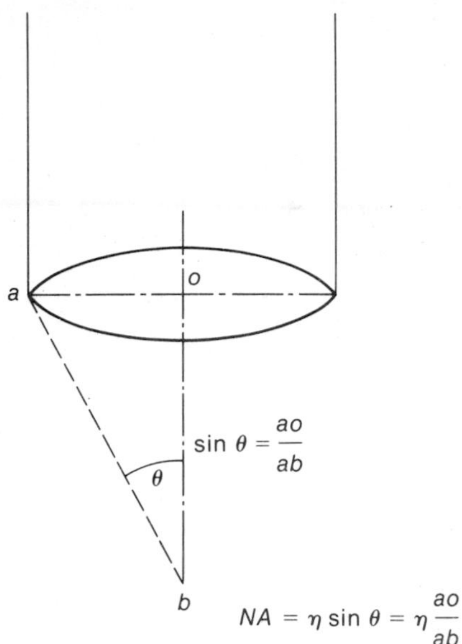

FIG. 4–6 A diagrammatic representation of numerical aperture.

Another important feature of modern-day instruments is the property of *parfocal.* Stated simply, this means the changing of objectives without major focusing adjustments. Thus, if a higher magnification is needed during the course of examining a specimen, one would just rotate the desired higher objective into place and make some minor focusing adjustment to bring the specimen into view.

The oil-immersion lens is an especially important tool for studying microorganisms. The highest-magnification objective used in general microbiology courses, it can magnify specimens about 100 times. To obtain the best possible results, the objective is immersed in a medium that has approximately the same index of refraction as glass, 1.6. One medium commonly employed for this purpose is cedarwood oil. Other materials containing mineral oil also are in common use. Oils have the advantage of not evaporating when exposed to air for long periods of time. Further, since its index of refraction is the same as that of glass, oil does not bend the light rays entering the front lens of the oil-immersion objective (Figure 4–7). If air rather than oil is present between the specimen and the objective, some light is lost. The image observed is usually fuzzy, and the finer details cannot be seen (Figure 4–8). The resolving power of the oil-immersion objective is definitely enhanced by the oil medium.

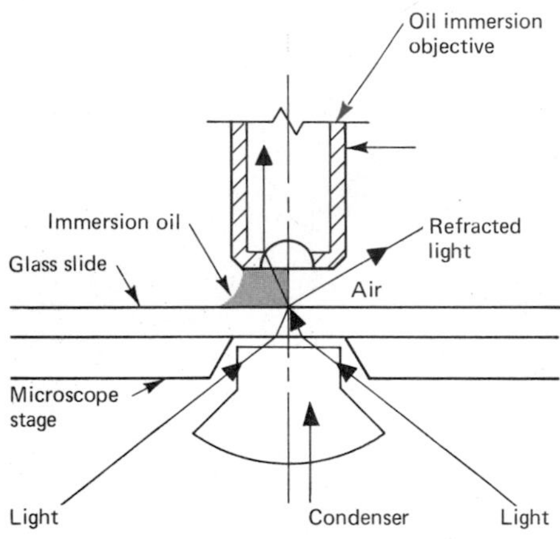

FIG. 4–7 Comparison between the effects of oil and air on the passage of light rays from a specimen to the front lens of the oil-immersion objective. *Adapted from Carpenter, P. L.* Microbiology. *Philadelphia: W. B. Saunders, 1967.*

Individuals using the oil-immersion objective for the first time tend to use large quantities of oil. One good drop is usually sufficient. To preserve the microscope component, all oil should be removed from the objective and all other parts after use. Lens paper is used for this purpose.

THE CONDENSER AND IRIS DIAPHRAGM

A condenser is found under the microscope stage between the source of illumination and the specimen or object to be viewed. This component frequently is called a *substage condenser.* One of the most commonly used is the Abbé condenser (Figure 4–11). It consists of two lenses that illuminate specimens with transmitted light. The condenser is important to high-resolution microscopy. Microscopic examinations of specimens with either high-power or oil-immersion objectives require adequate illumination. The condenser serves this purpose. In addition to the Abbé, variable-focus and achromatic condensers are also commonly used.

Occasionally, too much light may pass through the specimen and into the objective lens, significantly decreasing the contrast of the specimen. Microscope condensers are generally equipped with an *iris diaphragm* to control light intensity. This component functions to control the amount of light entering the condenser. When unstained material, such as living protozoa or hanging-drop preparations of bacteria, is to be examined, the opening of the iris diaphragm generally is reduced. This component is regulated by the iris diaphragm lever. Many newer microscopes are equipped with fixed condensers and iris diaphragms, regulated for general use.

Micrometry

In certain aspects of microbiology, it is necessary to measure the dimensions of cells or, if possible, of their components. With light microscopy, this type of procedure can usually be performed with the aid of an ***ocular micrometer***, a special ocular containing a graduated scale, and a ***stage micrometer***. The latter device is a glass slide on which a millimeter scale is usually imprinted. Graduation of this scale is in hundredths of a millimeter.

The measurement procedure requires that the ocular micrometer first be calibrated with the stage device. This is done by replacing the normal eyepiece of the microscope with the ocular micrometer and determining the exact number of divisions, that is, hundredths of a millimeter, that correspond to those of the millimeter scale on the stage micrometer. The particular objective used should be noted, as this component is important to the accuracy of the measurements taken. The manipulation or exchange of these parts will change calibration values. With the calibration of the ocular micrometer complete, the stage micrometer is removed and the specimen to be measured is placed in position.

Photographic variations of this procedure are also used. With photography, permanent records of the dimensions of organisms can readily be made.

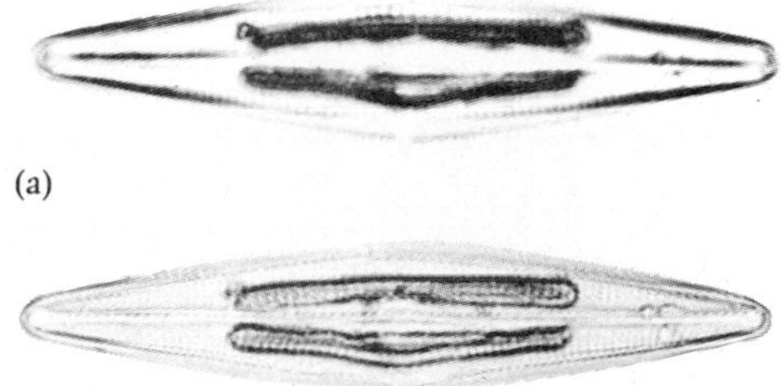

(a)

(b)

FIG. 4–8 A comparison of an observed image of a diatom when viewed with the oil-immersion objective. (a) No oil was used here. Air was present between the objective and the specimen. (b) The effect with immersion oil. Note the clearer image and the greater detail.

Specimen Preparation for Bright-field Microscopy

The procedures used to prepare microorganisms for microscopic examination are of two types. The ***hanging-drop*** and ***temporary wet-mount*** techniques are used with living organisms. The second type of procedure, ***staining***, employs **smears,** which are thin films of microorganisms spread on the surface of a clean glass slide that has been air-dried. The smear is then heat-fixed by passing the slide through the flame of a Bunsen burner. This step not only kills but coagulates the protein of cells and thereby fixes the organisms to the slide.

THE HANGING-DROP AND TEMPORARY WET-MOUNT TECHNIQUES

The direct examination of microorganisms in the normal, living state can be extremely useful in determining size and shape relationships, motility, and reactions to various chemicals or immune sera. The hanging-drop and temporary wet-mount techniques both maintain the natural shape of organisms and reduce the distorted effects that can occur when specimens are dried and fixed. Because the majority of microorganisms are not very different from the fluid in which they are suspended in terms of either color or refractive index, a low-intensity light source is used for viewing them.

Hanging-drop preparations (Figure 4–9) are made by placing a drop of a microbial suspension on the center of a cover slip, usually ringed with petroleum jelly or a similar material. This sealing material is used primarily to eliminate air currents and reduce evaporation. A depression slide (hollow-ground slide with a concave central area) in an inverted position is lowered onto the prepared cover slip. Slight pressure is applied to the slide in order to ensure contact between the cover slip and the depression slide. The finished preparation then is turned right side up and ready for examination.

Certain microorganisms, such as protozoa, move too quickly to be studied. A

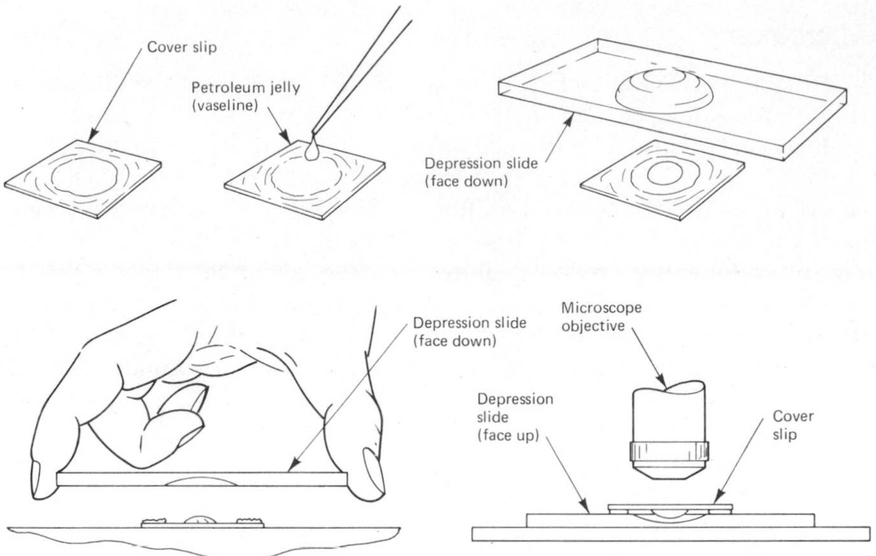

FIG. 4-9 A schematic representation of the steps in the hanging-drop preparation technique.

2 percent solution of carboxy-methyl-cellulose can be used to slow down such rapidly moving organisms. Another possible difficulty is actually locating the specimen. Making a wax-pencil mark close to the edge of the droplet of the microbial suspension and diminishing the intensity of the light source help greatly in eliminating most problems in locating specimens.

Temporary wet-mounts of specimens are prepared by placing a drop of microbial suspension on the center of a clean glass slide and placing a cover slip over it. The procedure for locating microorganisms in a specimen is similar to the one described for the hanging-drop technique.

STAINING

The microscopic study of live cells is limited, in that usually only the outline and structural arrangement of cells are revealed by bright-field microscopy. Stained preparations of fixed cells permit a greater visualization of cells, observation of internal cellular components, and, to some extent, a differentiation of microbial species.

The Nature of Dyes. Dyes used for staining are usually in the form of salts. They are of two general types, basic and acidic. The electric charge on the dye ion determines the type of dye it is. Basic dyes are positively charged. Substances of this kind stain or react with nuclear components. Acid dyes are negatively charged. Compounds of this type stain cytoplasmic material and certain kinds of granules and other related materials.

Simple Staining. Various bacteriological procedures utilize staining solutions that contain one and only one dye dissolved in either a dilute alcoholic solution or water. Such preparations are referred to as ***simple stains.*** The concentrations of the commonly used dyes are quite low, approximately 1 to 2 percent. Simple staining solutions include carbolfuchsin, crystal violet, methylene blue, and safranin.

This type of staining procedure involves applying the simple stain to a fixed bacterial smear for a length of time that may range from a few seconds to several minutes. Such stains should never be allowed to dry on the smear. Before the microscopic examination, preparations are rinsed to remove excess stain and dried by blotting between layers of filter paper or other appropriate material. Bacterial cells to which these simple staining solutions are applied take the color of the dye preparation (Color Photograph 9).

Simple stains can be used to demonstrate the shapes, arrangements, and sizes of microorganisms, to differentiate or distinguish bacterial cells from nonliving structures, and to show the presence of bacterial spores.

Differential Staining. The preliminary grouping of bacteria is usually based upon their general shape and the manner in which they react to certain staining techniques called **differential staining methods.** Procedures of this type use more than one dye preparation. When properly carried out, these techniques will divide nearly all bacteria into major groups. The two most widely used differential staining methods in bacteriology are the **Gram** and **acid-fast staining** techniques. The differentiation principle is also used to view bacterial structures inside or outside the cell—spores and capsules, for example.

Gram Stain. The Gram staining reaction was developed about 1883 by Hans Christian Gram, a Danish physician. He discovered this technique while trying to stain biopsy (pathologic) specimens so that microorganisms could be distinguished from surrounding tissue. Gram noted that some bacterial cells exhibit an unusual resistance to decolorization. He used this observation as the basis for a differential staining technique.

The Gram differentiation is based upon the color reactions of bacteria in a fixed smear when they are treated with the primary dye crystal violet followed by an iodine-potassium-iodide solution. Certain organisms lose the violet color rapidly when a decolorizing agent such as ethyl alcohol or a mixture of acetone and alcohol is applied. Others lose their color more slowly. After this decolorization step, a counterstain, usually the red dye safranin, is used. A standardized procedure listing the specific reagents and respective staining times is given in Table 4–3. Bacterial cells resistant to decolorization will retain the primary dye and exhibit a blue or purple color. They will not take the counterstain. Such organisms are referred to as *Gram-positive* (Color Photograph 10a). Those microorganisms unable to retain the crystal violet stain, the decolorized cells, will take the counterstain, and consequently exhibit a pink or red color (Color Photograph 10b). The term *Gram-negative* is used to describe these organisms. Several characteristics of the Gram-positive and Gram-negative groups appear to be correlated with their staining reactions. These include chemical composition, sensitivity to penicillin, and relative cell-wall thickness.

When properly performed, the Gram stain can be useful in the diagnosis of many infectious diseases. The reactions of a wide variety of bacteria, both pathogenic and nonpathogenic, are listed in Table 4–4.

In addition to the two major categories of bacteria, Gram-variables and Gram-nonreactives have also been recognized. The *Gram-nonreactive* category includes those microorganisms that do not stain, or that stain only poorly. Members of the genus *Mycobacterium* and various spirochetes may fall into this group.

Gram-variables are bacteria that under ordinary conditions may be Gram-positive and Gram-negative on the same slide. This variation in staining may also be due, in large part, to improper technique, such as lack of attention to decolorization, thick smears, or use of old cultures of Gram-positive bacteria. The Gram staining reactions listed in Table 4–4 and those most commonly listed elsewhere are those of 24-hour-old cultures. With certain organisms,

TABLE 4-3 A Representative Standardized Gram Staining Procedure

Reagents in Their Order of Application[a]	Length of Time Applied	Reactions and Appearance of Cells[b]: Gram-positives	Gram-negatives	Appearance
Crystal violet (CV)	1 minute	1. Dye is taken up by cells in two forms, bound and unbound 2. Cells appear violet	1. Same 2. Same	(G-) (G+) G- G+ G-
Iodine solution (I)	1 minute	1. Iodine reacts, i.e., fixes probably both the unbound and bound crystal violet[c] 2. A CV-I precipitate (CV-I complex) is formed 3. Cells remain violet in color	1. Same 2. Same 3. Same	G+ G+ G-
Decolorizer (ethanol or an acetone-ethanol mixture)	Applied cautiously drop by drop until a purple color no longer comes from the smear	1. The decolorizer causes the dissociation of the CV-I precipitate, CV-I = CV + I 2. The components of the complex are now soluble 3. Dehydration of the thick cell wall occurs 4. Diffusion of dye proceeds slowly	1. Same 2. Same 3. Dehydration of the thin cell envelope occurs 4. Diffusion of dye proceeds faster	G+ G-
Counterstain (safranin or a dilute solution of carbolfuchsin)	½–1 minute	1. Some displacement of CV may occur, but in general cells are not affected 2. Cells appear purple or blue	1. Displacements of any CV left occurs 2. Cells take up counterstain 3. Cells appear red or pink	G+ (purple) G- (red)

[a]Note that wash steps are used after the application of each reagent.
[b]Based on information provided by Bartholomew, J. W., T. Cromwell, and R. Gan, "Analysis of the Mechanism of Gram Differentiation by Use of Filter Paper Chromatographic Technique," *J. Bacteriol.* 90:766 (1965).
[c]Iodine is called a ***mordant*** in this capacity.

TABLE 4-4 Gram Stain Reactions of Various Bacterial Pathogens and Commonly Encountered Nonpathogenic Organisms

Microorganism	Gram Reaction	Morphology	Disease Caused or Habitat
Actinomyces bovis	+	Rod	Lumpy jaw, actinomycosis
Agrobacterium spp.[a]	–	Rod	Causes tumors (galls) in plants; widely distributed in soil
Alcaligenes spp.	–	Rod	Saprophytic inhabitant of intestinal tract of vertebrates
Azotobacter spp.	–	Rod	Inhabitants of soil water and leaf surfaces
Bacillus anthracis	+	Rod	Anthrax

Microorganism	Gram Reaction	Morphology	Disease Caused or Habitat
B. subtilis	+	Rod	Saprophytic organism widely distributed in nature; recently associated with abscesses after tooth extraction
Bacteroides spp.	–	Rod	Members of normal flora in gastrointestinal tract; causes brain abscesses and wound infections
Bifidobacterium spp.	+	Rod	Inhabitant of the intestinal tracts of a variety of animals
Bordetella pertussis	–	Rod	Whooping cough
Branhamella (Neisseria) catarrhalis	–	Coccus	Normal inhabitant of the upper respiratory tract; however, has been known to cause meningitis
Brucella melitensis	–	Rod	Brucellosis (Malta fever)
Clostridium botulinum	+	Rod	Botulism (fatal food poisoning)
C. tetani	+	Rod	Tetanus (lockjaw)
Corynebacterium diphtheriae	+	Rod	Diphtheria
Enterobacter (Aerobacter) aerogenes	–	Rod	Widespread in nature; nonpathogenic
Escherichia coli	–	Rod	Normal inhabitant of the intestinal tract; certain strains can produce infant (summer) diarrhea
Francisella tularensis	–	Rod	Tularemia in humans and several other warm-blooded animals
Hemophilus aegyptius	–	Rod	Pink-eye
Klebsiella pneumoniae	–	Rod	Pneumonia; urinary tract infections
Micrococcus (Sarcina) lutea	+	Coccus	Widely distributed in nature; nonpathogenic
Mycobacterium leprae	+[b]	Rod	Leprosy
M. tuberculosis	+[b]	Rod	Tuberculosis
Neisseria gonorrhoeae	–	Coccus	Gonorrhea
N. meningitidis	–	Coccus	Meningitis; upper respiratory tract infection
Pseudomonas aeruginosa		Rod	Can cause infections of the respiratory and urogenital systems
Rickettsia rickettsii	–	Rod	Rocky Mountain spotted fever
Salmonella typhi	–	Rod	Typhoid fever
Serratia marcescens	–	Rod	Widespread in nature; has been the cause of respiratory infections
Shigella dysenteriae	–	Rod	Bacterial dysentery
Staphylococcus aureus[c]	+	Coccus	Causes boils, carbuncles, pneumonia, and many other types of diseases
Streptococcus lactis	+	Coccus	Sours milk
S. pneumoniae	+	Coccus	Lobar pneumonia
Treponema pallidum	–[d]	Spirochete	Syphilis
Vibrio cholerae	–	Vibrio	Asiatic cholera
Yersinia (Pasteurella) pestis	–	Rod	Plague

[a]The abbreviation *spp.* stands for "several species."
[b]The significance of the Gram stain reaction is debatable here. However, the fact that these organisms are acid-fast is of diagnostic importance.
[c]Pathogenic staphylococci usually are detected on the basis of a positive coagulase test. The details of this procedure are discussed in Chapter 28.
[d]The staining of this organism requires special techniques. Dark-field microscopy and even stained tissue preparations produce more convincing indications of infection.

Gram-positivity disappears in older cultures—possibly leading to this kind of Gram-variability.

Customarily, each reagent (the primary dye, the iodine solution, the decolorizer, and the counterstain) is removed after its period of application by rinsing with water. Excessive washing, however, can remove the dye or dye-iodine complexes within the cells and consequently greatly affect the overall staining reaction. As the decolorization step is probably the most critical, it should be performed with special care. A common control is the use of a mixed smear of cultures of a Gram-positive coccus and of a Gram-negative rod on an area of the same slide containing an unknown specimen. Appropriate positive and negative reactions of the known cultures indicate proper technique. The results of the unknown specimen can then also be considered accurate. The final step in the procedure, application of the counterstain, must be performed very carefully. Given too much exposure time, the counterstain will replace the primary dye in Gram-positive organisms, thus affecting the stained appearance of these cells.

Since Gram's original work, many investigators have tried, with little success, to find the mechanism involved in Gram differentiation. The explanations offered for the Gram-positive state can be grouped in at least three categories: (1) the existence of a specific chemical material that reacts Gram-positively; (2) different affinities for the primary dye crystal violet by Gram-positive and Gram-negative cells; and (3) permeability differences between Gram-positive and Gram-negative microorganisms.

At the present time, Gram differentiation appears to be a permeation phenomenon. Both the thickness of an organism's cell wall and the size of the spaces in these structures, the pore size, are important to the final outcome of the Gram stain procedure.

Acid-fast Stain Procedure. This staining technique was developed by Paul Ehrlich in 1882. Acid-fastness is a resistance of cells stained with a basic dye to decolorize in a 3 percent solution of acid alcohol—a hydrochloric acid (HCl) and ethyl alcohol mixture. Acid-fastness is the most important property differentiating mycobacteria from other bacterial species. Among the better-known members of this acid-fast group are *Mycobacterium leprae,* which causes leprosy, and *M. tuberculosis,* the cause of tuberculosis.

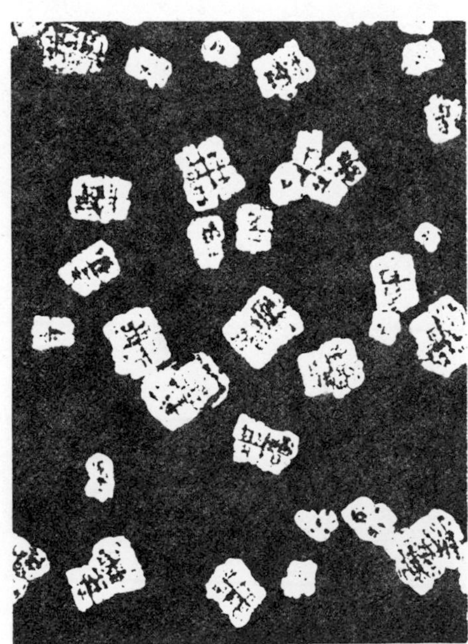

FIG. 4-10 A photomicrograph showing the dark-field image produced with bacteria. Note the bright appearance of cocci (spherical cells) against the dark background. *Koyama, T., M. Yamada, and M. Matsuhashi,* J. Bacteriol. 129:*1518–1523 (1977).*

Most bacterial cells can be easily stained by general techniques. However, certain microorganisms have cell walls with substantial quantities of fatty or waxy substances. Staining or decolorizing them by the usual methods can prove to be difficult. This difficulty prompted Ehrlich to develop the acid-fast staining procedure. The Ziehl-Neelsen procedure, a modification of Ehrlich's method, is the one now used in laboratories to identify acid-fast organisms.

The acid-fast staining procedure is performed by applying the primary dye, carbolfuchsin, to a heat-fixed bacterial smear. Next, the preparation is steamed for approximately 5 minutes. More dye is added as needed to prevent drying. After heating, the slide is allowed to cool, and then it is rinsed gently in running tap water. Acid alcohol, the decolorizing agent, is applied to the smear drop by drop, until a red color (the primary dye) no longer runs off from the smear. The preparation is rinsed again immediately and then is covered with the counterstain, methylene blue. After one minute, this reagent is rinsed from the slide. On microscopic examination, acid-fast cells are red (Color Photograph 11a) and non-acid-fast cells (Color Photograph 11b) are blue.

The mechanism of the acid-fast staining reaction is unclear at the present time. Some researchers believe that mycolic acid (a fatty acid) alone is responsible for the property of acid-fastness. However, there is no conclusive evidence to support this view. One general requirement for the reaction to occur appears to be intact cells. Disrupted cells of normally acid-fast organisms become non-acid-fast.

Spore Stain. Bacterial spores are known for their resistance to high temperature, radiation, desiccation (drying), chemical disinfection, and staining. These structures, which are formed within the cell **(endospores),** cannot be stained by ordinary methods, such as those described earlier. The dyes do not penetrate the spore's wall. Stained smears of spore-containing cells appear to have oval holes, or colorless spheres, within them. Drastic procedures are needed to demonstrate the presence of spores. A modified Ziehl-Neelsen method (Color Photograph 12b) can be used for this purpose, but the Schaeffer-Fulton procedure is more commonly employed (Color Photograph 12a). In this procedure the primary stain, malachite green, is applied to a heat-fixed smear and heated to steaming for approximately 5 minutes. The steaming is done to enhance the penetration of the dye into the relatively inpermeable spore coats. Next, the preparation is washed for approximately 30 seconds in running water. The wash step mainly removes the malachite green from cellular parts other than the spores. A counterstain, safranin, is then applied to the smear. This compound displaces any residual primary dye in the vegetative, or nonsporulating, cells, but not in the spores. In adequately prepared smears, one can readily observe green spores within red or pink cells, as well as free green spores (Color Photograph 12a).

Spore-staining techniques are of taxonomic importance in that they can be used to help identify spore-producing bacteria belonging to the genera *Bacillus* and *Clostridium*. The genus of *Bacillus* includes the causative agent of anthrax, *B. anthracis,* while the genus of *Clostridium* contains a wealth of human pathogens, including *C. botulinum, C. perfringens,* and *C. tetani.* These organisms cause botulism (fatal food poisoning), gas gangrene, and tetanus (lockjaw), respectively. The intracellular location, shape, and size of endospores are relatively constant and characteristic for a given bacterial species (Color Photograph 12b). Consequently, they can be used to establish the identity of a newly isolated, unknown organism.

Dark-field Microscopy

Specimens examined by ***dark-field microscopy*** are usually seen as bright objects against a black or dark background (Figure 4–10). This is an effect opposite to the one obtained with bright-field microscopy, in which specimens usually appear darker than the light background. The dark-field procedure is commonly performed by fitting an Abbé condenser with an opaque disk or "dark-field stop" (Figure 4–11). This dark-field stop is placed below the condenser, thus eliminating all light from the central portion of the condenser. A thin cone of illumination reaches the specimen at an angle to the objective lens. Light is scattered by the specimen, which thus acts as a light source. It appears as a glowing object against a dark background.

The microscope slides and cover slips used in dark-field examinations must be absolutely free from dirt, dust, and scratches. Unwanted objects and marks can reflect light and could easily brighten the background.

Dark-field microscopy is used for examination of unstained microorganisms, the contents of hanging-drop preparations and colloidal solutions. This procedure has diagnostic importance, especially in the case of syphilis (Figure 2–11b).

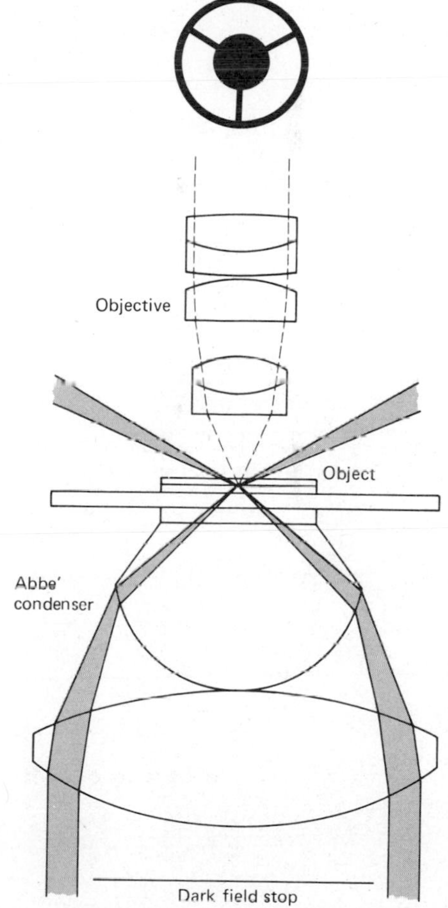

FIG. 4–11 Dark-field microscopy. Because of the application of the dark-field stop, the specimen is illuminated only by oblique rays of light. An Abbé condenser is also shown, as well as a typical dark-field stop. *Courtesy of Bausch & Lomb Incorporated, Rochester, N.Y.*

Fluorescence Microscopy

An early-twentieth-century advance, ***fluorescence microscopy*** is used for examining various cell types and cellular structures (Color Photograph 16),

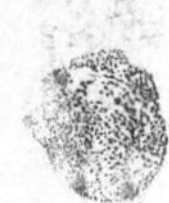

locating chemical components in cells and tissues, and for the rapid diagnosis of otherwise difficult disease states. This type of microscopy provides a means of studying structural details and other properties of a wide variety of specimens. Instruments used in fluorescence microscopy do not differ optically or mechanically from conventional microscopes, but they do require special filter systems. The different types of specimens differ in "fluorescing power" from their surroundings. This property of **fluorescence** is obvious when a substance becomes luminous upon exposure to ultraviolet light. With certain substances, including some dyes, fat, oil droplets, and uranium ores, exposure to this form of radiation causes them to absorb the energy of the invisible ultraviolet light waves and reemit the energy as visible light waves. Many living tissues fluoresce naturally, absorbing ultraviolet radiation and emitting green, yellow, or red light (Color Photograph 16). Selective combinations of natural fluorescence with fluorescent dyes makes possible identification, location, and counting of cell types and differentiation of cell parts. Fluorescence of cells can be measured and used to compute the concentration of chemical components present.

Fluorescent dyes used in this way include acridine orange R (Color Photograph 16), auramine O, primulin, and thiazo-yellow G. These substances apparently have a selective action for microorganisms and their components. For example, the fluorescent dye auramine O is used in a detection procedure for *Myobacterium tuberculosis*. The dye, which glows yellow when exposed to ultraviolet light, has a strong selective action for the wax-like substances present in this organism. Auramine O is applied to a smear of a sputum specimen suspected of containing *M. tuberculosis*. Excess dye is removed by washing. Then the stained preparation is examined with the aid of the fluorescence microscope. The presence of the tubercle bacilli is indicated by the bright yellow organisms against a dark background. (Although the effect produced is similar to that observed with a dark-field microscope, the principles involved differ significantly.)

Immunofluorescence is another adaptation of this type of microscopy. Fluorescent dyes, such as fluorescein isothiocyanate and lissamine rhodamine B, are employed to react chemically with blood serum proteins, called antibodies, and thereby "label" or tag them. The former compound produces an apple-green color, and the latter an orange one. Antibodies are noted for their ability to react with protein or protein-polysaccharide components or products of various types of cells, including bacteria (Color Photograph 15). Such chemical substances that react with antibodies are known as **antigens.**

Antibodies can be obtained by injecting antigens into a suitable animal. After a sufficient length of time, the injected animal is bled to obtain the antibodies that it produced. A fluorescent dye such as fluorescein is combined with these antibodies, thus creating a fluorescein-labeled antibody preparation. When this material is applied to a specimen smear containing the antigen responsible for the initial production of the antibody, a specific antigen-antibody reaction occurs. The antibody fluoresces when a treated smear is examined by fluorescent microscopy. The details of antibody production and fluorescent antibody methods can be found in Chapters 23 and 24, respectively.

Immunofluorescence techniques have several important uses, including the detection of disease agents in tissues, cells, and other specimens and the detection of the products of various types of microorganisms. The chemical structure of cells can be effectively investigated by such procedures.

Phase Microscopy

Phase microscopy is sometimes useful in examining the internal structures of transparent, living cells or in demonstrating their presence in certain fluid

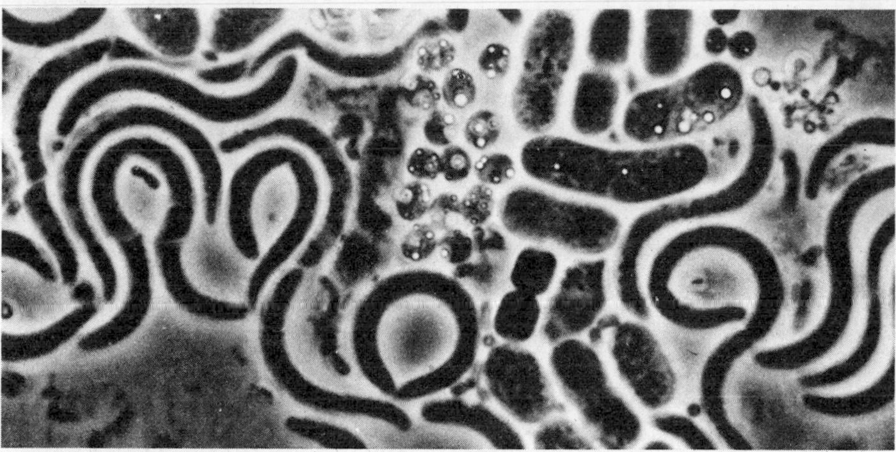

FIG. 4–12 A phase-contrast micrograph showing a variety of bacterial cells comprising a microbial community in a Michigan Lake. Cocci (spherical forms), rods (somewhat rectangular and oval), and spirals (wormlike) are evident. *Reproduced by permission of the National Research Council of Canada from Caldwell, D. E., and J. M. Tiedje,* Can. J. Microbiol. 21:*377–385 (1975).*

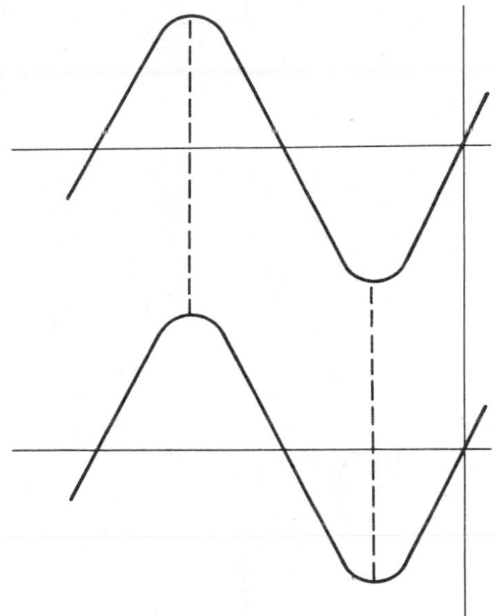

FIG. 4–13 The properties of light wave amplitude and frequency with respect to phase. (a) Two light waves of equal frequency and amplitude in phase. (b) Light waves showing the same properties of amplitude and frequency but out of phase. The phase-contrast microscope transforms this difference into a visible phenomenon. *After Wren, L. A.,* Understanding and Using the Phase Microscope. *Newton Highlands, Mass.: Unitron Instrument Company, 1963.*

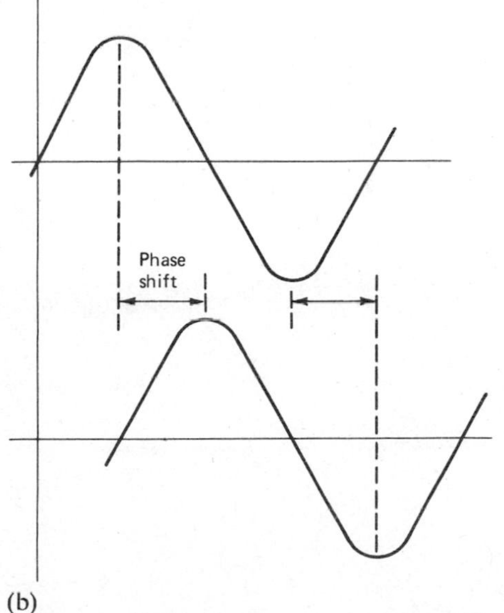

environments (Figure 4–12). The phase-contrast microscope can also be used to estimate concentrations of substances within cells or cellular regions. Phase microscopy takes advantage of the fact that different parts of cells have different densities. Cells are also denser than the material surrounding them. However, in the living state, cells are difficult to see because of their transparent quality. Use of the phase-contrast principle distinguishes cells and their structures from the background so that their shapes, sizes, and other features can be studied.

The phase-contrast principle was discovered by Fritz Zernike, who was recognized for his achievement by being awarded the Nobel Prize in physics in 1953. As discussed earlier, light waves have several variable characteristics, including frequency and amplitude. Two light waves with the same amplitude and frequency may be traveling so that their troughs and crests pass a given point at the same time. In this case they are said to be *in phase* (Figure 4–13a). They are *out of phase* when their crests pass a given point at different instants (Figure 4–13b). A special optical device called a *condenser* makes these phase differences visible to the human eye (Figure 4–14).

In a phase-contrast instrument, and sometimes in a regular compound microscope, the condenser has a special *annular diaphragm*. This component allows only a ring of light to pass through the condenser and strike the specimen being viewed. The microscope objective also contains a transparent disk, called the *phase-shifting plate* or *phase-shifting element*. A ring on this disk is used for focusing the light from the annular diaphragm. Depending on its composition, this ring can alter the phase of light waves passing through it by either delaying or advancing them. By briefly slowing one wave, the disk forces it out of phase with one that has not been delayed.

Electron Microscopes

The Transmission Electron Microscope

The realization that the light microscope had reached its limit of resolution (0.2 μm), with further improvements unlikely, prompted the development of the electron microscope. "It was inevitable," says physicist R. Wyckoff, "that

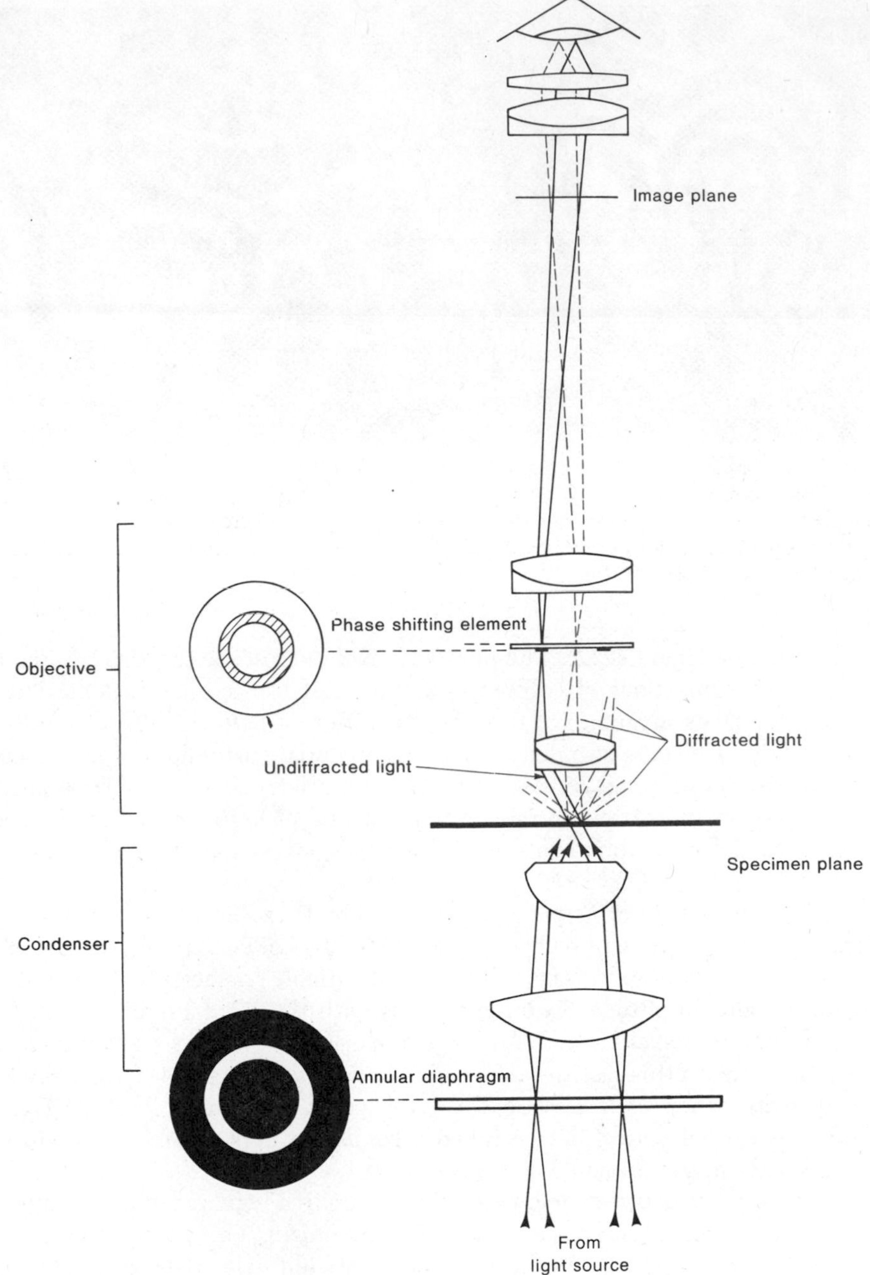

FIG. 4–14 The operation of the phase-contrast principle.

the realization of the exceedingly short wavelength of electrons would give microscope research quite a new direction." Electrons are very small negatively charged particles that behave in many respects like light waves. Accelerating electrons through 50,000 volts, for example, produces a wavelength of approximately 0.05 Å, much shorter than even ultraviolet light. In actual practice, the resolving power achieved in the electron microscope is about 4 Å, or 0.0004 μm.

Most ***transmission electron microscopes*** are similar in basic design to the light microscope (Figures 4–15 and 4–16). However, certain distinct differences exist (Table 4–5). The basic components of the transmission electron microscope include a source of illumination, optical, viewing, and vacuum systems, and electronic systems designed to hold the electron voltage (wavelength) stable.

TABLE 4-5 Differences Between the Ordinary Light Microscope and a Typical Transmission Electron Microscope

Property or Procedure	*Light Microscope*	*Transmission Electron Microscope*[a]
Source of radiation for image formation	Visible light	Electrons
Medium through which radiation travels	Air	Vacuum (approx. 10^{-4} mm mercury)
Specimen mounting	Glass slides	Thin films of collodion or other supporting material on copper grids
Nature of lenses	Glass	Magnetic fields or electrostatic lenses
Focusing	Mechanical (i.e., raising or lowering objectives)	Electrical, i.e., the current of the objective lens coil is changed
Magnification adjustments	Changing objectives	Electrical, i.e., changing current of the projector lens coil
Major means of providing specimen contrast	Light absorption	Electron scattering

[a]Most of these properties are also true for scanning instruments. Specimens, however, are supported on the round, solid surfaces of stubs (Figure 4–17).

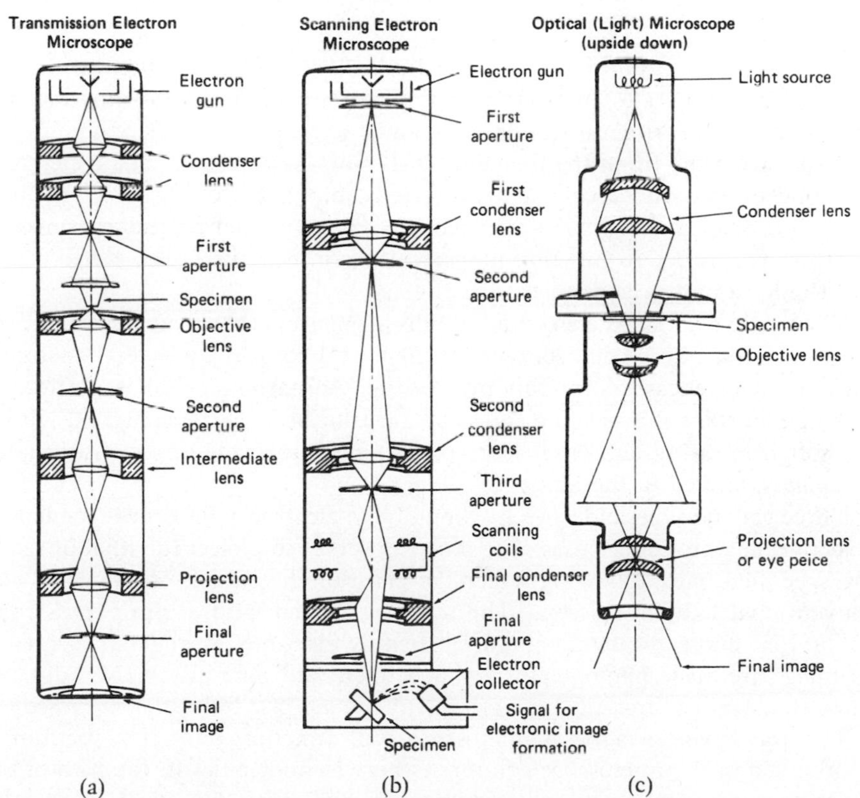

FIG. 4-15 A comparison of (a) the transmission electron microscope, (b) the scanning electron microscope, and (c) the optical, or bright-field, microscope.

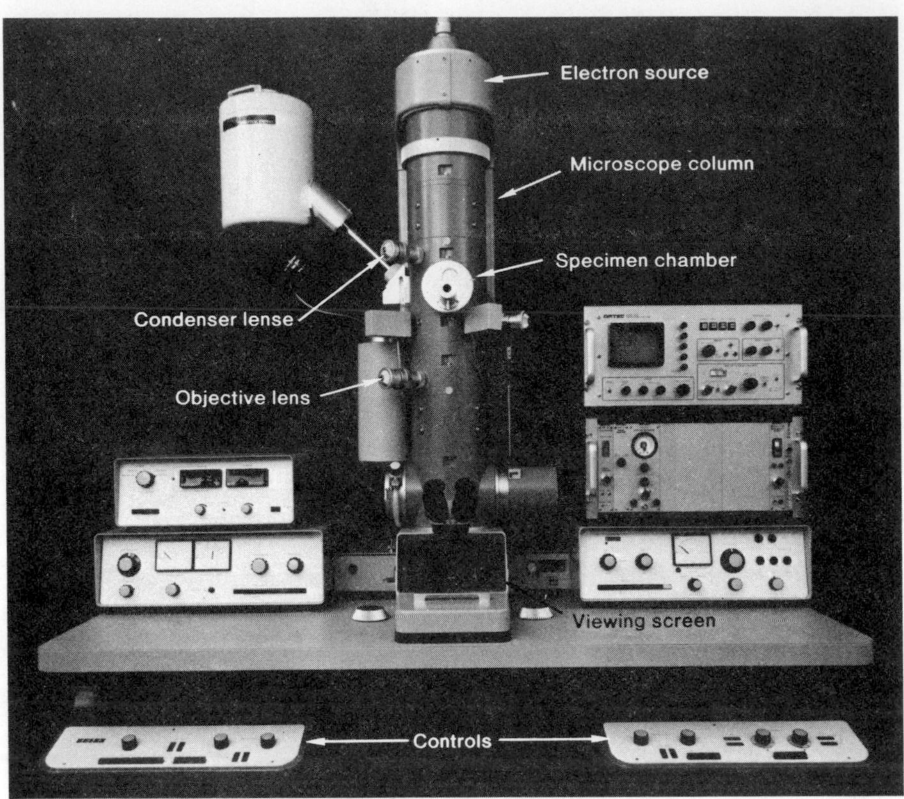

FIG. 4-16 One of the large number of currently available electron microscopes. *Courtesy of Carl Zeiss, Inc., New York.*

The source of illumination for the transmission electron microscope, the electron gun, generates an electron beam from a thin, V-shaped tungsten filament. This metal wire must be heated enough to release a sufficient quantity of electrons from the tip of the filament by thermionic emission. These electrons are concentrated and accelerated by other components of the electron gun, producing a fast-moving narrow beam of electrons. In order for the transmission electron microscope to function properly, the components of the electron gun and the lenses must be aligned with one another.

The lens system for the electron beam is magnetic rather than glass. The lens of an electron microscope consists of a lens coil formed by several thousand turns of wire encased in a soft iron casing. A magnetic field is created by passing a current through the coil. The electron beam is concentrated within the soft iron casing and other lens components also made of soft iron, called ***polepieces***, located in the lens coil.

Three general types of lenses are found in an electron microscope: condenser, objective, and projector lenses. The projector serves to project the final image of the specimen onto a viewing screen, in place of the ocular, or eyepiece, of a conventional light microscope. The screen is coated with a phosphorus compound that fluoresces upon being irradiated by electrons. Permanent records of an image are made photographically. Specimens are generally viewed directly through clear, lead-treated thick glass with the aid of a binocular microscope.

The transmission electron microscope will function only if a vacuum is maintained in the microscope column. Otherwise molecules in the path of the electrons can deflect them and interfere with the image.

Further details of operation and related subjects can be found in the books listed in the Suggested Readings at the end of this chapter.

Specimen Preparation for Electron Microscopy

SPECIMEN VIEWING AND CONTRAST

As electrons pass through a specially treated specimen being studied, the denser portions of the specimen scatter electrons more readily than those that are less dense. The resulting contrast creates an image of the specimen. The image is focused on a fluorescent screen or photographic emulsion.

When an untreated biological specimen is placed on the usual type of metal grid (Figure 4–17) coated with a plastic support film and is viewed in an electron microscope, the contrast between the specimen's electron image and its supporting film is very poor. This is principally because biological materials are mainly composed of the elements carbon, hydrogen, nitrogen, and oxygen. Because these elements have low atomic weights, their ability to scatter, or deflect, electrons is poor. Thus, in order to see specimens such as isolated macromolecules of protein or nucleic acid, or to study the structural features of cells, special techniques are necessary to make specimens stand out against the supporting film. Three such specimen preparation techniques are shadow casting, replicas, and electron staining.

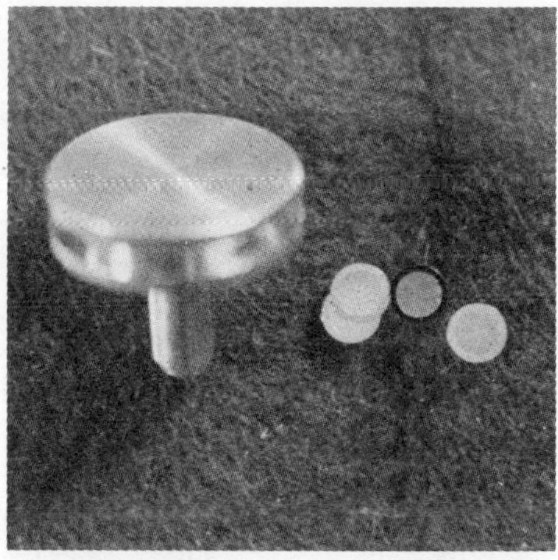

FIG. 4–17 A comparison of specimen holders used in electron microscopy. A specimen stub used for scanning electron microscopy and a number of metal specimen grids used in transmission electron microscopy studies.

SHADOW CASTING

In the ***shadow-casting*** procedure, a thin film of an electron-dense material is deposited at an angle on a specimen (Figure 4–18). Substances employed for this purpose are heavy metals (chromium, nickel, platinum, uranium, or alloys of gold and palladium or platinum and palladium). The metal to be used is placed on a tungsten filament or other device, which is heated to cause the electron-dense material to evaporate from the surface.

The shadow-casting technique decidedly increases the specimen's contrast. This is illustrated by the electron micrograph shown in Figure 4–19.

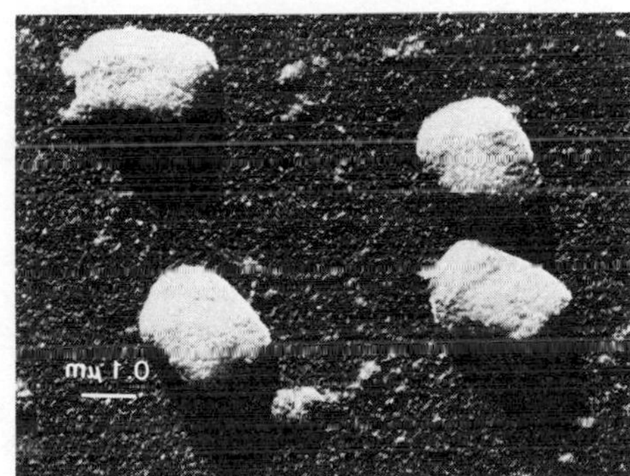

FIG. 4–19 An electron micrograph demonstrating the effect of shadow casting. The specimen here is vaccinia virus. This microorganism is used in vaccination against smallpox. *Courtesy of Dr. Robley C. Williams and the Virus Laboratory, University of California, Berkeley.*

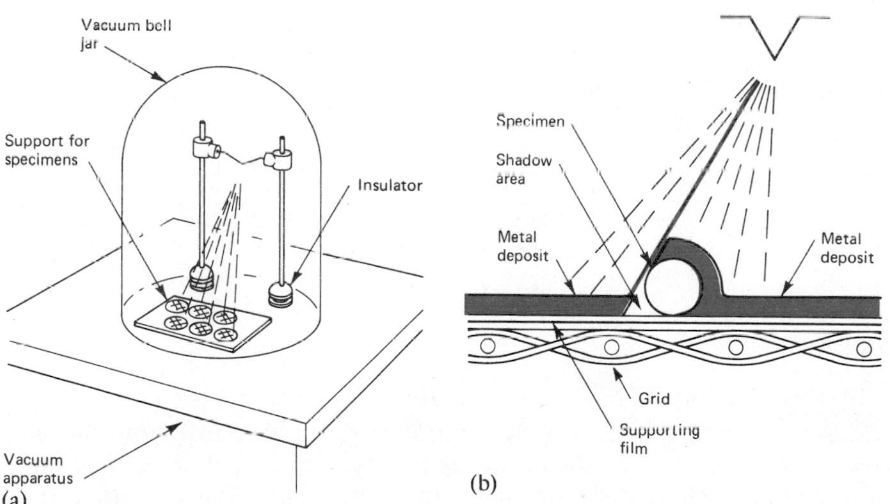

FIG. 4–18 (a) A diagrammatic representation of the shadow-casting apparatus. (b) The distribution of metal evaporated onto a specimen. The shadow area is transparent and consequently appears light in viewing the specimen. Because most electron micrographs are printed as negatives, it registers as a dark region in electron micrographs.

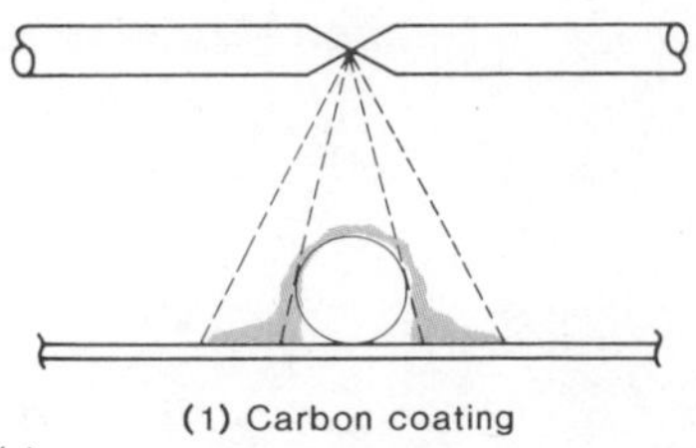

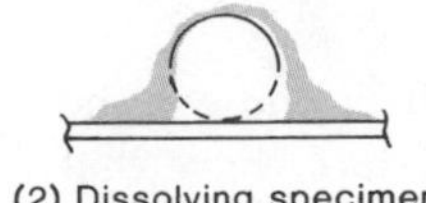

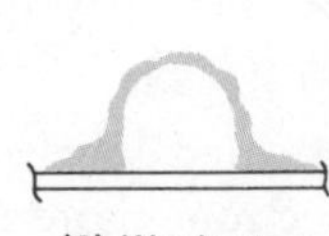

(a)

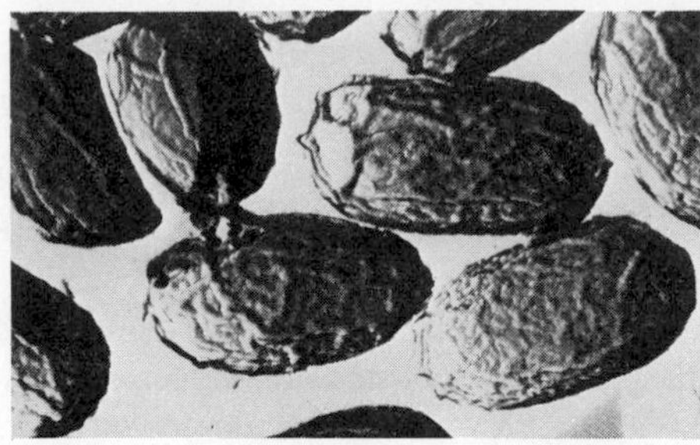

FIG. 4–20 (a) Surface replicas. (b) The result of carbon replication showing the surface of resting spores of *Bacillus megaterium*. Note the clear surface detail. *Unpublished electron micrographs by L. J. Rode and Leodocia Pope, Department of Microbiology, The University of Texas at Austin, Austin, Texas 78712.*

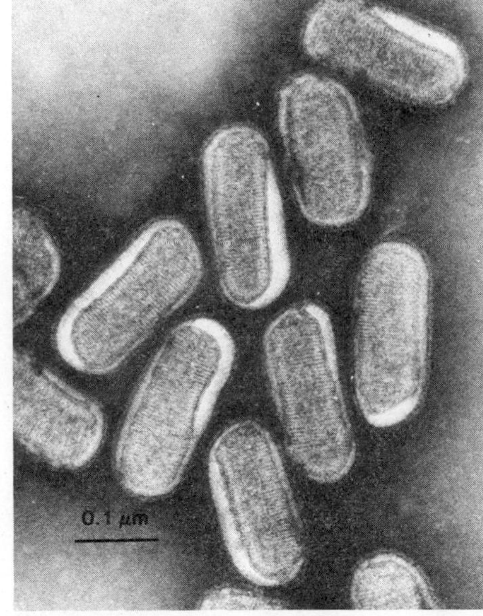

(a)

FIG. 4–21 Two different negative staining procedures involving sowthistle yellow vein virus. (a) The appearance of the virus when stained with phosphotungstic acid. (b) A similar viral preparation stained with uranyl acetate. The surface proteins of the virus are quite evident. *Courtesy of D. Peters and E. W. Kitajima.*

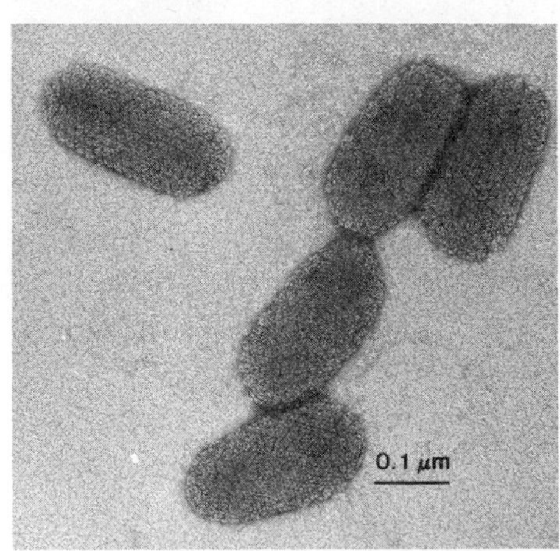

(b)

SURFACE REPLICAS

Surface replicas have been widely used in areas of microbiology involving the surfaces of specimens such as algae, bacterial spores, and viruses. Surface replicas are generally prepared by a single-stage technique (Figure 4–20a). In this technique, a thin layer of a low-molecular-weight material such as carbon is deposited on the surface of a specimen *in vacuo*. The newly coated specimen is then floated onto a water surface from which it is transferred to a strong acid or alkali solution capable of dissolving away the specimen without damaging the replica. The resulting cleaned replica is washed in water and placed on a specimen grid for viewing in the electron microscope (Figure 4–20b). Replicas are generally shadow-cast in order to emphasize certain aspects of surface detail.

ELECTRON STAINING

Electron stains are solutions that contain heavy metal elements, for example, osmic tetroxide, phosphotungstic acid (PTA), and uranyl acetate. These preparations are used to increase the contrast of specimens. Most electron stains function either by being absorbed on the surface or by combining with specific chemically reactive groups of the specimen. Two general types of staining techniques are known—positive and negative staining. *Positive staining* makes electron-transparent particles visible against a relatively transparent background, while ***negative staining*** sets specimens against an electron-dense background. In 1959, while studying preparations of turnip yellow mosaic virus, S. Brenner and R. W. Horne introduced this simple negative-contrast technique into general use for electron microscopy. The procedure provides a high resolution for the examination of viruses (Figure 4–21) and other specimen types. One advantage of this technique is that it does not require any specialized vacuum equipment. Negative staining in electron microscopy is often used as a quantitative device to determine numbers of viruses, as well as being used as a diagnostic tool.

THIN SECTIONING (MICROTOMY)

Many biological specimens are too thick for direct examination in the electron microscope. To make them suitable for investigation, either surface replication or thin sectioning (slicing) is employed (Figure 4–22). *Thin sectioning,* or *microtomy,* seems applicable to a larger variety of specimens. By this technique, structural arrangements of tissue (cellular interconnections), the internal organization of cells, developmental cycles of microorganisms, and many other items of biological interest can be effectively studied. Figure 4–23 compares the information obtained by thin sectioning with that obtained from electron staining.

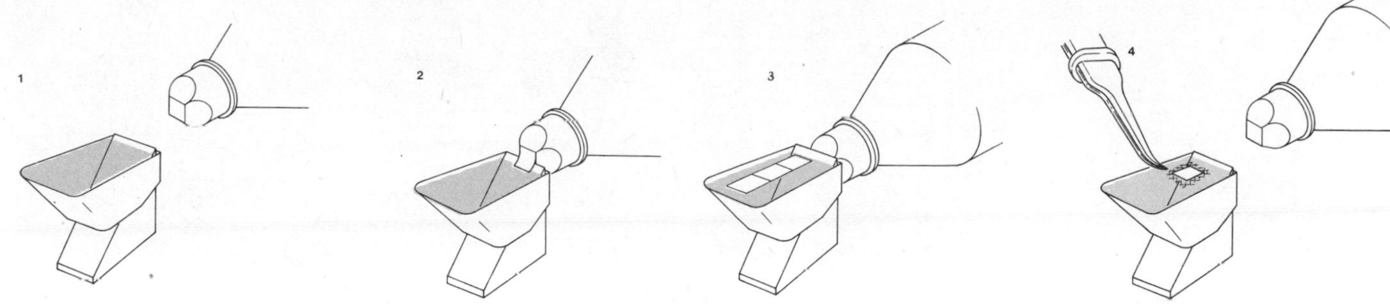

FIG. 4-22 A representation of how ultrathin sectioning is performed: (1) The specimen approaches the surface of the glass knife. (2) The beginning of a section. (3) The appearance of several sections. (4) The removal of a specimen for viewing on a coated grid.

Before sections or slices of biological material can be prepared, the specimen must be treated in some manner to preserve a specific structure or structures. Preservation of biological structures involves fixation, dehydration, and embedding in plastic. The reliability of the final appearance of a preparation depends upon these steps, as the reagents used may easily affect the physical and chemical properties of the specimen.

FREEZE-FRACTURE

The more recent technique of **freeze-fracture** is most welcome in the biological sciences, since it avoids fixation, embedding, and sectioning of speci-

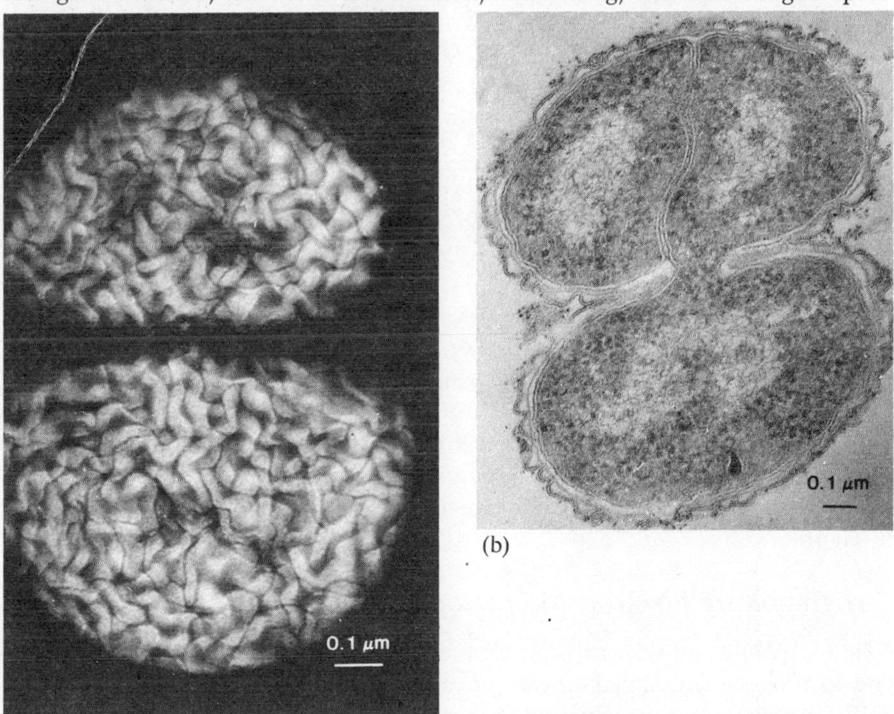

FIG. 4-23 Electron micrographs of *Veillonella* sp. comparing two techniques used in electron microscopy. (a) A negatively stained whole cell preparation. Note the convoluted surfaces of the diplococci. (b) A thin section. Note the internal appearance of the organisms as well as their convoluted outer regions. The cell on the right has developed a cross wall that will eventually result in division. *Mergenhagen, S. E., H. A. Bladen, and K. C. Hsu,* Ann. N.Y. Acad. Sci. 133:*279 (1966). © The New York Academy of Sciences; 1966; Reprinted by permission.*

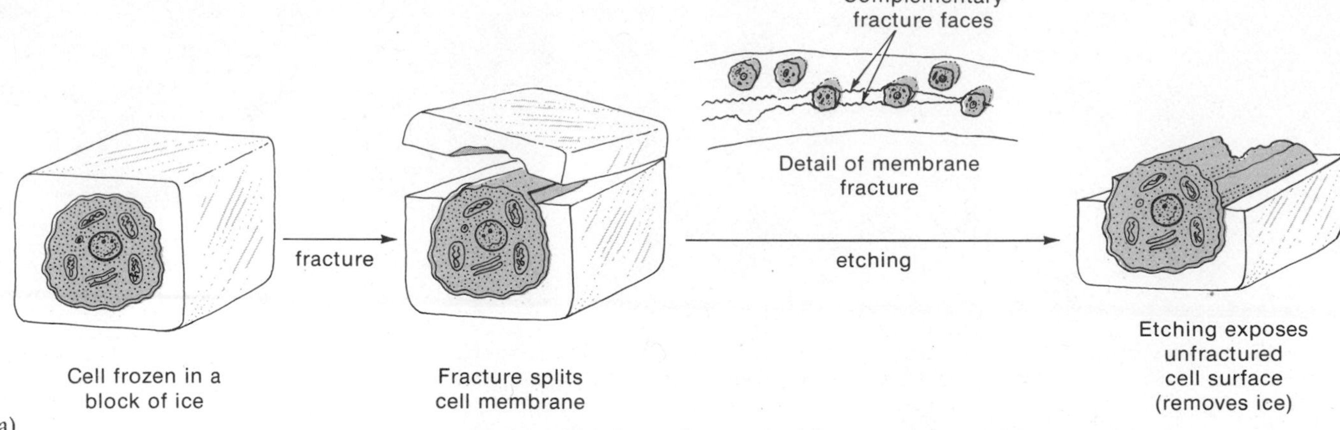

FIG. 4–24 The freeze-fracture and freeze-etching technique. (a) The frozen cell is fractured with a sharp blow by a blade or knife. The fracture line vary often runs through the interior of membranes, separating the two layers there by revealing membrane proteins that would otherwise remain buried. The last step allows for the etching of the membrane through the sublimation of surface ice. This exposes the unfractured membrane surface, thereby providing detail of the complementary fracture faces of the membrane. (b) An example of the freeze-fracture technique. With membranes, two complementary fracture faces are produced, OFF, the outer fracture face, and IFF, the inner (concave) fracture face. Both faces of this cell membrane of *Streptococcus faecalis* show particles. *Tsien, H. C., and M. L. Higgins,* J. Bacteriol. 118:725–734 *(1974).*

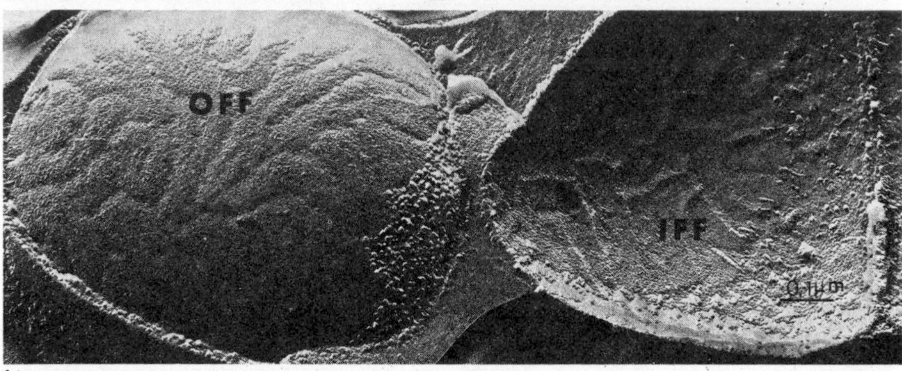

(b)

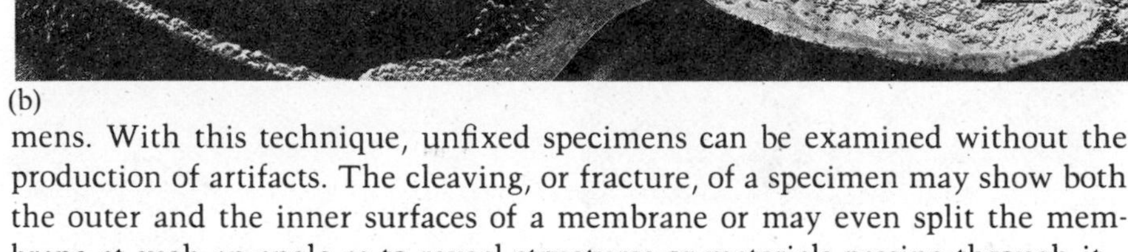

mens. With this technique, unfixed specimens can be examined without the production of artifacts. The cleaving, or fracture, of a specimen may show both the outer and the inner surfaces of a membrane or may even split the membrane at such an angle as to reveal structures or materials passing through it.

In freeze-fracture, cells are quick-frozen in water, split, or cleaved, and treated to expose their interior structures. Exposed surfaces are shadowed to provide contrast, and a replica is prepared. The procedure and results are shown in Figure 4–24.

High-voltage Electron Microscopy

The capability of transmission electron microscopes to show minute details and to produce functional images of preparations depends on the specimen's ability to scatter electrons passed through it. This passage of electrons is influenced by two factors, the thickness of the specimen and the energy of the electrons. The latter depends on the accelerating voltage used to generate the electrons. A new instrument, the ***high-voltage electron microscope,*** is similar to the general transmission microscope, except that its electron voltage is considerably greater. This feature of the microscope makes it possible to penetrate thicker specimens and to observe the three-dimensional relationships of cell components (Figure 4–25).

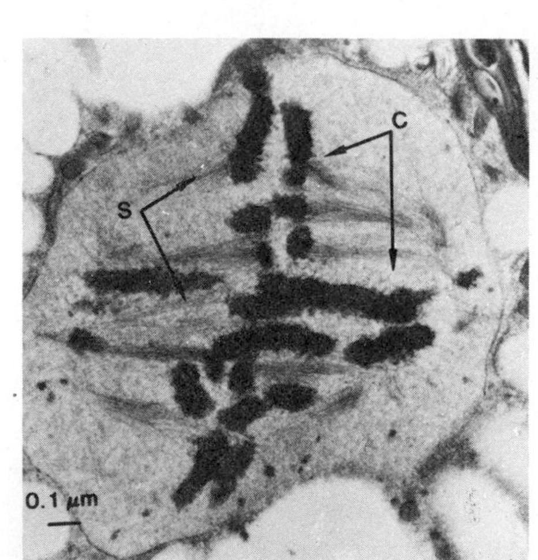

FIG. 4–25 A high-voltage electron micrograph of the stage of cell division called early anaphase in the green alga *Oedogonium cardiacum.* The chromosomes (C) and remains of the mitotic spindle (S) are well preserved. What advantages does this form of microscopy offer to the microbiologist? *Çoss, R. A., and J. D. Pickett-Heaps,* J. Cell Biol. 63:84–98 *(1974).*

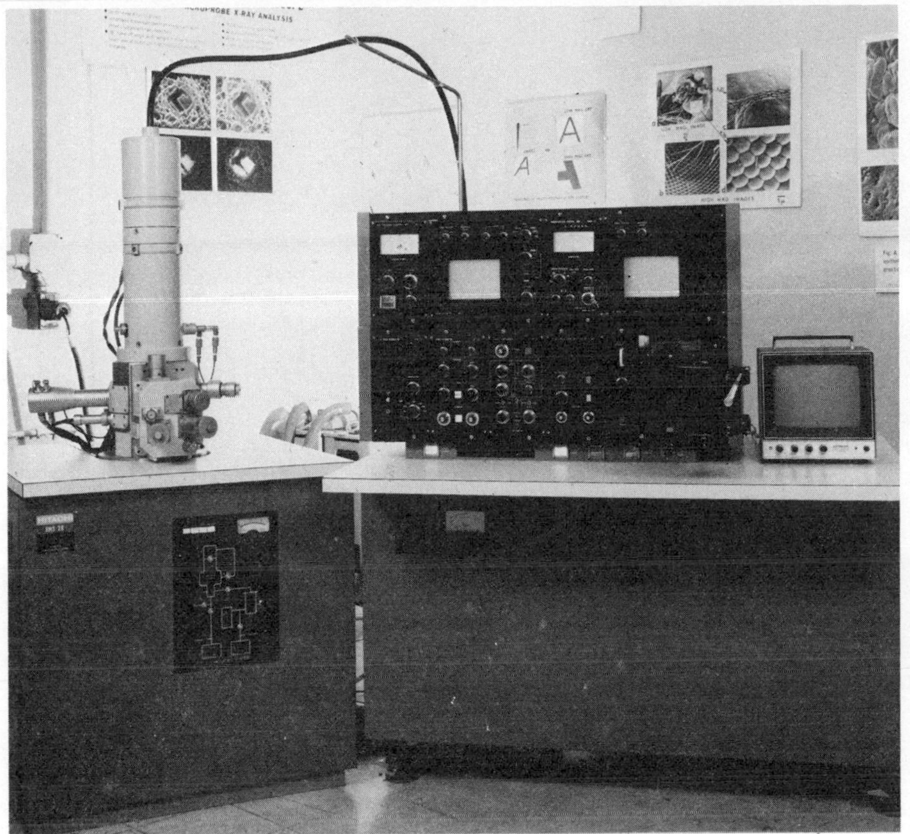

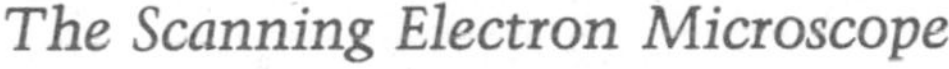

FIG. 4–26 The Hitachi Perkin-Elmer Model HHS-2R Scanning Electron Microscope. A television monitor (T), a photographic device (P), and related equipment are shown. *Courtesy The Perkin-Elmer Corporation, Scientific Instruments Department.*

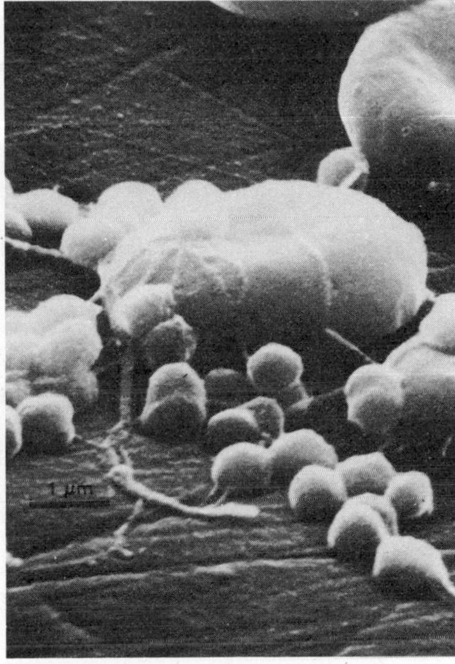

(a)

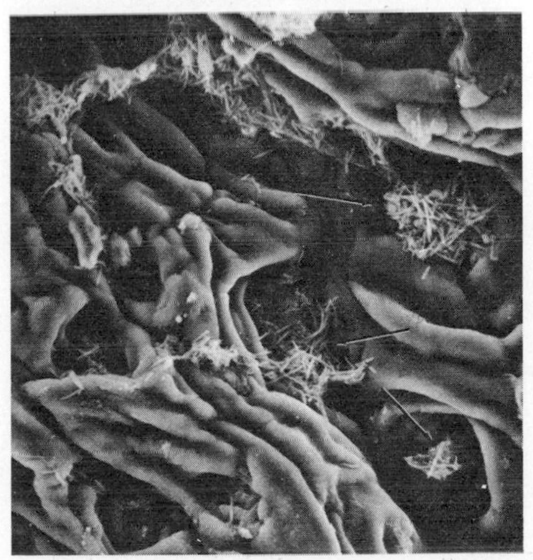

(b)

FIG. 4–27 (a) A scanning micrograph showing the clumping of red blood cells by cells of the bacterium *Neisseria catarrhalis*. Note the difference in size betwen the red blood cells and the bacteria. *Wistreich, G. A., and R. F. Baker,* J. Gen. Micro. 65:167 *(1971)*. (b) A scanning electron microscopic view of a crypt of Lieberkuhn in the colon of an adult mouse. Note that the opening to the crypt (arrows) is filled with masses of spiral- and spindle-shaped microorganisms. *Savage, D. C., and R. V. H. Blumershine,* Infect. Immun. 10:*240–250 (1974)*.

The Scanning Electron Microscope

The *scanning electron microscope* (Figure 4–26) is comparatively new and quite different in principle as well as in application from the conventional transmission electron microscope. The scanning electron microscope gives a three-dimensional quality to specimen images. It has been used a great deal to study the surfaces of specimens too thick for conventional transmission electron microscopy. Specimens for the scanning electron microscope require less preparation than those for transmission instruments. Furthermore, large portions of surfaces can be seen in detail with excellent contrast (Figure 4–27). Normally, the scanning microscope is operated by scanning, or sweeping, a very narrow beam of electrons (an electron probe) back and forth across a metal-coated specimen, revealing its surface features rather than its internal structure.

In microbiology, the scanning electron microscope is especially useful in studies of bacterial cells (Figure 4–27a), spores, and fungi. It is also becoming important in studies of morphological changes in tissues infected with microorganisms, and in studies of the organization and structure of microbial communities in various environments.

SUMMARY

Microscopes and Microscopy

1. Depending upon the magnification principle involved, microscopes fall in one of two categories: *light* (optical) or *electron.*
2. Light microscopes include *bright-field, dark-field, fluorescence,* and *phase-contrast* instruments.
3. Electron microscopes include the *transmission* and *scanning* instruments.

Units of Measurement

The basis of scientific concepts, laws, and theories requires careful measurement of lengths, volumes, weights, and other quantities.

1. *Le Système International d'Unitès,* or *SI system,* is a widely accepted system for measurement.
2. The units used for length, volume, mass, and temperature are the meter, liter, gram, and Celsius degree, respectively.
3. Commonly used metric units for the measurement of lengths include the meter (m), centimeter (cm), millimeter (mm), micrometer (μm), nanometer (nm), and Angstrom (Å).
4. The *bar marker* on photographs serves as a size reference and represents the length of a metric unit at a particular magnification.

Properties of Light

1. *Light waves* are described in terms of their amplitude, frequency, and wavelength.
2. *Amplitude* refers to the maximum displacement of a light wave from its equilibrium position.
3. *Frequency* is the number of vibrations that occur in one second.
4. *Wavelength* is defined as the distance between two corresponding points on a wave.
5. The *resolving power* of a microscope refers to its ability to reveal detail. It depends on the wavelength of light used.
6. The type of material or medium through which light passes during the operation of a microscope plays a major role in the image seen.

Light Microscopes

Bright-field Microscopy

1. Two types of bright-field microscopes are known, the *simple* (one-lens) microscope and the *compound* microscope.
2. A compound microscope consists of at least two lens systems: the *objective,* which forms and magnifies the image of the specimen, and the *eyepiece,* or *ocular,* which magnifies the image produced by the objective lens.
3. *Resolving power* (the ability to show details of specimens) and *parfocal* (changing objectives without major focusing adjustments) are two important microscope features.
4. The highest-magnification objective used in general courses is the oil-immersion objective, which for best results should be immersed in a medium having the same *index of refraction* as glass.
5. Condensers serve to concentrate light for specimen viewing. Most condensers are equipped with a shutterlike device, the *iris diaphragm,* to control light intensity.

Micrometry

Micrometry refers to procedures used to measure the dimensions of cells or, if possible, their parts.

Specimen Preparation for Bright-field Microscopy

1. *Hanging-drop* and temporary *wet-mount* techniques are used for the microscopic examination of living organisms. These procedures maintain the natural shape of the specimen and are useful in determining sizes, shapes, detection of movement, and reactions to various chemicals and immune sera.
2. General staining procedures involve the applications of dye-containing solutions to smears (thin films of microorganisms on glass slides, which have been air-dried and heat-fixed). These procedures permit greater observation of cells and, to some extent, a differentiation of microbial species.
3. Two general types of dyes are used for staining: basic dyes, which react with nuclear components, and acid dyes, which stain cytoplasmic and related materials.
4. *Simple staining* methods involve the application of only one dye solution. Such procedures provide information as to microbial size, shape, arrangement, and the presence or absence of spores.
5. *Differential staining* methods involve the application of more than one dye solution. Such procedures make possible the separation of bacteria into major groups and the identification of certain bacterial parts.
6. The two most widely used differential staining methods are the *Gram* and *acid-fast* staining techniques.
7. Based on resulting color reactions of the Gram stain, microorganisms are classified as either *Gram-positive* (purple) or *Gram-negative* (red).
8. Several bacterial properties appear to be correlated with Gram staining reactions; these include chemical composition, sensitivity to penicillin, and relative cell-wall thickness.
9. The acid-fast procedure is used mainly to differentiate mycobacteria from other bacteria. The decolorizing agent, acid alcohol, differs from the one used in the Gram stain.
10. *Spore-staining* techniques are of taxonomic importance in that they can be used to identify spore-forming bacteria.

Dark-field Microscopy

1. Specimens examined by *dark-field microscopy* usually appear as bright objects against a dark background.
2. Dark-field microscopy is useful with unstained preparations and may have diagnostic importance.

Fluorescence Microscopy

1. *Fluorescence microscopy* is used for examination of various cell types and cellular structures, the location of chemical components in cells, and the rapid diagnosis of certain diseases.
2. Ultraviolet light, fluorescent chemicals, and special microscope filter systems are required for this type of microscopy.

Phase Microscopy

1. *Phase microscopy* is of value in the examination or detection of living cells in certain fluid environments.
2. The *phase-contrast* principle makes cells and their parts stand out from the background.

Electron Microscopes

The Transmission Electron Microscope

1. Most *transmission electron microscopes* are similar in basic design to the light microscope.
2. The fundamental difference is that electron microscopes use electrons as the source of illumination. Therefore, they have different lens construction and specimen preparation procedures. They can produce higher magnification with better resolving power.

Specimen Preparation for Electron Microscopy

1. Because of their chemical composition, untreated biological specimens are difficult to see in the transmission electron microscope.
2. Special treatment procedures are used to increase the contrast of such specimens: these include shadow casting, replicas, and electron staining.
3. *Shadow casting* involves depositing, at an angle, a film of heavy metal on a specimen.
4. *Surface replicas* are surface impressions of specimens.
5. *Electron stains* are solutions that contain heavy metal elements that may combine with certain components of cells.
6. *Thin sectioning,* or *slicing,* is used with specimens that are too thick for direct examination in the electron microscope.
7. Thin sectioning can be used to study the internal organization, structural arrangement, and related properties of cells.
8. *Freeze-fracture* can be used to study biological specimens without the preparation associated with other techniques.

High-voltage Electron Microscopy

This form of microscopy makes it possible to penetrate thicker specimens and to observe three-dimensional relationships among cell components.

The Scanning Electron Microscope

1. This instrument provides a three-dimensional quality to the images of the specimens viewed.
2. Large portions of specimen surfaces can be seen in detail with excellent contrast.
3. Specimens are metal-coated for examination.

QUESTIONS FOR REVIEW

1. Define or explain the following:
   a. simple microscope
   b. Gram-variable
   c. compound microscope
   d. wet-mount
   e. micrometer
   f. scanning electron microscope
   g. nanometer
   h. contrast
   i. acid alcohol
2. Distinguish between resolving power (RP) and magnification.
3. What is parfocal?
4. What are the functions of the following microscope components?
   a. condenser
   b. iris diaphragm
   c. low-power objective
   d. ocular
5. Compare the types of microscopy listed below with respect to (1) source of illumination, (2) specimen preparation, (3) limits of magnification, and (4) general uses. The construction of a table with these categories would be quite helpful.
   a. bright-field microscopy
   b. fluorescence microscopy
   c. dark-field microscopy
   d. transmission electron microscopy
   e. phase-contrast microscopy
   f. scanning electron microscopy
   g. high-voltage electron microscopy
6. Compare the results that can be obtained in using the hanging-drop procedure with those associated with simple stains.
7. Give the equivalent metric units specified for the following:
   a. 10 μm = ________ nm
   b. 10 mm = ________ μm
   c. 1 m = ________ nm
   d. 100 nm = ________ Å
8. What is the purpose of differential staining procedures? What are common examples of this type of technique?
9. What are the functions of the different reagents used in the Gram stain?
10. What factors play prominent roles in determing Gram-positivity?
11. What are the specific color characteristics of the cell types or microbial structures listed below after the performance of the standard Gram, acid-fast, and spore stains?
    a. *Staphylococcus aureus*
    b. *Escherichia coli*
    c. Gram-positive bacteria
    d. *Mycobacterium leprae*
    e. Gram-negative bacteria
    f. acid-fast bacteria
    g. spores and associated vegetative cells
    h. Gram-variable organisms
    i. non-acid-fast cells
    j. Gram-nonreactives
12. What factors contribute to the resolving power of a microscope?
13. What is the purpose of using immersion oil? How is this material applied?
14. Indicate the general range of sizes of the following microorganisms.
    a. bacteria
    b. protozoa
    c. rickettsia
    d. viruses
    e. fungi
15. What is an acid dye?
16. What types of cellular structures are stained by a basic dye?

SUGGESTED READINGS

Bradbury, S., *The Optical Microscope in Biology*. London: Edward Arnold Ltd., 1976. *A short, simple text on the theory of microscopy and various techniques of microscopy.*

Burrells, W., *Microscope Technique, A Comprehensive Handbook for General and Applied Microscopy*. New York: John Wiley & Sons, 1977. *In-depth discussions of light microscopy are provided by this general reference. Techniques available to light microscopists and an introduction to electron microscopy are also included.*

Hayat, M. A., *Introduction to Biological Scanning Electron Microscopy*. Baltimore: University Park Press, 1978. *Provides a functional treatment of the operation, design, and uses of the scanning electron microscope. It is well written and contains many references and illustrations.*

Lennette, E. H., E. H. Spaulding, and J. P. Truant, eds., *Manual of Clinical Microbiology*. 2nd ed. Washington, D.C.: American Society for Microbiology, 1974. *Several chapters deal with different types of microscopy, for example, bright-field, dark-field, and fluorescent, as well as appropriate specimen preparations.*

Lillie, R. D., *H. J. Conn's Biological Stains: A Handbook on the Nature and Uses of the Dyes Employed in the Biological Laboratory*. 9th ed. Baltimore: Williams & Wilkins, 1977. *An internationally accepted publication that contains the most complete and physical information on biological dyes and their application.*

Meek, G. A., *Practical Electron Microscopy for Biologists*. New York: John Wiley & Sons, 1976. *A comprehensive coverage of principles of electron optics, instrument operation, and specimen preparation.*

Wren, L. A., *Understanding and Using the Phase Microscope*. Newton Highlands, Mass.: Unitron Instrument Company, 1963. *Principles and use of phase-contrast microscopy are presented in an understandable manner.*

Introduction to Biochemistry

CHAPTER 5

To understand life you must know something of the relationship between living things and chemical elements. The way microorganisms function and their role in disease and in normal life processes are all reactions involving biochemical substances. Chapter 5 discusses basic chemical concepts and describes biologically important substances such as carbohydrates, lipids, nucleic acids, and proteins.

After reading this chapter, you should be able to:

1. **Define atom, element, molecule, and compound.**
2. **Describe the formation of ionic, covalent, and hydrogen bonds.**
3. **List eight common functional groups and the reactions that yield esters and peptides.**
4. **Describe the concept of oxidation-reduction.**
5. **Define pH, the pH scale, and buffers.**
6. **List the basic chemical characteristics and biological functions of lipids, carbohydrates, nucleic acids, and proteins.**
7. **Define enzymes and describe their function in cellular reactions.**

Microbiology is so intimately involved with biochemistry that it is often difficult to separate the two. Microorganisms are composed of and use many of the same compounds characteristically used by other life forms. Many aspects of their cellular physiology resemble those of plant and animal cells. For this reason, microorganisms have been used in many studies of biochemistry, biophysics, genetics, and physiology intended to uncover the secrets of life.

This chapter discusses biochemical compounds. Pertinent details will be introduced wherever possible in these discussions, but space limitations preclude detailed discussion of any one topic. Mastering this subject matter should enable you to understand many of the principles and mechanisms discussed in the chapters that follow. For a more complete treatment of compounds, metabolism, and their relationship to normal functioning and to disease states, refer to the Suggested Readings at the end of the chapter.

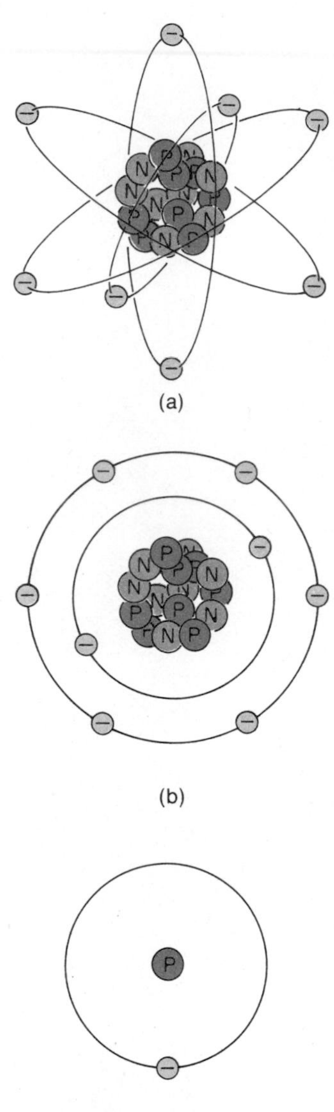

FIG. 5-1 Three ways of showing the components of atoms. (a) A generalized scheme illustrating a central atomic nuclear region consisting of neutrons (N) and protons (P), which is circled by electrons (−) at varying distances from the center. The electrons move in orbital paths. (b) The oxygen atom. Note the eight protons, eight neutrons, and eight electrons. The electrons form shells around the atom's nucleus. (c) The hydrogen atom. How many protons, neutrons, and electrons are there in this chemical element's atom?

Basic Chemistry Review

Atoms: The Particles of Matter

In describing the basic units of matter, the early Greek philosopher Democritus (460–370 B.C.) used the term ***atom*** for the ultimate, smallest particles. His usage of the word implied "that which cannot be further divided." Modern research, however, has demonstrated that atoms are divisible into smaller particles that are arranged as a central nuclear core surrounded by moving units (Figure 5-1). The three most important types of atomic particles are ***protons*** (positively charged), ***electrons*** (negatively charged), and ***neutrons*** (electrically neutral). The **nucleus,** or center of an atom, which accounts for most of its total mass, contains protons and neutrons. Electrons whirl around the nucleus at varying distances from it. An atom is electrically neutral because the number of protons it contains is equal to the number of its electrons. What distinguishes one type of atom from another is its characteristic number and arrangement of electrons, neutrons, and protons (Figure 5-1).

The number and arrangement of electrons in various orbitals forming electron shells around the nucleus determines the characteristics of the atom, which include the degree to which it will react with other atoms. For example, hydrogen has one electron. However, the possible number of electrons its particular orbital can hold is two. Thus hydrogen is reactive. A heavier element is most often stable if it can fill its outermost shell, for example, get eight electrons in its outermost orbital. Oxygen, which has six electrons in its outermost shell, needs two electrons; it is therefore reactive.

Elements

A substance consisting of atoms that all have the same numbers of protons and electrons is called an ***element.*** Over one hundred such elements are known. These elements have particular chemical and physical characteristics that account for their different activities. Carbon (C), hydrogen (H), nitrogen (N) oxygen (O), and phosphorus (P) are all elements that are present in living systems and participate in processes vital to life. The letters C, H, N, O, and P are the atomic symbols for these elements. This is essentially a means of chemical shorthand that is handy when you need to discuss or write the composition of a substance containing many different atoms.

Compounds, Molecules, and Macromolecules

The physical-chemical joining of two or more different kinds of atoms results in the formation of a ***compound.*** The smallest unit of a compound that is representative of its composition and properties is called a ***molecule.*** There are two kinds of compounds: **organic** compounds, containing carbon in a form other than carbonates (CO_3), and **inorganic** compounds, generally not containing carbon.

The number and types of atoms in a molecule are indicated by a *chemical formula.* For example, the formula for sodium chloride, ordinary table salt, is NaCl. It is made up of sodium (Na) and chlorine (Cl) atoms held together by a *chemical bond.* These two atoms react with one another because they both need electrons. The outer orbit of sodium contains one electron, whereas chlorine has seven electrons in its outer orbit. In this case chlorine needs one electron to stabilize the orbit at eight electrons. Thus, as sodium loses one and chlorine gains one, the reaction occurs and these atoms are bonded. This type of bond is called an *ionic bond* because an electron was transferred, producing two *ions,* electrically charged atoms. The sodium atom lost an electron and became a positive ion, while the chlorine atom gained an electron and became a negative ion. These ions are written as Na^+ and Cl^-. Ionically bonded compounds are held together because of the opposite charges of the components. However, ionic bonds dissociate (break) in water and are therefore not strong enough to hold living systems together.

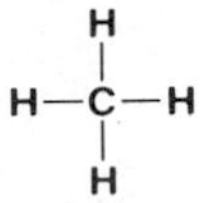

The kind of bond required for protoplasm is the *covalent bond.* This type of bond occurs when electrons are *shared* by the atoms making the bond. Therefore, ions are not generated and these compounds do not dissociate in water. Natural gas, or methane, is a good example of covalent bonding. Hydrogen has one electron to share, and carbon needs four electrons to stabilize its orbit. Four hydrogen atoms, therefore, share their electrons with one carbon atom, producing methane, chemically noted as CH_4 or as shown in Figure 5-2.

H
H—C—H
H
Methane

FIG. 5-2 The chemical formula for methane. Methane, or natural gas, is an example of covalent bonding.

Many molecules involve the sharing of four or even six electrons between two atoms. Carbon dioxide (CO_2) is one such molecule. Each oxygen atom shares a total of four electrons with carbon, forming *double bonds.* These are symbolized by two dashes: O=C=O.

Covalent bonds allow the formation of large molecules, or *macromolecules,* that are relatively stable. Many cellular activities involve the synthesis, or manufacture, of these macromolecules, while other processes break them down.

Another common bond found in biological molecules is the *hydrogen bond.* This results from the nature of hydrogen to form *polar molecules.* In a polar molecule there are regions of positive and negative charge in an overall neutral molecule. An excellent example is water, H/O\H in which the oxygen atom has some negative charge and the hydrogen atoms some positive charge. Thus, in water, the oxygen atom of one molecule is attracted to and loosely bonded to a hydrogen atom of another molecule (Figure 5-3). This, in part, gives water its cohesiveness and accounts for its surface tension and unusually high boiling point. The same phenomenon occurs in many biological molecules and accounts for some of the characteristic structures of large molecules. In contrast to ionic and covalent bonds, hydrogen bonds are relatively weak and easily broken. The usual representation of hydrogen bonds as dashed, rather than solid, lines suggests this weakness.

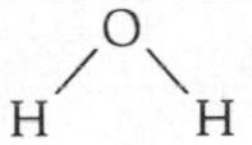

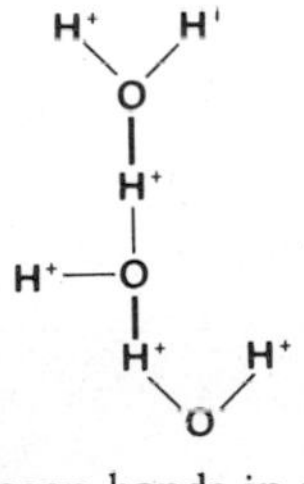

FIG. 5-3 Hydrogen bonds in water.

Functional Groups

A typical cell is an incredibly complex array of chemical molecules. Moreover, cells manufacture a wide variety of organic compounds. The main types of compounds contained in and synthesized by cells are **carbohydrates, lipids, nucleic acids,** and **proteins.** Some of these are used as components of cell parts; others provide energy for cellular activities; and still others are of particular importance to the regulation of cellular chemical activities **(metabolism).** Such organic molecules contain certain recurring assemblies of atoms called *functional groups.* Each group has its own characteristics, including solubility in aqueous or nonaqueous materials and ability to react with other functional groups. It is the arrangement of these groups in a biological molecule that gives that molecule its specific and characteristic chemical properties. Some common functional groups are shown in Table 5-1. Two particularly common bonding arrangements are peptide bonds and ester formation, shown in Table 5-2.

TABLE 5-1 Common Functional Groups

Functional Group	*Formula*
Aldehyde	—C(=O)—H
Amino	N(—H)(—H)
Carbonyl	—C(=O)—
Carboxyl (acid)	—C(=O)—O—H
Hydroxyl	—O—H
Methyl	—C(H)(H)—H
Phosphate	—P(=O)(=O)—O
Sulfhydryl (thiol)	—S—H

Oxidation-Reduction

Whenever an atom, molecule, or ion loses one or more electrons, the process is called **oxidation** and the particle is said to have been *oxidized.* The name suggests that oxygen is involved in the process, but this is not necessarily so.

The electrons that have been lost by an oxidized molecule do not float randomly. They are reactive and are readily picked up by another molecule. The resulting gain of one or more electrons is referred to as **reduction.** The second molecule has been *reduced.*

Certain molecules readily either lose or gain electrons. Those that lose electrons supply them to molecules to be reduced and are therefore called *reducing agents.* In the same way, those that gain electrons are obtaining them from molecules being oxidized and are therefore called *oxidizing agents.*

Oxidation and reduction in biological systems are intimately associated with

TABLE 5-2 Two Common Bonding Arrangements

Reaction Type	*Functional Groups*	*Reaction*[a]	*Biological Significance*
Peptide bond	—N(—H)—H (amino); —C(=O)—O—H (carboxyl)	R—CH(NH₂)—C(=O)OH (amino acid) + HN(H)—CH(R)—C(=O)OH (amino acid) → R—CH(NH₂)—C(=O)—N(H)—CH(R)—C(=O)—OH (peptide) + H_2O	Peptide bonds serve to form proteins by linking various amino acids together.
Ester formation	—O—H (hydroxyl); —C(=O)—OH (carboxyl)	R—OH (alcohol) + HO—C(=O)—R (acid) → R—O—C(=O)—R (ester) + H_2O	Ester formation is the means by which components of fats, oils, and other lipids are bonded. A comparable reaction between hydroxyl groups and phosphate is the basis for the linking of nucleic acids.

[a]The symbol R in each organic chemical represents a general chemical group that varies among molecules of the related chemicals.

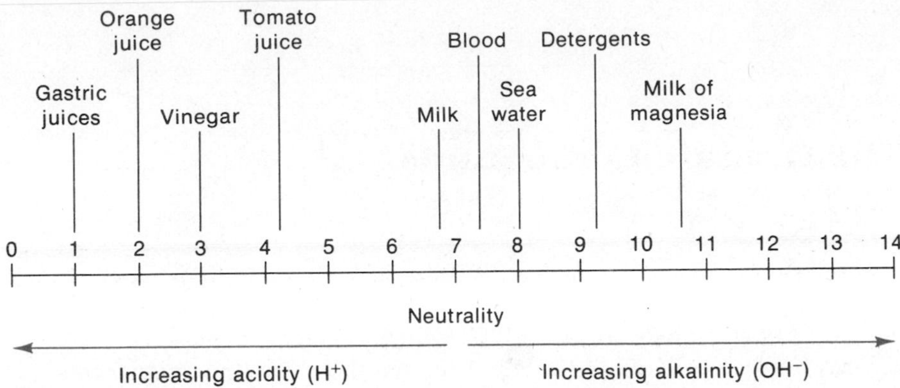

FIG. 5-4 The pH scale. The pH values of some common materials are also shown in this diagram.

the many metabolic reactions necessary for life. In particular, they are associated with energy production by cells.

pH and Buffers

Situations involving exchanges of hydrogen ions (H^+) are called *acid/base reactions.* **Acids** supply hydrogen ions, while **bases** combine with and neutralize solutions containing hydrogen ions. Basic substances also supply hydroxyl ions (OH^-). Certain compounds are either acid or basic *(alkaline)* (Figure 5–4). Others, such as water, can react as an acid or a base.

Reactions that take place in cells, tissues, and many organ systems, particularly those involving organic catalytic agents called **enzymes,** are quite sensitive to changes in acidity. The acidity of various compounds is determined by the number of hydrogen ions produced. Strong acids, such as hydrochloric acid (HCl), produce a high concentration of H^+ ions:

$$HCl \rightarrow H^+ + Cl^-$$

In the same sense, the alkalinity of a substance depends upon the concentration of hydroxyl (OH^-) ions it produces. The degree of acidity or alkalinity of a substance is expressed as its *pH.* When equal numbers of H^+ and OH^- ions are present, the substance is neutral and has a pH value of 7. Changes in the two ion concentrations move the pH value either toward an acid range (pH 0 to 6.9) or toward an alkaline range (pH 7.1 to 14). The pH scale is shown in Figure 5–4.

Acids and bases are produced as waste products of metabolism. In the form of acids or bases, waste products are more water soluble and are more easily eliminated from the cell by diffusion through the cell membrane. However, too much acid or base in a cell can be harmful. Fortunately, cells have mechanisms to control pH changes. One such mechanism is the **buffer** system, a chemical or mixture of chemicals that will react with H^+ and OH^- and regulate the pH of a solution. An example of a buffer in human blood is carbonic acid-bicarbonate system (H_2CO_3-HCO_3^-). When H^+ is added to the buffer, it reacts with HCO_3^- to form H_2CO_3 and is not available to make the solution more acid. When OH^- is added to the buffer, it reacts with H_2CO_3 to form H_2O and HCO_3^- and does not drastically change the pH. Any buffer system performs only within certain pH limits. When too much H^+ or OH^- has been added, its protective effect can be impaired or destroyed.

The Organic Compounds

Lipids

The term **lipid** usually refers to any substance soluble in organic solvents such as acetone, benzene, carbon tetrachloride, chloroform, and ether. Lipids include fatty acids, fats, oils, waxes, phospholipids, and steroids.

These molecules serve as (1) important cellular structural components; (2) sources of energy; (3) insulation and padding; (4) lubricants for mammalian gastrointestinal tracts; (5) certain hormones; and (6) protection.

FATTY ACIDS

Naturally occurring **fatty acids** are even-numbered carbon chains (of from 4 to 30 carbon atoms) with an acid group (—COOH). They may be *saturated* or *unsaturated*. Saturated fatty acids do not contain double bonds in their chains, whereas unsaturated fatty acids have one or more double bonds (see Table 5–3).

FATS, OILS, AND WAXES

Fats and *oils* are *esters* formed by reaction of the carboxyl group of fatty acids and the hydroxyl (OH) group of glycerol. *Waxes* are esters of fatty acids with long-chained alcohols. The basic difference between fats and oils is that fats are solid at normal room temperature and oils are liquid. This characteristic is determined by the degree of saturation. The compound containing unsaturated fatty acids is the liquid.

A fat may consist of glycerol esterified with one, two, or three different fatty acids. Tristearin is an example of a simple triglyceride (see Figure 5–5). Linolenyl-oleylstearin is an example of a mixed triglyceride. As shown in Figure 5–6, this compound is formed from glycerol (a), linolenic acid (b), oleic acid (c) and stearic acid (d). Saturated fatty acids such as stearic acid have no double bonds (=) between their carbon atoms. Unsaturated fatty acids, including linolenic and oleic acids, have one or more double bonds. Those fatty acids with more than one double bond are also called *polyunsaturated* fatty acids.

Waxes occur in a wide variety of materials, including beeswax, carnauba wax, lanolin, and the cutin on surfaces of leaves and fruits.

TABLE 5–3 Representative Saturated and Unsaturated Fatty Acids

Saturated Fatty Acid		*Unsaturated Fatty Acid*	
Compound Designation	*Chemical Formula*	*Compound Designation*	*Chemical Formula*
Butyric acid (found in butter)	$CH_3(CH_2)_2—COOH$	Oleic acid (olive oil)	$CH_3(CH_2)_7—CH{=}CH(CH_2)_7COOH$
Caproic acid (found in butter)	$CH_3(CH_2)_3—COOH$	Linoleic acid (linseed oil)	$CH_3(CH_2)_7—CH{=}CH—CH_2CH{=}CH(CH_2)_4COOH$
Stearic acid (found in animal and plant fats)	$CH_3(CH_2)_{16}—COOH$		

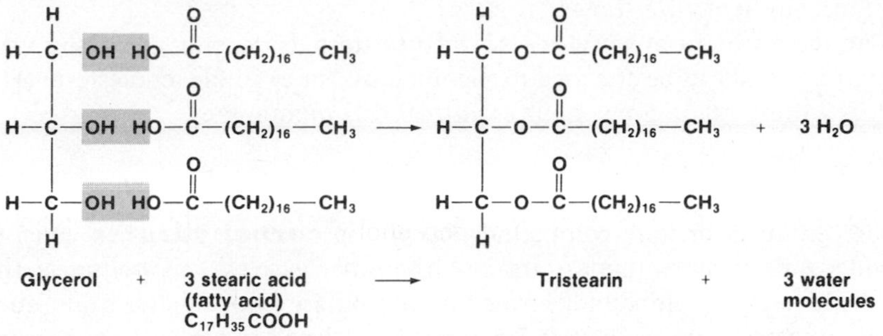

FIG. 5-5 The formation of the simple triglyceride tristearin.

PHOSPHOLIPIDS

Phospholipids play an important role in the cell because they contain groups that generally do not dissolve in water (*hydrophobic* groups), like those in lipids, as well as functional groups that do dissolve in water (*hydrophilic* groups). This dual nature appears to be a key factor to the function of the cell membrane.

There are several groups of phospholipids. One group, the *lecithins*, is of particular importance in mammalian physiology. Their composition includes choline, fatty acids, glycerol, and phosphoric acid. Choline (Figure 5-7) functions as an essential *metabolite* in mammalian physiology, being involved with both fat metabolism and nerve impulses.

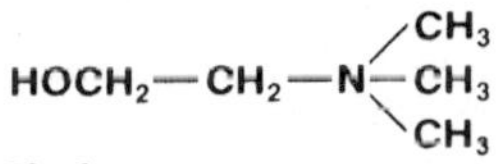

FIG. 5-7 Choline.

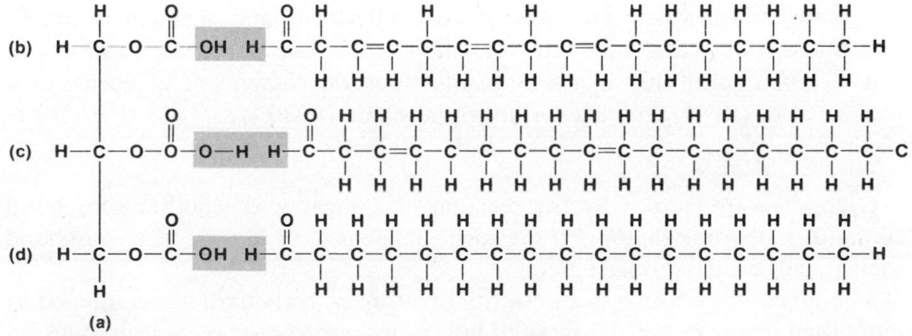

FIG. 5-6 The mixed triglyceride linolenyl-oleylstearin.

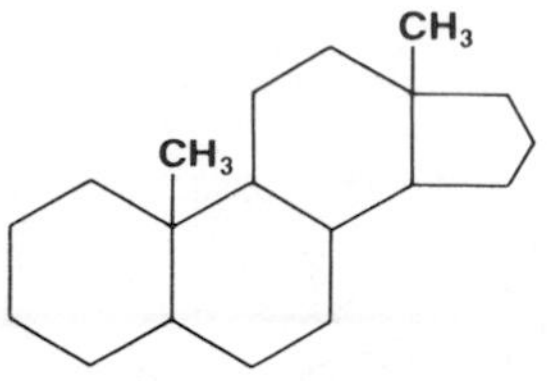

STEROIDS

Steroids are important forms of lipids that do not contain fatty acids. Many are physiologically important substances, and include bile acids, cholesterol, cortisone, ergosterol, and several hormones. The basic structure of steroids is the four-ring structure shown in Figure 5–8.

The wide variety of activities ascribed to steroids depends upon the various side groups that can be attached to the nucleus. For example, cholesterol (Figure 5–9) is an important component of animal cell membranes.

FIG. 5–8 The basic four-ring structure of steroids.

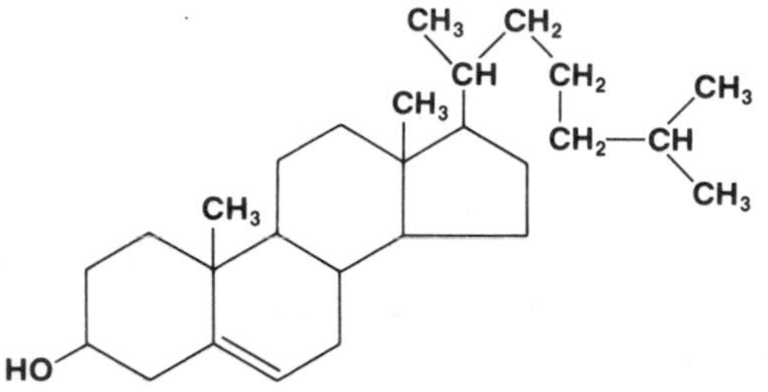

FIG. 5–9 Cholesterol.

Carbohydrates

The group of organic compounds known as **carbohydrates** consists of a wide variety of simple sugars and their derivatives and *polymers* (high-molecular-weight compounds formed by combinations of smaller units) such as starch, glycogen, and cellulose. For the sake of brevity, we will only discuss a few representative carbohydrates.

For the most part we will use the Fischer system to present the structure of these compounds. In this system, the molecule is drawn with the aldehyde (HC=O) or ketone (C=O) group at the top of the carbon skeleton, the primary alcohol (CH_2OH) at the bottom, and hydrogen (H) and hydroxyl (OH) groups at right angles to the carbon backbone of the compound. As examples, four aldo sugars (sugars containing an aldehyde group) and one keto (ketone-containing sugar) are shown in Figure 5–10. These compounds are referred to as triose, tetrose, pentose, and hexose, or as three-, four-, five-, and six-carbon sugars, respectively.

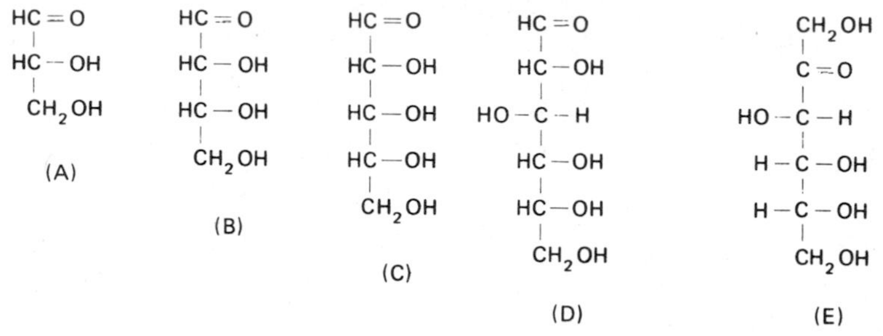

FIG. 5–10 Structural formulas of representative aldo sugars and a keto sugar. (a) Glyceral-dehyde. (b) Erythrose. (c) Ribose. (d) Glucose. (e) Fructose (a keto sugar).

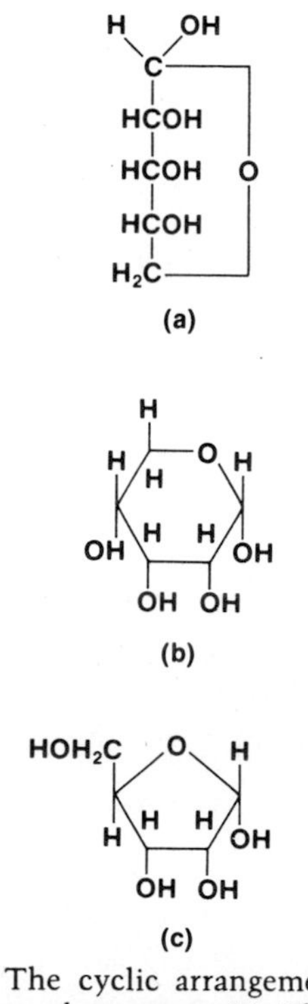

Pentoses and hexoses can also exist in cyclic form, and different cyclic arrangements can be drawn. Figure 5–11 shows the cyclic arrangements of ribose, a five-carbon sugar that is a significant structural component of coenzymes, nucleic acids (RNA), and adenosine triphosphate (ATP).

FIG. 5–11 The cyclic arrangements of ribose, a five-carbon sugar. (a) The Fischer system representation. (b) The pyran ring. (c) The furan ring. Parts (b) and (c) are representations of the Haworth system.

GLYCOSIDES

Glycosides are formed by the reaction of a sugar with another compound containing a hydroxyl group. If the sugar happens to be glucose, the compound then is called a **glucoside.**

The glycosidic linkage is an essential feature of carbohydrates composed of more than one sugar unit: disaccharides, trisaccharides, and polysaccharides. In chained polysaccharides, the linkage between the sugar monomers is commonly expressed as 1, 4 or 1, 6, based upon the attachment points between the sugar units. Numbering the ring carbons clockwise starting at the ring oxygen of the sugar molecule, we get the diagram shown in Figure 5–12. The disaccharide maltose is formed by 1, 4 glycosidic linkage of two molecules of glucose (Figure 5–13). In writing this equation, we have used a convention common in organic chemistry. Where no substituent is shown, as on the bonds to the mannose ring, hydrogen is assumed. We shall use this convention later with a variety of ring compounds.

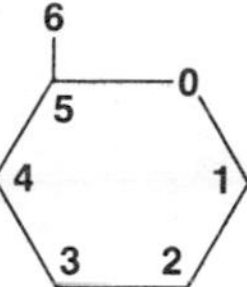

FIG. 5–12 The clockwise numbering system for sugar molecules.

MONOSACCHARIDES

Probably the most important **monosaccharides** (simple sugars) are the six-carbon hexoses. Among the common hexoses are fructose, galactose, glucose, and mannose. Glucose is the primary energy source for nutrition, but mammals metabolize all four hexoses similarly.

Deoxyribose (Figure 5–14), found in the genetic material deoxyribonucleic acid (DNA), is a derivative of the pentose *ribose*. In the sugars discussed earlier, the number of oxygen atoms equals the number of carbon atoms: glucose, $C_6H_{12}O_6$, and ribose, $C_5H_{10}O_5$. In contrast, deoxyribose is characterized by having one fewer atom of oxygen than of carbon: $C_5H_{10}O_4$.

Other important monosaccharides include amino sugars, sugar acids, and sugar alcohols. Representative monosaccharides of these types are shown in Figure 5–15. The amino sugars are found in mucoproteins, in chitin, and as components of some antibiotics. Glucuronic acid represents one type of sugar acid found in certain polysaccharides. The sugar alcohols occur in polysaccharides and phospholipids.

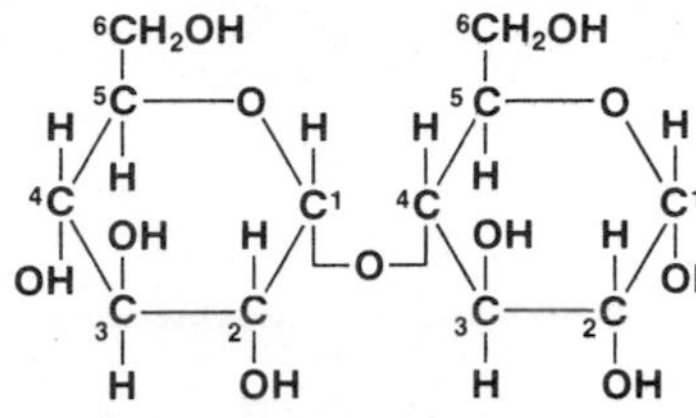

FIG. 5–13 The disaccharide maltose.

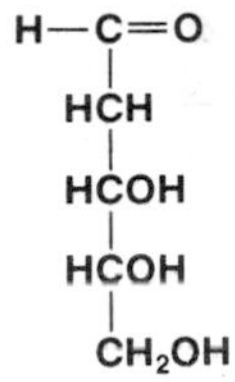

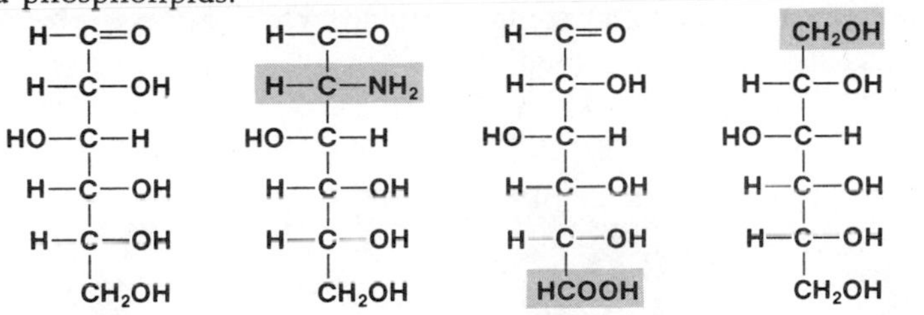

Glucose (a)	Glucosamine (b)	Glucuronic Acid (c)	Glucitol (sorbitol) (d)
H—C=O	H—C=O	H—C=O	CH_2OH
H—C—OH	H—C—NH_2	H—C—OH	H—C—OH
HO—C—H	HO—C—H	HO—C—H	HO—C—H
H—C—OH	H—C—OH	H—C—OH	H—C—OH
H—C—OH	H—C—OH	H—C—OH	H—C—OH
CH_2OH	CH_2OH	HCOOH	CH_2OH

FIG. 5–15 Structural formulas of different forms of the monosaccharide glucose. (a) General formula for glucose. (b) The amino form, glucosamine. (c) The uronic acid form, glucuronic acid. (d) The alcohol form, glucitol or sorbitol.

H—C=O
HCH
HCOH
HCOH
CH_2OH

FIG. 5–14 The monosaccharide deoxyribose.

DISACCHARIDES

Disaccharides are molecules composed of two monosaccharides. Usually they can be split to yield simple sugars. The three most common disaccharides are lactose, maltose, and sucrose. Lactose, or milk sugar, a prime component of milk, consists of glucose and galactose molecules. Maltose is made up of two glucose molecules, as noted earlier. It is produced by the breakdown of starch molecules. Sucrose, composed of glucose and fructose, is the natural sugar found in pineapple, sugar beets, and sugar cane.

POLYSACCHARIDES

Polysaccharides, the long-chain polymers (combinations) of sugar, may consist of only one type of sugar molecule or of different ones. *Starch,* which is the main food storage product in plants, is composed entirely of glucose units. It is of two basic types, *amylose* and *amylopectin.* The amylose molecule has a linear arrangement of units; amylopectin is a branched molecule with some side chains. The linear structures of starch are essentially chains of maltose units with 1,4 linkages. Amylopectin contains linear 1,4 linked chains that are attached by 1,6 linkages to the backbone polymer at intervals along the main chain.

The chief animal polysaccharide is ***glycogen***. It is structurally similar to amylopectin in that it contains 1,4 linked glucose units cross-connected with 1,6 linkages.

Cellulose, the main structural component of wood, is yet another polysaccharide of glucose units connected by 1,4 linkages. This component of plants has a different 1,4 linkage from that found in starch, which makes it resistant to the effects of mammalian enzymes. It is therefore indigestible to humans. However, various microorganisms present in certain animal digestive systems are able to cleave the molecule into utilizable sugar units. It is because of these microbes that ruminants (such as cattle, sheep, and goats) and termites are able to digest cellulose.

Nucleic Acids

Nucleic acids are found in all microorganisms, plants, and animals with the exception of mature mammalian red blood cells. They contain the cell's storehouse of information to govern activities such as protein synthesis and reproduction.

Nucleic acids are polymers of subunits called **nucleotides.** These smaller components in turn are made up of nitrogen-containing bases **(purines** and **pyrimidines),** phosphate, and a five-carbon sugar. The pentose classifies nucleic acids into two main classes: ribonucleic and deoxyribonucleic acids. **Ribonucleic acid (RNA)** contains ribose, while **deoxyribonucleic acid (DNA)** has deoxyribose (Figure 5–16).

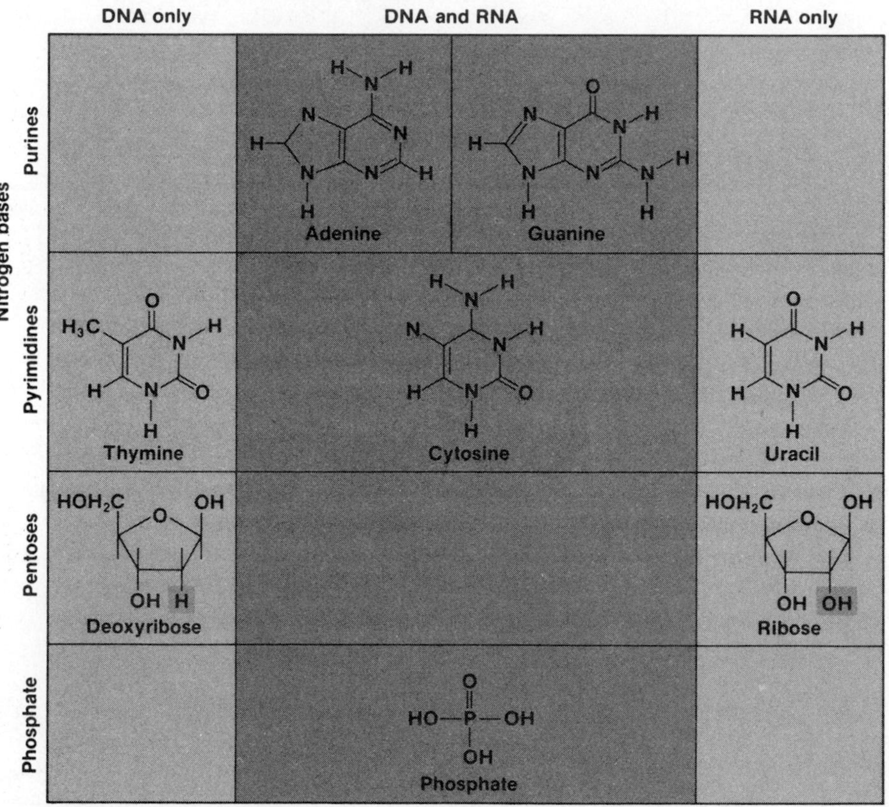

FIG. 5–16 The components of nucleic acids. Both purines are found in DNA and RNA. The pyrimidines cytosine and thymine are found in DNA; cytosine and uracil are found in RNA. DNA contains the pentose deoxyribose, while RNA contains ribose. Phosphate is found in both DNA and RNA.

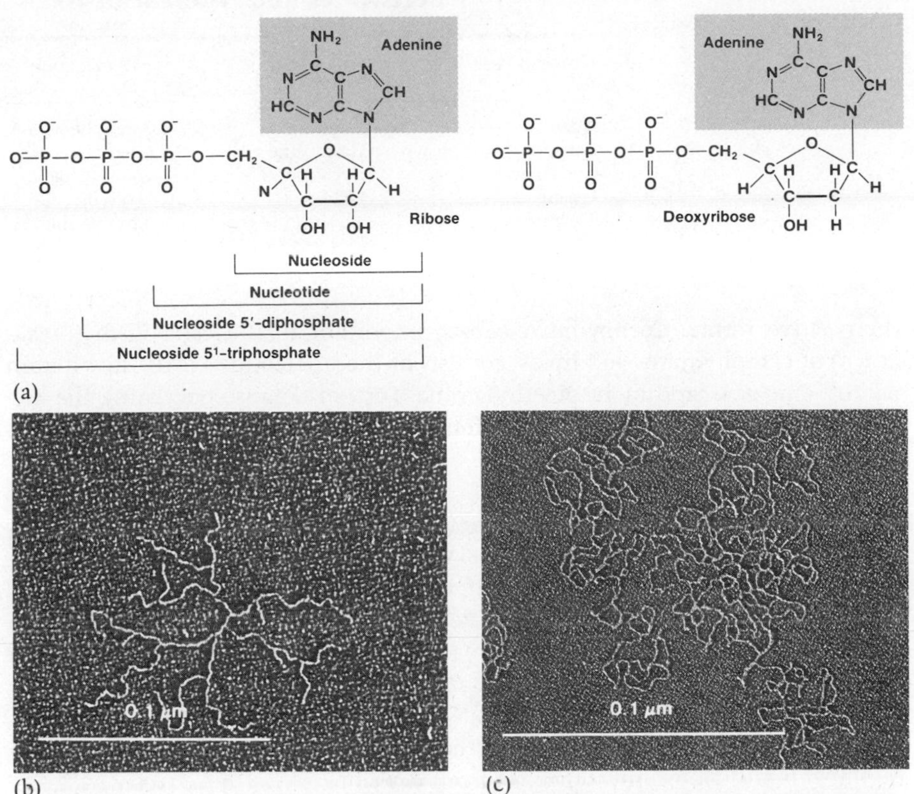

FIG. 5-17 *The building blocks of nucleic acids.* (a) Using the purine adenine, the construction of a nucleotide (purine + five-carbon sugar + PO_4) and related compounds can be visualized. Note that adenine is common to both DNA and RNA. A nucleoside consists of a purine or a pyrimidine and a five-carbon sugar. (b) An electron micrograph showing nucleotide units of adenine. (c) The appearance of deoxyribonucleic acid molecules. *The photos used are through the courtesy of H. Bujard, Universitat Heidelberg.*

The primary nitrogenous bases found in RNA are adenine, guanine, cytosine, and uracil. Adenine and guanine are purines; cytosine and uracil are pyrimidines. DNA (Figure 5–17) also contains adenine, guanine, and cytosine, but the pyrimidine thymine replaces uracil.

When a purine or pyrimidine is linked with ribose or deoxyribose, the resulting molecule is called a **nucleoside.** With the attachment of a phosphate group, the molecule becomes a *nucleotide*. An example of a ribose nucleoside is adenosine (adenine + pentose), shown in Figure 5–17. The corresponding nucleotide would be adenylic acid (adenine + pentose + phosphate), also known as adenosine monophosphate (AMP). This compound is involved in energy metabolism and protein synthesis. The addition of a second phosphate yields adenosine diphosphate (ADP). Adding a third phosphate forms **adenosine triphosphate (ATP),** the high-energy-containing compound in the cell. The names of various nucleosides and nucleotides are presented in Table 5–4.

Other nucleoside triphosphates are important in some metabolic reactions. For example, the triphosphates of uridine, cytidine, and guanosine are essential to the synthesis of polysaccharides. Various nucleotides are also involved in other cellular activities. Four molecules responsible for oxidation-reduction reactions are nicotinamide adenine dinucleotide (NAD), nicotinamide adenine dinucleotide phosphate (NADP), flavin adenine dinucleotide (FAD), and flavin mononucleotide (FMN). They contain the vitamins niacin and riboflavin in

TABLE 5-4 Common Nomenclature of Nucleosides and Nucleotides

Nitrogen Base	*Nucleoside*	*Nucleotide*
Adenine	Adenosine	Adenylic acid
Guanine	Guanosine	Guanylic acid
Cytosine	Cytidine	Cytidylic acid
Uracil	Uridine	Uridylic acid
Thymine	Thymidine	Thymidylic acid

their active forms. Coenzyme A (CoA), important to the catabolism (breakdown) of carbohydrates and lipids, consists of the nucleotide AMP, the vitamin pantothenic acid, and mercaptoethylamine. Further details concerning the biochemistry of these structures can be found in the reference works listed at the end of this chapter.

ADENOSINE TRIPHOSPHATE (ATP)

Adenosine triphosphate (Figure 5–18) is involved in the mobilization of energy. ATP would not be required if all of the oxidation-reduction reactions and energy-yielding as well as energy-requiring reactions occurred close to one another. However, because these events occur in various regions throughout a cell, ATP serves as a high-energy-containing compound that can be formed in several locations and can easily be made available to cellular areas requiring it. ATP is a versatile compound that can be utilized for various purposes, including movement, bioluminescence, and cell division.

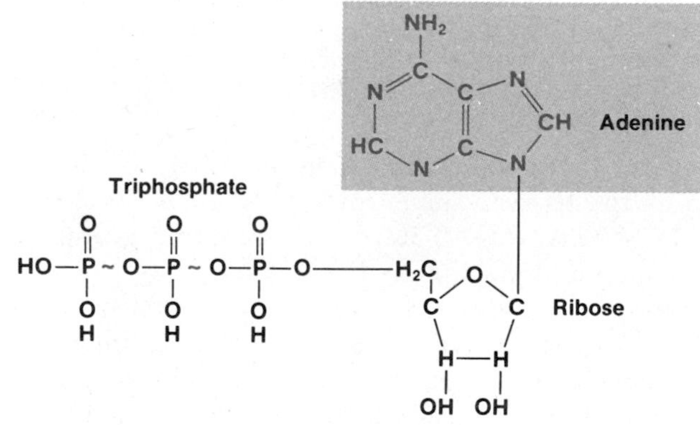

FIG. 5–18 Adenosine triphosphate (ATP). Note that the components of this compound, adenine, ribose, and phosphate groups, can also serve as portions of coenzymes and structural parts of nucleic acids.

Adenosine triphosphate and other such high-energy phosphate compounds are unique in that they have one or more so-called high-energy phosphate bonds. These bonds enable ATP to hold much greater quantities of energy than compounds having ordinary linkages. It is customary to indicate high-energy phosphate bonds by the symbol ~, and ordinary bonds by — . Thus, the relationship of various components of ATP could be represented by

Adenosine — Phosphate ~ Phosphate ~ Phosphate

Compare this with adenosine monophosphate, which does not have a high-energy phosphate bond:

Adenosine Phosphate

When the activities of a cell require energy, a ***hydrolytic*** reaction occurs, splitting a high-energy bond. The hydrolysis is controlled by the enzyme adenosine triphosphatase (ATP-ase). For each high-energy bond broken, one molecule of inorganic (i) phosphate is produced:

$$\text{ATP} \rightarrow \text{ADP} + \text{i phosphate}$$

DEOXYRIBONUCLEIC ACID (DNA)

By virtue of its purine and pyrimidine composition, DNA contains the genetic information necessary to control and direct various activities of a cell. The studies of James D. Watson and Francis H. C. Crick in 1953 and of several other investigators led to our present understanding of how this genetic information is coded. The Watson and Crick model of a DNA molecule (Figure 5–19) shows a double-stranded helical structure (similar to a spiral ladder) linked together by pairs of nitrogen bases. In these pairs adenine is always linked to thymine and cytosine is always linked to guanine. These purine and pyrimidine combinations are called ***base pairs***.

FIG. 5–19 The nucleic acids. (a) The double helix of deoxyribonucleic acid (DNA). Note the kinds of purines (adenine = A and guanine = G) and pyrimidines (cytosine = C and thymine = T) in this macromolecule. Adenine is always paired to thymine and cytosine to guanine by means of hydrogen bonds. The sugar phosphate backbone of the DNA molecule is not shown. The distance between base pairs in the DNA chain is 3.4 Å; the total width of the molecule is 10 Å. (b) The formation of new DNA strands. When the two strands of DNA unwind, each acts as a pattern, or template, on which to assemble purines and pyrimidines from the immediate cellular environment. The end result is usually a perfect duplicate of each strand. (c) The clover-leaf model for one type of RNA.

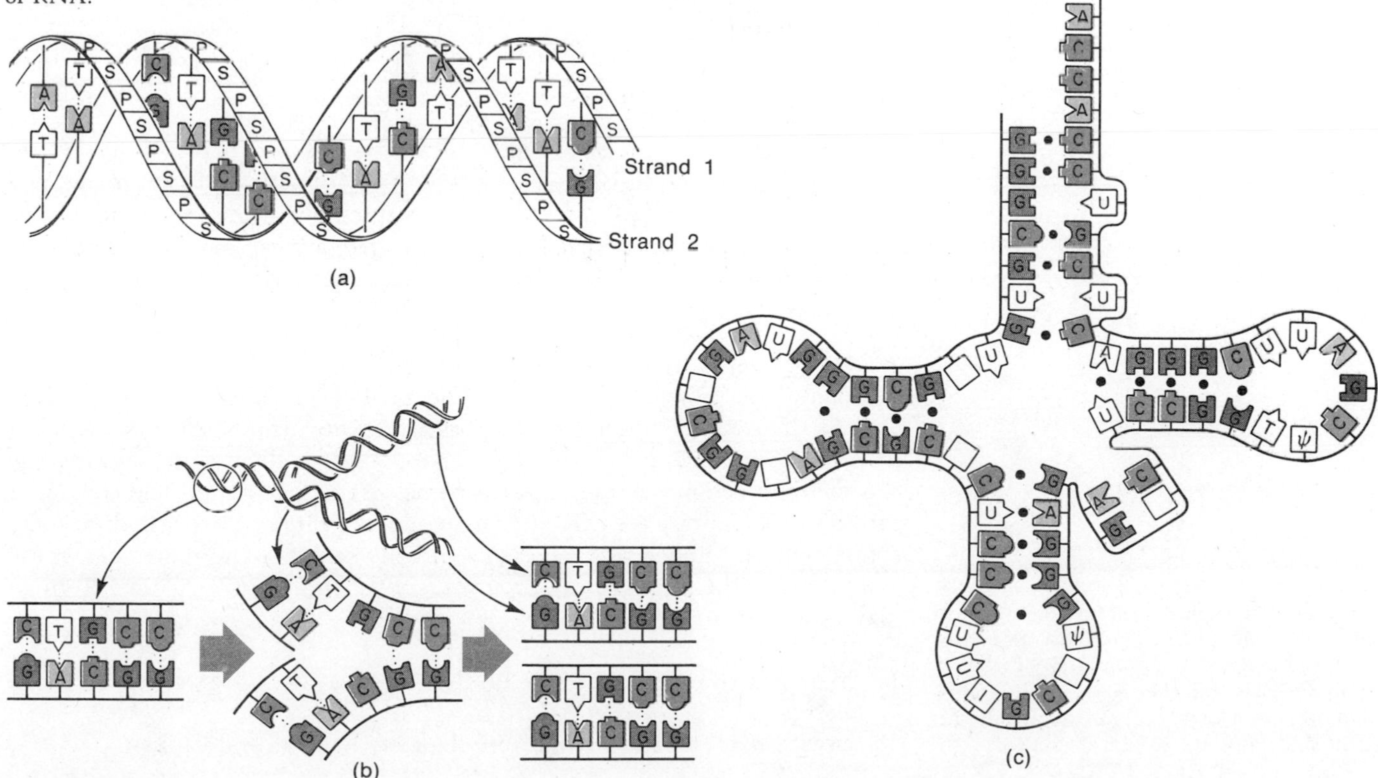

The *base pairing*, or *complementarity*, of adenine-thymine and guanine-cytosine has proved useful as a guide to taxonomic relationships in the biological world. In practice, DNA is extracted from different organisms and analyzed for the four nitrogenous bases. Then the total percent of guanine and cytosine is calculated and compared. Studies have shown remarkable similarity in the amounts of guanine and cytosine between apparently "unrelated" species and even genera.

The DNA molecule is threadlike with a definite diameter. All of the nitrogenous bases are attached to sugar molecules. The spiral shape results from the hydrogen bonding of bases of one strand to those of the other.

The purines and pyrimidines and their arrangement in the backbone of the double-stranded helical DNA molecule hold the information, or blueprint, on which the characteristics of an organism are based. In short, groups of bases function as letters in an alphabet to form the chemical language of life, or what has simply been labeled the **genetic code.** The information contained in a DNA molecule, along with the aid of three types of RNA molecules, controls the formation of proteins and related compounds.

The formation of new DNA strands involves the unwinding of the helical structure and the partial separation of the two strands. Each strand then acts as a pattern on which specific nucleotides from the cellular environment are assembled. The result is usually two perfect duplicates of the DNA molecule (Figure 5–19b), although permanent changes and "errors" known as **mutations** can occur naturally in replication. Various chemicals and radiation are also known to cause such mutations.

RIBONUCLEIC ACID (RNA)

Unlike the DNA found in most forms of life, RNA is single stranded. Moreover, thymine is replaced by uracil in this nucleic acid (Figure 5–16). Three different types of RNA are found in cells. They are messenger RNA (mRNA), transfer RNA (tRNA), and ribosomal RNA (rRNA), depending on their location and function. Ribosomal RNA is a major component of the cellular structures known as ribosomes. All three types of ribonucleic acid are important to protein synthesis.

Proteins

Proteins are among the largest molecules known. They are found in all forms of life and are involved in a wide variety of cell functions. For example, proteins are important constituents of cellular structures such as membranes, cilia, flagella (the structures involved with movement), and ribosomes. Enzymes are all proteins, as are certain hormones and protective agents in the body, namely antibodies (immunoglobulins).

THE STRUCTURE OF AMINO ACIDS

Proteins are polymers of smaller functional units called **amino acids.** Carbon, hydrogen, oxygen, and nitrogen are the major elements found in amino acids and proteins. Other elements appear in small amounts, sulfur being the one most commonly found. As its name suggests, an amino acid contains a carboxylic acid group (—COOH) and an amino group (—NH_2). Both of these components are linked or bonded to a carbon skeleton. The remainder of the amino acid is the radical, or R, group, as shown in Figure 5–20. The R group may be any of the following:

1. hydrogen (H), as in the case of glycine, or a methyl group (CH_3), as in alanine;
2. larger carbon chains, such as in isoleucine, leucine, and valine;

```
      NH2
      |
  R—C—COOH
      |
      H
```

FIG. 5–20 The typical structure of an amino acid, the basic unit of proteins. Note the presence of an amino group (NH_2), carboxyl group (COOH), and the radical, or R, group. The latter is a carbon chain to which the amino and carboxyl groups are linked.

3. an alcohol group (CH_2OH), as in serine and threonine;
4. sulfur (S), as in cysteine, cystine or methionine;
5. acid or basic in nature, as in glutamic acid or lysine, respectively;
6. heterocyclic, as in the amino acids histidine, hydroxyproline, proline, and tryptophan, which have a ring structure in which at least one atom is not a carbon atom (Figure 5-21);
7. benzene ring, as in the aromatic amino acids phenylalanine and tyrosine (Figure 5-22).

Structural formulas of ten amino acids are shown in Table 5-5.

Cystine and cysteine are especially significant amino acids in that their structures permit the formation of disulfide linkages (S—S) between thiol groups (—SH) in proteins. Such bonds contribute to the ultimate shape of the protein molecules and in this way are important to the activity of enzymes. The disulfide bridge is shown in the cystine molecule in Table 5-5.

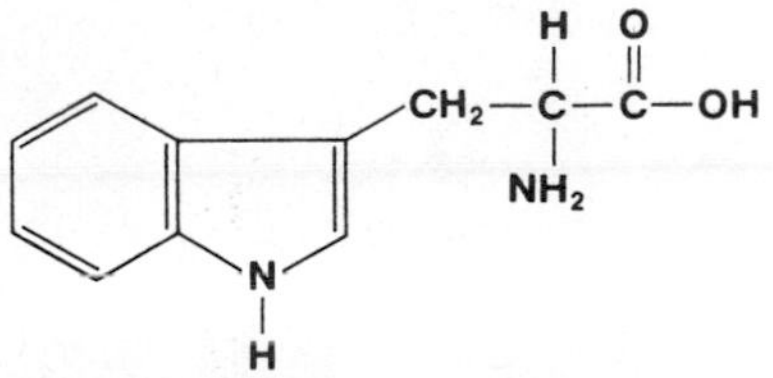

FIG. 5-21 An example of a heterocyclic R group.

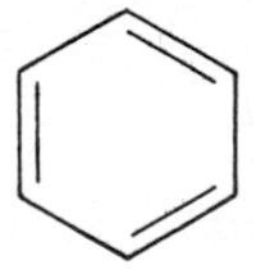

FIG. 5-22 An example of the benzene ring.

PROTEIN STRUCTURE AND FORMATION

The formation of proteins from amino acids involves the bonding of amino acids by a type of linkage referred to as the **peptide bond.** When such a bond is formed, the acid group of one amino acid reacts with the amino group of another with the removal of one molecule of water (H_2O) (Figure 5-23). The protein molecule is constructed from this general type of reaction repeated many times. When two amino acids are joined, they form a dipeptide; three, a tripeptide; several, a polypeptide. Finally, the linking together of large numbers of polypeptides and larger amino acid combinations produces a protein molecule. It should be noted that in living organisms, this process of protein synthesis involves several enzymes and the expenditure of energy. Additional types of bonding both within and between peptide chains include disulfide bonds, hydrogen bonds, and ionic linkages. All three types of bonds result in the coiling or folding of a protein molecule containing them.

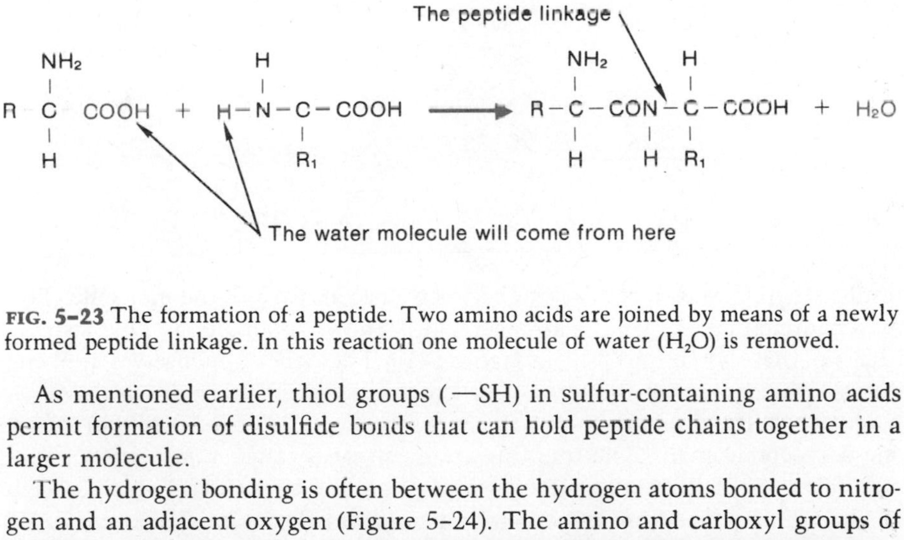

The peptide linkage

The water molecule will come from here

FIG. 5-23 The formation of a peptide. Two amino acids are joined by means of a newly formed peptide linkage. In this reaction one molecule of water (H_2O) is removed.

As mentioned earlier, thiol groups (—SH) in sulfur-containing amino acids permit formation of disulfide bonds that can hold peptide chains together in a larger molecule.

The hydrogen bonding is often between the hydrogen atoms bonded to nitrogen and an adjacent oxygen (Figure 5-24). The amino and carboxyl groups of peptide bonds are often involved in hydrogen bonding. The ionic linkages are between various positive and negative charges on amino acids.

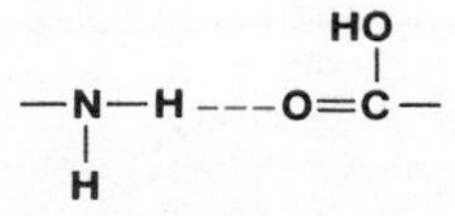

The structures of protein are usually described as either primary, secondary, tertiary, or quaternary. The *primary structure* refers to the sequence of amino acids held together by peptide bonds in the macromolecule. The *secondary structure* is the coiled, or twisted, chain shape, often helical (springlike), that

FIG. 5-24 An example of hydrogen bonding.

TABLE 5-5 Structural Formulas of Representative Amino Acids

R Group	*Amino Acid Group*	*Name*
H—	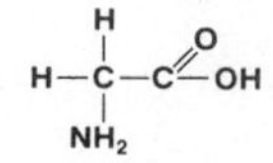 $-\overset{H}{\underset{NH_2}{C}}-COOH$	Glycine
CH_3—	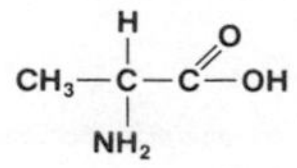 $-\overset{H}{\underset{NH_2}{C}}-COOH$	Alanine
$(CH_3)_2CH$—	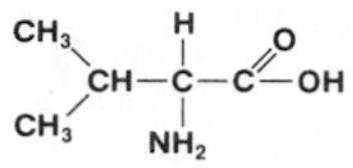 $-\overset{H}{\underset{NH_2}{C}}-COOH$	Valine
HO—CH_2—	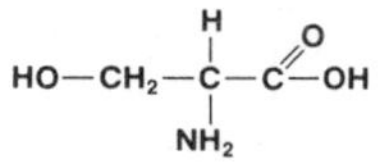 $-\overset{H}{\underset{NH_2}{C}}-COOH$	Serine
HS—	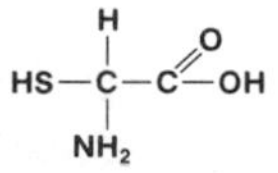 $-\overset{H}{\underset{NH_2}{C}}-COOH$	Cysteine
S—CH_2— / | / S—CH_2—	$-\overset{H}{\underset{NH_2}{C}}-COOH$ (each)	Cystine
HO—C(=O)—CH_2—	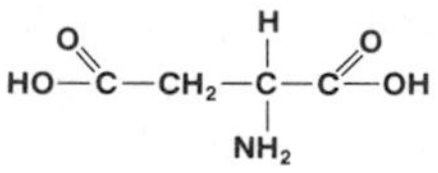 $-\overset{H}{\underset{NH_2}{C}}-COOH$	Clutamic acid
$H_2N-CH_2-CH_2-CH_2-CH_2$—	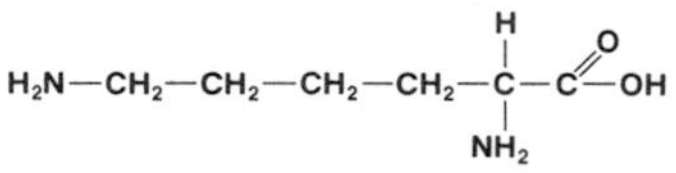 $-\overset{H}{\underset{NH_2}{C}}-COOH$	Lysine
HC=C—CH_2— (imidazole ring: N, NH, C—H)	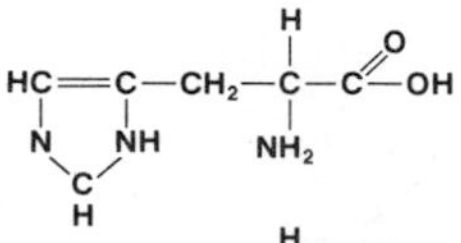 $-\overset{H}{\underset{NH_2}{C}}-COOH$	Histidine
C_6H_5—CH_2—	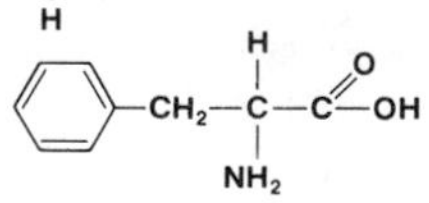 $-\overset{H}{\underset{NH_2}{C}}-COOH$	Phenylalanine

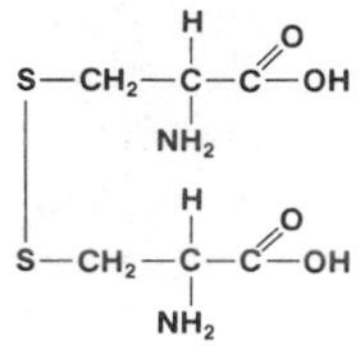

results when hydrogen bonds form between adjacent parts of the molecule. The most common type of coiling arrangement is known as an alpha helix, a structure like that shown for DNA in Figure 5–19. The helices themselves are bent into a globular form in the *tertiary structure*. Several globular proteins such as hemoglobin (the respiratory pigment) and some enzymes consist of more than one polypeptide chain. The resulting arrangement is called a *quaternary structure*. Figure 5–25 illustrates the variations of protein structure.

The primary structure of a protein determines the manner in which the protein will fold. Changes in the pattern of protein folds can alter chemical reactions. Thus a change in sequence may produce an overall change in the shape of the protein and a change in the spatial arrangement (configuration) of the protruding R groups on each of the amino acid residues. The sequence of the amino acids and the manner in which these sequences are folded produce an almost infinite variety of proteins.

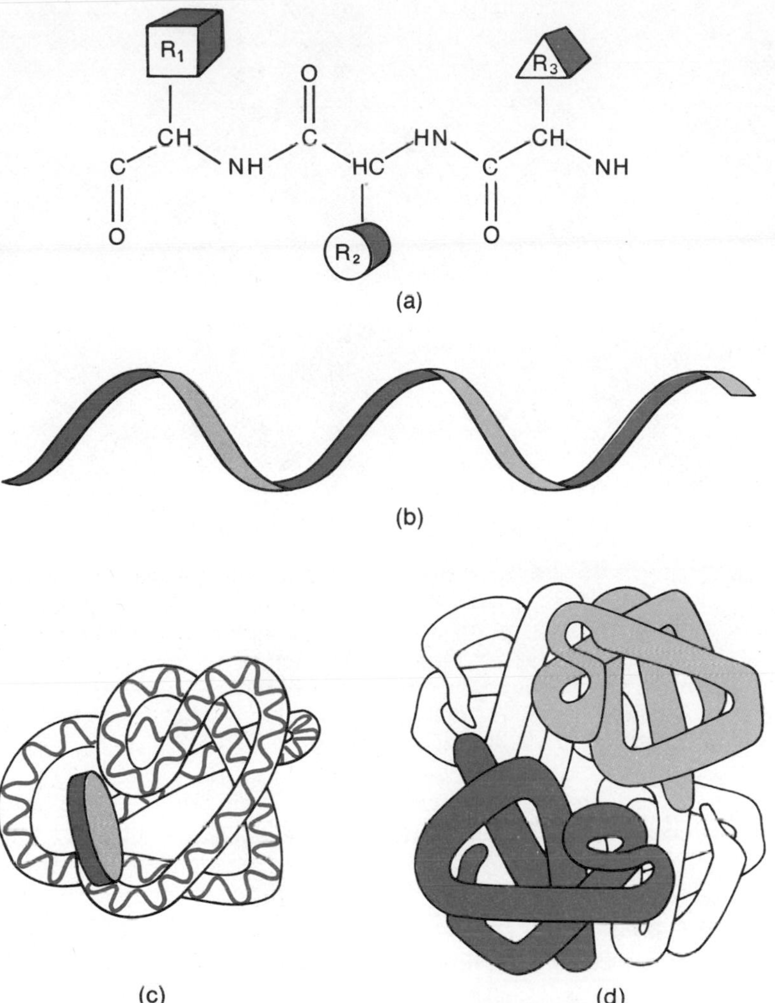

FIG. 5-25 A diagrammatic representation of protein structure. The connecting link or bond between amino acids is the peptide bond. The arrangement of chains of amino acids determines protein structure. (a) The primary structure. (b) The secondary structure. (c) The tertiary structure. (d) The quaternary structure.

Since the bonds associated with the secondary and tertiary structures of globular proteins are not very strong chemically, they are easily ruptured, thereby causing a change in the compound's shape and often destroying its original properties. This process, called **denaturation,** may be produced by several factors including heat. The cooking of an egg and the sterilizing of surgical instruments both involve denaturation. The spatial arrangement of protein is severely altered, causing the coagulation of the egg protein and the destruction of any infectious material on the instruments.

ENZYMES

Proteins also function as **enzymes,** the biological, or organic, catalysts (Figure 5-26). Enzymes are associated with metabolic reactions, respiration, the conversion and transfer of energy within living systems, and the formation of various macromolecules and cellular components. It has been estimated that the human body contains 150,000 different kinds of working enzymes. Although no one knows exactly the total number of enzymes produced by all kinds of organisms, the possibilities seem infinite.

Chemical reactions occur between compounds when molecules collide,

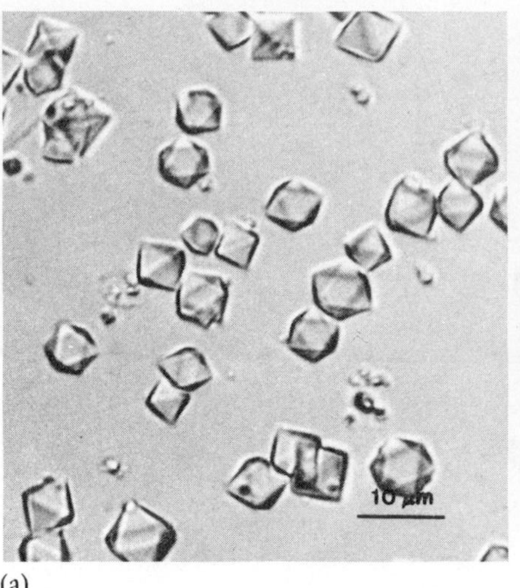

(a)

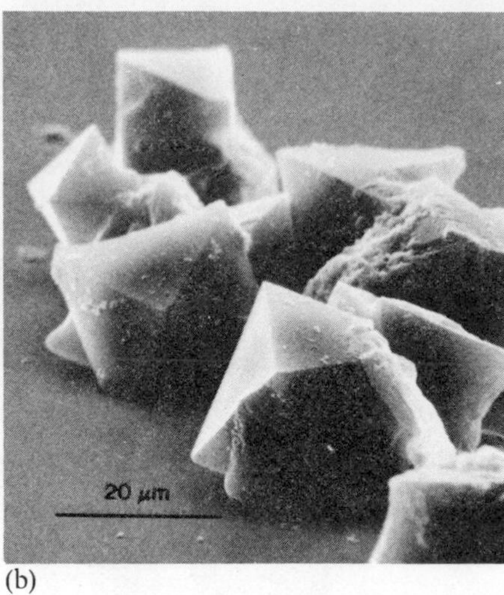

(b)

FIG. 5-26 What does an enzyme look like? Chemists and biochemists have rather remarkable insights about the shapes of enzyme molecules. With the aid of a scanning electron microscope, the actual appearance of certain organic substances can be viewed. The two photographs show a crystalline preparation of the enzyme isocitrate dehydrogenase. This protein is an important factor in energy-producing cellular activities. (a) A light micrograph. (b) A scanning micrograph. Note the eight-sided, or octahedral, geometry. *Burke, W. F., et al.*, Science *181:59–60 (1973).*

make contact with one another, and have sufficient energy. Therefore, any condition that increases the collision frequency between molecules also increases the rate at which chemical reactions occur. Among the conditions that will do this are increases in pressure, temperature, and the concentrations of the reacting substances. Some substances can speed a reaction by increasing the contact between molecules or lowering the energy requirement for a reaction (the activation energy). A substance that achieves those effects without being permanently altered in the process is known as a **catalyst.**

Biological systems continually show evidence of very high rates of chemical reactions: the rapid growth of seeds, the almost visible growing of young animals, and the almost unbelievable rate at which bacteria can reproduce. These changes require rapid chemical reactions for energy production and cell formation. Such reactions do not proceed at a sufficient speed under normal environmental conditions, which can vary from moment to moment. For reactions to occur fast enough to be suitable for biological systems, they would have to occur at temperatures too high or at a pH too extreme for life. Biological systems, therefore, require catalysts that can function under conditions compatible with life. These catalysts are enzymes.

Many enzymes are entirely or primarily protein (Figure 5–26) and are called **simple enzymes.** Those that contain a nonprotein group are called **conjugated enzymes.** The protein portion is called an *apoenzyme,* meaning incomplete, and is inactive. The nonprotein portion, which may be organic or inorganic, is known as a *coenzyme, cofactor,* or *prosthetic group.* A cofactor is an inorganic or organic compound that is needed to activate an enzyme and that is easily removed from the enzyme. Examples of cofactors are metallic ions such as copper, iron, and zinc and some vitamins. A coenzyme is an organic factor. Many coenzymes are derived from dietary vitamins. Vitamin deficiency diseases are thus related to the decreased ability of certain enzymes to function in normal metabolic activities. Prosthetic groups differ from coenzymes and cofactors in that they are bound more tightly and are therefore more difficult to

TABLE 5-6 Selected Enzymes and Their Catalytic Actions

General Enzyme Type	*Catalytic Action*	*Specific Example*
Deaminase	Removes amino (NH_2) groups	Alanine deaminase
Decarboxylase	Causes the release of carbon dioxide (CO_2)	Pyruvate decarboxylating enzyme complex
Dehydrogenase	Causes removal and transfer of hydrogen to acceptor compound	Isocitric dehydrogenase
Oxido-reductases	Causes oxidation-reduction reactions	Cytochrome oxidase
Phosphorylase	Causes the incorporation of phosphate (PO_4) groups	ATP synthesizing enzymes

remove from the enzyme. No matter what the accessory group is called, its function concerns the activity of the particular enzyme involved.

FACTORS AFFECTING ENZYME ACTIVITY

Earlier we discussed the fact that enzymes function under conditions compatible with life. Thus, conditions that affect life undoubtedly do so by exerting some effect on enzyme activity. Being protein in composition, enzymes are sensitive to pH, temperature, osmotic pressure, radiations, heavy metals—that is, to anything that will denature or inactivate the protein. However, enzymes have particular conditions of pH and temperature under which they function best. Each enzyme has a more functional or optimal pH and temperature. In general, the optimal pHs occur in the range of 4.5 to 8.5. Optimal temperatures occur in several categories, depending on the optimal temperatures for the organism, approximately 10°, 35°, or 60°C. Each enzyme has its particular optimum somewhere within one of these temperature categories.

Because various denaturing chemicals (including acids), radiation, and extremes of temperature inhibit or destroy enzymes, these conditions are of value in the control of microorganisms. More subtle factors affecting enzyme activity, which involve the enzyme itself and the reaction that the enzyme is regulating, are discussed in a later chapter.

Enzymes are usually unaltered by the process they promote. Thus they can be used over and over again by the cell. Some enzymes are quite specific, often catalyzing only one particular reaction (Table 5-6). An enzyme frequently is named after the material, or **substrate,** on which it acts. For example, amylose, a major component of starch, is the substrate for the enzyme amylase. Enzymes are also named for their associated actions. Thus the enzyme dehydrogenase removes hydrogen, and a decarboxylase removes carbon dioxide. Note the ending *ase* that identifies almost all enzyme names.

The mechanism by which an enzyme and its substrate interact is frequently compared to a lock and key. It is thought that the large protein component of the enzyme molecule contains an active site where the substrate molecule becomes attached and the reaction takes place. The enzyme's specificity corresponds to a specific key that will only open a lock for which the key is exactly matched. The lock and key arrangement can be illustrated by considering the enzyme maltase, important in carbohydrate metabolism. Maltase converts the disaccharide maltose into two glucose molecules. Figure 5-27 illustrates how a maltose molecule could be held in a position to allow the breaking of the glycosidic bond with the incorporation of water. The enzyme, maltase, reacts with the substrate, maltose, and water to produce a complex that leads to the forma-

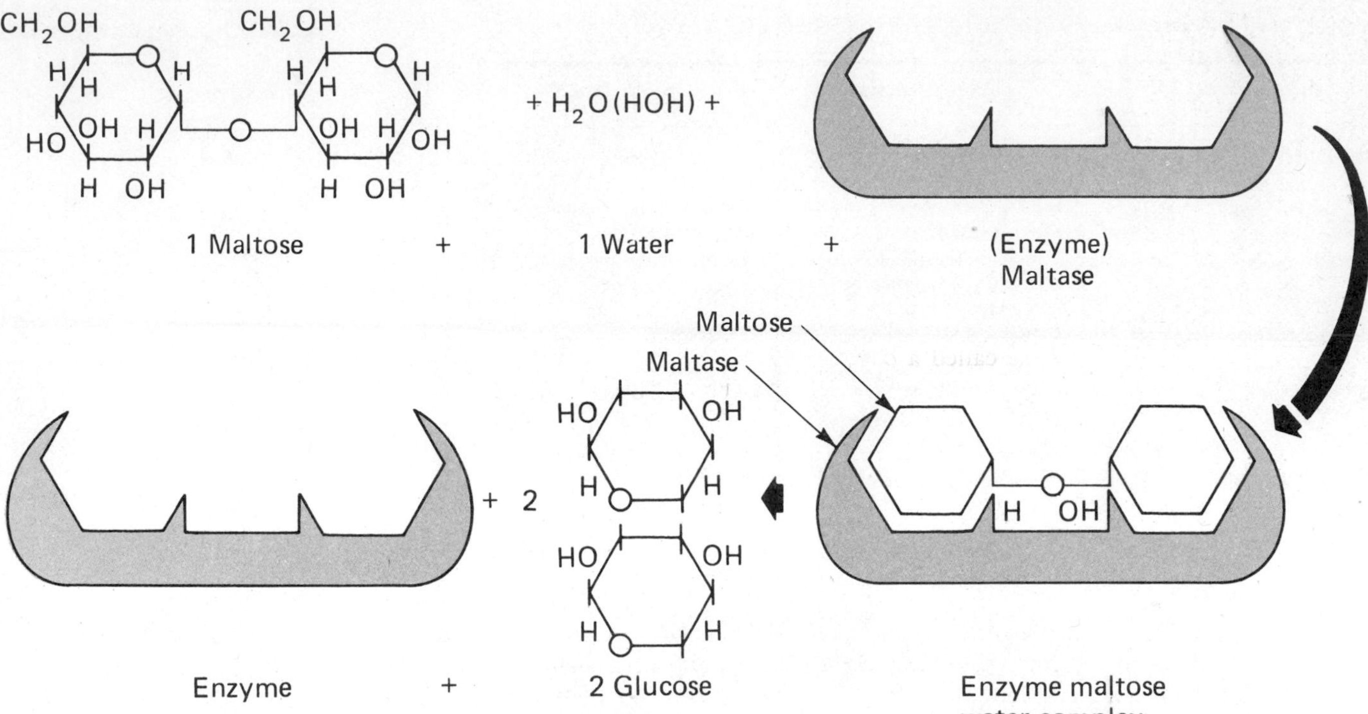

FIG. 5-27 A diagrammatic representation of enzyme substrate interaction between the enzyme maltase and the sugar maltose.

tion of glucose and the regenerated enzyme.

It is important to note here that enzymes do not cause reactions to occur that otherwise would not. Their function is only to speed reactions that would otherwise proceed very slowly.

SUMMARY

Basic Chemistry Review

Atoms: The Basic Particles of Matter

The atom is the smallest particle of an element; it is made up of a nucleus, which contains protons and neutrons, and orbiting electrons.

Elements

An element consists of atoms all having the same number of protons and electrons.

Compounds, Molecules, and Macromolecules

1. A compound is the result of the physical-chemical joining of two or more different kinds of atoms.
2. The smallest unit of a compound that is representative of its composition and properties is a molecule.
3. *Ionic* and *covalent bonds* hold atoms together in a molecule.
4. Ionic bonds occur when atoms that have developed opposite charges attract and form molecules. These molecules are relatively unstable in water.
5. Some atoms share electrons to form very stong covalent bonds requiring a great deal of energy to break. They are stable in water and allow the formation of long-chained macromolecules characteristic of life.
6. One means by which molecules may be held to other molecules is the *hydrogen bond.*
7. Some regions in molecules may be *polar,* that is, charged. These charges can attract and form linkages that hold subunits of large molecules together or hold a single large molecule in a particular shape.

Functional Groups

1. Different chemical arrangements account for the particular chemical activity and characteristics of biologically important molecules.
2. Two common reactions between functional groups are formation of the peptide bond important in proteins, and ester formation important in lipids and nucleic acid synthesis.
3. The removal of water (dehydration) from a molecule of an organic acid and an alcohol, or from two amino acids, results in the formation of an ester or peptide, respectively.

Oxidation-Reduction

This is a common paired reaction in which one molecule loses electrons and is oxidized while the other molecule gains the electrons and is reduced.

pH and Buffers

1. pH refers to the degree of acidity or alkalinity of a substance. The pH scale extends from 0 to 14, 0 being highly acid and 14 being highly alkaline.

2. A buffer is a chemical or mixture of chemicals that can react with H^+ and OH^- to minimize drastic changes in pH that may be lethal to the cell.

The Organic Compounds

Lipids

Lipids are soluble in organic solvents. They include fatty acids, fats, oils, waxes, phospholipids, and steroids. They serve as structural components of membranes, take part in cell metabolism, and are reserve sources of energy for the cell.

1. *Fatty acids* are naturally occurring organic acids with even-numbered carbon chains. These compounds may be unsaturated or saturated.
2. *Fats* and *oils* are esters of fatty acids and glycerol. *Waxes* are esters of fatty acids with long-chained alcohols.
3. In addition to having the usual hydrophobic characteristic of lipids, *phospholipids* also have functional groups that are hydrophilic.
4. *Steroids* have as their basic unit the four-ring structure shown in Figure 5–8.

Carbohydrates

Examples of this group of chemicals include simple sugars and polysaccharides. Some of these compounds serve a structural role in plants in the form of cellulose, and as starch and glycogen they provide for food storage in various organisms.

1. *Glycosides* are carbohydrates formed by the reaction of a sugar with another compound containing a hydroxyl group.
2. *Monosaccharides* are simple, or basic, sugars.
3. *Disaccharides* are carbohydrates composed of two simple sugars joined by a glycosidic linkage.
4. *Polysaccharides* are carbohydrates composed of long chains of simple sugars joined by glycosidic linkages.

Nucleic acids

Nucleic acids are compounds composed of pentoses, phosphate, and a nitrogenous base.

1. *Adenosine triphosphate (ATP)* is a high-energy-containing compound that is a nucleotide.
2. ATP is used for many of the energy-requiring metabolic processes in the cell.
3. *Deoxyribonucleic acid (DNA)* is formed from deoxyribose, phosphate, thymine, adenine, guanine, and cytosine.
4. DNA is the storage material for the information the cell needs to perform all its functions.
5. *Ribonucleic acid (RNA)* contains ribose, phosphate, uracil, adenine, guanine, and cytosine.
6. One form of RNA, messenger RNA, is the carrier of genetic information to the cell's cytoplasm for use in protein synthesis.

Proteins

Proteins are macromolecules that are important constituents of cellular structures, such as membranes, mitochondria, cilia, flagella, and ribosomes.

1. Chemically, proteins are composed of smaller units called *amino acids*.
2. Amino acids contain a carboxyl group and an amino group.
3. The basic structure of all amino acids is the same, with differences depending upon the nature of the side chain.
4. The *primary* structure of a protein is determined by the linkage of amino acids held together by peptide bonds.
5. Additional forms of protein structure are *secondary, tertiary,* and *quaternary* configurations.
6. Enzymes are primarily protein substances that act as catalysts to speed up and regulate most chemical reactions in the cell.
7. Each enzyme is specific, that is, it acts on one particular kind of reaction.
8. Enzymes are sensitive to pH, temperature, osmotic pressure, radiation, and heavy-metal ions, all of which will denature or inactivate the protein.
9. For every enzyme there are optimal conditions of pH and temperature.

QUESTIONS FOR REVIEW

1. Define the following terms: *atom, element, molecule,* and *compound.*
2. Describe the formation of ionic, covalent, and hydrogen bonds.
3. List and give molecular formulas for eight common functional groups.
4. Describe the reaction required to form an ester.
5. Describe the reaction required to form a peptide.
6. What is meant by oxidation-reduction? What are reducing and oxidizing agents?
7. Define pH, and describe the pH scale.
8. What is meant by the term *buffer?* Why is it significant in biological systems?
9. What are the basic organic chemical groupings associated with lipids, carbohydrates, proteins, and nucleic acids?
10. Differentiate between:
    a. phospholipid and wax
    b. glucose and fructose
    c. ribose and deoxyribose
    d. RNA and DNA
    e. nucleotides and nucleosides
    f. starch and cellulose
    g. polypeptide and protein
11. What are the major radical, or R, groups of amino acids?
12. Identify several amino acids that contribute to secondary protein structure.
13. Describe a possible mechanism of enzyme action and protein structure.
14. What is meant by "enzyme specificity"?
15. How might enzyme specificity be used in clinical medicine?
16. Why is ATP considered a critical compound?

SUGGESTED READINGS

Frienden, I., "The Chemical Elements of Life," *Sci. Amer.* 227: 52–60 (1972). *An interesting article describing the functions of chemical elements and their involvement in life processes.*

Kendrew, J. C., "The Three-dimensional Structure of a Protein Molecule," *Sci. Amer.* 205:96–110 (1961). *Description of the approach to determine, as well as the arrangement of, amino acids in a large protein molecule.*

Koshland, D. E., "Protein Shape and Biological Control," *Sci. Amer.* 229:52–64 (1973). *The importance of enzymes in the control of life processes is emphasized.*

Lehninger, A., *Biochemistry.* 2nd ed. New York: Worth Publishing Co., 1975. *A well-written, highly detailed, complete account of biochemistry.*

Miller, O. L., Jr., "The Visualization of Genes in Action," *Sci. Amer.* 228:34–42 (1973). *An electron-microscopic view of genetic information being transcribed into messenger RNA, which in turn is translated for the manufacture of proteins. Numerous diagrams and electron micrographs are included.*

Watson, J. D., *The Double Helix.* New York: Atheneum, 1968. *An easy-to-read personal account of the discovery of the structure of deoxyribonucleic acid.*

Watson, J. D., *The Molecular Biology of the Gene.* 3rd ed. New York: Benjamin, 1976. *An extremely popular treatment of the structure and function of genes in protein synthesis by one of the co-discoverers of DNA structure.*

PART TWO

The World of Microorganisms

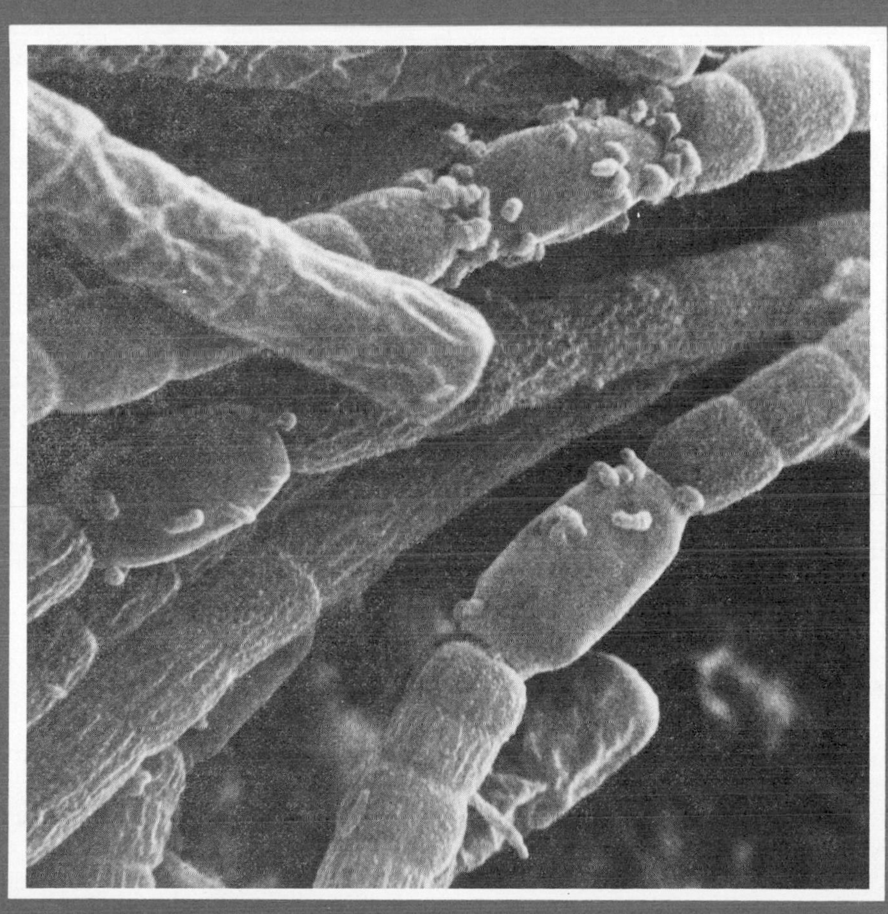

CHAPTER 6

The Structures of Typical Animal and Plant Cells

Cells are found in a great variety of sizes and shapes. They range in size from the smallest bacteria, only about 0.5 μm, to certain algae and bird eggs with diameters of several centimeters. Cells vary in internal organization as well. As a result, no "typical" cell exists. Nevertheless, there are certain features common to all cells. This chapter deals with the organization and structure of higher animal and plant cells, with emphasis on the similarities and differences between such eucaryotic cells. Because many of the features of animal and plant cells are also found in microorganisms, this chapter provides a basis for comparing the organization of all microbial groups.

After reading this chapter, you should be able to:

1. **Explain how the cell is the basic unit of life.**
2. **Describe general differences between eucaryotic and procaryotic cellular organization.**
3. **Describe how cellular components interact with one another.**
4. **Differentiate among eucaryotic cell components as to structure, function, and chemical composition.**
5. **Distinguish between cell wall and cell membrane.**
6. **List the major organelles of animal and plant cells and their associated functions.**
7. **Summarize the similarities and differences between the major organelles of animal and plant cells.**
8. **Identify animal and plant organelles in electron micrographs.**

The basic unit of all living organisms is the cell. In certain cases, as with microorganisms, the cell itself *is* the organism and performs all the complex functions essential for life. In other situations, the cell serves as a component part of a multicellular animal or plant and becomes specialized to perform specific functions in the organism. Whether cells exist as single independent units or as the building blocks of multicellular organisms, they apparently have similarities in organization, structure, and function. This should not be surprising, since all cells must perform similar activities and tasks during some phase of their existence.

The Cell's Role in Life

Cells are considered the basic biological units of structure and function. However, these microscopic units can live and survive only under rather limited conditions of pH, temperature, water content, and so forth. If these conditions change so greatly that the cells cannot readily adjust to them, the cells die. Cells must contain mechanisms not only to control their internal activities, such as growth, metabolism, and reproduction, but also to adjust to various external events and forces.

With the development of the electron microscope, we have learned a great deal about the organization of cells. The task of defining the functions of newly discovered cellular components remains. In later chapters we will discuss the structural components (together with their known functions) that contribute to the distinctive architecture of representative microorganisms. Here we shall study characteristic features of cells of higher animals and plants. We are taking this approach to microbial *cytology* (the study of cells) for two reasons. First, it will enable us to see the basic structural differences between higher forms of life and microorganisms, and second, it will provide a basis for understanding certain features of resistance and pathologic processes presented in later chapters.

The Cell Theory

In 1665, pioneer microscopist Robert Hooke observed that cork consists of small, boxlike units that reminded him of the living quarters of monks. He named these microscopic spaces *cells*, from the Latin word *cella*, meaning "small enclosure." What Hooke saw was the remains of cells—their cell walls. The fact that living cells contained "juices" became evident from other studies he performed.

Several years passed before microscopes were advanced enough to yield more detailed information about cells. Until 1833, a plant cell was thought to be composed of a wall and green-colored bodies (now called **chloroplasts**). In that year the English biologist Robert Brown discovered that all the cells he observed, whether animal or plant, contained a large oval-to-round structure, which he called the nucleus. Within a short time, the German botanist Matthias Schleiden uncovered a smaller body inside the nucleus. This intranuclear structure was named the **nucleolus** (Figure 6–1).

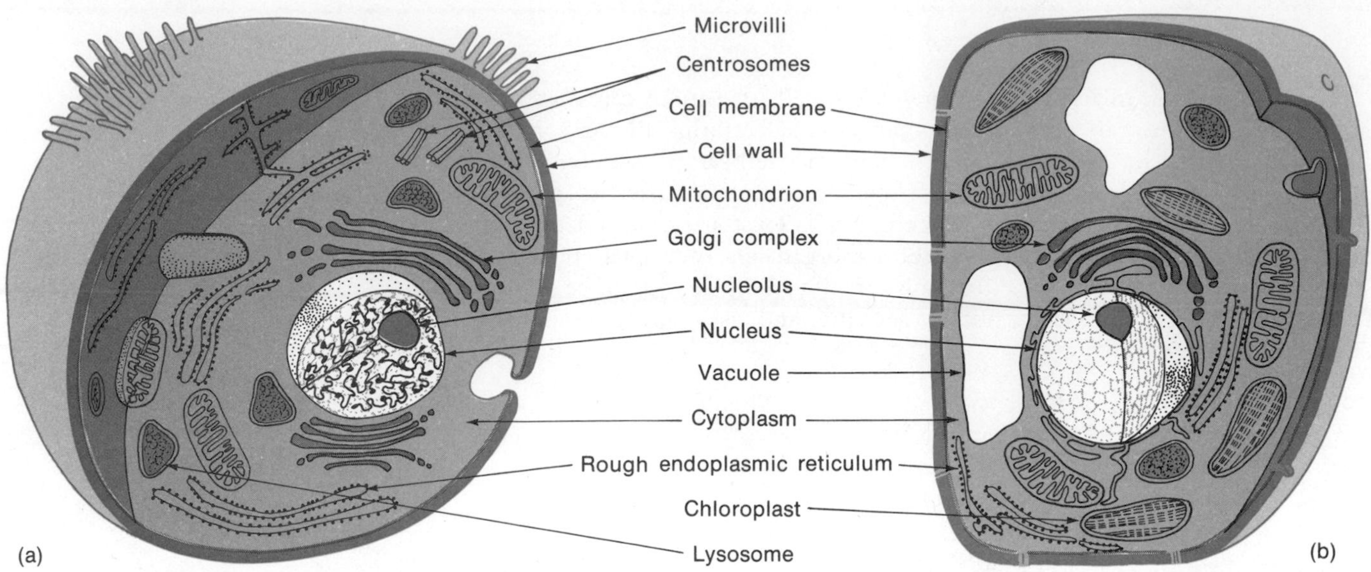

FIG. 6–1 A comparison of eucaryotic animal (a) and plant (b) cells, showing the individual components of each. Compare these diagrams with the electron micrographs shown in Figures 6–2, 6–11, and 6–15.

Schleiden is also known for his contribution to the formulation of the cell theory. In discussions with Theodor Schwann, a zoologist, he developed the concept that all organisms consist of cells. This theory, which with some exceptions (such as viruses) is accepted today, also held that the cell represents a fundamental unit of both structure and function.

The formulation of the cell theory gave rise to an important question—namely, where do cells come from? The answer was provided in 1855 by Rudolf Virchow, who generalized the situation by stating that "cells come only from cells." In other words, new cells can only come into being through the division of previously existing cells.

During this time, interest grew in the basic living substance that composed cells and was essential for life, **protoplasm.** This clear, apparently uniform material seemed to fill the cells.

Although the cell theory and understanding of cellular composition were substantially correct at the turn of the century, better procedures and instruments developed through the years uncovered additional cellular properties. These findings changed the general concept of cells. For example, the term *protoplasm* lost its original meaning. Now the cellular material surrounding a nucleus is called **cytoplasm,** while the material contained within the nucleus is referred to as **nucleoplasm.** Cells are now known to contain highly organized and specialized structures called **organelles** (Figures 6–1 and 6–2).

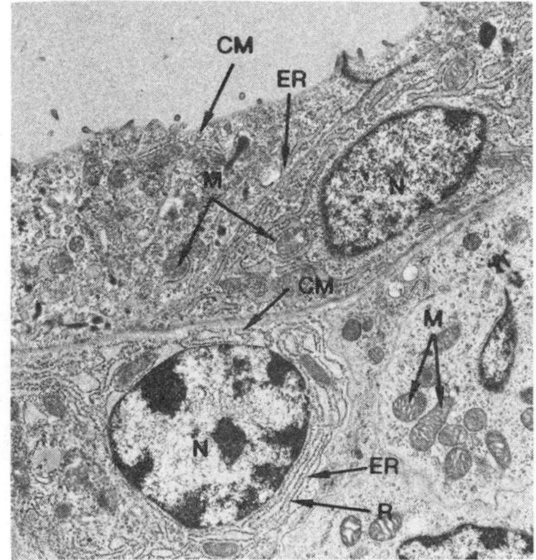

FIG. 6–2 An electron micrograph showing various organelles of eucaryotic cells. Note the presence of the cell membrane (CM), endoplasmic reticulum (ER), mitochondria (M), nucleus (N), and ribosomes (R). *Kalderon, A. E., et al.,* Lab. Invest. *5:487 (1977).*

Types of Cellular Organization

There are two different and distinct levels of cellular organization, eucaryotic and procaryotic. Eucaryotic cells (Figures 6–1 and 6–2) normally have a discrete nucleus surrounded by a nuclear membrane, a nucleolus, and various membrane-bound organelles. During **mitosis** (asexual division) and during **meiosis** (the preparatory cellular stages to sexual reproduction), eucaryotes exhibit definite stainable chromosomes (Color Photograph 18 and Figure 6–5b). Procaryotic cells, such as bacteria (Figure 3–1c), lack well-defined nuclei, mitotic apparatus, stainable chromosomes, and most other permanent structures and features characteristically associated with eucaryotes.

The Anatomy of Animal Cells

The cell is far from simple, yet it is the basic unit of organization for relatively independent biological activity. Individual animal cells differ substantially in various properties, including function, shape, size, and structural components (Color Photographs 8 and 17). Nevertheless, certain organelles are common to most cells (Figures 7–1 and 7–2). These and other cellular components, together with their functions and chemical composition, are discussed in the following section. Most of these structures are also characteristic of plant cells.

The main parts of an animal cell are (1) the cell membrane and cytoplasm (2) the nucleus and nucleolus, (3) internal membrane-associated structures, and (4) microtubules, which include cilia and flagella. The cells of higher animals and the cells of plants are organized and differentiated into specific tissues (Color Photographs 7 and 8).

The Cell Membrane and Cytoplasm

The outer surface of an animal cell is bounded by a sharply defined elastic covering, sometimes referred to in a general sense as "skin." This portion of the cell, which can be called the ***plasma membrane***, the ***cytoplasmic membrane***, or just ***cell membrane***, is an integral functioning structure.

Membranes partition the cellular space into compartments in which biochemical reactions occur. Structures similar to, if not identical to, the cytoplasmic membrane also surround intracellular organelles such as the nucleus, mitochondria, and endoplasmic reticulum. The plasma membrane of a eucaryote is continuous, or interconnected, with the cell's internal membrane systems.

The cell membrane regulates the passage of molecules into and out of cells in a selective or differential manner. It acts sometimes as a *passive* barrier and sometimes as an *active* barrier. When a cell membrane acts as a passive barrier, substances pass through it by simple diffusion, moving from an area of greater concentration to one of lesser concentration until an equilibrium is reached. Recent studies have shown that the membrane contains certain regions capable of performing work to "pump" certain molecules into or out of the cell against a difference in concentration. This so-called "osmotic work" involves the expenditure of energy and is generally referred to as **active transport** (Figure 6–3a). Cells involved in the transport of substances, such as certain ones in the intestine, frequently have elongated, slender extensions of the membrane called *microvilli* (Figure 6–1). These formations greatly increase the surface area, aiding absorption.

There is also a third type of transport—the cell's ability to "trap" small quantities of the solution or liquid surrounding it. This process, called **pinocytosis** or "drinking-in," enables a cell to acquire high-molecular-weight compounds, such as proteins. The pinocytic mechanism begins by the invagination (folding-in) of the membrane, resulting in the formation of a sac, referred to as a *vacuole* or *vesicle* (Figure 6–3b). In time, these vacuoles release their fluid contents, which become mixed with other substances in the cytoplasm. Certain drugs and viruses gain entrance to cells by pinocytosis. Like active transport, this phenomenon requires energy expenditure. Reverse pinocytosis is referred to as *exocytosis*. This type of process may be involved in cellular secretion.

With the development of ultrathin sectioning and appropriate staining proce-

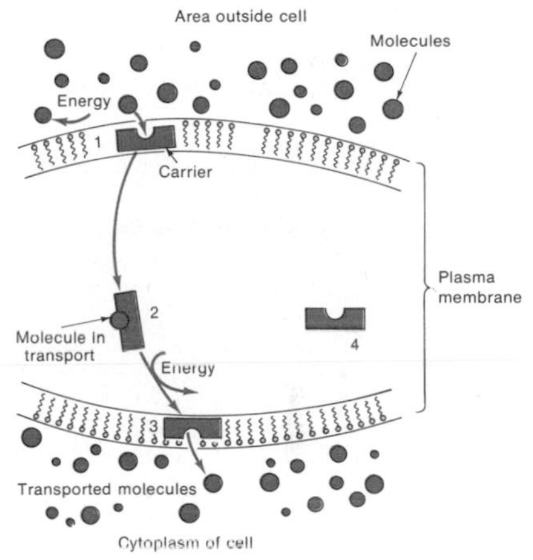

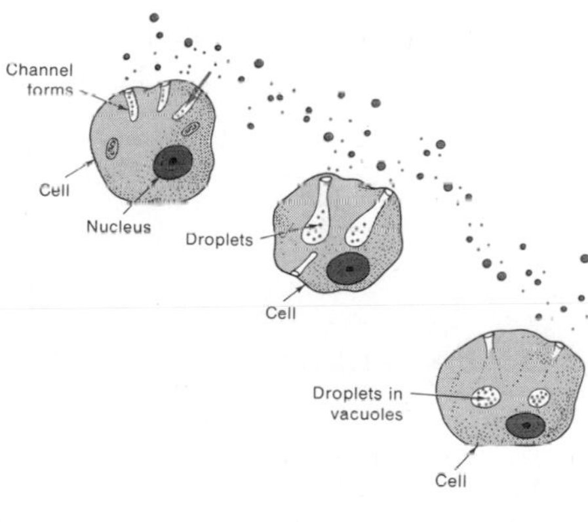

FIG. 6–3 Active processes involving the movement of substances (molecules) across the cell membrane. (a) Inactive transport, substances are carried across membranes from an area of lower concentration to one of higher concentration with the expenditure of energy. Energy is involved at various stages of the process. A carrier located in the membrane picks up a molecule to be transported (1), carries it through the membrane (2), releases the molecule into the cell's cytoplasm (3), and then becomes available to perform the transporting activity again (4). (b) In pinocytosis, an ingested substance gains entrance to the cell through a channel that is formed by the membrane. This channel develops into a vacuole.

dures, biologists obtained direct visual evidence for the structure of membranes. According to a theory proposed in final form by Hugh Davson and James Danielli in 1954, the membrane is a three-layered (protein-lipid-protein) sandwich. X-ray diffraction and electron microscopy support this model. Electron micrographs show two electron-dense lines, each approximately 2.5 nm (25Å) wide, enclosing a much lighter layer of the same width. This membrane would be 7.5 nm (75 Å) thick. Recent studies of membranes with the newly perfected freeze-etching technique, which does not employ chemical fixatives, support the three-layered structure for membranes with the central lipid portion actually a double layer (*bilayer*) of lipid molecules.

Some alternative structures, however, have been proposed by several investigators with respect to the position and arrangement of proteins to the lipid bilayer. It has been suggested that protein molecules are not arranged in an orderly array upon the lipid bilayer (Figure 6–4) but that they actually penetrate into the lipid region and may extend through it completely. Further, the protein molecules continually move and reorganize their molecular shape.

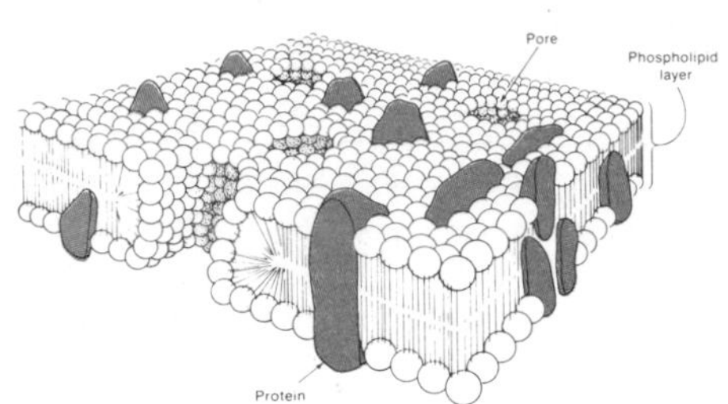

FIG. 6–4 The current model of the plasma membrane, showing the relationship of the phospholipid layer and protein molecules. An enlarged view of plasma membrane showing the relationship between the phospholipid layer and protein molecules is also shown.

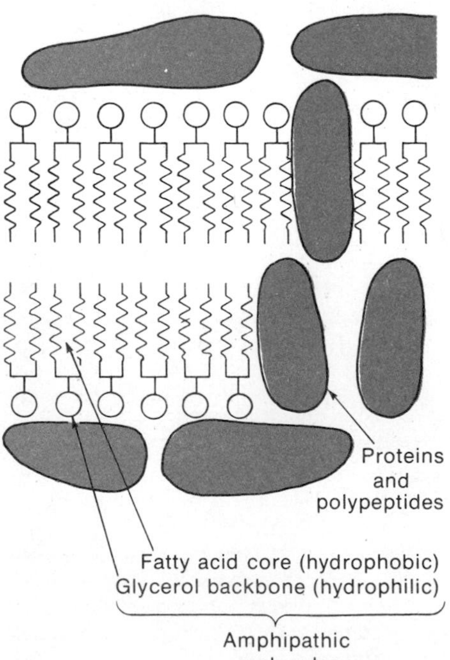

The proteins of the cell membrane are enzymes that perform specific roles: the selective permeability property of membranes is one of them. The lipids provide strength and other structural properties for the membrane. Membrane lipids are *phospholipids*. These molecules are amphipathic, because they consist of regions that are spatially separated so that one end is repelled by water (hydrophobic) and the opposite end is attracted to water (hydrophilic). The hydrophilic end, which carries an ionic charge and is polar, consists of glycerol attached to phosphate and other chemical groups. The nonpolar, hydrophobic end consists of hydrocarbon chains of fatty acids (Figure 6–4).

Membranes differ chemically among different cell types. Analyses have clearly shown differences in the types of lipids and in the protein-lipid ratios of membranes obtained from different kinds of cells. The enzyme compositions also vary considerably.

Membrane systems have many biological functions, including (1) active transport across the membrane, (2) protein synthesis, (3) phagocytosis (a process involving engulfment of foreign matter), (4) pinocytosis, (5) wound healing, and (6) aiding the movement of small molecules across the membrane. These systems are also involved in drug sensitivity, tumor (abnormal growth) behavior, and the immune response (reaction to foreign materials by the body).

The Nucleus and Nucleolus

The shape of the nucleus (Color Photograph 8) generally resembles that of the cell in which it is found. During their maturation, certain cell types, for example, mammalian red blood cells, or erythrocytes (Color Photograph 17), lose this organelle. Some cells of the liver and stomach contain more than one nucleus; that is, they are *multinucleate*.

Structurally, animal cell nuclei are similar to those of the plant cells. The nuclear sap, the ***karyolymph*** or ***nucleoplasm***, is separated from the surrounding cytoplasm by a delicate ***nuclear membrane*** that resembles a two-layered plasma membrane but has large gaps. These "nuclear pores" (Figure 6–5a) provide for easier passage of cellular substances. Chemically, the nuclear membrane is lipid and protein.

Slender threads of nuclear material called chromosomes occur within the karyolymph. These structures are usually evident during specific stages of mitosis. Chromosomes are composed of submicroscopic hereditary factors known as *genes*. They, in turn, are composed of deoxyribonucleic acid (DNA) and certain closely associated proteins.

The nucleus is the control center for all the cell's physiological processes. Included in these activities are the synthesis of nucleic acids, cell growth, and duplication.

The karyolymph of a cell that is not undergoing reproduction usually contains one or more small bodies called nucleoli (singular, nucleolus). The electron micrograph shown in Figure 6–5b shows these structures well. It is interesting to note that the total volume of the nucleoli within a nucleus is relatively constant. For example, if only one nucleolus is present, it is generally quite large. If more than one such structure is present, the total volume of all nucleoli is approximately that of a single nucleolus. Chemically, the nucleoli consist of protein and ribonucleic acid (RNA). Functionally, they are sites for ribosome formation. Ribosome RNA is processed here.

Internal Membrane-associated Structures

MITOCHONDRIA

Mitochondria were first observed around the turn of the century by the German cytologist R. Altmann. The mitochondria (singular, mitochondrion) are primarily concerned with energy conversion and for this reason are often called the cell's powerhouse. Chloroplasts, another type of specialized structure concerned with this cellular activity, are discussed in the section on plant cells. Mitochondria appear as filaments (Figure 6–6b), granules, or spheres (Figure 6–2). Although larger mitochondria can be viewed by light microscopy, the electron microscope is necessary for investigation of their ultrastructure.

Mitochondria are bound by a double membrane, the outer layer of which separates it from the surrounding cytoplasm. The inner layer is folded repeatedly into parallel ridges or plates called *cristae.* These structures may extend to meet other cristae and actually fuse with them. Recent electron microscopic studies have demonstrated the presence of stalked particles, or so-called "lollipops," at approximately 10-nm (100-Å) intervals along cristae surfaces (Figure 6–6c). These particles consist of a hollow stalk or stem portion, 3.0 to 3.5 nm (30 to 35 Å) wide and 4.5 to 5.0 nm (45 to 50 Å) long, and a spherical head of 7.5 to 8.0 nm (75 to 80 Å) diameter. Although the exact function of these particles is not known, they are believed to contain the enzymes needed for a series of reactions in which energy-containing compounds are formed and released.

The inner compartment of the mitochondrion contains a semifluid material, referred to as a **matrix**. Certain of the enzymes involved with the oxidation of fatty acids and those associated with the Krebs (citric acid) cycle are found here. The location of the enzymes as well as the functions of mitochondria have been determined to a large extent by biochemical procedures. Biochemists can separate these organelles from other cellular components by differential high-speed centrifugation. The rupturing of mitochondria and the subsequent separation of their components provides additional material for analysis. From such studies it has been found that mitochondria produce a number of proteins and that they consume fat and respire. Their primary function, however, still remains the release of usable energy. Mitochondria consist primarily of lipids, protein, and nucleic acids, including DNA. Recent studies have shown that mitochondria replicate independently within dividing cells.

ENDOPLASMIC RETICULUM, RIBOSOMES, AND POLYSOMES

The cytoplasm of cells actively engaged in protein synthesis has been found to contain an extensive and complicated system of membranes known as the endoplasmic reticulum. Other types of cells also have endoplasmic reticulum components, but fewer of them. This membranous labyrinth consists of canals and vesicles extending from the cell membrane deep into the interior of the cell (Figure 6–2). Like other membranes, it is composed of proteins and lipids. The endoplasmic reticulum has been shown to be connected with cer-

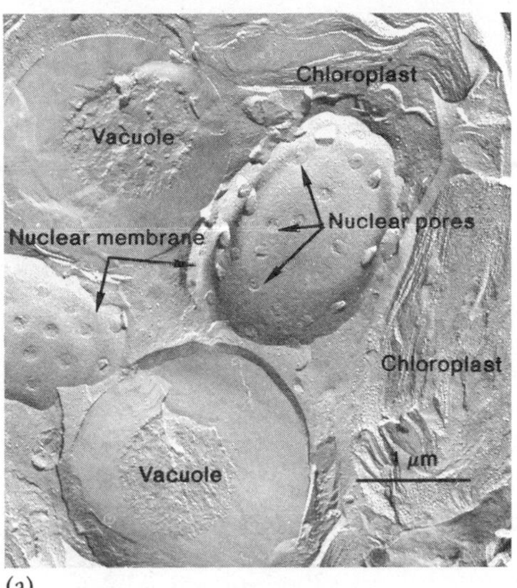

(a)

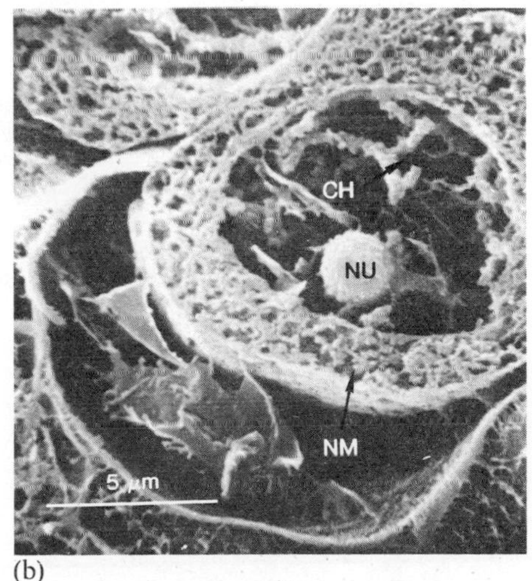

(b)

FIG. 6–5 The nucleus. (a) Nuclear pores (NP) within the nucleus (N) revealed by freeze-fracture techniques. The nuclear membrane (NM) and vacuole (V) are also visible. *Severs, N. J., and E. G. Jordan,* Ultrastruct. Res. *52:85–99 (1975).* (b) The components of a nucleus shown *in situ* by scanning electron microscopy. This three-dimensional micrograph shows the nuclear membrane (NM), nucleolus (Nu), and chromosomes (Ch). *Reproduced by permission of the National Research Council of Canada from Whelan, E.D.P., et al.,* Can. J. Botany *52:1438–1440 (1974).*

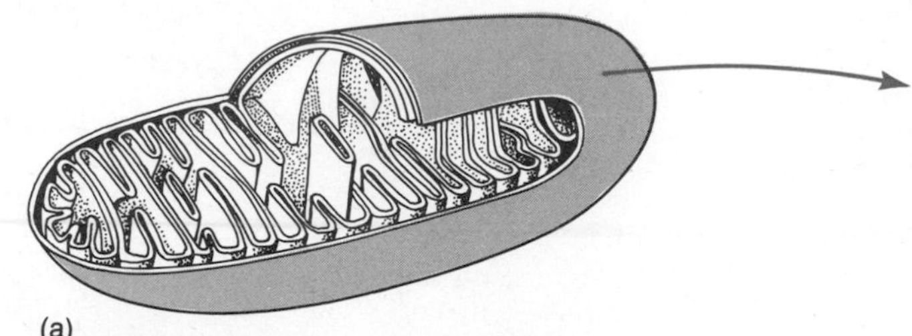
(a)

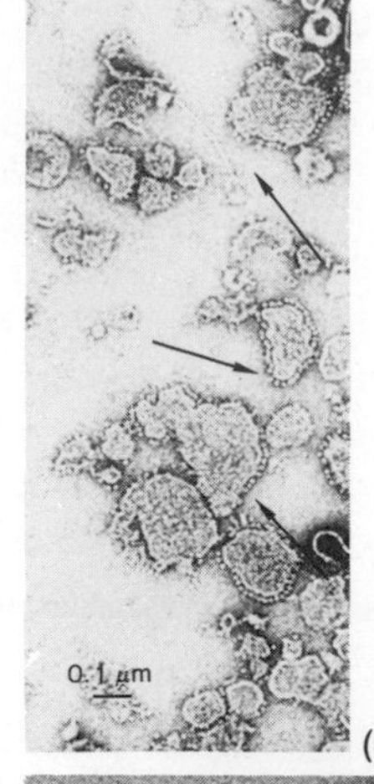

(c)

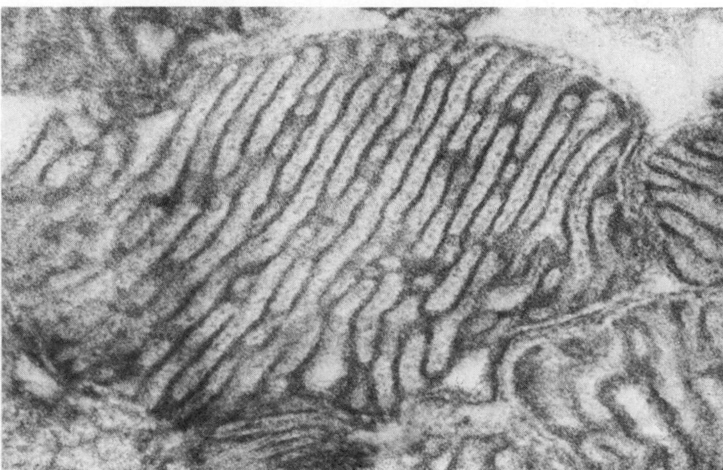
(b)

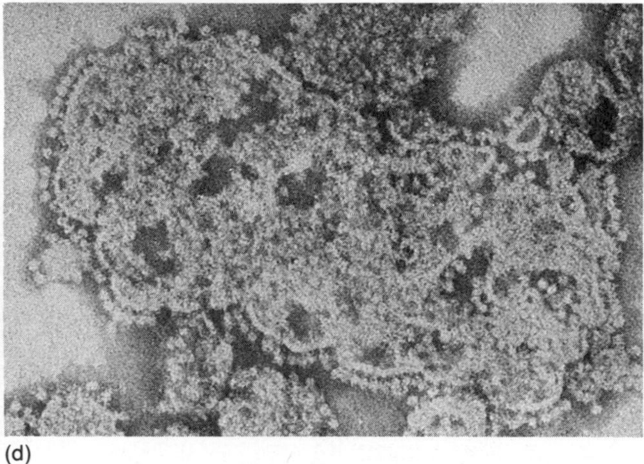
(d)

FIG. 6–6 The mitochondrion, the eucaryotic cell's powerhouse, shown diagrammatically (a) and in an electron micrograph (b). Note how the cristae stand out, with high contrast, against the surrounding matrix. *Sjostrand, F. S.,* J. Ultra. Res. *59:292 (1977).* (c) A freeze-fracture preparation shows the surface particles of a mitochondrion's outer membrane surface. Recent studies have shown that the mitochondrial membranes are structurally and functionally different from one another. *Sjostrand, F. S., and R. Z. Cassel,* J. Ultra. Res. *63:138 (1978).* (d) Submitochondrial particles associated with cristae are shown by negative staining and transmission electron microscopy. *Christiansen, R. O. et al.,* J. Biol. Chem. *244:4428 (1969).*

tain other cellular components, for example, the double nuclear membrane and the golgi complex.

Two general types of endoplasmic reticulum are known: rough-surfaced, or *granular,* and smooth-surfaced, or *agranular.* Smooth endoplasmic reticulum consists primarily of membranes; rough endoplasmic reticulum, in addition to membranes, also contains many small ribonucleoprotein particles called *ribosomes.* These particles are bound to the endoplasmic reticulum on the side facing the cytoplasm. Both types of endoplasmic reticulum may be present in the same cell, and both are involved in secretion.

Ribosomes may be associated with the endoplasmic reticulum or they may exist free in the cytoplasm (Figure 6–2). Chemically, ribosomes are approximately one half RNA and one half protein. Physically, they are made up of two different-sized components.

Functionally, ribosomes are important in protein synthesis. The most active ribosomes are those in clusters of four or more, called a **polysome** or *polyribosome* (Figure 6–7). The individual components of such aggregations are held together by a strand of another type of ribonucleic acid referred to as messenger RNA. The ribosomes "collaborate" with this nucleic acid to form protein molecules.

GOLGI COMPLEX

Named after the Italian cytologist Camillo Golgi, the ***golgi complex*** (or golgi apparatus), a tightly packed assemblage of "membrane-limited vesicles" or sacs, is generally found near the cell's nucleus. The number of golgi complexes per cell varies. These vesicles usually occur in two forms—as small spheres and as broad, flattened structures, frequently referred to as ***cisternae*** (singular, ***cisterna***). In electron micrographs of ultrathin tissue sections, the cisternae appear as networks of elongated, parallel, membrane-enclosed spaces stacked closely on each other (Figure 6–8a). The membranous portions of the golgi apparatus are always smooth. That is, they do not have associated ribosomes. A major role of the golgi complex is to form secretory vesicles whose membranes bond to the cell membrane (Figure 6–8b). Some of the vesicles may function as discrete cell components (lysosomes and condensing vacuoles, for example) before their contents are discharged at cell surface.

In most eucaryotic cells, secretory activities involve several cellular components, including the endoplasmic reticulum, golgi complex, nuclear envelope, and derived vesicles. These structures work together as a unified cytoplasmic membrane system. The golgi apparatus assists in the transfer of proteins, membrane components, and certain other cellular materials from the endoplasmic reticulum to the plasma membrane and ultimately to a secretory cell's exterior. Depending on the cell type, secretory vesicles derived from the golgi apparatus may contain a wide variety of macromolecules, including complex carbohydrates, glycoproteins, enzymes, lipoproteins, structural proteins, and pigments. It is important to note that these cellular substances are not manufactured exclusively within the golgi complex, but may be simply modified or transformed there.

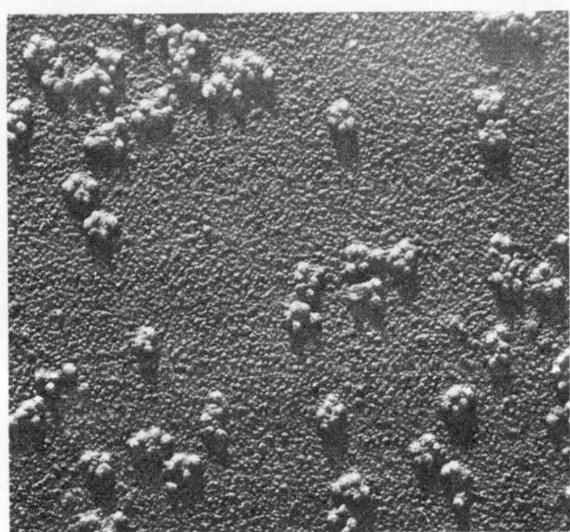

FIG. 6–7 An electron micrograph of polyribosomes isolated from rabbit reticulocytes that were engaged in the synthesis of hemoglobin. ***Courtesy of Dr. Alexander Rich, Massachusetts Institute of Technology, Cambridge, Mass.***

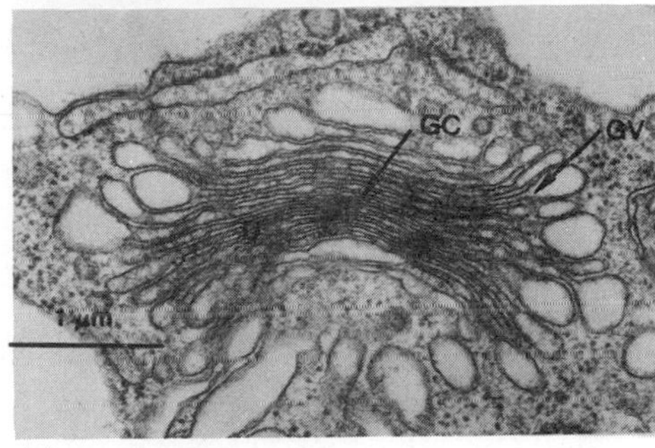

(a)

FIG. 6–8 The golgi complex. (a) An electron micrograph showing the following components: golgi cisternae (Gc), individual parallel cisternae (Ipc), and golgi vesicles (Gv). ***Eyden, B. P., J. Protozoology 22:336–344 (1975).*** (b) Secretion by the golgi apparatus, endoplasmic reticulum, plasma membrane, and ribosomes. The formation of secretory vesicles, their release, and their eventual transport out of a cell is shown.

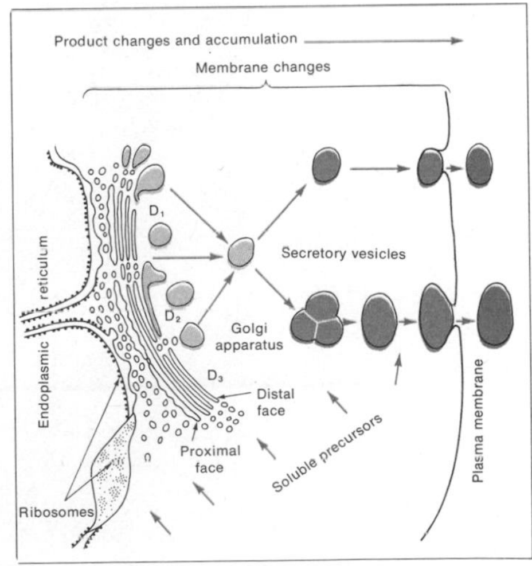

(b)

LYSOSOMES

It has recently been found that among their membrane-bounded organelles, animal cells have small vesicles containing a number of hydrolytic enzymes. These enzymes are capable of breaking down, or degrading, nucleic acids, proteins, and other macromolecules. In a normal, intact cell these enzymes are segregated in spherical vesicular structures called ***lysosomes*** (Color Photograph 16) to prevent them from digesting cellular components. When a lysosome ruptures, the enzymes are released and proceed to participate in the disruption, or lysis, and digestion of dying or dead cells. This type of activity is believed to be part of several processes, including phagocytosis and the destruction of toxic substances that may enter the body.

MICROBODIES OR PEROXISOMES

Microbodies arise from the flattened sacs, or saccules, of the endoplasmic reticulum. Microbodies contain a number of specialized enzymes including some that break down peroxides, such as hydrogen peroxide (H_2O_2), which are potentially harmful to the cells. Because early studies demonstrated the presence of peroxide-degrading enzymes in microbodies, they are also referred to as ***peroxisomes***. Peroxisomes function in cooperation with other organelles and are involved in amino acid and carbohydrate utilization.

Microtubules

Recent electron microscope studies have revealed a class of organelles, the ***microtubules***, found in a variety of eucaryotic cells. They are long, straight cylinders with a diameter of 180 to 250 A and a hollow core approximately

150 Å in diameter. The walls of microtubules are composed of protein subunits called ***tubulins*** (Figure 6–9).

Microtubules are involved in many cell processes. Their major functions include transport of material within a cell, ciliary and flagellar movement, and the movement and positioning of chromosomes during mitosis. Microtubules are often grouped into two broad classes, based on sensitivity to antimitotic agents, temperature, pressure, or other treatments. Easily disrupted tubules, ***labile microtubules***, include those that form the spindle fibers during mitosis and are randomly distributed throughout the cytoplasm during other stages of the cell cycle. ***Stable microtubules*** (those that are more difficult to disrupt) are the usual components of cilia, flagella, centrioles, and related structures (Figure 6–10). Some viruses have been shown to use microtubules for their own replication.

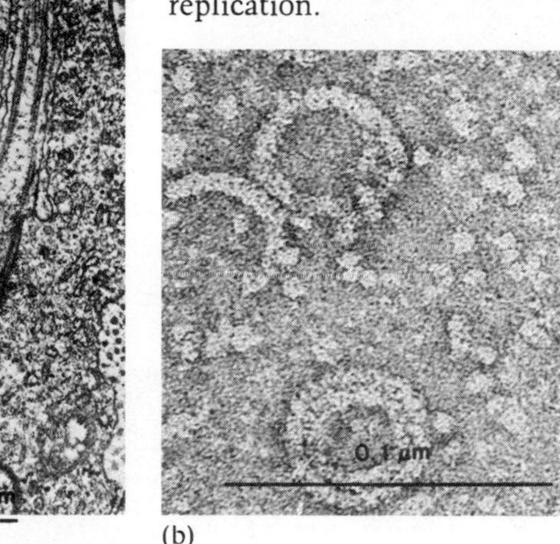

(a)

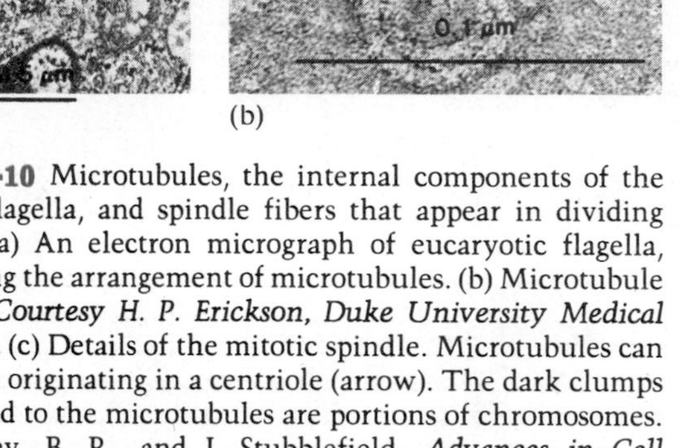

(b)

FIG. 6–10 Microtubules, the internal components of the cilia, flagella, and spindle fibers that appear in dividing cells. (a) An electron micrograph of eucaryotic flagella, showing the arrangement of microtubules. (b) Microtubule rings. *Courtesy H. P. Erickson, Duke University Medical Center.* (c) Details of the mitotic spindle. Microtubules can be seen originating in a centriole (arrow). The dark clumps attached to the microtubules are portions of chromosomes. Brinkley, B. R., and J. Stubblefield, *Advances in Cell Biology*. 1.(d) A diagrammatic representation of flagellar or ciliary organization.

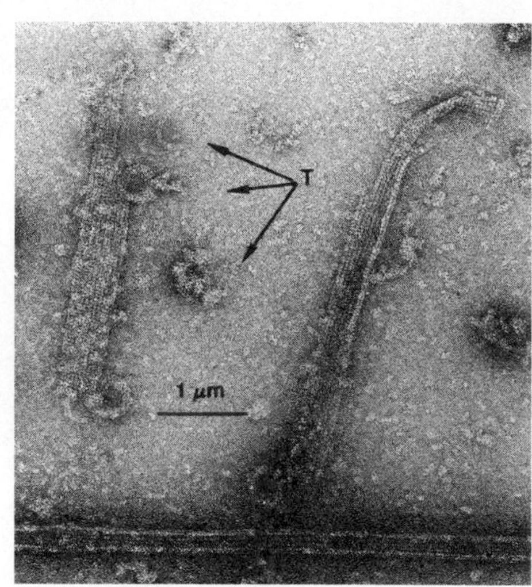

FIG. 6–9 An electron micrograph of negatively stained microtubules and their components. Note the subunits and tubulin rings (T). *Erickson, H. P.,* Ann. N. Y. Acad. Sci. *255:60 (1978).*

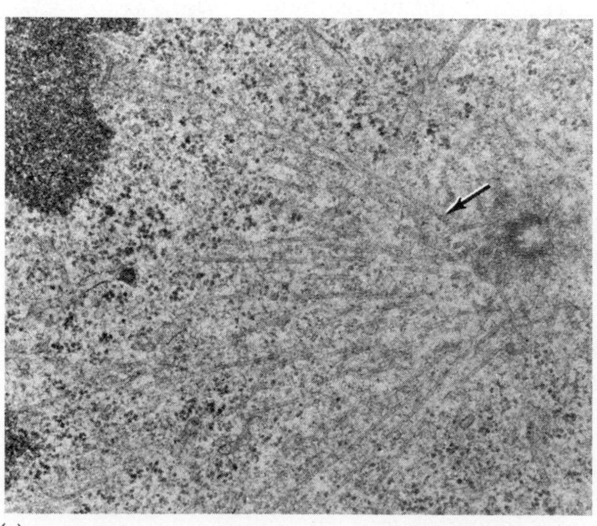

(c)

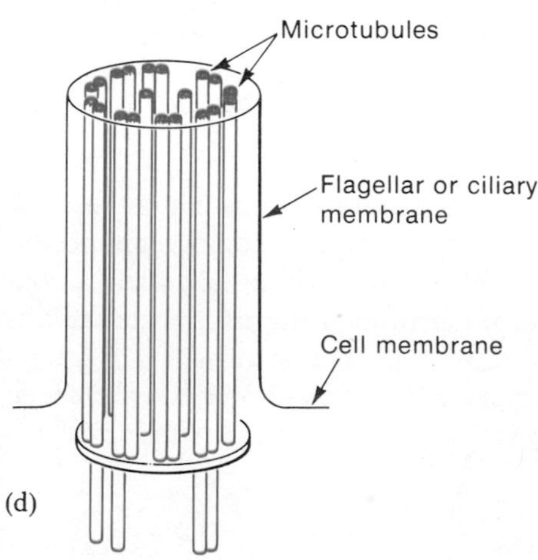

(d)

Plant Cells and Tissues

The cells of land plants and of some not as highly developed plants (Figures 6–1 and 6–11) have several of the same organelles found in animal cells. Plant cells are also organized and differentiated into tissues with different structures and functions. In various parts of plants, these tissues merge into one another. This arrangement enables the plant to perform essential processes such as excretion, photosynthesis, reproduction, and transportation of various materials from one region to another. Representative light-microscopy stained preparation of plant cells are shown in Color Photographs 7 and 20 and in Figure 6–11.

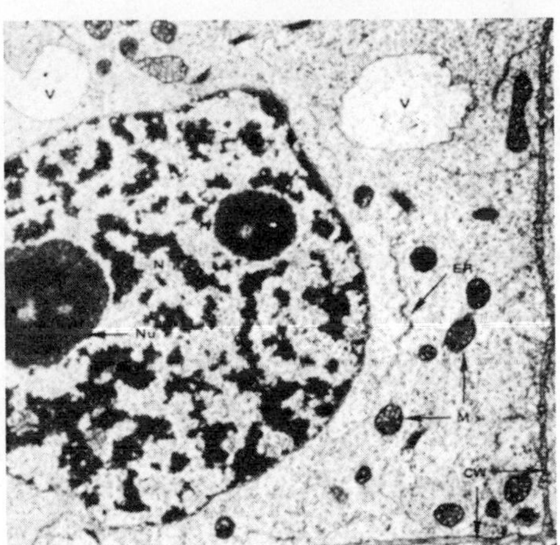

FIG. 6–11 The plant cell. Ultrathin section of an onion root cell. The various components of this cell include the cell wall (CW), endoplasmic reticulum (ER), mitochondria (M), nucleus (N), nucleolus (Nu), and vacuoles (V). *Courtesy of Dr. R. B. Park, Department of Botany, University of California, Berkeley.*

Cell Wall

Plant cells characteristically have an outer structure called a **cell wall** (Figure 6–12) that encloses the plasma membrane and the various organelles within it. Cell walls vary in both structure and chemical composition, depending upon the age and type of cell. For example, the structure surrounding a young cell is single and is referred to as a *primary* wall. It is thin (approximately 1 to 4 μm thick) and relatively elastic. Its elasticity enables the cell to grow. In older cells, as growth ceases, a *secondary* wall forms between the primary wall and the remainder of the cell. This newly formed structure differs in chemical composition and physical properties from the primary wall. Secondary walls provide additional strength. Most plant cells have primary walls, but not necessarily secondary ones. Tissues that transport substances through a plant are made up of cells having both. The ultrastructures of cell walls, as demonstrated by electron microscopy, are composed of strands, or *microfibrils* (Figure 6–13), within a complex mixture of compounds called a *matrix*. A common layer between the primary walls of cells, known as the *middle lamella*, serves to hold groups of cells together. Pits, small holes in the cell walls, permit passage of materials from one cell to another.

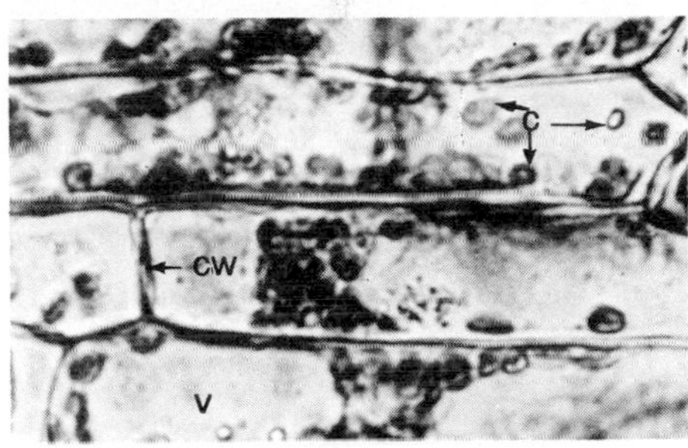

FIG. 6–12 A temporary wet-mount preparation of a leaf of the common water plant *Elodea*. Certain cellular components evident in this preparation for light microscopy include ones that distinguish plant cells from animal cells: cell wall (CW), chloroplasts (C), and sap vacuole (V).

Chemically, the polysaccharide cellulose is the major structural component of cell walls—especially of the primary wall of young cells and the middle lamella. Additonal compounds found in these structures include derivatives of other six-carbon sugars called *hexuronic acids*. Secondary walls contain lignin, which imparts rigidity and strength. It should be noted that the cell wall is not a living component of the plant cell.

Plasma Membrane

The plasma membrane surrounds the cytoplasm of a plant cell, separating it from the cell wall (Color Photograph 19). The plasma membrane differs substantially from the wall in chemical composition, function, and structure. These differences are summarized in Table 6–1.

Plastids

Most plant cells contain specialized structures involved in the synthesis and storage of nutrients. These cellular bodies, called **plastids,** include chromoplastids, leucoplastids, and chloroplastids (chloroplasts).

CHROMOPLASTIDS

Chromoplastids contain the pigments that account for the colors of flowers, fruits, and leaves and are important in photosynthesis.

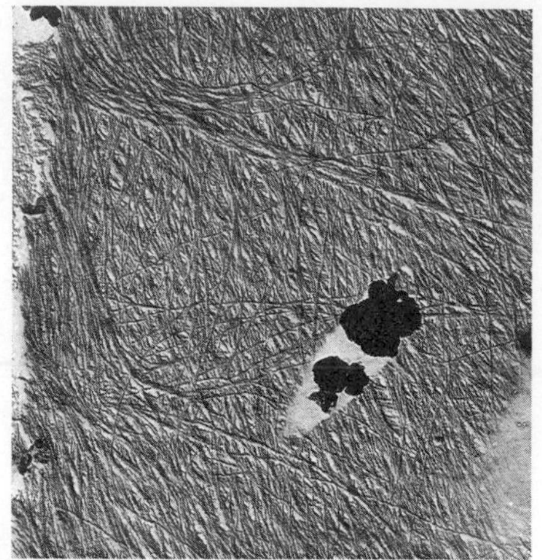

FIG. 6-13 A shadow-cast specimen, showing the microfibrils of a plant cell wall. *Noel, A. R. A.*, Ann. Bot. *38:495-504 (1974).*

TABLE 6-1 Differences between a Plant Cell Wall and its Plasma Membrane

Property	*Cell Wall*	*Plasma Membrane*
Chemical composition	Primarily carbohydrate; secondary walls contain lignin	Lipid and protein
Function	Imparts rigidity and strength to the cell	Regulates the passage of substances into and out of cell, maintaining the integrity of the cell
Structure	Rigid and relatively thick; primary walls range from 1 to 3 μm, while secondary structures exhibit thickness of 5 to 10 μm	Flexible and thin, approximately 7.5 nm (75 Å)[a]

[a]Other structural features of plasma membranes are described in the earlier section dealing with animal cells.

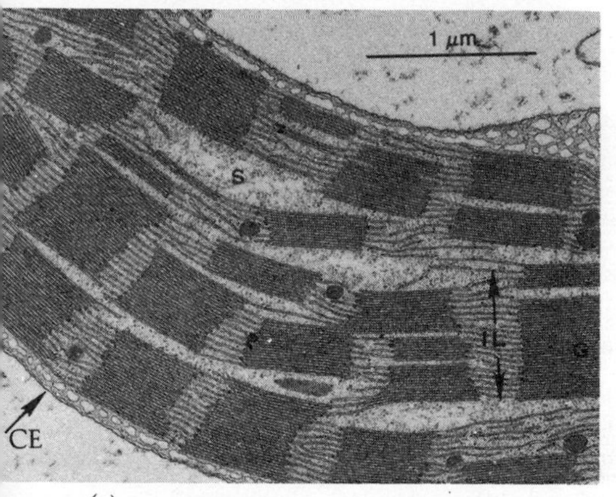

(a)

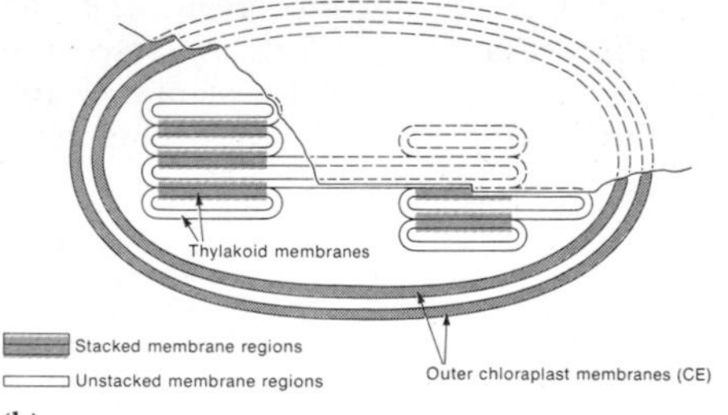

(b)

FIG. 6-14 (a) An ultrathin section of a chloroplast from a corn leaf *(Zea mays)*. Note the closely packed lamellae that form the grana (G). The light reaction of photosynthesis is associated with the lamellae, or thylakoids. Other portions of the chloroplast shown include the envelope or membrane (CE), the lamellae of the intergranum (IL), and the stroma (S). The substances needed for the dark reaction of photosynthesis are found in the stroma. *Courtesy of L. K. Shumway, Genetics and Botany, Washington State University.* (b) A diagrammatic representation of the chloroplast.

LEUKOPLASTIDS

In general, *leukoplastids* are colorless components of cells not exposed to light, which serve as storage centers for starch and related compounds. They are found in the cells of roots and underground stems. Starch-containing leukoplastids are called *amyloplasts.*

CHLOROPLASTS

Chloroplasts are probably the best-known plastids of higher plants. Leeuwenhoek was the first to observe these "green-colored bodies" in plant cells. Structurally, chloroplasts (Figures 6–12 and 6–14) are disc-shaped and measure approximately 2 to 4 μm in diameter and 0.5 to 1.0 μm in thickness. Ultrathin sections of these organelles reveal an elaborate internal organization. Within individual chloroplasts, chlorophyll pigment is concentrated in discrete regions called *grana,* which in turn are embedded in an optically clear region, the *stroma* (Figure 6–14a). Each granum is composed of a stack of parallel membrane layers. These platelike subunits, which are found throughout this organelle, are referred to as **thylakoids** or *lamellae.* The membranes in the stroma that connect the grana are called *stroma thylakoids* or *intergranum thylakoids.* A double membrane bounds the chloroplast.

The internal arrangement and structure of chloroplasts differ among the various species. Generally, the type of chloroplast shown in Figure 6–14 (that is, structures with a double limiting membrane, thylakoids, and grana) is common to seed plants, mosses, and ferns. The chloroplasts of green, brown, and red algae are similar but lack grana. Blue-green bacteria and other photosynthetic bacteria have structures that contain photosynthetic pigments but are not enclosed by double membranes and are quite different from the chloroplasts of higher plants (Figure 7–5b).

Chloroplasts primarily contain lipids, pigments, protein, RNA, and DNA. The pigments are perhaps the most distinctive of these compounds. These substances, which are found in all plants, are of major importance in photosynthesis. Two major classes of pigments are usually present: the *chlorophylls* and the *carotenoids.* Carotenoids are yellow pigments, quite different in molecular structure from the green chlorophylls. Animals utilize carotenoids as a source of Vitamin A. A third class of pigments, *phycobillins,* are also present in certain organisms. These compounds are accessory photosynthetic pigments.

Chloroplasts have one main function—they participate in photosynthesis. This process, the most important set of reactions in plant cells, converts light

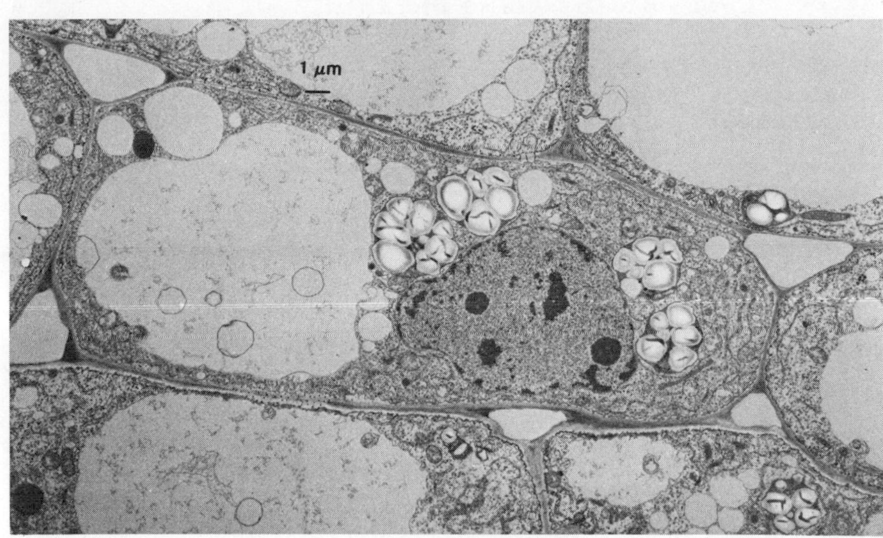

FIG. 6-15 An electron micrograph of a parenchymal cell from a cotton plant. Note the granules (G), nucleus (N), vacuoles (V), and thin cell wall (CW). *Courtesy of Dr. R. B. Park, Department of Botany, University of California, Berkeley.*

energy to chemical energy by synthesizing carbohydrates from carbon dioxide, photosynthetic pigments, and water.

Photosynthesis

The overall photosynthetic process by which organic molecules are produced and molecular oxygen is released into the environment is represented by the following chemical equation:

$$6\,CO_2 + 6\,H_2O \xrightarrow{\text{absorbed light energy}} C_6H_{12}O_6 + 6\,O_2$$

The sequence of reactions that make up this overall reaction can be divided into two successive series of reactions. In the first reaction, known as the rapid ***light reaction,*** chlorophyll drives the synthetic mechanism by capturing light energy and converting it into the chemical energy of carbohydrate bonds. In the course of the light reaction, oxygen is generated and released into the atmosphere. The second, slower portion of photosynthesis is referred to as the ***dark reaction,*** as it is not light dependent. Here the trapped chemical energy is used to incorporate carbon dioxide in various organic compounds such as carbohydrates. Further details of the photosynthetic process can be found in several of the references listed at the end of this chapter.

Vacuoles

In the majority of mature plant cells, most of the central areas are occupied by bubblelike cavities called ***vacuoles*** (Figure 6–15). These cellular components are bordered by a vacuolar membrane, which resembles the plasma membrane in both structure and function: it regulates the passage of materials into and out of the vacuole. In general, vacuoles are small in young plant tissue. However, they enlarge substantially as cells mature. Because these vacuoles are located near the center of the cell, their expansion pushes the general compo-

TABLE 6-2 Eucaryotic Organelles and Their Functions and Activities

Organelle	*Associated Functions and Activities*
Cell membrane	1. Transport of substances into and out of cells 2. In some cells, engulfment of foreign material (phagocytosis) 3. Pinocytosis
Cell wall	1. Found only in plants, imparts shape and strength to the cell 2. Protection against certain osmotic imbalances
Chloroplast	Photosynthesis
Cilium	Motion, or movement of substances past the ciliated cell
Endoplasmic reticulum	Protein synthesis
Flagellum	Propulsion
Golgi apparatus	1. Transfer of proteins and other cellular components to a secretory cell's exterior 2. Storage and packing structure for cellular products
Microbody, or peroxisome	Enzymatic activities
Microtubule	1. Cell transport of materials 2. Development and maintenance of cell shape 3. Cell division 4. Ciliary and flagellar movement
Mitochondrion	Synthesis of the energy-rich compound adenosine triphosphate (ATP)
Nucleolus	Major site for the formation of ribosomal components
Nucleus	1. Control of cellular physiological process 2. Transfer of hereditary factors to subsequent generations
Ribosome	Protein synthesis
Vacuoles	1. Locations of water 2. Storage site for certain amino acids, carbohydrates, and proteins 3. Dumping ground for cellular wastes

nents of the cytoplasm out against the cell wall (Figure 6–15). Vacuoles contain mostly water, but other substances, such as soluble waste products, are sometimes found.

Inclusions

Cell ***inclusions*** are a large and diverse group of chemicals. These substances are usually organic and may appear or disappear at various times during the life of the cell. One form of inclusion, called ***granules***, may be evident in the cytoplasm of plant cells (Figure 6–15). These granules are storage centers of various solids, including fat, protein, and starch.

Major cell components and their functions and activities are summarized in Table 6–2.

SUMMARY

The Cell's Role in Life

1. The cell is the basic biological unit of structure and function.
2. Cells must possess the mechanisms needed to control their own activities as well as to adjust to various external events and forces.

The Cell Theory

1. All organisms consist of cells, and new cells come only from previously existing cells.
2. The cellular material surrounding a nucleus is called *cytoplasm,* while the material within the nucleus is referred to as *nucleoplasm.*
3. Highly organized and specialized cellular parts are known as *organelles.*

Types of Cellular Organization

Two different and distinct levels of cellular organization exist, *eucaryotic* and *procaryotic.*

The Anatomy of the Animal Cell

The principal parts of an animal cell include the cell membrane and cytoplasm, the nucleus and nucleolus, internal membrane-associated structures, and microtubules.

The Cell Membrane and Cytoplasm

1. The cell membrane is the outer surface of an animal cell.
2. It is continuous with the cell's internal membrane system.
3. The membrane's semipermeable nature serves to regulate passage of certain substances. Materials pass through membranes by several processes including *passive transport, active transport,* and *pinocytosis.*
4. The plasma membrane is composed of proteins and a lipid bilayer.
5. Membrane systems are involved with many other functions such as phagocytosis, tumor formation, drug sensitivity, and reactions to foreign materials.

The Nucleus and Nucleolus

1. The parts of the nucleus include the nuclear membrane, nucleoplasm, nucleoli, and genetic material (DNA), com prising the chromosomes.
2. Functionally, the nucleus controls the cell's physiological and reproductive processes.
3. The nucleolus is the site for ribosome formation.

Internal Membrane-associated Structures

1. *Mitochondria* consist of a smooth outer membrane and a folded inner membrane. The inner folds are called *cristae.* These structures are called "powerhouses of the cell" because ATP is produced in them.
2. The *endoplasmic reticulum* is a network of parallel membranes continuous with the plasma membrane and the nuclear membrane. These membranes function in chemical reactions, transportation, and storage.
3. A rough endoplasmic reticulum has attached ribosomes. A smooth endoplasmic reticulum does not contain ribosomes.
4. *Ribosomes* are small spherical bodies that are the sites of protein synthesis.
5. The *golgi complex* consists of flattened channels stacked on each other. It is prominent in secretory cells.
6. *Lysosomes* are spherical structures containing digestive enzymes. They are found in large numbers in particle-ingesting (phagocytic) white blood cells.

Microtubules

Microtubules consist of small protein tubules composed of tubulin. They form the internal framework of cilia, flagella, and mitotic spindle fibers.

Plant Cells and Tissues

The cells of higher plants have several of the same organelles found in animal cells, including cell membrane, nucleus, nucleolus, mitochondria, and endoplasmic reticulum.

Cell Wall

1. The outermost structure of plant cells is the cell wall.
2. Cell walls vary in both shape and chemical composition, depending upon the age of the cell.
3. Cell walls are composed of strands called *microfibrils.* Cellulose, a complex polysaccharide, is a major component of these structures.

Plasma Membrane

The *plasma membrane* surrounds the cytoplasm of a plant cell, separating it from the cell wall.

Plastids

1. Most plant cells contain specialized structures called *plastids,* which are involved in the formation and storage of nutrients.
2. Examples of plastids include pigment-containing *chromoplastids* and *chloroplasts,* as well as the colorless *leukoplastids,* which serve as storage centers for starch and related compounds.
3. Chloroplasts have one primary role, namely, participation in photosynthesis. They consist of parallel membrane layers known as *thylakoids,* or *lamellae.* Densely packed lamellae within the chloroplast are called *grana.*

Photosynthesis

Photosynthesis is a process involving two series of reactions, the *light reaction* and the *dark reaction.*

Vacuoles

The majority of mature plant cells contain bubblelike cavities called *vacuoles.* Their contents can include wastes, certain amino acids, and proteins.

Inclusions

1. Plant cell inclusions are a large and diverse group of chemicals.
2. One form of inclusion is the granule, the most common of which consists of starch. Granules can be storage centers for fat and protein.

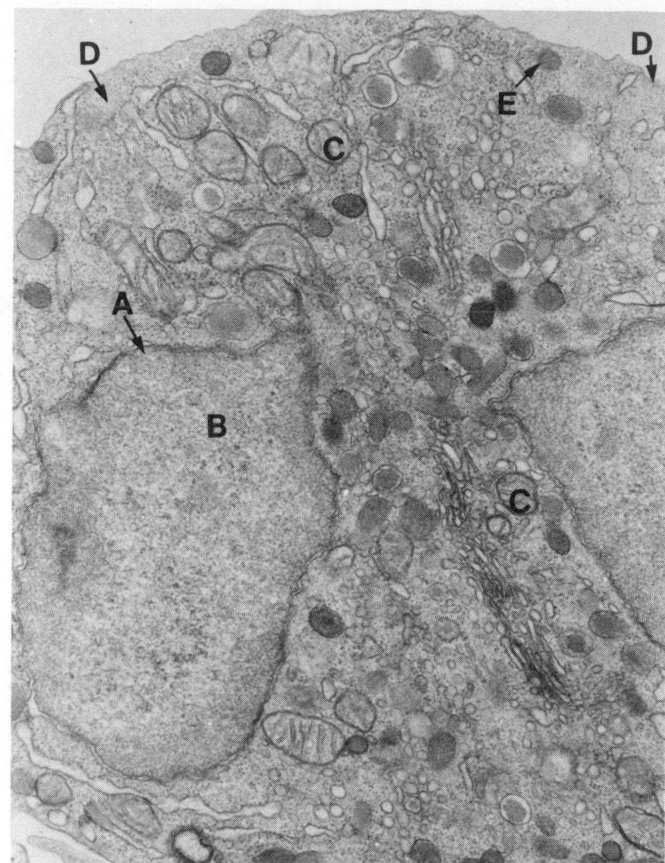

FIG. 6–16 *Photograph from Schmucker, D. C., et al.,* J. Cell Biol. *78:319 (1978).*

QUESTIONS FOR REVIEW

1. Compare structural similarities and differences between a typical plant cell and an animal cell.
2. Construct a table listing the functions and chemical composition of the following organelles:
   a. chloroplast
   b. cell wall
   c. polyribosomes
   d. cell membrane
   e. endoplasmic reticulum
   f. nucleus
   g. mitochondrion
   h. nucleolus
   i. microtubule
3. Describe the organization of the cell membrane according to the most recent theories.
4. Identify and then give the functions of each labeled structure in the electron micrograph shown in Figure 6–16.

SUGGESTED READINGS

Avers, C. J., *Cell Biology.* New York: D. Van Nostrand Company, 1976. *An advanced, well-illustrated text that provides a perspective on structure and function within both eucaryotic and procaryotic cells. The importance of observation, experimentation, and interpretation of data are stressed throughout.*

Bryan, J., "Microtubules," *Bioscience* 24:701–711 (1974). *An excellent description of the formation, structure, and functions of microtubules.*

Dyson, R. D., *Essentials of Cell Biology.* Boston: Allyn & Bacon, 1976. *A basic textbook on the cell, including topics on mitochondria, membranes and transport, genes, and cell division.*

Fox, C. F., "The Structure of Cell Membranes," *Sci. Amer.* 226: 31–38 (1972). *An excellent article describing the chemical composition, activities, and functions of the thin, sturdy envelope of the living cell.*

Maclean, N., *The Differentiation of Cells.* Baltimore: University Park Press, 1977. *This book gives an introduction to the differentiation of living cells and how the many types of cells in the same organism all arise from the same fertilized egg.*

Novikoff, A. B., and E. Holtzman, *Cells and Organelles.* New York: Holt, Rinehart & Winston, 1976. *A well-written, understandable treatment of the general state of knowledge concerning cells and their organelles.*

Threadgold, L. T., *The Ultrastructure of the Animal Cell.* 2nd ed. New York: Pergamon Press, 1976. *An excellent book with several electron micrographs of animal cells. Many details of organelles within the cell are also discussed.*

CHAPTER 7

The Procaryotes, Their Structures and Organization

In this chapter we shall present a fairly detailed account of procaryotes, including their shapes, their organization and arrangement, and their distinctive structures. Throughout the chapter emphasis is on those features that distinguish bacteria from other microbial types.

After reading this chapter, you should be able to:

1. **Describe the size range, organization, cellular arrangements, and distinctive structures and associated functions of procaryotes.**
2. **Compare the biochemical, structural, and functional properties of procaryotes with those of other microorganisms such as algae, fungi, protozoa, and viruses.**
3. **Identify the cellular structures of bacteria in different types of micrographs.**
4. **Define or explain the following:**

a. pilus	**f. sporulation**
b. mesosome	**g. endospore**
c. flagellum	**h. conidium**
d. plasmid	**i. cyst**
e. capsule	**j. heterocyst**

Bacteria, first discovered by Leeuwenhoek, are among the most widely distributed forms of life. They are found in air, water, the upper layers of soil, and internal and external regions of the human body and lower animals and plants. Well over 1700 species are known at the present time. As later chapters will show, these procaryotes are almost completely at the mercy of their environment. Temperature, the availability of suitable nutrients, and the presence of toxic substances greatly affect the activities and survival of bacteria and other microorganisms. This chapter describes the structural organization of procaryotes. In this text the procaryotes known as blue-green algae will be treated as bacteria. Various studies have clearly shown that these procaryotes are sufficiently similar to bacteria as to be placed in the same microbial category.

Bacterial cells are distinguished by morphological features such as size, shape, patterns of cell arrangement, and ultrastructure, the fine structural detail of the cell. Many of these properties are important in identifying particular bacterial species and in correlating the various intracellular structures with the overall functioning of the organism.

Bacterial Size

The small size of bacterial cells is obvious from microscopic examination. The dimensions of the smallest procaryote species border on the limits of resolution of the bright-field microscope. Most disease-causing bacteria range in size from approximately 0.2 to 1.2 μm in diameter and 0.4 to 14 μm in length.

The relative size of bacteria compared to the cells of higher forms of life and to various cell compounds are shown in Figure 7–1. Note that bacterial cells are about the size of mitochondria.

Shapes and Patterns of Arrangement

Individual bacteria have one of three shapes: spherical, rodlike (cylindrical) or spiral.

Spherical bacteria, called **cocci** (singular, **coccus**) can assume a wide variety of arrangements (Figure 7–2 and Color Photograph 9b). Among the most common are

1. diplococci: pairs of cells (Color Photograph 13)
2. streptococci: chains of four or more cells
3. tetrad: four cocci in a boxlike, or square, arrangement
4. sarcinae: cubical packet consisting of eight cells
5. staphylococci: irregular, grapelike clusters of cocci (Figures 7–2 and 7–3a and Color Photograph 10a).

Rodlike bacteria, or *bacilli* (singular, *bacillus*), are cylindrical, or relatively long, ellipsoids (Figures 7–2 and 7–3b and Color Photograph 9a). These cells may occur singly, in pairs (diplobacilli), or in chains (streptobacilli). The cells of certain species appear to be small, rounded rods, difficult to distinguish

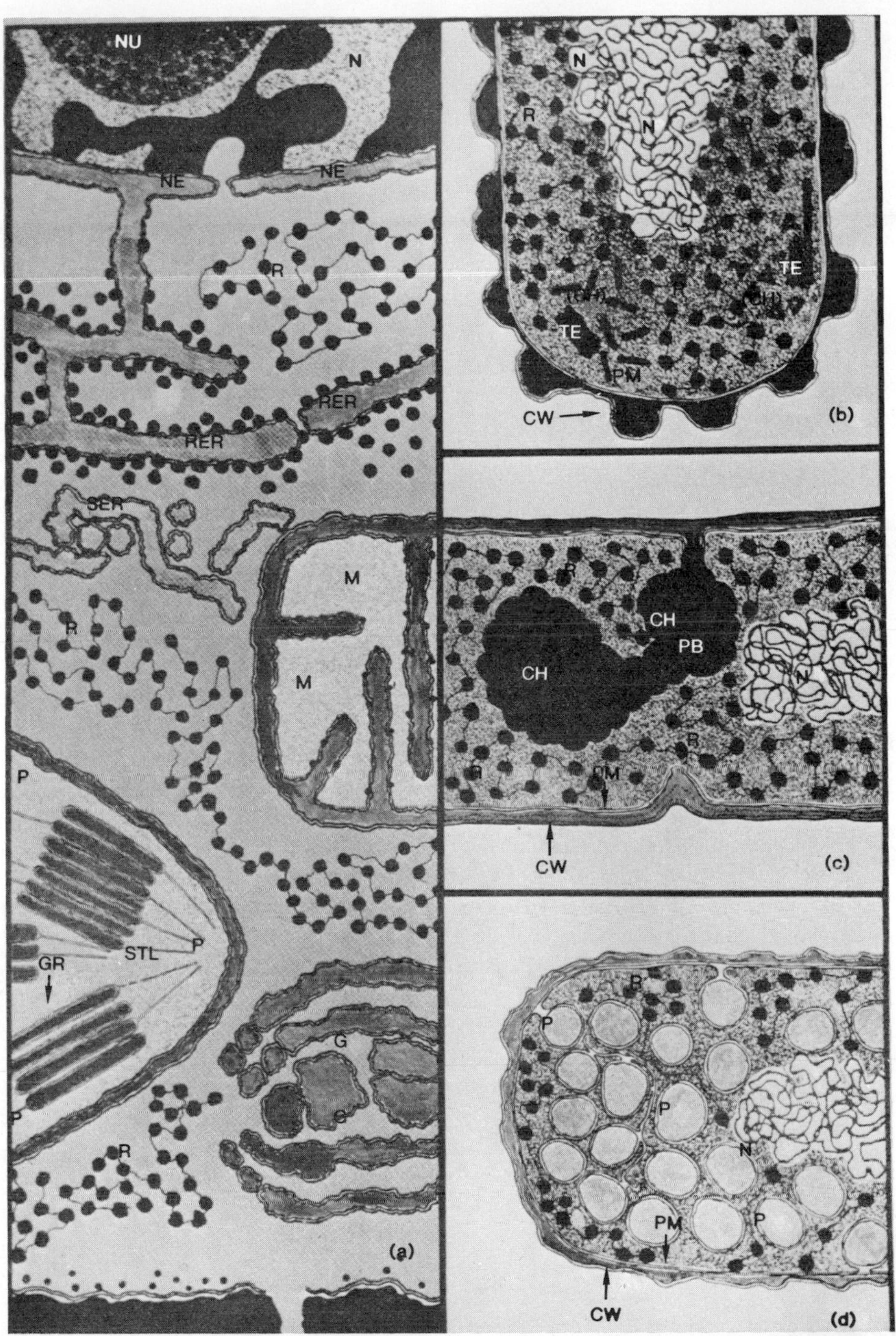

FIG. 7-1 Drawings of a typical cell of a higher form of life and a bacterium. Structures are drawn to scale. (a) A generalized eucaryotic plant cell. (b) A Gram-negative bacterium treated with tellurite. (c) A Gram-positive rod. (d) A photosynthetic bacterium. Symbols: CW, cell wall; Gr, granum of chloroplast; GC, golgi complex; M, mitochondrion; N, nucleus; NE, nuclear envelope; Np, procaryotic nuclear region; Nu, nucleolus; PB, peripheral body; P, plastid; PM, plasma membrane; RER, rough and endoplasmic reticulum; SER, smooth endoplasmic reticulum; R, ribosomes; StL, stroma lamellae. *Van Iterson, W.*, Bact. Rev. *29:299–325 (1965).*

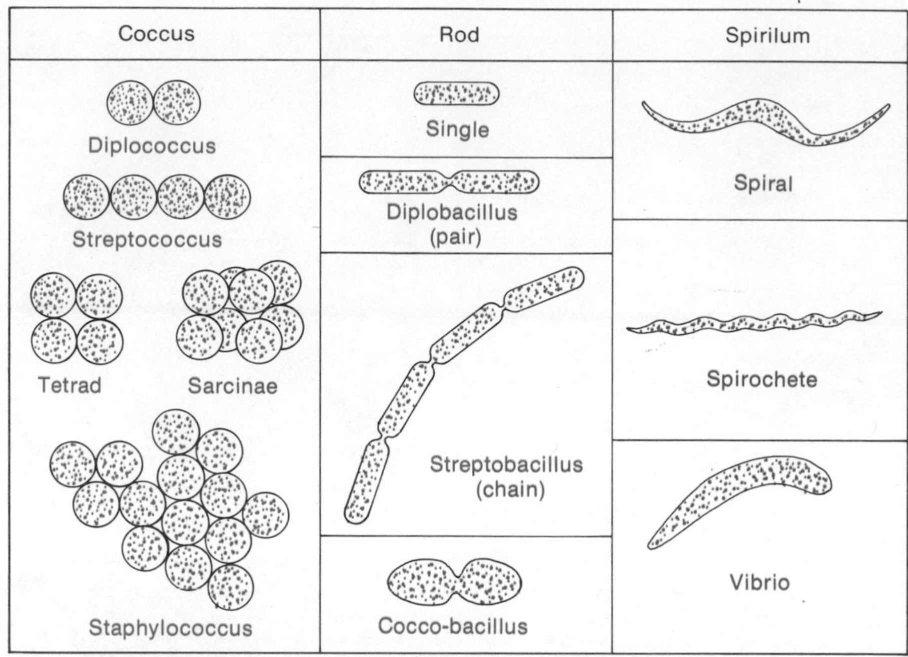

FIG. 7-2 Characteristic bacterial cell structures and arrangements.

clearly from cocci. Such cells are referred to as *cocco-bacilli* (Figure 7-2).

Certain bacterial species may produce unique groupings of their cells. *Corynebacterium diphtheriae* is one example of this. The arrangement of its cells to resemble a picket fence (palisading) is well known. Spiral organisms, known as *spirilla* (singular, *spirillum*), exhibit significant differences as to the number and fullness of spirals and the length and rigidity of the spiral turns, or coils, depending on the species. *Vibrios* (Figure 7-2 and Color Photograph 10b) are bacteria that consist of only a portion of a spiral. Other organisms possess several loose turns (Figure 7-3c). The agent that causes syphilis, *Treponema pallidum* (Color Photograph 27 and Figure 2-11b), has the corkscrew appearance of coils.

Most bacteria, as well as other microorganisms, vary in shape and size in response to external conditions.

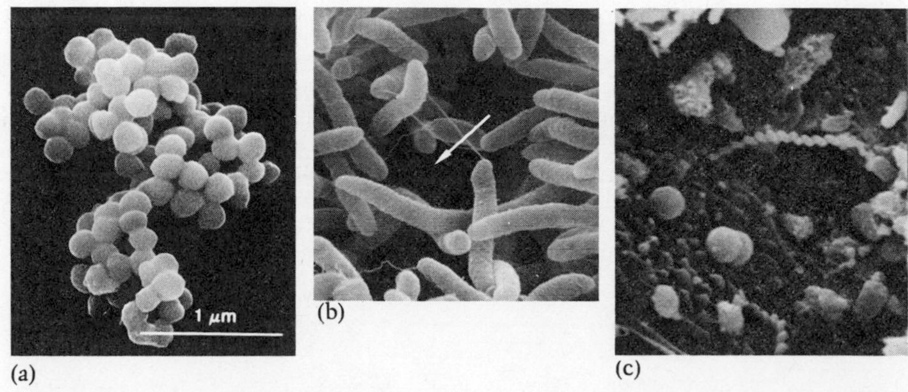

FIG. 7-3 Scanning micrographs of morphological arrangements. (a) The staphylococci pattern. *Yamada, M., et al.,* J. Bacteriol. *123:678-686 (1975).* (b) Rods. Note the flagella on some cells. *Tago, Y., and K. Aida,* Appl. Environ. Microbiol. *34:308-314 (1977).* (c) The corkscrew spirochete. *Bauchop, T., et al.* Appl. Microbiol. *30:668-675 (1975).*

Structures and Functions

Before microbiologists could begin to investigate the molecular architecture of cells and the functional interrelationships of cellular components (Figure 7–4), they needed to know the chemical composition of the cell and the arrangement of cell parts. This information came from extremely sensitive microanalytical chemical procedures and from electron microscopic examinations of intact cells and isolated intracellular components.

Several procedures are used to disrupt microorganisms and obtain the cell components to be studied. In general, mechanical means of cell disintegration are successful for such purposes. Techniques of this type include (1) grinding or violent agitation with abrasive materials, for example, alumina, glass beads, or sand, (2) pressure cell disintegration, by forcing cells under pressure through a cooled needle valve, and (3) sonic and ultrasonic disintegration. The centrifugation and washing of resulting preparations remove unwanted substances, such as abrasives. The separation and isolation of particular cellular components, such as cell membranes, cell walls, enzymes, and ribosomes, can be achieved through the use of different centrifugation speeds (differential centrifugation).

The Bacterial Surface

In recent years, the surfaces and structures of bacterial cells (Figure 7–4) have been the focus of much attention. Many intriguing studies have furthered

FIG. 7–4 Two procaryotic cell types. (a) The ultrastructural features of a general bacterial cell. (b) A blue-green procaryote (cyanobacterium). Certain structures, such as capsules, flagella, mesosomes, pili, and photosynthetic apparatus have not been found with all procaryotes.

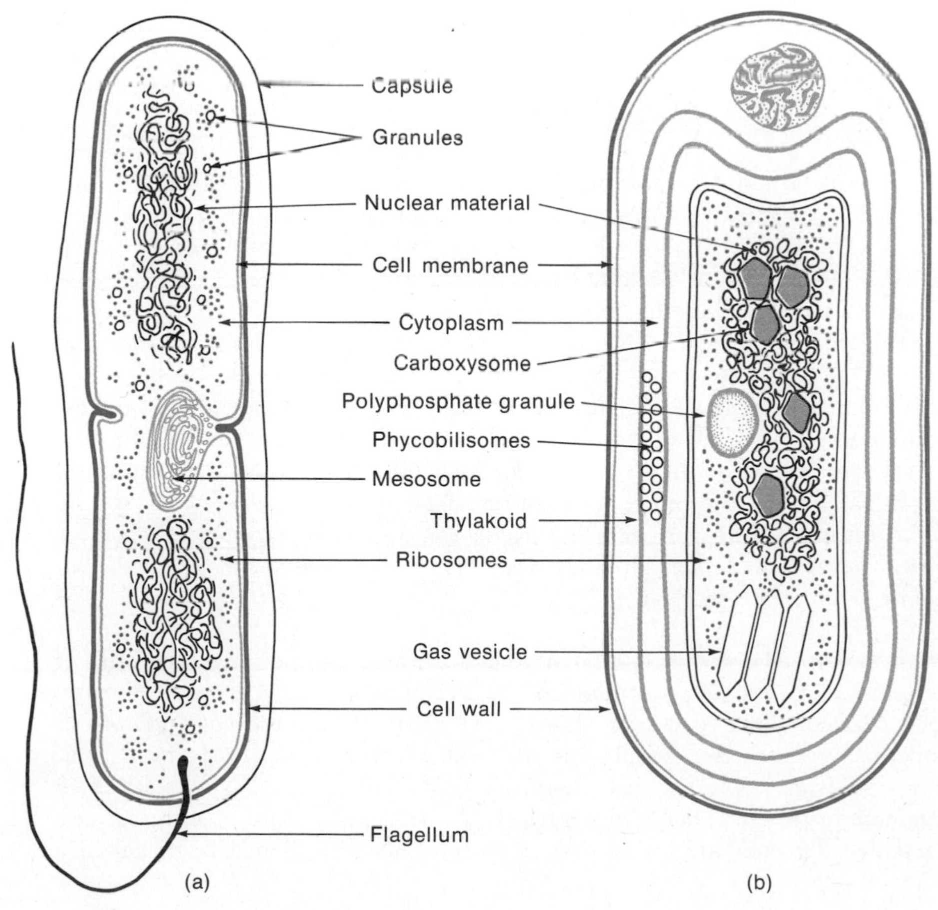

our understanding of transport across surface barriers, formation of surface structures, effects of antibiotics, and the roles of bacterial surface components in the causation, diagnosis, and prevention of infectious diseases. This section describes the currently recognized surface and closely related structures. They are (1) surface appendages, namely, flagella, pili, and spines, (2) surface adherents, consisting of capsules and slimes, (3) cell walls, and (4) protoplasts and spheroplasts.

The bacterial surface-associated structures flagella, pili, and spines (Figures 7–5 through 7–9) differ both in function and in overall appearance. However, they do share certain common properties.

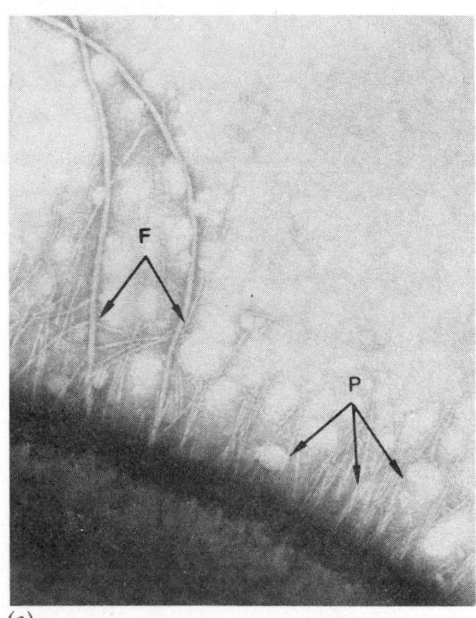

(a)

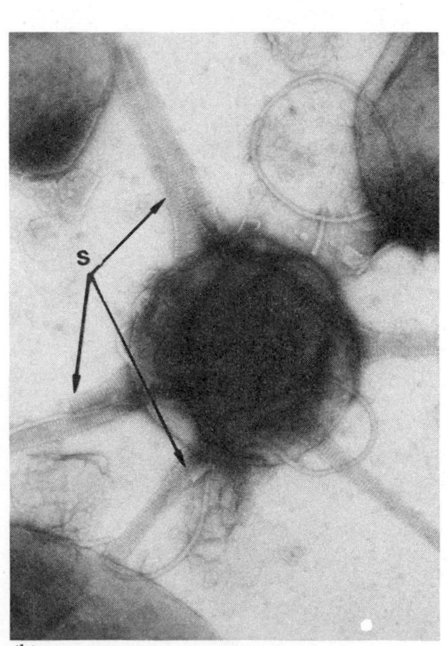

(b)

FIG. 7–5 A comparison of surface appendages. (a) A negatively stained preparation showing a clear distinction between the thin pili (P) and the thicker flagella (F) of *Proteus* spp. (b) An electron micrograph showing spines (S) with cone-shaped bases attached to bacterial surfaces. Flagella (F) also are present. *Willison, J. H. M., et al.,* Can. J. Microbiol. *23:258–266 (1977).*

FLAGELLA

The surface filaments known as **flagella** are responsible for the motility of bacteria. In addition to being observed under the microscope, motility can be demonstrated in various semisolid agar-containing media. Motile organisms are recognized by the visible spread of their growth pattern throughout the medium.

Motility can be significant in identifying a bacterial species. However, care must be taken to distinguish true movement from the quivering to-and-fro motion known as **Brownian movement.** The latter is caused by a bombardment of the bacteria by various molecules of the fluid in which they are suspended.

The presence of flagella and their associated activity do not necessarily correlate with other bacterial physiological properties. However, it appears that flagellation does bear a direct relationship to growth rate. Several factors may affect flagellation, among them the chemical composition of the medium, the pH, and the liquid or solid state of the medium. More flagellation occurs in liquid preparations. This finding also holds true for the formation of another type of filamentous appendage, the pili (fimbriae).

The existence of locomotor organelles such as flagella had been suspected since the mid-1800s. Yet it was not possible to see them without the aid of electron microscopy and the special flagella stain developed by Einar Leifson that is used in light microscopy (Figure 7–6).

Flagellar Shape and Arrangement. Flagella are extremely delicate structures that are readily detached from their bacterial cells. Flagella in a stained preparation (Color Photograph 14) are long and slender with an undulating shape. Their shape is fairly uniform for most bacterial species.

The thickness of flagella, however, varies from species to species, ranging from 12 to 15 nm, much thinner than those of protozoa. They also vary in number and arrangement (Figure 7–6). Some organisms possess no flagella, a condition referred to as *atrichous;* others may have one *(monotrichous)* or several *(multitrichous).* The flagella may also be arranged in several ways. The tufted arrangement of Figure 7–6b is *lophotrichous* flagellation; distribution of flagella all around the cell is *peritrichous* flagellation.

Organisms having peritrichous flagella can spread in large numbers over media surfaces. Such spreading zones involve the movement of bullet-shaped microcolonies, or rafts (Figure 7–7).

Flagellar Ultrastructure. Bacterial flagella are much thinner than the cilia of vertebrates or the flagella of protozoa. A typical flagellum is of relatively uniform diameter along its length. However, where it attaches to a ***basal granule,*** or ***body,*** just beneath the cytoplasmic membrane, a thickened, hook-shaped portion, the ***basal hook,*** can be observed (Figure 7–8). Flagella are believed to originate in the basal body. In negatively stained preparations of some species, basal flagellar ends are found to be connected to a broadened body, called a

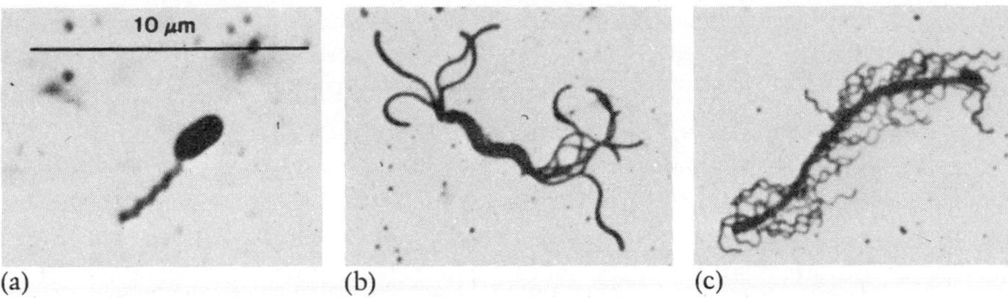

(a) (b) (c)

FIG. 7-6 Bacterial flagella. (a) *Pseudomonas diminuta* has a single flagellum at one end (polar monotrichous flagellation). The wavelength of the flagellum is quite short and very unusual. (b) A fresh-water isolate, *Spirillum* sp. It represents the tufted, or lophotrichous, form of flagellation. (c) *Flavobacterium* sp. showing flagellation all around the cell (peritrichous). The magnification is the same for all preparations. Preparations were stained by the Leifson flagella-staining procedure. *All micrographs are through the courtesy of E. Leifson.*

collar, which in turn is connected by a constricted region, or neck, to a disc- or cup-shaped part (Figure 7-8b). The latter structure, which may have a paired disc appearance, is believed by some microbiologists to be a detached section of the basal body. The collar is believed to be a cell wall fragment. It should be noted here that a flagellum originates in the cytoplasmic region and pierces the cell wall as it emerges from the bacteria. It is *not* part of the cell wall.

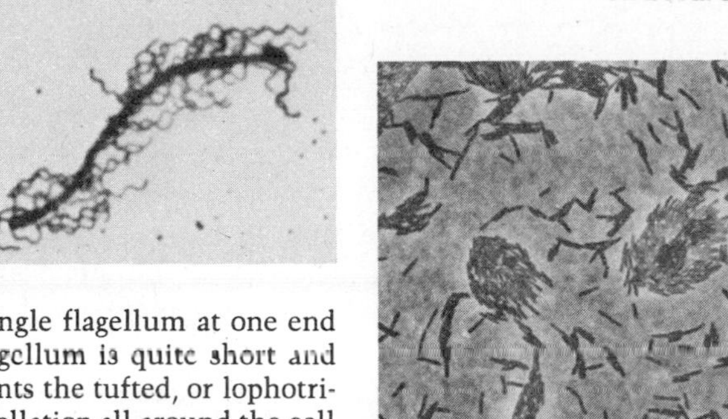

(a)

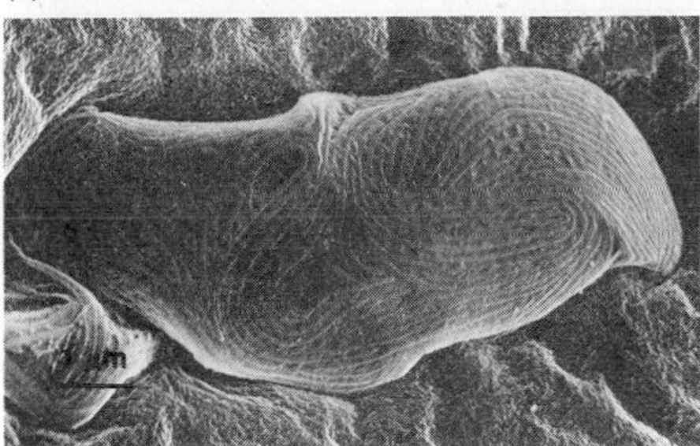

(b)

FIG. 7-7 The swarming of bacteria. (a) A light micrograph showing the outer swarming zone. The inset is of a heavily flagellated cell from this zone. *Henrichsen, J.,* Bacteriol. Revs. *36:478-503 (1972).* (b) A scanning micrograph showing the bullet-shaped microcolonies of swarming organisms. Note the large number of cells. *Reproduced by the permission of the National Research Council of Canada from Williams, F. D., and G. E. Vandermolen,* Can. J. Microbiol. *23:107-112 (1976).*

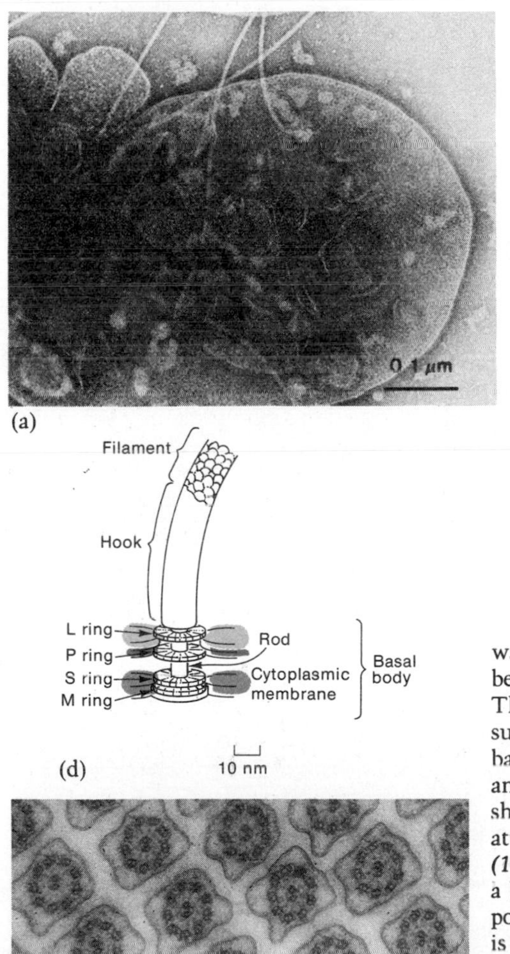

(a) (d)

(b) (c) (e)

FIG. 7-8 Negatively stained preparations of *Proteus mirabilis,* showing the bases of flagella and other components of bacterial cells. (a) An electron micrograph of an osmotically shocked bacterial cell (suspended in distilled water after treatment with penicillin). Most of the cytoplasmic content of the cell has been eliminated, except for remnants of the plasma membrane (P) and basal bodies (B). The relatively fine structure of the cell wall (CW) and portions of the plasma membrane surrounding the basal bodies can be seen. (b) A micrograph showing the relationship of a basal body to its flagellum. Note the presence of a collarlike structure (C) on the flagellum and a narrowing region where the flagellum is attached to the basal body (B). A disc-shaped structure can be seen there (D). (c) The flagellar collar (C), narrowed region of attachment, and disc-shaped structure (D). *Hoeniger, J. F. M., et al.* J. Cell Biol. *31:603-618 (1966).* (d) Flagellar structure. In Gram-positive bacteria, only the lower (S and M) rings of a basal body are present. Apparently, the upper pair is not required to support the rod portion of the flagellum as it passes through the relatively thick cell wall. This difference is significant, since it implies that only the S and M rings are essential for flagellar activity. (e) An electron micrograph of a cross-section through the cilia of a eucaryotic ciliated cell. Note the presence in each cilium of an outer ring of nine pairs of fibrils surrounding two centrally located fibrils, characteristic of higher animals and plants. Procaryotic flagella have dimensions similar to the two central fibrils. *Courtesy L. E. Roth and Y. Shigesaka, Kansas State University.*

Electron micrographs show that the flagella of bacteria consist of three parallel protein fibers intertwining in a triple helical structure. These fibers are composed of a protein called *flagellin*. The molecular weight of flagellin is relatively low, approximately 20,000 to 40,000. An amino acid not found elsewhere has been identified in this protein compound. It is ϵ (epsilon)-N-methyl-lysine. Although there is a similarity in the amino acid composition and molecular weight among the flagellins of different bacterial species, these compounds are by no means identical. This fact is demonstrated by the immunological specificity, that is, the production of different antibodies in response to flagella preparations from different bacterial species, subspecies, and strains. Such differences are important in the identification of certain pathogens.

The motility of flagellated bacteria is believed to be associated with mechanical changes in the basal body. Apparently, the rotation of the curved flagellum propels the cell through the medium. In cells that possess more than one flagellum, the rotation of the different flagella must be coordinated in some way in order for purposeful motion toward or from a stimulus to occur. The mechanism for this coordination is still unknown.

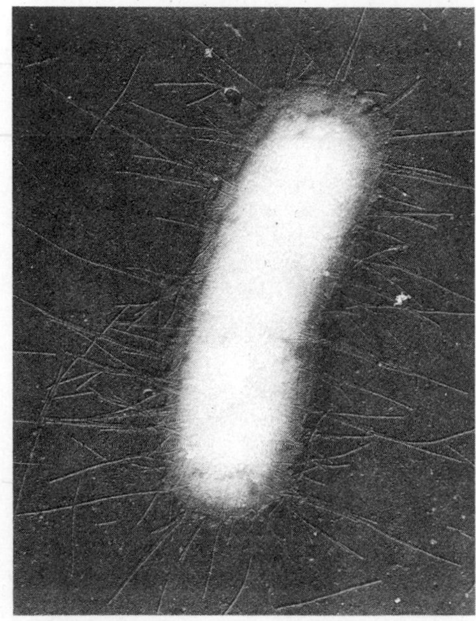

FIG. 7–9 Bacterial pili (fimbriae) Type 1 piliated *Escherichia coli*, strain K-12F. *Courtesy of Drs. C. C. Brinton, Jr., and J. Carnahan, University of Pittsburgh.*

Function. Bacterial cells benefit from flagella in the following ways: (1) they can migrate toward environments favorable for growth and away from those that might be harmful; (2) they can increase the concentration of nutrients or decrease the concentration of poisonous materials near the bacterial surfaces by causing a change in the flow rate of environmental fluids; and (3) they can disperse flagellated organisms to uninhabited areas where colony formation can be achieved. It has also been suggested that flagellated pathogens may more easily penetrate certain host defense barriers, such as mucous secretions.

PILI (FIMBRIAE)

Pili (singular, **pilus**), or *fimbriae*, are surface filaments of varying diameters and lengths. Their presence on bacterial cells can be detected directly by such electron microscopy procedures as shadow casting (Figure 7–9) and negative staining (7–5a) or indirectly by hemagglutination tests (Figure 4–27a).

Hemagglutination involves the clumping (agglutination) of red blood cells from humans and a variety of laboratory animals. Hemagglutination tests alone are not always a reliable indicator of pili, as the reaction can be caused by mechanisms other than those associated with pili. Moreover, certain fimbriated organisms are known not to produce this reaction.

In general, pili differ from bacterial flagella in several properties, including (1) their smaller diameter, (2) the absence of the snakelike appearance so characteristic of flagella, and (3) the apparent lack of association with an organism's true motility.

Chemical analyses of pili show them to be mainly protein. Specific homogeneous protein subunits called *pilin* interlock and form the rigid, helical, tubelike pilus. The production of pili is under genetic control.

These filamentous surface structures have been found primarily in Gram-negative bacteria. Included in this group are members of the following genera: *Branhamella, Escherichia, Klebsiella, Neisseria, Pseudomonas, Shigella,* and *Vibrio.* There have been reports of pili in numerous strains of the Gram-positive organism *Corynebacterium renale.*

Function. The functions of pili include (1) adherence to most surfaces, cellular or otherwise, (2) attachment of two bacteria prior to the transfer of DNA from one cell to the other, (3) formation of surface films of organisms *(pellicles)*, which could enhance microbial growth in still-culture situations when the oxygen supply is limited, and (4) use as receptor sites for bacterial viruses. A correlation between a twitching movement of bacteria and the presence of polar pili has recently been established. This special type of surface activity may lead to spreading growth on media poor in certain nutrients.

SPINES (SPINAE)

Certain marine Gram-negative bacteria have been found to bear unusual appendages known as *spines,* or *spinae* (Figure 7–5b). These structures consist of hollow shafts with expanded cone-shaped bases by which they are attached to the outer cell wall surface. The function of spines is not known.

CAPSULES AND SLIMES

Bacterial **capsules** have been described as organized accumulations of gelatinous material on cell walls, in contrast to *slime layers,* which are unorganized accumulations of similar material. The presence of capsules usually is indicated when colonies are mucoid (Figure 7–10a), that is, when they exhibit a stringy consistency when touched with an inoculation loop. With the aid of India ink or negative stains and bright-field microscopy, capsules can usually be demonstrated as uncolored halos (clear zones) between the opaque background and the individual bacterial cells (Color Photograph 13).

Common procedures utilize suspensions of bacteria and India ink as either wet-mounts or smears. The wet-mount procedure tends to provide a more accurate indication of the true shapes and sizes of capsules. Special staining, immunologic procedures, and electron microscopy (Figure 24–xb) are also used for the demonstration of these structures.

The production of capsules is determined largely by genetic as well as environmental conditions. Consequently, a wide range in density, thickness, and adhesiveness exists among strains of organisms. Capsule formation also depends on the presence or absence of capsule-degrading enzymes and on various growth factors. Electron micrographs of capsules generally do not show any specific structural features; however, many of the "true capsules," as opposed to slime layers, have been shown to possess definite borders (Figure 7–10b).

Capsules have varying chemical composition. Complex polysaccharides, either alone or in combination with nitrogen-containing mucinlike substances and polypeptides, are the most common constituents of bacterial capsules. Uronic acid is one type of compound commonly found in capsules but not in cell walls. The characteristics of capsules associated with particular pathogenic microorganisms will be given in later chapters.

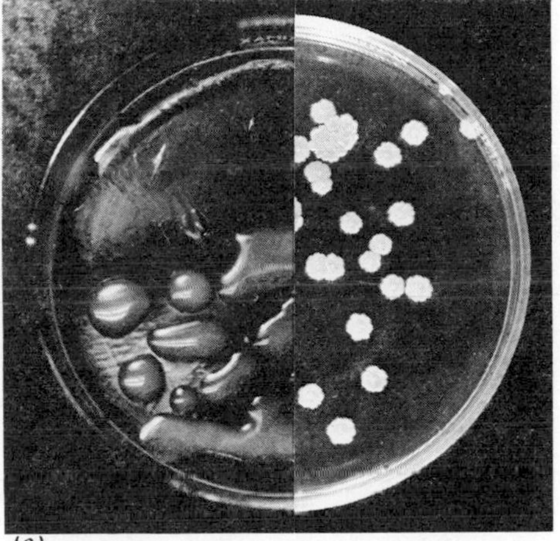

(a)

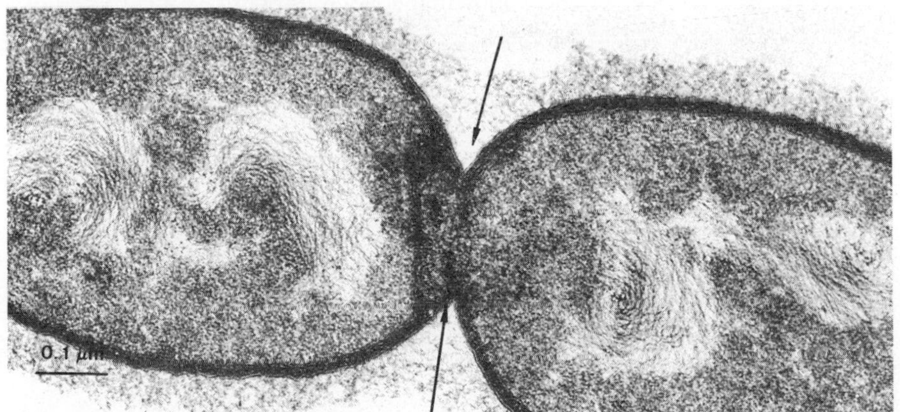

(b)

FIG. 7–10 Bacterial capsules. (a) On the left are shown rather sticky, mucoid colonies of capsule-forming organisms; on the right the rough, or coarse, colonies of non-capsule-formers are evident. *Chai, T. J., and R. E. Levin,* Appl. Microbiol. *30:450–455 (1975).* (b) An ultrathin section of *Klebsiella pneumoniae,* a capsule (Ca)-forming bacterium. Other bacterial components shown include: the cell wall (CW), ribosomes (R), and nuclear area (NU). Note the constricted area (arrows) of cell separation where the capsular material is scanty. *Cassone, A., and E. Garaci,* Can. J. Microbiol. *23:684–689 (1977).*

Encapsulation (capsule production) is important to certain pathogenic bacteria, as it influences their disease-producing capabilities. Capsules protect pathogens against phagocytosis and bactericidal factors in the body fluids of the host. The loss of the capsule-producing property often results in reduction or disappearance of disease-causing capacity. Many pathogens will form capsules on their initial laboratory isolation from a diseased individual. Examples of bacteria whose virulence is associated with encapsulation include *Bacillus anthracis* (the cause of anthrax), *Clostridium perfringens* (gas gangrene), and *Streptococcus pneumoniae* (lobar pneumonia) (Color Photograph 13).

CELL WALLS

The presence of cell walls was implied in Leeuwenhoek's descriptions of bacteria. Apparently he recognized the need for some type of structure that would not only preserve a bacterium's shape, but would also hold its cellular contents together.

The rigid cell wall is the main structural component of most procaryotes. Its presence was first demonstrated by placing bacterial cells in a very concentrated sucrose solution. The cellular membrane and its contents were seen to shrink away from an outer, bounding, rigid envelope as water from the inside of the cell diffused out into the sucrose under the influence of osmotic pressure. Thus the bacterial cell's outer structural limit was defined.

Some of the functions of the cell wall are (1) to prevent rupture of bacteria due to osmotic pressure differences between intracellular and extracellular environments, (2) to provide a solid support for flagella, and (3) to maintain the characteristic shape of the microorganism. The sites of attachment of most bacterial viruses (bacteriophages) are on the cell wall.

The cell wall accounts for 20 to 40 percent of a bacterium's dry weight. Several factors affect this percentage, including the organism's stage of growth and its nutritional deficiencies.

In recent years, the development of various types of equipment and techniques for isolating and characterizing bacterial cell walls has provided much information on their chemical composition and ultrastructure. The first chemical analysis of bacterial cell walls was carried out in 1887 by L. Vincenzi. His studies showed the presence of substantial amounts of nitrogen, indicating that bacterial cell walls were not made of cellulose, the common component of plant cell walls. During the 1950s and later years, M. R. J. Salton and others performed analyses that led to the following general properties for bacterial cell walls:

1. The cell walls contain two simple sugars related to glucose, N-acetylglucosamine (NAG) and N-acetylmuramic acid (NAM) (Figure 7–11). NAM occurs only in bacteria, which include the cyanobacteria and the rickettsia (Figure 8–12). NAG and NAM are interconnected to form the mucopeptide or peptidoglycan layer of the wall (Figure 7–13d).
2. Cell walls may contain a variety of natural or common amino acids that form proteins. Included in this group are alanine, glycine, glutamic acid, and lysine. Differences exist between the amino acid composition of Gram-positive and Gram-negative cell walls.
3. Bacterial cell walls also contain certain uncommon amino acids, the atoms of which are arranged differently in space than those of most natural amino acids.
4. Certain organisms contain a compound called diaminopimelic acid (Figure 7–12). It is found only in these bacteria in walls lacking lysine.

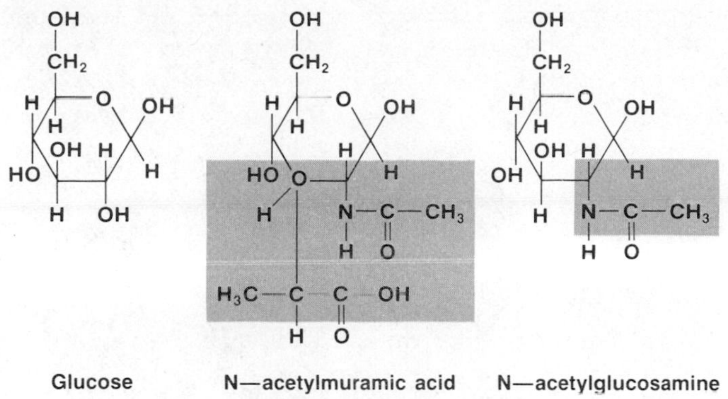

FIG. 7-11 The amino sugars found in bacterial cell walls. For comparison, glucose is included. The encircled portions of N-acetylmuramic acid (NAM) and N-acetylglucosamine (NAG) indicate where these compounds differ from glucose. *Sharon, N.*, Sci. Amer., *220:92 (1969)*.

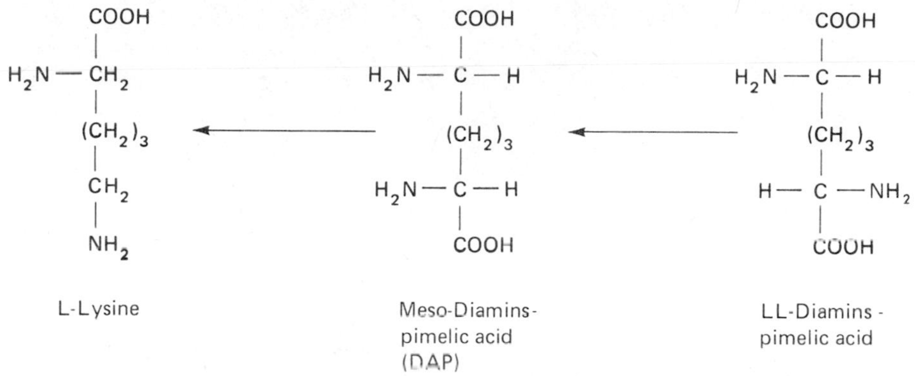

FIG. 7-12 L-lysine and meso- and LL-diamino-pimelic acids. Certain organisms utilize LL-DAP in their cell walls; others convert its derivative meso-DAP into lysine for wall formation.

Certain chemical differences exist between the walls of Gram-positive and Gram-negative bacteria. The cell walls of Gram-negative bacteria are more complex and contain a wider range of amino acids and significant amounts of lipid, polysaccharide, and protein constituents. Combinations of these components, for example, lipoprotein and lipopolysaccharide, are also present (Figure 7-13d). Such compounds have antigenic and toxic properties.

The cell walls of Gram-positives are relatively thick (15 to 18 nm). Moreover, they are uniformly dense (Figure 7-13a). The walls of Gram-negative bacteria are thinner (approximately 10 nm) (Figures 7-1b and 7-13d).

A "backbone" layer in both types of walls imparts the mechanical rigidity to these structures. It is the innermost part of the cell wall, next to the cell membrane, and is composed of NAG and NAM. The term ***murein sacculus*** has been given to the rigid backbone layer (Figure 7-13c). Additional layers composed of proteins and lipopolysaccharides apparently cover this cell wall component of Gram-negative organisms (Figure 7-13d). The Gram-positive bacteria may have special polysaccharides such as teichoic acids associated with their cell walls.

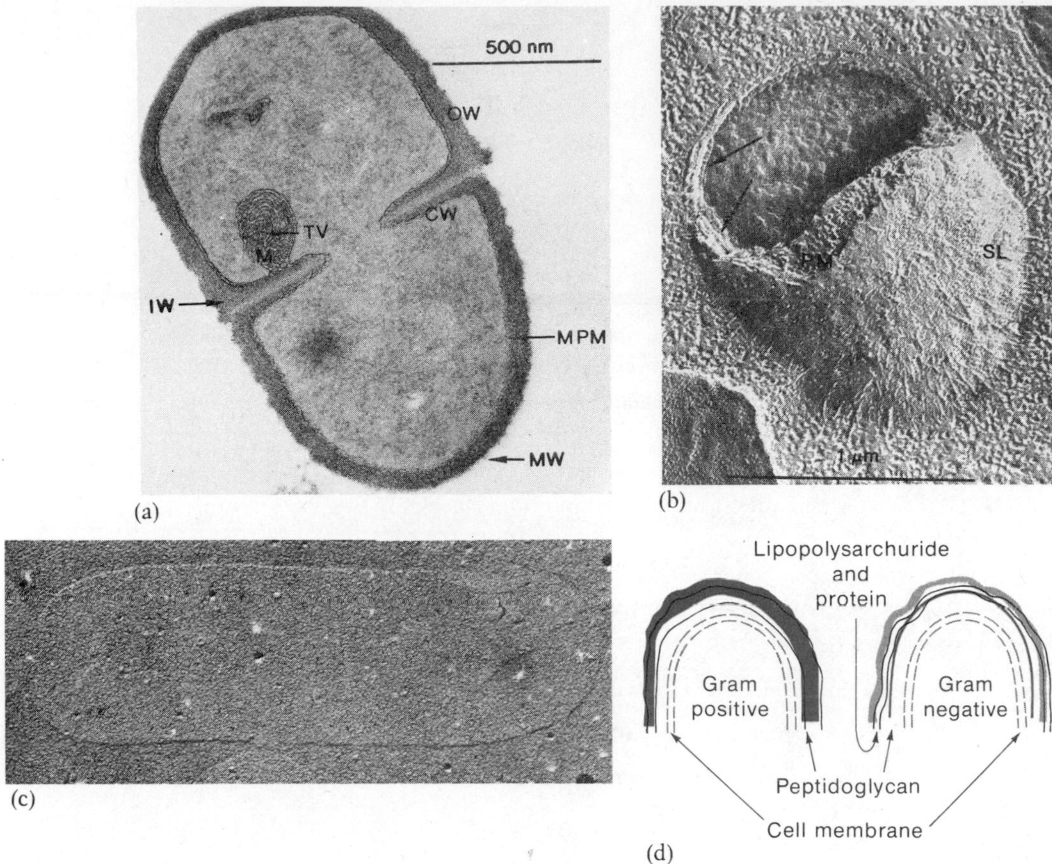

FIG. 7–13 (a) An electron micrograph of dividing cells of *Lactobacillus casei*, showing thick outer walls (OW) and middle cell walls (MW) extending into the areas of cross wall or septum formation (CW). The darkly stained inner cell wall (IW) of the cell on the lower right is seen in the peripheral region but not in the cross wall. The cell membrane (MPM) of the cell on the upper left is closely applied to the wall and cross wall and can be seen to extend into and surround the mesosome (M) boundary. Mesosomes, their tubular-vesicular (TV) components, and ribosomes (R) are quite evident. *Courtesy of Thorne, K. J. I., and D. C. Barker,* J. Gen. Microbiol. *70:87–98 (1972).* (b) A freeze-etched preparation showing the relationship of a multilayered cell wall (arrows) to the plasma membrane (PM). The outer surface of the wall is covered with material (SL) from which numerous pili radiate outward. *Horisberger, M.,* Arch. Microbiol. *112:297–302 (1977) and through the courtesy of Dr. M. Horisberger, Nestle Products Technical Assistance, Research Department.* (c) An electron micrograph of a normal rod-shaped murein sacculus or peptidoglycan layer. *Courtesy of Schwarz, U., and W. Leutgeb,* J. Bacteriol. *106:588–595 (1971).* (d) A comparison of organization of the cell walls of Gram-positive and Gram-negative bacteria. The relationship of the cell wall to the cell membrane is also shown.

PROTOPLASTS AND SPHEROPLASTS

Under certain conditions, bacterial cells may lose all or a portion of their walls. Three general conditions can bring about this state, namely, the presence of a poisonous substance, such as penicillin, the lack of essential nutrients needed for formation of cell walls, and treatment with enzymes capable of hydrolyzing linkages in the murein sacculus of bacterial walls. When the cytoplasmic membrane is found either to contain only trace amounts of cell wall or to be completely free of such material (Figure 7–14), the term ***protoplast*** is usually used to denote the remaining unit. This designation customarily refers to Gram-positive organisms. If the cell wall material is not completely removed from the bacterium, the structure is called a ***spheroplast***. This term is usually applied to rounded Gram-negative organisms that have developed as a consequence of the treatment mentioned above.

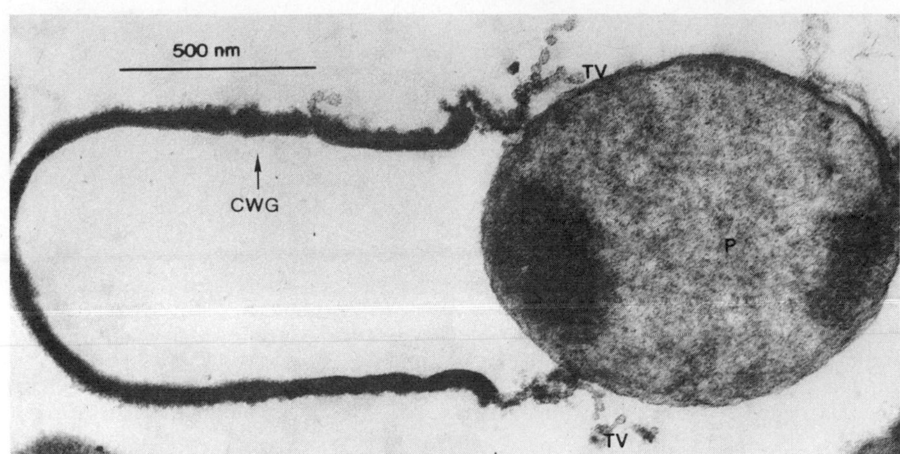

FIG. 7–14 A protoplast (P) of *L. casei*. Note the absence of a cell wall and of mesosomes. The tubular-vesicular (TV) components of the mesosomes are attached to the cell wall ghost (CWG) with protoplast formation. *Courtesy of Thorne, K. J. I., and D. C. Barker,* J. Gen. Microbiol. *70:87–98 (1972).*

Penicillin, when introduced in proper concentrations and under appropriate culture conditions, can transform growing cells of several species into spheroplasts. The antibiotic functions in this manner by inhibiting cell wall synthesis at a particular point in the process.

The enzyme lysozyme has been used by numerous investigators to produce cells either completely or almost free of wall material. Rod-shaped cells are converted by such treatment into osmotically sensitive spherical structures. To prevent the destruction of such cells, procedures are performed in stabilizing solutions, such as polyethylene glycol or sucrose. These precautionary measures are necessary regardless of the method used for protoplast or spheroplast production.

The cytoplasm of isolated protoplasts does not contain the membranous organelles called mesosomes that are often present at or near the site of division in whole cells.

L-forms. Certain bacteria can spontaneously give rise to variants that can replicate in the form of small cells with defective or absent cell walls. These **L-forms,** which are small enough to pass through most filters, can also be formed by several other species when their cell wall synthesis is inhibited or impaired. Penicillin and other antibiotics, specific immunoglobulins, and lysosomal enzymes that degrade cell walls can create the environment necessary for L-form production in the tissues of a suitable host. The role of these organisms in causing disease is unclear. However, L-forms have been isolated from several disease states in humans, lower animals, and plants.

L-forms are structurally equivalent to protoplasts and spheroplasts (Figure 7–14). However, the designation L-form refers only to cells that can multiply. Some L-forms revert to normal cell-wall-containing cells in a suitable host or a favorable medium, whereas others maintain their morphological property. Special media must be used for the isolation and growth of all L-forms.

Structures Interior to the Cell Wall

PLASMA MEMBRANE

The plasma membrane lies just beneath the bacterial cell wall (Figure 7–15). In addition to serving as an osmotic barrier that passively regulates the passage

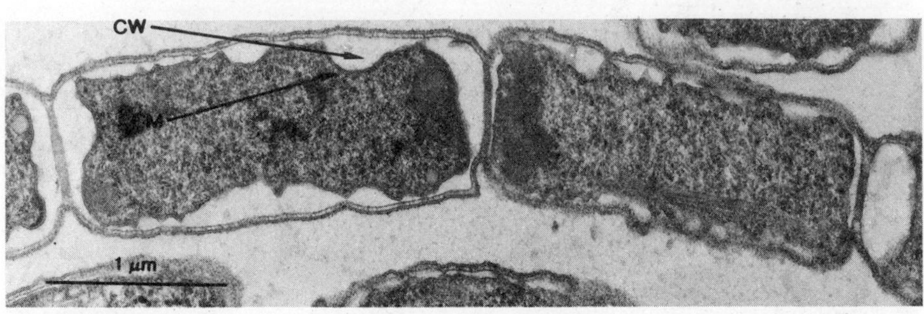

FIG. 7-15 An ultrathin section of the Gram-negative *Thermothrix thioparus.* This electron micrograph clearly shows the organism's cell membrane (CM), which was separated from the cell wall (CW). *Reproduced with the permission of the National Research Council of Canada from Caldwell, D. E., et al.,* Can. J. Microbiol. *22:1509–1517 (1976).*

of materials into and out of the cell, the plasma membrane participates in the active transport of various substances into the bacterial cell. Active transport provides bacteria with certain advantages, including the ability to maintain a fairly constant intracellular ionic state in the presence of varying external ionic concentrations and the means with which to capture nutrient materials present in low concentrations in media. Membranes contain several types of transport systems for such substances as amino acids, mineral ions, sugars, and related compounds.

The bacterial plasma membrane also participates in the outward transport of molecular waste products, substances necessary in the formation of surface structures, and **exoenzymes.** The membrane and membrane-associated structures, such as mesosomes, are important to the energy-producing reactions of the cell.

Chemically, the plasma membrane of bacteria consists of both proteins and lipids. Sterol, a high-molecular-weight lipid, is not found in the bacterial membranes, but it is a common constituent of higher forms. The exact structural arrangement of bacterial membranes remains undetermined at this time. However, they range from 5 to 8 nm in thickness and comprise 10 to 20 percent of a bacterium's dry weight.

AXIAL FILAMENTS

Spirochetes, which have flexible cell walls, move by unique structures called *axial filaments.* Electron micrographs show that each filament is composed of two fibrils identical in structure to flagella. The fibrils originate at each end of the organism and extend toward the other end between the two layers that make up the cell wall (Figure 7–16). Apparently the fibrils overlap in the organism's mid-region.

MESOSOMES

The bacterial membranous structures called **mesosomes** were observed in *Mycobacterium avium* (the cause of tuberculosis in birds) by Shinohara, Fukushi, and Suzuki in 1957. Since then, many other investigators have found similar organelles in various bacterial species. Mesosomes occur primarily in species of various Gram-positive bacteria. In this group of organisms are species of *Bacillus, Lactobacillus* (Figure 7–13a), *Staphylococcus,* and *Streptococcus.* Membranous structures similar to the mesosomes of Gram-positives are seldom seen in Gram-negative bacteria. The appearance of their organelles differs substantially. Mesosomes in Gram-positive bacteria generally appear as pocketlike structures that contain tubules, vesicles (Figure 7–13a), or lamellae (folded membrane arrangement). Gram-negative organisms primarily exhibit the lamellar form.

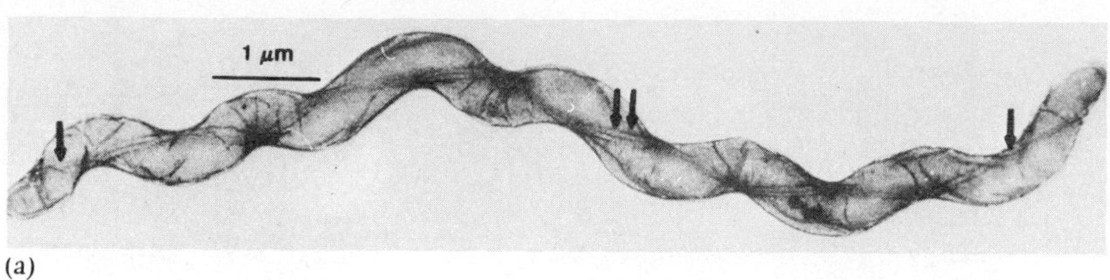

(a)

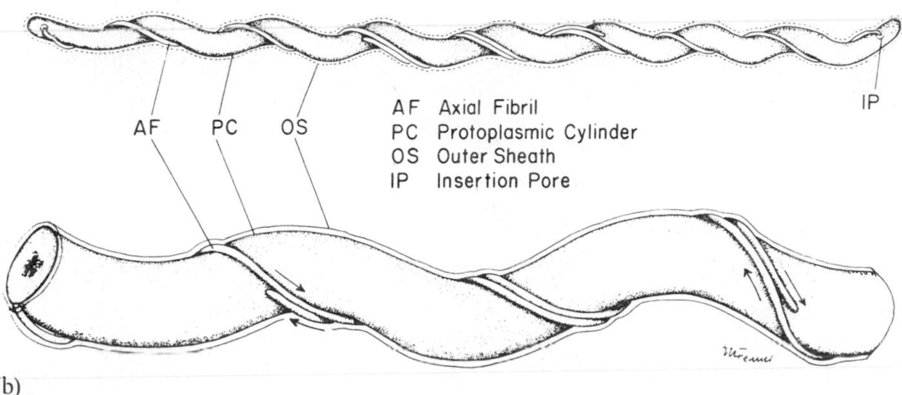

(b)

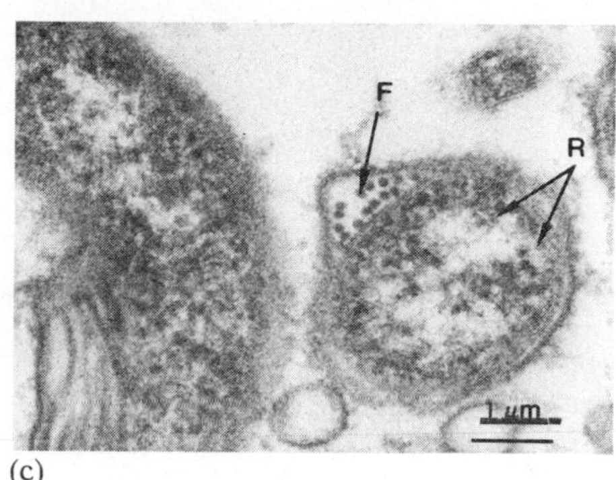

(c)

FIG. 7-16 Axial fibrils. (a) An electron micrograph showing axial filaments extending for most of the spirochete's length. *Holt, S.,* Microbiol. Revs. *42:114–160 (1978).* (b) The anatomical parts of spirochetes showing axial fibrils (AF) and outer sheath (OS). *Holt, S.,* Microbiol. Revs. *42:114–160 (1978).* (c) This thin section shows the location of fibrils (AF) between the outer membrane and the plasma membrane. Ribosomes (R) within the cell are also evident. *Hougen, K. H.,* Acta Path. Microbiol. *Scand. Sect. B, 82:799–809 (1974).*

Mesosomes are apparently involved in several bacterial processes. They function essentially to increase the cell's membrane surface, which in turn increases enzymatic content. A relationship seems to exist between the enzymatic needs of cells and the formation of new mesosomes.

The activities with which mesosomes have been associated include (1) cell wall synthesis, (2) division of nuclear material, (3) respiration, and (4) spore formation. Mesosomes do not seem to be essential for nuclear division, which involves the segregation of DNA, and cell wall synthesis. These activities have been observed in the absence of mesosomes.

PROCARYOTIC NUCLEOIDS, OR GENOME, NUCLEOPLASM REGION, AND PLASMIDS

Procaryotic cells lack the distinct nucleus of eucaryotic cells. They also lack other features and structures characteristic of higher forms, such as a mitotic apparatus, nuclear membrane, and nucleolus. The essential genetic information, or ***genome,*** of a procaryotic cell is contained within a single chromosome composed of a single DNA molecule. This structure is located in the ***nucleoplasm region*** of the cell (Figure 7–10b). The chromosome is not surrounded by a nuclear membrane and exists in the form of a closed loop. In electron micrographs, nucleoplasmic areas, or nucleoids, may appear as coarse, dense areas or as bundles of relatively fine fibrils.

Many bacteria contain additional genetic information in extrachromosomal circular DNA molecules, known as **plasmids** (Figure 7–17). These extrachromosomal components are capable of independent replication and carry genetic information for a variety of different functions, such as drug resistance. As a general rule, extrachromosomal DNA is not essential to the life of an organism.

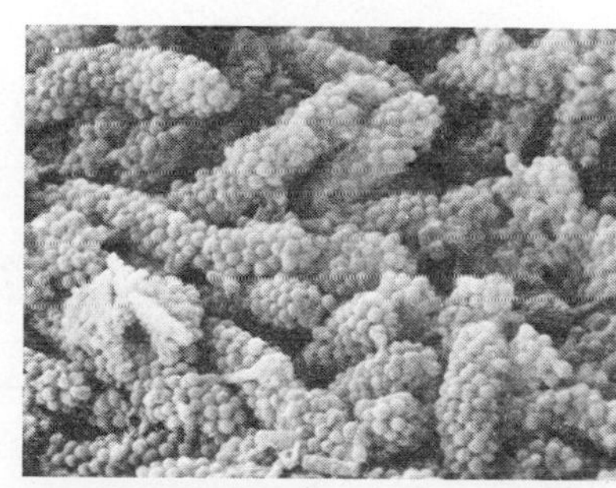

FIG. 7-17 A plasmid DNA from *Vibrio parahaemolyticus.* These extrachromosomal structures contain genes that can provide additional capabilities to the bacterium. *Guerry and Codwell,* Inf. Imm. *16:328 (1977).*

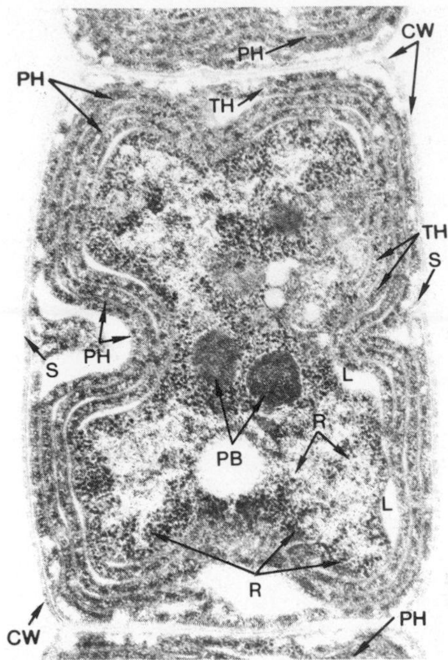

FIG. 7–18 The photosynthetic machinery of procaryotes. (a) Ultrastructure of the blue-green bacterium *Plectonema boryanum*. Note the following structures: cell wall (CW) nucleoid (N) containing DNA, phycobilisomes (Ph), polyhedral carboxysome (PB), ribosomes (R), developing septum (S), and thylakoids (Th). *Kessel, M., et al.*, Can. J. Microbiol. *19:831–836 (1973)*. (b) An electron micrograph of a thin section of *Ectothiorhodospira mobilis* showing its general internal arrangement. Included are multilayered cell wall (CW), photosynthesizing membrane, stacks (LS), nucleoplasm (N), plasma membrane (PM), and ribosomes (R). This organism is classified as a photosynthetic, Gram-negative, motile bacterium. *Remsen, C. C., et al.*, J. Bacteriol. *95:2374–2392 (1968)*.

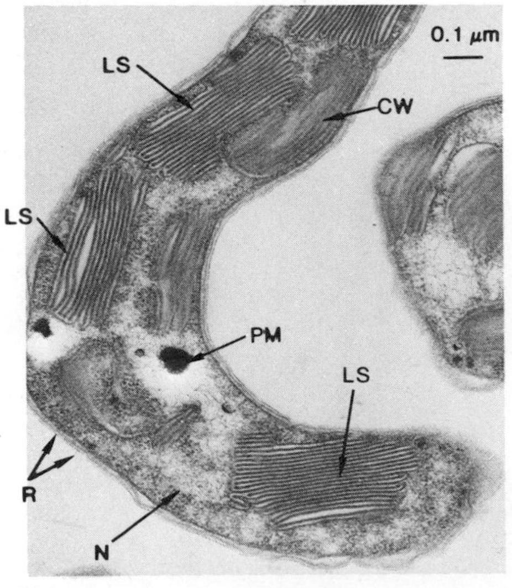

(b)

RIBOSOMES

Ribosomes are free in bacterial cytoplasm (Figures 7–10b, 7–13a, and 7–16c). Ultrathin sections show these submicroscopic structures as fine granules within the cells. By weight, bacterial ribosomes are somewhat smaller than those of eucaryotic cells and other microbial types. They are estimated to account for approximately 40 percent of a bacterium's dry weight.

Chemically, ribosomes are approximately 40 percent protein and 60 percent RNA; 90 percent of a bacterial cell's total RNA is associated with these structures.

As in other forms of life, bacterial ribosomes are important to the protein-synthesizing process. Groups of ribosomes, held together by strands of messenger RNA, that is, polyribosomes or polysomes, are the sites for protein synthesis.

PHOTOSYNTHETIC MACHINERY

Purple and green bacteria as well as blue-green bacteria (Color Photograph 29) carry out the essential steps of photosynthesis using specific light-harvesting pigments and cellular components different from the complex eucaryotic organelle, the chloroplast (Figure 6–14a). The photosynthetic pigments of purple bacteria are incorporated in a complex cell membrane system (Figure 7–18b). In green bacteria, such pigments are housed in special organelles called ***chlorobium vesicles***. In blue-green bacteria, the major photosynthetic pigments, phycobiliproteins, are localized in specialized structures known as ***phycobilisomes***. These components are attached to the outer surfaces of membranes known as thylakoids (Figures 7–4b and 7–18a). Other distinguishing properties of these photosynthesizing procaryotes are given in Table 8–4.

SELECTED CYTOPLASMIC INCLUSIONS

During growth cycles, bacteria can accumulate several kinds of reserve materials, both water-insoluble and water-soluble. Such accumulations, which are nonliving bodies, are called ***inclusions*** and include lipids, polysaccharides, and certain inorganic substances. Some of these cellular inclusions are common to a wide variety of microorganisms, while others appear to be limited to a few and can therefore be extremely useful in the identification of certain bacterial species. For example, structures called ***metachromatic granules*** are conspicuous in *Corynebacterium diphtheriae* (Figure 7–19), the cause of diphtheria. These inclusions can be shown by several methods. The choice of procedure is generally determined by the chemical nature of the inclusion in question.

Cytoplasmic inclusions are divided into two major groups based on the presence or absence of a surrounding membrane.

NON-MEMBRANE-ENCLOSED INCLUSIONS

Metachromatic Granules. These inclusions are found in several types of microorganisms, including algae, bacteria, fungi, and protozoa. Their name (***meta***, meaning "change" and ***chromatic***, meaning "color") derives from the fact that they become red on staining with aged methylene blue solution. The actual chemical composition of metachromatic granules (also called ***Babes-Ernst granules*** or ***volutin***) has been disputed for some time. Certain investigators hold that they are polymerized inorganic phosphate. Others contend that the granules are composed of nucleic acid, lipid, and protein. Metachromatic granules are believed to serve as temporary storage of reserve food. Unstained, the inclusions appear refractile in the light microscope and opaque in the electron microscope (see Figure 7–20).

Polysaccharide Granules. Glycogen and starch are two common types of ***polysaccharide granules***. Iodine solutions have been used to distinguish between them. Those areas producing a bluish color contain starch. Those with the reddish brown color of the iodine solution are designated as glycogen.

MEMBRANE-ENCLOSED INCLUSIONS

The barrier surrounding membrane-enclosed inclusions is not a double-layered membrane. Current evidence indicates it is composed entirely of protein. Examples of these inclusions include carboxysomes, lipid inclusions, sulfur-containing globules, and gas vacuoles.

Carboxysomes. Nonunit membrane organelles called ***carboxysomes*** contain the enzyme responsible for carbon dioxide fixation in photosynthesis. The enzyme appears always to be present in the vegetative cells of cyanobacteria and has a polyhedral (many-sided) profile.

Lipid Inclusions. Lipid droplets have been reported in many bacteria, including species of the genera ***Azotobacter, Bacillus, Corynebacterium, Microbacterium, Mycobacterium,*** and ***Spirillum.*** Generally speaking, fat granules appear most regularly in Gram-positive species and become more prominent as the cell ages. Lipids may take the form of either neutral fats or granules of polymerized β-hydroxybutyric acid (Figure 7–21). The latter is the only food storage lipid for certain organisms.

For light microscopy, lipid or poly-β-hydroxybutyrate granules can be stained

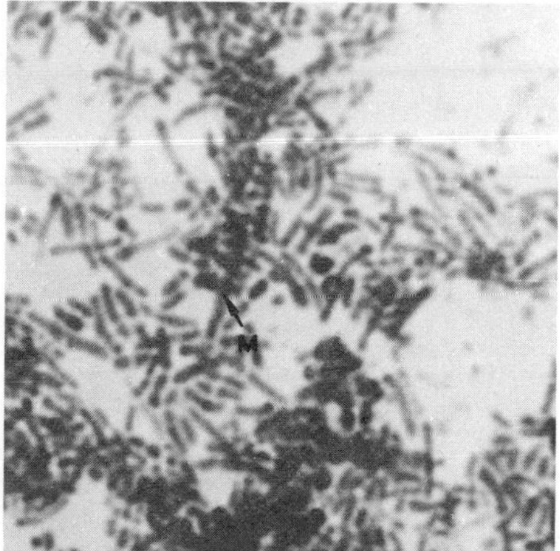

FIG. 7–19 A preparation of *Corynebacterium diphtheriae* stained by an aged methylene blue solution, showing mesachromatic granules (M). The characteristic arrangements of the bacterial cells shown here are associated with members of the genus *Corynebacterium. Courtesy of J. Mosley, East Los Angeles College.*

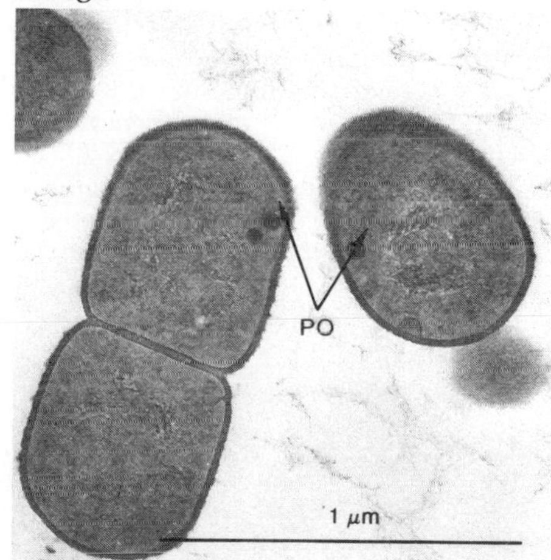

FIG. 7–20 A section of *Microbacterium thermosphactum* showing polymetaphosphate inclusions (PO), large reserves of inorganic phosphate. *Davidson, C. M., et al.,* J. Appl. Bact. *31:551–559 (1968).*

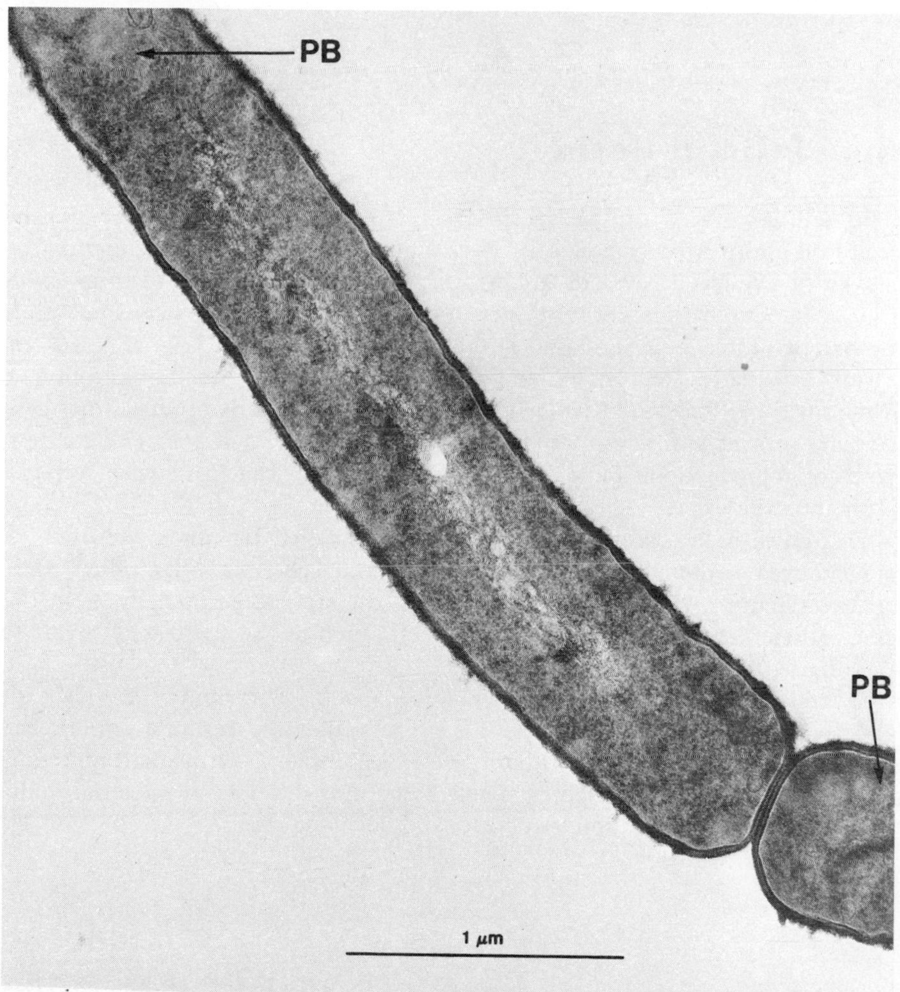

FIG. 7–21 A section of *Microbacterium thermosphactum* showing poly-β-hydroxybutyrate inclusions (PB). This bacterial species is frequently isolated from pork sausages. *Davidson, C. M.,* J. Appl. Bact. *31:551–559 (1968).*

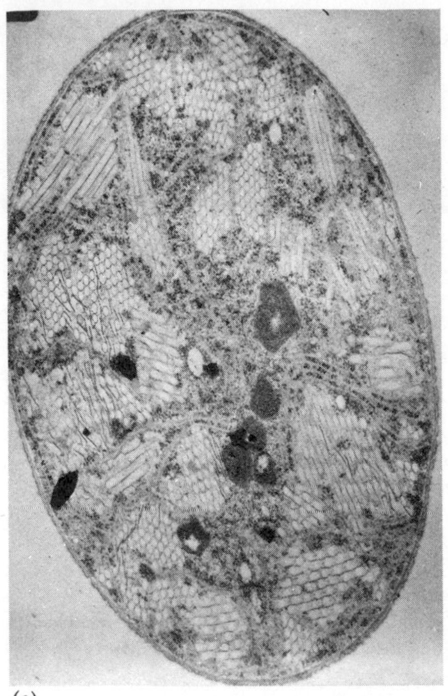

(a)

FIG. 7-22 Gas vesicles. (a) An electron micrograph showing typical blue-green bacterial cell inclusions, gas vacuoles (G), and polyhedral (many-sided) bodies (PB). Note the great number of gas vacuoles. *Kessel, M. J.,* Ultrastruct. Res. *62:203–212 (1978).* (b) Collapsed gas vesicles of the blue-green bacterium *Anabaena flos-aquae,* negatively stained × 200,000. *Courtesy of Branton, D.,* Bact. Revs. *36:1–32 (1972).*

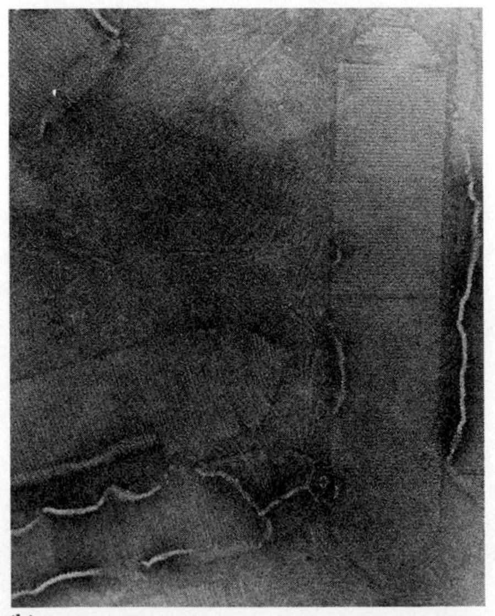

(b)

TABLE 7-1 Selected Characteristics of Bacterial Dormant Structures

	Structures		
Property	*Endospores*	*Cysts*	*Conidia (Heat-susceptible Spores)*
Heat resistance	Characteristically present	Absent	To a limited degree
Cortex	Present	Absent	Absent
Dipicolinic acid (DPA)	Present	Absent	Absent
Number formed per cell	1	1	Formed in chains

easily with fat-soluble dyes such as the Sudan series. In simple-stained (one-stain) preparations, these lipid inclusions appear as colorless areas.

Gas Vacuoles. Many aquatic procaryotes, including the photosynthetic blue-green, green, and purple sulfur bacteria, contain gas-filled structures known as *gas vacuoles* (Figure 7–22a). Electron microscopic examination shows that each gas vacuole consists of several individual gas vesicles (Figure 7–22b). These vesicles are hollow cylinders with conical ends bounded by a layer of protein. These vesicles are arranged in regular rows in the vacuoles. Among the functions attributed to vacuoles are provision and regulation of cell buoyancy, light shielding, surface-to-volume regulation, and various combinations of these functions.

Specialized Cells

The cellular events in the cycles of certain procaryotes may change and lead to the formation of new cell types. This type of activity is *differentiation* at a primitive level. In bacteria, *dormant,* or resting, structures of three kinds can be produced: heat-resistant **endospores, cysts,** and heat-susceptible **conidia** (Table 7-1). Endospores (Figure 7–23) and cysts (Figure 7–26) are formed asexually, that is, without the union of nuclear material from two different types of cells. Usually only one such structure is produced per cell. Conidia present a different situation, as several are formed and used for purposes of reproduction. Table 7–2 lists some bacteria that form each type of dormant structure.

Blue-green bacteria can produce cystlike cells called **heterocysts,** which are believed involved in nitrogen fixation, and sporelike cells called **akinetes** (Figure 7-27). The differentiation event may be permanent, as in the case of heterocysts, while differentiated cells such as the spore may revert to the original.

Several species of bacterial genera are capable of forming heat-resistant endospores (Table 7-1). However, this property is more common among the members of *Bacillus* and *Clostridium.* Some cyanobacteria form small reproductive cells also called endospores. These structures differ from bacterial endospores in mode of formation, structure, and development.

TABLE 7-2 The Occurrence of Dormant Structures in Bacterial Genera

	Structures	
Heat-resistant Endospores	*Cysts*	*Conidia (Heat-susceptible Spores)*
Bacillus	*Azotobacter*	*Actinomyces*
Clostridium	*Myxococcus*	*Micromonospora*
Desulfotomaculum	*Sporocytophaga*	*Nocardia*
Sporosarcina		*Streptomyces*
Thermoactinomyces		*Streptosporangium*

Bacterial Endospores

An **endospore** is a dormant structure formed inside an individual bacterial cell, or *sporangium,* during the spore formation, or **sporulation,** period (Figure 7–23b). Disintegration of the parent cell releases the endospore (Color Photograph 12a). The terms *exospore* and *free spore* are used to describe such released structures (Figure 7–23a).

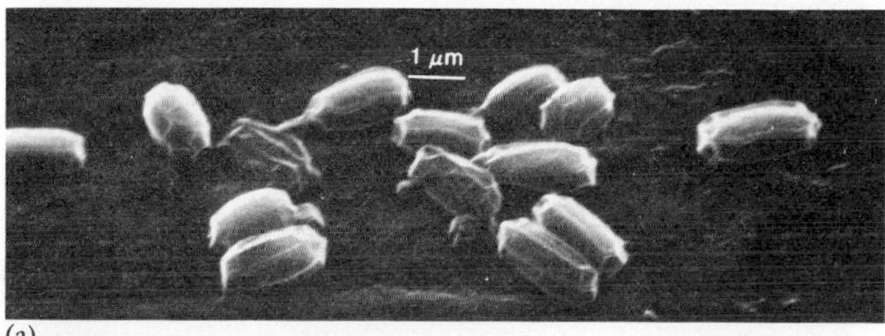

(a)

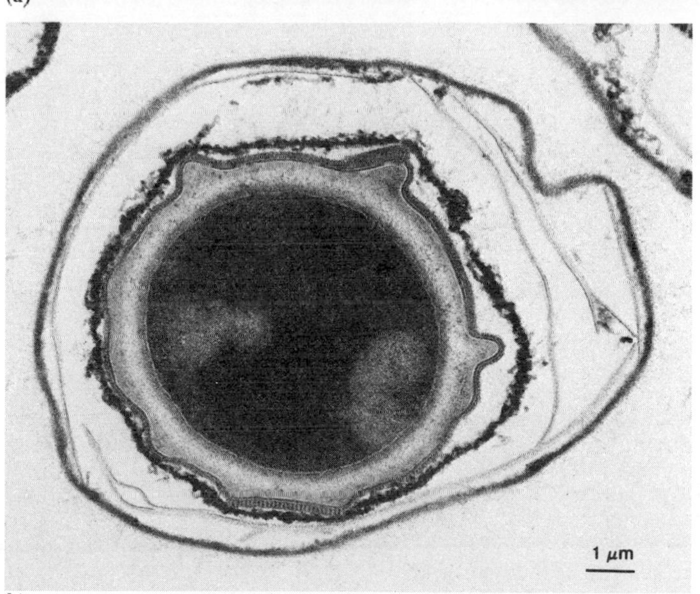

(b)

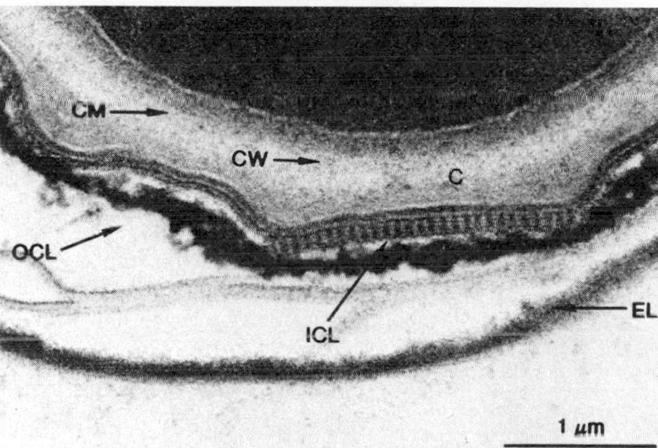

(c)

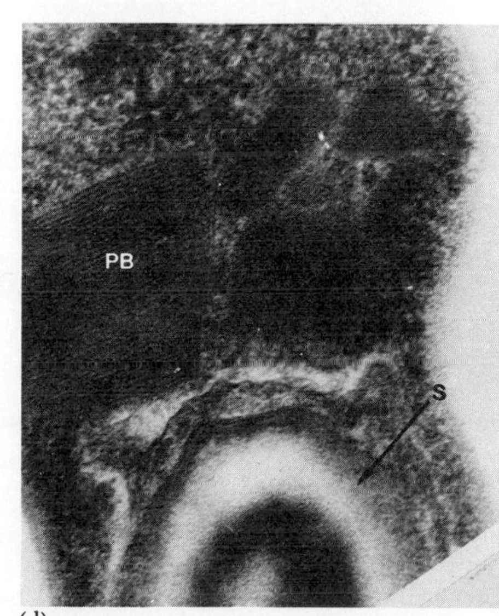

(d)

FIG. 7–23 The bacterial spore. (a) A scanning micrograph showing the spores of *Bacillus polymyxa. Murphy, J. A., and L. L. Campbell,* J. Bacteriol. *98:737 (1969).* (b) A thin-sectioned spore of the insect pathogen *Bacillus thuringiensis.* (c) An enlarged portion of *B. thuringiensis* spore. Note the relationships of core membrane (CM), core wall (CW), cortex (C), inner spore coat layer (ICL), outer spore coat layer (OCL), nucleoplasm (N), and the exosporium layer (EL). *Gerhardt, P., et al.,* Appl. Environ. Microbiol. *32:438–440 (1976).* (d) An ultrathin section showing both a spore (S) and parasporal body (PB) of *B. thuringiensis. Courtesy of Drs. J. R. Norris and H. M. Proctor, Shell Research Ltd., Milstead Laboratory of Chemical Enzymology, Sittingbourne, England.*

A bacterial dehydrated spore resembles dried protein in its density and ability to bend light rays. Spores have characteristic resistance to the effects of heat, drying, chemical disinfection, and radiation and an impermeability to common stains. Several of these characteristics can be used not only to detect the presence of spores but also to determine when these structures develop into bacterial cells—**germination.**

Dormancy, Sporulation, and Germination

DORMANCY

The **dormancy** of bacterial spores is well documented. Spores of *Bacillus anthracis,* for example, have been found to survive for 60 years in soil at room temperature. Meat that was canned for 118 years was found to contain spores of a thermophilic bacillus. What's more, examination of ancient materials has uncovered the presence of certain sporeformers, such as *Bacillus circulans.* In the abdominal regions of well-preserved mummies in Bohemia, approximately 180 to 250 years old, were found several species of *Clostridium*—species not found on the surface of the mummies, on their coffins, or in the ground.

SPORULATION

Sporulation, or spore formation, is a survival mechanism and may also be a primitive mechanism by which a portion of a cell's cytoplasm and genetic material can be separated from the rest of the cell's contents and segregated into a distinct package, the spore.

During the 1880s, Behring viewed sporulation as an intermediate stage in the normal development of the bacterial cell, a process that may be partially or completely inhibited by some physiological injury short of total prevention of growth. This concept still serves as a good description of sporulation, since it does not attempt to explain the purpose of sporulation beyond defining it as a natural step in the life cycle of certain bacteria. Sporulation represents an extremely complex process of differentiation. In most vegetative cells, the process leads to the formation of a new cell type totally different from the parent cell in chemical composition, fine structure (Figure 7–23), and physiological properties.

Specific genetic information and a suitable physiological environment, both internal and external, are necessary for sporulation. The following physical factors are needed: (1) a narrow temperature range that approximates the optimum for vegetative growth, (2) a narrow pH range, about the same optimum level as for vegetative growth, and (3) increased oxygen when cells such as those of *Bacillus* spp. begin to sporulate.

The following chemical substances appear to be required for sporulation: (1) glucose, (2) particular amino acids, and (3) growth factors such as vitamins and minerals, including folic acid (for *B. coagulans*), phosphate, calcium, manganese, and bicarbonate.

Spore Characteristics. Several stages can be observed in sporulation (Figure 7–25). A variety of biochemical and physical activities are associated with each stage.

The first definite indication of the beginning of sporulation is formation of a cross wall, or septum, near one end of the cell (stages a, b, and c in Figure 7–24). This structure separates the cytoplasm and the DNA of the smaller cell from the rest of the cell contents. The larger cell engulfs the smaller one to produce a *forespore* (stage d). This particular sporulation phase is called the *point of commitment;* the organism has reached a point from which it has no alternative but to complete the process.

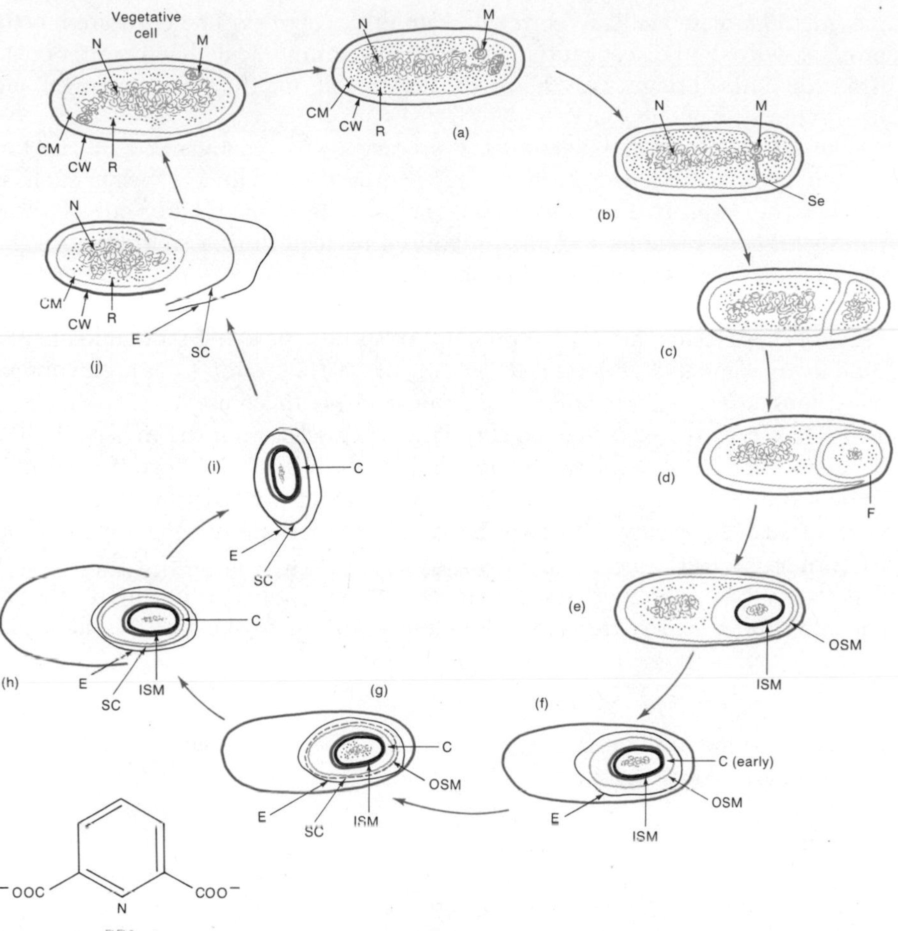

FIG. 7–24 The stages of bacterial sporulation. Portions of the vegetative cell and spore shown include cell membrane (CM), cell wall (CW), cortex (C), exosporium (E), forespore (F), inner spore membrane (ISM), mesosome (M), nuclear material (NM), outer spore membrane (OSM), septum (Se), and spore coat (SC). Note the formula for dipicolinic acid (DPA), a factor in the heat resistance of spores.

Following the development of the forespore, rapid formation of the new spore-associated structures takes place (stages e and f in Figure 7–24). These structures include the ***cortex***, which develops between the two concentric sets of membrane of the forespore (the inner and outer spore membranes), and the ***spore coat***, which forms outside the outermost membrane (stage g in Figure 7–24). In certain species an additional thin layer, the ***exosporium***, forms outside the spore coat (Figure 7–23c and stage f in Figure 7–24). After endospore formation, the parent cell disintegrates, and the dormant structure becomes an ***exospore*** (free spore) (stage i in Figure 7–24). A mature spore is shown in Figure 7–23. The central area is the ***core***, or ***spore cytoplasm***. The core wall (CW) and cell membrane (CM) become the cell wall and cytoplasmic membrane of the cell that appears upon germination (stage j in Figure 7–24). The appearance of the spore under light microscopy and its imperviousness is attributed to the cortex and spore coats.

Chemical Makeup and Thermal Resistance. Chemically, the spore has very little free water. Calcium dipicolinate makes up about 10 percent of the structure's dry weight. The core region contains a characteristic quantity of DNA but relatively small amounts of enzymes and RNA. No messenger RNA is present. The spore wall and cortex contain glycopeptides. The coats are mostly proteins with a high concentration of cystine amino acid that permits cross-linkages. These bridges may be partly responsible for the heat resistance and imperviousness of the spore.

The onset of sporulation for many procaryotes is accompanied by the formation of protein-related antibiotic substances. In certain organisms such as *Bacillus thuringensis*, a protein crystal inclusion is formed. Only one of these *parasporal bodies* (Figure 7–23d) is produced per cell during sporulation. Parasporal bodies are used to control certain insects.

The thermal resistance of spores appears to be due to a variety of factors. Some of these factors are (1) the presence of specific heat-resistant components, such as thermostable enzymes, (2) an absence of free water, (3) a high content of various minerals, particularly calcium, and (4) the presence of dipicolinic acid (DPA) (Figure 7–24). A good correlation exists between the massive intake of calcium ions (Ca^{2+}), the production of dipicolinic acid, and heat resistance. If spore-forming bacteria are grown in media deficient in calcium, the level of heat resistance appears to be correspondingly low. A similar phenomenon has been observed with spores grown in a manner that results in a dipicolinate deficiency. At the present time, evidence seems to indicate that high mineral and dipicolinic acid content is more closely related to the heat resistance of bacterial spores.

GERMINATION OF SPORES

The transition of the resting spore to an actively dividing vegetative bacterial cell is **germination** (Figure 7–25). The state of dormancy is broken by an overall process consisting of activation, germination, and outgrowth.

Phase I: Activation. Dormant structures may fail to develop even when placed in an environment that allows vegetative growth. Under such conditions, a spore will germinate if it is exposed to some triggering or germination agent, either physical or chemical. Physical triggering agents include a few minutes of heat treatment at 60° to 70°C, mechanical treatment, and refrigeration at 42°C for some time. Chemical factors include surface wetting agents, inorganic materials such as chloride, cobalt, manganese, phosphate, and zinc, and various normal metabolic compounds, such as adenosine, alanine, calcium dipicolinate, carbon dioxide, glucose, lactic acid, and tyrosine.

Regardless of the agent involved, activation appears to involve (1) a breaking down of permeability barriers by activation of lytic enzymes, (2) physical disruption of the spore coat and/or the cortex material, and (3) a subsequent activation of carbohydrate metabolism. Thus *activation*, or Phase I, represents a lag period during which the spore emerges from dormancy.

Phase II: Germination. Germination is the transition of a heat-resistant, refractile, impervious structure into one that has lost these characteristics. Phase II appears to be initiated by the formation of a germination groove in the spore coat. This groove may serve as the means by which water and nutrients enter the spore. Several events occur with water uptake: (1) a significant increase in oxygen consumption and glucose oxidation, (2) swelling of the spore (Figure 7–25b), and (3) the excretion of approximately 30 percent of the spore's dry weight. The excreted solids are about equal amounts of calcium dipicolinate, various proteins, amino acids, and glycopeptide (Figure 7–25c). At this point, the spore is considered to have germinated, based on four major criteria: (1) sensitivity to heat, (2) stainability with simple dyes, (3) loss of refractility, as determined by its phase-contrast appearance, and (4) decrease in the optical density of the spore suspension.

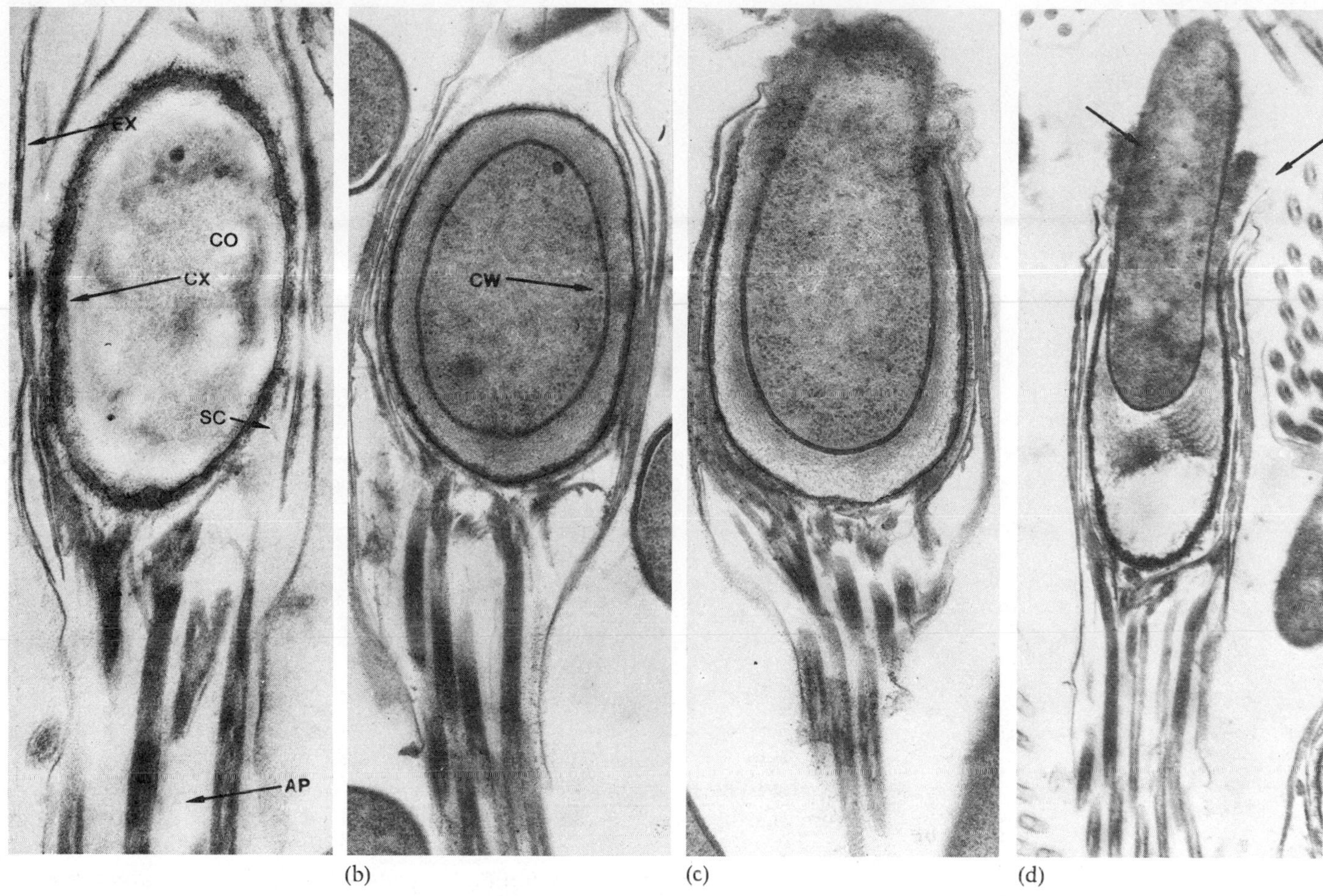

FIG. 7–25 Spore germination and bacterial cell outgrowth. (a) A thin section of a dormant spore of *Clostridium bifermentans*. The components include appendages (AP), core (CO), cortex (CX), spore coat layers (SC), and exosporium (EX). (b) The early stage of germination. The cortex has been changed into a region without any visible ultrastructure inside the core wall (CW). (c) and (d) The stages of elongation and outgrowth. In (c), the bacterial cell is constricted by the spore coat as it emerges. In (d), cortex material (arrows) is squeezed from the remains of the spore. *Samsonoff, W. A., et al.*, J. Bacteriol. *101:1038–1045 (1970)*.

Phase III: Outgrowth. Once the spore has been activated and germinated, ***outgrowth*** may occur (Figure 7–25d). A complete growth medium is now required, or the germinated cell will not be able to reproduce. The initial stages of outgrowth include visible swelling of the spore within its spore coat and a rapid formation of a vegetative cell wall and plasma membrane. The newly formed vegetative cell emerges from the spore coat, and elongates. If an antibiotic such as chloramphenicol, a potent inhibitor of protein synthesis, is added during Phase II, germination will occur without subsequent outgrowth. Figure 7–25 shows spore germination and outgrowth in *Clostridium bifermentans*, as shown by electron microscopy.

Bacterial Cysts

The cysts produced by ***Azotobacter*** spp. and various myxobacteria are usually spherical with contracted cytoplasm and a thick wall. The cytoplasm of *Azoto-*

bacter spp. usually contains evident nuclear material, lipid globules, and electron-dense bodies (Figure 7–26). The thick wall of this organism consists of an inner layer, or **intine,** and an outer layer, or **exine.** Cysts of *A. agilis* are not heat resistant, while those of another species, *A. chroococcum,* have considerable resistance. Cysts are resistant to drying and are formed singly within vegetative cells.

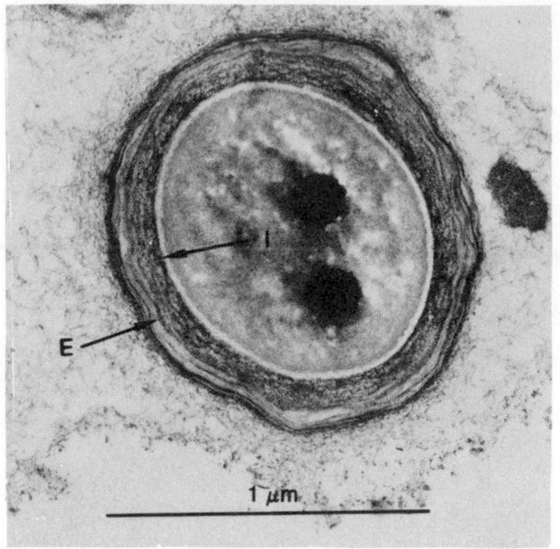

FIG. 7–26 An ultrathin section through a cyst of *Azotobacter vinelandii.* This preparation has been stained with ruthenium red, which demonstrates capsular material. The cyst coat shown clearly demonstrates the outer exine (E) and inner intine (I) layers. Note the lamination visible in the exine layer. *Pope, L. M., and O. Wyss,* J. Bacteriol. *102:234–239 (1970).*

Heat-susceptible Spores, Conidia

The dormant structure of the funguslike actinomycetes is an asexual spore that is formed at the end of special surface (aerial) cells by a process of fragmentation. These resting bodies are called *conidia.* Mild thermal resistance seems to be the only characteristic shared by some conidia and bacterial spores. Among the differences between these two types of dormant bodies are absence of a cortex, absence of dipicolinic acid (DPA), and a lack of refractility.

Heterocysts and Akinetes

Blue-green bacteria grow in either filamentous or nonfilamentous form. The filamentous forms produce chains of vegetative cells (Figure 7–27a) known as **trichomes** in an enclosing gelatinous sheath. The filamentous blue-greens reproduce by the break-up of filaments into short segments called **hormogonia.** Fragmentation, which may be caused by the wave action of water or the feeding habits of aquatic animals, results in a population increase of cells. Blue-green bacteria can also reproduce by forming differentiated cells called *heterocysts* and *akinetes,* which occur singly at intervals along the filament (Figure 7–27a). Nondividing heterocysts are involved in the nitrogen-fixing process. The heterocyst is similar in size to vegetative cells but differs from them in having a thickened wall (Figure 7–27b) and two swollen points called *papillae.* Akinetes (Figure 7–27c) are usually larger than most vegetative cells.

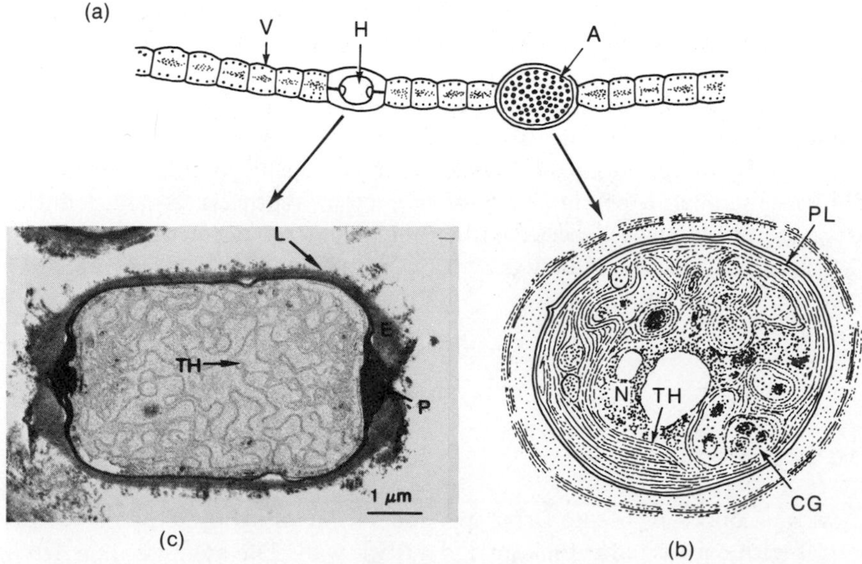

FIG. 7–27 Heterocysts and akinetes. (a) The filament of a blue-green bacterium. A blue-green filament showing vegetative cells (V), heterocysts (H), and akinetes (A). (b) An ultrathin section of a heterocyst of *Anabaena cylindrica.* Note the large concentration of pigment-bearing membranes (TH), the envelope (E), the many layers of the envelope (L), and the pore (P) in this structure. *Yamamoto, Y. and K. J. Suzuki,* Gen. Appl. Microbiol. *23:285–295 (1977).* (c) An akinete showing a cyanophycin granule (CG), plasma membrane (PL), nuclear region (N), and thylakoid membrane (TH).

Table 7–3 summarizes the procaryotic structures, their properties, functions, and chemical composition.

TABLE 7–3 Procaryotic Structures, Their Properties, Functions, and Activities and Chemical Composition

Structure	*Properties, Functions, Activities*	*Major Chemical Components*
Akinete	1. Limited protection? 2. Resting cell (spore) 3. Nitrogen fixation?	General components of a blue-green procaryotic cell
Axial filament	Movement in spiral types of organisms	Protein
Capsule	Protection against phagocytosis and certain drugs	Polysaccharides, polypeptides
Carboxysome	Utilization of carbon dioxide	Protein
Cell membrane	1. Selective barrier between the cell's interior and exterior 2. Biosynthesis 3. Chromosome separation	Protein, fatty acids, no sterols
Cell wall	1. Encloses procaryotic cell 2. Provides shape and mechanical protection 3. Contains bacterial virus receptor sites	Amino sugar (N-acetylglucosamine and N-acetylmuramic acid), protein, lipopolysaccharides
Chlorobium vesicle	Photosynthesis	Protein, lipid, photosynthetic pigment
Cyst	1. Limited protection? 2. Resting stage	General components of procaryotic cell
Endospore	1. Protection against physical heat, pH changes and drying 2. Cellular differentiation 3. Reproduction, for some blue-green bacteria[a]	General components of procaryotic cell plus calcium and dipicolinic acid DPA
Flagellum	Movement	Protein
Gas vesicle	1. Regulates buoyancy 2. Light shielding	Protein, common gases
Genome (nuclear region, or nucleoplasm)	Contains all of the genetic information of the procaryote	Deoxyribonucleic acid
Heterocyst	Nitrogen fixation	Protein, lipid
Mesosome	1. Nucleoplasm division 2. Sporulation 3. Biosynthesis 4. Cell wall formation	Protein, lipid
Metachromatic granules	Storage of reserve nutrients	Nucleic acids, lipid, protein, phosphate
Plasmid	Carries genetic factors associated with drug resistance and certain metabolic enzymes	Extrachromosomal DNA
Pilus	1. Attachment 2. Transfer of genetic material 3. Receptor sites for viruses	Protein
Ribosome	Protein synthesis	Protein, ribosomal RNA
Spine	Unknown	Protein
Thylakoid	Photosynthesis	Protein, lipid, photosynthetic pigment

[a]Endospores of blue-green bacteria differ both in chemical composition and function from those of other procaryotes.

SUMMARY

Morphological properties of bacteria are important because they can be used to identify bacterial species, locate specific structures and their functions, and show the relationships of structures to the overall function of the organism.

Bacterial Size
The dimensions of bacteria border on the limits of the resolution of the bright-field microscope.

Shapes and Patterns of Arrangement

1. Bacteria have one of three principal shapes: *coccus (spherical)*, *rodlike (cylindrical)*, or *spiral*.
2. Cocci can appear as pairs *(diplococci)*, chains *(streptococci)*, fours in a square arrangement *(tetrad)*, cubical packets *(sarcinae)*, and irregular clusters *(staphylococci)*.
3. Rods may occur singly *(bacilli)*, in pairs *(diplobacilli)*, or in chains *(streptobacilli)*.
4. Small, rounded rods are *cocco-bacilli*.
5. Spiral bacteria vary as to the number and amplitude of spirals and the length and rigidity of their coils.
6. *Vibrios* are bacteria that consist of only a portion of a spiral.

Structures and Functions

1. Procedures used for cell disruption include, (1) grinding or violent shaking with abrasives, (2) pressure cell disintegration, (3) sonic and ultrasonic disintegration.
2. The separation and isolation of cellular parts can be obtained with different centrifugation speeds.

The Bacterial Surface
Recognized structures associated with the bacterial cell surface include (1) surface appendages *(flagella, pili,* and *spines)*, (2) surface adherents *(capsules* and *slimes)*, (3) the *cell wall*, and (4) protoplasts and spheroplasts.

1. Flagella are responsible for bacterial motility.
2. Differences as to the thickness, number, and arrangement of flagella exist among bacterial species.
3. Organisms without flagella are referred to as *atrichous*, those with one as *monotrichous*, and others with several as *multitrichous*.
4. Spreading rapidly or swarming over media surfaces involves microcolonies, or rafts, of bacteria with flagella surrounding the cell.
5. Flagella originate in the cell's cytoplasm from a *basal body*.
6. Bacterial flagella are thinner than those of eucaryotic cells and composed of a protein called *flagellin*.
7. Flagella give bacteria the ability to migrate toward favorable environments and a means with which to either increase nutrients or decrease poisonous substances near the cell surface.
8. Pili (fimbriae) can be seen only with the aid of special techniques and electron microscopy.
9. Pili differ from bacterial flagella in several ways: smaller diameter, general appearance, and a general lack of association with an organism's true motility.
10. Pili are composed of a specific protein called *pilin*.
11. Pili enable bacterial cells to stick to surfaces, attach to other bacteria prior to the transfer of DNA, and form surface films.
12. Pili provide receptor sites for bacterial viruses.
13. Certain marine Gram-negative bacteria bear hollow-shaft, cone-shaped appendages called *spines*.
14. *Capsules* are orderly accumulations of polysaccharide and/or polypeptide material adhering to cell walls.
15. Slimes are unorganized accumulations of similar material.
16. Colonies of capsule-producing organisms appear as sticky, mucoid growths.
17. Capsule production is influenced by genetic and environmental factors.
18. *Encapsulation* protects pathogenic organisms against certain drugs, phagocytosis and bactericidal factors in a host's body.
19. The functions of *cell walls* include (1) protection against rupture due to osmotic pressure differences between intracellular and extracellular environments, (2) support for flagella, (3) maintenance of characteristic shape of organisms.
20. Bacterial cell walls contain (1) two simple unique sugars, N-acetylglucosamine and N-acetylmuramic acid, (2) a variety of naturally occurring amino acids, and (3) "unnatural" forms of amino acids.
21. Some bacterial walls contain diaminopimelic acid.
22. Certain chemical and physical differences exist between the walls of Gram-positives and Gram-negatives.
23. The murein sacculus or peptidoglycan layer is the backbone layer of bacterial cell walls.
24. Bacterial cells treated with or cultured in the presence of certain antibiotics or enzymes may lose all or a portion of their walls.
25. *Protoplasts* are bacterial cells with little or no cell wall material.
26. *Spheroplasts* are cells having some cell wall material.
27. *L-forms* are morphologically equivalent to protoplasts and spheroplasts. However, they revert to cells with normal cell walls in a suitable environment.

Structures Interior to the Cell Wall

1. The *plasma membrane* lies just beneath the cell wall.
2. It functions as an osmotic barrier and an aid for the outward transport of wastes, and it is important to the cell's energy production.
3. Spirochetes move by unique structures called *axial filaments*.
4. These filaments are composed of two fibrils identical in structure to flagella.
5. *Mesosomes* have been reported primarily for Gram-positive species.
6. The activities with which mesosomes have been associated include (1) cell wall formation, (2) division of nuclear material, (3) cellular respiration, (4) spore formation.

7. Procaryotes lack the distinct nucleus of eucaryotes and the associated structures and features such as mitotic apparatus, nuclear membrane, and nucleolus.
8. Essential genetic information, the ***genome,*** of a procaryote is contained within a single chromosome, which is composed of a single DNA molecule.
9. Many bacteria contain additional genetic information in the form of extrachromosomal circular DNA molecules, known as ***plasmids.***
10. Plasmids can replicate independently and carry genetic information for functions that are not essential to the life of an organism.
11. ***Ribosomes*** in procaryotes are free in the cytoplasm.
12. Ribosomes are composed of protein and RNA.
13. Ribosomes are important in protein synthesis.
14. In purple bacteria, ***photosynthetic*** pigments are incorporated into a complex cell membrane system.
15. Green bacterial pigments are housed in ***chlorobium vesicles.***
16. Major blue-green bacterial photosynthetic pigments, phycobiliproteins, are localized in ***phycobilisomes,*** which are attached to outer surfaces of ***thylakoids.***
17. ***Inclusions*** are accumulations of reserve materials.
18. Cytoplasmic inclusions can be divided into two major groups, non-membrane-enclosed and membrane enclosed. The former include ***metachromatic granules*** and ***polysaccharide granules.***
19. Membrane-enclosed inclusions include ***carboxysomes, lipid inclusions,*** and ***gas vacuoles.***

Specialized Cells

1. Examples of differentiated cells include ***heat-resistant endospores, cysts, heat-susceptible conidia,*** and the ***heterocysts*** and ***akinetes*** of blue-green bacteria.
2. Differentiation may be permanent as with heterocysts or temporary, as with the spore.

Bacterial Endospores

1. An endospore is a ***dormant*** structure formed within an individual bacterial cell. Endospores appear within a parent cell as spore formation occurs.
2. Spores can exist outside of the cells that formed them.
3. Bacterial spores exhibit unusual resistance to heat, drying, chemical disinfection, and radiation and an impermeability to common stains.
4. The spore formation process is called ***sporulation.*** The development of spores into vegetative bacteria is ***germination.***

Dormancy, Sporulation, and Germination

1. A spore is a dormant, or resting, cell. It can remain in this state for many years.
2. Specific physical factors, including temperature and pH, as well as nutrients such as glucose, particular amino acids, vitamins, and minerals, are needed for sporulation to occur.
3. A mature spore has a central area, or ***core,*** a ***cortex,*** a spore wall, and a membrane.
4. Chemically, the heat-resistant spore has very little water but a high content of dipicolinic acid and calcium, which seems to correlate with heat resistance.
5. The change of a resting spore into an actively dividing vegetative cell involves stages of ***activation, germination,*** and ***outgrowth.***

Bacterial Cysts

Members of the genus *Azotobacter* produce distinctive resting cells called ***cysts.*** These structures are resistant to drying but not to heat.

Heat-susceptible Spores, Conidia

1. The dormant structure of the actinomycetes is an asexual spore (sometimes called ***conidium***) formed at the end of cells by fragmentation.
2. These spores are not heat resistant.
3. Specific conditions are necessary for germination.

Heterocysts and Akinetes

1. Some blue-green bacteria form rounded specialized cells known as ***heterocysts.*** These cells arise from ***vegetative*** cells and are the major sites for the utilization of atmospheric nitrogen (nitrogen fixation).
2. Akinetes, or spores, protect blue-green bacteria that form them against drying and freezing.

QUESTIONS FOR REVIEW

1. Distinguish between procaryotic and eucaryotic cells and give representative examples of each.
2. Compare structural similarities and differences between a typical plant cell and a photosynthetic procaryote.
3. Construct a table listing the functions and chemical composition of the following organelles:
   a. bacterial cell wall
   b. capsule
   c. mesosome
   d. pilus
   e. bacterial cell membrane
   f. cilium
   g. bacterial flagellum
   h. thylakoid
   i. phycobilisome
   j. endoplasmic reticulum
   k. ribosome
   l. nucleolus
   m. polyribosome
   n. mitochondrium
   o. gas vacuole
4. Compare the cell walls of Gram-positive and Gram-negative bacteria.
5. Describe the different arrangements found in bacteria. Can these arrangements be utilized for purposes of classification?
6. Identify the morphological arrangements shown in Figure 7–28. Identify any labeled structures as well.

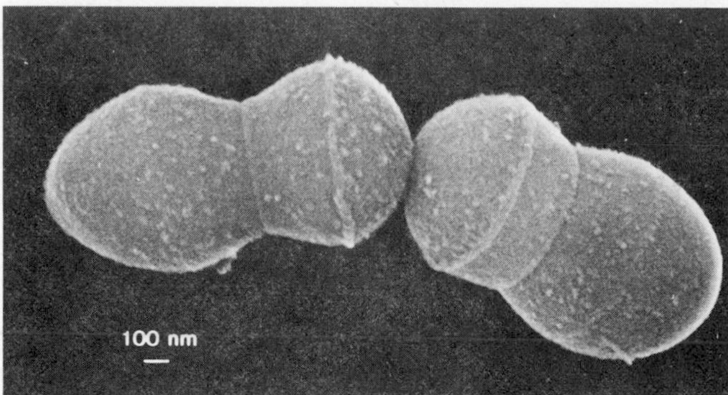

(a)

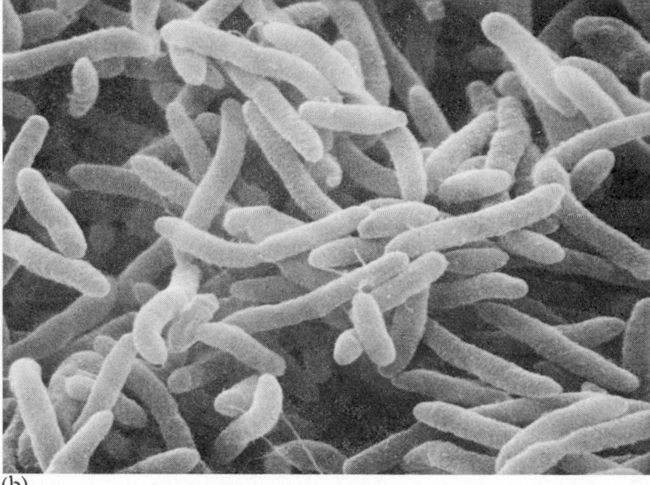

(b)

FIG. 7-28 (a) From *Amako, K. and A. Umeda,* J. Ultrastruct. Res. *58:34–40 (1977).* (b) *Courtesy of Y. Tago, H. Kuraishi, and K. Aida.*

7. What procedure or procedures are necessary to observe the following organisms or organelles?
   a. bacterial spores
   b. cell membranes
   c. flagella
   d. ribosomes
   e. capsules
   f. endoplasmic reticula
   g. mesosomes
   h. mitochondria
8. How does the structure containing the genetic information of bacteria differ from that of a typical animal cell?
9. Compare a bacterial flagellum to one of a eucaryotic cell.
10. a. What is a bacterial spore?
    b. Describe the process of sporulation.
    c. How can bacterial spores be destroyed?
11. Differentiate between a protoplast and a spheroplast.
12. What is the importance of each of the following structures to the virulence of a microorganism, disease transmission, or diagnosis?
    a. bacterial flagella
    b. capsules
    c. pili
    d. cell walls
    e. spores
    f. ribosomes
13. How could one obtain a preparation of cell walls from a bacterial culture?
14. What are L-forms?
15. Identify the bacterial structures indicated in the electron micrograph shown in Figure 7-29.

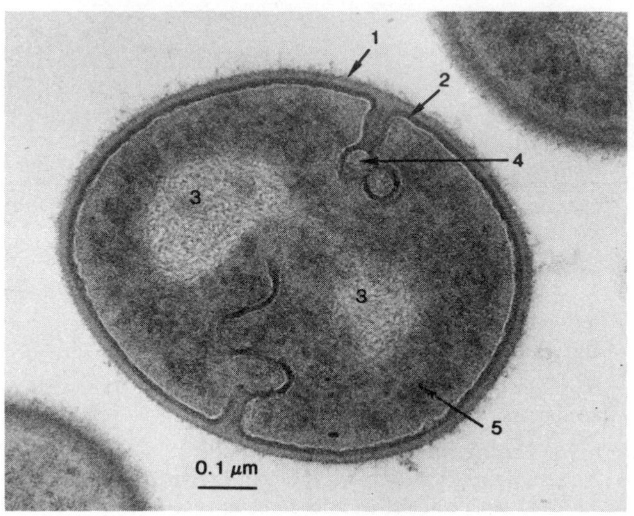

FIG. 7-29 An ultrathin section of *Staphylococcus aureus. Popkin, T. J., et al.,* J. Bacteriol. *107:907 (1971).*

SUGGESTED READINGS

Adler, J., "The Sensing of Chemicals by Bacteria," *Sci. Amer.* 235:40 (1976). *Describes chemotaxis, the capability of motile bacteria to move toward some chemicals and away from others by chemosensors in the cell envelope that can detect chemicals and cause the cell to respond.*

Berg, H. C., "How Bacteria Swim," *Sci. Amer.* 234:36 (1975). *Describes how the bacterial flagellum, a thin helical filament, moves the bacterium, not by waving or beating, but by rotating like propellers driven by a reversible rotary action at their base.*

Canale-Parola, E., "Motility and Chemotaxis of Spirochetes," *Ann. Rev. Microbiol.* 32:69–99 (1978). *A discussion of the unique cellular anatomy and distinctive movement of spirochetes.*

Costerton, J. W., G. G. Geesey, and K. J. Cheng, "How Bacteria Stick," *Sci. Amer.* 239:86 (1978). *Tells how in nature bacteria are covered with a "sheath" of fibers that stick to surfaces and other cells. This adhesion may be prevented by a new kind of antibiotic.*

Salton, M. R. J., and P. Owen, "Bacterial Membrane Structure," *Ann. Rev. Microbiol.* 30:451–482 (1976). *A detailed presentation of the current knowledge and understanding of bacterial membranes and associated transport processes.*

Schwartz, R. M., and M. O. Dayoff, "Origins of Prokaryotes, Eukaryotes, Mitochondria and Chloroplasts," *Science* 194: 395–403 (1978). *A highly detailed article that describes a biological evolutionary tree based on biochemical information that extends back to the earliest of records.*

Walsby, A. E., "The Gas Vacuoles of Blue-green Algae," *Sci. Amer.* 237:90 (1977). *Discussion of how gas vacuoles of the tiny, bacteriumlike blue-green algae help to regulate their buoyancy. The structure and function of these vacuoles is discussed.*

CHAPTER 8 A Survey of Procaryotes

In this chapter we will build upon the information of Chapter 7 by describing a variety of representative bacteria together with their distribution, classification, and activities. Because the cultivation of microorganisms is important in microbiology and several other areas of biology and medicine, we will begin with a brief discussion of the approaches to bacterial cultivation. We will also consider the sources of energy used by bacteria.

After reading this chapter, you should be able to:

1. **List and describe the distinguishing features of the major types of procaryotes.**
2. **List some of the beneficial and harmful effects of bacteria.**
3. **Identify the principal sources of energy used by bacteria.**
4. **Discuss obligate intracellular parasitic procaryotes and their effects on host cells.**
5. **Select and describe the life cycle of one obligate intracellular parasitic procaryote.**
6. **List at least four different environments and describe the types of bacteria found there.**
7. **Define or explain**
   - **a. autotroph**
   - **b. heterotroph**
   - **c. facultative**
   - **d. microaerophilic**
   - **e. chlamydia**
   - **f. colony**
   - **g. culture**
   - **h. medium**
   - **i. chemolitotrophs**
   - **j. algal bloom**

Throughout its history, microbiology has focused on the identification and control of microorganisms and the discovery of their functions. Through the years it has become apparent that many of the metabolic processes of microorganisms such as bacteria are similar to those of cells in higher forms of life. Today it is not unusual to find these rapidly dividing organisms used as models, or "microscopic guinea pigs," in studies of genetics and metabolism. This has stimulated further interest and research directed toward finding new areas in which to apply the wide range of metabolic and other capabilities of microorganisms.

Cultivation of Bacteria

Bacteria grow and reproduce when they are provided with a favorable environment. In the laboratory, cultivation of bacteria involves maintaining appropriate conditions of oxygen, pH, and temperature and supplying nutrients in a usable form. The growth, or *culture,* as it is called, appears after a sufficient incubation period. The resulting accumulation of bacteria on a solid nutrient is called a *colony* (Figure 8–1). Often the physical appearance of a colony—its color or shape—distinguishes a bacterial species (Color Photographs 21 through 26). The ability or inability of bacteria to break down compounds contained in a growth medium may also identify the species (Color Photographs 62, 63 and 65). Later chapters deal with the uses of media in the isolation, growth, and identification of bacteria. Certain bacteria require living cells (hosts) for their activities and survival and are referred to as *obligate intracellular parasites.* In the laboratory, living cells are provided in the form of tissue cultures or whole animals and plants.

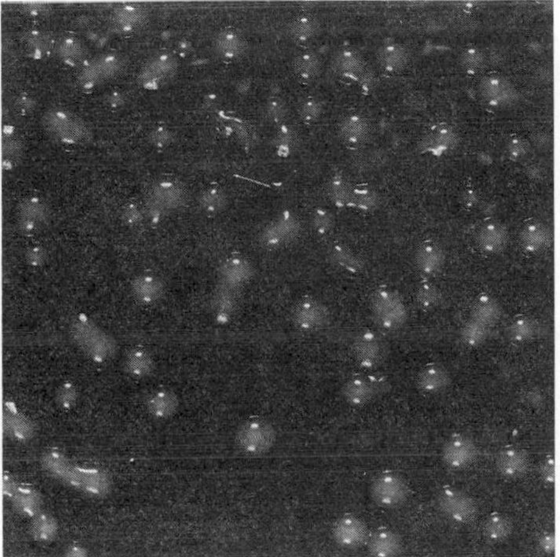

(a)

FIG. 8–1 Bacterial colonial morphology. (a) Colonies of clover nodule bacteria growing on a solid medium in a Petri dish. Each colony is composed of several million bacteria. *Courtesy of The Nitragin Company, Inc.* (b) A scanning electron micrograph of colonial growth showing the arrangement of bacterial rods at the edge of a colony. *Afrikian, E. G., et al.,* Jr. Appl. Microbiol. *26:934–937 (1973).*

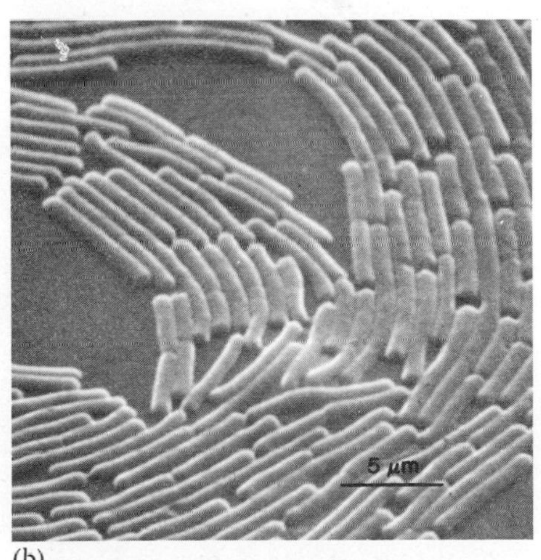

(b)

Representative Procaryotes

Chapter 7 described the differences in structure and organization between bacteria and other forms of life. Here we shall discuss a number of species and their activities to show the widespread distribution and major contributions of this microbial group.

In their natural habitats, bacteria associate with other bacteria or with different microbial types (Figure 8–2). Such relationships may be either beneficial or harmful to the forms of life involved. Fortunately, most bacteria are harmless, and many perform functions that are favorable to humans and other forms of life. These include

1. aiding the digestive processes of animals
2. decomposing organic material
3. producing and flavoring foods
4. returning chemical elements to the soil for use by plants.

The functions of bacteria are so important that if they were to stop, all animals and plants would soon become extinct.

There are several detailed classifications of bacteria. One of these, the 1974

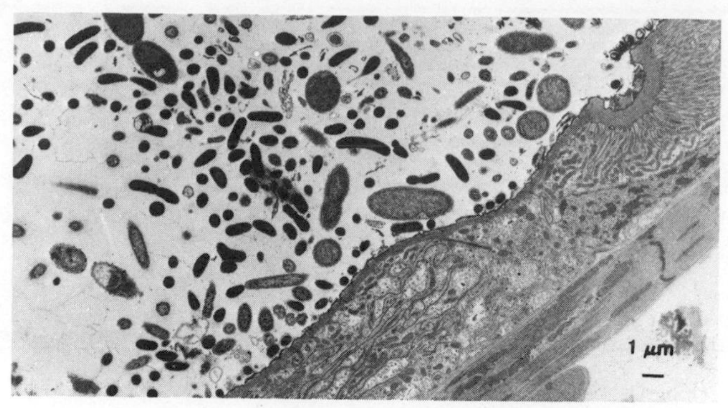

FIG. 8-2 A wide variety of bacteria are closely associated with the digestive system of a termite. Such an association is believed to enable the termite and the bacteria to exchange nutrients to the benefit of both. *Breznak, J., and H. S. Pankrantz,* Appl. Environ. Microbiol. *33:406-426 (1977).*

edition of ***Bergey's Manual of Determinative Bacteriology,*** lists 1576 recognized species belonging to 245 genera. These organisms and hundreds more of unknown taxonomic status are divided into 19 parts. Table 8-1 shows this arrangement together with descriptions of the bacteria belonging to each part. (A

TABLE 8-1 A Description of the Bacteria

Part[a]	*Category*	*General Description*	*Number of Genera*	*Representative Genera*[b]
1	Phototrophic bacteria	Gram-negative, spherical or rod-shaped bacteria; multiplication is by binary fission and/or budding; they are photosynthetic without producing oxygen; pigments are purple, purple-violet, red, orange-brown, brown, or green	18	*Chromatium, Rhodomicrobium*
2	Gliding bacteria	Gram-negative rods typically embedded in a tough slime coat; they are capable of a slow gliding movement; reproduction is by binary fission; gliding bacteria sometimes form colorful fruiting bodies	27	*Beggiatoa, Cytophaga, Leucothrix*
3	Sheathed bacteria	Gram-negative rods that occur in chains within a thin sheath; they sometimes have a holdfast cell for attachment to surfaces	7	*Crenothrix, Leptothrix, Sphaerotilus*
4	Budding and/or appendaged bacteria	Bacteria with rod-, oval-, egg-, or bean-shaped filamentous growth; multiplication is by budding or binary fission; these bacteria sometimes have a holdfast cell	17	*Caulobacter, Hyphomicrobium*
5	Spirochetes	Slender, flexible, coiled cells; they may occur in chains and exhibit transverse fission	5	*Borrelia,*[b] *Cristispira, Leptospira,*[b,c] *Treponema*[b,c]
6	Spiral and curved bacteria	Rigid, helically curved rods with less than one complete turn to many turns	6	*Bdellovibrio,*[c] *Campylocabacter,*[c] *Microcyclus, Spirillum*[c]
7	Gram-negative aerobic rods and cocci	Rods that are usually motile, with polar flagella; bluntly rod-shaped to oval cells, some of which are motile by polar or peritrichous flagella and some of which are cyst formers; and rods and cocci that require high concentrations of sodium chloride for growth	20	*Acetobacter, Alcaligenes,*[c] *Agrobacterium, Azotobacter,*[b] *Bordetella,*[b,c] *Brucella,*[b,c] *Francisella,*[b,c] *Halobacterium, Pseudomonas*[b,c]
8	Gram-negative facultatively anaerobic rods	Straight and curved rods; some are nonmotile; others are motile by polar or peritrichate flagella; all members are non-sporeformers; some have special growth requirements	26	*Citrobacter,*[c] *Edwardsiella, Enterobacter,*[c] *Escherichia,*[b,c] *Haemophilus,*[b,c] *Klebsiella,*[b,c] *Pasteurella,*[b,c] *Salmonella,*[b,c] *Serratia,*[b,c] *Shigella,*[b,c] *Streptobacillus,*[c] *Vibrio,*[b,c] *Yersinia*[b,c]
9	Gram-negative anaerobic rods	Strict (obligate) anaerobic, non-spore-forming organisms; some members are motile; pleomorphism (variation in shape) occurs	9	*Bacteroides,*[b,c] *Desulfovibrio, Fusobacterium,*[b] *Leptotrichia*
10	Gram-negative cocci and coccal bacilli	Cocci, characteristically occuring in pairs; adjacent sides of the cells may be flattened; organisms are not flagellated	6	*Acinetobacter,*[c] *Branhamella,*[c] *Moraxella,*[b,c] *Neisseria*[b,c]

more detailed classification can be found in Appendix A and in some of the texts listed in the Suggested Readings for this chapter.) Not only have more bacteria now been found and classified, but various studies have shown the remarkable similarity between bacteria and the procaryotic blue-green algae, or cyanobacteria. The growing trend is to consider both procaryotic groups of bacteria and to classify them into a new kingdom, namely Procaryotae.

Different procaryotes use different compounds to supply their needed carbon and energy. At one end of the spectrum are the **heterotrophs.** These are organisms that require certain preformed organic compounds for their nutrition. At the other end are the **autotrophs.** Autotrophs are noted for their ability to exploit specialized and often unconventional sources of carbon and energy. Autotrophs that use inorganic compounds such as carbon dioxide as their carbon source thrive best in soil and aquatic environments. Heterotrophs grow well in any habitat having a source of organic and other nutrients.

Certain heterotrophic bacteria can invade, multiply in, and carry out their life processes at the expense of a susceptible animal, plant, or other microorganism. These organisms may grow in the presence of free oxygen (aerobic), or in the absence of free oxygen (anaerobic). **Facultative** bacteria are able to adjust to various environmental conditions.

Part[a]	*Category*	*General Description*	*Number of Genera*	*Representative Genera*[b]
11	Gram-negative anaerobic cocci	Cocci of variable size and characteristically in pairs; they are not flagellated	3	*Veillonella*[c]
12	Gram negative chemolithotrophic bacteria	Pleomorphic rods; these organisms use inorganic materials for energy	17	*Nitrobacter,*[b] *Nitrococcus,*[b] *Thiobacillus*[b]
13	Methane-producing bacteria	Rods or cocci; some members are Gram-positive, others are Gram-negative; all are anaerobic and produce methane	3	*Methanobacterium,*[b] *Methanococcus, Methanosarcina*
14	Gram-positive cocci	Various arrangements of cocci that are aerobic, facultative, or anaerobic	12	*Aerococcus,*[c] *Micrococcus, Peptococcus, Sarcina, Staphylococcus,*[b,c] *Streptococcus*[b,c]
15	Endospore-forming rods and cocci	Members are aerobic, facultatively anaerobic, or anaerobic; most members are Gram-positive	6	*Bacillus,*[b] *Clostridium,*[b,c] *Sporosarcina*
16	Gram-positive asporogenous (non-spore-forming) rod-shaped bacteria	Members may be aerobic, facultatively anaerobic, or anaerobic	4	*Erysipelothrix,*[c] *Lactobacillus,*[b] *Listeria*[b,c]
17	Actinomycetes and related organisms	Rods or pleomorphic rods, with filamentous and branching filaments; included are aerobic, facultatively anaerobic, and anaerobic rods; these organisms are usually Gram-positive, and some are acid-alcohol-fast (acid-fast)	39	*Actinomyces,*[c] *Arachnia, Arthrobacter, Bifidobacterium,*[b,c] *Corynebacterium,*[b,c] *Mycobacterium,*[b,c] *Nocardia,*[c] *Propionibacterium, Streptomyces*[b]
18	Rickettsia	The majority of cells are Gram-negative coccoid or pleomorphic rods; most are obligate intracellular parasites transmitted by arthropods	18	*Chlamydia,*[b,c] *Cowdria, Coxiella,*[b,c] *Ehrlichia, Neorickettsia, Rickettsia,*[b,c] *Rickettsiella, Rochalimaea,*[c] *Symbiotes*
19	Mycoplasma	Highly pleomorphic, Gram negative organisms that contain no cell wall; they reproduce by fission, by production of many small bodies, or by budding; members may be aerobic, facultatively (adaptable) anaerobic, or anaerobic	4	*Acholeplasma, Mycoplasma,*[b,c] *Spiroplasma, Thermoplasma*

[a]Based on the divisions and descriptions in Buchanan, R. E., and Gibbons, N. E., eds., *Bergey's Manual of Determinative Bacteriology.* 8th ed. Baltimore. Williams & Wilkins, 1974.
[b]Genera discussed in various chapters of this text.
[c]Medically important species are contained in this genus.

Heterotrophic Bacteria

Procaryotes that require organic compounds as sources of energy comprise a large and diverse group. Heterotrophic bacteria show a wide variety of shapes, sizes, colonial forms (Figure 8–3 and Color Photographs 21 and 23), cellular structures, cellular arrangements, and means of movement. Many heterotrophs have been studied extensively and are known to exert a profound influence on their environments.

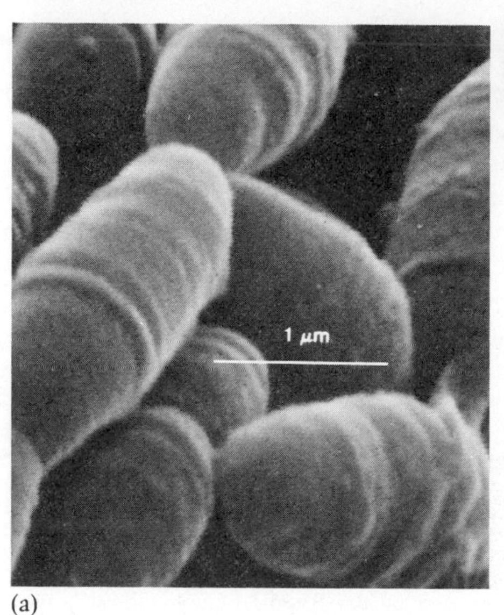

(a)

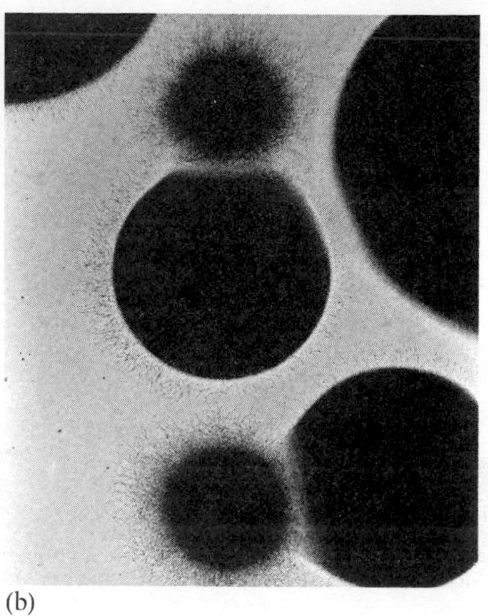
(b)

FIG. 8–3 Some unusual features of heterotrophic bacteria. (a) A scanning micrograph of the anaerobe *Bifidobacterium bifidum*, a normal inhabitant of the human intestine. Note the shape and general appearance of individual cells. The ridges on cells represent cross wall formations. *Bauer, H., et al.,* Can. J. Microbiol. *21:1305–1316 (1975).* (b) Unusual colonies of *Oerskovia xanthineolytica*. The branched appearance of these colonies is due to rodlike elements, which are Gram-positive and motile. Sources of this heterotrophic organism include soil, dry grass cuttings, and medically associated environments. *Sottnek, F. O., et al.,* Internat. J. Syst. Bacteriol. *27:263–270 (1977).*

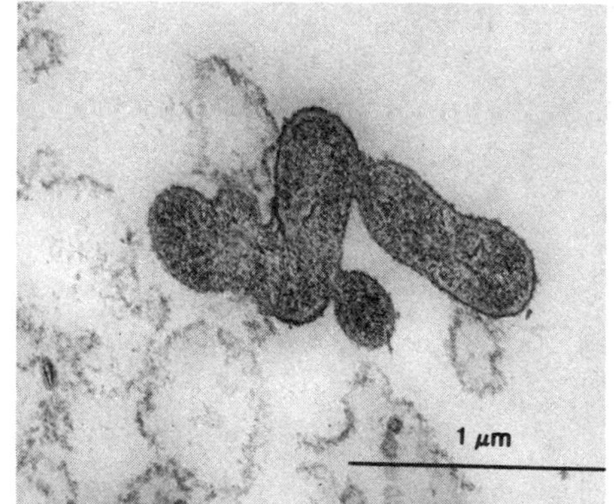

FIG. 8–4 The appearance of *Mycoplasma* HT grown in tissue culture. Note the variation in shape—rod, oval, and spherical. Refer to Color Photograph 00 for the appearance of *Mycoplasma* colonies. *Dmochowski, L., et al., The University of Texas, M. D. Anderson Hospital, and Tumor Institute at Houston Texas Medical Center,* Ann. N.Y. Acad. Sci. *143:578–607 (1967). © The New York Academy of Sciences; 1967; Reprinted by permission.*

The Mycoplasma and Related Organisms

The term **mycoplasma** refers to a group of microorganisms previously known as pleuropneumonia-like organisms, or PPLO. The many different isolates of this group have been separated from other bacteria in the class Mollicutes and catalogued into the genera *Acholeplasma, Anaeroplasma, Mycoplasma, Spiroplasma, Thermoplasma,* and *Ureaplasma* (T-strains) (Table 8-2). Mycoplasmas are medically important microorganisms, as they include the causative agents of a variety of animal and plant diseases. For example, *Mycoplasma pneumoniae* is the cause of one form of pneumonia. Mycoplasmas have been found in soil, sewage, rumens of cattle and sheep, hot and highly acidic coal piles, and as contaminants in tissue cultures used for virus studies and vaccines.

The mycoplasmas, among the smallest and simplest self-replicating procaryotes, are distinguished from all other bacteria by the absence of a cell wall (Figure 8–4). The mycoplasma cell is bounded by a single lipoprotein cell membrane and contains only the minimum set of organelles essential for growth and replication. Different species in this group have characteristic shapes.

These microorganisms use amino acids, carbohydrates, and other growth factors. Species of *Anaeroplasma, Mycoplasma, Spiroplasma,* and *Ureaplasma* require blood serum, a source of sterols such as cholesterol, which they cannot manufacture themselves (Table 8–2). The sterols help stabilize cell membranes and protect the organisms against osmotic destruction. With agar media, the mycoplasma grow down into the preparation, often producing colonies that look rather like fried eggs (Color Photograph 23).

TABLE 8-2 Genera of the Class Mollicutes

Genus	*Habitat*	*Sterol Required For Growth*
Mycoplasma	Animals	Yes
Acholeplasma	Saprophyte[a]	No
Ureaplasma (T-strains)	Animals	Yes
Spiroplasma	Plants, insects	Yes
Thermoplasma	Burning coal refuse piles	No
Anaeroplasma	Animals	Yes

[a]Obtains its nutrients from rotting and decaying organic matter.

Gliding Bacteria

Heterotrophs are not the only procaryotes that show a gliding form of movement. Some autotrophs glide, including photosynthesizers such as blue-green and green bacteria and nonphotosynthesizers such as ***Thiothrix***. Gliding motility is slow, occurs only when organisms are in contact with a solid surface, and usually involves secretion of a slime track. A number of filament-forming bacteria (organisms consisting of individual cells in a common outer cell wall) exhibit this type of movement. These include the genera of ***Flexibacter*** and ***Leucothrix*** (Figure 8-5a and c). Both groups of organisms are found in marine environments.

Although the mechanism of gliding motility is not known, a number of hypotheses have been proposed. Recent studies have show the presence of long fibers with goblet-shaped units ***(goblets)*** (Figure 8-5b) on the surfaces of gliding ***Flexibacter***. These may be important to the movement of these organisms or to the sticking of cells to solid surfaces.

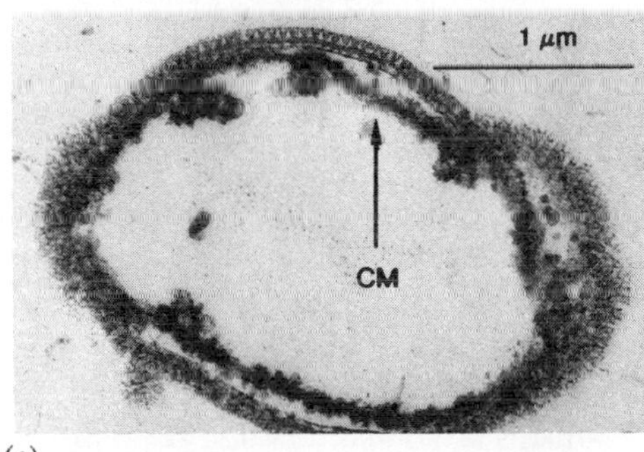

(a)

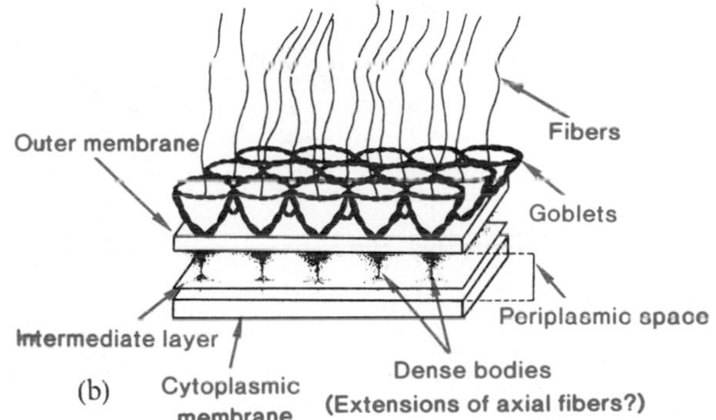

(b)

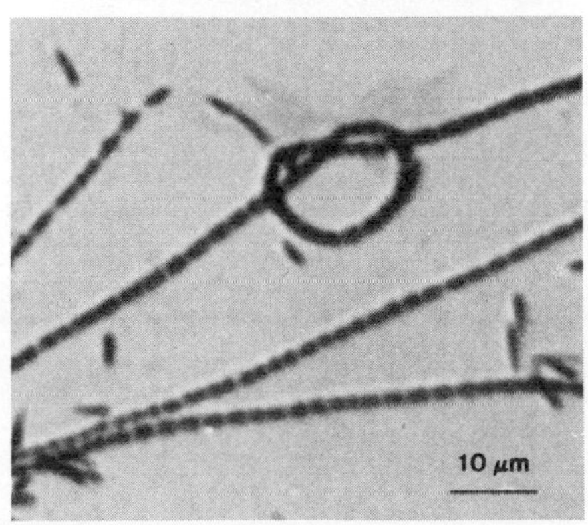

(c)

FIG. 8-5 Gliding bacteria. (a) An outer array of goblet shaped subunits ***on Flexibacter***, which serve as a continuous source of sticky fibers. These units and their associated secretions play a role in bacterial attachment and possibly in the gliding movement. The cytoplasmic membrane (CM) of the organism is also shown. (b) A diagrammatic representation of the goblets and long fibers. ***Reproduced with the permission of the National Research Council of Canada from Ridgeway, H. F., et al.***, Can. J. Microbiol. *21:1733–1750 (1975)*. (c) Filaments of ***Leucothrix*** may form knots when nutrients are plentiful, causing the filament to grow rapidly. ***Raj, H. D.***, CRC Critical Rev. Microbiol. *5:271–304 (1977)*.

Sheathed Bacteria

A limited number of aquatic procaryotes form a specialized covering known as a **sheath** (Figure 8–6a). The presence of a sheath enables organisms to attach themselves to solid surfaces and offers protection against predators. Several bacterial genera are noted for sheath-forming ability. These include *Chlonothrix, Crenothrix, Lieskeella, Phragmidiothrix, Sphaerotilus,* and the *Sphaerotilus-Leptothrix* group (Figure 8–6b). The bacteria of this last group often form sheaths surrounded by a slime layer. This outer layer is closely connected with their iron-accumulating and storing capacity (Figure 8–6c) and with their use of manganese for energy and growth. When environmental conditions become unfavorable, the sheathed bacteria form rounded cells known as *gonidia* (Figure 8–6d). These are released from the end of cellular filaments.

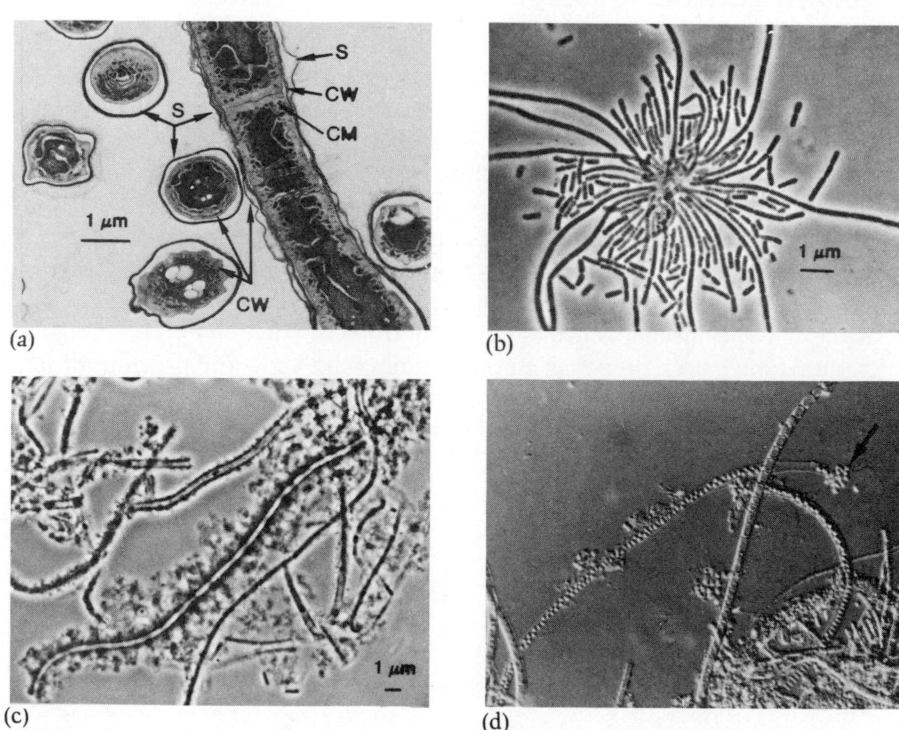

FIG. 8–6 Sheathed bacteria. (a) The relationship of the sheath (S), cell wall (CW), and cell membrane (CM) are clearly shown from different views of these organisms. *Deinema, M. H., S. Henstra, and E. W. von Elgg,* Antonie van Leeuwenhoek *43:19–29 (1977).* (b) Many trichomes of *Leptothrix lopholea* radiating from common holdfasts. (c) *Leptothrix cholodnii* sheaths covered with ferric chloride. *(b and c) van Veen, W. L., et al.,* Microbiol. Revs. *42:329–356 (1978).* (d) The masses of cell filaments of this bacterium *Crenothrix polyspora* can block water pipes and wells. The sheaths surrounding the cells (gonida) of the filaments are visible here. *Volker, H., et al.,* J. Bacteriol. *131:306–313 (1977).*

Sheathed bacteria are widely distributed in nature. They are found in sewage, soil, and water. Some of these organisms are noted for their contamination of water pipes and the formation of slimy masses of cell filaments.

Stalked and Budding Procaryotes (The Prosthecate Bacteria)

Several procaryotes with complex structures and morphologically distinctive cell cycles are found in fresh- and salt-water environments. Among the most interesting of these are bacteria with cell wall extensions that contain cytoplasm. These projections (Figure 8–7a), which appear during cell cycles, are called *prostheca.* In organisms such as *Caulobacter* species, the prosthecae help to attach the bacteria to cells or to nonliving substances and surfaces. Sticky material on the prosthecate structure, or stalk, aids in the cellular attachment.

The cell cycles of several prosthecate bacteria result in the formation of different cell types.

CAULOBACTER

The division cycle of *Caulobacter* differs significantly from those typical of most bacteria. Stalked cells divide to produce two structurally different cells (Figure 8–7b). One cell keeps the stalk; the other becomes a flagellated swarmer cell without a stalk. After separation, the swarmer cell does not divide until it, too, has developed a stalk.

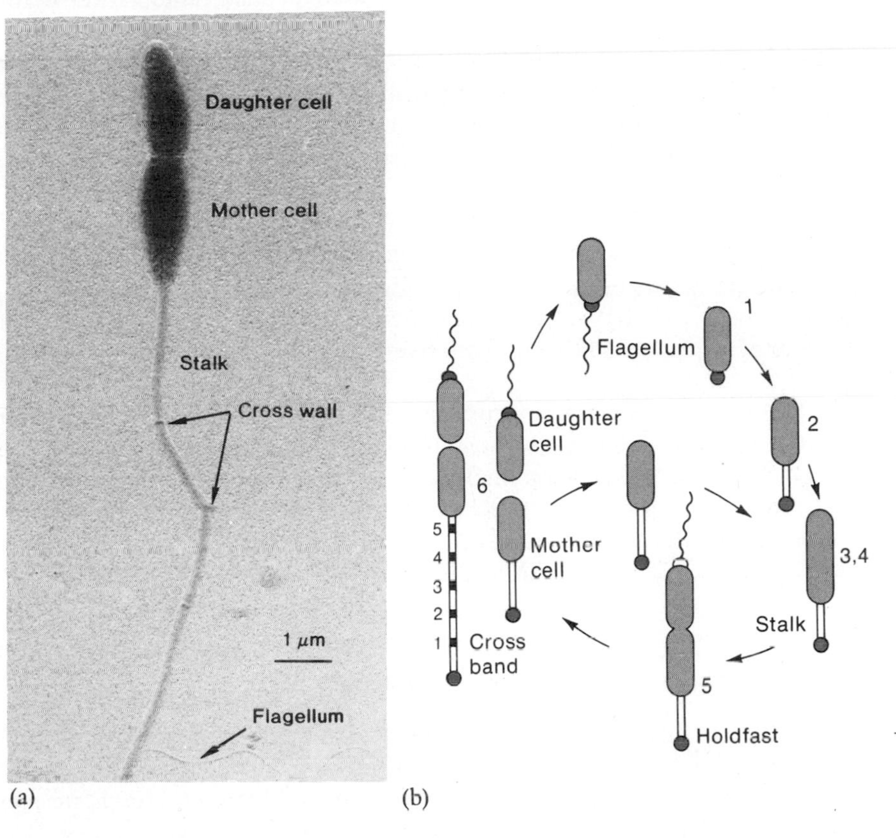

FIG. 8–7 The *Caulobacter* and related species. (a) An electron micrograph showing the various components of a *Caulobacter* species. (b) The cell cycle of *Caulobacter*, starting with the motile swarm cell stage. Note the loss of the flagellum (1), stalk formation (2), swarm cell production (3, 4), flagellum and holdfast synthesis (5), and cell division to produce a stalked cell and a swarm cell (6). *Whittenbury, R., and C. S. Dow,* Bacteriol. Rev. *41:754–808 (1977).*

HYPHOMICROBIUM (A BUDDING PROCARYOTE)

Species of *Hyphomicrobium* and of the related photosynthetic *Rhodomicrobium* have a division cycle different from that of *Caulobacter.* Reproduction of these organisms occurs by the formation of a bud either directly from the main, or mother, cell or at the tip of a filament (Figure 8–8). Buds are flagellated and normally detach from the main cell. Upon separation, only one cell has a filament.

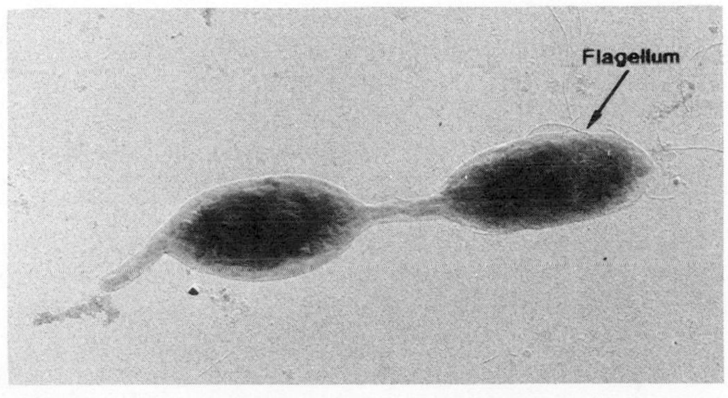

(b)

FIG. 8–8 A budding bacterium *Rhodomicrobium vannielii.* (a) An electron micrograph showing the components of a budding organism. (b) A cell cycle starting with a swarm cell. Note that a filament forms before each and every daughter cell. Specific stages show the formation of a thin outgrowth (1), the enlargement of the outgrowth or the formation of a bud (2), the formation of flagella by the bud (3), the breaking away of the flagellated bud (4), the swimming away of the flagellated bud to start cycle again (5), and a new bud formation on the original cell that began the cycle (6). *(a and b) Whittenbury, R., and C. S. Dow,* Bacteriol. Rev. *41:754–808 (1977).*

Spiral and Curved Bacteria

Spiral bacteria are heterotrophic organisms with a unique cellular anatomy and distinctive forms of movement. Spirochetes (Figure 8–9), spirilla, and curved rods such as *Campylobacter* species are such procaryotes. These organisms grow in a wide range of natural habitats including fresh and marine bodies of water, mud, and internal and external body surfaces of humans and other animals. A small number of spiral bacteria cause diseases such as leptospirosis, syphilis (Color Photograph 27), and relapsing fever.

A spirochete is a flexible helical bacterium with a coiled protoplasmic cylinder that consists of the cytoplasmic and nuclear regions surrounded by a plasma–cell wall complex. Wound around the cylinder are axial fibrils (Figure 7–16). Because of their particular structure, spirochetes can move in liquid environments without being in contact with solid surfaces. Some spirochetes also exhibit a creeping or crawling movement on solid surfaces, similar to the locomotion of gliding bacteria.

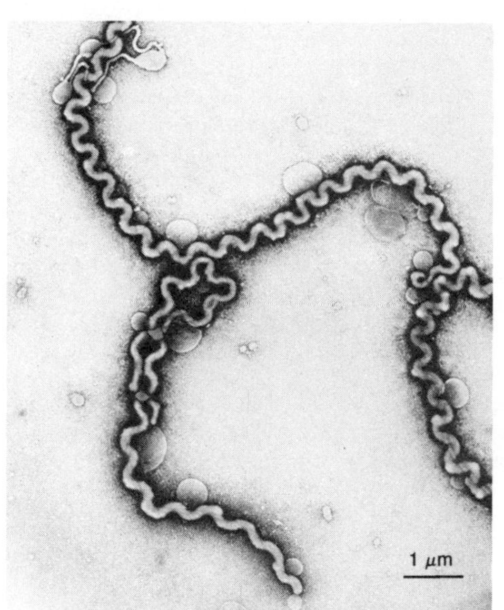

FIG. 8–9 Negatively stained cells of *Leptospira canicola*. Note the smooth, coiled shape of these organisms. *Anderson, D. L., and R. C. Johnson*, J. Bacteriol. *95:2293–2309 (1968).*

Despite basic similarity of structure, many differences exist among spirochetes. Spirochetes can be aerobic, facultatively anaerobic, or strictly anaerobic. The general properties of five genera of spirochetes are given in Table 8–3.

Spirilla have rigid cell walls and one or more flagella at one or both ends (Color Photograph 14). Most spirilla are free-living, but one species is a human pathogen.

Members of *Campylobacter* are curved, spiral rods. Some species form chains and appear ribbon-shaped. These organisms are Gram-negative, require small amounts of oxygen *(microaerophilic)*, have a single flagellum at one or both ends of their cells, and move with a characteristic corkscrew motion. They are found in the mouths and intestines of humans and other animals. One species is known to cause abortion in cattle and a variety of disease in humans.

The Obligate Intracellular Procaryotes

Many bacteria require other living cells for their development and reproduction. Some species require eucaryotic animal and plant cells, while other species utilize procaryotes. The properties of a few well-known groups are presented here.

TABLE 8–3 General Properties of Spirochete Genera

Genus	*Properties*
Borrelia	Generally anaerobic or microaerophilic; species cause relapsing fever in humans and other animals; lice or ticks spread the disease agents
Cristispira	Large spirochetes, usually found in the digestive tracts of many fresh-water and marine molluscs[a]
Leptospira	Strictly (obligate) aerobic; usually found free-living in soil or surface waters or in association with humans and other animals; some species cause disease
Spirochaeta	Most are anaerobic; usually found as free-living forms in aquatic environments
Treponema	Anaerobes; found in genital areas, the intestinal tract, or mouths of humans and other animals; many species are normally present in healthy individuals; others are disease producing

[a]The genus *Pillotina* is a recently proposed designation for the large spirochetes normally present in termite intestinal tracts.

BDELLOVIBRIOS

In 1962, an interesting parasitic relationship between bacteria was observed. *Bdellovibrio bacteriovorus*, an aerobic, flagellated, Gram-negative vibrio (comma-shaped) was found to attack certain host bacteria for its benefit. The generic name for this attacking bacteria indicates the organism's behavior. *Bdello* comes from the Greek word referring to "leech." These organisms are now known to be widely distributed in soil and sewage.

Bdellovibrio attacks its prey by striking the host cell surface at a high velocity (Figure 8–10). It penetrates the cell wall with a spinning motion and with the aid of cell wall digestive enzymes. In the process, the parasite's flagellum is left behind. The invading organism situates itself between its host's cell wall and plasma membrane. Here the *Bdellovibrio* uses partially degraded host components to grow and reproduce. Newly formed offspring leave the host cell to find new susceptible bacteria in which to repeat this parasitic cycle. In cultures containing hosts and parasites, *Bdellovibrio* destroys the host cells. This results in clear, circular areas known as plaques (Color Photograph 28).

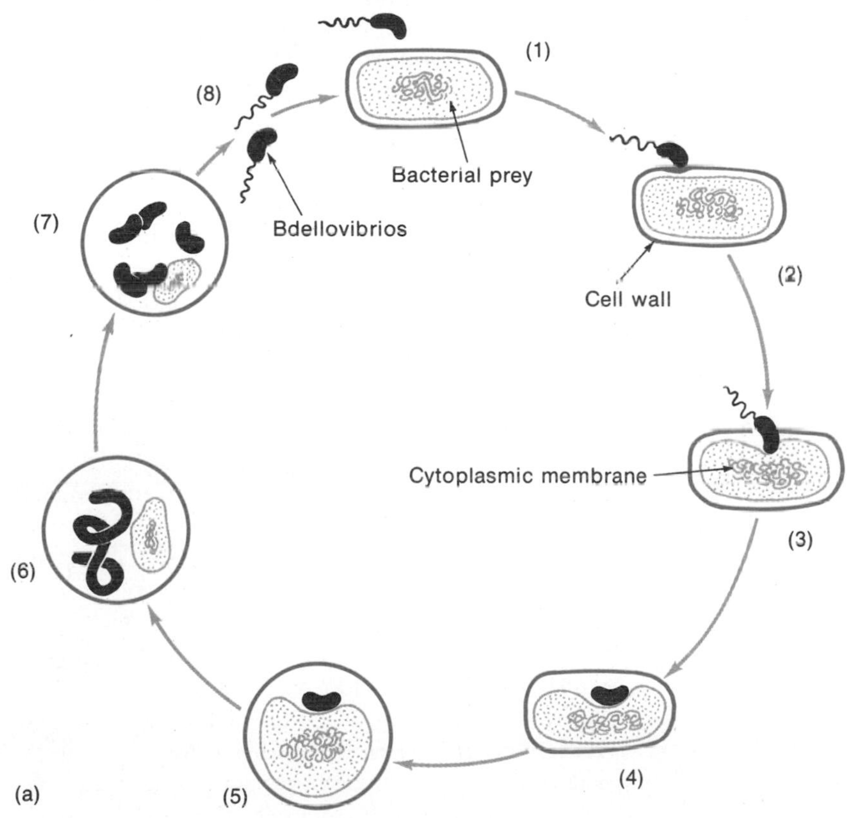

FIG. 8–10 *Bdellovibrio*. (a) The stages in the life cycle of this parasitic bacterium. See Color Photograph 28 for the appearance of plaques, the evidence of host cell destruction. The stages of the cycle show the approach to the susceptible host (1), *Bdellovibrio* attachment (2), penetration of host cell by the invading *Bdellovibrio* (3), the situation of the invader in the host bacterium between the host's cell wall and plasma membrane (4 and 5), the use of the host for the production of new *Bdellovibrio* cells (6 and 7), and the release of newly formed *Bdellovibrio* cells (8).

(b) After the parasite has penetrated its host (H), it will use the nutrients there for reproductive purposes. Eventually the host will break open, releasing newly formed *Bdellovibrio*. *Abram, et al.*, J. Bacteriol. *118:663 (1974)*.

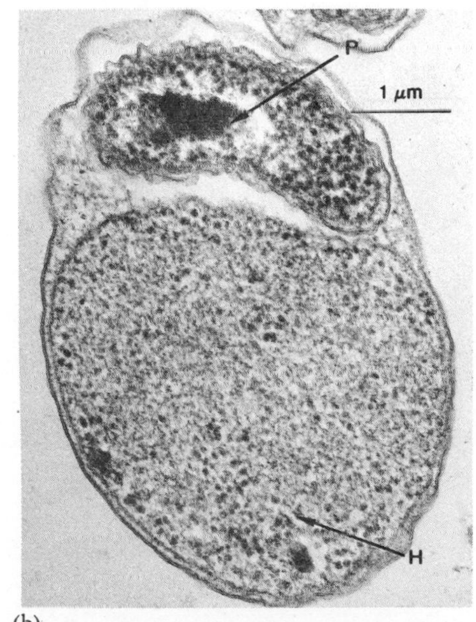

(b)

CHLAMYDIAE

The genus *Chlamydia* consists of procaryotic microorganisms that invade and use eucaryotic cells for their own survival (Figure 8–11). Because of this parasitic property, these microbes were once considered viruses. However, they are different from viruses in that chlamydia use their own ribosomes and enzymes for the formation of protein and nucleic acids; they depend on their host cells only for certain growth factors. Viruses, on the other hand, are totally dependent on host cells for their development.

Because they can survive only by parasitism and because of their ability to infect humans and other animals, chlamydia cause a number of diseases. These include the respiratory infection psittacosis, or parrot fever, trachoma, a leading cause of blindness in the world, and the venereal disease lymphogranuloma venereum. *Chlamydia psittaci* is the causative agent of respiratory infections; different strains of *C. trachomatis* cause the other diseases mentioned. A chlamydial organism is also the suspected cause of the famous Legionnaire's disease (Figure 8–11b and Color Photograph 22).

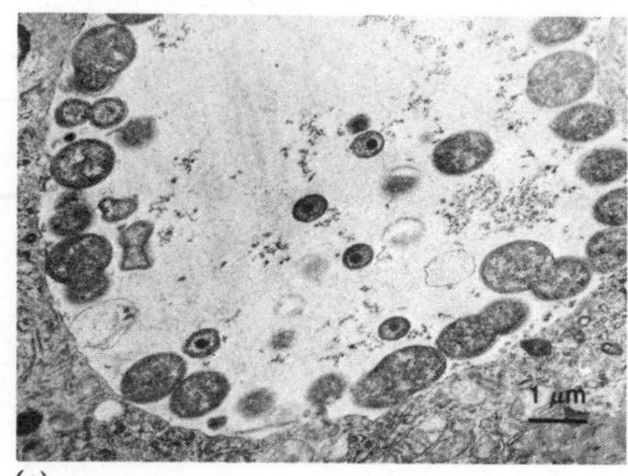

(a)

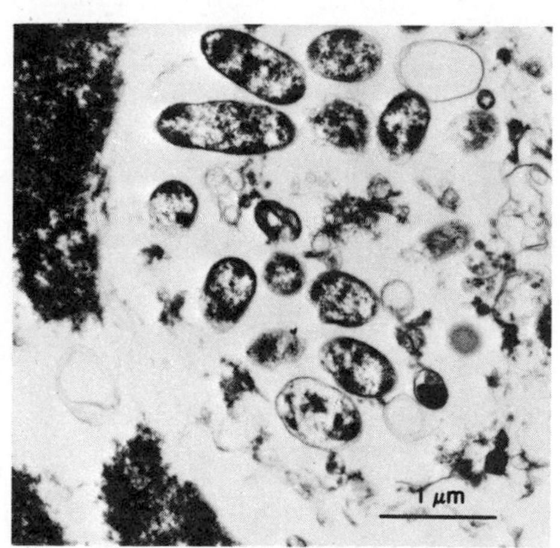

(b)

FIG. 8–11 Chlamydia develop only in the cytoplasm of eucaryotic cells, a property resembling that of animal and plant viruses. (a) This electron micrograph shows the appearance of *Chlamydia trachomatis* in a eucaryotic cell. *Becker*, Y., Microbiol. Revs. *42:274–306 (1978)*. (b) Another chlamydia, the cause of Legionnaire's disease. Note the intracellular location of these bacteria. *Courtesy Center for Disease Control, Atlanta, Georgia.*

Chemical and morphological analyses show that chlamydiae are Gram-negative coccoid forms, inhibited by a variety of antibiotics including penicillin. In addition, the cycle of this particular group was found to be unique among procaryotes. This cycle is started by extracellular, sporelike particles with a rigid cell wall, known as ***elementary bodies***. After entering the host cell, usually through phagocytosis, the elementary body develops into a second form, known as the ***initial***, or ***reticulate***, body. Proteins, nucleic acids, and other macromolecules are produced in these bodies, leading to the formation of a new group of infectious elementary bodies. These agents reinitiate the infection cycle. In the laboratory, tissue cultures are used for their cultivation.

RICKETTSIA

Rickettsia have been responsible for the deaths of millions of people during times of war and natural disasters. It has been claimed that Napoleon's defeat in Russia in 1812 was brought about by typhus fever (a well-known rickettsial disease). This infection struck again during World War I, killing more than 3 millon soldiers and civilians. Even during World War II and the Korean conflict, epidemics threatened the outcome of several military operations.

These microscopic forms were named after Howard Taylor Ricketts, who first isolated the agent causing Rocky Mountain spotted fever. He died in Mexico City in 1910, while studying typhus fever. The genus designation for most of these procaryotes is *Rickettsia*. At one time rickettsia were classified somewhere between bacteria and viruses. However, within the last fifteen years, it has become clear that they are a very special form of bacteria having definite requirements. All rickettsia, with the exception of the causative agent of Trench fever, *Rickettsia quintana*, are obligate intracellular parasites; that is, they must have living, susceptible cells for growth and multiplication (Figure 8–12). This property distinguishes them from most other bacteria.

Rickettsia can infect a wide range of natural hosts including arthropods (fleas, mites, and ticks) (Figure 3–4b), birds, and mammals. Members of the genera *Cowdria, Ehrlichia*, and *Neorickettsia* are pathogenic for some mammals. For example, *E. canis* causes a serious disease in dogs (Figure 3–4a). *Cowdria* species cause heartwater, a blood disease of cattle, goats, and sheep. *Neorickettsia* are involved in a complicated worm-borne disease of canines. Characteristically, most of these microorganisms are transmitted from vertebrate host to vertebrate host by an arthropod, referred to as a **vector.** Some rickettsia may be passed on from one generation of arthropods to the next, by introduction into eggs. The public health dangers posed by rickettsia have stimulated research in the production of antibiotics, insecticides, and vaccines.

Although many rickettsia are pathogenic, there are also several apparently nonpathogenic species. Rickettsia belonging to the genera of *Rickettsiella* and *Symbiotes* do not harm their insect hosts and appear to be essential for development and reproduction. This situation may be due to the establishment of a mutually beneficial relationship **(mutualism).** Relatively little is known about these nonpathogenic rickettsia.

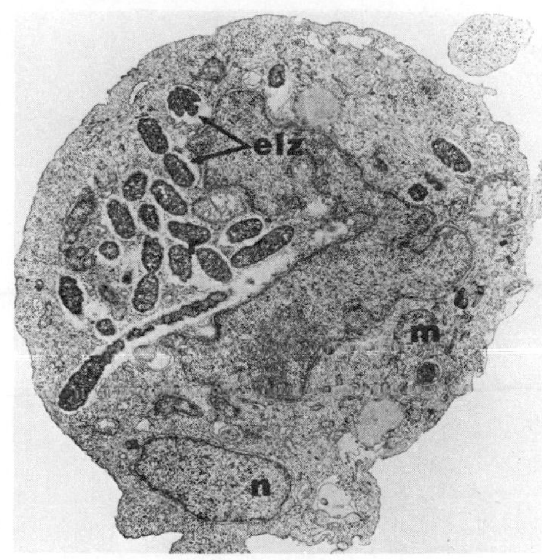

FIG. 8-12 A tissue culture cell infected with *Rickettsia prowazeki* (R) the cause of the rickettsial disease typhus fever. *Courtesy of Drs. David J. Silverman and Charles L. Wisseman, Jr., Department of Microbiology, University of Maryland School of Medicine.*

Autotrophs

Organisms that can obtain the energy they need for growth from inorganic compounds are called **chemoautotrophs** or **chemolitotrophs.** They require very specific inorganic materials, such as ammonia, ferrous iron (FE^{2+}), molecular hydrogen, nitrate (NO_3^-), and various forms of sulfur. These microorganisms are found in a wide variety of environments (Figure 8–13 and Color Photograph 66).

Related procaryotes include methylotrophs (Figure 3–11) and phototrophs. The methylotrophs can use methane and other one-carbon compounds. Phototrophs are noted for their photosynthetic activity.

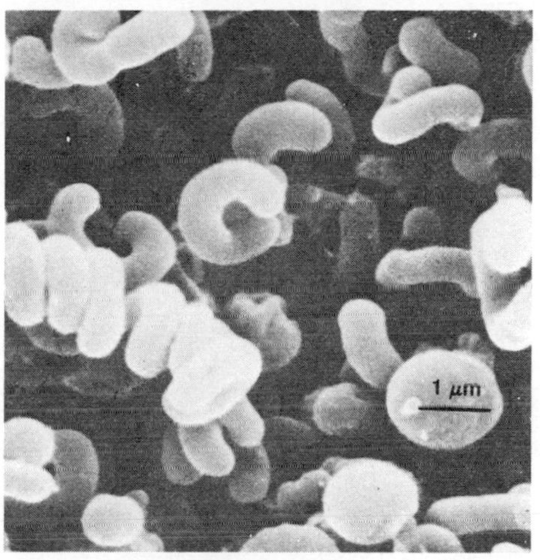

FIG. 8-13 A scanning micrograph of the ring-forming bacteria *Microcyclus marinus.* These "doughnut-shaped," Gram-negative, marine bacteria are widespread in nature. *Raj, H. D.,* Internat. J. Syst. Bacteriol. *26:528–544 (1976).*

The Phototrophs

The phototrophic procaryotes include those bacteria that are capable of using environments that contain inorganic sources of carbon. Three distinct and well-defined groups of Gram-negative phototrophs are recognized: the cyanophyta (blue-green bacteria), the green bacteria, and the purple bacteria. The photosynthetic pigments of these three groups distinguish them.

Photosynthesis by green and purple bacteria (Figure 8–14) or by other related anaerobic organisms does not produce oxygen **(anoxygenic photosynthesis).** The blue-green bacteria, on the other hand, do produce oxygen as a by-product of photosynthesis. Table 8–4 lists other differences between these phototrophic groups.

BLUE-GREEN BACTERIA (CYANOBACTERIA)

Blue-green bacteria (cyanobacteria) represent the largest, most diverse, and most widely distributed group of photosynthetic bacteria. The cyanobacteria are found in a wide variety of environments. Some grow freely in snow on high mountain tops. Others thrive in thermal springs, such as those found in Yellowstone National Park, where the temperature may be as high as 85°C

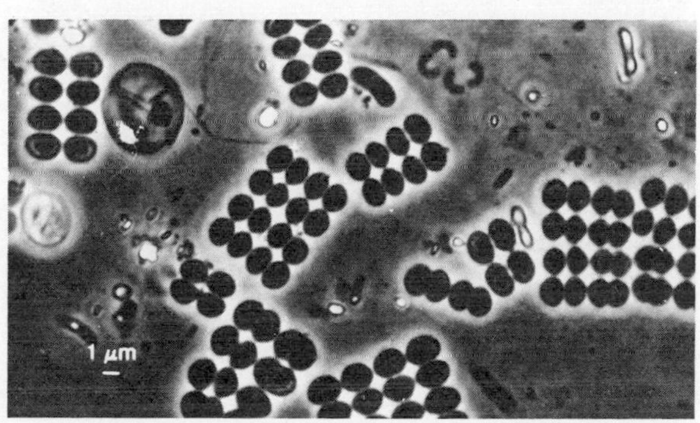

FIG. 8-14 A green sulfur bacterial community. *Reproduced with the permission of the National Research Council of Canada from Caldwell, D. E., and J. M. Tiedje,* Can. J. Microbiol. *21:377–385 (1975).*

TABLE 8-4 Basic Differences betwen Cyanobacteria and the Green and Purple Bacteria

Property	Cyanobacteria (Blue-green Bacteria)	Procaryotes Green Bacteria	Purple Bacteria
Motility	Gliding	Nonmotile and gliding forms	Motile
Nitrogen fixation	Occurs in some species	Absent	Absent
Oxygenic photosynthesis[a]	Present	Absent	Absent
Major photosynthetic pigment[b]	Chlorophyll and phycobiliproteins	Bacteriochlorophylls *a,b,c,d,* or *e*	Bacteriochlorophylls *a,b,c,d,* or *e*
Reserve nonnitrogenous organic material	Glycogen	Absent	Glycogen and poly-B-hydroxybutyrate

[a]Oxygen produced as a product of photosynthesis.
[b]All of these organisms contain carotenoid pigments.

(185°F). Still others are found in marine and fresh waters, in soil, and even in wet flower pots. Certain blue-green bacteria can grow on volcanic rock where most plant life fails to develop. The explanation lies in the ability of these microorganisms to utilize gaseous nitrogen, carbon dioxide, and water vapor from the air for their nutritional needs. This use of elemental nitrogen to form nitrogen-containing compounds is called **nitrogen fixation.** It is a process that introduces nitrates into soil and maintains soil fertility. Occasionally, when water temperature, nutrients (usually pollutants), and other factors reach a favorable level, certain blue-green bacteria multiply very rapidly, resulting in a microbial bloom (Color Photograph 4a). When this occurs, the waste products of such organisms accumulate and may seriously affect the other forms of water life and even humans.

The cellular properties of blue-green bacteria are clearly unlike those of any eucaryotic algal group; their only common property is procaryotic cellular organization.

Many subgroups of cyanobacteria are unicellular (Figure 8–15), although new cells produced by division may remain connected to form aggregates. Blue-green bacteria may be spherical, rod-shaped, or spiral (Figure 8–15c). Their cells are 1.5 to 2 μm in diameter. Small reproductive cells, a type of endospore, called *baeocytes* (Figure 8–15b) are formed from the multiple splitting of vegetative cells.

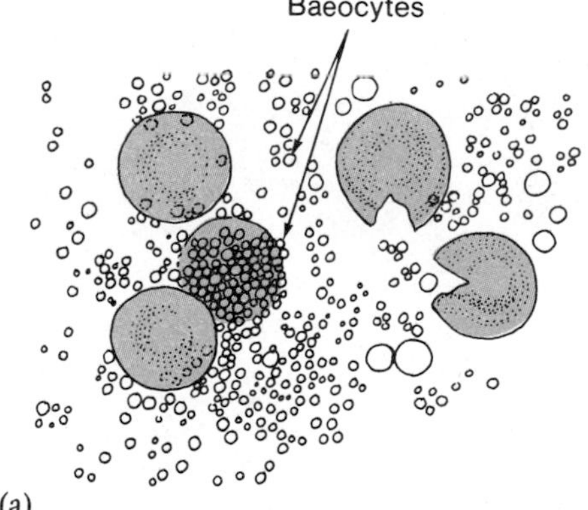

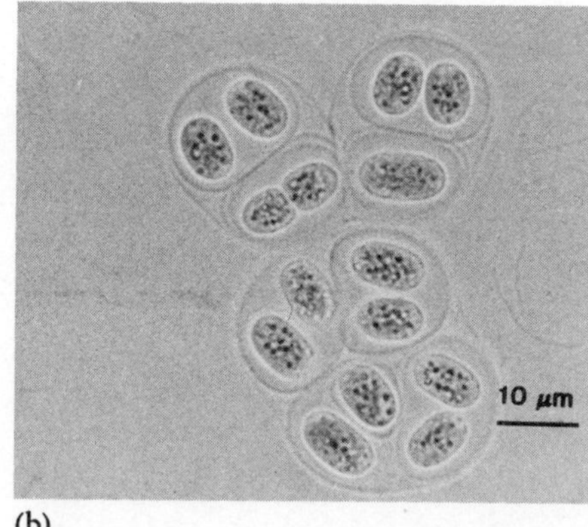

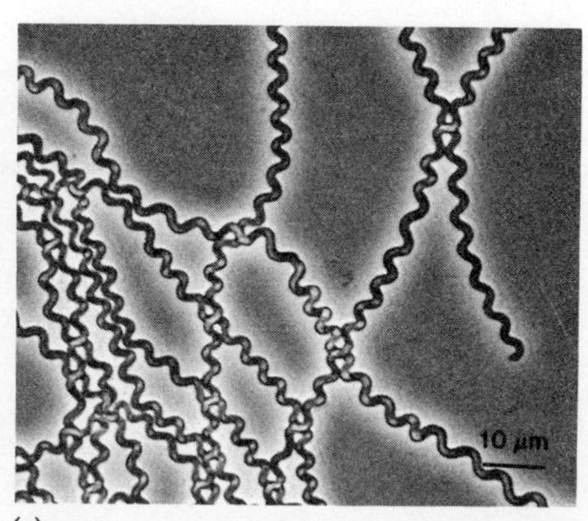

FIG. 8–15 Cyanobacteria. (a) A drawing of *Dermocarpa.* Spherical cells of varying size are filled with reproductive spores known as baeocytes. The formation of spores distinguishes this organism from other cyanobacteria. (b) Young aggregates of the coccal cyanobacterium, *Myxosarcina.* Note the cubical packets of cells. (c) The spiral, loosely coiled cells of *Spirulina. Courtesy of R. Rippka.*

In other subgroups, the unit of structure is the filament, in which cells are bound together in a common sheath (trichome). Reproduction occurs by breakage of these trichomes into shorter chains of cells, called ***hormogonia*** (Figure 8–16).

Heterocysts and akinetes are produced by certain filamentous cyanobacteria (Figures 7–27a and b). These cells can also be distinguished from vegetative cells from a structural standpoint (Figure 7–18a). By its involvement in nitrogen fixation, the heterocyst enables blue-green bacteria to survive and develop in nitrogen-deficient environments.

Blue-green bacteria may actually be green (Color Photograph 29), purple, red, yellow, or even colorless. These variations are brought about by different kinds and amounts of pigments (Table 8–4). The photosynthetic pigments of cyanobacteria are contained in structures known as phycobilisomes, which are attached to the outer surfaces of thylakoids (Figure 7–18a).

The cyanobacteria constitute one of the largest and most diverse subgroups of Gram-negative procaryotes known today.

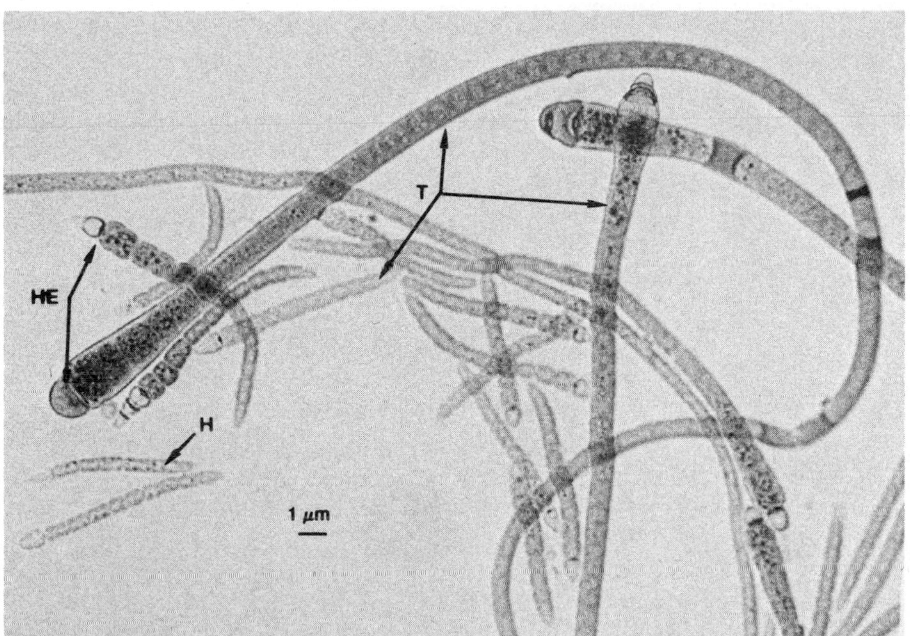

FIG. 8–16 Trichomes and hormogonia. This photo of the cyanobacterium *Calothrix* shows the long trichomes (T), containing many cells in a common sheath, and the shorter cell chains, the hormogonia (H). Heterocysts (He) can be seen at the end of the trichomes. *Courtesy of R. Rippka.*

SUMMARY

Cultivation of Bacteria

1. In the laboratory, bacteria are supplied with the nutrients required for growth in the *culture medium.*
2. Choice of a particular medium is determined by the growth needs of an organism.
3. Resulting growth of bacteria after a suitable period of incubation is called a *culture.*
4. Accumulation of bacteria on a solid medium is called a *colony.*
5. Certain bacteria require living cells for their activities and survival. General laboratory systems that provide for such needs include tissue culture systems.

Representative Procaryotes

1. In their natural habitats, bacteria are generally associated either with other bacteria or with other microbial types.
2. Most bacteria are harmless and may perform beneficial functions, such as aiding digestive processes of animals, producing and flavoring foods, and returning chemical elements to the soil for use by plants in their growth and other basic processes.
3. Detailed classifications of 1576 recognized bacterial species are contained in the 1974 edition of *Bergey's Manual of Determinative Bacteria.* These organisms are divided into 19 taxonomic parts.
4. There is a growing trend to consider bacteria and blue-green *(cyanobacteria)* algae as one group of procaryotes.
5. Procaryotes differ widely in the range of compounds that support their need for carbon and energy.
6. *Heterotrophs* require preformed organic compounds for their nutrition.
7. *Autotrophs* can utilize inorganic compounds such as carbon dioxide as their carbon source.
8. Certain heterotrophs can invade, multiply, and carry out their life processes at the expense of a susceptible animal, plant or other microorganism.

Heterotrophic Bacteria

The Mycoplasma and Related Organisms

1. The genus *Mycoplasma* contains procaryotes that normally do not have cell walls.
2. Blood serum, which contains sterols, is required for the growth and reproduction of these organisms.

Gliding Bacteria (The Gliders)

1. *Gliding* motility is found among both heterotrophs and autotrophs.
2. This form of movement is slow, occurs only when organisms are in contact with a solid surface, and involves a secretion of a slime track.
3. A number of filamentous bacteria exhibit gliding motility. These include *Flexibacter* and *Leucothrix.*
4. The mechanism of gliding motility is not known.

Sheathed Bacteria

1. A limited number of aquatic bacteria form specialized coverings known as *sheaths.*
2. The sheath has both ecological and nutritional consequences for the organisms that form them.
3. The sheathed bacteria include *Clonothrix, Crenothrix, Lieskeella, Phragmidiothrix, Sphaerotilus,* and the *Sphaerotilus-Leptothrix* group.
4. When environmental conditions become unfavorable, rounded cells known as *gonidia* are formed.
5. Sheathed bacteria are found in sewage, soil, and water.

Stalked and Budding Procaryotes (The Prosthecate Bacteria)

1. Several procaryotes found in aquatic environments have complex fine structures and morphologically distinct cell cycles.
2. Cell wall extensions containing cytoplasm are called *prostheca.*
3. Some organisms, such as species of the *Caulobacter,* use prosthecae called *stalks* for attachment purposes. These structures contain sticky material at the tip, known as a holdfast.
4. The prosthecate bacteria have cell cycles that involve formation of new cell types and are significantly different from those of typical bacteria.
5. *Hyphomicrobium* and the related photosynthetic *Rhodomicrobium* are budding bacteria that have extensions known as *filaments.* Bud formation can occur at the tip of such structures.

Spiral and Curved Bacteria

1. *Spiral bacteria* are heterotrophs with unique cellular anatomy and motion.
2. Examples of these procaryotes include spirochetes, spirals, and curved rods.
3. Spirals occur in a wide range of natural habitats. A small number cause diseases of humans and lower animals.
4. Despite similarities in morphology, spirochetes differ in their physiology, activities, and distribution.
5. Most spirilla are free-living bacteria with rigid cell walls and flagella at one or both ends.
6. Curved, spiral rods of the genus *Campylobacter* are *microaerophilic,* have a single flagellum at one or both ends, and move with a characteristic corkscrew motion. One species causes disease in lower animals and humans.

The Obligate Intracellular Procaryotes

1. Several bacterial species require living eucaryotic animal, plant, or microbial cells for development and reproduction.
2. Examples of such parasitic procaryotes include *Bdellovibrio, Chlamydia,* and *Rickettsia.*
3. Each genus of obligate intracellular bacteria has distinctive features of its cycle, including transmission, penetration of host cells, reproduction and release of progeny, and cultivation.

Autotrophs

The Phototrophs

1. Photosynthetic procaryotes use inorganic sources of carbon.

2. Three distinct groups of Gram-negative organisms are recognized as phototrophs: *cyanobacteria (blue-green bacteria)* and the *green* and *purple bacteria.*
3. The green and purple bacteria do not produce oxygen as a product of their photosynthetic activity (anoxygenic photosynthesis) and contain pigments different from those of the blue-green bacteria.
4. Blue-green bacteria are the largest, most diverse, and most widely distributed group of photosynthetic bacteria.
5. Certain cyanobacteria form heterocysts where *nitrogen fixation* occurs.
6. Blue-green bacteria, in the presence of various nutrients, temperature, and other factors, can multiply rapidly to form an algal bloom.
7. Morphologically, many subgroups of cyanobacteria are unicellular; others may appear as long filaments of cells bound together in a common sheath *(trichomes).*
8. Reproduction in blue-green bacteria, depending on the species, can occur by the breakage of trichomes or by the formation of reproductive cells, *baeocytes* or *endospores.*
9. Heterocysts and akinetes are produced by certain filamentous cyanobacteria.
10. The photosynthetic pigments of cyanobacteria are contained in structures known as phycobilisomes that are attached to outer surfaces of *thylakoids.*

QUESTIONS FOR REVIEW

1. How are bacteria cultured in the laboratory?
2. How do the energy needs or sources of the following procaryotes differ from most others?
   a. rickettsia
   b. blue-green bacteria
   c. mycoplasma
   d. *Bdellovibrio*
   e. *Chlamydia*
3. Compare the steps involved in the life cycles of the following procaryotes:
   a. *Chlamydia* and budding bacteria
   b. *Bdellovibrio* and stalked bacteria
4. List and explain at least two distinguishing properties of the following procaryotes:
   a. sheathed bacteria
   b. gliding bacteria
   c. *Bacillus* species
   d. methane-producing bacteria
   e. spirochetes
   f. green bacteria
   g. purple bacteria
   h. blue-green bacteria
5. What beneficial functions or activities are performed by the various procaryotes discussed in this chapter?
6. What is an algal bloom? How does it form?
7. How do the mycoplasma differ from most other heterotrophic bacteria?

SUGGESTED READINGS

Becker, Y., "The Chlamydia: Molecular Biology of Procaryotic Obligate Parasites of Eucaryocytes," *Microbiol. Revs.* 42:274–306 (1978). *A functional approach to defining the molecular structure and processes associated with the cycle of infection of* Chlamydia psittaci *and* C. trachomatis. *Basic differences between these two chlamydial agents and other microbes are also discussed.*

Holt, J. G., ed., *The Shorter Bergey's Manual of Determinative Bacteriology.* Baltimore: Williams & Wilkins, 1977. *As the title indicates, this book is a shorter version of a standard reference used for bacterial identification and classification. It contains descriptions of all genera, keys and tables for species identification, and an outline to bacterial classification.*

Krieg, N. R., and P. B. Hylemon, "The Taxonomy of the Chemoheterotrophic Spirilla," *Ann. Rev. Microbiol.* 30: 303–325 (1976). *A useful article describing the general features of these rigid helical bacteria that have fascinated investigators since the early history of bacteriology.*

London, J., "The Ecology and Taxonomic Status of the Lactobacilli," *Ann. Rev. Microbiol.* 30:279–301 (1976). *An up-dated coverage of the bacteria that form the lactic acid group. Attention is given to their ecology, cell wall structure, activities, and classification.*

Pfennig, N., "Photographic Green and Purple Bacteria: A Comparative Systematic Survey," *Ann. Rev. Microbiol.* 31:275–290 (1977). *A concise discussion of the properties of two clearly different physiological-ecological groups of phototrophic bacteria.*

Razin, S., "The Mycoplasmas," *Microbiol. Revs.* 42:414–470 (1978). *A review that focuses on new developments in the areas of mycoplasma physiology, structure, pathogenicity, and viruses.*

Rippka, R., J. Deruelles, J. B. Waterbury, M. Herdman, and R. Y. Stanier, "Generic Assignments, Strain Histories and Properties of Pure Cultures of Cyanobacteria," *J. Gen. Microbiol.* 111:1–61 (1979). *An excellent, well-illustrated comparative study of 178 strains of cyanobacteria. Revised definitions of several genera also are proposed.*

Stanier, R. Y., and G. Cohen-Bazire, "Phototrophic Prokaryotes: The Cyanobacteria," *Ann. Rev. Microbiol.* 31:277–274 (1977). *A comprehensive treatment of three aspects of the biology of cyanobacteria: major patterns of development, cellular structure and organization, and metabolism.*

Tachibana, D. K., "Microbiology of the Foot," *Ann. Rev. Microbiol.* 30:351–375 (1976). *An interesting consideration of this area of the body, which appears to provide a unique habitat for microbes. Diseases of the foot, as well as the problem of foot odor, are among the topics discussed.*

CHAPTER 9

Fungi

The fungi constitute an extremely important and interesting group of microorganisms. In this chapter we shall discuss their distribution, structure, and organization, as well as the way they interact with other forms of life and their commercial importance.

After reading this chapter, you should be able to:

1. **Describe the general characteristics of fungi and the position they occupy in the biological world.**
2. **List the distribution and features of the major classes of fungi.**
3. **Explain how fungi differ from other types of microorganisms.**
4. **Outline the features of fungal reproduction.**
5. **Identify the structures of fungi.**
6. **Describe the methods used to grow fungi.**
7. **List and describe the major beneficial and destructive activities of fungi.**
8. **Define or explain the following:**
   a. **antibiotic**
   b. **hyphae**
   c. **mycelia**
   d. **aflatoxin**
   e. **fungal spores**
   f. **yeast**

Fungi (singular, fungus) are larger than bacteria and structurally more complex. Like animals, protozoa, and most bacteria, they require organic nutrients as sources of energy. Since fungi contain no photosynthetic pigments, they depend on other structures and enzyme systems for energy to carry out their various activities.

The fungi are a distinctive life form of great practical and ecological importance. This unique group of eucaryotic, nonphotosynthetic microorganisms contains more than 80,000 species and includes the large conspicuous mushrooms, puffballs, and woody bracket forms (Color Photographs 30 through 33), as well as the smaller molds and yeasts (Color Photographs 34, 35, and 36).

Distribution and Activities

Fungi are widespread in nature (Figures 9–1 and 9–2). They grow well in dark, moist environments and in habitats where organic material is available. Thus fungi are found in soil and in aquatic environments.

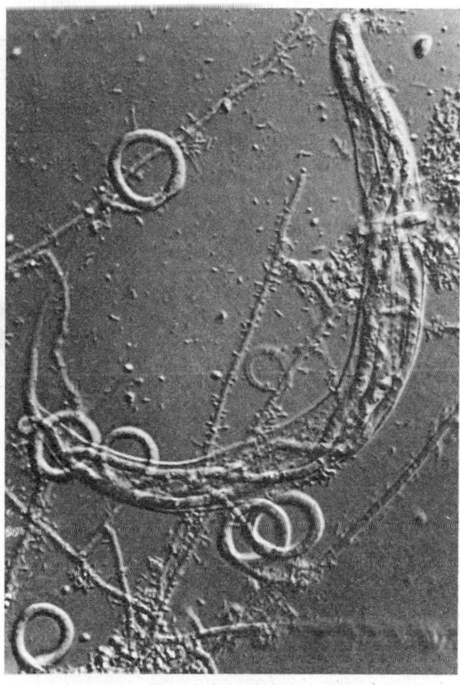

FIG. 9–1 A nematode-trapping fungus. Here the ringed hyphae of *Arthrobotrys anchonic* grasp and eventually immobilize the unsuspecting roundworm (× 400). Barron, G. L.: *The Nematode Destroying Fungi* (1977).

FIG. 9–2 An infected root system of mycorrhiza is generally beneficial to both the fungus and the host plant. The extent of invasion by fungus is usually kept in check to prevent injury to the plant rootlet. (a) A scanning micrograph showing the fungus cell or hypha penetrating into the plant cell. (b) A transmission micrograph of the association. Note the eucaryotic organization of the fungus. Components of the plant cell host include the cell wall (PCW). Hyphal structures shown include cell wall (HCW), nucleus (N), and vacuoles (V). *Reproduced by permission of the National Research Council of Canada from Kinden, D. A., and N. F. Brown,* Can. J. Microbiol. *21:1768–1780 (1975).*

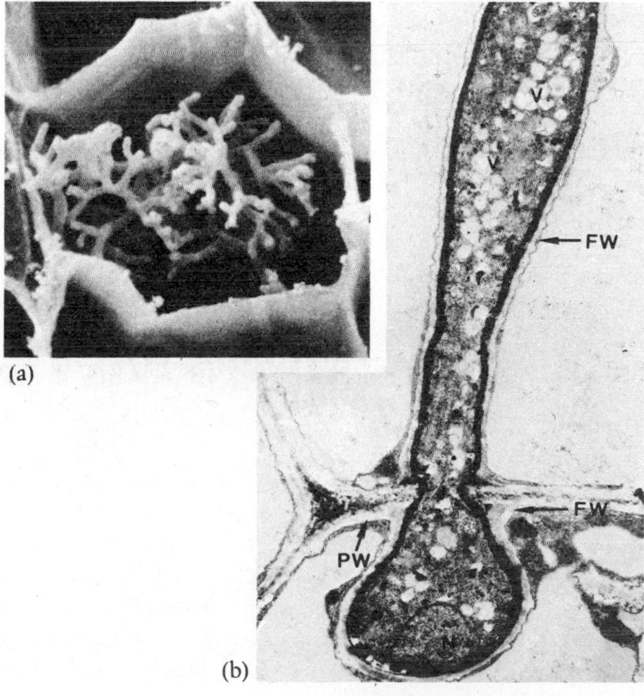

Since fungi do not contain chlorophyll, they are dependent upon the organic products of other organisms, either living or dead, as sources of energy. Therefore, fungi are heterotrophic and are usually referred to as *saprobes* or *saprophytes*. Many of these organisms are active producers of enzymes that enable them to break down complex substances for their use. The production of such digestive enzymes has several beneficial effects, such as the recycling of elements to the soil, making it more suitable for plant growth and enabling certain plants to obtain minerals. However, these enzyme systems can also have undesirable effects. Some fungi are known for their parasitic and destructive effects on plants and lower animals (Figure 9–3 and Color Photographs 38 and 40). Mold spoilage of food is a familiar problem to the marketer of agriculture produce. Each year millions of dollars in fruits and vegetables are lost to damage caused by fungi (Color Photograph 3b). Fortunately, most fungi that spoil foods do not invade the tissues of humans and lower animals.

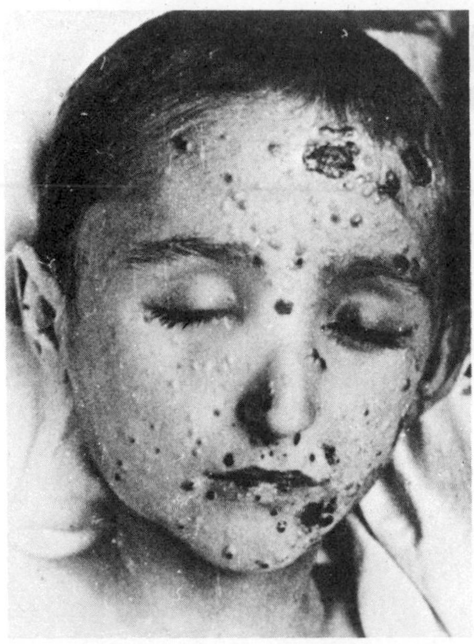

(a)

FIG. 9–3 (a) The destructive effects of the yeast pathogen *Cryptococcus neoformans*, cryptococcosis of the face. *Photograph given to Dr. Zimmerman by Bilgisi Sheseti, Istanbul, Turkey. Courtesy of the Armed Forces Institute of Pathology, Neg. No. 55-8225.* (b) The fungus disease of dry beans, called bean rust. The causative agent, *Uromyces phaseola typica*, produces destructive lesions on the plant's leaves. *Courtesy of the U.S. Department of Agriculture's Bureau of Plant Industry.*

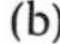

(b)

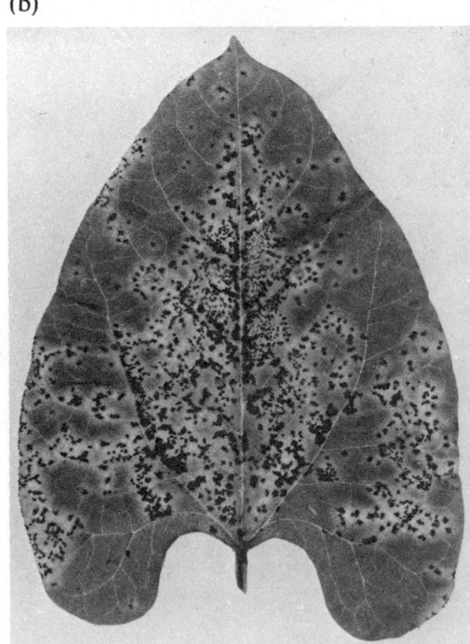

Structure and Function

Fungi differ from bacteria in several ways including their size (fungi are larger), structural development, cellular organization, and methods of reproduction. It is important to note that the term *fungus* is a general term that includes the two different forms **molds** and **yeasts.**

Molds

Although molds do not have true roots, stems, or leaves, they do show differentiation (Figure 9–4). Most molds, for example, consist of tubular, branching eucaryotic cells called **hyphae** (Figure 9–5c). Filaments of these cells are often subdivided by crosswalls (septa) into multicellular hyphae (Figure 9–5d). In species that do not contain septa between the two or more nuclei of the hyphae (the coenocytic state), the contents of the hyphae can move freely throughout the filament.

As molds continue to grow, the hyphae branch, intermingle, and often fuse to eventually form a visible cobweblike aggregation like that seen on moldy bread or fruit. These structures, which are analogous to bacterial colonies, are called **mycelia** (singular, **mycelium**) (Figure 9–5a). These hyphal masses appear dry and powdery (Color Photographs 34 and 41). This is often the result of the formation of various types of reproductive spores. In some instances the mycelium is made up of two general regions (Figure 9–17). One of these regions extends below the surface of the medium in which the mycelium is growing for the purpose of food collection. This part of the mycelium is called the *vegetative mycelium*. Certain species possess rootlike structures called *rhizoids* that obtain food and also serve as anchoring devices. The part of the fungus that is above the substrate is the *aerial mycelium*. It is the reproductive portion of the microorganism, with specialized branches that produce spores (Figures 9–4 and 9–5b).

Yeasts

The fungi known as yeasts are oval, spherical, or elongated cells (Figure 9–6) that form moist, shining colonies. (Color Photographs 35a and 35b.) Yeasts also have an eucaryotic organization and a thick cell wall. In some yeasts, such as *Cryptococcus neoformans*, a capsule surrounds the cell wall.

Certain yeasts reproduce asexually by a process of division (fission) that results in the formation of a new *bud*, or *daughter cell* (Color Photograph 36). The

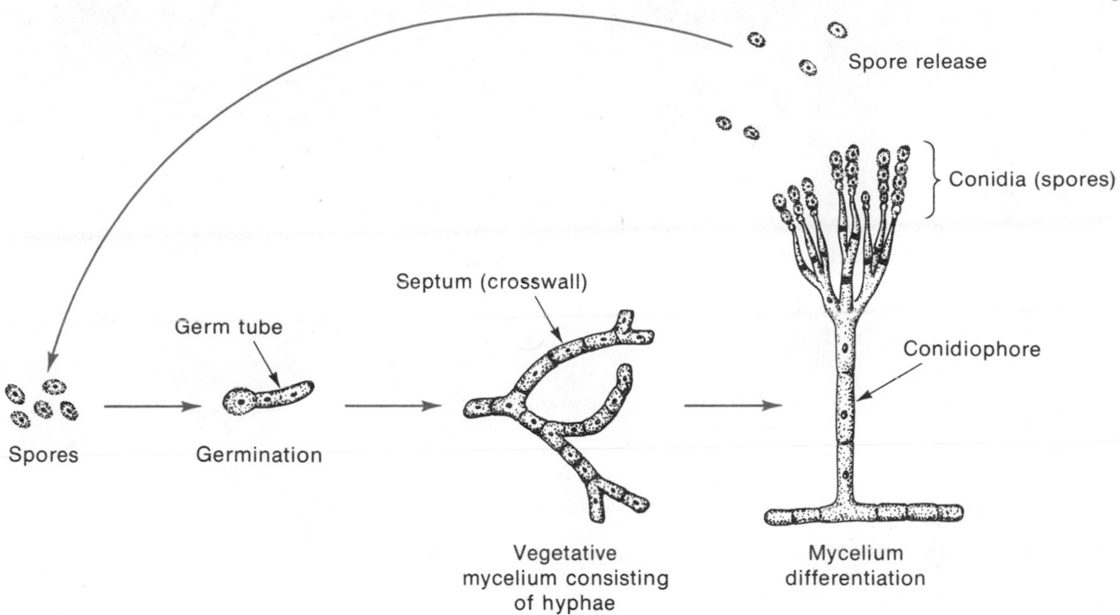

FIG. 9-4 The asexual life cycle of the common fungus *Penicillium* sp., showing several typical structures and their arrangements. Spores, hyphae, vegetative mycelium, and crosswalls (septa) are indicated. The germination of the spore into a hypha starts the development of the fungus. Refer to Color Photograph 34 for the coloration of this organism's mycelium.

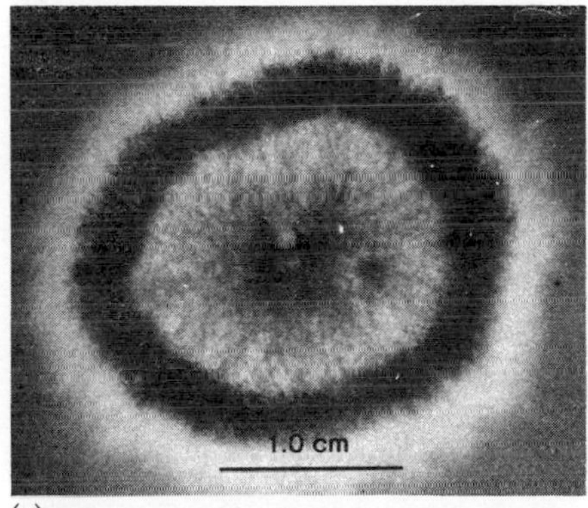

(a)

FIG. 9-5 Components of molds. (a) The cottony mycelium.

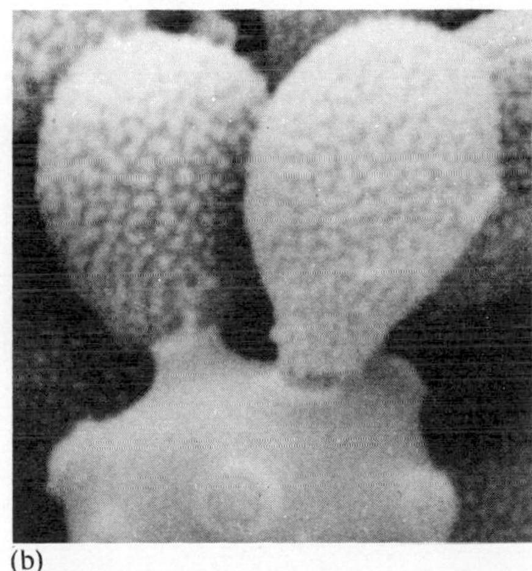

(b)

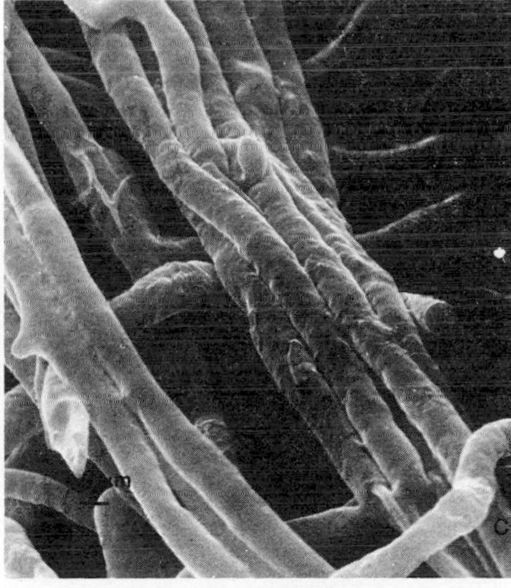

(c)

(b) A scanning micrograph of spores and their attachment to the fungal structure from which they arose. *Courtesy of P. Jeffries and J. W. K. Young.* (c) The tubular hyphae, or threads, that form most of the fungal mycelium. *Photos (a) and (c) reproduced by permission of the National Research Council of Canada from Ellis, D. H., and D. A. Griffiths,* Can. J. Microbiol. *21:442-452 (1975).*

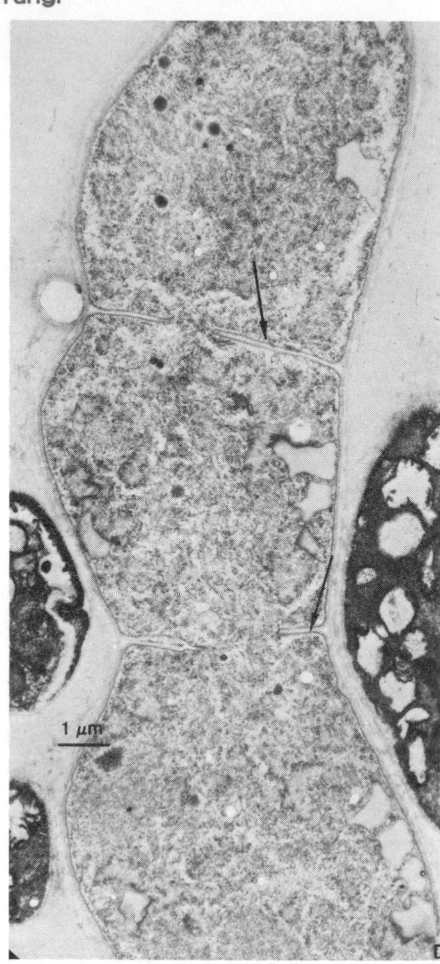

(d) An ultrathin section of hyphal cells showing the crosswalls, or septa (arrows), that are characteristic of specific fungi. *Photo (d) reproduced by permission of the National Research Council of Canada from Ellis, D. H., and D. A. Griffiths,* Can. J. Microbiol. *21:442–452 (1975).*

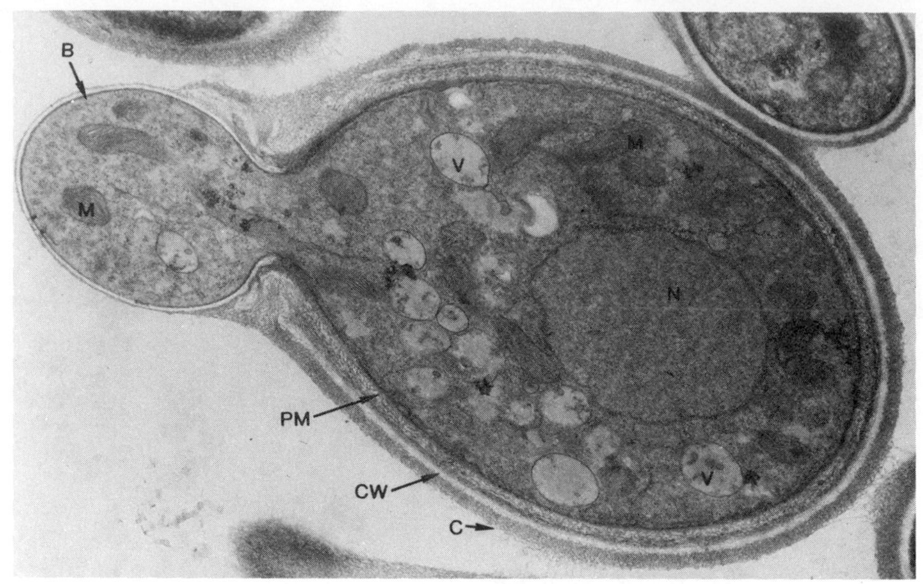

(a)

FIG. 9–6 (a) An electron micrograph showing the eucaryotic organization of a yeast cell and its bud. Note the presence of the bud (B), capsule (C), cell wall (CW), mitochondria (M), nucleus (N), plasma membrane (PM), and vacuole (V). *Reproduced by permission of the National Research Council of Canada, from Peterson, E. M., R. J. Hawley, and R. A. Calderone,* Can. J. Microbiol. *22:1518–1521 (1976).*

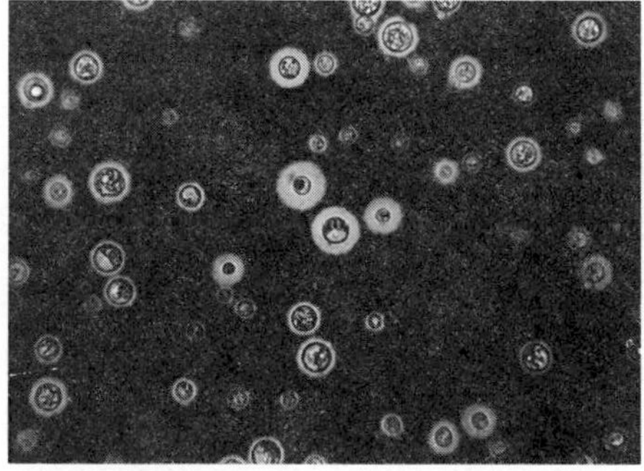

(b)

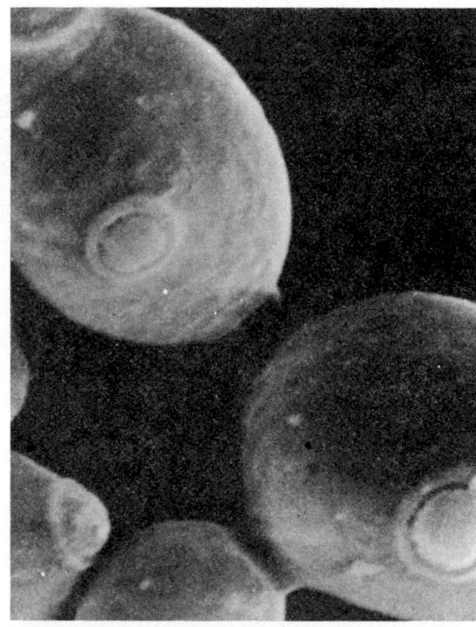

(c)

(b) ***Cryptococcus neoformans*** stained with Nigrosin clearly shows the capsular regions surrounding the cells. Note also the presence of buds on some cells (see arrows). *Courtesy of Dr. M. Silva-Hutner, Columbia University, College of Physicians and Surgeons, N.Y.* (c) Various stages in the formation of buds on yeast cells. Birth scars (S), sites left by buds on the main cells, and the corresponding scars (B) on buds can also be seen. *Watson, K., and Arthur, H.,* J. Bacteriol. *130:312–317 (1977).*

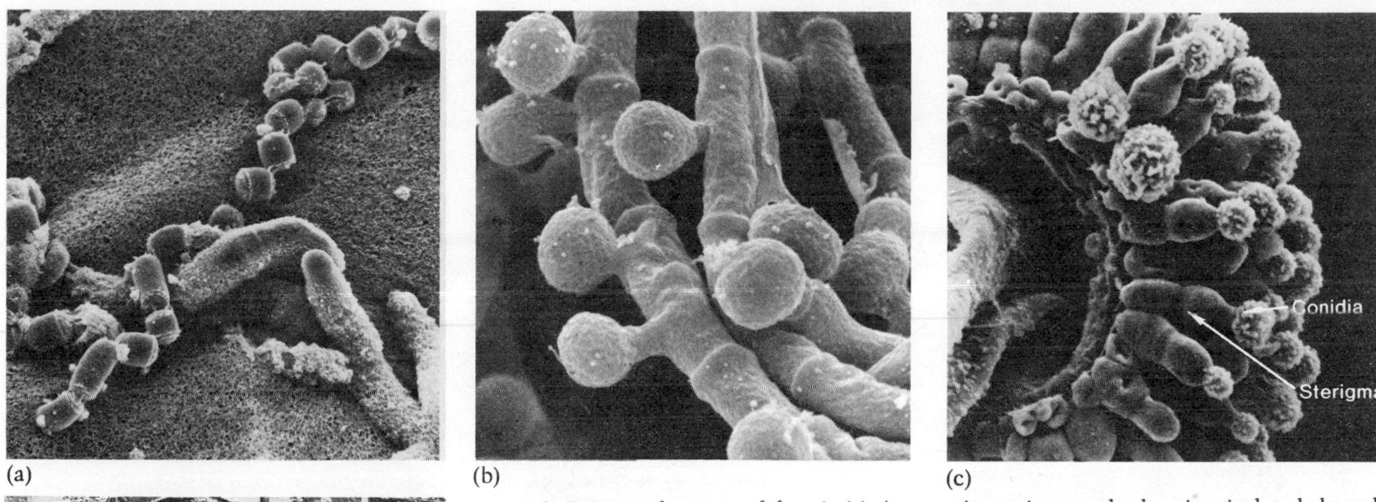

(d)

FIG. 9–7 Asexual spores of fungi. (a) A scanning micrograph showing isolated, barrel-shaped arthrospores of ***Trichophyton mentagrophytes***, a ringworm-causing fungus (see Color Photograph 40). These spores break off from the hyphae. The bar market measures 5 μm. (b) Microconidia developing from hyphae. These spores emerge directly from the tubular hyphae of the fungus. The bar marker measures 1 μm. ***Photographs (a) and (b). Bibel, D. J., D. A. Crumrine, K. Yee, and R. D. King,*** Inf. Imm. *15:958–971 (1977).* (c) Conidia of ***Aspergillus. Tokunaga, M., J. Tokunaga, and K. Harada,*** J. Elect. Micro. *22:27–38 (1973).* (d) An electron micrograph of a freeze-etched fungal spore (conidium) showing its internal organization. Note the thickness of the spore wall (SW), of the typical eucaryotic organelles, and the association of the endoplasmic reticulum (ER) with the plasma membrane (PM), many vesicles (V), mitochondria (M), and the nuclear membrane (NM). ***Sekiguchi, J., G. M. Gaucher, and J. W. Costerton,*** Can. J. Microbiol. *21:2048–2058 (1975).*

mother cell bears a bud scar at the region where separation took place; the bud has a birth scar (Figure 9–6). In some species the newly formed cells do not separate. These connected yeasts cells are called *pseudomycelia* (Figure 9–6e).

Dimorphism

Several disease-causing fungi are **dimorphic,** exhibiting two different forms under two different environmental conditions. Under certain environmental conditions these organisms exhibit their normal type of saprobic form, but in animal tissues or when grown on rich nutrient preparation at higher temperatures, they appear as yeasts. The term **saprophytic form** has been suggested for the mold phase, **parasitic form** for the yeast stage.

Reproduction and Spores

The type of spore produced and the manner of sporulation are both important in the identification and classification of fungi. These specialized structures function as reproductive cells, but usually they are no more resistant than any other type of fungal cell.

Asexual Spores

Depending on the species, both asexual and sexual spores or only asexual spores are produced (Table 9–1). Asexual spores (Figure 9–7) include ***arthrospores, blastospores, chlamydospores, conidia, sporangiospores,*** and ***zoospores.*** Some fungi have the ability to form two types of asexual spores. Asexual spores vary in color, shape, and size and may have one or several nuclei. Many of the properties of these reproductive cells are summarized in Table 9–1.

TABLE 9-1 Properties of Fungal Spores

Spore Type	Site and/or Type of Formation	Single or Multicellular	Shape	Resistance to Environment	Examples of Genera that Form Spore Type[a]
Asexual					
Arthrospore	Fragmentation of hyphae (Figure 9-7a)	Single	Cylindrical to round	Usually none	*Coccidioides, Geotrichum, Trichosporon*
Blastospore (buds)	Formed on main cell	Single	Round to oval	Usually none	*Candida, Saccharomyces*
Chlamydospore	Enlargement of terminal hyphal cells	Single	Considerable variation but usually round	These thick-walled cells exhibit unusual resistance to drying and heat	*Candida, Mucor*
Conidium (conidiospore)	Borne on specialized hyphal branches, conidiophores	Single (microconidia)	Round to oval	Usually none	*Aspergillus, Cephalosporium, Penicillium*
		Multicellular (macroconidia)	Long and tapering	None	*Alternaria, Microsporum, Trichophyton*
Phialospore (modified conidium)	Borne on specialized hyphal branches, conidiophores, phialides	Single	Round to oval	Usually none	*Philalophora*
Sporangiospore	Formed within sacs, sporangia, at end of hyphal cells	Single	Round	None	*Absidia, Coccidioides, Mucor, Rhizopus*
Zoospore	Formed within sacs, sporangia, at end of hyphal branches	Single, flagellated	Round	None	*Saprolegnia*
Sexual					
Ascospore	Formed within sac-like cells, asci, after cellular and nuclear union	Single (usually 8 per ascus)	Round to oval	None	*Allescheria, Neurospora*
Basidiospore	Formed at end of club-shaped structures, *basidia* (Figure 9-13)	Usually single (usually 4 in number)	Round to oval	None	*Amanita, Agaricus, Coprinus*
Oospore	Developed within a fertilized egg cell, *oogonia*	Single (usually 1 to 20 per oogonium)	Round	More resistant than most asexual spores	*Saprolegnia*
Zygospore	Formed after cellular and nuclear fusion (Figure 9-9)	Large, thick-walled, single structure	Round to oval	None	*Rhizopus*

[a]Certain fungi can form more than one type of spore.

Under suitable conditions of nutrition, moisture, pH, and temperature, fungal spores germinate and produce one to several filamentous structures called *germ tubes* (Figures 9-4 and 9-8). These usually penetrate through thin or weakened portions of the spore *(germ pores)*. The fungal germ tubes develop by elongating and branching to form the hyphae.

Sexual Spores

Sexual spores (Figure 9-9) are produced by nuclear fusion. Reproductive cells of this type include *ascospores, basidiospores, oospores,* and *zygospores.* In general, sexual spores are observed less often than asexual ones. Certain environmental conditions must be provided before sexual sporulation can be induced. Table 9-1 lists several properties of sexual spores.

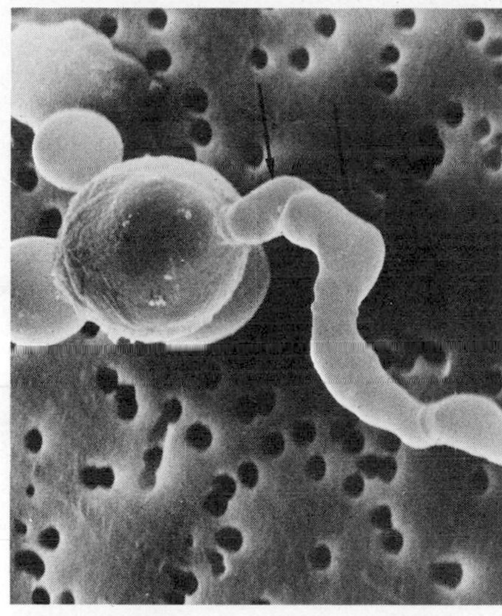

FIG. 9–8 A scanning micrograph showing germ tube formation by an arthrospore. Separate, newly formed hyphal cells can also be seen. *Queener, S. W., and L. F. Ellis,* Can. J. Microbiol. *21:1981–1996 (1975).*

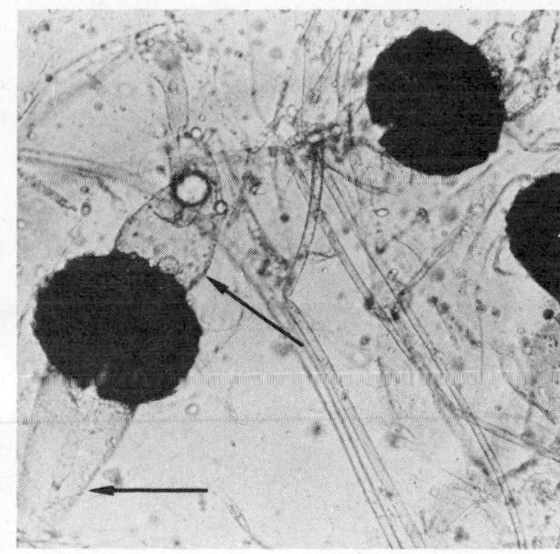

FIG. 9–9 A representative zygospore of *Rhizopus* spp. Note the two hyphal branches (arrows).

The Ultrastructure of Fungi

Both yeasts and molds are eucaryotic (Figures 9–2b, 9–5d, 9–6b and 9–7d). Their cells usually contain membrane-bound organelles, including endoplasmic reticula, mitochondria, and well-defined nuclei. The membranes surrounding the nuclear material of the cells contain sterols such as cholesterollike compounds. Sterols, with the exception of bacteria such as the mycoplasma, are not found in procaryotes but only in the structures of higher forms of life. Since the fungi resemble higher plants and animals both in their cellular complexity and in their organelles, only the cell wall and fimbriae will be discussed here.

As in bacteria, the cell wall lies immediately external to the fungal cell's cytoplasmic membrane (Figure 9–10). Under the electron microscope the

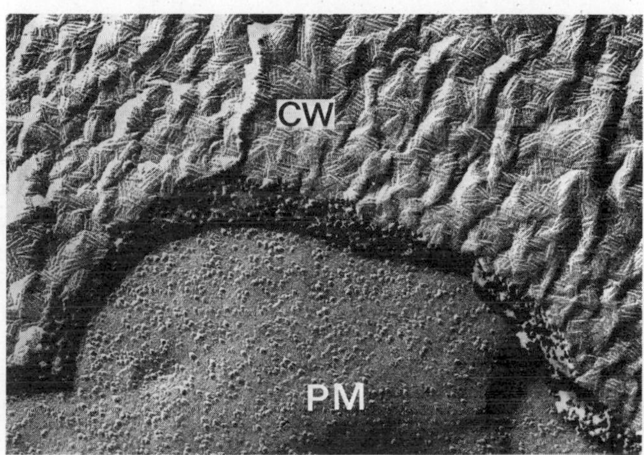

FIG. 9–10 An electron micrograph showing the appearance of interlacing microfibrils. The relationship of the cell wall (CW) to the plasma (cell) membrame (PM) is also shown. *Caputo, R., M. Innocenti, and M. Shimono,* J. Ultrastruct. *59:149–157 (1977).*

walls of filamentous fungi appear to be composed of thin, threadlike structures called **microfibrils** (Figure 9–10). These measure approximately 15 to 25 nm in diameter and are arranged in a type of thatchwork. Chemically, the microfibrils in many fungi are composed of **chitin,** a polymer of N-acetylglucosamine (Figure 7–11) that is also the principal structural substance in the exoskeletons of crayfish, crabs, and related forms. Cellulose, the major component of plant cell walls, has also been found in the hyphal walls of filamentous fungi.

The chemical composition of yeast cell walls is quite different. They contain approximately equal quantities of the highly branched, insoluble polysaccharide glucan and the soluble polysaccharide mannan. Other compounds found in the cell wall include lipids, proteins, and the amino sugar glucosamine.

The surfaces of fungi are important to several interactions, including the joining of cells for sexual reproduction **(conjugation)** and the uptake and excretion of molecules. Recent ultrastructural studies have revealed the presence of pili, or fimbriae (Figure 9–11), on the surfaces of various yeasts. These structures, which are remarkably similar in several respects to those of bacteria (Figure 7–9), originate below the cell wall. They may be necessary to complete conjugation.

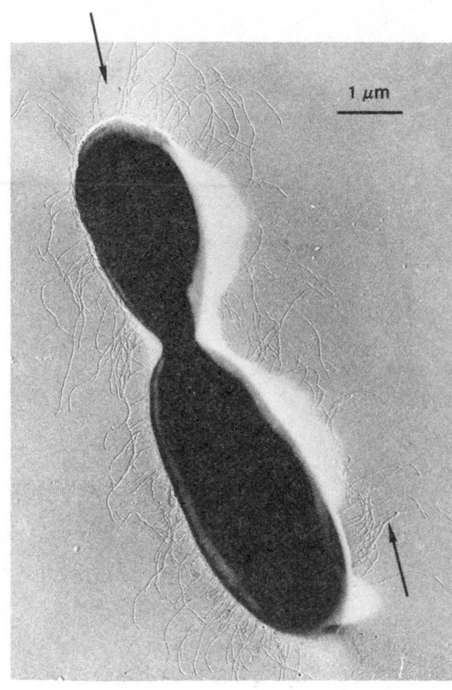

FIG. 9–11 The fimbriae of fungi. These surface hairlike appendages have been found on several yeasts and are believed to be involved in sexual reproduction. Some fimbriae produce knobs. *Poon, N. H., and A. W. Day.* Can. J. Microbiol. 21:537–546 (1975).

Cultivation of Fungi

Molds and yeasts can be grown and studied by cultural methods similar to those used for many bacteria. Most fungi are able to grow under aerobic conditions, but many grow more slowly than bacteria. Consequently, media that can support both bacteria and fungi are apt to become overgrown with bacteria. In working with fungi, therefore, it is advisable to use culture media that limit the growth of other microbial types. Ingredients that can be added to media for this purpose include antibiotics (such as chloramphenicol, gentamicin, penicillin, and streptomycin), dyes (such as crystal violet), and high concentrations of sugar. Another important property of preparations for fungal cultivation is their acidity, pH 5.6 to 6.

When it is necessary to prevent or suppress the growth of unwanted fungi, cyclohexamide (Actidione), another type of antibiotic, can be incorporated into the medium.

Nearly all of the culture media used for fungi can be obtained in the dehydrated state from commercial sources. Most can be used in either the liquid or solid state. The solid form can be made, in many instances, by simply adding agar to the liquid medium.

Types of Media

In general, three basic types of media can be used in fungus cultivation: natural, dehydrated (basic), and synthetic (chemically defined) preparations. Natural media are not widely used in the laboratory. Examples of such cultivation materials include slices or infusions of animal tissues, fruits, and vegetables. For example, carrot plugs and potato slices have been used.

Dehydrated, or basic, media contain, in addition to dextrose (glucose) and/or sodium chloride, a wide assortment of organic ingredients such as peptones, beef extract, and corn meal, which have variable compositions. One of the most commonly used of these preparations is Sabouraud (Sab) dextrose or maltose medium, which also contains peptone, agar, and distilled water. After sterilization, it can be used in the form of slants or plates for the isolation and identifi-

TABLE 9-2 Selected Characteristics of the Major Classes of Fungi

Class	Type of Mycelium	Spores: Asexual — Site of Formation	Spores: Sexual — Site of Formation	Representative Groups
Ascomycetes	Septate	At the tips of hyphae	Within sacs	Common antibiotic-producing fungi (e.g., *Pencillium* spp.), yeasts
Basidiomycetes	Septate	At the tips of hyphae	On a surface of a basidium	Poisonous mushrooms (*Amanita* spp.), mushrooms, rusts, smuts
Deuteromycetes (Fungi Imperfecti)	Septate	At the tips of hyphae	None present	Most human pathogens
Oomycetes	Aseptate	In sacs	Within a unicellular female sex organ (oogonium)	Some aquatic forms, pathogens responsible for powdery mildew, blights of plants and fish infections
Zygomycetes	Almost completely aseptate (coenocytic)	In sacs	In mycelium	Bread mold (*Rhizopus nigricans*), aquatic species

cation of a wide variety of molds (Color Photographs 34 and 41) and yeasts (Color Photograph 35a). Incorporation of the dye trypan blue in Sabouraud agar permits rapid detection and tentative identification of several species of yeast (Color Photograph 35b). Other examples of basic media include blood agar, brain agar, corn meal agar, and thioglycollate broth.

Synthetic media—those for which the exact composition is known—are used for the isolation of saprophytic and pathogenic fungi. Most saprophytic fungi grow at room temperature and are unable to grow at 37°C, but most pathogens grow readily at 37°C.

Distinctive Mycelia

Several fungi can be identified by the appearance of their mycelia. Color, diffusion of pigment, and texture are but a few of the important features. Cultures of these fungi are generally prepared by inoculating the center of a particular medium. After a suitable incubation period at the appropriate temperature, the distinctive mycelium should have developed (Color Photographs 34 and 41). The under-surfaces of certain pathogenic fungi also exhibit a characteristic appearance. A trained worker usually has little difficulty in identifying typical fungal species.

Classification

Several properties of fungi are important to their classification and identification. These include method of reproduction, mycelial formation, and cellular structure and formation (Table 9–2). On the basis of the methods of reproduction, five major classes of fungi are recognized: **Ascomycetes, Basidiomycetes, Deuteromycetes** (Fungi Imperfecti), **Oomycetes,** and

Zygomycetes. The general properties of these groups and of the slime molds (Myxomycetes), their ecological roles, and their economic importance are presented in the following sections.

Ascomycetes

Several species of Ascomycetes, also known as *sac fungi,* are biologically and economically important. Some members of the group live in aquatic or moist land environments. Others are parasitic or live with other microorganisms or plants in a mutually beneficial association. The asexual spores by which Ascomycetes reproduce are produced at the ends of hyphae. The spores germinate to form new mycelia.

Ascospores are the characteristic sexual spores of the Ascomycetes, formed following the fusion of tubelike structures from two neighboring cells. The two nuclei of these cells fuse and form a single nucleus. Daughter nuclei are subsequently produced through meiotic division. As many as eight nuclei may form. Each becomes surrounded by a dense protoplasmic layer and a spore coat, or

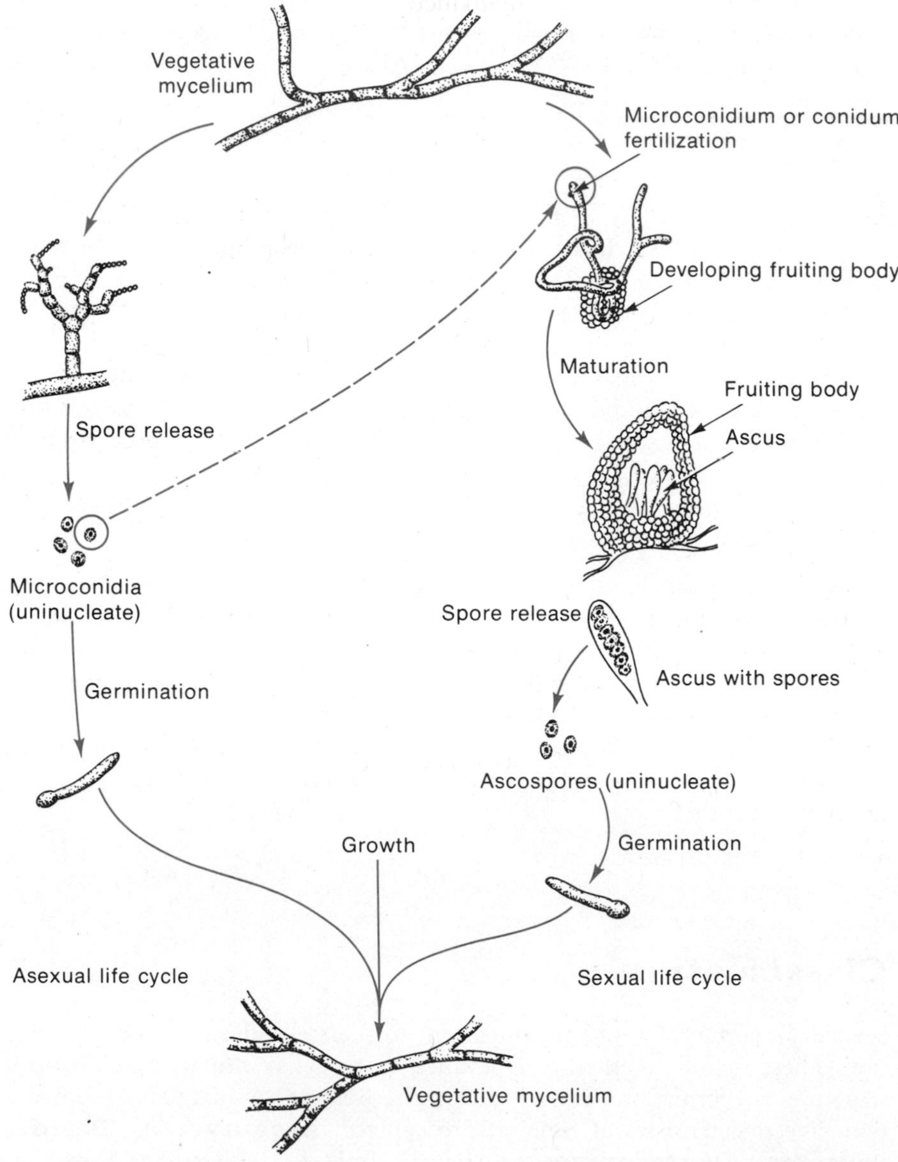

FIG. 9–12 The asexual and sexual life cycles of the ascomycete *Neurospora.*

wall, thus forming an **ascospore.** These reproductive structures are contained in the original wall formed during the initial union of the two neighboring cells. This enclosing sac is called an **ascus.** The life cycle of *Neurospora,* an ascomycete that has contributed greatly to genetic studies, is shown in Figure 9–12.

The yeasts, such as *Saccharomyces cerevisiae,* which leaven breads and ferment beer and wine, are also Ascomycetes. In the production of alcoholic beverages, carbon dioxide is a by-product of this fermentation. In baking, however, carbon dioxide is the essential ingredient. Yeasts are mixed with dough, where they multiply and produce sugar-fermenting enzymes. The fermentative activity of the yeasts produces alcohol and carbon dioxide. Tiny bubbles of carbon dioxide form in the dough and cause it to rise. Upon baking, the gas expands and the alcohol escapes.

Certain yeasts also serve as important sources of the B complex vitamins and ergosterol, which is used in the production of vitamin D.

Yeast cells reproduce asexually by *budding.* In this process the cell nucleus divides by mitosis, and one of the two nuclei becomes enclosed in a small projection, or *bud,* formed on the side of the parental cell (Figures 9–6b and d). Yeasts are also capable of sexual reproduction.

Two edible fungi are also ascomycetes. One of these is the mushroom-like morel. The other is the truffle (Color Photograph 37), a subterranean spherical fungus found around certain species of oak trees. The truffle mycelium, and possibly that of morels, grows in association with tree roots. The unique flavor of truffles and morels is highly valued by many cooks and gastronomes. The rarity and difficulty of harvesting truffles, which mainly grow only in certain regions of France and Italy, combined with their unique flavor places them among the most expensive of all foods, even though they have little nutritive value.

Several ascomycetes are known for their harmful activities. These include a variety of plant diseases such as apple scab, powdery mildew of roses and related plants (Color Photograph 3b); the production of the poisonous substance (toxin) *ergot* by *Claviceps purpurea* growing on rye and other cereals; and the production of substances related to ergot, such as the well-known hallucinogen LSD (lysergic acid diethylamide). On the other hand, substances derived from ergot, the ergotomine drugs, are used medically to treat vascular diseases such as migraine headaches.

Basidiomycetes

The Basidiomycetes include the bracket fungi of trees (Color Photograph 33), mushrooms (Color Photographs 31 and 32), puffballs, rusts, smuts, and toadstools. Of these various species, the most familiar is the often edible mushroom.

Commercial mushrooms, *Agaricus* species, are the only cultivated food crop of this group. Mushrooms are grown by "planting" the primary mycelia, known as *spawn,* in soil enriched with animal manure in a dark, cool place, such as a cave, basement, or similar environment.

Mushroom poisoning occurs frequently. When not caused by bacteria (botulism) in marinated mushroom preparations, it is most often attributable to species of the mushroom genus *Amanita* (Color Photograph 30). The species of *Amanita* can be identified by three characteristics: (1) the veil that covers the emerging mushroom; (2) white spores when the mushroom is mature; and (3) a distinctive cup at the base. However, mushrooms lacking these characteristics are not necessarily safe to eat.

The rusts and smuts, which are plant parasites, cause considerable damage and economic loss. This is especially true for grain plants such as corn, oats, and wheat. Each species of smut is restricted to a single host species. Some of these plant pathogens, such as the stem rust of wheat and the white pine blister rust, have complicated life cycles, passed in two or more different plants and involving the production of several kinds of spores.

The sexual spore-bearing structure of the basidiomycete is known as a basidium and grows out of an extensive underground mycelium (Figure 9–13). Each basidium is an enlarged, club-shaped hypha, at the tip of which four basidiospores develop. These spores, which develop outside of the basidium, are eventually released to develop into new mycelia under appropriate environmental conditions. The life cycle and other distinguishing properties of a mushroom are shown in Figure 9–13 and described in Table 9–2.

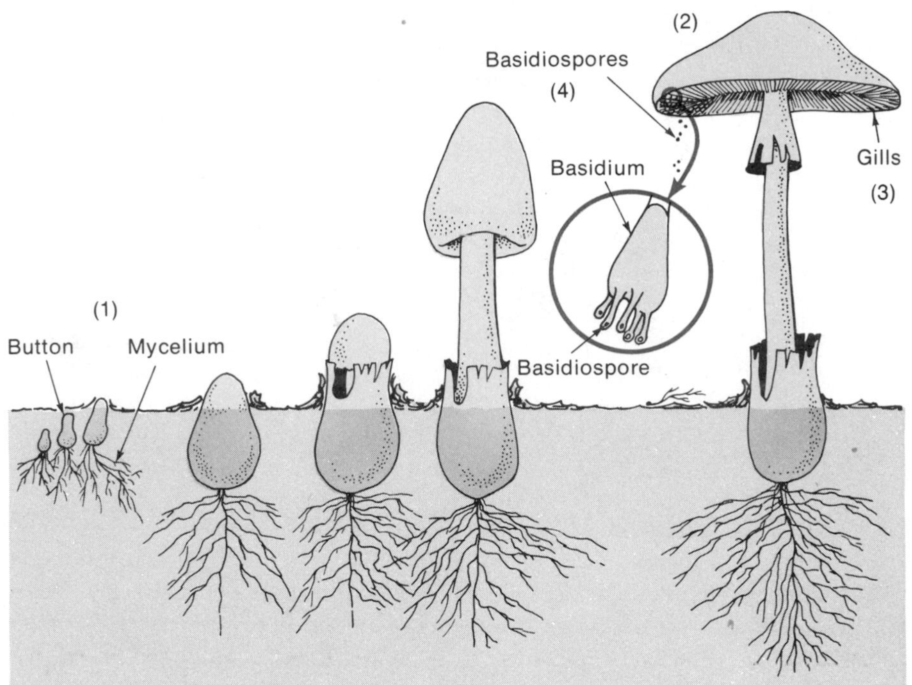

FIG. 9–13 Mushroom development stages from the hyphae masses (mycelium) to the completed mushroom. A compact button appears underground (1) and grows into the complete fruiting body, or mushroom (2). On the undersurface of the mushroom, thin perpendicular gills appear (3) on which specialized hyphae (basidia) develop and produce basidiospores (4). The spores are released, and in a favorable environment they germinate and give rise to new hyphae and mycelia.

Deuteromycetes (Fungi Imperfecti)

Deuteromycetes include all fungi in which sexual reproduction is unknown. These organisms reproduce only by means of asexual spores. Among the deuteromycetes are a number of important fungi that resemble the Ascomycetes in every respect except that they lack a sexual process.

Several deuteromycete species are commercially and medically important. Among the most important are members of the genus *Penicillium* (Figure 9–14a and Color Photograph 34). The distinctive flavor and soft consistency of Camembert and several other cheeses is caused by the enzymatic activities of specific fungi. The mycelium forms the white coat that covers the surface of the cheese. Eventually, the hyphae penetrate into the cheese, softening it by enzymatic action and imparting a unique flavor. The characteristic flavor and appearance of Roquefort and related blue cheeses are due to the activities of another *Penicillium* species.

Several *Penicillium* species are important sources of the antibiotic penicillin. Other commercially important fungi are discussed later in the text.

Pathogenic fungi belonging to the Deuteromycetes cause two types of human infections, namely those that involve the superficial tissues, such as hair, nails, and skin, and those that affect the deeper tissues and organs. Examples of the

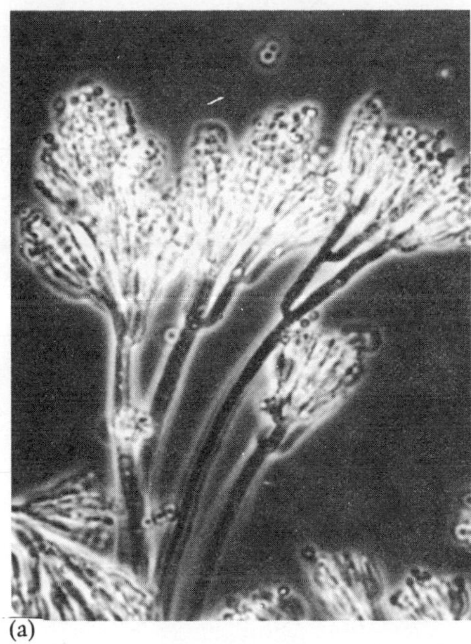
(a)

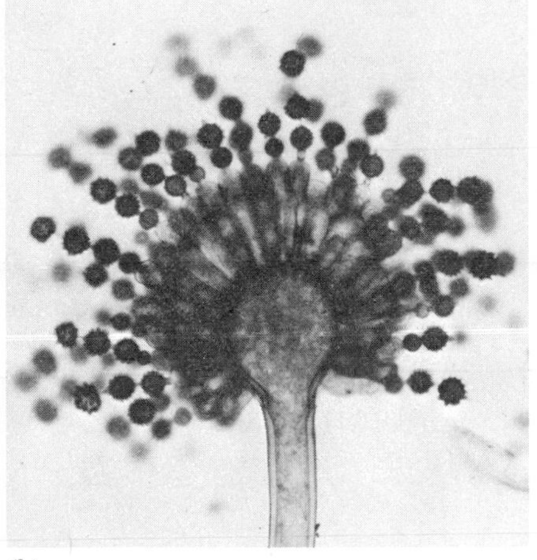
(b)

FIG. 9–14 The structures of common fungi. The typical microscopic appearances of fungal species are shown. (a) *Penicillium notatum*. The characteristic brushlike feature of this mold is quite apparent. *Courtesy of S. Stanley Schneierson, M. D., and Abbott Laboratories.* (b) *Aspergillus niger*. Note the free spores (arrows). *Courtesy of CCM: General Biological, Inc., Chicago.*

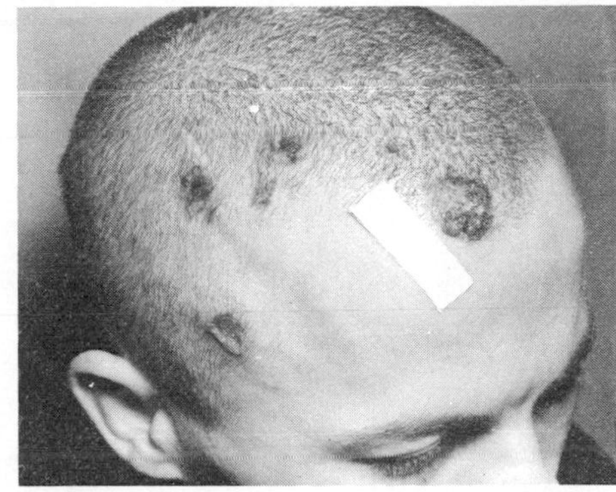

FIG. 9–15 Favus, a severe form of ringworm of the scalp. *Courtesy of the Armed Forces Institute of Pathology, Washington, D.C., Neg. No. B-535-1.*

former include the variety of infections called ringworm (Figure 9–15 and Color Photographs 41 and 42). Some Deuteromycetes cause only one of the general forms of disease states; others can produce both types of infection (Figures 29–8 and 31–5). Many of these mycotic infections are described in later chapters.

Certain Deuteromycetes produce poisons known as **mycotoxins** (Figure 9–16). Although most molds growing on foods are harmless, some are not. *Aspergillus flavus* and other fungi, which often grow on stored cereal products and nuts, produce one type of mycotoxin, **aflatoxins** from the terms **(A**spergillus **fla**vus **toxin),** which are quite toxic to many animal species. The real and potential danger of these toxins was dramatically shown in 1960 by a large-scale trout poisoning in commercial fish hatcheries. The fish had been fed rations later shown to be contaminated by fungi. Concurrent outbreaks of turkey X disease in England were traced to similar contamination.

The presence of mycotoxins in food is not too surprising considering the wide distribution of fungi and their growth during storage and handling of food and crops. The recognition of aflatoxins stimulated research that led to isolation and identification of many additional mycotoxins. Other mycotoxins were found not only to be toxic to many animal species, but also to cause cancer in the liver.

Poisoning by such fungal toxins assumes worldwide significance in view of population groups suffering from protein deficiency diseases. While being treated for malnutrition, affected individuals may suffer severe liver injury from mycotoxins. This poisoning occurs because the protein sources often used to correct malnutrition, peanuts and cereals, may be contaminated by mycotoxin-producing fungi. The World Health Organization (WHO) has been a leader in directing attention to the serious health hazards associated with fungus-contaminated foods.

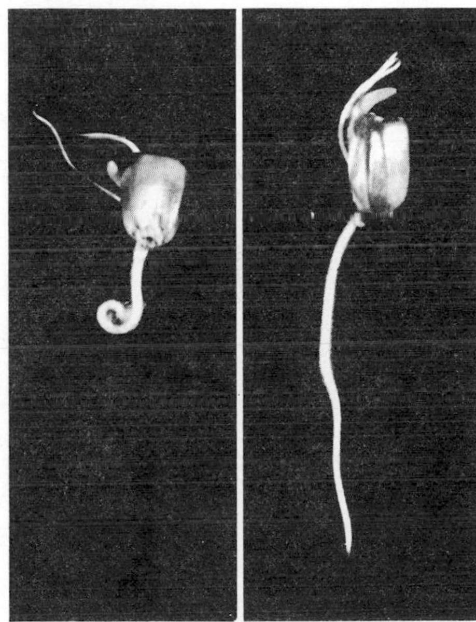

FIG. 9–16 Fungi produce a variety of compounds. Certain of these substances have antibiotic action for bacteria, but they may exert serious disturbances in other forms of life. The malformins are a group of compounds that affect plant growth. The corn plant on the left has been exposed to malformin from *Aspergillus niger*. The plant on the right has been exposed only to water. *Curtis, R. W., W. R. Stevenson, and J. Tuite,* Appl. Microbiol. *28:362–365 (1974).*

Oomycetes

Oomycetes are noted for the production of single-celled, motile asexual zoospores that can move only in water or moist environments. The life cycle of oomycetes includes two reproductive stages, one asexual and the other sexual, involving oospores.

Species of this fungal class cause some of the most destructive plant diseases known. These include downy mildew of grapes, which nearly ruined the French wine industry. It was finally brought under control by the invention of Bordeaux mixture, a mixture of copper sulfate and lime that is still a common fungicide. A far more serious disease caused by oomycetes is late blight of potatoes, which almost totally destroyed the potato crop in Ireland in 1845, 1846, and 1848. The destruction of potatoes resulted in widespread famine and death in Ireland during those years. Thousands fled the country and emigrated to other lands, especially to the United States.

Zygomycetes

The smallest class of fungi are the Zygomycetes. The hyphae of the Zygomycetes have few or no crosswalls; they form coencytic mycelia. Their asexual spores include chlamydospores, conidia, and sporangiospores. Sexual reproduction is by fusion of the hyphal tips of two different mating cell types, resulting in a zygote (Figure 9–17a).

A familiar, but unwelcomed, zygomycete is the common bread mold, *Rhizopus nigricans* (Figure 9–17). Bread becomes moldy when a spore of this

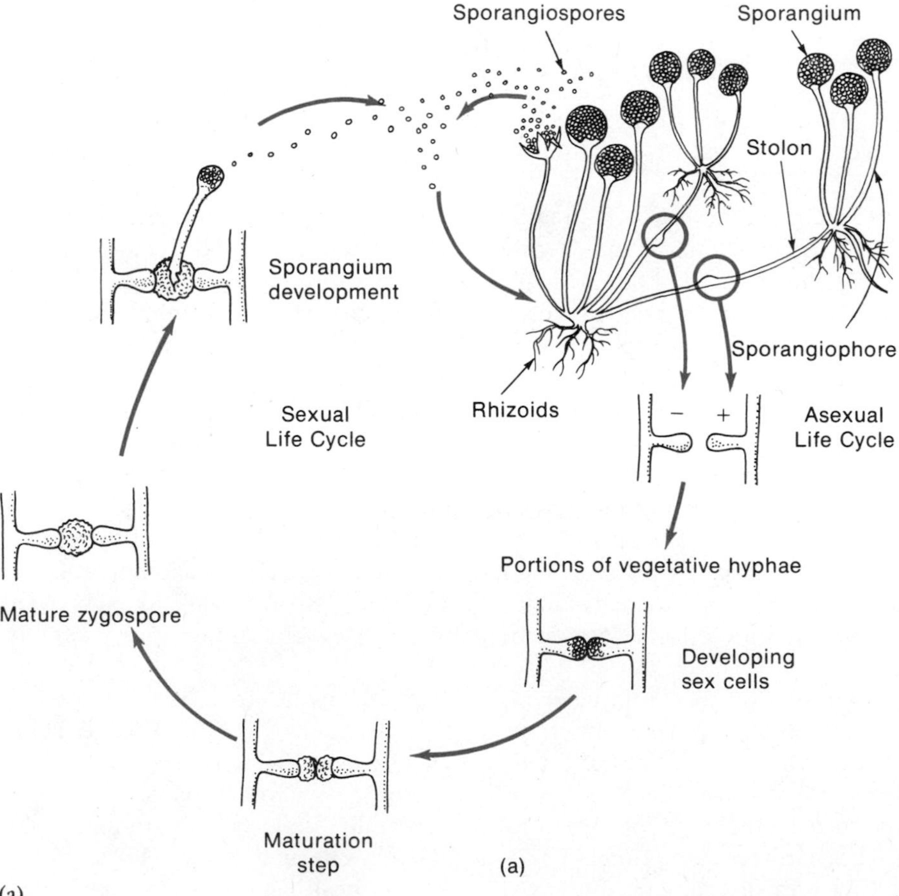

(a)

FIG. 9–17 The common bread mold ***Rhizopus nigricans.*** (a) The life cycle of this mold, showing the various structures of the mycelium.

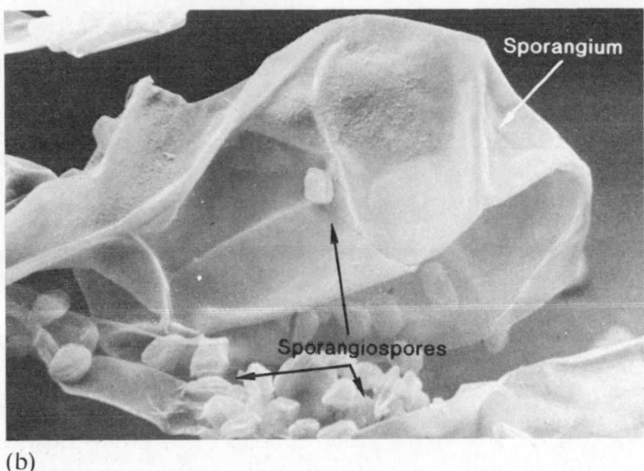

(b)

FIG. 9–17 (b) A scanning micrograph showing a collapsed sporangium and numerous sporangiospores. Note the thin texture of the saclike structure.

organism falls on it, germinates, and grows to form the mycelium that covers the bread surface. Some of the hyphae, the ***rhizoids***, penetrate the bread to obtain nutrients and anchor the mold. Others, the ***stolons***, spread horizontally with amazing speed. Eventually, certain hyphae grow upward and develop sacs, or ***sporangia***, at their tips. Clusters of brown to black spherical asexual spores develop within each sac (Figure 9–17b) and are released when the delicate spore sac ruptures. Growth of molds such as this one is usually prevented in commercial bakeries by the addition of preservatives to the bread dough before baking.

Certain Zygomycetes cause fungus infections in humans and other animals. Other parasitize roundworms (Figure 9–18) and arthropods.

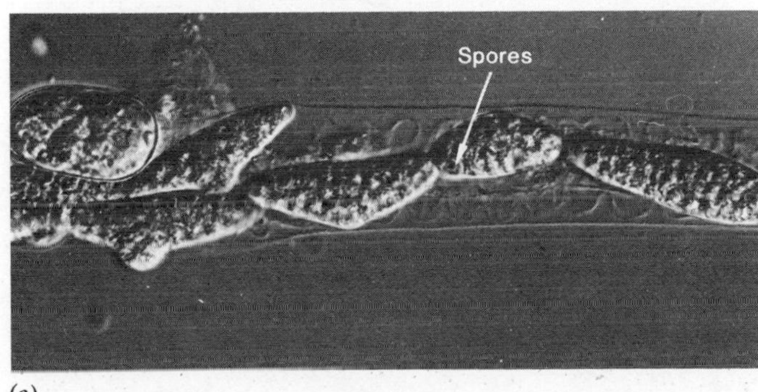

(a)

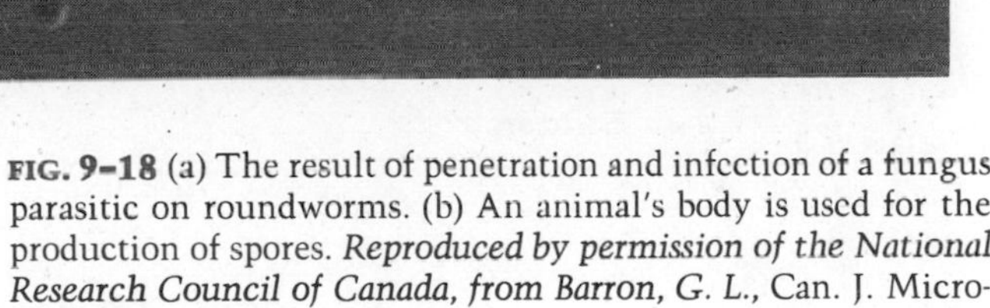

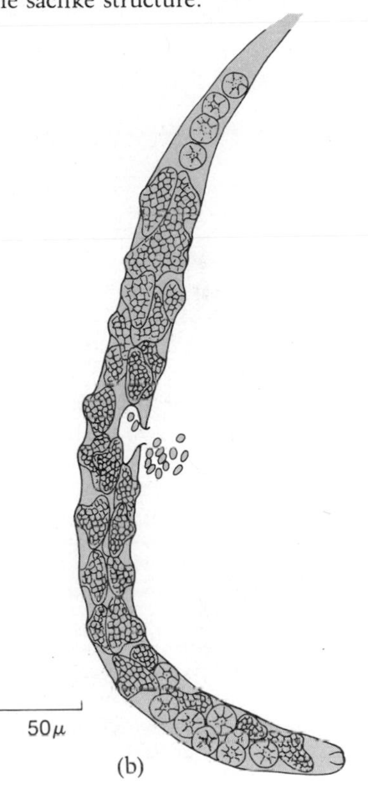

(b)

FIG. 9–18 (a) The result of penetration and infection of a fungus parasitic on roundworms. (b) An animal's body is used for the production of spores. *Reproduced by permission of the National Research Council of Canada, from Barron, G. L.,* Can. J. Microbiol. *22:752–762 (1976).*

Myxomycetes, the Slime Molds

The Myxomycetes are commonly called slime molds because of the slimy appearance of their vegetative forms, called ***slugs*** or ***plasmodia*** (singular, ***plasmodium***). Because these unique protists resemble both fungi and protozoa, slime molds have at times been classified as both fungi and protozoa. Their actively feeding vegetative structures are composed of masses of amoebalike cells without cell walls, and their fruiting (reproductive) structures resemble those of fungi. Approximately 500 species of slime molds are recognized. Usually they are saprophytic, feeding on decaying plant life, and can appear in various colors on decaying logs, dead leaves in dense, shaded forests, or in damp soil. Certain parasitic slime molds, such as *Plasmodiophora brassicae,* cause significant injury to food crops such as cauliflower, radish, rutabaga, and turnip. This organism causes club-root disease of plants, in which the roots of the plant increase in size and provide an environment for slime mold growth and development.

The slime molds can be divided into two groups, ***cellular*** and ***acellular*** slime molds. The vegetative forms of the cellular mold consist of single amoebalike cells. The acellular slime molds are masses of protoplasm of indefinite size and shape (plasmodia) in their vegetative forms.

One of the outstanding features of this group of microorganisms is their rather unique life cycle. The cycle of a cellular slime mold provides an example. (Sexual reproduction apparently does not occur in these forms, whereas it does in the acellular slime molds.) Cellular slime molds (Figure 9–19) live and multiply in soil habitats as amoebae with one nucleus. They use the bacteria in these environments as food. However, when the supply of bacteria is exhausted, the amoebae combine their efforts and collect into multicellular aggregates (pseudoplasmodia, or slugs) of 100,000 or more amoebae. The cells comprising this structure lose some of their individuality but do not fuse. The aggregation process is initiated by the production of acrasin, a chemical recently identified as cyclic adenosine monophosphate (cAMP). Each aggregate undergoes a complex development cycle resulting in the formation of a fruiting body. The latter structure consists of a base, a slender stalk, and a cluster of spores in a

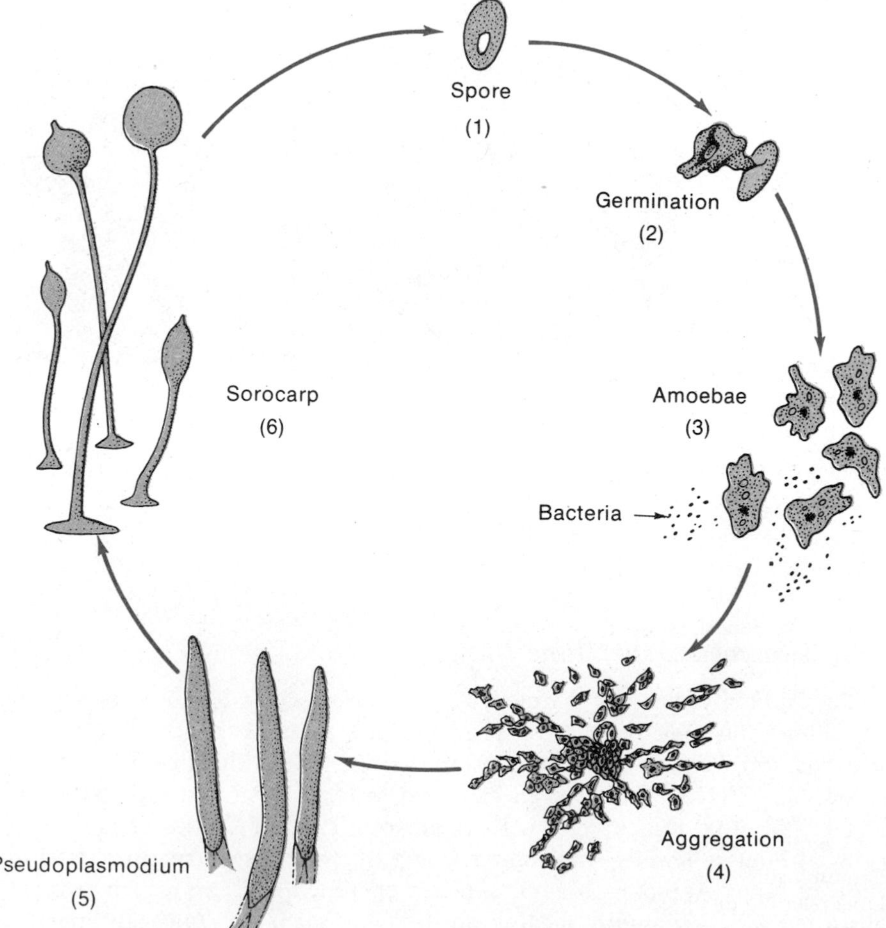

FIG. 9–19 The life cycle of the cellular slime mold *Dictyostelium discoideum*. In a suitable environment the spores (1) of this organism germinate (2) and give rise to amoebalike cells (3) that feed on bacteria, grow, and divide. When food sources decrease, some cells produce a hormonelike substance, a crasin, which causes other cells to stream toward a central area forming an aggregation (4). Next, aggregations form a pseudoplasmodium, or slug (5). At a particular stage of this organism's development, the cells of the slug differentiate into a spore-producing sorocarp (6) and the cycle starts again.

capsule at the head. The fruiting body is composed of two specialized types of cells. *Stalk cells* lift the spore mass off from the substratum, the surface on which the slime mold is situated. The *spores* are reproductive cells. Environmental factors apparently play an important role in the development of the fruiting structure.

When moistened, the spores of the slime mold germinate and give rise to the single cells called *myxamoebae*. These forms, which closely resemble typical protozoan amoebae, divide or reproduce by simple fission (splitting). Eventually, under the conditions mentioned earlier, pseudoplasmodia again are formed, and the development cycle begins once more.

SUMMARY

1. Fungi are eucaryotic and nonphotosynthetic.
2. Fungi are of great practical and ecological importance; they include mushrooms, puffballs, woody bracket fungi, molds, and yeasts.

Distribution and Activities

1. Fungi are widespread in nature, growing well in dark, moist environments where organic material is available.
2. These organisms are heterotrophic and are referred to as *saprobes*, since they utilize preexisting organic products.
3. Fungi produce digestive enzymes that, depending on the species, may be beneficial or destructive.

Structure and Function

1. Fungi differ from bacteria in size, structure, cellular organization, and methods of reproduction.
2. The term *fungus* is a general term that includes two different forms, molds and yeasts.

Molds

1. Molds do not have true roots, stems, or leaves, but do exhibit a differentiation of parts.
2. The structural unit of most molds is the *hypha*.
3. Strands, or filaments, of hyphae can be subdivided into multicellular forms by crosswalls, or septa.
4. Hyphae without septa are called coenocytic.
5. Mold growth resulting in a visible cobweblike aggregation of hyphae is called a *mycelium*.
6. Spores are the specialized reproductive cells of molds.

Yeasts

1. Yeasts appear as oval to spherical cells that form moist, shining colonies.
2. Some yeasts may produce capsules.
3. These microorganisms reproduce sexually by producing new *buds*, or *daughter cells*. Birth scars are carried by new cells, while main cells exhibit bud scars.
4. Newly formed cells that do not separate form *pseudohyphae*.

Dimorphism

Under certain environmental conditions some fungi exhibit two different forms, appearing as either molds or yeasts. This phenomenon is called *dimorphism*.

Reproduction and Spores

1. The type of spore and the sporulation process are both important to fungal identification and classification.
2. Fungal spores function as reproductive cells and are not more resistant to environmental factors than other cell types.

Asexual Spores

1. Spores are formed either through asexual or sexual processes. Depending on the species, both asexual and sexual spores or only asexual spores are formed.
2. Asexual spores include: *arthrospores, blastospores, chlamydospores, conidia, sporangiospores*, and *zoospores*.
3. Under appropriate conditions of nutrition, moisture, pH, and temperature, fungal spores germinate and produce one or more long structures called *germ tubes*. Germ tubes subsequently develop into *hyphae*.

Sexual Spores

Sexual spores are the result of nuclear fusion between two different cell types and include *ascospores, basidiospores, oospores*, and *zygospores*.

The Ultrastructure of Fungi

1. Both molds and yeasts exhibit eucaryotic cellular organization.
2. Cellular membranes contain sterols, a property that separates fungi from procaryotes.
3. The cell walls of filamentous fungi are composed of thin, threadlike structures called *microfibrils* (which are composed of *chitin*) and cellulose. Yeast cell walls contain the complex polysaccharides glucan and mannan, as well as lipids, proteins, and the amino sugar glucosamine.
4. Pili appear on the cell walls of various yeasts. These structures are similar to those of bacteria and may be involved with the sexual reproduction of yeasts.

Cultivation of Fungi

1. Molds and yeasts can be grown and studied by cultural methods similar to those used for many bacteria.
2. Media used for fungus cultivation are modified to limit the growth of other microbes. Ingredients used for this purpose include antibiotics, dyes, high concentrations of sugars, and compounds that lower the pH of media.

Types of Media

Three basic types of media are used: *natural* (carrot plugs, potato slices), *dehydrated* (Sabouraud dextrose agar), and *synthetic*.

Distinctive Mycelia

The appearance of and the diffusion of pigment from mycelia are used for identification purposes.

Classification

1. Several properties of fungi are used in fungus classification. These incude methods of reproduction, mycelial formation, and cellular structure and formation.
2. Five fungal classes are recognized on the basis of their method of reproduction: *Ascomycetes, Basidiomycetes, Deuteromycetes* (Fungi Imperfecti), *Oomycetes,* and *Zygomycetes.*

Ascomycetes

The Ascomycetes, or sac fungi, include a variety of economic and biologically important organisms. Members of this group can be found in a variety of environments including aquatic, land, and other forms of life. The Ascomycetes reproduce both asexually and sexually.

Basidiomycetes

The Basidiomycetes include the bracket fungi of trees, mushrooms, puffballs, rusts, smuts, and toadstools. These fungi are also economically and biologically important. Some members of the group, such as the species of the *Amanita,* are highly poisonous. The Basidiomycetes reproduce asexually and sexually.

Deuteromycetes (Fungi Imperfecti)

The Deuteromycetes represent a group of fungi in which sexual reproduction is unknown. Several members of the group are medically and commercially important. Some species are noted for their production of highly poisonous ***mycotoxins*** such as ***aflatoxins.***

Oomycetes

The Oomycetes are noted for their production of single-celled, motile asexual zoospores, which can move about only in water or moist environments. These fungi can also reproduce sexually. Certain species cause some of the most destructive plant diseases known.

Zygomycetes

The Zygomycetes contain the smallest number of species. They reproduce both asexually and sexually. Some members are parasitic.

Myxomycetes, the Slime Molds

1. Slime molds have at times been classified as both fungi and protozoa because of the cell types produced in their unique life cycle.
2. The slime molds can be divided into two groups, the cellular and acellular forms.
3. While most slime molds are saprophytic, feeding on decaying plant life, some can be parasitic and cause the destruction of various vegetable plants.

QUESTIONS FOR REVIEW

1. List three ways in which fungi differ from bacteria.
2. a. What type of cellular organization do fungi have?
   b. List at least six organelles found in fungi, and give their respective functions.
3. a. Differentiate between asexual and sexual spores.
   b. List and describe three examples of each type of fungal spore.
   c. What type of spore do yeasts produce?
4. Distinguish between aerial and reproductive mycelia.
5. Define or explain the following terms:
   a. hypha
   b. mycelium
   c. septum
   d. coenocytic
   e. bud
   f. basidium
   g. mold
   h. yeast
6. What is dimorphism?
7. Do the techniques used for the cultivation of fungi differ from those used with bacteria? Explain.
8. a. What criteria are used in the identification and classification of molds?
   b. Do such criteria differ from the ones used for bacterial classification? Explain.
9. List the major classes of fungi and give two beneficial and two harmful activities of each.
10. Identify and give the function of each of the labeled structures in Figure 9-20.
11. a. What are slime molds?
    b. How do slime molds differ from members of the Ascomycetes?

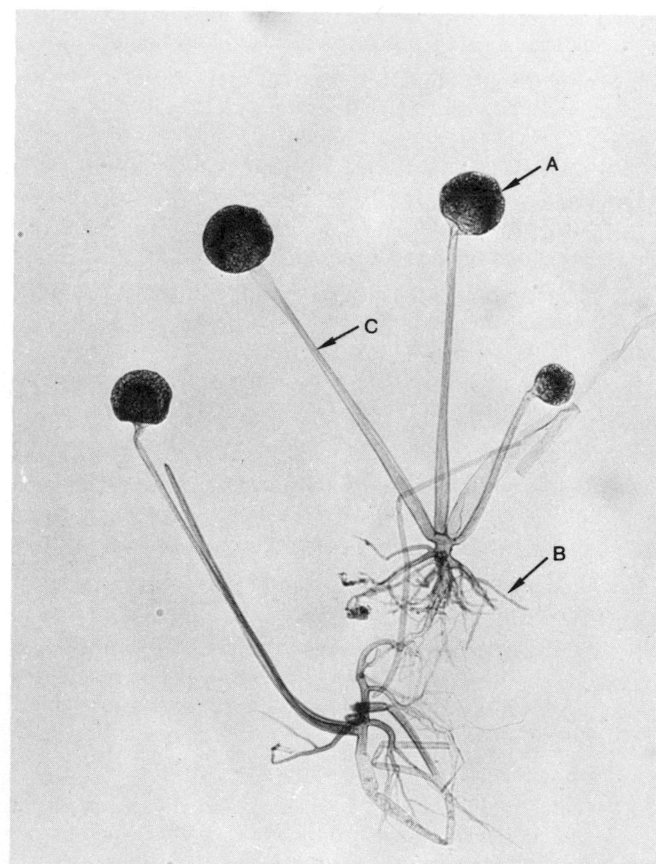

FIG. 9-20 *Courtesy Carolina Biological Supply Company.*

SUGGESTED READINGS

Ahearn, D. G., "Medically Important Yeasts," *Ann. Rev. Microbiol.* 32:59–68 (1978). *The ecology and physiology of pathogenic species and the conditions that predispose humans to yeast infections are discussed.*

Bigelow, H. E., *Mushroom Pocket Field Guide.* New York: Macmillan, 1974. *A superb, compact field guide with several excellent color photographs.*

Burnett, J. H., *Mycogenetics: An Introduction to the General Genetics of Fungi.* New York: John Wiley & Sons, 1975. *The genetics of fungi with topics such as genetic markers, recombination, segregation, and linkage of nuclei, extrachromosomal elements, population genetics, and applications are discussed.*

Cooke, R. C., *The Biology of Symbiotic Fungi.* New York: John Wiley & Sons, 1977. *This book attempts to outline all major symbiotic associations between fungi and either animals or plants and show how these various associations function.*

Gray, W. D., *The Relation of Fungi to Human Affairs.* New York: Holt, Rinehart & Winston, 1959. *A comprehensive treatment of the numerous ways fungi affect human life.*

Rose, A. H., and J. S. Harrison (eds.), *The Yeasts,* Vol. 3: *Yeast Technology.* New York: Academic Press, 1970. *Various aspects of the industrial applications of yeast are discussed by experts. The chapters on beer and wine yeasts are especially good.*

Sieburth, J. M., *Microbial Seascapes.* Baltimore: University Park Press, 1975. *A fascinating view of marine microorganisms and their respective environments as seen through the scanning electron microscope.*

Smith, J. E., and D. R. Berry (eds.), *The Filamentous Fungi,* Vol. 1: *Industrial Mycology.* New York: John Wiley & Sons, 1975. *The uses of filamentous fungi in the production of enzymes, organic acids, single-cell protein, and other industrially important products are reviewed.*

Wasson, R. G., *Soma, Divine Mushroom of Immortality.* New York: Harcourt Brace Jovanovich, 1967. *A fascinating discussion of the long history of the poisonous mushroom, Amanita. Numerous illustrations, some in color.*

Wogan, G. N., "Mycotoxins," *Ann. Rev. Pharmacology* 15:437 (1975). *Reports on the current status of mycotoxins and the areas thought to be most relevant to public health.*

CHAPTER **10**

Protozoa

Chapter 10 surveys the protozoa. We shall discuss their distribution, structure, and life cycles, as well as their beneficial and harmful activities.

After reading this chapter, you should be able to:

1. **Describe the general properties of protozoa and the position they occupy in the biological world.**
2. **Explain the basis of protozoan classification.**
3. **Identify protozoan structures and give their functions.**
4. **List and describe the distinguishing properties of the major groups of protozoa.**
5. **Explain how protozoa differ from other types of microorganisms.**
6. **Outline the general features of protozoan reproduction.**
7. **List and describe the major beneficial and destructive activities and functions of protozoa.**
8. **Describe the methods used for protozoan cultivation.**
9. **Define or explain the following:**
   a. trophozoite **c. contractile vacuole**
   b. cyst **d. conjugation**

Since their discovery by Anton van Leeuwenhoek in 1674, protozoa have been extensively studied and even put to work. Today, protozoa are of interest to biologists working in various fields: the dating of oil beds by means of the fossil remains of protozoa; chemotherapy of protozoan diseases such as malaria and toxoplasmosis; electron microscopy of protozoan structures; and use of protozoa as biologic indicators of pollution.

Protozoa are unicellular, eucaryotic microorganisms. Many are motile and

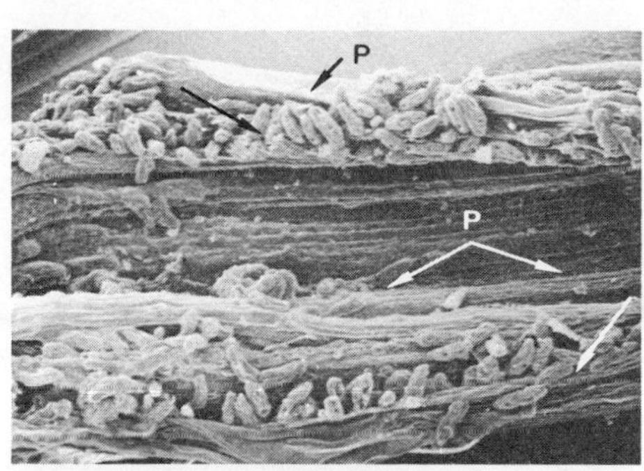

FIG. 10-1 A scanning micrograph showing the ciliate *Epidinium crawley* (arrows) attached to plant fragments (P) undergoing digestion in the intestinal tract of sheep. *Epidinium*, inhabitants of the digestive tract of sheep and cattle in various regions of the world, are known to ingest whole or damaged chloroplasts and starch grains. *Bauchop, T., and R. T. J. Clark*, Appl. Environ. Microbiol. *32:417–422 (1976)*.

many require organic food and obtain it from their environments. Because of properties such as these, protozoa have traditionally been considered animals. Modern systems that divide living organisms into more than two kingdoms classify protozoa as belonging to the Protista (Figure 3–2). At least 45,000 protozoan species have been described to date. These microorganisms vary widely in shape, size, structure, and physiological properties.

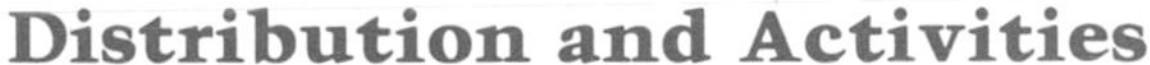

Distribution and Activities

Protozoa are found in many different environments. Some are present in bodies of water where they play an important role in the food chains of natural communities. Others have mutually beneficial *(symbiotic)* relationships with higher forms of animal life (Figure 10–1) or with other microorganisms (Figure 10–2). Protozoa contribute to soil fertility through their role in the decomposition of organic matter. They function as a natural control on microbial populations by feeding on various types of microorganisms.

Protozoa are also known for their harmful activities. African sleeping sickness, amoebic dysentery, malaria, and toxoplasmosis are but a few of the diseases associated with these microorganisms.

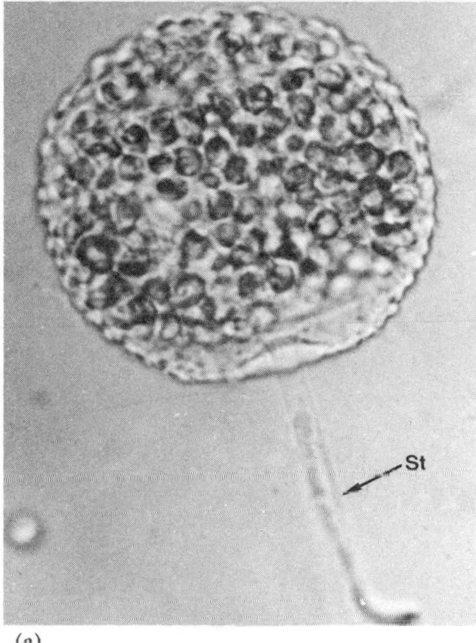

(a)

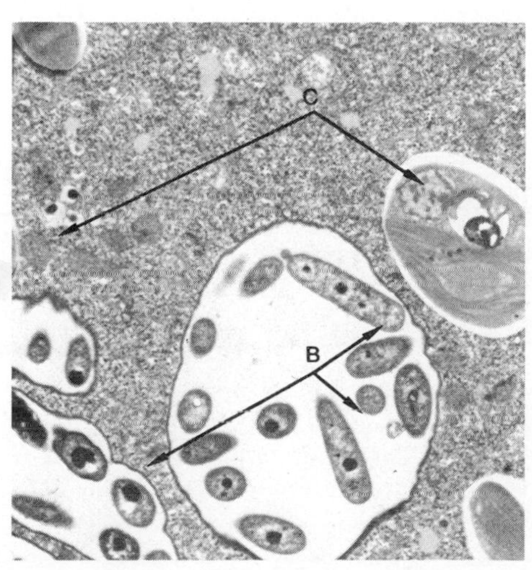

(b)

FIG. 10-2 Associations of protozoa with other forms of life. (a) A photomicrograph of a single green *Vorticella* with its stalks (ST). *Graham, L. E., and J. M. Graham*, J. Protozool. *25:207–210 (1978)*. (b) An ultrathin view of this protozoan shows the presence of not only endosymbiotic green algae, *Chlorella* (C), but intact bacteria (B).

Structure and Function

Even in protozoa, the complexity of essential functions requires division of labor among cellular parts. Different organelles are involved with movement, obtaining and utilizing nutrients, excretion and osmoregulation, reproduction and protection.

Locomotion

Three types of locomotor organelles occur among the protozoa: **pseudopodia, flagella,** and **cilia.** These structures are important to the classification of protozoa. Pseudopodia ("false feet") are temporary organelles commonly associated with amoebae. The cell moves as a whole when the organism extends an area of its protoplasm and then the rest of the cell flows into the extension. Pseudopodia also aid in capturing food. Several types of pseudopodia are found among amoebalike organisms (Figure 10–3). These include finger-shaped, round-tipped *lobopodia;* thin, pointed *filopodia;* branching, slender, pointed *rhizopodia;* slender *axopodia,* with several fibers forming an axial filament.

Protozoan flagella are delicate whiplike structures that beat to propel the organism. These organelles appear to respond to stimuli such as chemicals and touch. The structure and organization of flagella are approximately the same in all types of eucaryotic cells and organisms (Figure 6–10a). Internally an individual flagellum consists of two central microtubules, surrounded by nine double tubules. This 9 + 2 arrangement is characteristic of most cilia and flagella associated with all eucaryotic cells, from paramecia to humans. The outer covering, or sheath, of a flagellum is a continuation of the cell membrane. Each flagellum terminates beneath an organism's surface in a basal granule called a *kinetosome*. In some flagellates the flagellum may be buried in the cell membrane along much of its length, forming a finlike undulating membrane (Figure 10–16 and Color Photograph 5).

Cilia are miniature flagella. Like flagella, they are composed of two central and nine peripheral filaments (Figure 10–4) enclosed by a covering that is continuous with the cell membrane. These organelles may cover the surface of the protozoan, or they may be restricted to a particular region, such as the oral region. In some organisms cilia are fused in stiffened tufts called *cirri* (Figure 10–4). Such cirri may function as tiny legs. Ciliary structures have a coordinating network of fibers that lies just beneath the protozoan covering (Figure 10–4c and d).

Feeding and Digestion

Three major methods of obtaining nutrients are found among the protozoa. Some organisms are autotrophic, capable of synthesizing organic compounds from inorganic ones. Others are heterotrophic, requiring preformed organic substances from their environment. Some heterotrophs are **saprobic,** obtaining nutrients by absorbing what is needed through the cell surface, or **holo-**

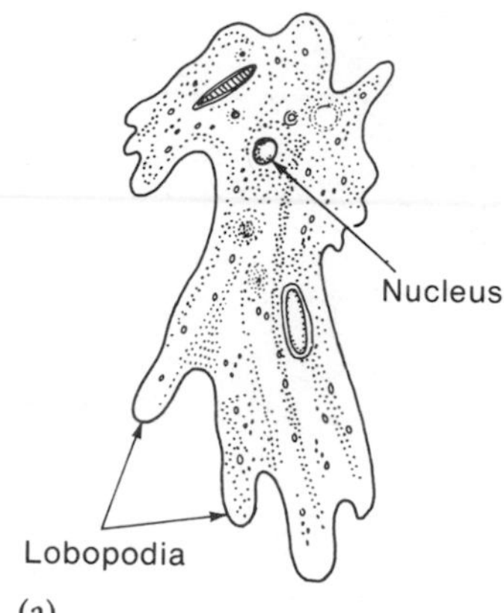

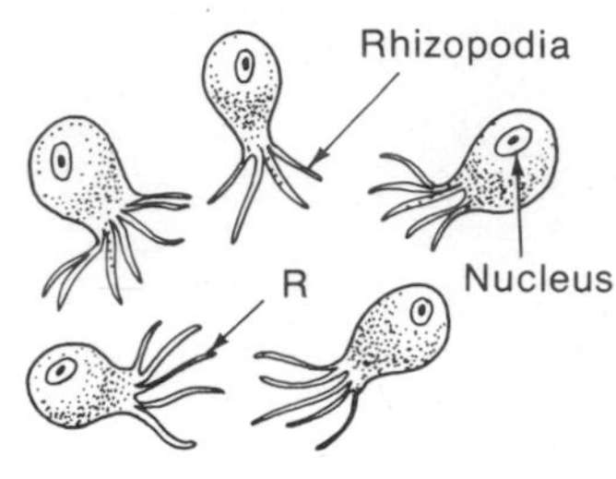

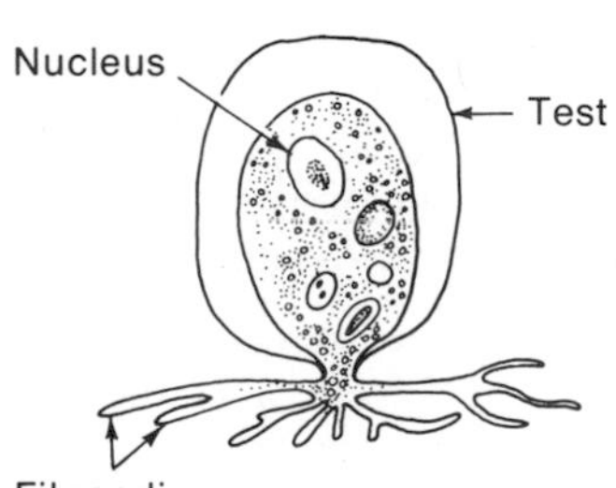

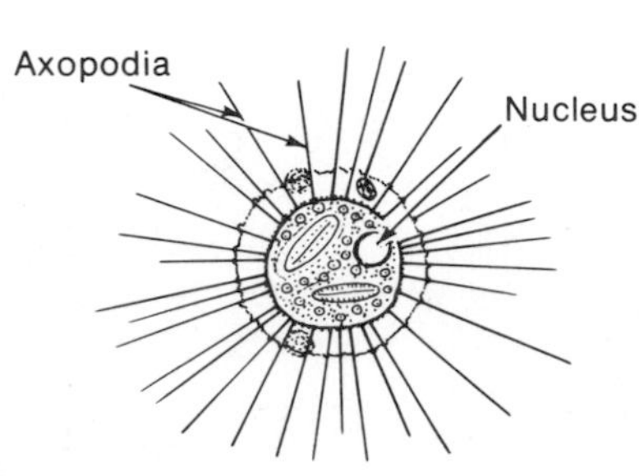

FIG. 10–3 Types of pseudopodia. (a) Lobopodia. (b) Filopodia. (c) Rhizopodia. (d) Axopodia. *After Meglitsch, P. A.,* Invertebrate Zoology. *London: Oxford University Press, 1967.*

FIG. 10–4 Ciliary structures of the protozoan *Gastrostyla steinii.* (a) A diagrammatic representation of a cirrus-bearing protozoan. (b) A view showing the rows of cirri. (c) Network of fibrils (A) and individual fibrils (B) just beneath the network. Numbering of triplet, instead of double, microtubules is shown for one kinetosome in (A). (d) Kinetsomes and internal fibrils from a cirrus. *Grim, J. N.,* J. Protozool. *19 (1):113 (1972).*

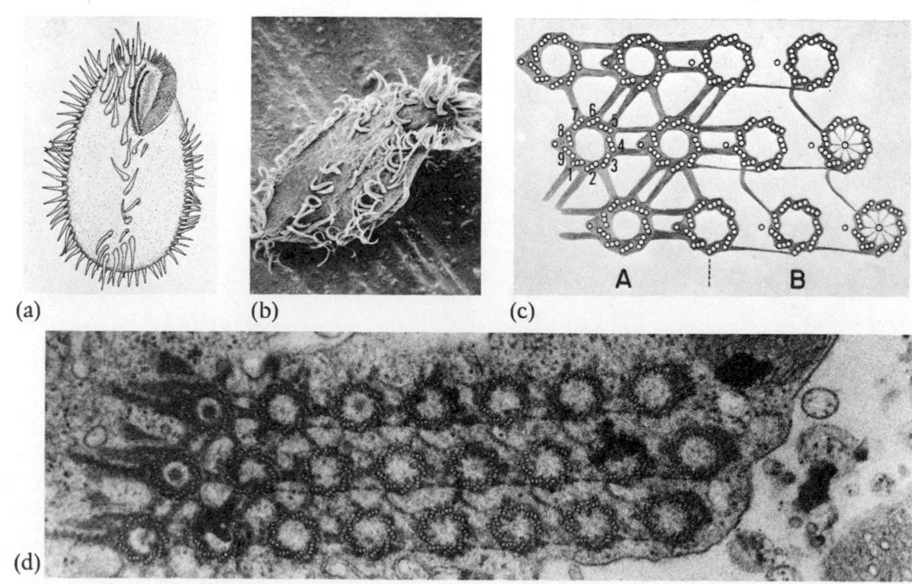

zoic, ingesting entire organisms (Figure 10–5) or smaller particles of food. Holozoic protozoa must have mechanisms for food capture. These include food cups (Figure 10–6), cytosomes (mouths) (Figure 10–7), and tentacles with which to trap prey (Figure 10–14b). Ingested food particles pass into intracellular digestive cavities known as *food vacuoles*. Indigestible material is voided either through a temporary opening or through a permanent opening, the *cytopyge*.

Excretion and Osmoregulation

The excretion of wastes occurs at the cell surface. Most protozoans excrete most of the nitrogen from protein degradation as ammonia. Other waste products produced by intracellular parasitic forms such as the causative agents of malaria (Color Photograph 00) are secreted and accumulated in the host cell. With the destruction of infected cells in the human, the release of waste products produces chills and high body temperatures.

In many protozoans, excretion and osmoregulation are the function of the **contractile vacuoles.** The contractile vacuole system separates a dilute *(hypotonic)* solution of water and electrolytes from the cytoplasm. Eventually it expels this solution from the cell through an opening in the cell surface called the *contractile vacuole pore* (Figure 10–8b). In some protozoa, such as amoebae, the pore is a temporary structure formed at the onset of each contraction (systole). In *Paramecium* (Figure 10–8a) and other ciliates, the pore is a permanent opening in the cellular covering *(pellicle)*. A membranous diaphragm keeps the vacuole closed during the expanding (diastole) period. Contractile vacuoles are well developed in protozoans from freshwater habitats but are usually absent from marine and parasitic protozoans.

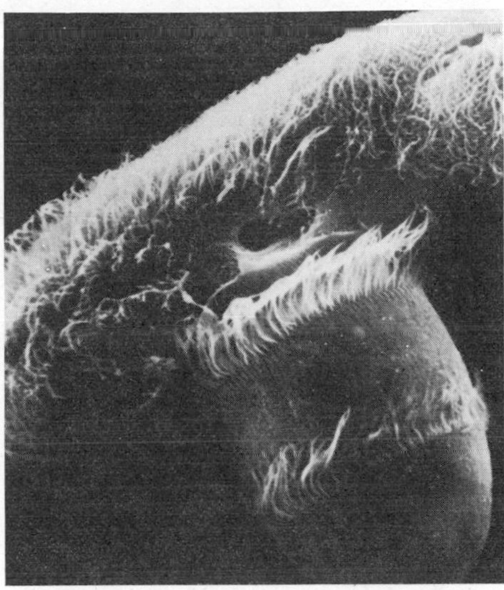

FIG. 10–5 A scanning micrograph showing an early stage in the ingestion of a *Paramecium* by another ciliate, *Didinium*. *Wessenberg, H., and G. Antipa,* J. Protozool. *17:250–270 (1970).*

Protective Structures

Protozoans are exposed to many environmental hazards. Much of their behavior is in response to toxic, life-threatening conditions. Therefore, the development and use of special protective devices help them to survive. Most of the protective structures of protozoans prevent mechanical injury or protect against drying, excessive water intake, and predators. They include several types of surface coverings and trichocysts (Figure 10–9). Other protozoans resort to encystment.

Several flagellates, some amoebae, and all ciliates (Figure 10–8a) have an outermost surface envelope known as a **pellicle.** This covering is stronger

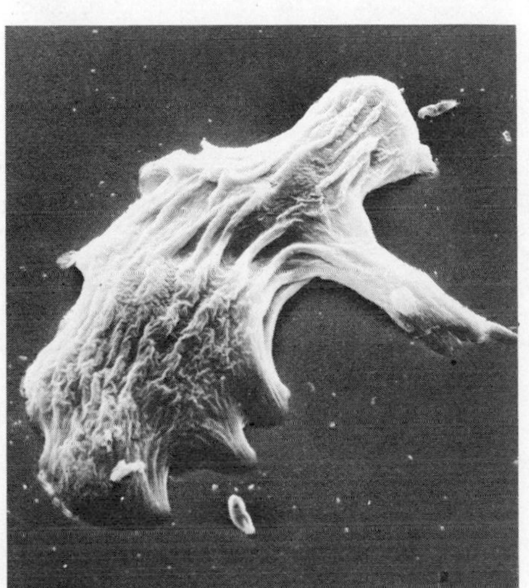

(a)

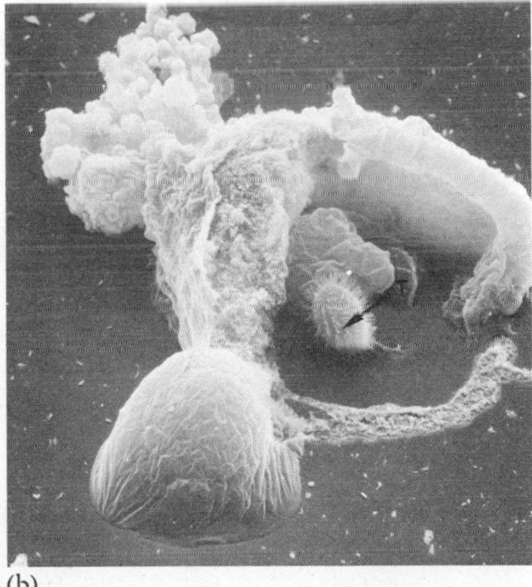

(b)

FIG. 10–6 The feeding action of an amoeba. (a) A nonfeeding amoeba beginning to extend itself in response to a potential food source. (b) An amoeba showing food cups, one of which is open. The inside surface of a food cup enclosing the ciliated protozoan *Tetrahymena* (T) is evident. *Jeon, K. W., and M. S. Jeon,* J. Protozool. *23:83–86 (1976).*

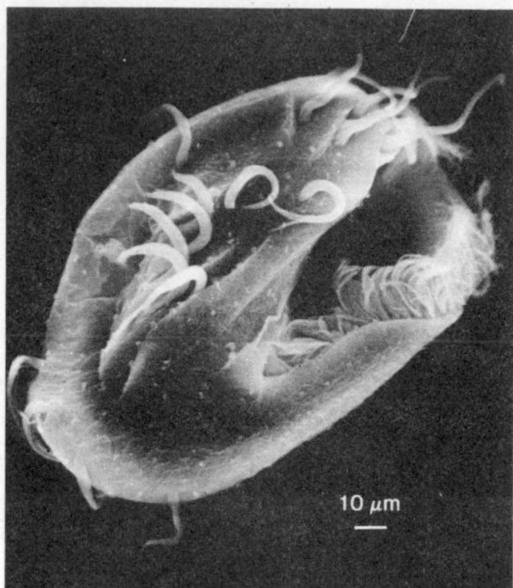

FIG. 10-7 A vegetative protozoan showing a prominent feeding apparatus, the cytosome (C), fringed by a row of cilia. *Kloetzel, J. A.,* J. Protozool. *22:385-392 (1975).*

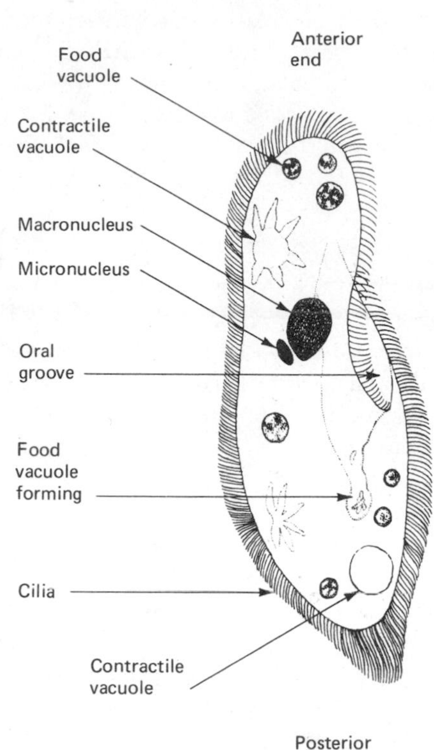

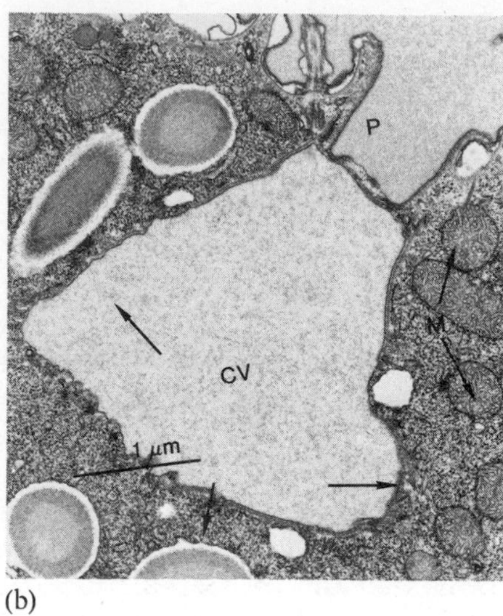

FIG. 10-8 (a) The ciliated *Paramecium.* This eucaryotic organism and other protozoa are several thousand times larger than bacteria. Paramecia have a specialized structure, the oral groove, or gullet, which is used for food ingestion. Liquid is excreted through the contractile vacuole. (b) This view shows a partially closed contracting vacuole. *McKanna, J. A.,* J. Protozool. *20:631-638 (1973).*

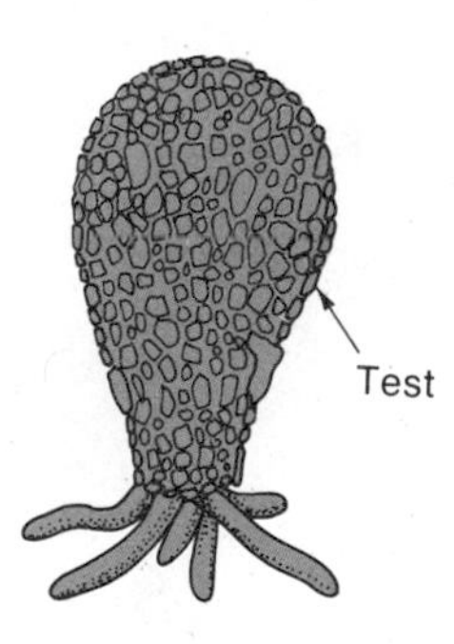

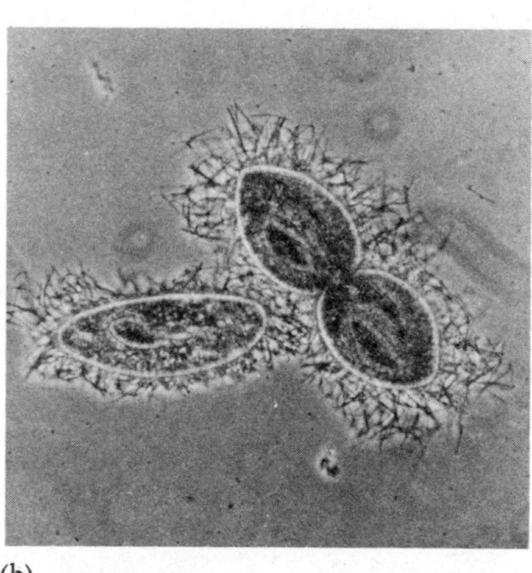

FIG. 10-9 Protective devices of protozoans. (a) *Difflugia,* a test-forming organism, belongs to the *Sarcodina.* (b) Paramecia with trichocysts discharged in response to an unfavorable environmental situation. *From Nyberg, D.,* J. Protozool. *25:107-112 (1978).*

than the cell membrane to which it is attached. Pellicles provide protection against chemicals, drying, and mechanical injury.

Many stationary and some free-living protozoans build coverings called **tests** or *shells* (Figure 10-9a). Some structures consist of sand grains or other foreign particles cemented together; others are composed of secretions of calcium carbonate or silica.

Trichocysts (Figure 10-9b) are specialized intracellular organelles used for defense or for the capture of food. Some ciliates discharge these structures in response to toxic environments.

Trophozoites and Cysts

In several parasitic species and free-living protozoans found in temporary bodies of water, the normal, active feeding form, known as the **trophozoite** (Figure 10–10 and Color Photograph 00), often cannot withstand the effects of various chemicals, food deficiencies, temperature or pH change, and other harsh factors in the environment. To overcome such conditions, many protozoans can secrete a thick, resistant covering and develop into a resting stage called a **cyst** (Figure 10–10). The conditions necessary for such encystment are not fully known, but the process definitely represents a type of cellular differentiation. In addition to providing protection, cysts may serve as sites for cellular reorganization and nuclear division followed by multiplication after the organism leaves the cyst. In the case of certain pathogens such as *Entamoeba histolytica,* which causes amoebic dysentery, cysts also aid in spreading the disease agent. The importance of the trophozoite and cyst stages in the diagnosis of disease is discussed in later chapters.

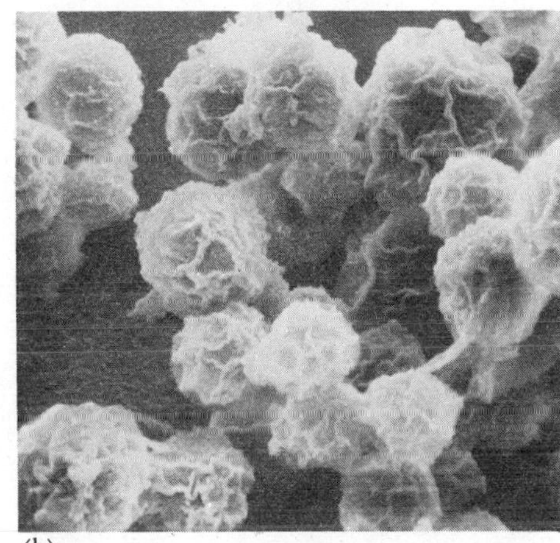

(b)

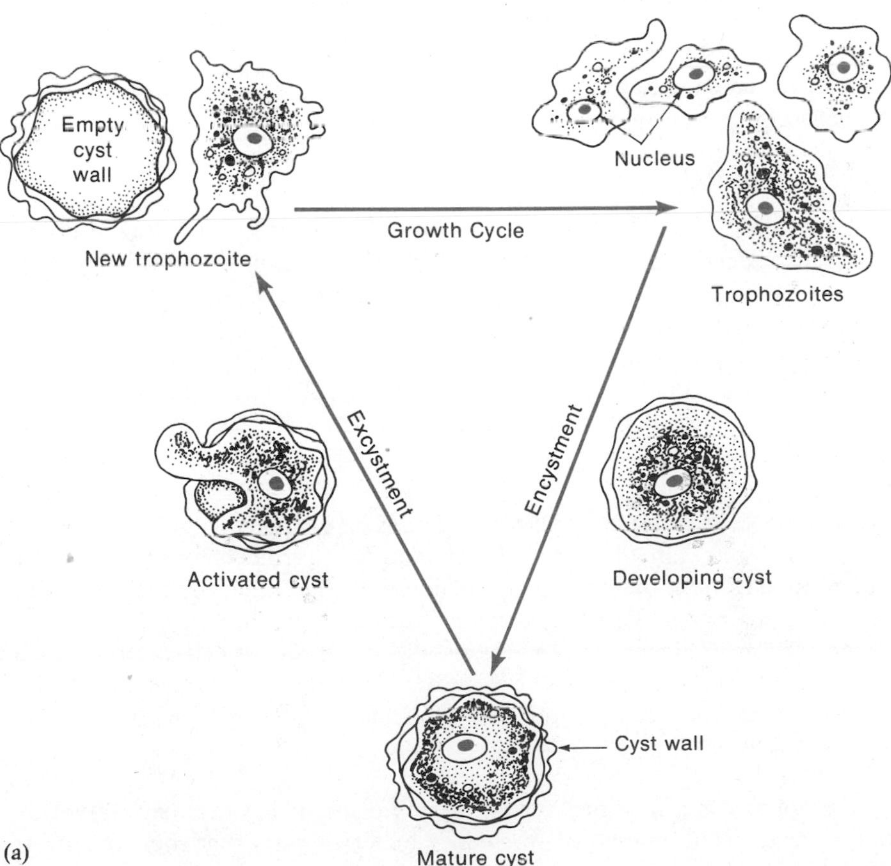

FIG. 10–10 Trophozoites and cysts. (a) The growth and differentiation cycle of protozoa having both trophozoite and cyst stages. In response to encystment stimuli, the vegetative stage, the trophozoite, undergoes metabolic changes to form the resting stage, or cyst. Such cells can withstand prolonged starvation and drying. (b) This scanning micrograph shows the cysts of *Acanthamoeba castellanii. Courtesy of J. J. Pasternak, J. E. Thompson, T. M. G. Schultz, and K. Zachariah.*

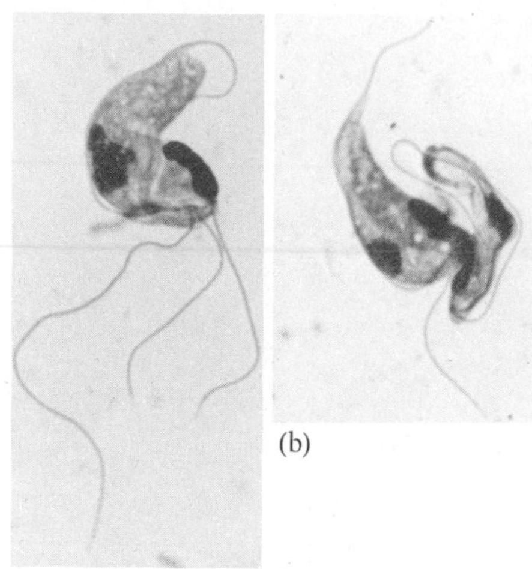

FIG. 10-11 Stages in the binary fission of the flagellate *Cryptobia salmositica*. This protozoan is commonly found in the blood of spawning salmon on the west coast of North America. A leech transmits it from fish to fish. (a) Before division. (b) After division. *Reprinted with the permission of the National Research Council of Canada from Woo, P. T. K.*, Can. J. Zoo. *56:1514–1518 (1978).*

Methods of Reproduction

Ciliated protozoans are multinucleate. They possess at least one *macronucleus* and one *micronucleus* (Figure 10–8a). The macronucleus, which varies in shape, regulates metabolic and developmental functions and maintains all visible traits. The micronucleus exerts an overall control over a cell's macronucleus and regulates cellular sexual and reproductive processes.

Asexual Reproduction

Both asexual and sexual reproduction occur among protozoans. Like certain other microbial types, some protozoa are capable of reproducing asexually only. In this process, the parent cell divides, either equally or unequally, to produce one or more offspring that eventually develop into mature forms. **Binary fission** (division in two parts) is the most common type of asexual reproduction (Figure 10–11). Division may be nuclear or cytoplasmic. Neither meiosis (reduction division) nor fertilization (sexual reproduction) takes place during binary fission.

In addition to binary fission, protozoa reproduce asexually by budding, multiple fission, and plasmotomy. In *budding*, a new individual is formed either at the protozoan's surface or in an internal cavity. **Multiple fission,** or *schizogony*, involves the formation of a multinucleate organism that undergoes division. Division produces a large number of single-nucleus-containing cells almost simultaneously. In multiple fission, the nucleus and other essential organelles divide repeatedly before the cytoplasm divides (cytokinesis). Multiple fission is characteristic of sporozoan parasites (Figure 10–20 and Color Photograph 85). Multinucleated protozoans sometimes divide into two or more multinucleated daughter cells. This type of asexual reproduction is known as *plasmotomy.*

Sexual Reproduction

Sexual reproduction may be relatively simple or complex. Although the production of sex cells (meiosis) apparently takes place, the details of this phenomenon are not well understood. Types of sexual reproduction include syngamy, conjugation, and autogamy.

In **syngamy,** the union of two different sex cells *(gametes)* results in the formation of a fertilized cell, or **zygote.** The zygote may undergo additional development. This type of reproduction is found in sporozoans such as malarial parasites (Figure 10–20).

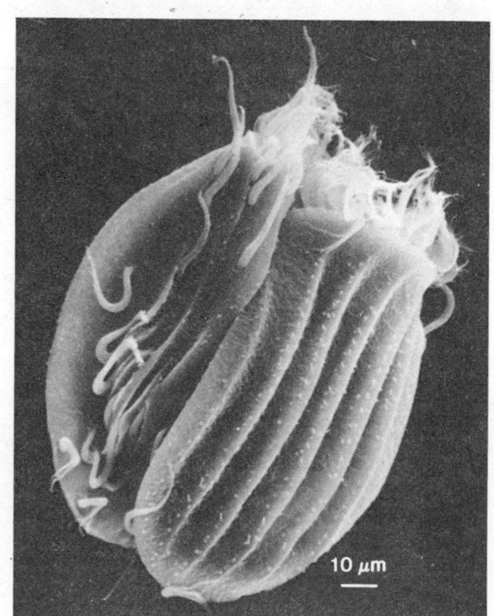

FIG. 10-12 Conjugation shown by scanning electron microscopy. The conjugating partners are joined by a bridge of cytoplasm (not seen here). The dorsal ridges and bristle rows are prominent in the protozoan *Euplotes* at the right. *Kloetzel, J. A.*, J. Protozool. *22:385–392 (1975).*

Conjugation characteristically takes place in ciliated protozoans (Figure 10–12). The process involves the partial union of two ciliates for the transfer of a micronucleus from one organism, the donor, to the other, the recipient. The donor nucleus unites with the recipient nucleus to form a zygote (fertilized) nucleus. To maintain normal conditions within the donor cell, a series of nuclear divisions occur, resulting in the formation of two transferable nuclei. One of these remains behind to ensure that new ciliates will have the normal structural composition.

Autogamy is a modified version of conjugation that occurs only within one protozoan. The micronucleus divides into two parts that then reunite to form a zygote nucleus. The protozoan then divides to yield two cells, each with its full complement of nuclear structures.

Regeneration

The regeneration of lost or damaged parts is a characteristic property of most protozoans. When a cell is cut in two, only the portion containing the nucleus regenerates.

Cultivation

The protozoans are a large and varied group. Their cultivation requirements—especially those of parasites—are also quite diverse. Here we shall present some basic considerations.

In general, free-living protozoans are best cultured under conditions of moderate light, temperatures ranging from 15° to 21°C, and a neutral to slightly alkaline pH. Artificial media used for general cultivation may contain rice, wheat grains, skim milk, hay, or lettuce. More specific growth media contain glucose, proteins and related substances, minerals, and yeast extract. Certain protozoans such as *Amoeba* species and ciliates, including *Didinium*, require the addition of other protozoa or microbes as food sources (Figures 10–5 and 10–6). Solid or semisolid preparations can also be used successfully (Figure 10–13a and b) with some species. Commercially prepared media are available for protozoan cultivation.

Parasitic protozoans have been cultured successfully in tissue culture preparations. In tissue culture, living cells of various animals serve as sites for development and reproduction (Figure 10–13c). Depending on the species, liquid or solid growth media can also be used.

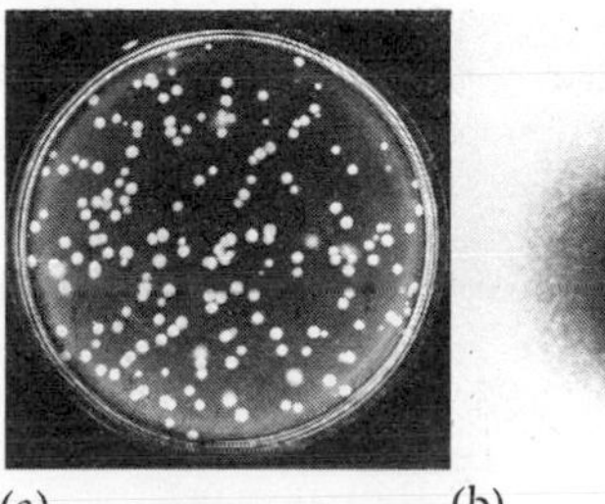

(a)

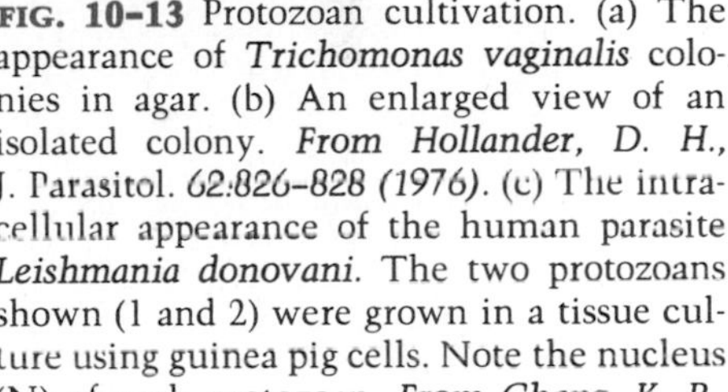

(b)

FIG. 10-13 Protozoan cultivation. (a) The appearance of *Trichomonas vaginalis* colonies in agar. (b) An enlarged view of an isolated colony. *From Hollander, D. H.,* J. Parasitol. *62:826–828 (1976).* (c) The intracellular appearance of the human parasite *Leishmania donovani.* The two protozoans shown (1 and 2) were grown in a tissue culture using guinea pig cells. Note the nucleus (N) of each protozoan. *From Chang, K. P., and D. M. Dwyer,* Science *193:678–680 (1976).*

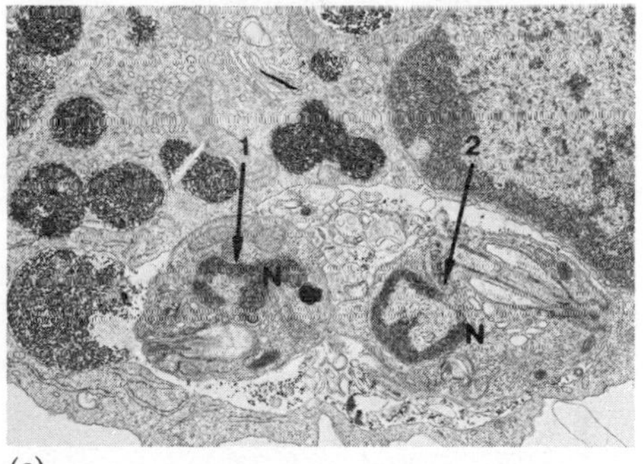

(c)

Classification

The principle subgroups of protozoa are distinctive and easily defined, but their classification is not without problems. This is largely because as new facts are discovered and new ideas grow out of them, the details of classification change. Various properties of protozoa are used in their classification. Among them are method of obtaining nutrients; method of reproduction; cellular organization, structure, and function; and organelles of locomotion. General features of the principle subgroups are described in the following sections and summarized in Table 10–1.

Ciliata

The Ciliata are characterized by their cilia, which function both in moving the organism and in obtaining food (Figure 10–5). The movement of the cilia is such that the cell revolves as it swims. The ciliata are found in both fresh and salt water. Some are free-living; others are either parasitic (Color Photograph 45) or ***commensal,*** the term used when two or more different organisms live together and one benefits while the other is neither benefited nor harmed.

Of all the protozoa, the members of Ciliata are the most specialized because they have organelles that carry out particular vital processes. One such organelle is the bottle- or rod-shaped trichocyst (Figure 10–9b). Depending on

TABLE 10-1 Description of the Protozoa

Subphylum	*Superclass*	*Means of Movement*	*Selected Differentiating Properties Method of Reproduction*		*Representatives*
			Asexual	*Sexual*	
Ciliophora[a]	Ciliata	Cilia	Transverse fission	Conjugation	*Balantidium coli*,[b] *Euplotes, Paramecium* spp., *Stentor Tetrahymena, Vorticella*
Sarcomastigophora	Opalinata	Cilia	Binary fission	Syngamy	*Opalina, Protoopalina*
	Sarcodina	Pseudopodia (false feet)	Binary fission	When present, involves flagellated sex cells	*Amoeba* spp., *Difflugia, Entamoeba histolytica*[b]
	Mastigophora	Flagella	Binary fission	None	*Chlamydomonas, Giarida intestinalis, Trichomonas* spp.,[b] *Trichomympha, Trypanosoma gambiense*,[b] *T. cruzi*[b]
Apicomplexa	Sporozoa	Generally nonmotile except for certain sex cells	Multiple fission	Involves flagellated sex cells	*Eimeria*,[c] *Plasmodium* spp.,[b] *Toxoplasma gondii*[b]

[a]Suctoria belong to this subphylum.
[b]Human parasite.
[c]Small animal pathogen.

the species, trichocysts may be discharged to serve as anchoring devices, weapons of defense, or tools with which to capture prey.

Suctoria

The Suctoria are ciliated protozoans. The young Suctoria are free-swimming. As they develop into adults, they lose their cilia and attach themselves to some object by means of a stalk or disc (Figure 10–14a).

Suctorians, which live in both fresh and salt water and on aquatic plants and animals, obtain food with delicate protoplasmic tentacles. Some of these are pointed and can spear unsuspecting prey. Others are rounded and function as suckers in catching food (Figure 10–14b). These protozoans reproduce by asexual budding.

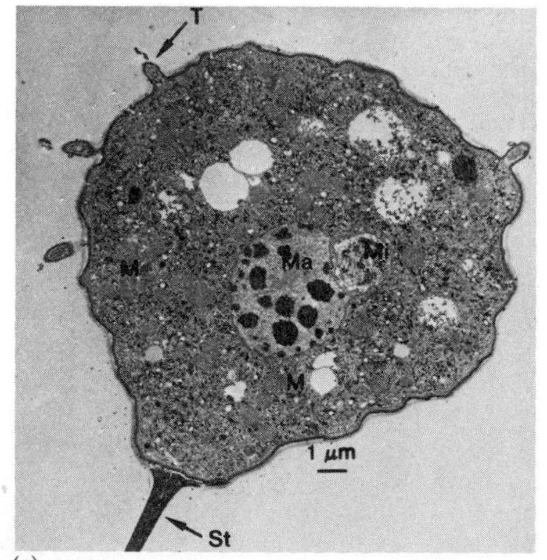

(a)

FIG. 10–14 The *Suctoria.* (a) An electron micrograph of the adult suctorian, *Tokophyra,* showing eucaryotic organization: macronucleus (Ma), micronucleus (Mi), mitochondria (M), tentacles (T), and a rod-like stalk (St). *Courtesy J. B. Tucker.*

Opalinata

The opalinates occur in the large intestines of frogs and toads. These protozoans have many cilialike organelles arranged in rows over their body surfaces. Some organisms have two or more nuclei. However, there is no differentiation of these structures into micro- and macronuclei. The opalinates reproduce by syngamy.

Sarcodina

For the Sarcodina, locomotion and food capture are both accomplished by means of pseudopodia (Figures 10–6 and 10–15). The amoebae, well known for this mode of action, are members of the Sarcodina. The Sarcodina are simpler in structure than the ciliates and flagellates, with fewer organelles (Figure 10–15).

The many kinds of protozoa that comprise the Sarcodina are found in all bodies of water. One of the most interesting is the large subgroup called the foraminiferida (approximately 18,000 different species, found mostly in salt water). These microorganisms form shells made of lime or of substances such as sand from the surrounding waters. Since foraminiferida have inhabited the seas for millions of years, their shells have accumulated on the ocean floors and form a large portion of certain layers of sedimentary rock. Deposits of these organisms form a grayish ooze that can be transformed into chalk under proper geologic conditions. The White Cliffs of Dover represent one such accumulation, and the pyramids near Cairo, Egypt, were carved from limestone deposits of the same origin. The presence of foraminiferida has also proved to be a guide to the petroleum geologist seeking new oil fields.

Other members of the Sarcodina, the parasitic amoebae, are known to occur in most kinds of animals. The most important form to attack humans is ***Entamoeba histolytica*** (Color Photograph 44), which causes amoebic dysentery. This disease presents a serious medical problem in tropical and subtropical regions and in occasional severe outbreaks in temperate regions. The disease is spread by ingestion of cysts (Figure 10–10) in contaminated food or water.

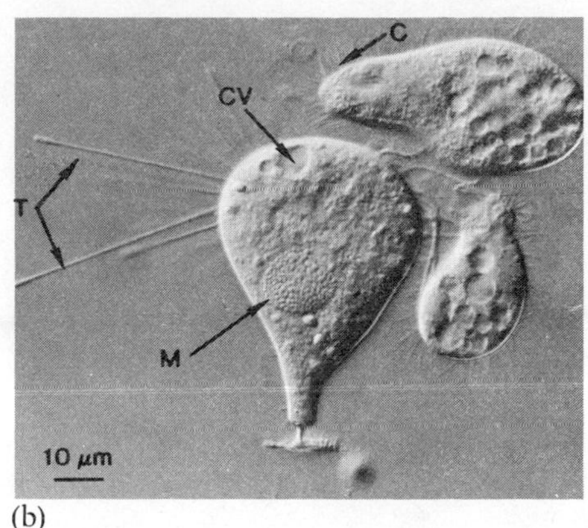

(b)

(b) ***Tokophrya*** feeding on two ***Tetrahymena*** (ciliates). The contractile vacuole (C), macronucleus (Ma), and feeding tentacles (T) are clearly shown.

Mastigophora

The Mastigophora, or flagellates, are mostly unicellular and usually possess at least one flagellum at some stage of their life cycle (Figure 10–16). These flagella are used for locomotion, for obtaining food, and as sense receptors.

The flagellates (Figure 10–17) are an extremely variable group and are believed to be the oldest of the eucaryotic organisms and the ancestors of the other major forms of life. In some classifications these protozoans are divided into two groups: the phytoflagellates (plantlike) and the zooflagellates (animallike). The phytoflagellates contain chlorophyll and are photosynthetic. The zooflagellates lack photosynthetic pigments and are heterotrophic.

Free-living Mastigophora are common in both fresh and salt water. Many others inhabit the soil or the intestinal tracts of some animals. Some Mastigophora are free-living, commensal, mutualistic, or parasitic. Certain parasitic flagellates are medically important. One disease caused by Mastigophora is African sleeping sickness (Figure 35–5). ***Trypanosoma gambiense*** (Color Photograph 5) and ***Trypanosoma rhodesiense*** are transmitted by the bite of the tse-tse fly. In an untreated case of the disease, the victim becomes drowsy and passes into a coma, which is followed by death.

Another genus of this group that is parasitic to humans and other animals is ***Leishmania***. The human skin disease known as cutaneous leishmaniasis is especially common in the Mediterranean region. Uncomplicated cases do not present any problems, and infected persons usually recover within one year's time. However, when bacteria complicate this condition, a tropical ulcer develops (Figure 10–18). The details of this disease, as well as others caused by mastigophorans, are discussed more fully in later chapters.

An interesting relationship exists between certain members of Mastigophora and termites (Figure 8–1). This association is a mutualistic one in which the two organisms live together for mutual benefit. The termite ingests wood but cannot digest the cellulose in it. Protozoa living in the intestine of the termite digest the cellulose, providing sugar for the nutrition of the insect as well as for themselves.

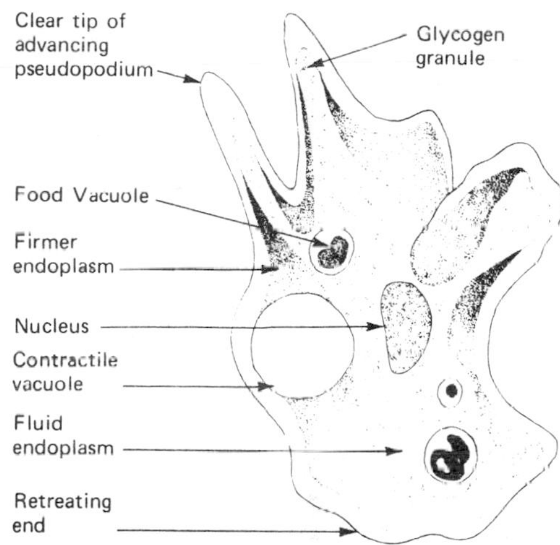

FIG. 10–15 The *Sarcodina*. A diagram of the components of *Amoeba* spp.

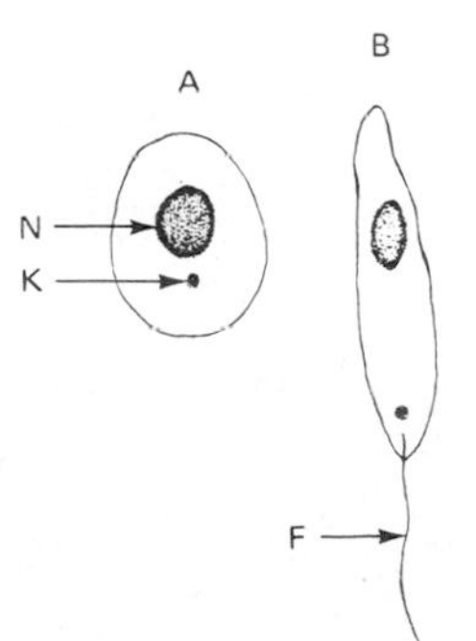

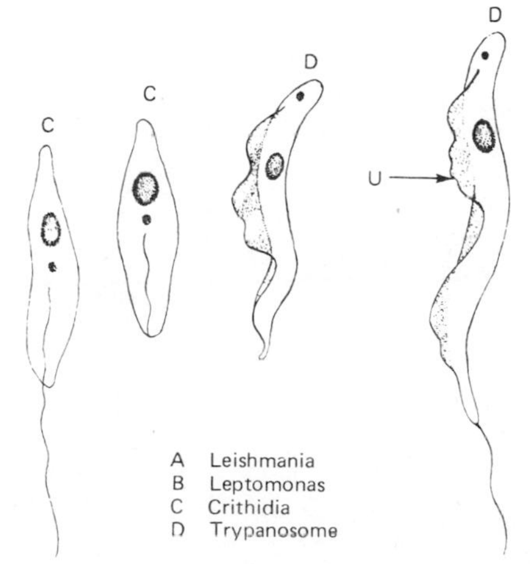

FIG. 10–16 Morphological stages of selected flagellates. (a) The leishmanial form is oval or round and contains a nucleus (N) and closely associated kinetoplast (K), the basal structure of a flagellum, but no flagellum or undulating membrane. (b) The leptomonad is elongated and possesses a kinetoplast and a free flagellum (F), but no undulating membrane. (c) The crithidial form is characterized by an elongated body, a kinetoplast near the nucleus, and a flagellum. (d) The trypanosomal form, in addition to the organelles of the crithidial form, has an undulating membrane (U).

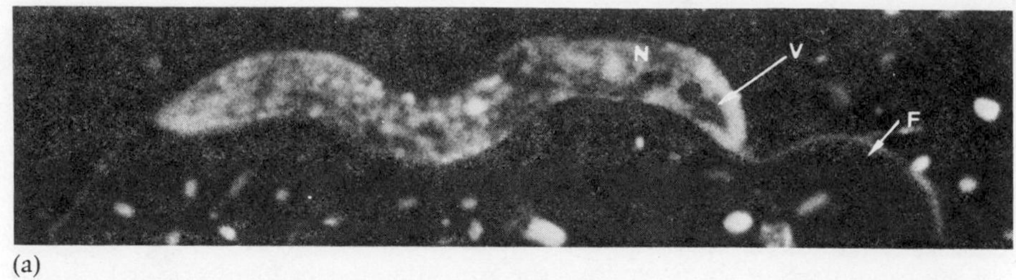

(a)

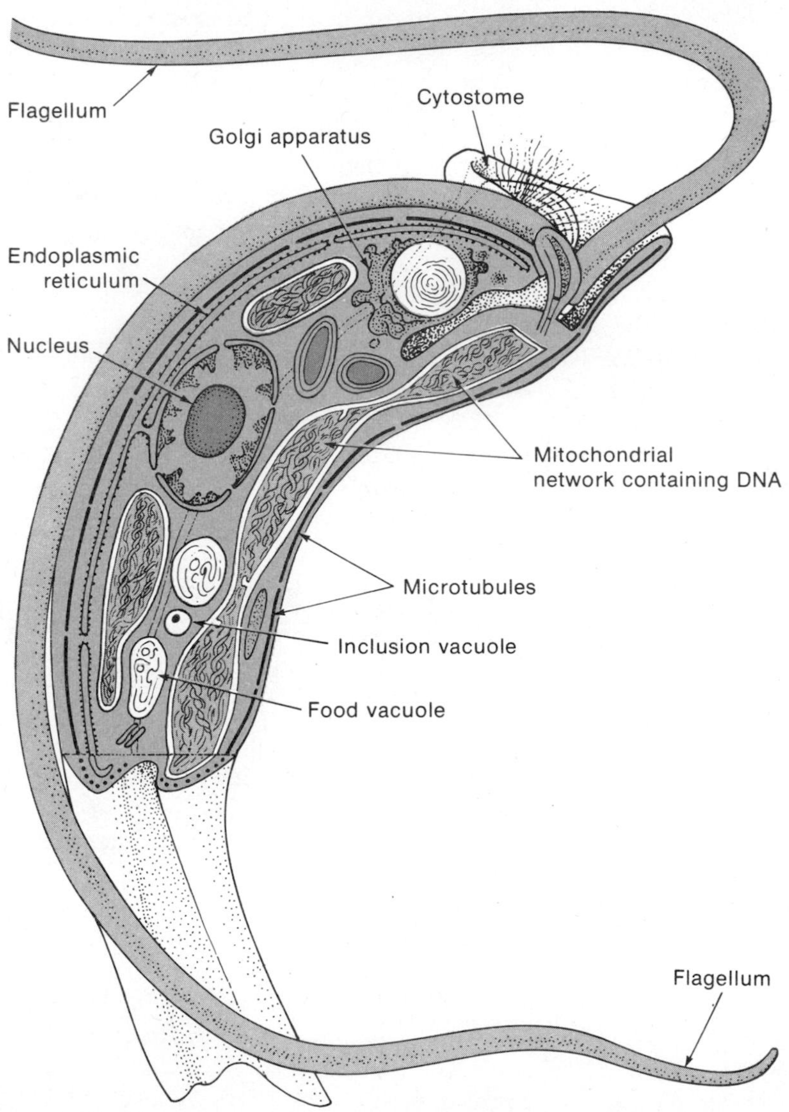

(b)

FIG. 10-17 Structural features of flagellates. (a) A phase-contrast micrograph showing the contractile vacuole (V), flagellum (F), and nucleus (N) of *Cryptobia*. (b) A drawing of this flagellate's cellular organization. *From Vickerman, K.,* J. Protozool. *24:221-233 (1977).*

Sporozoa

All sporozoans are parasitic, absorbing nutrients from their hosts (Figure 10–19). Some are intracellular, that is, they live within the host's cells (Color Photographs 43 and 85). Others live in body fluids or various body organs. Adult sporozoans have no locomotor organelles.

Both asexual and sexual reproduction occur among sporozoans. A number of sporozoans undergo sporulation, producing numerous small, infective spores called *oocysts*. Infective spores reach a susceptible host by way of food, water, or arthropod bites. Spores typically contain one or more smaller individual organisms called **sporozoites.** Many of the sporozoans have complicated life cycles, certain stages taking place in one host and other stages in a different one. An example of such a cycle involves mosquitoes and the different species of *Plasmodium,* which cause malaria not only in humans, but in several other animals including canaries, chickens, ducks, lizards, pigeons, mice, monkeys, rats, and snakes. The general life cycle of the malarial parasite is shown in Figure 10–20. The symptoms, treatment, and related topics are presented in Chapter 33.

A related protozoan, ***Toxoplasma gondii*** (Color Photograph 43), has generated considerable interest in recent years. The disease caused by this organism, toxoplasmosis, has been found in cats, cattle, dogs, humans, and sheep. This organism may enter a host by way of the nose or mouth. Toxoplasmosis gained public notice when it was revealed that this disease in a pregnant woman might also infect the fetus, causing serious defects or death.

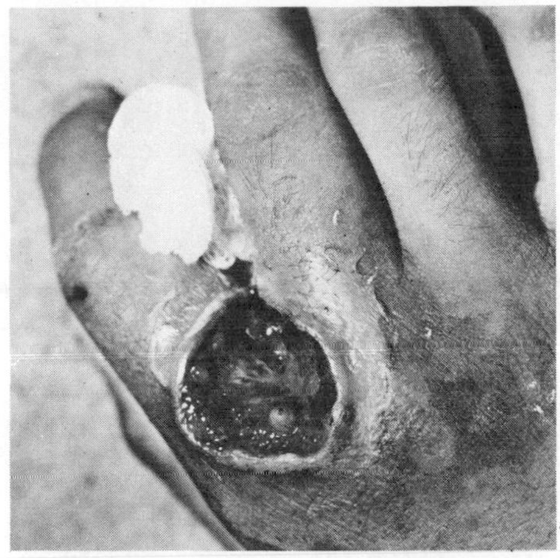

FIG. 10–18 Tropical ulcer of the hand. *Courtesy of the Armed Forces Institute of Pathology, Neg. No. A-43127-1.*

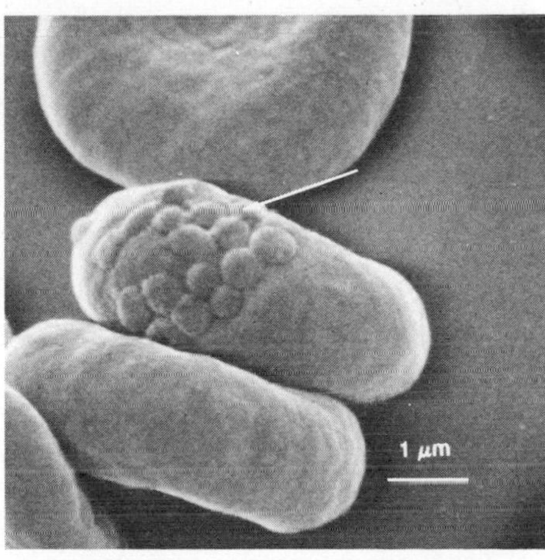

FIG. 10–19 A scanning micrograph showing the parasitic sporozoan ***Eperythrozoon wenyoni*** on red blood cells. This protozoan, which is found in cattle severely ill from other diseases, can cause significant red blood cell destruction. *Deeton, K. S., and N. C. Jain,* J. Parasitol. *50:867–873 (1973).*

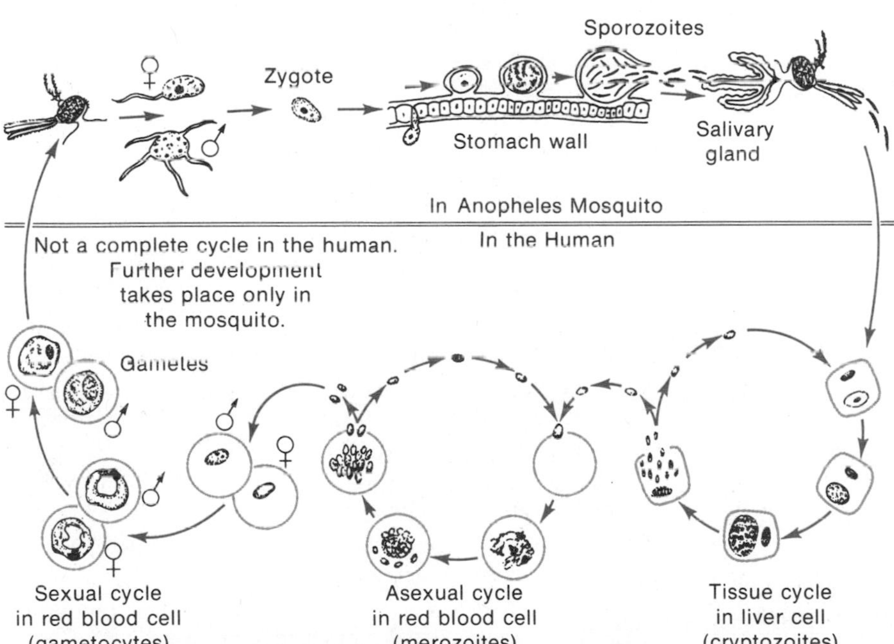

FIG. 10–20 The life cycle of *Plasmodium* in a mosquito and in the human. The human host is infected by small elongated infective cells, the ***sporozoites,*** produced in the ***Anopheles*** mosquito and which invade the salivary gland of the insect. The female mosquito introduces sporozoites into the human blood stream when she takes a blood meal. The newly introduced parasites are removed from the blood by organs such as the liver and spleen, where they multiply and produce other infective forms that are released into the blood stream to attack and carry out the asexual cycle in red blood cells. The outcome of this cycle is the formation of sex cells (gametocytes) and other infective units for red blood cells. If these sex cells are ingested by another female mosquito, they mature and participate in the sexual reproductive phase by forming a zygote. This fertilized cell undergoes developmental changes within the mosquito's intestine, where it enlarges and forms a large number of sporozoites. And the cycle can begin again.

Several other sporozoan species affect human well-being, not only because they cause infections in humans, but because they infect many domestic animals, causing losses of millions of dollars to agriculture every year.

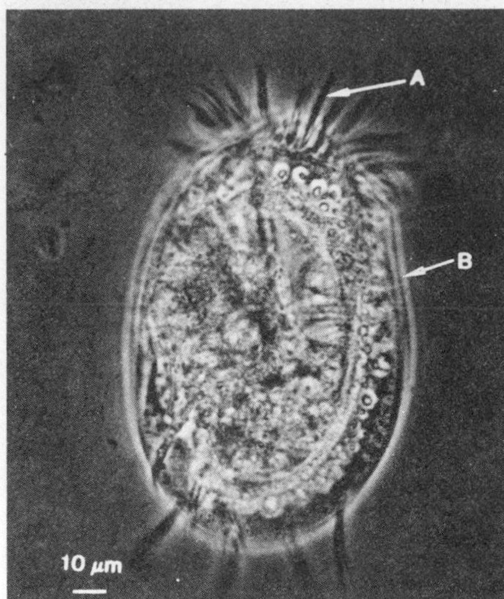

FIG. **10-21** A phase-contrast micrograph showing the ciliate *Euplotes eurystomus*. *Shigenaka, Y., K. Wantanabe, and M. Hareda,* J. Protozool. *20:414–428 (1973).*

SUMMARY

1. Protozoans are unicellular, eucaryotic microorganisms belonging to the kingdom of Protista.
2. Many protozoans are motile and require organic food sources.

Distribution and Activities

Protozoans are widely distributed and exhibit both beneficial and harmful symbiotic relationships.

Structure and Function

Locomotion

1. There are three basic types of organelles for movement among the protozoans: *pseudopodia, flagella,* and *cilia.* These structures are important to classification.
2. Individual flagella and cilia consist of two centrally located microtubules surrounded by nine double tubules. These organelles originate from a cytoplasmic basal granule or *kinetosome.* Modifications of both structures occur among protozoans.

Feeding and Digestion

1. Three major methods of obtaining nutrients are found among protozoa, classifying them as *autotrophic, saprobic,* or *holozoic* (the last two being heterotrophic forms).
2. Holozoic protozoans have various mechanisms for food capture, including food cups, cytosomes (mouths), and tentacles.

Excretion and Osmoregulation

1. Disposal of excretory wastes occurs at the cell surface.
2. Most nitrogen wastes from protein digestion are excreted as ammonia.
3. In the case of parasitic protozoans, waste products are released with the destruction of the host cells.
4. The *contractile vacuole* system is involved with osmoregulation.

Protective Structures

1. Most of the protective structures of protozoans function to prevent mechanical injury or to guard against drying, excessive water intake, and predators.
2. Examples of protective structures include the *pellicle,* a strong outer covering of ciliates and some amoebae, *tests,* or *shells,* coverings of calcium carbonate or silica, and *trichocysts,* specialized defense organelles.

Trophozoites and Cysts

1. The normal, active feeding form of free-living as well as several parasitic protozoans is the *trophozoite.*
2. Many protozoans can secrete a resistant thick covering that develops into a resting stage, a form known as a *cyst.*
3. Cysts also serve as sites for division and as a means for spreading pathogenic protozoans.

Methods of Reproduction

1. Ciliated organisms are mutinucleated. Usually one macronucleus and one micronucleus are present.
2. The macronucleus regulates metabolism and developmental functions and maintains all visible traits.
3. The micronucleus exerts overall control over the entire cell and its sexual and reproductive processes.

Asexual Reproduction

1. Both asexual and sexual reproduction occur among protozoans.
2. Some protozoans reproduce asexually only.
3. The forms of asexual reproduction include splitting, either equally or unequally, into two new cells *(binary fission), budding,* splitting into several new cells *(multiple fission),* and forming two or more multinucleated cells *(plasmotomy).*

Sexual Reproduction

The types of sexual reproduction include the union of two different types of sex cells *(syngamy),* the transfer of nuclear material from one cell to another through a temporary connection *(conjugation)*, and a modified version of conjugation known as *autogamy*.

Regeneration

Regeneration of lost or damaged parts is characteristic of protozoans. When a cell is cut in two, only the portion containing the nucleus regenerates.

Cultivation

Several protozoans can be cultured under a variety of natural or laboratory conditions. Both liquid and solid media also can be used for their cultivation.

Classification

Protozoa can be classified according to mode of nutrition, structures and associated functions, methods of reproduction, and means of movement.

Ciliata

1. Ciliata are protozoans that characteristically have short hairs called cilia that function in moving the organism and obtaining food.
2. Ciliates can be free-living, *commensal*, or parasitic.

Suctoria

1. Suctorians are ciliated during the early stages of their life cycles, but adults lose these organelles.
2. Adult forms develop a stalk for attachment to surfaces and delicate tentacles to obtain food.

Opalinata

1. The opalinates are found in the large intestines of frogs and toads.
2. These protozoans have cilialike structures arranged in rows on their body surfaces and two or more nuclei. They reproduce sexually by syngamy.

Sarcodina

1. Protozoans belonging to the group Sarcodina move and capture food by means of pseudopodia and are simpler in structure than ciliates.
2. Members of the Sarcodina are widely distributed in nature and can be free-living as well as parasitic.

Mastigophora

1. The organisms of Mastigophora are mostly unicellular and usually have one or more flagella at some or all stages of their life cycle.
2. Flagellates are widely distributed in natural environments. They are believed to be the oldest of eucaryotic organisms and the ancestors of other major forms of life.
3. These protozoans can be free-living, commensal, mutualistic, or parasitic.

Sporozoa

1. All of these protozoans are parasitic and obtain essential nutrients from their hosts.
2. Adult sporozoans do not have any organelles for movement.
3. The causative agents of malaria and toxoplasmosis belong to this group of protozoans.

QUESTIONS FOR REVIEW

1. List three characteristics that all protozoa have in common.
2. List at least three ways in which protozoa differ from fungi.
3. a. What type of cellular organization do protozoa exhibit?
   b. List at least six organelles found in protozoa, and give the functions of each.
4. a. Differentiate between a trophozoite and a cyst.
   b. What are the respective functions or activities associated with trophozoites and cysts?
   c. Do all protozoa have both trophozoites and cysts? Explain.
5. a. What criteria are used to identify or classify protozoa?
   b. Do such criteria differ from the ones used for bacterial and fungus classification? Explain.
6. a. How do protozoa reproduce?
   b. List and describe three reproductive mechanisms.
7. List the major groups of protozoa, and indicate at least one human disease agent from each group.
8. How are protozoa cultured?
9. Define or explain the following terms:
   a. pseudopodium
   b. contractile vacuole
   c. pellicle
   d. cirri
   e. macronucleus
   f. micronucleus
10. Do protozoa have any ecological value?
11. Figure 10–21 shows a phase-contrast micrograph of the ciliate *Euplotes eurystomus*. What organelles of this protozoan do you see?

SUGGESTED READINGS

Grell, K. G., *Protozoology*. New York: Springer-Verlag, 1973. *A well-illustrated, advanced text dealing with the biology of protozoa.*

Horgen, P. A., and J. C. Silver, "Chromatin in Eukaryotic Microbes," *Ann. Rev. Microbiol.* 32:249–284 (1978). *An interesting article dealing with the structure, function, and evolution of chromatin in eucaryotic microbes including protozoans.*

Jahn, T. L., and F. F. Jahn, *How to Know the Protozoa*. Dubuque, Iowa: William C. Brown, 1949. *Identification keys to the common protozoa.*

Levine, N. D., *Protozoan Parasites of Domestic Animals and of Man*. Minneapolis: Burgess Publishing Co., 1973. *An excellent reference, especially with respect to details of individual species.*

Noble, E. R., and G. A. Noble, *Parasitology, The Biology of Animal Parasites*. 4th ed. Philadelphia: Lea & Febiger, 1976. *An advanced text that provides detailed consideration of many important human parasitic diseases. It also serves as a ready reference of reasonably up-to-date information.*

Rudzinska, M. A., "Do Suctoria Really Feed by Suction?," *Bioscience* 23:87–94 (1973). *Concerned with the feeding habits of this most interesting group of protozoans.*

Scholtyseck, E., *Fine Structure of Parasitic Protozoa*. New York: Springer-Verlag, 1979. *An excellent combination of electron micrographs and diagrams showing the fine structural features of a number of representative protozoa.*

Trager, W., "Some Aspects of Intracellular Parasitism," *Science* 183:269–273 (1974). *An interesting short account of intracellular parasitism, with an emphasis on nutrition.*

CHAPTER **11** Algae

Algae

Chapter 11 describes the distinctive structural and organizational properties of algae. Because of their world-wide distribution and their beneficial activities, the algae are of great ecological and economic importance.

After reading this chapter, you should be able to:

1. **Describe the importance of algae to the functioning of the biological world.**
2. **Distinguish among the divisions of algae.**
3. **List the features of the divisions of algae.**
4. **Identify and give the associated functions of algal structures.**
5. **Compare algae with other types of microorganisms and explain how algae differ from them.**
6. **List and describe the major beneficial and destructive activities of algae.**
7. **Outline the general features of algal reproduction.**
8. **Describe the methods used for the cultivation of algae.**

In the early twentieth century, most aquatic plant life was lumped together and collectively referred to as *algae.* By the 1920s it became clear that the algae contained several related yet distinct groups of microscopic and massive forms of life.

Not only do algae serve as the basic source of food in the sea upon which other marine life depend, but they also fix, or capture, more carbon by photosynthesis than do all land plants. Moreover, they are valuable in illustrating the relationships between biological structure and function. These and other properties make the algae both fascinating and important to study.

Algae: "The Grass of the Waters"

Algae are photosynthetic aquatic protists. Most algal forms are free-floating and free-living. Certain species, however, participate in symbiotic associations, living together with other organisms. **Lichens** are a primary example of this type of mutualism.

Algae are frequently found in bodies of water used by humans—lakes, ponds, reservoirs, rivers, streams, and swimming pools. Unfortunately, in certain cases, algae may be quite troublesome, giving drinking water a disagreeable taste and odor and clogging water filtering systems. The occasional spurts of growth known as **algal blooms** (Color Photograph 4a) may disrupt aquatic communities by the increased accumulations of their waste products.

Algae constitute an important part of the **plankton** population, the microscopic forms of life floating near the surfaces of most bodies of water. The term *phytoplankton* is used to designate the algae of the group, while *zooplankton* is applied to the animallike organisms. Plankton are the basis of several food chains. These organisms are eaten by progressively larger forms of life, which in turn may be consumed by humans (Figure 11–1).

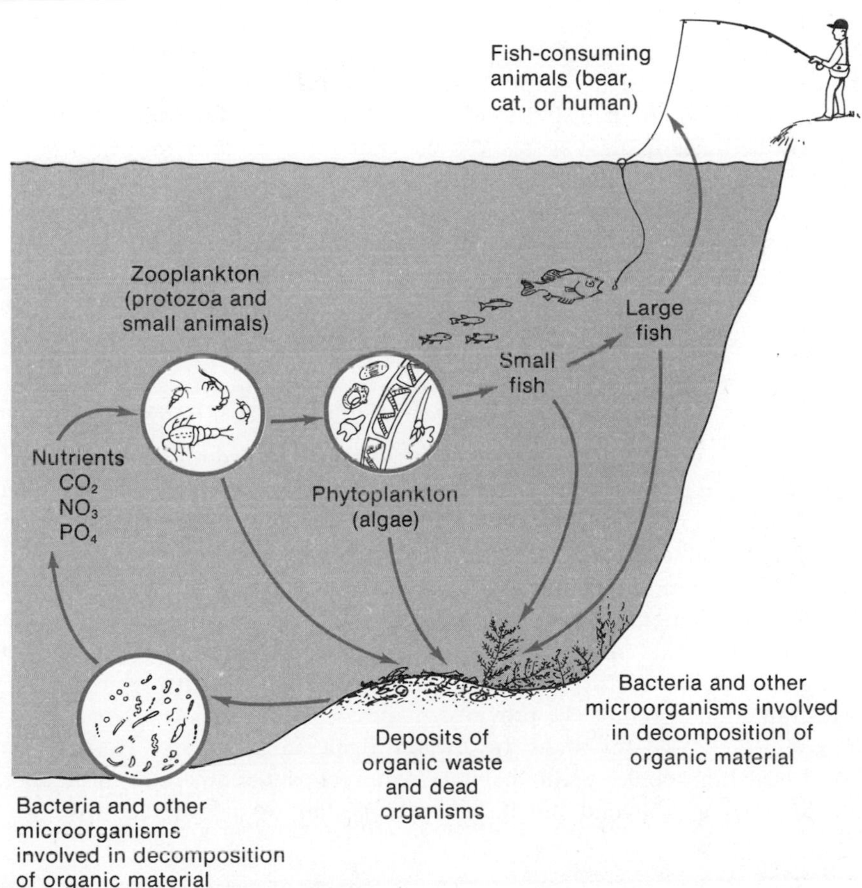

FIG. 11–1 An example of a food chain beginning with plankton and showing the position of algae in this most important chain of events. Additional information on such environmental situations is presented in Chapter 16.

Cell membrane
Chloroplast
Cell wall
Nuclear membrane
(a)

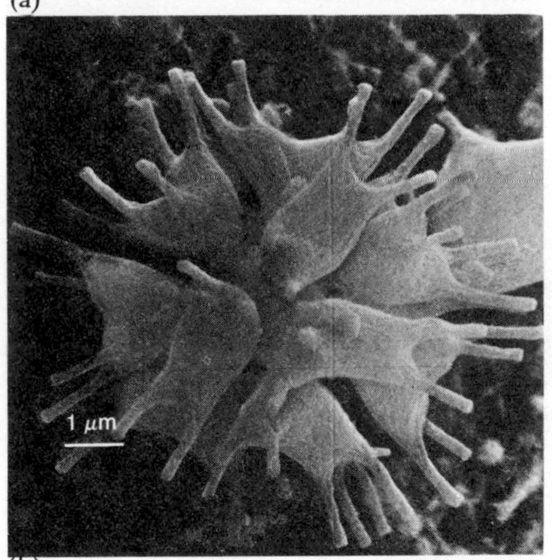

(b)

FIG. 11-2 Some unicellular and multicellular algae. (a) A scanning micrograph of the diatom *Melosira*. *Crowford, R. J.,* J. Phycol. *9:50–61 (1973).* (b) A micrograph of the colony-forming green alga, *Sorastrum*. Colonies of this organism can contain between four and sixty-four cells arranged as a sphere. The outward directed horns of *Sorastrum* give a rather dramatic appearance to the organism. *Marchant, H. J.,* J. Phycol. *10:107–120 (1974).*

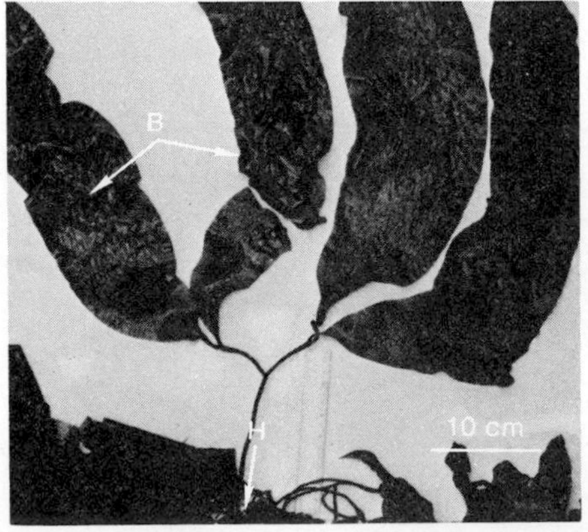

FIG. 11-3 The more plantlike appearance of algae. This brown alga has a blade (B) and rootlike holdfasts (H). *Sambonsuga, Y., and M. Neushul,* J. Phycol. *14:214–224 (1978).*

Structure and Organization

Algae are eucaryotic organisms having a wide range of sizes and shapes (Color Photographs 48 and 49). They range in size from microscopic dimensions to lengths of 60 meters. Some algae are unicellular; others are highly differentiated and multicellular. The unicellular species may be curved, rodlike, or spherical (Figure 11–2). Multicellular algae assume many filamentous or colonial arrangements with shapes of varying complexity. Some algae may even have rootlike organs, stems, and leaves (Figure 11–3). Because cellular shape, arrangement, and organization vary so much among the different divisions of algae, further consideration will be given to these topics in later sections dealing with specific groups.

Means of Reproduction

Algae may reproduce either asexually or sexually. At the cellular level, sexual reproduction can involve the union of cells *(plasmogamy)* (Figure 11–4), the union of nuclei *(karyogamy)*, and the reduction of chromosome number **(meiosis).** As later sections will show, some algal species have complicated life cycles.

Means of asexual reproduction among the algae include production of unicellular spores that germinate without fusing with other cells; fragmentation of filamentous forms; and cell division by splitting to form new individuals like the parent cell. Many algal spores, especially those of aquatic forms, have flagella (Figure 11–5), are motile, and lack a cell wall. These motile forms are called **zoospores.** Nonmotile spores known as **aplanospores** and other types are produced by various algae and will be discussed later.

Cultivation

Many years ago the study of algae in laboratories depended on collecting fresh samples or preserving specimens. New approaches to algae cultivation have led to the development of various types of liquid and solid (agar-based) nutrient media. Many media contain exact amounts of substances required for growth, such as vitamins, and inorganic as well as organic sources of nitrogen, phosphorus, and other elements. Other preparations used may be composed mostly of undefined ingredients including soil, rice grains, and split peas. Depending on the algae, either marine or fresh water is used to support cultures. Proper pH and illumination also must be provided.

Temperatures used for many freshwater algal cultures range from 19° to 21°C. Algae from colder ocean habitats require lower temperatures. Some of the references at the end of this chapter pertain to additional aspects of cultivation.

Classification

Classification has undergone many changes since the time of Linnaeus, when only fourteen genera were recognized. At the present time, at least six eucaryotic algal divisions are recognized. To draw attention to the algal level of organization, the names of these divisions include the root *phyco*, from the Greek *phykos*, meaning "seaweed."

Algal divisions are distinguished by several characteristics, including cellular organization, cell wall chemistry and physical properties, flagellation or its absence, pigmentation, reserve storage products, and reproductive structures and methods. Table 11–1 summarizes these and other properties of the six major divisions. Selected features of these groups are presented in the following sections.

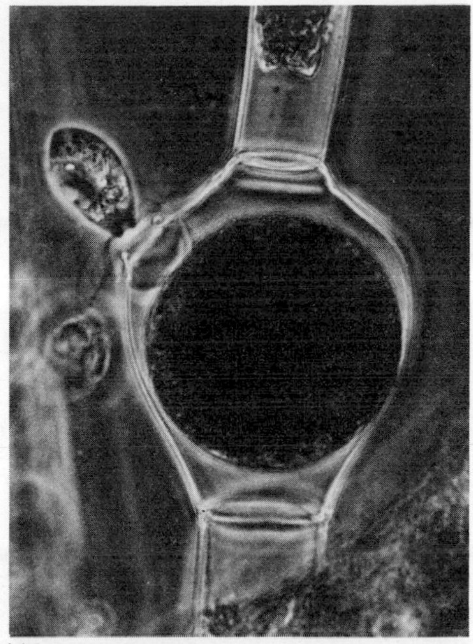

(a)

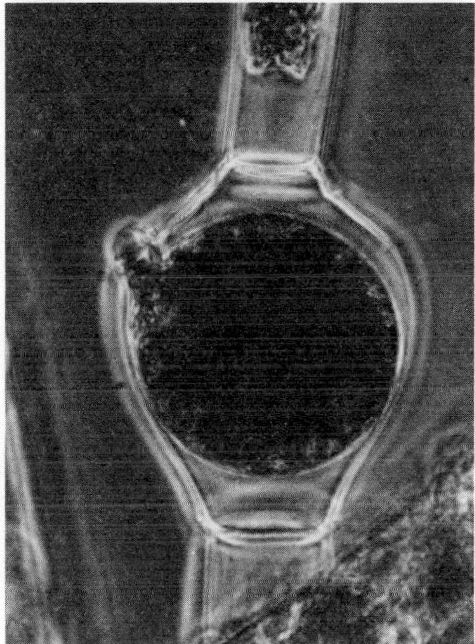

(b)

FIG. 11–4 A view of the fertilization process with *Oedegonium*. (a) The small sperm cell is shown making its initial contact with the larger egg cell. *Hoffman, L. R.*, J. Phycol. *9:62–81 (1973)*. (b) A later view showing the fusion of nuclear material of both cells. *Hoffman, L. R.*, J. Phycol. *9:296–301 (1973)*.

The Green Algae (Chlorophycophyta)

Over six thousand species of green algae are known today. Many are unicellular (Color Photograph 4b), while some are multicellular filaments or aggregated colonies (Figure 11–6). Like other algae, green algae are found in abundance in the upper portions of aquatic environments. All the essential nutrients for growth and reproduction are right at hand, dissolved in the surrounding areas. Few of these microorganisms are found at depths greater than 8 meters, largely because sunlight does not penetrate to that depth. Many green algae are found growing in freshwater and terrestrial environments such as on rocks (Color Photograph 47), on the bark of trees and on soil. The freshwater varieties grow submerged in shallow pools or deeper bodies of water as free-floating or free-swimming (planktonic) forms. Some green algae are found growing in the cells of various protozoa or lower animal forms such as coelenterates (hydrae) and sponges. Because they are found in animal life, such algae are said to be *endozoic* (Figure 11–7). Some of these algae have been found to contain viruslike particles (Figure 11–7b), suggesting that algae may help transmit these viruses.

Structure and Organization

Green algae are thought to be closely related to higher forms of plant life because of their similar features (Figure 11–8). These shared properties include cell walls containing cellulose, a complex polysaccharide; a definite nucleus; chlorophylls *a* and *b* and other pigments in well-defined chloroplasts; and the production of starch as the means for storing the excess products of photosynthesis. Most green algae produce cellular bodies called *pyrenoids* (Figure 11–9), which are centers of starch formation. Some botanists believe that land plants evolved from green algae.

Reproduction

The green algae have several methods of asexual reproduction. Various algae undergo fragmentation of filamentous forms, zoospore formation (Figure 11–5), and simple division, or mitosis (Figure 11–9a and b). They may also reproduce sexually by fusion between morphologically and physiologically similar or different sex cells *(gametes)*. Fertilization is accomplished by the release of flagellated sex cells into a water environment, where they fuse with other gametes (Figure 11–5).

Economic and Ecological Importance

The green algae have an important impact on various human affairs. Photosynthesis by green algae contributes significantly to the concentrations of oxygen in the atmosphere and in water supplies. In addition, while relatively few algal species are used directly for human consumption, the green algae found in phytoplankton contribute to human food supplies indirectly. Such algae form the basis for many food chains and food pyramids. Green algae is also used in animal feed. Added to grain feed at a concentration of about 10 percent, algae have been found to be a valuable food for cattle, sheep, and swine.

Certain green algae have been used in the breakdown and purification of sewage and waste; as indicators of particular water conditions, such as nitrogen and phosphorus concentrations, and sewage pollution; and as a source of antibiotics.

The activities of green algae are not all beneficial, however. Several species are responsible for clogging various waterways and filter systems and for causing the poisoning, and in some cases the death, of various types of aquatic life by production of algatoxins (Color Photograph 4b).

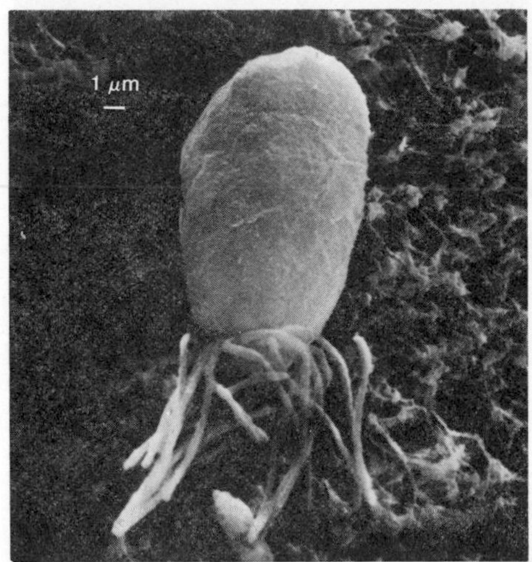

FIG. 11-5 A scanning micrograph of a motile algal zoospore. These flagellated (F) cells exhibit a typical eucaryotic organization. Zoospores are usually produced from the contents of a vegetative algal cell. *Markowitz, M. M.,* J. Phycol. *14:289-302 (1978).*

The Golden Brown Algae and the Diatoms (Chrysophycophyta)

The Chrysophycophyta group is highly diverse in pigmentation, cell wall chemistry, and flagellation (Table 11-1). The golden algae, the yellow-green algae, and the diatoms are included in this division. Because of space limitations, we shall concentrate here on the diatoms.

The large floating populations in fresh and salt water referred to as ***plankton*** are in large part diatoms. This accumulation of organisms is composed of trillions of algae which as a group produce more food through photosynthesis than all the rest of the plant world combined. Diatoms are found abundantly even in arctic regions (Color Photograph 48).

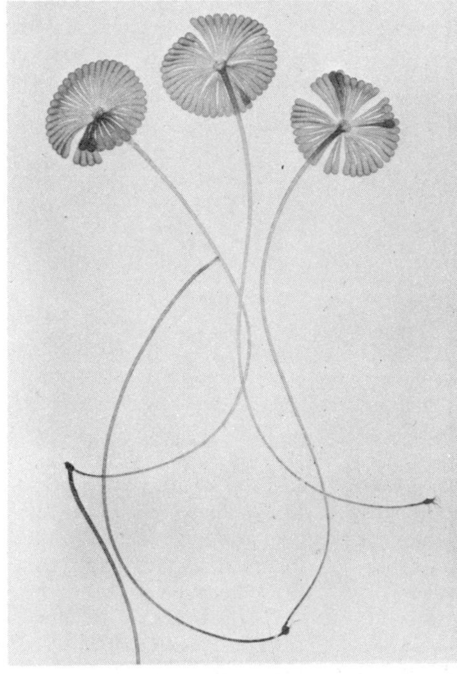

FIG. 11-6 The green algae. (a) A marine green alga, *Acetabularia crenulata*, the mermaid's wine glass. This organism has been used in numerous experiments associated with nuclear and cytoplasmic relationships. *Courtesy of Carolina Biological Supply Company.*

Structure and Organization

An obvious characteristic of diatoms is the intricately sculptured bilateral and radial patterns of their cell walls (Figures 11-10a and b). Diatoms are usually classified on the basis of the shape, symmetry, and structure of their cell walls, called **frustules.** The walls of diatoms consist of two halves, referred to as *valves,* which fit together much like the parts of a pillbox (Figure 11-13). The larger upper half is the ***epivalve;*** the lower one is the ***hypovalve.*** The organisms with circular valves (Figure 11-10a) are called *centric* diatoms, while those characterized by boat-shaped structures like that in Figure 11-11 are the *pennate* diatoms. The structural details of these skeletons provide a basis for more detailed classification.

Cell wall markings help distinguish diatoms from certain green algae. These may be holes *(puncta)* arranged in rows *(striae)* (Figure 11-11c) or ridges. The valves of some diatoms also have a long, narrow opening called a ***raphe*** (Figure 11-11b and c).

Diatoms are chemically unique in that their cell walls contain large concentrations of silicates. These substances are the basic components of glass, granite, and sand. Diatoms continually absorb silicates and deposit them in their cell walls. When a diatom dies, the silica in the cell wall begins to dissolve rapidly. However, under favorable conditions, these glassy structures accumulate and form deposits of fossil diatoms called **diatomaceous earth.** Such deposits have been gathering for thousands of years, and in some parts of the world deposits 900 meters thick have been found. Locations of such deposits include the city of Lompoc, in California, and various sites in Maryland and Virginia.

Centric diatoms are capable of forming resting spores (Figure 11-12). These spores serve as the major means by which diatoms survive unfavorable growth conditions. Resting spores can be produced singly, in pairs, or in groups of four. They usually consist of two valves.

TABLE 11-1

Division	*Common Name*	*Habitat*	*General Structural Arrangement*	*Pigments Contained*	*Selected Reserve Materials*	*Motility*	*Method of Reproduction*
Chlorophy-cophyta	Green algae	Fresh water and moist environments	Unicellular to multicellular	Chlorophylls *a* and *b*, carotenes, xanthophylls	Starch, oils	Mostly nonmotile	Asexual by multiple fission; spores sexual
Chrysophy-cophyta	Golden algae (includes diatoms)	Fresh and salt water	Mainly unicellular	Chlorophylls *a* and *c*, special carotenoids, xanthophylls	Oils, leucosin, chrysolamin-arin, oils	Unique move-ment with diatoms; others utilize flagella	Asexual and sexual
Euglenophy-cophyta	Euglenoids[a]	Fresh water	Unicellular	Chlorophylls *a* and *b*, carotenes, xanthophylls	Fats, paramylum	Motile by means of flagella	Asexual only by binary fission
Phaeophy-cophyta	Brown algae	Salt water (cool en-vironment)	Multicellular	Chlorophylls *a* and *c*, special carotenoids, xanthophylls	Fats, laminarin	Motile	Asexual by motile zoo-spores (Figure 11–5); sexual by motile sex cells (gametes)
Pyrrophy-cophyta	Dinoflagel-lates[b]	Fresh and salt water	Unicellular	Chlorophylls *a* and *c*, carotenes, xanthophylls	Starch, oils	Motile	Asexual; sexual rare
Rhodophy-cophyta	Red algae	Salt water (warm en-vironment)	Multicellular	Chlorophyll *a*, phycobillins, carotenes, phy-coerythrin, xanthophylls	Starch, oils	Nonmotile	Asexual by spores; sexual by sex cells (gametes)

[a]These microorganisms possess characteristics of both animals and plants. Euglenoids seem intermediate between algae and protozoa.
[b]One genus, *Gonyaulax*, occurs in algal blooms referred to as the "red tide."

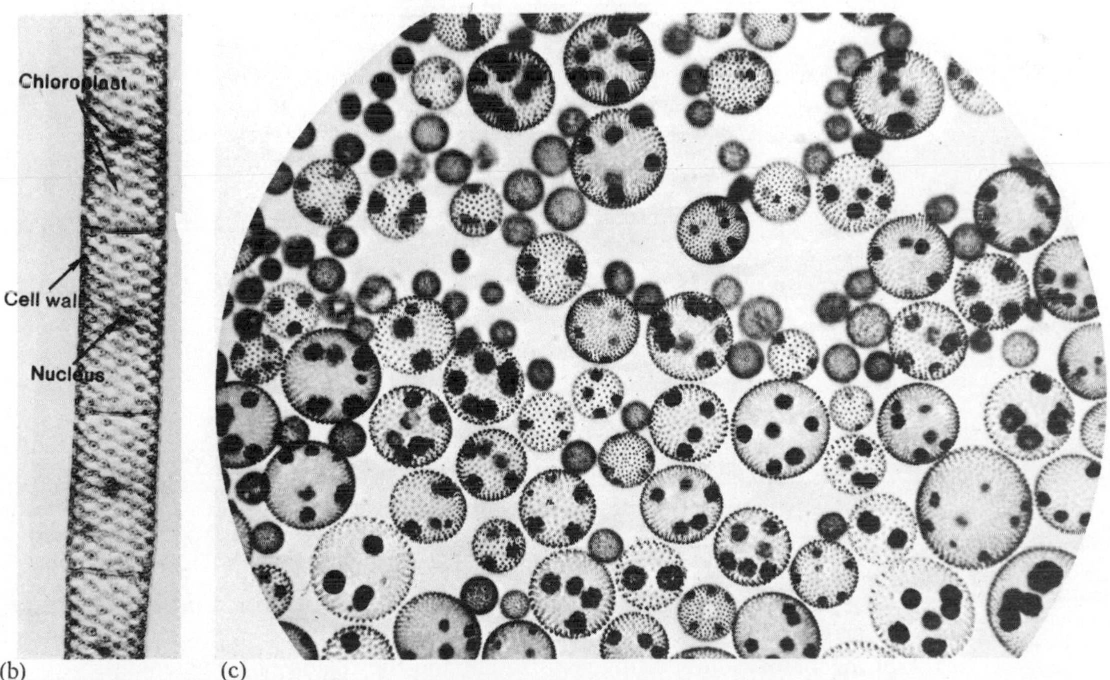

FIG. 11-6 (b) A filamentous green alga, *Spirogyra*. This organism is commonly seen in the surface scums of ponds and slow-moving bodies of water. The cells of *Spirogyra* show its unusual spiral-shaped chloroplasts. *Courtesy of Carolina Biological Supply Company.* (c) *Volvox*, a colonial aggregation of cells belonging to the green algae. *Courtesy CCM: General Biological, Inc., Chicago.*

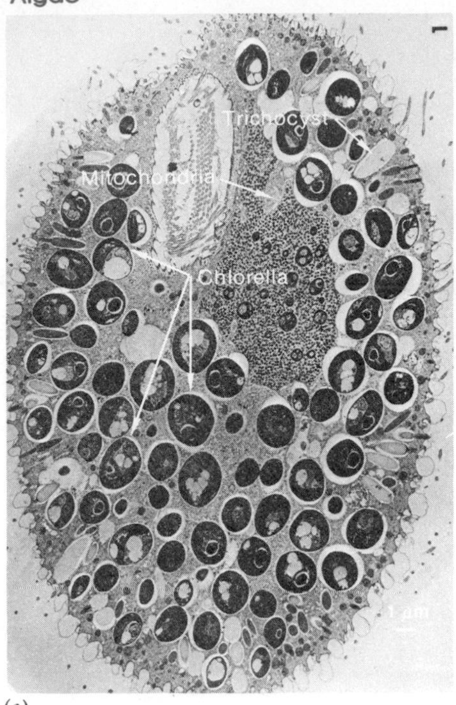

(a)

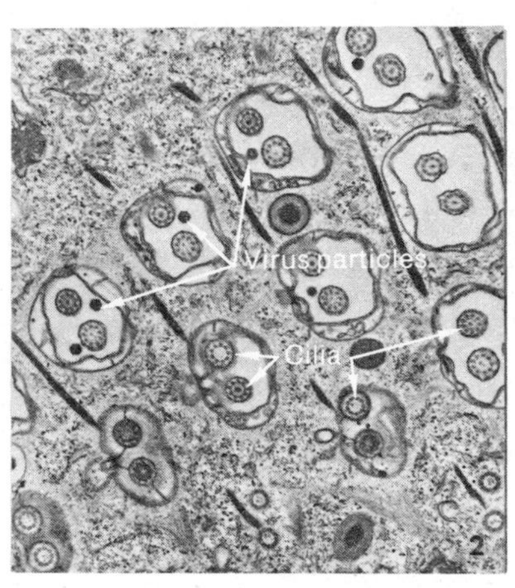

FIG. 11-7 A view of a symbiotic system involving algae, viruses, and protozoa. (a) An ultrathin preparation of *Paramecium* containing many green algae of the genus *Chlorella* (arrows). *Kawakami, H., and N. Kawakami,* J. Protozool. *25:217-225 (1978).* (b) Several infective virus particles found in the intracellular symbiotic algae. *Kawakami, H., and N. Kawakami,* J. Protozool. *25:217-225 (1978).*

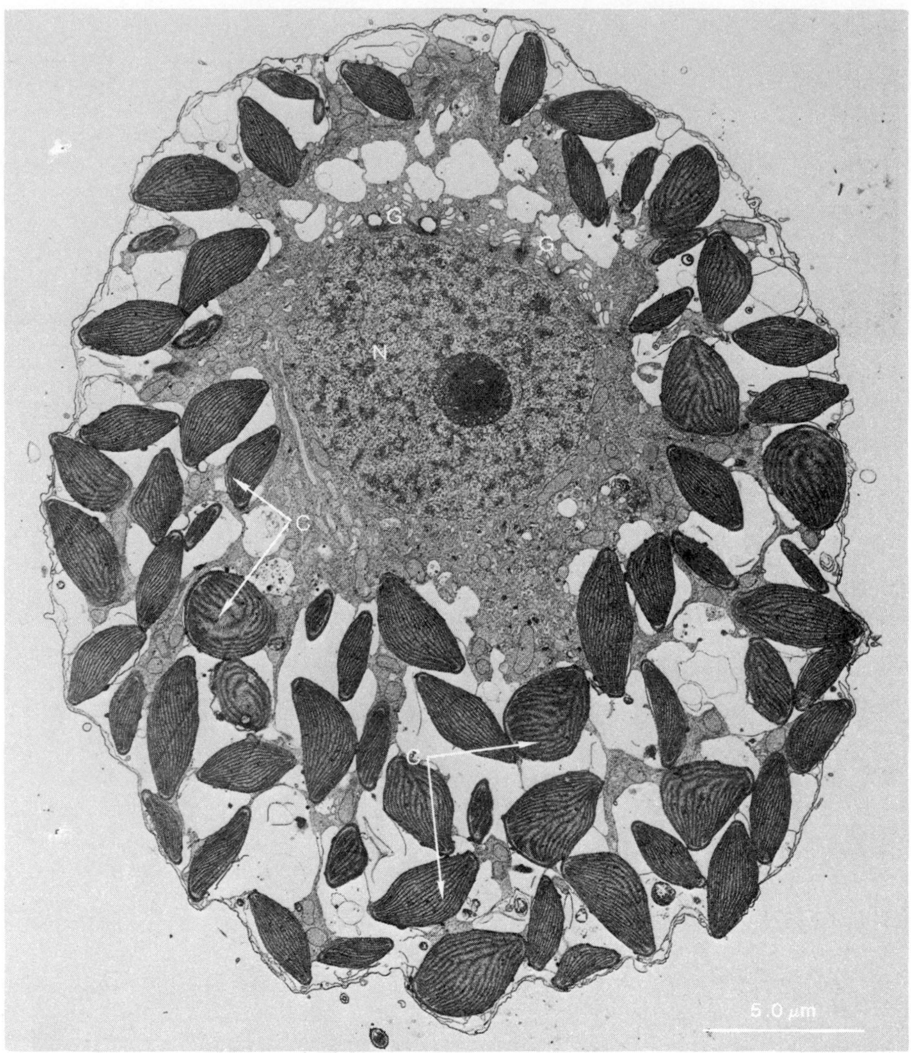

FIG. 11-8 An electron micrograph of the green alga *Vacuolaria virescens,* showing the large number and distribution of its chloroplasts (C). These photosynthesizing organelles occupy most of the dense cytoplasmic region surrounding the nucleus (N). A nucleolus (Nu) and golgi apparatus (G) are also evident in this view. *Heywood, P.,* J. Phycol. *13:68-72 (1977).*

Reproduction

Asexual cell division is the usual method of reproduction in diatoms (Figure 11-13). During the process, the two valves of the parent cell separate and serve as epivalves for the two newly formed products of division. One of the new cells is therefore always slightly smaller than the parent. Figure 11-13 shows this feature as well as other aspects of the process.

Sexual reproduction does not result in size reduction. Instead it is the means by which maximum cell size can be attained. The types of sexual reproduction found among other algal groups are also found among diatoms. That is, they may reproduce sexually by several means. Certain diatoms produce a unique sexual spore known as the ***auxospore***. Such spores can be produced by a number of mechanisms, including conjugation and the fusion of two gametes.

Economic and Ecological Importance

Diatomaceous earth has many important applications. For example, because of its abrasive quality, it is used as a polishing agent in toothpastes and metal polishes. It is also used in the manufacture of insulating materials and dynamite sticks. Other industries use diatomaceous earth for the filtration of beer, oil, and other fluids.

Because diatoms possess photosynthetic pigments, these organisms, as well as the golden algae and the yellow-green algae, produce and store the reserve food substances, chrysolaminarin and oils. It is believed that these algae have been significant sources of petroleum.

Aside from their present commercial value, diatoms are particularly interesting to scientists as members of food chains and indicators of various geological changes. Diatoms have been used to trace the pattern of glacier formation in northern Europe and as indicators of industrial water pollution.

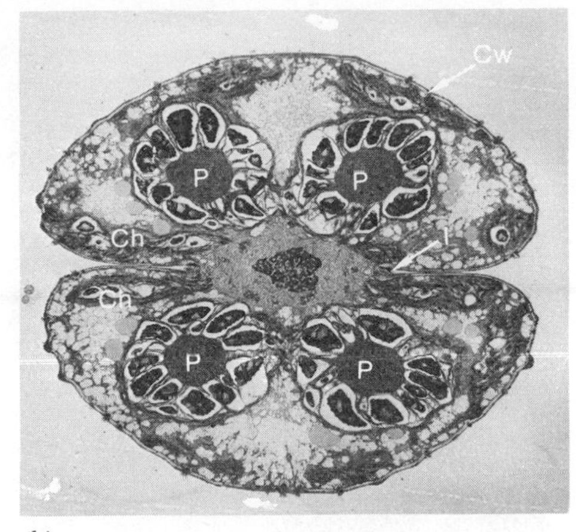

(b)

FIG. 11-9 (b) An ultrathin view of *Cosmarium* cells showing the area of constriction or isthmus (I), cell wall (CW), chloroplast (Ch), and pyrenoids (P). *Pickett-Heaps, J. D.,* J. Phycol. *8:343–360 (1972).* (c) Sexual reproduction of the green alga *Spirogrya.* Conjugation tubes (arrows) between participating algae are shown. Some cells contain zygotes (Z). *Courtesy of Carolina Biological Supply Company.*

The Euglenoids (Euglenophycophyta)

Euglenoids are a small group of eucaryotic, unicellular microorganisms (Figure 11–14) that have a curious combination of animal and plant properties. For example, like animal cells, they lack any cell wall and have the ability to ingest food particles. Like plants, they possess photosynthetic pigments, apparently identical to those found in the green algae (Table 11–1). All euglenoids are bounded by an outer thickened cell membrane, known as a *pellicle,* composed of spiral ridges (Figure 11–14c).

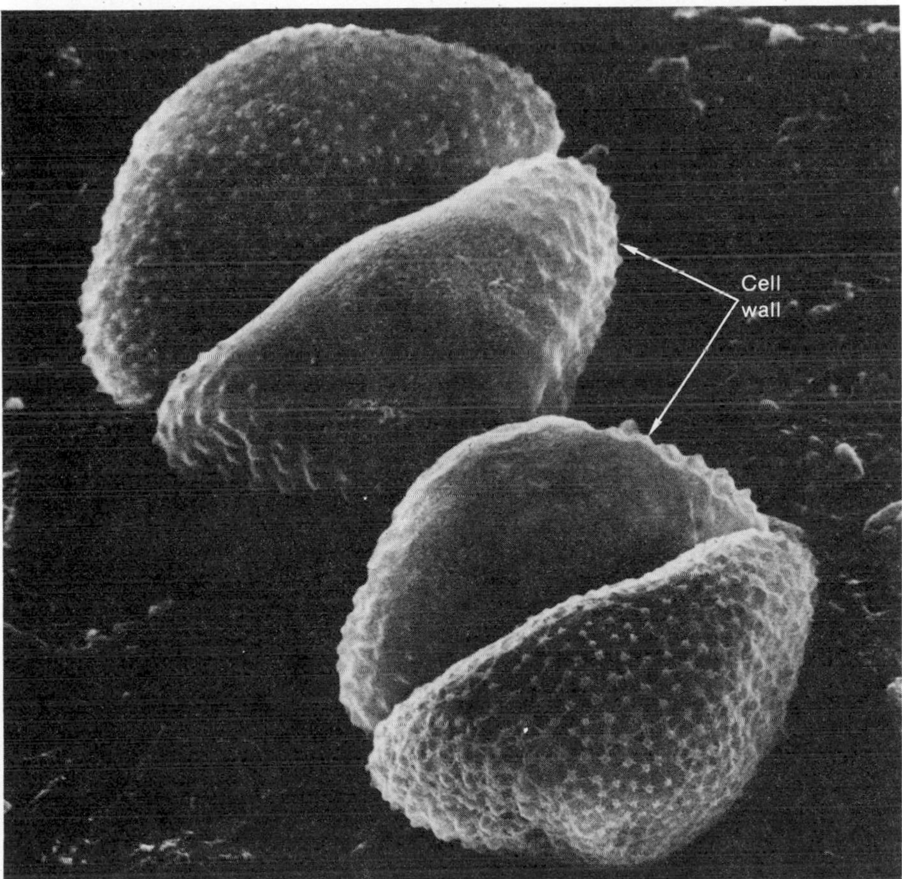

FIG. 11-9 Green algae reproduction. (a) A scanning micrograph of new asexually formed, curved cells of *Cosmarium.* The cell walls of desmids such as the ones shown are composed of two halves of different ages and origins. Note the surface appearance of the cells in each pair.

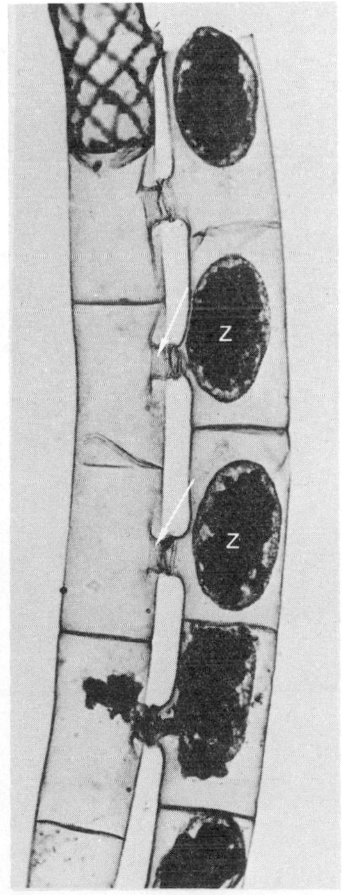

(c)

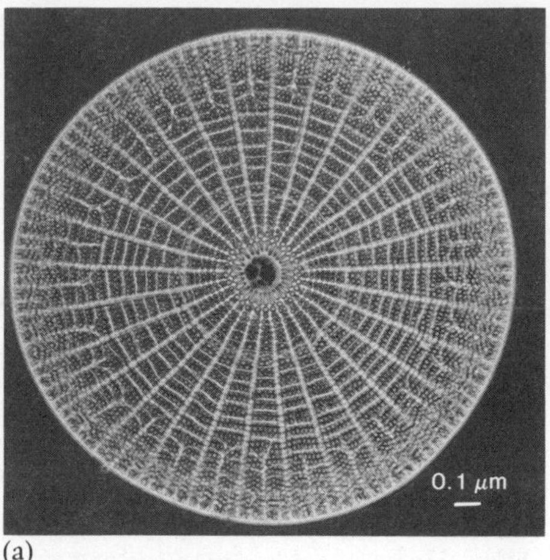

(a)

FIG. 11-10 Representative diatoms from the orders of Centrales and Pennales. (a) *Arachnoidiscus*, a marine centric diatom. (b) *Navicula*, a marine pennate diatom. *Courtesy of Dr. Paul E. Hargraves, Narragansett Marine Laboratory, Kingston, Rhode Island.*

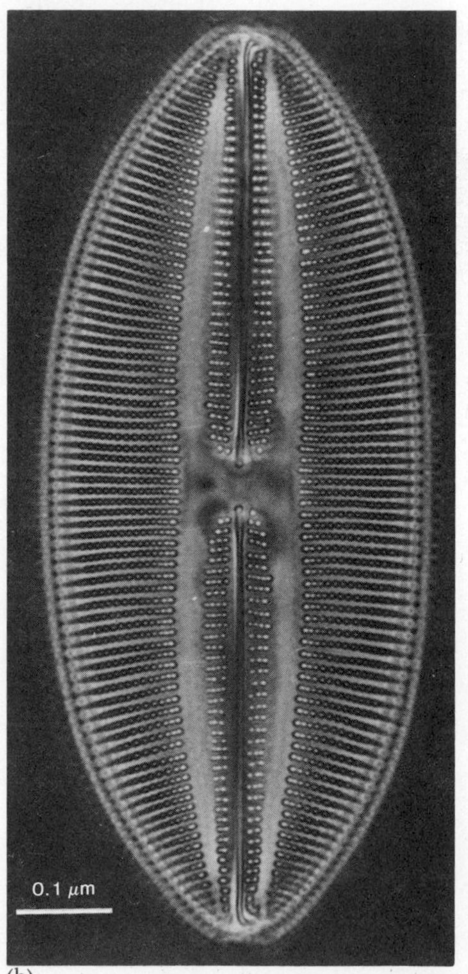

(b)

Some euglenoid cells move about by means of a flowing, contracting and expanding motion known as ***euglenoid movement***. Others are flagellated.

Some euglenoids have an eyespot that enables cells to respond to light stimuli and a contractile vacuole that is used to discharge excess water and wastes. Some species are even able to form resistant structures, ***cysts***, against unfavorable environments. Euglenoids reproduce asexually by simple cell division.

These microorganisms with their unique mixture of animal, plant, and microbial features present an interesting challenge to taxonomists.

The Brown Algae (Phaeophycophyta)

The Phaeophycophyta, commonly called the brown algae, include members ranging from simple filamentous forms to the massive kelp *Macrocystis*, the largest known marine plants (Figure 11–15). In California, about 150,000 metric tons of the giant kelp are harvested annually. It is the source of the substance ***algin***, which is used in adhesives and plastics and also in various dairy products such as cream cheese, ice cream, sherbet, and whipping cream to break up fats.

Most of the brown algae are exclusively marine (Color Photograph 50), found in open waters, rocky coastlines, and in regions where a large river meets the sea. Many are attached to rocks, muddy bottoms, shells, and other nonliving surfaces.

Structure and Organization

The brown algae are a highly specialized group (Table 11–1). The more complex forms possess conspicuous tissues that transport nutrients and reach treelike dimensions. Most algal bodies have definite forms (Figure 11–6). Although there is little tissue specialization, many of the brown algae have recognizable structures: flat expanded leaf portions, or ***blades;*** attachment devices known as ***holdfasts;*** and stalks, or ***stipes*** (Figure 11–15). Various large brown algae, the kelps, have ***gas-filled floats***, or ***air bladders***, which are located on the stipes or blades and which allow the major photosynthetic portion of the plant to float near the surface of the water. Although chlorophyll is their photosynthetic pigment, the distinctive color of brown algae is due to the predominance of other pigments, namely beta-carotene and fucoxanthin, a type of xanthophyll. Brown algal cells store food as the carbohydrate laminarin, the alcohol mannitol, and sometimes as lipids. No starch is formed.

All brown algae lack an internal air system to aid the exchange of gases within their body structure; and most significantly for their survival, they lack a waterproof covering to prevent water loss.

Reproduction

The brown algae reproduce asexually by zoospores. They may also reproduce by fusion between morphologically and physiologically similar or different gametes.

Economic Value and Importance

The brown algae have many important uses. Several species of kelp are used as a direct food source by Oriental peoples. In other countries brown algae are used as a vitamin source in pet foods and simply as a food source for domestic animals. Kelp farms are being organized to grow large quantities of brown algae to provide a new food source for the undernourished people of the world. Many brown algae have important medicinal uses as components of greaseless lubricating jellies and ointments and components of medical gauze.

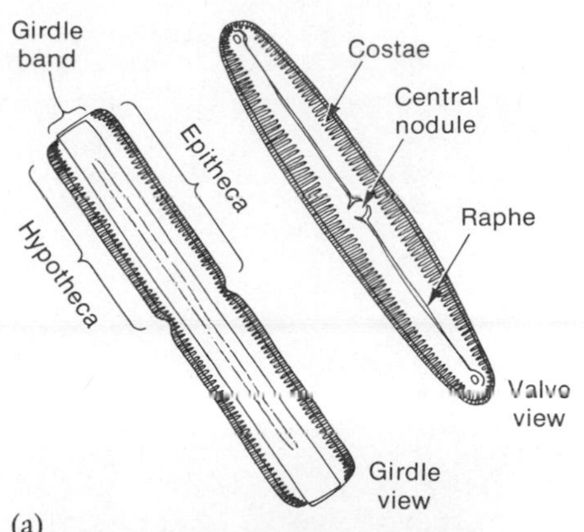

(a)

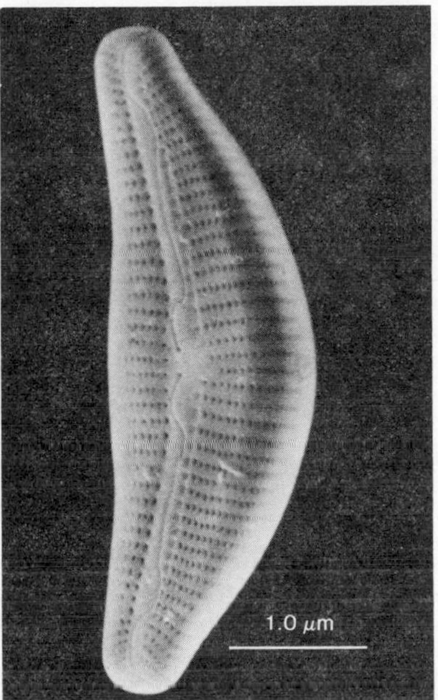

(b)

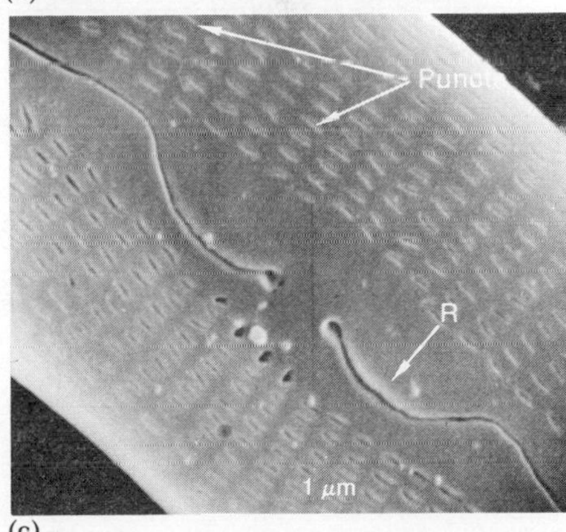

(c)

FIG. 11–11 The structure of a pennate diatom. (a) A drawing of a pennate diatom, *Pinnularia* sp. (b) A scanning micrograph of the cell wall, or *frustule*, of *Cymbella cistula*. (c) A higher magnification of the frustule, showing distinct puncta and raphe (R). Such ornamentation of the cell wall is extremely important to diatom classification. *Hufford, T. L., and G. B. Collins,* J. Phycol. *8:192–195 (1972).*

The Dinoflagellates (Pyrrophycophyta)

The dinoflagellates comprise a diverse group of biflagellated (Figure 11–16) and nonflagellated eucaryotic, unicellular organisms. For many years they were considered protozoans because of their motility and, in certain cases, their ability to ingest solid food particles. Further study of the group identified nonmotile and photosynthetic representatives, thereby establishing the dinoflagellate's relationship to algae.

The dinoflagellates occupy a variety of aquatic environments. They are found in both marine and freshwater habitats, where they exhibit parasitic, saprobic, and symbiotic relationships.

Structure and Organization

Most individual dinoflagellates have a heavy cell wall, or ***theca***, composed of cellulose-containing plates. Both the armored and unarmored (naked) organisms are circled by a transverse groove (Figure 11–16b). In motile cells two unequal flagella extend from a pore at a point along this groove.

Reproduction

The most common form of reproduction in dinoflagellates is by cell division. Some dinoflagellates reproduce by fragmentation. Others form zoospores and nonmotile spores called ***aplanospores***. Sexual reproduction has also been observed in a number of dinoflagellates.

Economic and Ecological Importance

Dinoflagellates are widely recognized as important members of food webs in the oceans and in some freshwater environments. They provide a basic food source. Aside from this beneficial function, most of the activities of dinoflagellates are of an unpleasant or harmful nature.

Many dinoflagellates impart an offensive odor and taste to water. Several members of this division also produce "red tides," a type of algal bloom. In this situation, environmental conditions are right for a sudden increase in the concentration of cells, which color the ocean in the immediate area red, brown, or yellow. Warm water, large concentrations of iron and phosphate, and other factors contribute to algal reproduction.

Most blooms of dinoflagellates produce toxic effects that may kill fish or invertebrates or contribute to paralytic shellfish poisoning (PSP) in humans. Paralytic shellfish poisoning results from eating clams, mussels, oysters, scallops, or other filter-feeding molluscs that have concentrated toxins of *Gonyaulax catenella* and related species (Figure 11–16b). The toxin of *G. catenella*, saxitoxin, affects the nervous system and is said to be 100,000 times as potent as cocaine.

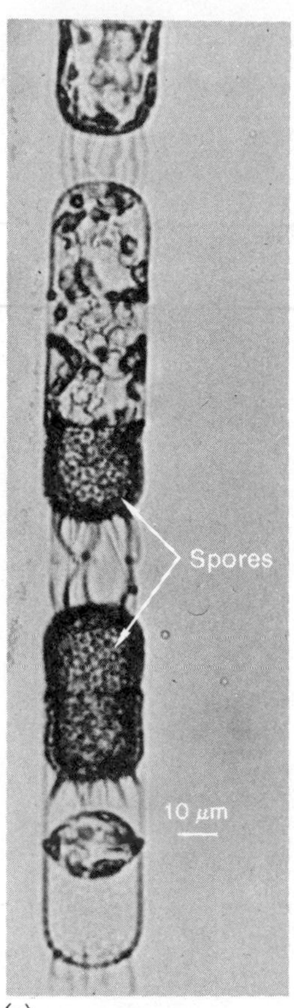

(a)

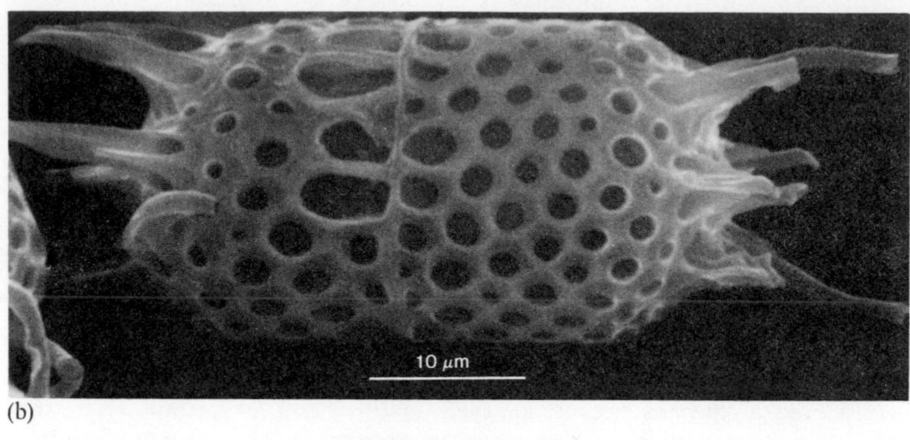

(b)

FIG. 11-12 Resting spores of the centric diatom *Stephanopyxis turris.* (a) Resting spore formation. (b) A scanning micrograph of an entire resting spore. Note the extensions on each end of the spore. *Hargraves, P. E.,* J. Phycol. *12:18–128 (1976).*

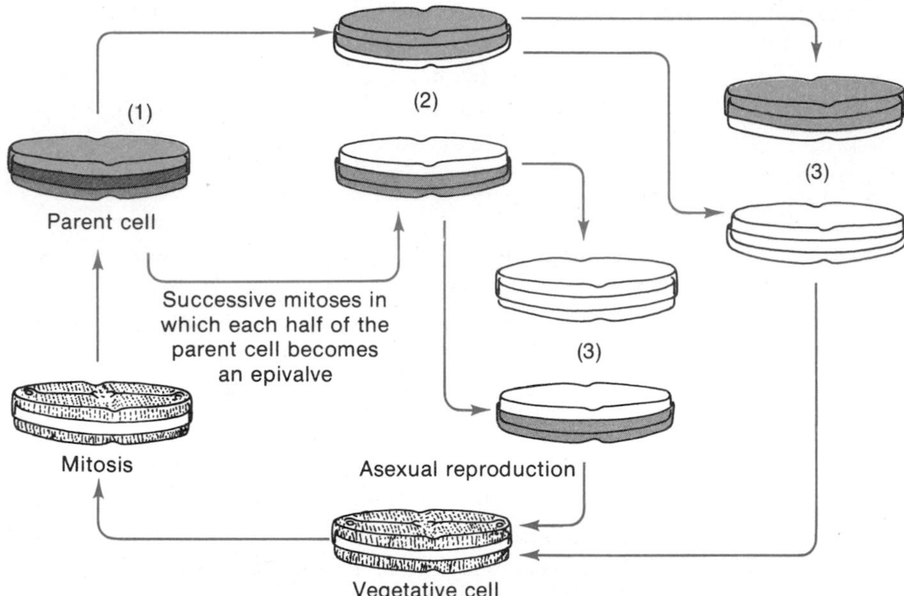

FIG. 11-13 Asexual reproduction of diatoms. During the process, the two parent valves (1) separate (2) and serve as respective epivalves for the daughter diatoms. The process continues with the newly formed pennate diatoms (3).

The Red Algae (Rhodophycophyta)

The red algae, of which there are some 4000 species, belong to the division of Rhodophycophyta (Figure 11–17a). Many are found at great depths in marine environments (Color Photograph 49). One of the most common rhodophycophyte species is *Bactrachopermum,* a red alga that ranges in color from gray-green to olive. It appears as branched masses attached to sticks and stones in flowing bodies of water and quiet pools. Red algae usually attach themselves to surfaces of other algae. Some are parasitic on closely related species.

The color of red algae comes from the red pigment ***phycoerythrin***. Red algae may also contain a blue pigment, often giving them a deep blue-green or blackish color.

The vegetative cells of most red algae are uninuclear and contain most of the organelles found in most other related eucaryotic algae (Figure 11–17b).

The red algae reproduce asexually by nonmotile spores. Their sexual process involves the fusion of well-differentiated male and female sex cells.

The red algae contribute significantly to the world's economy. The red algae *Gelidium* and *Gracilaria* produce the agar, widely used in culturing microorganisms.

Lichens

Many interesting relationships exist between various microorganisms. One of these is the symbiotic association between certain blue-green bacteria or green algae and fungi, the combination of which is called a *lichen* (Color Photographs 51 and 52). In the resulting plant body, called a **thallus,** the hypha of the fungus produces a tightly interwoven mycelium (Figure 11–18). Algal cells are usually housed and protected within this basic structure. The function of algae, according to one view, is to provide nutrients through the photosynthetic process. Fungi absorb from their environment water and minerals that are utilized by the companion algae. Since lichens are capable of living in environments that cannot support most other forms of life (for example, on rocks and in the arctic), it may be that this association is formed as a matter of utmost necessity for survival of the microorganisms forming the association.

Although lichens are remarkably resistant to drying, cold, heat, and other environmental conditions, they are extremely sensitive to air pollutants and quickly disappear from heavily polluted urban regions. Apparently, lichens absorb the pollutants from rain water. Because they have no means of excreting them, lethal concentrations of toxic air pollutants gradually build up.

At least 15,000 different lichen species have been identified. The fungal

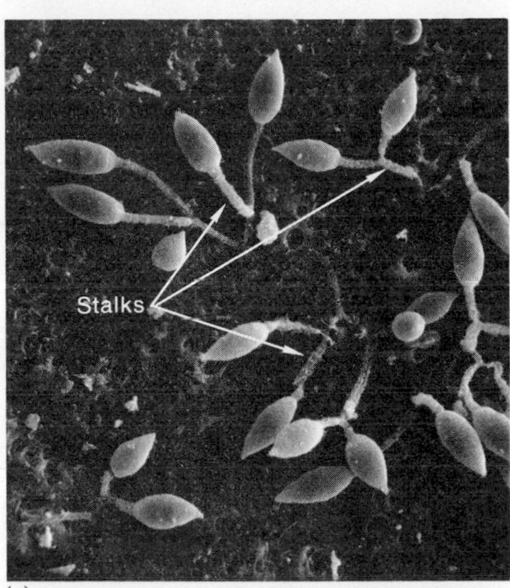

(a)

FIG. 11–14 The Euglenoids. (a) A scanning micrograph of stalked cells of *Colacium mucronatum*. Species of *Colacium* grow on a variety of aquatic animals such as free-living worms and protozoa, as well as on mud and in fresh water attached to aquatic plants. *Colacium* cells attach to surfaces by means of a sticky stalk. *Rosowski, J. R., and R. L. Willey,* J. Phycol. *13:16–21 (1977).* (b) An enlarged view of the ridged surface (pellicle) of *Euglena*. This micrograph also shows the microorganism's flagellum with hairs. *Rosowski, J. R.,* J. Phycol. *13:323–328 (1977).*

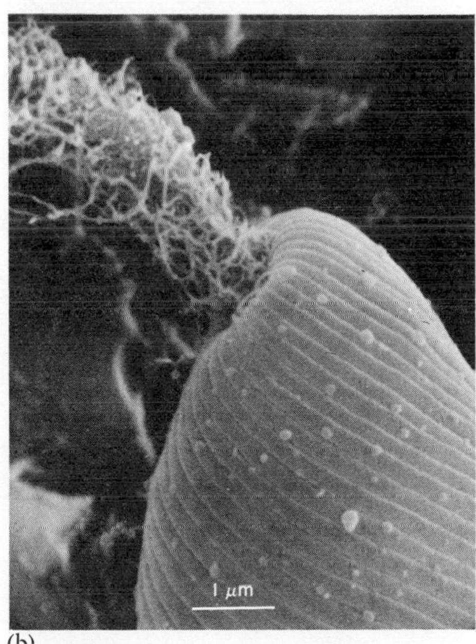

(b)

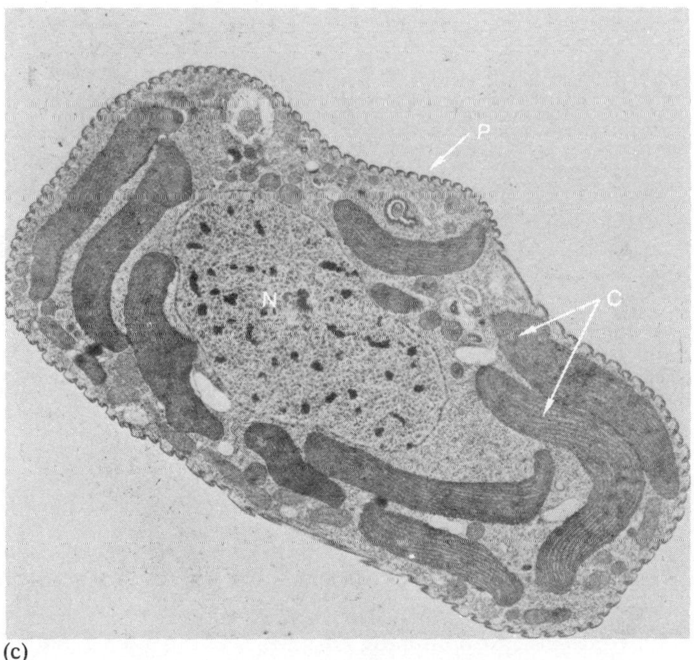

(c)

FIG. 11–14 (c) Features of *Euglena* as seen through transmission electron microscopy. This ultrathin section shows the following structures: ridged pellicle (P), nucleus (N), and chloroplasts (C). *Cook, J. R., and T. C. Li,* J. Protozool. *20:652–653 (1973).*

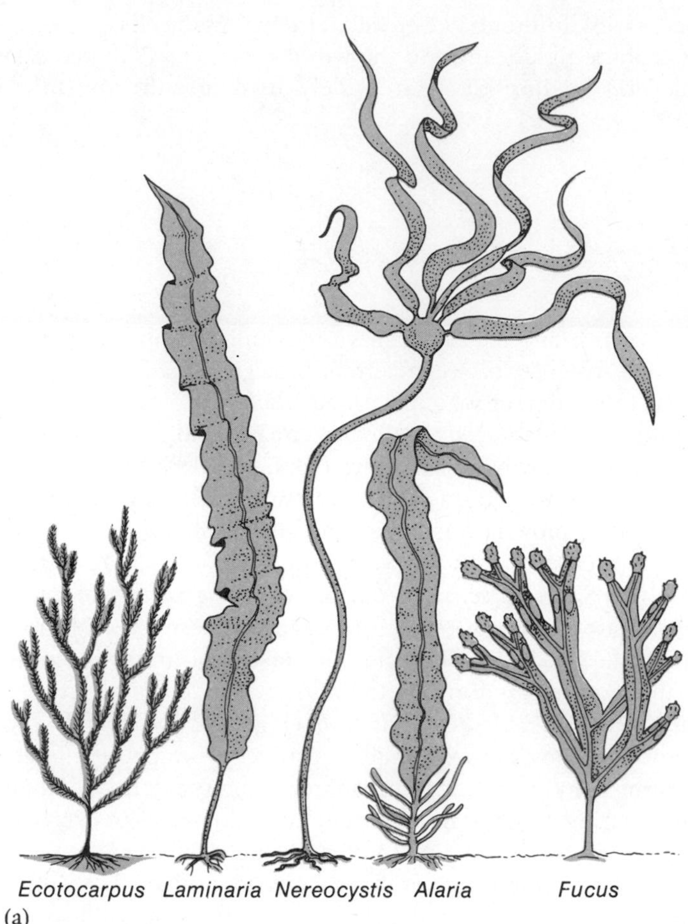

FIG. 11–15 The brown algae, or kelp. (a) Some species found in marine environments (not to scale). Each mature alga develops from a young organism with a single flat blade. (b) The giant, or vine, kelp and its parts.

member of the lichen is always a member of the class Ascomycetes. The other member may be one of many blue-green bacteria or green algae. Fungi are usually the dominant organisms and therefore determine the shape and size of the basic structure.

Many different arrangements and colors are displayed by lichens. These differences largely determine their type, or category. Three major types of lichens are recognized. *Crustose* (crustlike) lichens are usually found on rocks or bark as irregular, flat patches. The colors include black, gray, green, yellow, and brown (Color Photograph 52). *Foliose* (leaflike) lichens are curled, leafy, and usually greenish gray, possessing rootlike structures for attachment and the absorption of minerals. *Fruticose* (shrublike) lichens are highly branched and either hang from different tree parts or originate in the soil (Color Photograph 52b).

Lichens are ecologically and economically important. They serve as food for arctic caribou and reindeer and are used in the preparation of litmus paper, a well-known indicator in chemistry and related sciences. Recently certain lichens have been shown capable of producing antibiotics. From such reports it appears that lichens may have great potential in the treatment of certain bacterial and fungal diseases. Another role of lichens, one that is sometimes overlooked, is their contribution to the organic content of soil. Quite often the activity of their rootlike structures aids in the decomposition of rocks. The decaying remains of dead lichens become intermixed with the small rock particles, providing nutrients and a foundation for plant development.

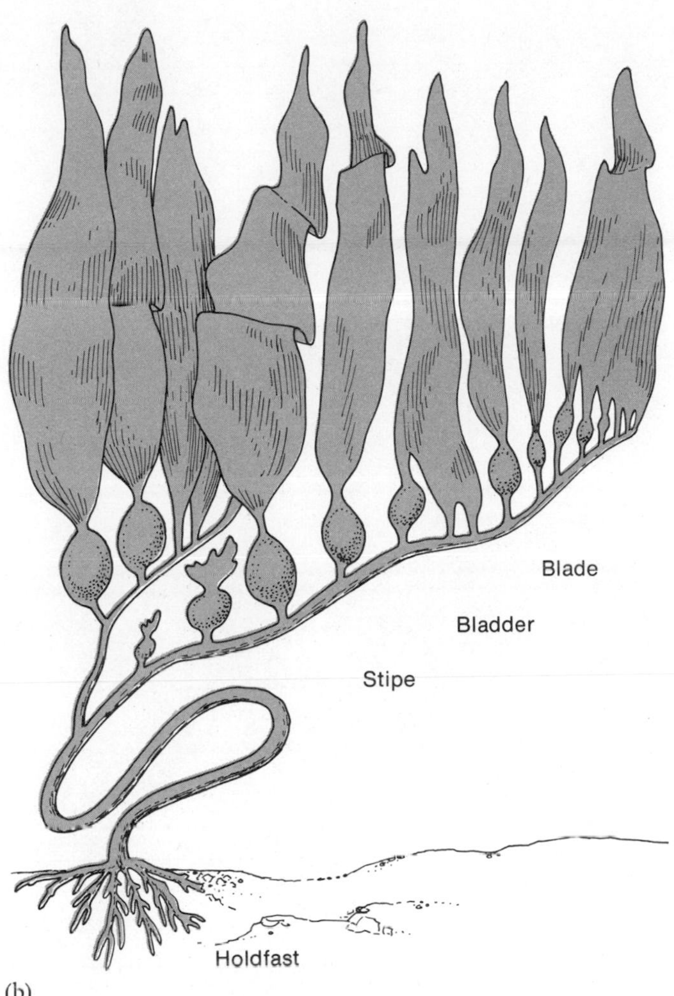

(b)

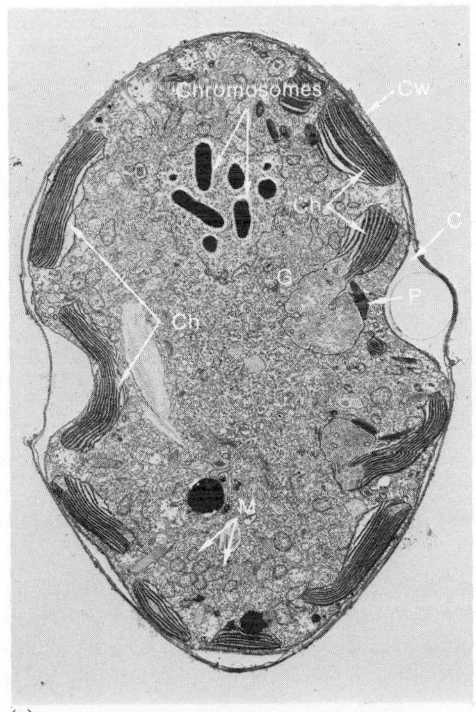

(a)

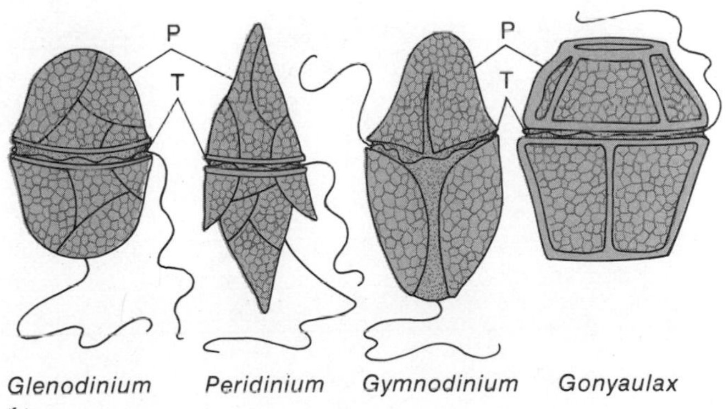

(b)

FIG. 11-16 (a) An internal view of the dinoflagellate, *Cachonina illdefina.* This cell shows its eucaryotic organization and the cell membrane (C), cell wall (CW), chloroplasts (Ch), golgi bodies (G), mitochondria (M), characteristic chromosomes (Chr), and pyrenoids (P). *Herman, E. M., and B. L. Sweeney*, J. Phycol. *12:198–205 (1976).* (b) Four dinoflagellate species. Note the plates (P) that enclose the single-celled organism. The presence of two flagella, one of which is located in the transverse groove (T), is another characteristic feature of these organisms.

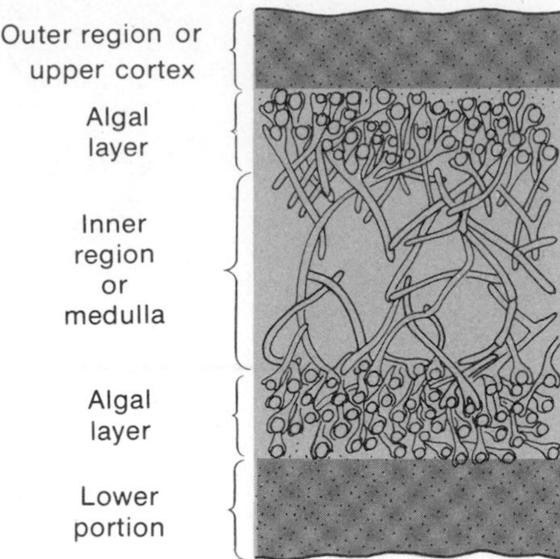

FIG. 11-18 A cross section of one type of lichen, fruticose. Note the algal layer and the fungus-containing medulla and cortex layers. (See Color Photographs 51 and 52.)

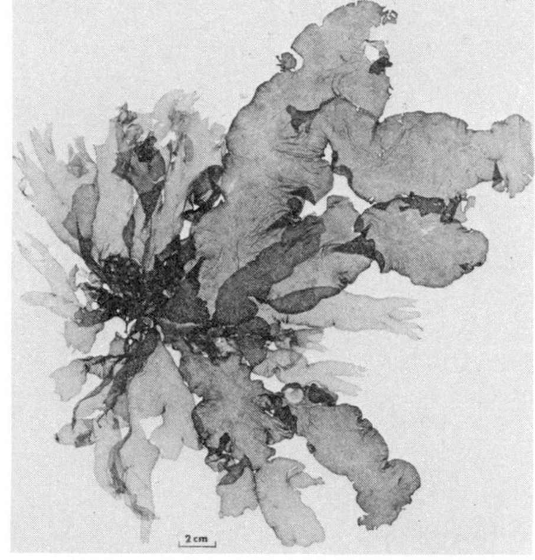

(a)

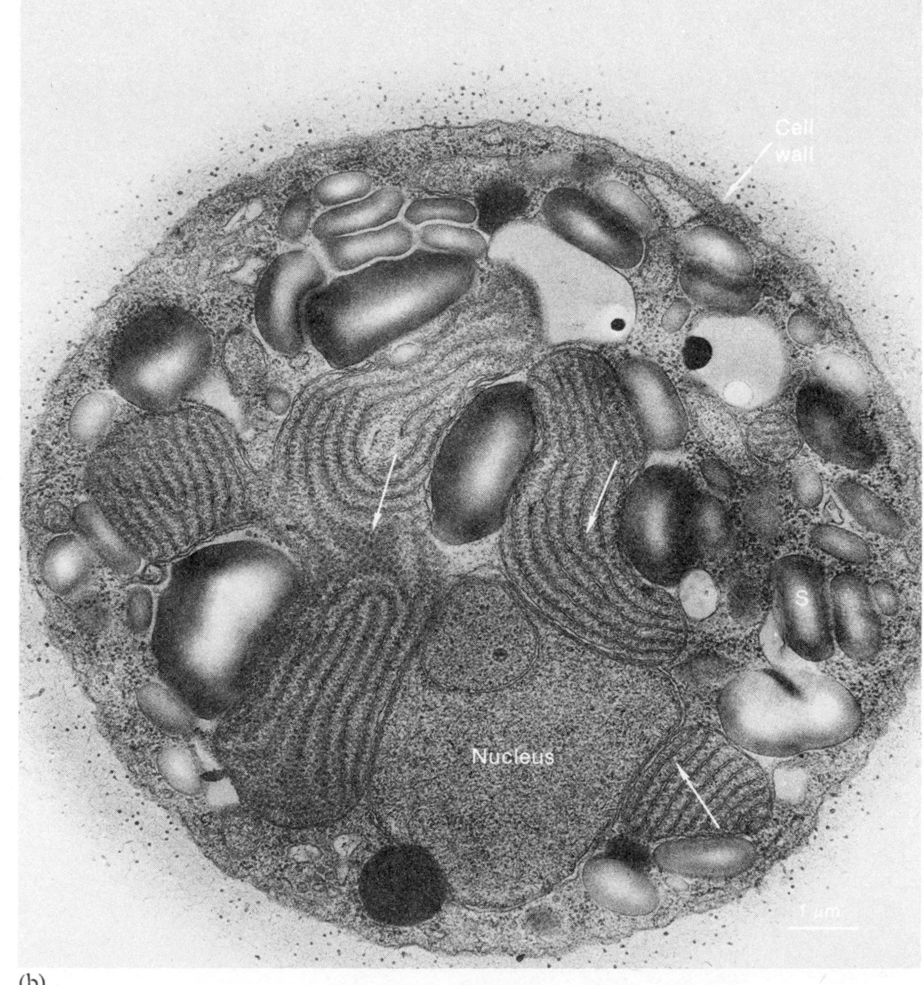

(b)

FIG. 11-17 Red algae. (a) The tropical *Platoma abbotiana*. Note its leafy features. *Norris, J., and K. Bucher,* J. Phycol. *13:155–162 (1977)*. (b) An ultrathin section of the red alga *Porphyridium cruentrum*. Small granules (arrows) are attached to the chloroplast lamellae (C). These granules have a diameter of about 35 nm. Other structures shown include a nucleus (N), cell wall (CW), and the storage product, starch granules (S). *Gant, E., and S. F. Conti, Dartmouth Medical School, Hanover, N. H.* J. Cell Biol. *25:423–434 (1966)*.

SUMMARY

Algae: The Grass of the Waters

1. Algae are photosynthetic aquatic organisms. Many are important members of several food chains. Others, such as algal blooms, pose environmental problems.
2. Many algae are free-floating and free-living. Some species live together with other organisms.

Structure and Organization

1. Algae are eucaryotic forms that exhibit a wide range of sizes and shapes.
2. Algae range in size from microscopic dimensions to lengths of 60 meters.
3. Cellular shape, organization, and arrangement vary considerably among algae divisions.

Means of Reproduction

1. Algae may reproduce either sexually or asexually. Some have rather complicated life cycles.
2. Asexual reproduction includes production of a variety of unicellular spores, fragmentation of filaments, and division by cellular splitting.

Cultivation

A variety of liquid or solid nutrient preparations are available for cultivation of fresh algal specimens.

Classification

1. At least six eucaryotic algal divisions are recognized.
2. The names of the divisions include the root *phyco* ("seaweed") to draw attention to the algal level of organization.
3. Algal divisions differ from one another in several respects, including cellular organization, cell wall chemistry, flagellation, pigmentation, reserve storage products, and means of reproduction.

The Green Algae (Chlorophycophyta)

These organisms exist in a variety of arrangements, including unicellular forms, filaments, and colonies.

Structure and Organization

The green algae resemble higher forms of plant life in several ways such as cellular chemistry and organization and pigmentation.

Reproduction

The green algae have several methods of asexual reproduction. They may also reproduce sexually by fusion between sex cells.

Economic and Ecological Importance

While most species are beneficial, some are responsible for the clogging of water systems and the production of harmful algatoxins.

The Golden Brown Algae and the Diatoms (Chrysophycophyta)

1. This division contains a highly diverse group of algae.
2. Diatoms form a major part of floating algal populations world wide.

Structure and Organization

Obvious distinguishing characteristics of diatoms are their intricately sculptured cell walls, or *frustules*, which contain large concentrations of silicates, the basic components of sand and glass.

Reproduction

Asexual cell division is the usual method of reproduction in diatoms. It results in two cells, with one of the new cells always slightly smaller than the parent. Sexual reproduction does not result in size reduction.

Economic and Ecological Importance

Diatoms have several important commercial applications, such as in polishes and filters. They can also serve as indicators of industrial water pollution.

The Euglenoids (Euglenophycophyta)

These eucaryotic unicellular forms exhibit a curious combination of animal and plant properties.

The Brown Algae (Phaeophycophyta)

The brown algae include simple filamentous forms as well as the massive kelp, which is among the largest of marine plants.

Structure and Organization

The more complex forms of brown algae possess conspicuous tissues that transport nutrients and reach treelike dimensions. Although there is little tissue specialization, many of the brown algae have recognizable structures.

Reproduction

The brown algae reproduce asexually by zoospores. They may also reproduce by fusion between gametes.

Economic and Ecological Importance

These algae serve as sources of food, greaseless lubricating jellies, and medicinal ointments.

The Dinoflagellates (Pryrrophycophyta)

This group contains biflagellated as well as nonflagellated forms.

Structure and Organization

The dinoflagellates have a characteristic transverse groove that divides cells into halves.

Reproduction

The most common form of reproduction in dinoflagellates is by cell division. Other methods of reproduction are fragmentation, formation of spores, and sexual reproduction.

Economic and Ecological Importance

Dinoflagellates are important members of food webs in aquatic environments. Some of these algae are also known for harmful effects such as red tides and toxin production.

The Red Algae (Rhodophycophyta)

1. These organisms are widely distributed in marine environments. Many are of economic importance.
2. Agar, the solidifying agent used in bacteriological media, is extracted from species of red algae.

Lichens

1. Lichens consist of the symbiotic association between certain blue-green bacteria, or green algae and fungi.
2. The fungus component provides a tightly woven foundation of water and minerals for the association, while the algae provide nutrients by means of photosynthesis.
3. Three major types of lichens are recognized: crustose (crustlike), foliose (leaflike), and fruticose (shrublike).

4. Lichens serve as sources of food for arctic animals, contribute to the organic content of soil, and are used in litmus indicator production.

QUESTIONS FOR REVIEW

1. Do algae resemble any other microbial type? Explain.
2. a. How are algae classified?
   b. What properties or features do algae have that are not found in any other microbial group? List at least three.
   c. List six criteria used in algal classification.
3. How do algae reproduce? Explain.
4. List four algal divisions and describe the distinguishing features of each one.
5. What is unique about the cell walls of diatoms?
6. Of what commercial value are algae?
7. Compare the cellular organization and photosynthetic process of green algae with that of photosynthetic bacteria.
8. List some of the beneficial and detrimental effects of algae.
9. a. What are lichens?
   b. What beneficial functions do they have?
10. Define or explain the following:
    a. food chain
    b. agar
    c. phytoplankton
    d. algal bloom
    e. zoospore
    f. frustule
11. Photographic Quiz
    a. What type of alga is shown in Figure 11–19a?
    b. Identify the labeled structures of the green alga in Figure 11–19b.

SUGGESTED READINGS

Bold, H. C., and M. J. Wynne, *Introduction to the Algae, Structure and Reproduction*. Englewood Cliffs, N.J.: Prentice-Hall, 1978. *An excellent traditional introduction to the structural and reproductive features of algae.*

Collins, M., "Algal Toxins," *Microbiol. Revs.* 42:725–746 (1978). *A review of the toxins produced by algae, with specific reference only to those that are harmful to multicellular organisms.*

Dawson, E. Y., *Marine Botany*. New York: Holt, Rinehart & Winston, 1966. *Especially recommended for its comprehensive coverage of marine algae.*

Hale, M. E., Jr., *The Biology of Lichens*. 2nd ed. London: Arnold, 1974. *A modern treatment of all aspects of lichens.*

Lewen, R. A. (ed.), *The Genetics of Algae*. Berkeley: University of California Press, 1976. *A detailed treatment of the divisions of algae, their genetics, and the various processes associated with them.*

Round, F. E., *The Biology of the Algae*. 2nd ed. New York: St. Martin Press, 1973. *Especially recommended because of its wide coverage on the structure, ecology, geographical distribution, and physiology of algae.*

Sumich, J. L., *An Introduction to the Biology of Marine Life*. Dubuque, Iowa: William C. Brown, 1976. *An introductory text dealing with the biology of marine animals, plants, and microorganisms. Various aspects of marine ecology and physiology are also incorporated throughout the text.*

Tippo, O., and W. L. Stern, *Humanistic Botany*. New York: W. W. Norton & Company, 1977. *An easy-to-read text that provides functional, up-to-date information on the various uses of plants in everyday life. Chapter 13 presents a well-illustrated description of algae and their impact on humans.*

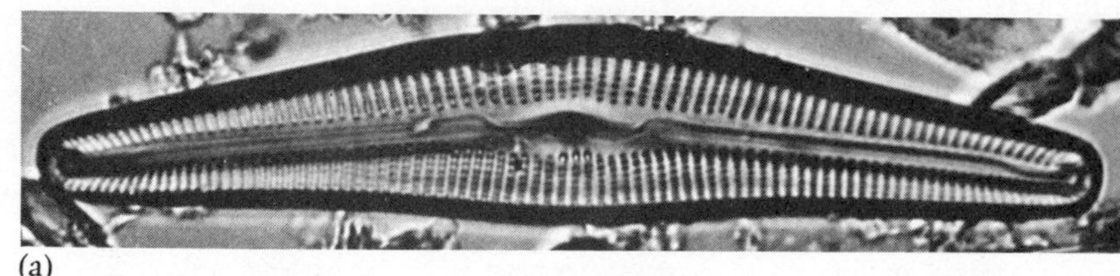

(a)

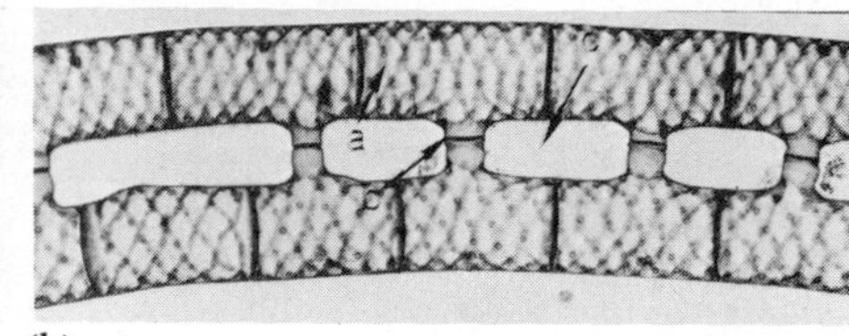

(b)

FIG. 11–19 (a) *Hufford, T. L., and G. B. Collins,* J. Phycol. *8:192–195 (1972).* (b) *Carolina Biological Supply Company.*

CHAPTER 12

Virus Structure, Organization, and Cultivation

True microorganisms, however small and simple, are cells. Unicellular microorganisms such as certain algae, bacteria, fungi, and protozoa always contain deoxyribonucleic acid as their storehouse of genetic information and have their own machinery for the production of energy and macromolecules such as carbohydrates, lipids, proteins, and nucleic acids. Viruses are totally different. They represent the ultimate in parasitism. This chapter surveys the structure and function of these most unusual submicroscopic organisms.

After reading this chapter, you should be able to:

1. **Outline the differences between viruses and other types of microorganisms.**
2. **Describe the size, range, organization, and distinctive structures and associated functions of viruses.**
3. **Describe the replication cycle of viruses.**
4. **Identify viral structures in electron micrographs.**
5. **List and describe the methods used for the cultivation of viruses.**
6. **Discuss the bases for virus classification and how they differ from those for other microbial types.**
7. **List the differences that exist among viruses with respect to structure, replication cycle, and host range.**
8. **Define or explain the following:**
   - a. **virion**
   - b. **viroid**
   - c. **lysogeny**
   - d. **tissue culture**
   - e. **cytopathic effect**
   - f. **plaque**

Virtually every kind of life can be parasitized by viruses—vertebrate and invertebrate animals, plants, procaryotes, and eucaryotic microorganisms, such as fungi, protozoa, and certain algae. There are even some "satellite" viruses, which are considered in a sense parasites on other viruses. This chapter will discuss viruses in terms of their hosts—animals, plants, procaryotes, and eucaryotic microorganisms. Aspects of specific human viral infections are presented in later chapters.

What is a Virus?

Viruses are unlike any other form of microorganism. This is obvious not only from their submicroscopic size, but from other differences related to the way they function (Table 12–1). They are so different, in fact, that for years the question was argued whether or not they are actually living. A completely satisfactory definition of a virus has yet to be agreed upon.

A suitable functional definition would distinguish viruses from all other biological forms. The definition proposed by A. Lwoff and P. Tournier in 1962 lists the following five specific properties of a mature virus particle, or ***virion:*** (1) the possession of only one type of nucleic acid, either DNA or RNA; (2) the replication of viral particles directed by the viral nucleic acid; (3) the absence of the binary fission characteristic of bacteria and related microorganisms; (4) the lack of any energy-harnessing metabolic cycle like those in other life forms; and (5) dependence on the ribosomes of the host cell for synthesis of proteins (Figure 12–1). The structures and activities of organisms that meet this definition are detailed in the following sections.

Basic Structure of Extracellular Viruses

In a typical viral life cycle, intracellular and extracellular phases occur. In the intracellular phase, replication of viral components leads to the formation of mature virus particles. The extracellular phase involves the mature infective particles, the **virion,** by which the virus invades other cells. Most mature infective viruses have a characteristic structure. Electron microscopy and x-ray diffraction analysis show the virions to consist of a nucleic acid inner core surrounded by a protein outer coat, called a **capsid** (Figures 12–2 and 12–3).

The Nucleic Acid of the Mature Virion

The viral nucleic acid, whether DNA or RNA, contains the viral genetic material, or **genome.** The nucleic acid may be either single-stranded or double-stranded and assumes a long, filamentous, folded or coiled form (Figure 12–4). The specific form and arrangement of the nucleic acid varies according to the virus. While most viruses have either single-stranded RNA or double-stranded DNA, some of these agents may possess double-stranded RNA or single-stranded DNA. In most cases the nucleic acid is found to be a single molecule. (Some large RNA-containing viruses are exceptions to this finding.) The length of the nucleic acid molecule varies among different viruses, but it is constant for a particular type. The DNA of several viruses is circular or cyclic, but in some DNA-containing agents and in all RNA viruses, the nucleic acid of the mature virus particle is linear, or noncyclic.

The Nucleocapsid

The protein coats of simple viruses are constructed from protein molecules *(structural subunits)*, which in clusters form the subunits referred to as **capsomeres** (Figure 12–5). In electron micrographs, these capsomeres are the visible portions of viruses, appearing in several recognizable forms. The covering of the nucleic acid core is made up of these capsomeres assembled to form the *capsid*. The capsid, together with its viral nucleic acid core, comprises the **nucleocapsid** (Figure 12–2b).

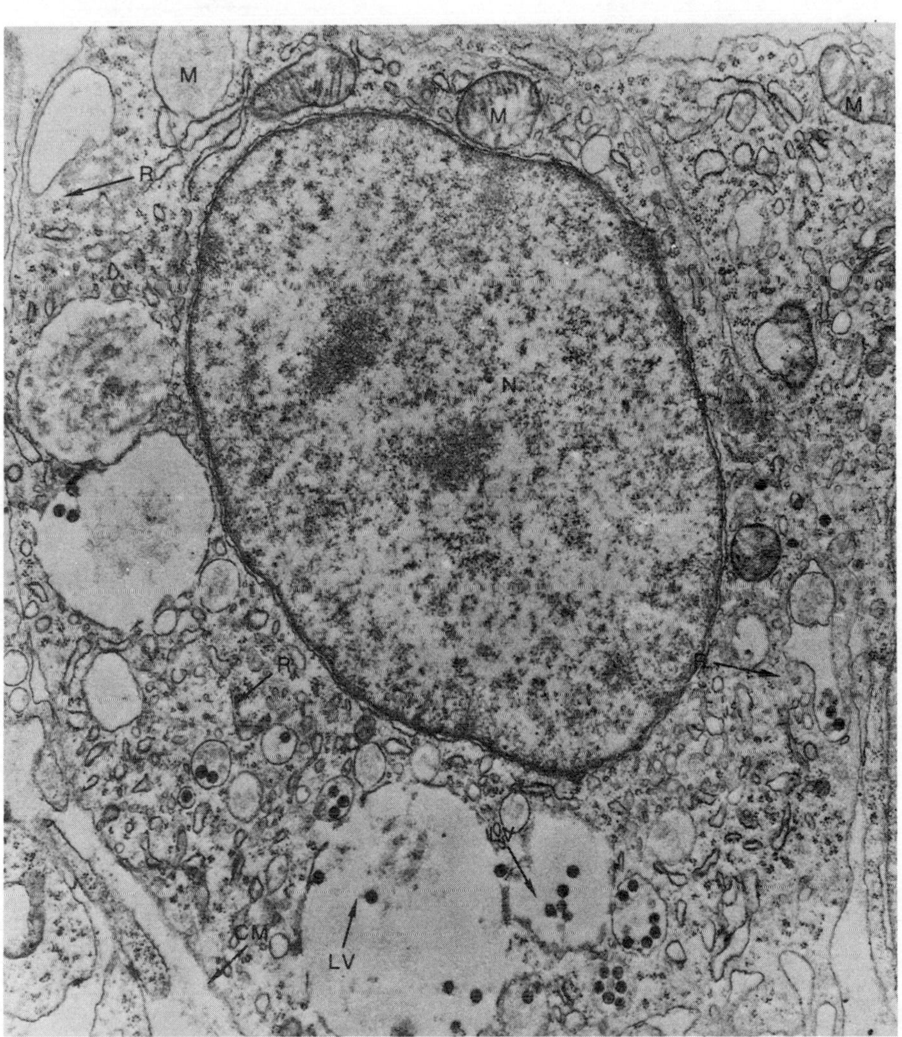

FIG. 12–1 An electron micrograph showing the presence of fowl leukosis virus (LV) in a cell from a nine-day-old chick embryo. This virus is the cause of a form of leukemia in birds. Note the relative size of the virus, the various parts of this cell, and the complete lack of a cellular organization in the viral particles. Shown here are cell membrane (CM), mitochondria (M), nucleus (N), and ribosomes (R). *Courtesy of the U.S. Department of Agriculture.*

TABLE 12-1 Properties of Viruses and Other Microorganisms

Microbial Group	*Microbial Components*				*Growth Requirements*		
	Cell Wall	*Internal Membrane Parts, i.e., Mitochondria*	*Ribosomes*	*DNA and RNA*	*Artificial Media*	*Living Cells*	*Sensitivity to Antibiotics*
Algae	Present	Present	Present	Present	Present	Absent	Variable
Bacteria	Present	Absent	Present	Present	Present	Some	Present
Fungi	Present	Present	Present	Present	Present	Absent	Variable
Protozoa	Absent	Present	Present	Present	Present	Some	Variable
Viruses	Absent	Absent	Absent[a]	Absent[b]	Absent	Present	Absent

[a]One group of viruses, the *Arenaviruses*, which cause natural infections in rodents, contain host cell ribosomes.
[b]Individual virus particles contain either DNA or RNA, never both.

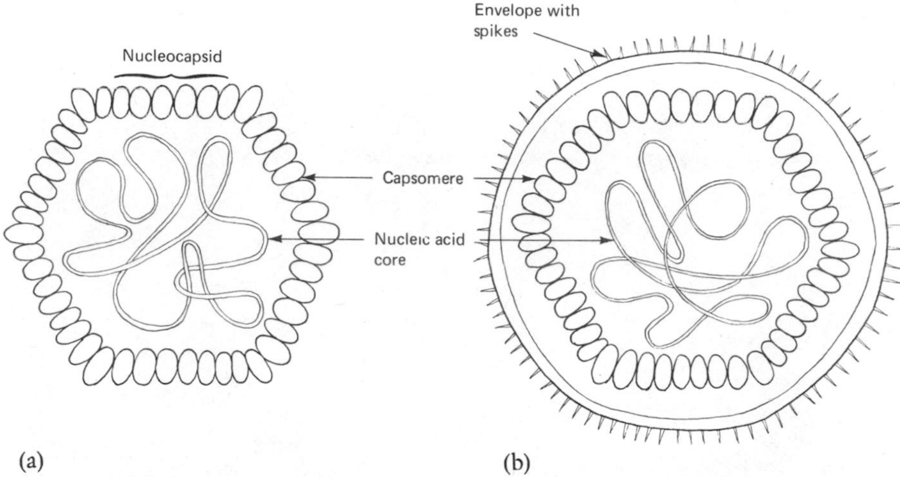

FIG. 12-2 Viral architecture. (a) A "naked" virus particle. Note the folding of the nucleic acid and the capsomeres. (b) An enveloped nucleic-acid-containing capsid. The envelope itself has spike structures. *Modified from Davis, et al.,* Microbiology, *Scranton, PA: Hoeber Medical Division, Harper & Row Publishers, 1968.*

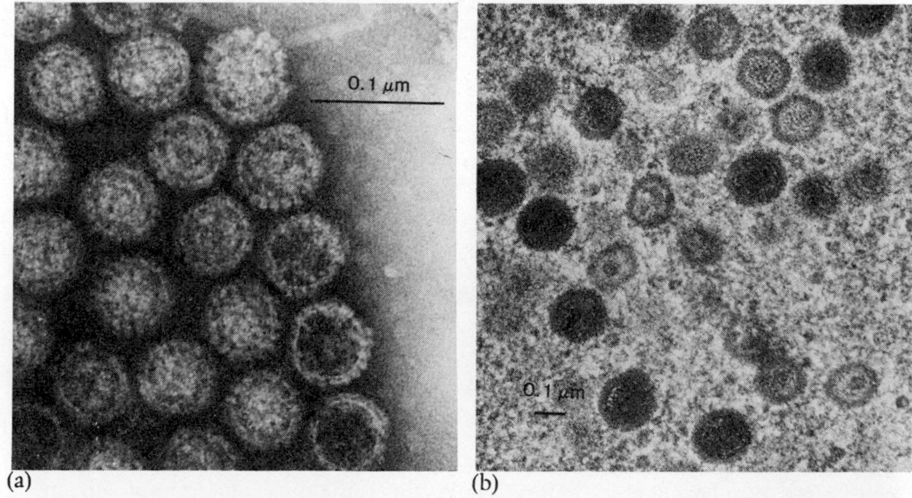

FIG. 12-3 (a) A negatively stained preparation of wound tumor virus. This plant virus contains RNA. Note the coiled appearance of the nucleic acid in individual viral particles. *Courtesy of L. M. Black and R. Markham.* (b) An electron micrograph of an iguana virus-infected cell. Several stages of capsid formation are shown. *Ziegel, R. F., and H. F. Clark,* Inf. Imm. 5*:570–582 (1972).*

The virus particle has one of several forms. Among the possible basic shapes are the cubic (Figure 12–6a), the helical shape (Figure 12–6b), and combinations of shapes known as binal (Figure 12–6c), bullet-shaped (Figure 12–6d), and filamentous. Many virus particles lacking an obvious discernible symmetry are called *complex* (Figure 12–6e).

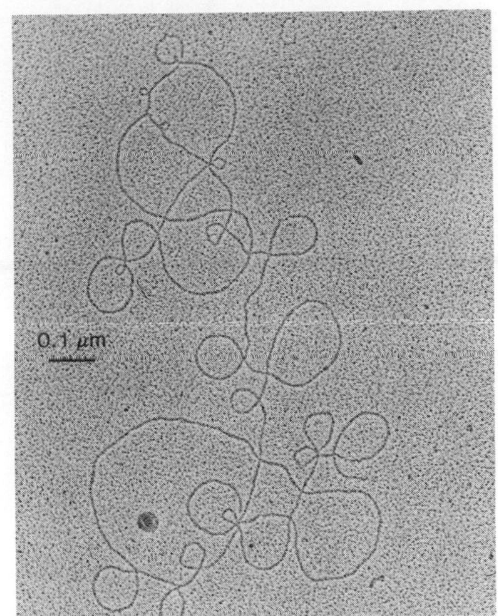

FIG. 12-4 An electron micrograph of the DNA molecule released by osmotic shock of a bacterial virus. Only one ghost (remains of the virus particle) is found near the nucleic acid, thus indicating that the virus contains a single DNA molecule. *Courtesy of Misra, D. N., R. K. Sinha, and N. N. Das Gupta,* Virology *39:183 (1969).*

Enveloped Viruses

Several animal virus particles, as a consequence of their intracellular development pattern, acquire an outer coat, or covering, from the cytoplasmic and/or nuclear membranes of infected cells as they pass through or are extruded from them (Figure 12–7). The term **envelope** has been given to this outer coat (Figure 12–2b). Viruses lacking such envelopes are commonly referred to as "naked." Envelopes are chemically composed of carbohydrates, lipids, and proteins. The molecular organization of these structures remains largely unknown. They usually range in thickness from 10 nm to 15 nm. Depending on the viral agent, the envelope may be covered with projecting spikes (Figure 12–2b and 12–7a), which in profile appear as knobs or a fringe (Figure 12–8a). The physical characteristics of such fringes differ among viral groups and can be used for identification purposes. The ability of viruses such as influenza to attach and clump red blood cells is associated with these spikes.

Shape and Size

Virions vary not only in size, but also in shape. The capsomeres of different viruses are arranged in definite geometric patterns. In the case of tobacco mosaic virus, the morphological units form a helical structure. This arrangement is shown diagrammatically in Figure 12–6b. The virus particle itself is a long rod and is referred to as a *helical virion.*

Several animal, plant, and bacterial viruses have polyhedral shapes, that is, they are many-sided (Figures 12–5 and 12–6). Their capsids are commonly icosahedral, having twenty triangular faces (Figure 12–5c). Such viral particles are called *icosahedral virions.* The size of this type of virus is determined by the number of capsomeres it has.

When either helical or icosahedral virions are enclosed by envelopes, they are described as enveloped helical or enveloped icosahedral. An example of the latter is herpes simplex virus, the causative agent of fever blisters (Figure 12–7). The viruses that cause influenza (Figure 12–6e) and mumps are typical enveloped helical forms.

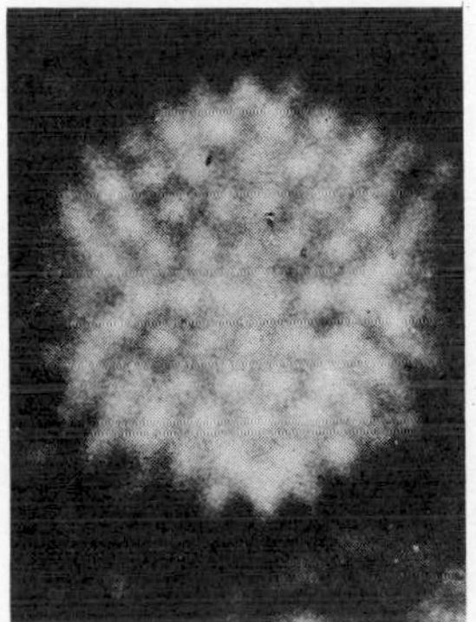

(a)

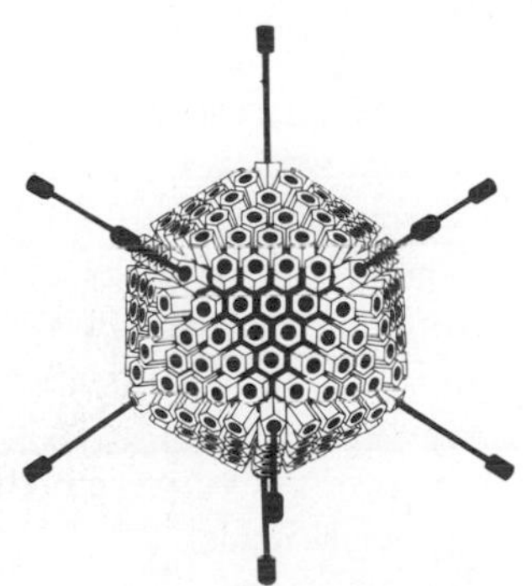

(b)

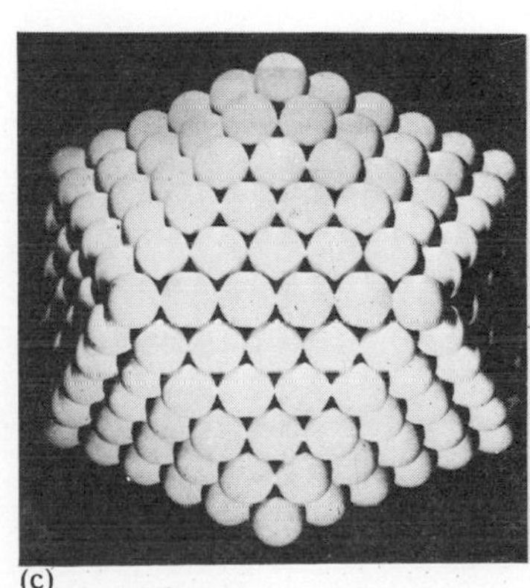

(c)

FIG. 12-5 (a) An electron micrograph showing the capsomere structure of adenovirus, type-5, in a negatively stained preparation. (b) A capsomere model of an adenovirus. *Courtesy of Dr. R. W. Horne, The John Innes Institute, Electron Microscope Laboratory, Norwich, England.* (c) An icosahedron (twenty-sided figure).

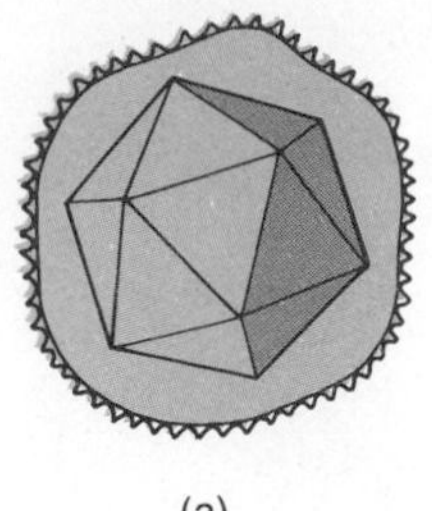
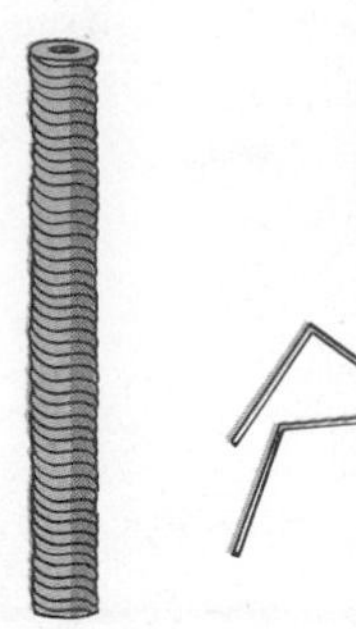
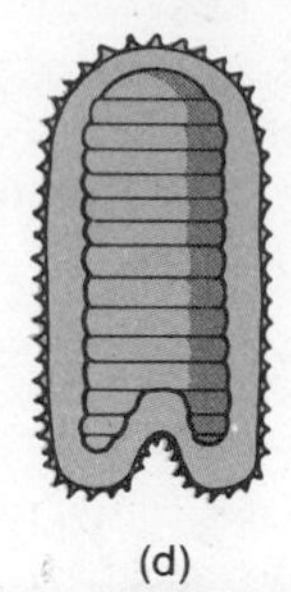
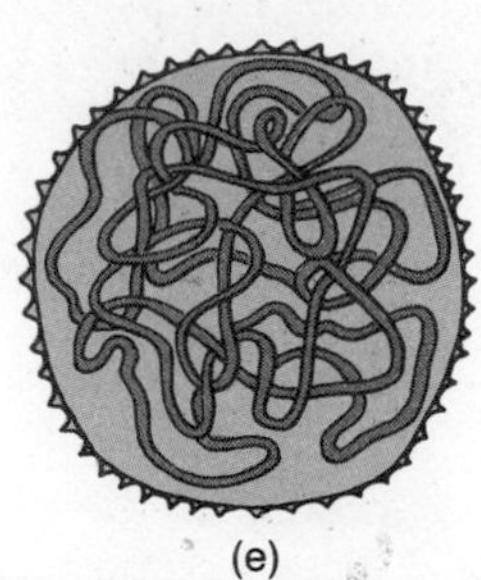

FIG. 12-6 A diagrammatic representation of the shapes of selected viruses. (a) Herpesviruses. (b) Plant viruses such as tobacco mosaic viruses. (c) T (type)-even bacteriophages. (d) Rabies virus and certain plant pathogens. (e) Mumps virus.

Classification

Viral classification is still in its infancy compared to the classifications of procaryotes or of higher forms of life. However, some of the newer and more sensitive approaches to the classification of viruses show a new refinement in determining the relationship between different forms of life.

Through the years, viruses have been grouped in several ways—according to the host normally infected, the particular tissue attacked, and even the general symptoms associated with a disease state. Although such approaches were useful, they were not very scientific or reliable. Not only could several different viruses cause similar disease symptoms, but one type of virus could produce quite different diseases depending on the host and the environment. Thus, it became apparent that a useful system of classification must be based on the basic properties of the virus itself. The constant chemical and structural properties of viruses lend themselves to such a precise system.

Several classification systems for viruses have been proposed. One of the most accepted systems uses Latinized binomial names like those used for other forms of life and is based on the characteristics of viruses as defined by Lwoff and Tournier in 1962. Under this system, viruses are classified according to the following properties of the virions:

1. *Capsid organization*
   (a) Shape and general size of virus particle
   (b) Number of capsomeres
   (c) Presence or absence of an envelope
   (d) General symmetry of nucleocapsid
2. *Nucleic acid chemistry*
   (a) Type of nucleic acid (whether DNA or RNA)
   (b) Number of strands (whether single or double)
   (c) Molecular weight of nucleic acid
   (d) Manner in which genetic information is translated into proteins
   (e) Presence of a **transcriptase** (an enzyme involved in the formation of nucleic acids)

Special features, such as cellular location for viral development and synthesis of viral parts, and host-parasite interactions, are used for further subdivision. Representative examples of this system are shown in Table 12–2.

(a)

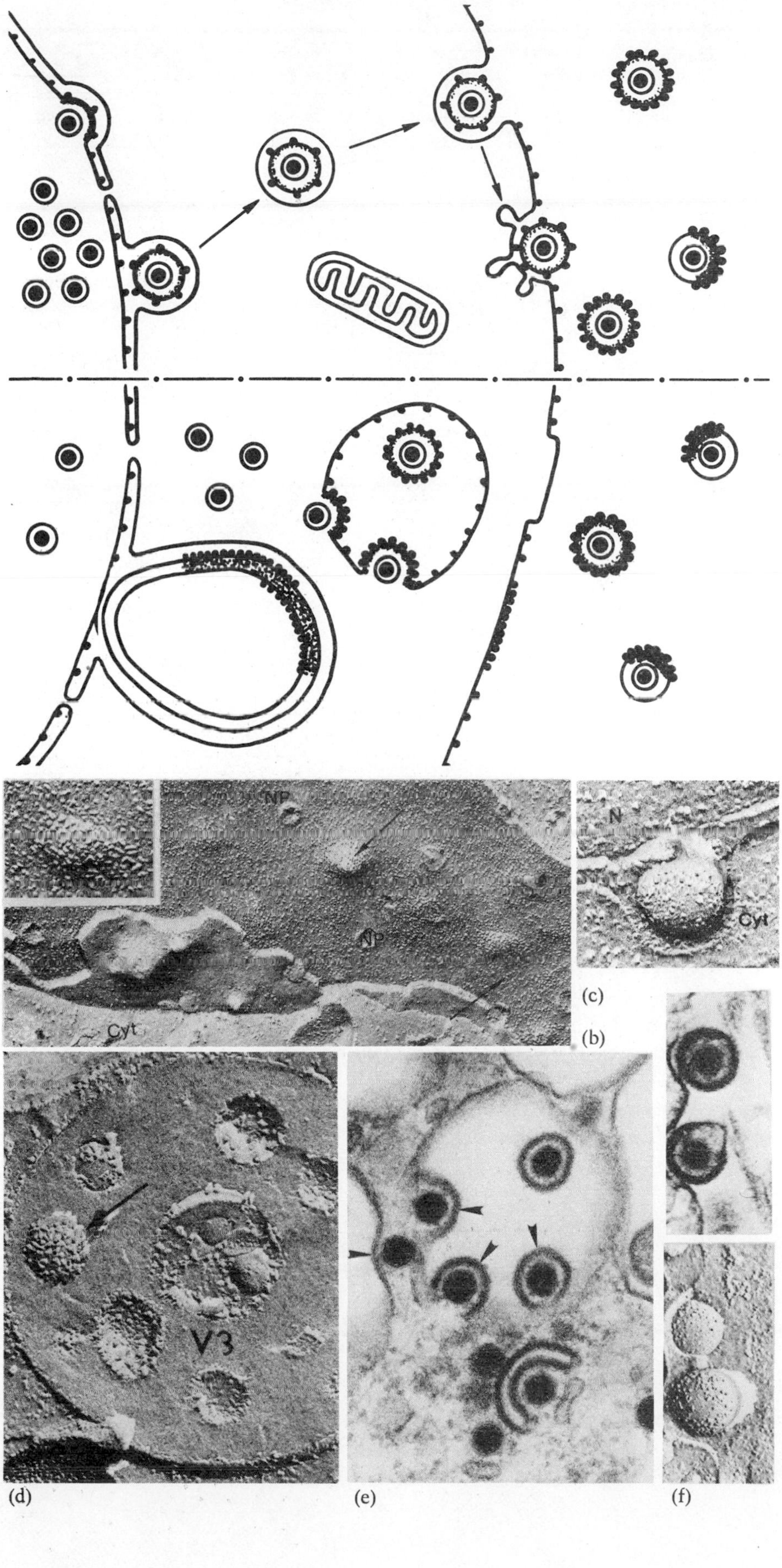

(b)

(c)

(d)

(e)

(f)

FIG. 12-7 The development of an enveloped herpes simplex virion. (a) A diagrammatic summary. In the intranuclear development (upper portion), virus particles are budding through the nuclear membrane (1) or being released into the space directly around the nucleus (2). In both cases they acquire an envelope composed of host membranes. Resulting enveloped viruses travel through the cytoplasm within smooth vacuoles (3). At the cell membrane enveloped virions are released by a process of reverse phagocytosis (4) followed by the folding of the membrane around released virions into vesicles (5). In the lower portion, the major cytoplasmic features are shown, including the virus budding in cytoplasmic vacuoles (6), extracellular viruses with significant amounts of intramembranous particles (7), virus particles with incomplete envelopes (8), and an area in which nuclear membrane and cytoplasmic vacuoles are fused (9). Virus particles developing in area 9 will have more intramembranous particles than those from other cellular sites. *Courtesy of Rodriguez, M., and M. J. Dubois-Dalcq,* Virol. 26:*435–447 (1978).* (b) Virions (arrows) protruding through the nuclear membrane. The inset shows a higher magnification of a virion with intramembranous particles. The nuclear pore (NP) and cytoplasm (Cyt) are shown. (c) A virion budding through the nuclear membrane. The nucleus (N) and cytoplasm (Cyt) are shown. (d) Cytoplasmic virion development (arrows) in a vacuole. (e) Thin slices of virus particles. (f) Two views of virus particles soon after release. Note the close contact between the virions and the presence of envelopes *(b,c,d,e,f) Rodriguez, M., and M. J. Dubois-Dalcq,* Virol. 26:*435–447 (1978).*

TABLE 12-2 Representative Characteristics Used in the Classification of Viruses

Nucleic Acid (NA)	*Double or Single-Stranded*	*Symmetry of Capsid*	*Number of Capsomeres*	*Size of Capsid in Ångstroms*	*Enveloped or Naked*	*Host Range of Viruses*			
						Animal	*Bacterial*	*Insect*	*Plant*
DNA	Single	Helical		50 × 8000	Naked		Coliphage fd		
	Double	Helical		90–100	Enveloped	Poxviruses			
	Single	Polyhedral	12	220	Naked		Coliphage ϕX-174		
	Double	Polyhedral	72	450–550	Naked	Polyoma and Papilloma			
			252	600–900	Naked	Adenoviruses			
			812	1400	Naked			Tipula iridescent virus	
			162	1000	Enveloped	Herpetoviruses			
		Binal (a combination of polyhedral and helical components)		Polyhedral head 950 × 650 Helical tail 170 × 1150	Naked		Coliphages $T_2T_4T_6$		
RNA	Single	Helical		175 × 3000	Naked				Tobacco mosaic virus
				90	Enveloped	Myxoviruses			
				180	Enveloped	Paramyxoviruses			
		Polyhedral		200–250	Naked		Coliphage f_2		
			32	280	Naked	Picornaviruses			Turnip yellow mosaic virus and tomato bushy stunt virus
	Double	Polyhedral	92	700	Naked	Reoviruses			Wound tumor virus

Bacteriophages (Bacterial Viruses)

Almost all of the large group of readily cultivable bacteria serve as hosts for ***bacteriophages,*** or bacterial viruses. The host range of a bacteriophage (also called ***phage***) may involve a single specific bacterial species or several bacterial genera. Viruses have been found to attack several blue-green bacterial species. Their morphological features greatly resemble those of other bacterial viruses (Figure 12–9).

Many bacterial viruses have proved useful in research on the mechanisms of cellular infections. Other phages have been valuable in the identification of bacterial pathogens and epidemiological investigations. For this reason, the bacterial viruses and their cultivation have been intensively studied.

The Basic Structure of Bacteriophages

Bacterial viruses may contain either DNA or RNA. In most DNA phages the nucleic acid is double-stranded, while in RNA bacteriophages the nucleic acid is single-stranded. The nucleic acid of most bacterial viruses (except for one phage group) is in a polyhedral capsid, frequently referred to as the "head" (Figure 12–9b). In many cases this capsid is attached to a helical protein structure called a "tail," which with its additional parts aids the phage in adsorbing onto a susceptible bacterial host (Figure 12–9c).

At the present time, many basic structures have been recognized among bacteriophages, with no particular form of phage being restricted to a specific bacterial genus. Bacteriophages are thought to show greater variation of form than any other viral group. The most common basic morphological types are illustrated in Figure 12–10. A newly discovered helical bacteriophage isolated from mycoplasma is shown in Figure 12–11.

Because most bacteriophage research has been carried out with agents that attack the Gram-negative bacterium *Escherichia coli*, we shall concentrate on this group. In addition, because more is known about the structures involved in the adsorption of bacterial viruses to hosts than is known about other viruses, this topic will also be discussed.

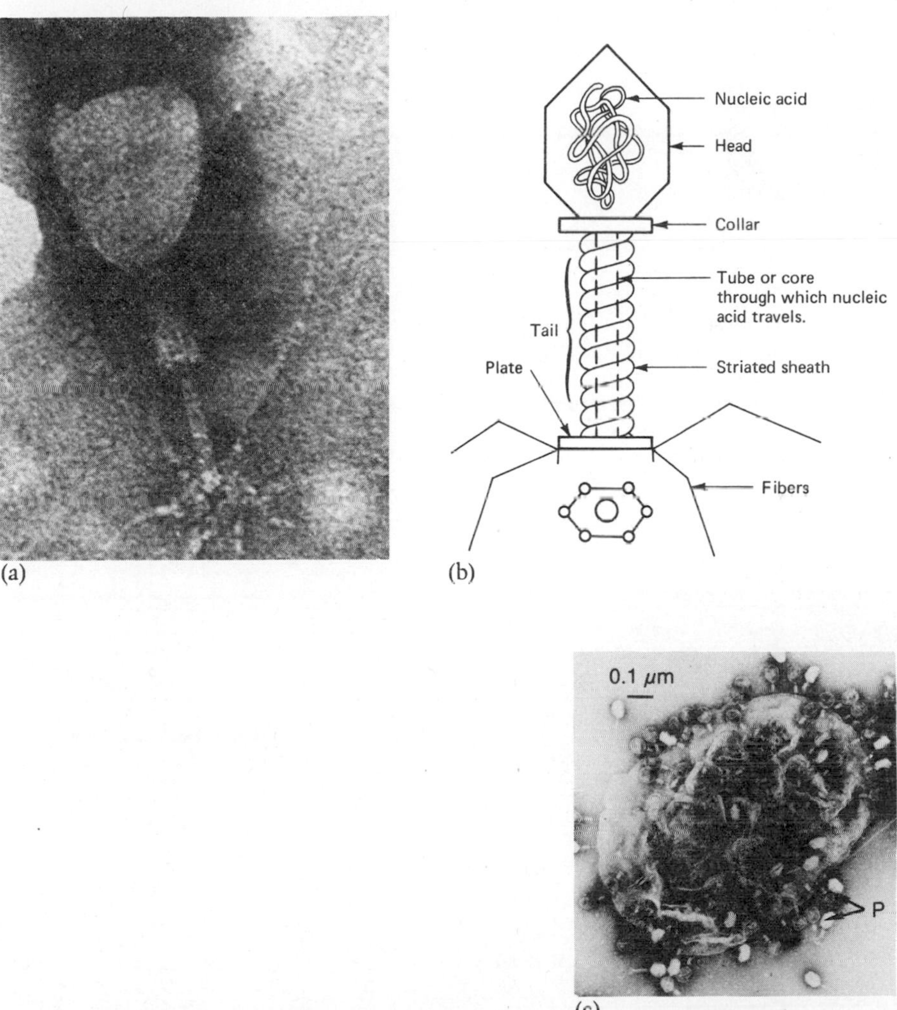

FIG. 12–9 Bacterial viruses. (a) A negatively stained type T_2 bacteriophage. Note the head, the striations in the tail, and the fibers attached to an end plate. *Anderson, T. F., and Stephens, R.*, Virology *23:113–116 (1964).* (b) A diagram showing the various components of a T_2 phage. The plate of this virus is hexagonal and contains a pin at each of its corners, with long, thin tail fibers connected to it. (c) An electron micrograph showing T_{4r} phages normally adsorbing onto *E. coli.* The cell wall of the organism has been severely damaged. This negatively stained preparation clearly shows the attachment of the virus to the bacterium. Note the contracted state of the viral sheaths. Numerous phage heads are clear, while others are opaque. Which ones still have their nucleic acid? *Simon, L. D., et al.*, Virology 41:77 *(1970).*

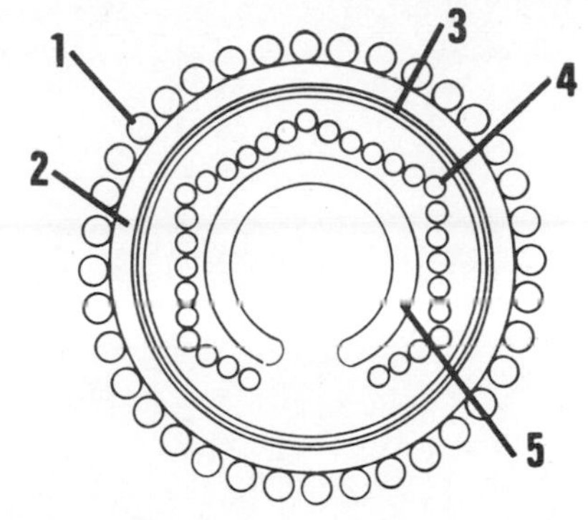

(a)

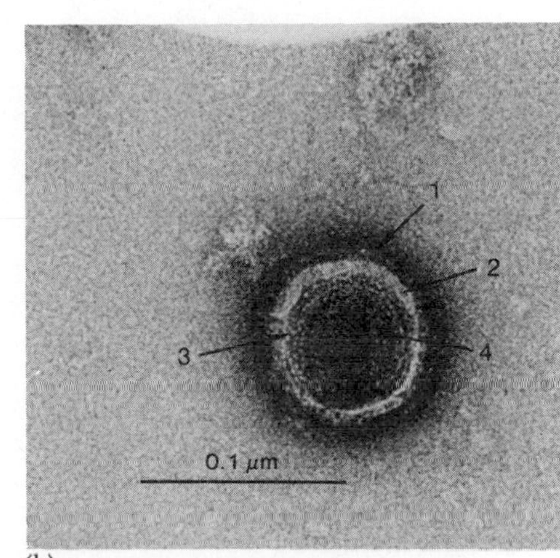

(b)

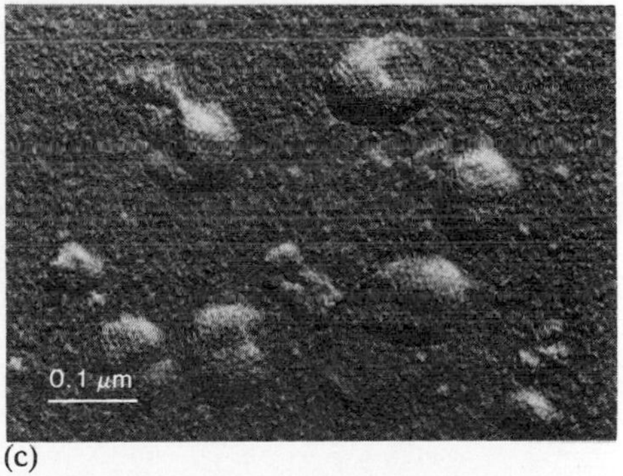

(c)

FIG. 12–8 Virus structure of mouse leukemia virus. (a) A sketch of virus structure and organization showing surface knobs or projections (1), viral membrane (2 and 3), capsid composed of individual capsomeres (4), and the nucleic acid core (5). The knobs and viral membrane form the viral envelope. (b) Negatively stained virions. (c) A shadow-cast preparation showing the surface. *Courtesy Dr. H. Frank, Max-Planck—Institute für Virusforschung.*

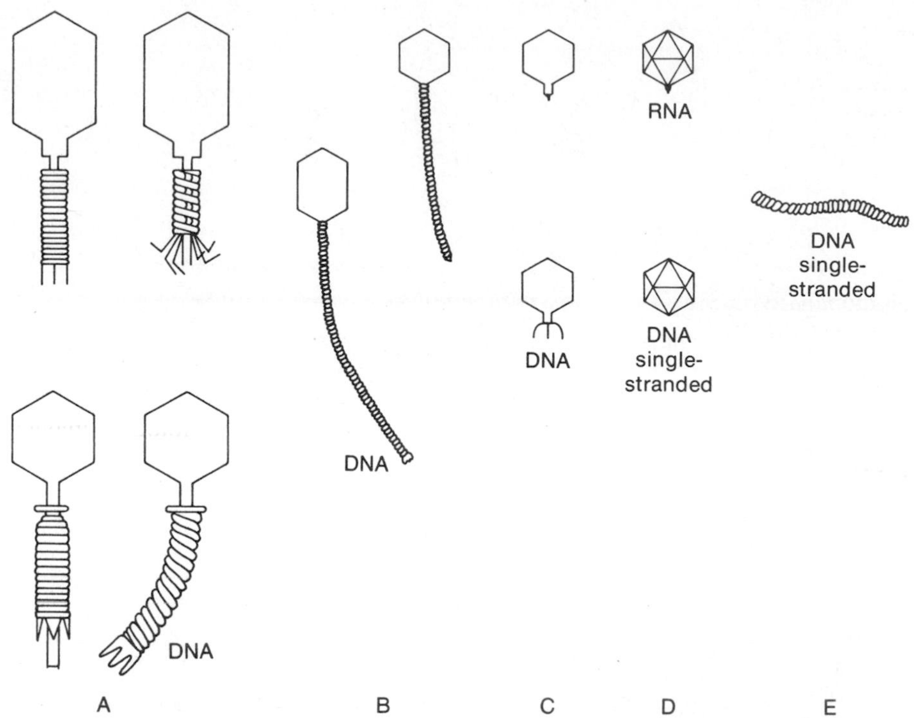

FIG. 12-10 Representative basic morphological features of bacteriophages together with their types of nucleic acid. Note the similarity of virus heads and the differences in the tails. (a, b, and c) Phages with variations in head shapes and tail structures. (d) Tailless heads. (e) A filamentous bacteriophage. *After Bradley, D. E., "A Comparative Study of the Structure and Biological Properties of Bacteriophages," in K. Maramorsch and E. Durstak, eds.,* Comparative Virology. *New York: Academic Press, 1971, pp. 207–253.*

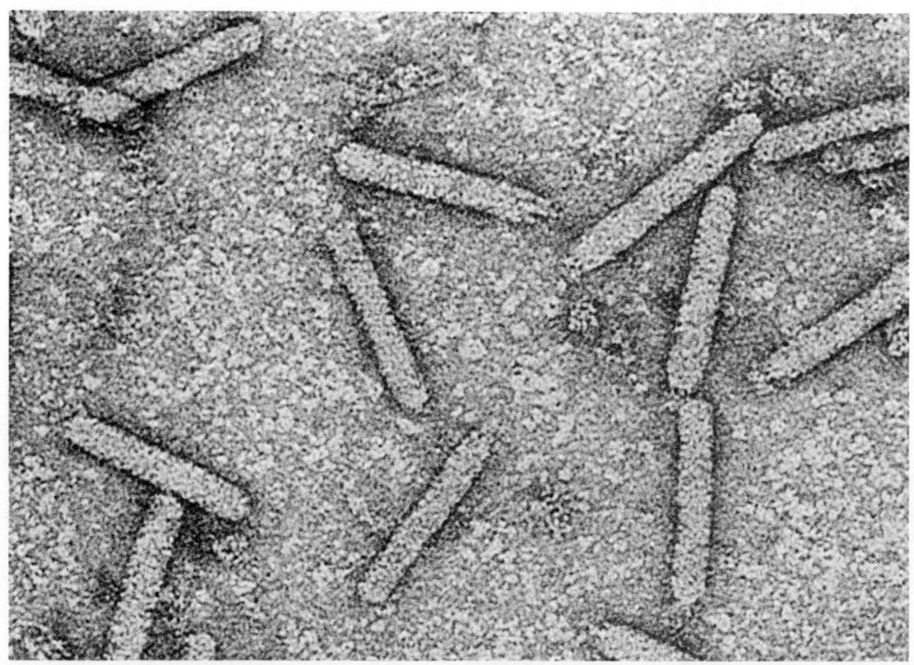

FIG. 12-11 Purified Mycoplasmatales virus, *laidlawii* 2, negatively stained with uranyl acetate. *From Gourlay, P. N.,* J. Gen. Virol. 12:65–67 *(1971).*

Filamentous Bacteriophages

The filamentous viruses, discovered in 1963, are among the smallest viruses known to date. They are the lone exception to the polyhedral form of bacteriophages. Filamentous viruses are long deoxyribonucleoproteins measuring approximately 5.5 nm in diameter. Purified preparations of DNA from these microorganisms have been found to exhibit single-stranded form. Two different lengths have been reported for filamentous viruses: approximately 870 nm and about 1300 nm.

Gram-negative bacteria, including *Escherichia coli, Pseudomonas aeruginosa, Salmonella typhimurium, Vibrio parahemolyticus,* and *Xanthomonas oryzae* are hosts for filamentous viruses. Adsorption of bacterial cells takes place at the ends of threadlike bacterial sex *pili* (Figure 15–6). Recently a binal-shaped, pilus-dependent phage was described (Figure 12–12).

Filamentous viruses have focused attention on a form of symbiotic behavior previously unrecognized in bacteria. Unlike other bacterial viruses, whose mode of replication destroys their respective hosts, filamentous viruses are released from dividing and growing bacteria without any apparent marked injury to the host cells. In short, this is a nonlytic form of viral release. Electron microscopic observations of infected bacteria tend to support the idea of nondestructive filamentous virus infections. Research suggests that filamentous viruses are assembled during their extrusion from the host. This resembles the mode of replication found in certain animal viruses. Some virologists believe that filamentous viruses may serve as excellent models in studies concerning the development and effects of *oncogenic* (cancer-inducing) viral agents.

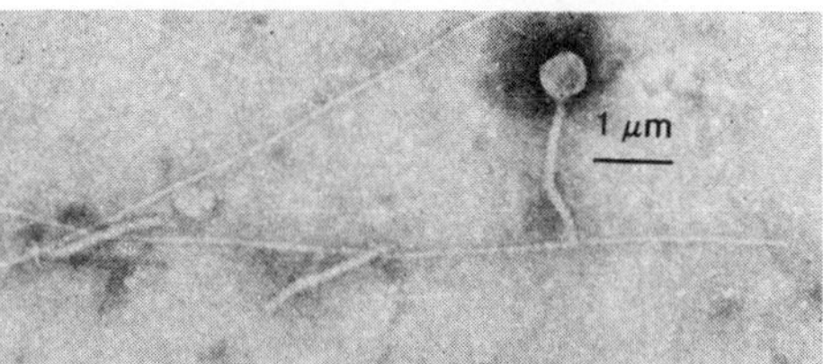

FIG. 12–12 *Pseudomonas aeruginosa* bacteriophage. Note the long tail of the phage and the additional headless tails attached to the pili (P). *Bradley, D. E.,* J. Virol. 12:*1139–1148 (1973).*

The Cultivation of Bacteriophages

In general, the cultivation of bacteriophages is relatively uncomplicated and neither expensive nor very time-consuming. Phages are commonly propagated on appropriate, actively growing young bacterial cells. Either broth or agar cultures are used for this purpose. In liquid cultures, the destruction of enough susceptible bacteria by the replicating viruses will cause the nutrient medium to clear. When agar plates are used, the presence of bacterial viruses is indicated by the development of transparent **plaques** against the dense background of bacterial growth on the medium's surface (Figure 12–13).

Various types of bacterial viruses can be isolated from natural sources such as dairy products, diseased tissues, feces, sewage, soil, and water. In principle, the presence of such viruses and their bacteriolytic action can be demonstrated by a fairly straightforward procedure. Fluid samples of any of the above materials are passed through a filter that retains bacteria but not viruses. The resultant filtrate material is then tested for the presence of phage. This usually involves introducing a small amount, such as 1 milliliter (ml), of the test material into approximately 10 ml of an appropriate fresh culture of a test host organism. Another tube, without the addition of the suspected phage-containing sample, is used as a control. Both tubes are then incubated under optimum environmental conditions. If the tube to which the test material was added (the inoculated tube) shows clearing, or at least less turbidity than the control tube, then the presence of phages in the original sample is indicated.

Unfortunately, the demonstration of bacterial viruses from natural sources is not always in practice so easy as this description suggests. In many studies, more involved procedures are required. Moreover, many samples of natural substances may not yield bacterial viruses.

Once a new phage is found, its characterization is usually undertaken. This

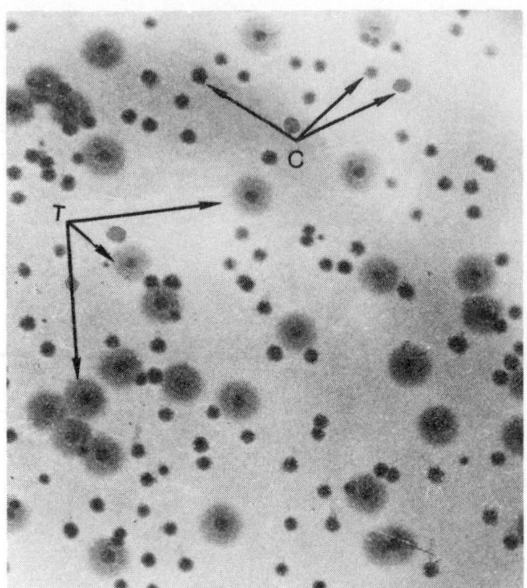

FIG. 12-13 The appearance of plaques produced by a mixture of bacteriophages. Smaller, sharp-edged, clear plaques (C), produced by one type of lytic virus, can be distinguished from the larger turbid (T) ones produced by others. Plaque appearance can be used in classification. *Courtesy of Follansbee, S. E., et al.,* Virology *58:180–198 (1974).*

involves determining its chemical and physical properties, uncovering its mechanism of action, and demonstrating its basic differences from and similarities to other bacterial viruses.

Enumeration of Phages

Several methods can be used to estimate the number of virus particles in a sample accurately. One of the most useful and most commonly employed procedures is the plaque count assay, which is simple and accurate and yields highly reproducible results. It was originally introduced by F. D'Herelle, a French Canadian who coined the term ***bacteriophage*** from the Greek word ***phagein***, meaning "to eat."

The phage suspension to be assayed is added to a tube containing 2.0 ml of melted soft agar kept at 45°C. One drop of an appropriate fresh bacterial culture is also introduced. The contents of the tube are mixed and quickly poured onto the surface of a dried, hard agar layer contained in a Petri dish. This plate is rocked gently back and forth to distribute both the bacteria and the phage mixture evenly over the agar surface before the soft agar hardens. Viral particles diffuse through the medium, infect, multiply, and lyse susceptible bacteria, leaving plaques on the agar. Those bacterial cells not infected grow, multiply, and form a cloudy, or turbid, layer over the hard agar surface. The number of viral particles in the original sample is determined by the number of plaques multiplied by the dilution factor, the reciprocal of the dilution. This product is expressed as the number of plaque-forming units (PFU) per milliliter of the initial sample.

The quantitative determination of virus particles contained in a particular specimen can also be made by electron microscopy.

Phage Typing

Bacterial viruses continually propagated in a specific bacterial species can become adapted to that particular bacterial host. Such viruses exhibit the phenomenon called ***host-controlled modification***. They will primarily infect and lyse a specific bacterial species or cells of associated strains. This adaptation is the basis for ***phage typing*** (Color Photograph 77), used to identify strains within certain bacterial species such as *Salmonella typhi* and *Staphylococcus aureus*. This is an extremely important procedure in tracing the sources of epidemics and distinguishing between pathogenic bacterial strains that cannot be differentiated by other means.

Phage typing is performed by growing the unknown bacterial culture—isolated from a patient, for example—on an agar plate. Known phages are systematically spotted onto the "lawn" of bacteria. After a suitable incubation period, zones of lysis appear if the appropriate phage is present. From the phage or phages that produce plaques, the bacterial host can be identified. Plastic plates with grid patterns embossed on their bottom surfaces (Figure 12–14) are available to simplify the procedure.

FIG. 12-14 An 'Integrid' Petri plate, an example of a Petri dish that can be used to systematically conduct phage-typing procedures. The grids are used to locate a particular phage or host. *Courtesy of Falcon Plastics, Division of BioQuest, Los Angeles.*

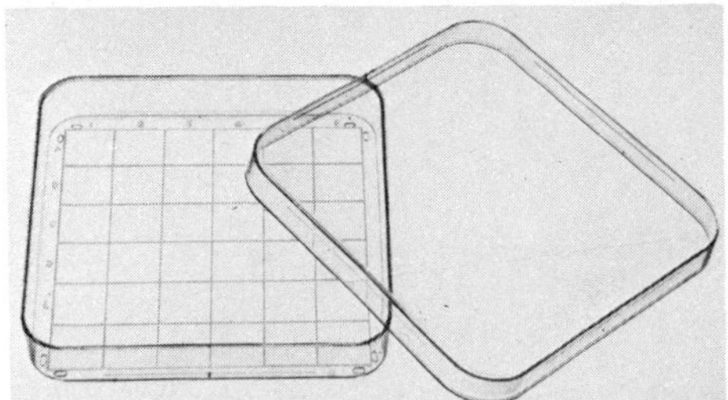

Replication Cycle of Bacteriophages

Phages that regularly infect, replicate, and complete their life cycles in bacterial hosts and that ultimately cause the destruction of bacterial cells are called *virulent* or *lytic* viruses. Not all infections of bacteria proceed in this manner for some viruses establish an entirely different relationship with a host cell. These viruses may replicate and bring about the host cell destruction, or their DNA may be incorporated into that of the host (host DNA) so that it is passed on to succeeding generations of the host cell. Such viruses are said to be *temperate,* and their integrated form is referred to as a *prophage.* A bacterial cell containing a prophage is **lysogenic.**

Lysogeny

When a temperate bacteriophage infects a host cell, two possibilities exist. The lytic cycle characteristic of virulent viruses may occur, or the cell, once infected, may harbor the virus in a noninfectious state as a *prophage.* During the prophage phase, the host cell may undergo significant changes in colonial morphology, antigenicity, and toxin production (Figure 12–15). These effects, called *lysogenic* or *viral conversion,* are discussed in Chapter 15.

Occasionally, a prophage can be activated to undergo a lytic cycle. Exposure of a lysogenic culture to ultraviolet light increases the rate of such prophage activation significantly. This is one means of determining if a given culture is lysogenic. The interrelationship of lytic and temperate viral cycles is represented in Figure 12–16. Lytic and temperate viral activities can usually be differentiated on the basis of the appearance of plaques that develop when bacterial hosts are plated. When relatively few viruses are mixed with many sensitive bacteria and placed on the surface of solid media, the plaques that develop after a suitable incubation period (Figure 12–13) will be clear for a lytic virus and turbid for a temperate one.

The clear plaque represents virulent viral activity in all infected cells, resulting in the death and subsequent lysis of such cells. In the turbid plaque, only some of the infected bacteria have undergone a lytic cycle and the surviving bacterial cells can and will reproduce, unaffected by the virus under the existing conditions.

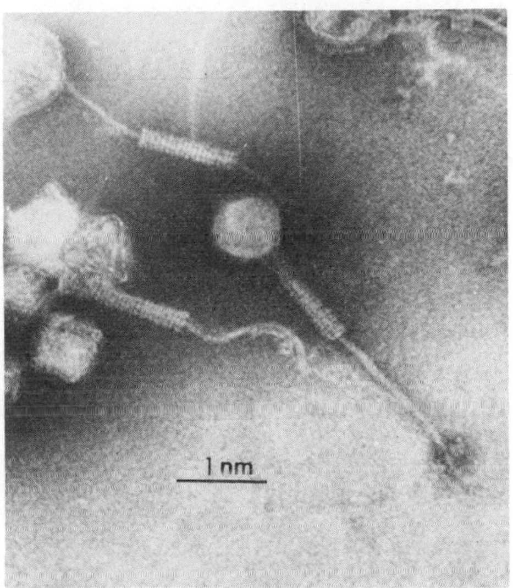

FIG. 12–15 An electron micrograph of *Clostridium botulinum* type $1D^{tox+}$ bacteriophage. This virus has recently been shown to influence the host bacterium's production of botulism toxin. *Eklund, M. W., and F. I. Poysky,* Appl. Microbiol. *27:251–258 (1974).*

During the lysogenic cycle, the occasional bursting of cells liberates free viruses into the general culture containing lysogenic bacteria. Even though additional viruses may be adsorbed and infection occasionally occurs with some bacteria in such lysogenic cultures, a lytic cycle usually cannot occur. Bacteria harboring a virus as a prophage, that is, lysogenic bacteria, are immune to infection by other phages of the same or similar type.

Another form of bacterial cell immunity occurs when a mutation alters the chemistry or structure of a receptor site in such a way as to prevent further viral adsorption. This phenomenon is called *resistance.*

The Lytic Cycle

The lytic cycle has been studied extensively in certain phages for which *Escherichia coli* and other bacteria were the hosts. Details of the structural and molecular properties of these viruses, designated T_2, T_4, and T_6 (or collectively, T even), are well enough known to allow construction of a general model of the processes of phage infection and host cell destruction. The steps in such a T-even cycle (Figure 12–16) include *adsorption, penetration, replication* of new viral DNA, *maturation,* and release of mature viruses (Figure 12–17).

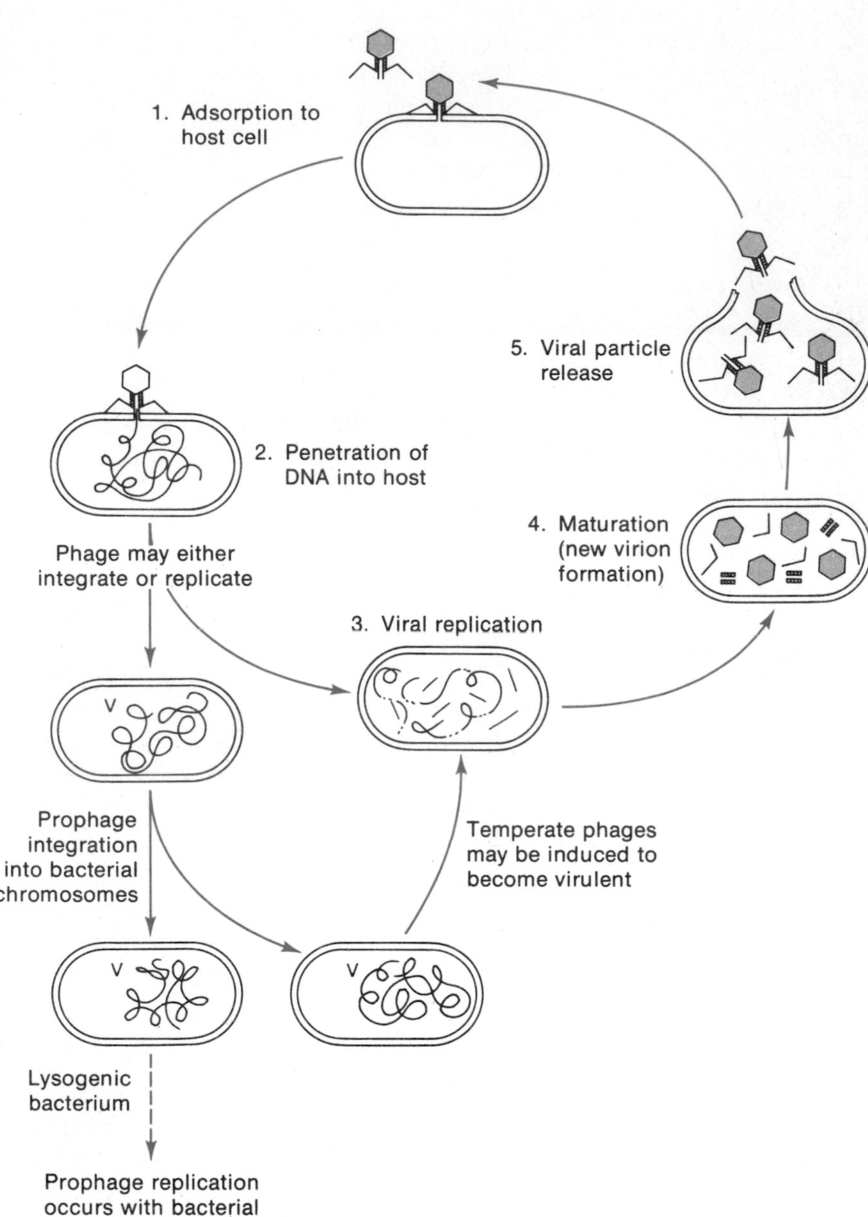

FIG. 12-16 Replication cycle of a temperate bacteriophage. The lysogenic portion of the cycle is shown on the lower left. The virulent, or lytic, segment is on the right. The viral DNA is represented by V.

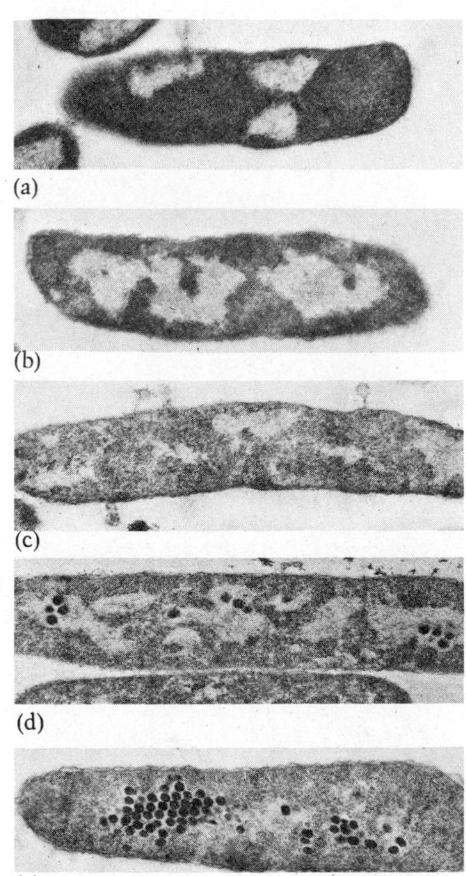

FIG. 12-17 The intracellular development of virus T_2 in *Escherichia coli.* (a) Time of infection shows *E. coli* with normal DNA (light areas). Adsorbed viruses are not evident. (b) Two minutes after infection. The appearance of the DNA has changed. (c) Ten minutes after infection. DNA has become more diffuse. Empty viral heads are evident on cell wall. (d) Twelve minutes after infection. First phages appear. (e) Thirty minutes after infection. Cell is nearly ready to burst. *Jacob, F., and E. L. Wollman, 'Viruses and Genes,'* Sci. Amer. *204:93 (June 1961). Micrographs by E. Kellenberger and A. Ryter.*

ADSORPTION AND PENETRATION

Adsorption is a specific event, since only certain viruses are able to infect particular bacterial host cells. The phage tail fibers (Figure 12-9b) function as *adsorption* sites that bind to specific *receptor* sites on the host bacterium's cell wall.

Once the bacteriophage has attached, an enzyme, *lysozyme,* is released from within the phage tail and digests a small portion of the host's cell wall. Following this step, the virus's tail sheath contracts, and the tail core, or central tube, mechanically penetrates the cell wall, preparing the way for a viral DNA injection. The phage DNA, located in the head component, is introduced from the open tip of the tail through the bacterial cell wall, across the cell membrane and into the host cell's interior. The exact mechanism of this injection process is unknown.

For phages of the T-even viruses, the protein capsid remains outside the host. For filamentous, single-stranded DNA phages, the capsid enters the host. Although a small amount of cytoplasmic leakage can occur after perforation of the cell wall, the bacterial host does not appear to experience any great difficulty. If, however, the ratio of virus particles to bacterial cells, the ***multiplicity of infection***, is great, sufficient injury to the cell wall results to cause lysis. This phenomenon is generally called *lysis from without*, to differentiate it from lysis that would normally occur upon release of viruses at the end of the lytic cycle.

VIRAL NUCLEIC ACID REPLICATION

Following the injection of phage DNA, there is an ***eclipse***, or latent period, during which no whole infective viruses can be observed (Figure 12–28). Once infection begins, the cellular synthesis of the host's own nucleic acids and protein ceases. Certain components of the host cell, such as ribosomes and enzymes, still function, but they are utilized for the replication of viral components. During this period, a portion of the viral DNA, upon reaching the host's cytoplasmic region, is immediately used for the formation of "early" viral messenger RNA (vmRNA). This nucleic acid contains the necessary information for the formation of viral proteins. The information of the newly formed vmRNA is translated by the host's ribosomes, resulting in the synthesis of specific viral enzymes, including those necessary for phage nucleic acid replication, protein capsid formation, and virus particle assembly.

MATURATION

During viral maturation, viral DNA is used to form other essential viral components, including the capsomeres of the capsid. As these capsid subunits accumulate, viral DNA molecules combine with a specific protein and become tightly packed into polyhedral units. The capsomeres crystallize on the surfaces of the polyhedrons to form mature bacteriophage heads. By continuing activity, the remaining subunits of the viruses are synthesized and assembled into complete ***virions***. The stepwise assembly process is controlled by certain viral genes described as ***morphopoietic*** (from the Greek *morphe*, meaning "form," and *poiein*, meaning "to make").

LIBERATION OF VIRUS PARTICLES

As in other phases of the lytic cycle, the liberation process differs among bacteriophages, but basically it includes the following sequence of events. As the maturation period of virus particles comes to an end, another viral protein product appears and steadily increases in concentration. This substance, known as ***bacteriophage lysozyme***, disrupts the chemical bonds holding together the components of the cell wall's rigid layer. The wall becomes progressively thinner. Eventually it ruptures from an osmotic pressure imbalance that causes water to flow into the cell from the surroundings *(plasmoptysis)*. The virus particles and remaining contents of the cell are thus released into the immediate environment. The lytic cycle is complete, and infectious viruses are once more available to begin the cycle.

Growth Curve

From events of the lytic bacteriophage cycle, it is possible to experimentally obtain a growth curve for bacterial viruses. This type of experiment is used to

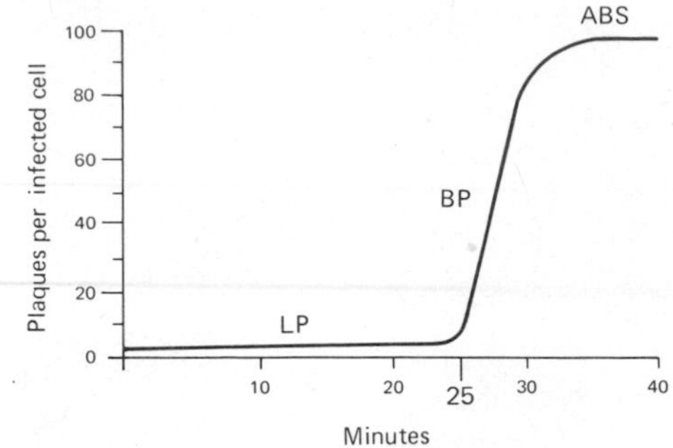

FIG. 12-18 A typical one-step viral growth curve. This representation shows the length of the latent period (LP), burst period (BP), and average burst size (ABS).

determine the time lapse between injection and the release of mature virus particles and to estimate the approximate number of these agents produced per cell, called the *burst size*. This *one-step growth curve* experiment shows how viral development differs from the growth cycle in cellular systems.

In this procedure, a virus suspension is added to bacteria at a low multiplicity of approximately 0.1 to 0.01 (one viral particle for each 10 to 100 bacterial cells). The low multiplicity of infection is needed to reduce the chance of several viruses infecting a single bacterium and producing abnormal results. After a short period of incubation to allow adsorption, nonadsorbed viruses are removed. Thus, the opportunity for subsequent infection of additional bacteria is substantially reduced, but so, too, is the possibility of more than one virus attacking a bacterium. Next the bacterial suspension is diluted to a desired concentration in fresh media. Samples are removed periodically and the number of free virus particles and infected bacteria is determined by plaque count. The virus-containing samples are mixed with a suspension of sensitive bacteria. The number of plaques produced by each sample is plotted and results in the formation of a curve such as the one shown in Figure 12–18.

The plaque count usually remains constant for a period of time. This phase of the growth curve is referred to as the *latent stage*, or *period*. The designation is misleading in the sense that significant viral activity is going on even though the plaque count does not indicate it. The lysis of infected bacteria and the subsequent release of viral particles are evidenced by an abrupt increase in plaque number. This stage, called the *burst period*, continues until all infected cells have lysed. Again, the plaque count reaches a more or less constant level, even if uninfected bacteria are present. In the diluted bacterial suspension, used cells are so widely separated that newly liberated phages cannot spread to uninfected bacteria. By knowing the number of infected bacteria at time zero, the number of plaques obtained at various intervals can be calculated in terms of PFU (plaque-forming units) per infected cell by dividing the number of plaques present after the burst period by the number present before. In Figure 12–18, the burst size was found to be 100 PFU. This is comparable to the burst size that would be found with virus T_2 shown in Figure 12–17e.

Cyanophages

In 1963, R. S. Safferman and M. E. Morris discovered a virus that attacks and lyses several species of blue-green bacteria. These viruses are the **cyanophages** now known to be present in nearly all bodies of fresh water.

Several of the cyanophages isolated thus far have been given names that correspond to their hosts. Phage groups have been designated by the initials of the generic names of the hosts, to which Arabic numerals are added to signify specific subgroups. For example, LPP phages attack three different filamentous blue-green bacterial genera, *Lyngbya, Phormidium,* and *Plectonema* (Figure 12–19a). Because using host specificity as a criterion for classification poses some problems, morphological properties and antigenic specificities are preferred for classification of cyanophages.

Cyanophages are very similar to other bacterial viruses both in structure (Figures 12–19b and c) and in infection cycle. LPP phages, one of the most extensively studied cyanophages, have virions of the head-tail type. All the nucleic acids of these viruses isolated to date are found to be linear, double-stranded DNAs.

The hosts of cyanophages, the blue-green bacteria, are widespread in the aquatic environment and often occur in great numbers in the form of blue-green bacterial or algal blooms (Color Photograph 4a), which sometimes result in fish poisonings. The discovery of cyanophages has led several investigators to consider these viruses as possible agents for the biological control of algal blooms.

Cyanophage Cultivation and Enumeration

Techniques for the cultivation and enumeration of cyanophages have been developed. The conditions, media, and procedures used for the preparation of suitable hosts (and subsequently for cyanophages) differ significantly from those used for bacteriophages. For example, most bacterial hosts and phages are stable from pH 5 to 8, whereas many blue-green algae and cyanophages are stable within the range of pH 7 to 11. As in bacteriophage culture, evidence of infection is provided by plaque formation, or electron microscopy may be used. Many of the studies involving cyanophages are complicated by the fact that their hosts are filamentous.

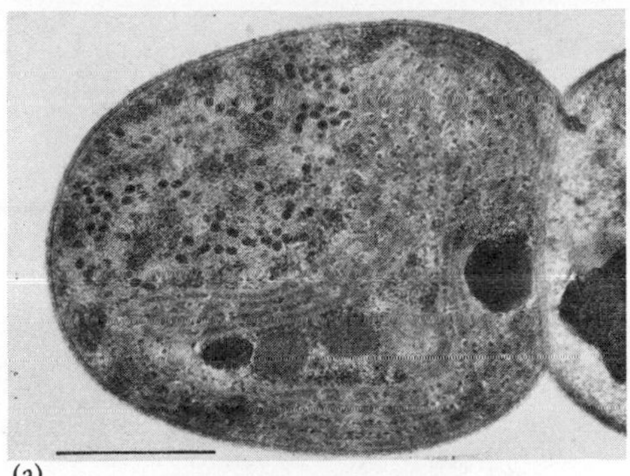

(a)

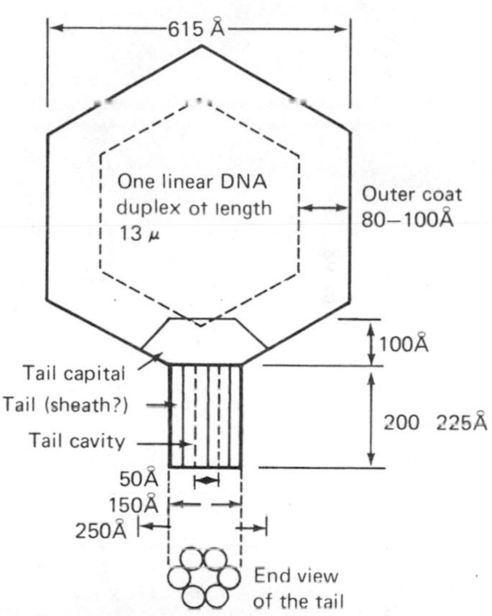

(b)

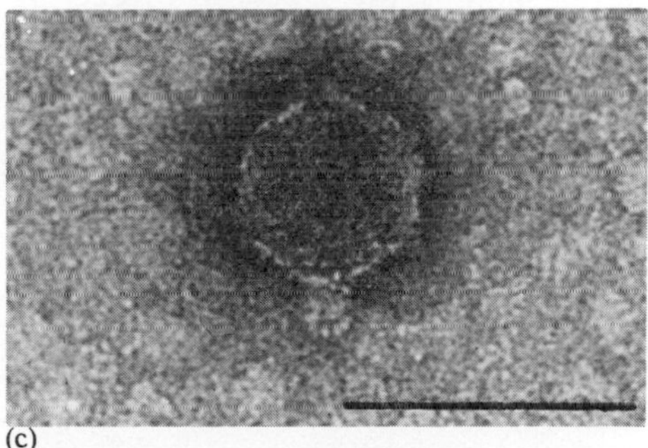

(c)

FIG. 12–19 The cyanophages. (a) The blue-green bacterium *Plectonema* infected with LPP-1G cyanophage. Note the photosynthetic lamellae (layers) and the numerous viral heads. (b) A model of the LPP-1 cyanophage. (c) A mature virus particle. *Courtesy of Paden, E., and M. Shilo,* Bact. Revs. 37:*343–370 (1973).*

Animal Viruses

Disease

Many human diseases now recognized as caused by viruses, such as smallpox (Figure 12–20a) and yellow fever, have been known for centuries. Several additional major illnesses of humans and other animals are also viral in nature (Table 12–3). These include canine distemper, chickenpox (Figure 12–20b), foot-and-mouth disease, influenza, measles, mumps, poliomyelitis, rabies, and various types of encephalitis. In 1911, P. Rous discovered the ability of viruses to produce malignant tumors (Rous sarcoma) in chickens. This finding was the first of many to recognize the viral nature of such tumors in both animals (Figure 12–21) and plants. The effects of animal viral agents can range from the production of mild skin rashes and upper respiratory symptoms to tissue destruction and death. Several of the later chapters discuss the various viral infections.

It has been found that many insects are attacked by viruses (Figure 12–22). A wide variety of such diseases are known. Some are of economic importance, as they involve insects such as honeybees and silkworms. Still other viruses attack pests and consequently may be of value as control devices.

In many insects, viral infections cause the formation of specific intracellular protein products or inclusions. These inclusions may be either granular or polyhedral (Figure 12–22b). Diseases associated with them are referred to as ***granuloses*** or ***polyhedroses***, respectively. A polyhedral inclusion may be formed in either the cytoplasmic or nuclear region of the cells of infected animals. Granular inclusions, which may be either capsules or oval grains of protein, are generally found in the cytoplasm.

Animal Virus Replication

Studies on the replication of animal and plant viruses, although less extensive than those on bacterial viruses, are sufficient to show that the sequence of events in replication is similar for all viruses. Animal virions attach to specific chemical receptor sites on the host cell (Figure 12–23). The projections of envel-

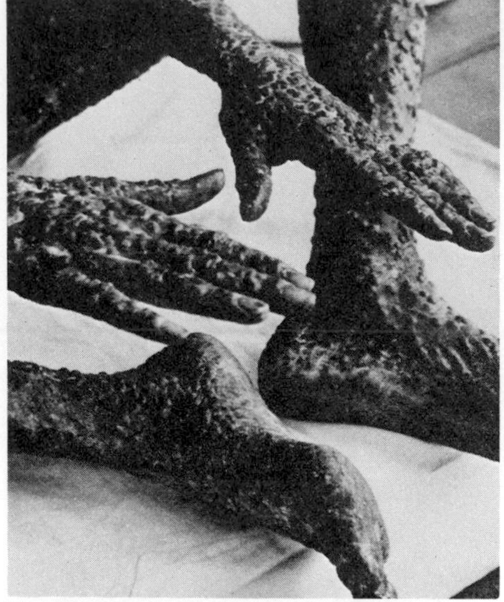

(a)

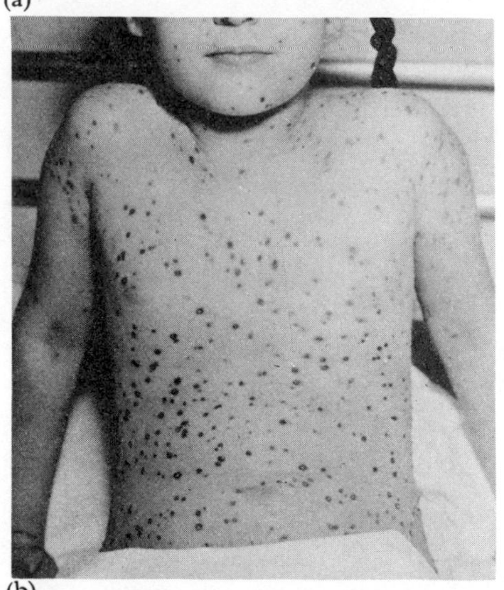

(b)

FIG. 12-20 Human viral diseases. (a) Confluent smallpox. "Confluent" refers to situations in which pocks are extremely close together. *Photo Government Ivoirien, courtesy of the World Health Organization.* (b) A typical case of chickenpox. *Courtesy of the Armed Forces Institute of Pathology, Washington, D.C., Neg. No. AMH-10529E.*

TABLE 12-3 Properties of Major Animal Virus Groups

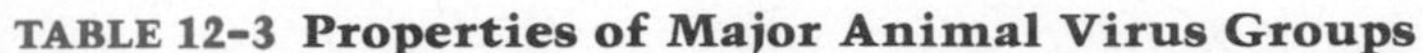

Virus Group[a]	*Type of Nucleic Acid*	*Single- or Double-Stranded*	*Enveloped*	*General Properties*
Adenovirus	DNA	Double	No	Found in several animal species, including humans; associated with respiratory infections and with tumors in laboratory animals
Herpetovirus	DNA	Double	Yes	Important causative agents of human disease such as chickenpox, infectious mononucleosis, and infections of the skin and mucous membranes
Papovavirus	DNA	Double	No	Causes warts; used in the study of tumor development
Parvovirus	DNA	Single	No	Satellite viruses that are incapable of replication except in presence of a helper virus
Poxvirus	DNA	Double	No	Found in several animal species, including humans; examples of infections include smallpox and molluscum contagiosum; all viruses affect the skin
Arenavirus	RNA	Single	Yes	Particles contain cellular ribosomes; viruses cause natural inapparent infections of rodents
Bunyavirus	RNA	Single	Yes	Viruses are spread by a variety of arthropods (arboviruses)
Coronavirus	RNA	Single	No	Includes several agents of the common cold
Orthromyxovirus	RNA	Single	Yes	Includes the influenza viruses
Paramyxovirus	RNA	Single	Yes	Many produce human childhood diseases such as measles and mumps and localized respiratory infections
Picornavirus	RNA	Single	No	Includes several agents of diseases such as poliomyelitis, rashes, meningitis, and mild upper respiratory infections
Reovirus	RNA	Double	No	All are spread by arthropods; many have yet to be associated with specific diseases
Retrovirus	RNA	Single	No	Group includes tumor- and cancer-causing agents
Rhabdovirus	RNA	Single	Yes	Group includes large bullet-shaped viruses such as the agents for rabies and vesicular stomatitis
Togavirus	RNA	Single	Yes	Arthropod-spread diseases, including yellow fever and several nervous system diseases

[a]Several new viruses, as well as some unclassified viruses, may require the formation of new groups.

oped virions serve as attachment devices. These microorganisms are carried inside the host cell by phagocytosis or pinocytosis. Once inside the cell, the virus remains in a phagocytic vacuole or similar structure for a short period of time. During this time, a variety of mechanisms come into action. The viral envelope and the capsid are removed from the nucleic acid, a process called *uncoating*. Replication of viral nucleic acid and synthesis of other viral components follow. The entire process is like an assembly line, in which various parts of the virus are made separately and then efficiently assembled into complete virions in the maturation stage.

Replication of enveloped viruses requires the active participation of the host cell. Before replication occurs, the viral nucleic acid is surrounded by a protein capsid, which in turn is enclosed by the host cell membrane (the envelope). In certain cases the envelopment occurs through a budding process (Figure 12–7a). When envelopment is complete, the newly formed viral particles are released, a process that may continue for hours or even days. The method of release varies according to the virus involved. Host cell death may or may not occur with viral release.

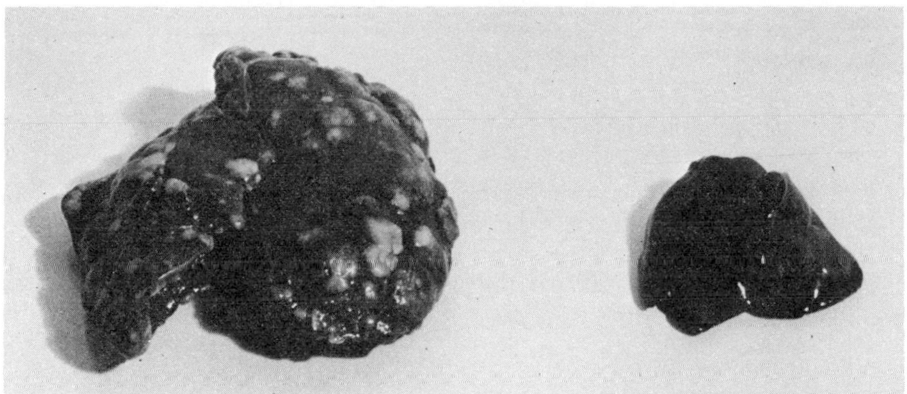

FIG. 12–21 The effects of tumor-causing viruses (Rous sarcoma). A greatly enlarged diseased liver (left) shows many tumorous growths. The liver on the right is from an unaffected chicken of the same age. *U.S.D.A. photograph by Madeleine Osborne.*

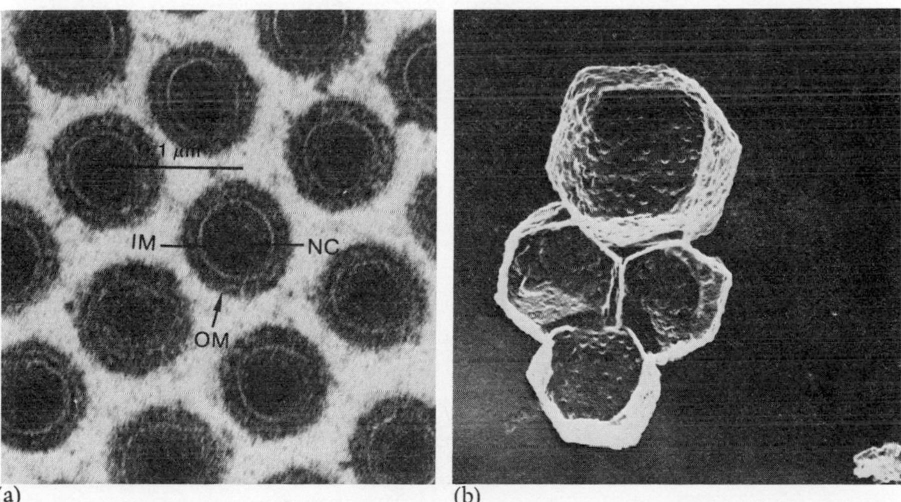

FIG. 12–22 Insect viruses. (a) Viruslike particles in the salivary gland of the tsetse fly. Note the nucleocapsid (NC) and surrounding inner membrane (IM) and outer membrane (OM). *Jaenson, T. G. T.,* trans. Roy. Soc. Trop. Med. Hyg. 72:*234–238 (1978).* (b) An electron micrograph of a cytoplasmic polyhedrosis virus. Spherical viral particles can be seen in the polyhedra shown. *Courtesy of Dr. R. Markham, Agricultural Research Council, Cambridge, England.*

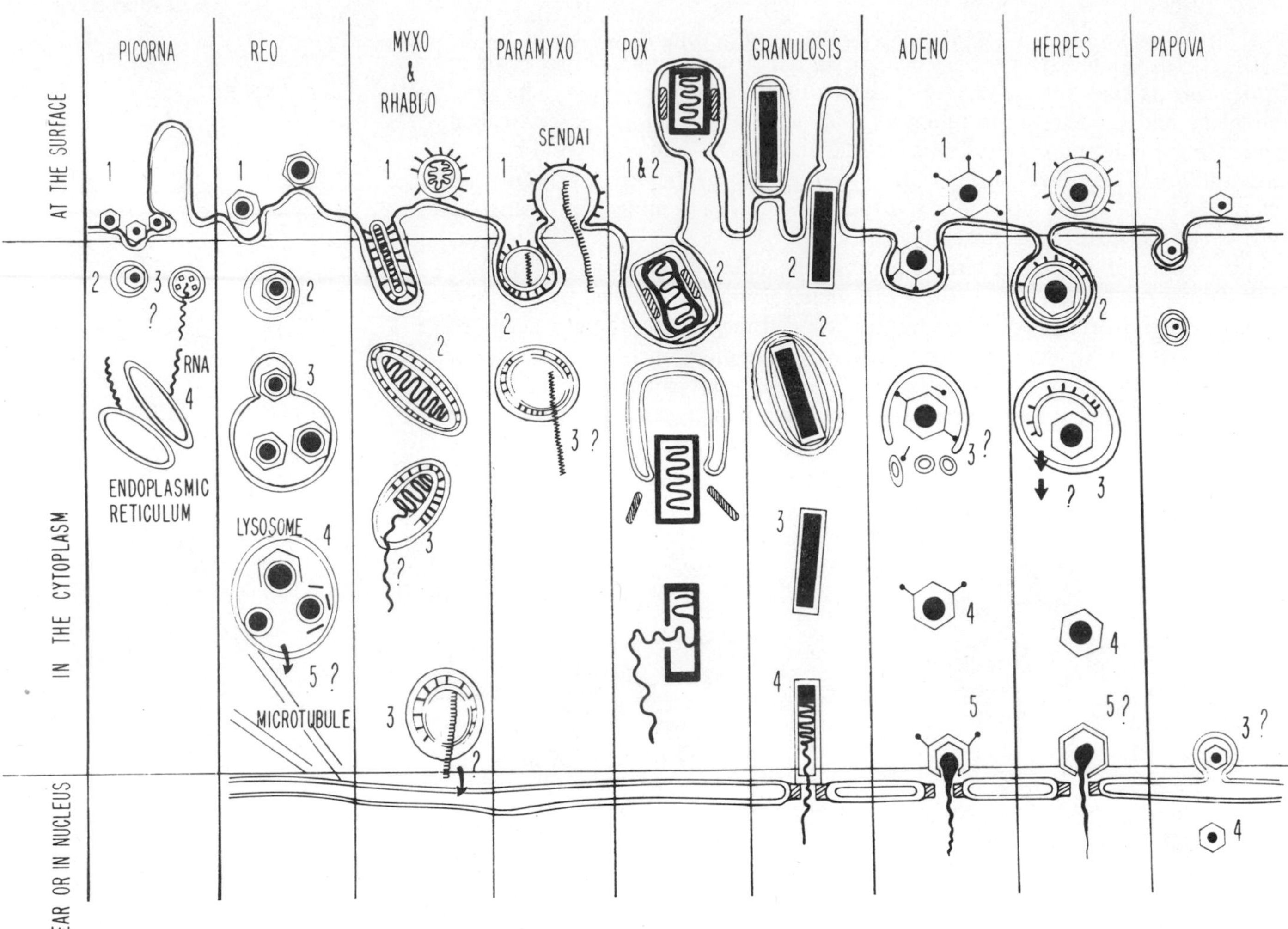

FIG. 12–23 Selected early aspects of animal virus replication in several viruses, including the processes of attachment (1), penetration (2), and uncoating (3, 4, and 5). Before the formation of different parts of new viruses can take place, the removal of the nucleic acid of the infecting virus from its capsid must occur. In some cases this uncoating begins in the phagocytic or pinocytic vesicle and ends in the host cell's cytoplasm. Certain viruses actually penetrate in the cell's nuclear region. *Dales, S.,* Bacteriol. Revs. *37:103 (1973).*

Animal Virus Cultivation

The early attempts to grow animal viruses were performed in susceptible animals. These included rhesus and other species of monkeys, hamsters, mice, and rats. Although these efforts were quite successful, other means had to be found to meet the needs of viruses and yet keep laboratory expenses within working limits. We will now describe some current procedures for cultivating animal viruses.

EMBRYONATED EGGS

The introduction of ***embryonated eggs*** as a suitable medium for the growth of viruses provided an invaluable means of obtaining large quantities of viruses for the preparation of vaccines and diagnostic reagents, as well as for viral studies.

There are many advantages of using embryonated eggs: their availability in virtually unlimited quantities; the relative ease of handling them; the presence of a naturally constant environment within the confines of the egg's components (the embryo as it ordinarily comes from the hen is sterile); the general inability of the embryo to produce antibodies against the viruses used as **inocula;** and the availability of eggs with a relatively uniform genetic constitution from flocks that have been imbred for several generations.

The embryonated eggs used for virus cultivation are fertilized chicken eggs that have undergone a normal embryonic development in the hen. Usually they are put into an incubator shortly after laying so that development can continue to the desired age, which might be 6 or 8 days.

Embryonated eggs used for the cultivation of viruses are usually *candled* first (Figure 12–24) to determine if the embryo is alive and to locate the blood vessels and other parts of the animal. Living embryos usually make spontaneous jerking movements (probably in response to the intensity of the strong light) and show well-developed, translucent, floating blood vessels. Dead embryos are immobile, their blood vessels barely visible.

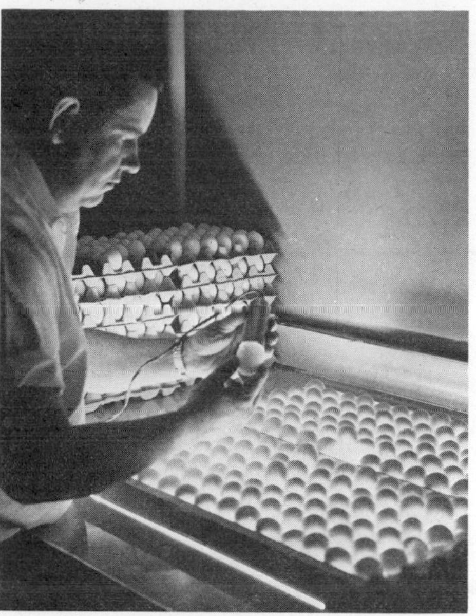

FIG. 12–24 The candling process. Eggs are incubated at 37°C until the embryos are 9 days old. They are then removed and checked for fertility and normal development, determined by subjecting them to a concentrated source of light and noting the shadow cast on their shell. Suitable eggs are inoculated. *Courtesy of Chas. Pfizer & Company, Inc., N.Y.*

Before inoculation of the chick embryo, the surface of the eggshell to be used is sterilized with an iodine solution. This may be followed by wiping with an alcohol solution (Figure 12–25). Surgical instruments and drills for boring into the shell are sterilized by standard methods such as autoclaving, and normal sterile precautions are observed in the working area. In addition, the inocula usually contain antibiotics to guard against bacterial and fungal contamination.

Several portions of the embryonated egg are used for viral cultivation, including the allantoic and amniotic cavities, the yolk sac, the chorioallantoic membrane (Figure 12–26), and the embryo itself. The particular region used depends on the virus to be cultured, as certain viral agents are capable of proliferating only in some parts of the embryo. Mumps and Newcastle disease viruses, for example, replicate particularly well in the allantoic cavity.

SIGNS OF VIRUS INFECTION

Besides being used to produce large numbers of viruses, embryo inoculation techniques are also used for studying the morphological features of viruses, isolating viruses from specimens, determining the effectiveness of drugs on viruses (chemotherapy), investigating the mechanism of viral infection, and providing viral infection.

Virus infection in chick embryos may appear in several ways. Certain viral agents produce local lesions called *pocks* that vary in size, shape, and opacity (Color Photographs 53a and 53b). However, it is difficult to identify a particular agent on the basis of this effect alone. Additional signs of infection are the death of the embryo and the demonstration of a blood clumping reaction, or **hemagglutination,** associated with the allantoic or amniotic fluid. Virus infection can sometimes be shown by detection of the virus or related agents by light or electron microscopy. However, it is also possible that there will be *no* obvious signs of viral infection.

Tissue Culture Cultivation of Viruses

Although the technique of tissue culture is almost as old as the study of viruses, early virologists could not use this technique because of problems of contamination by bacteria and fungi. It was only after three advances in virology that tissue culture gained routine acceptance for the cultivation of viruses and other agents requiring a living cell. The three advances were the

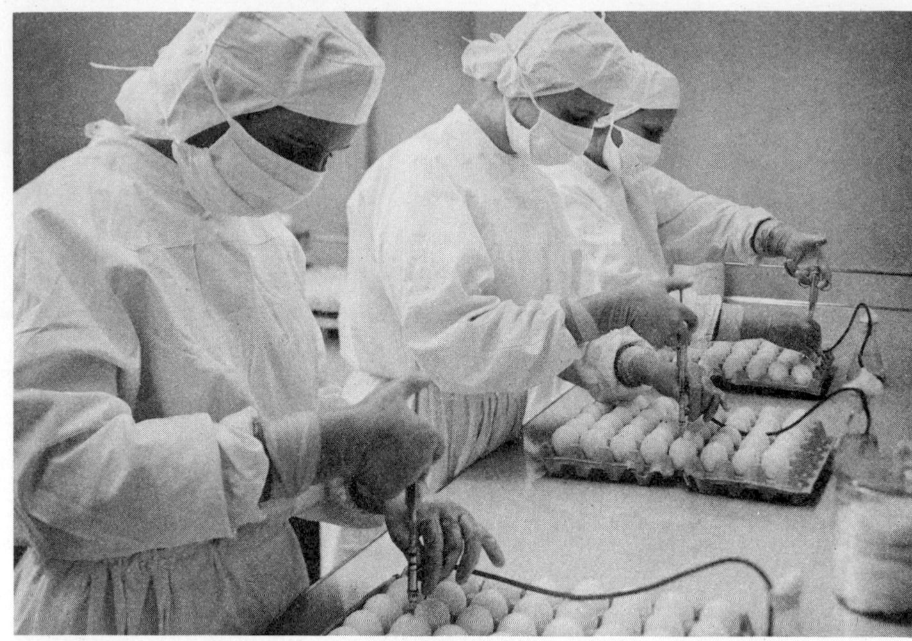

FIG. 12-25 Influenza vaccine production. Eggs that have been incubated, tested for fertility, and prepared for virus inoculation are punctured with a small drill and then seeded with influenza virus. Special instruments are used that break the shell but not the inner membrane. The eggs are then sealed with collodion gelatin and returned to the incubator. *Courtesy of Chas. Pfizer & Company, Inc., N.Y.*

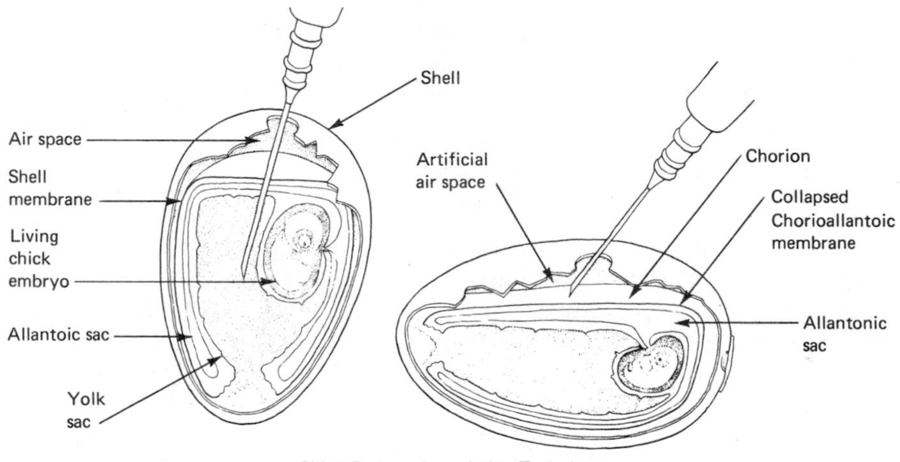

FIG. 12-26 Anatomical components of the chick embryo and possible inoculation sites. (a) Yolk sac inoculation. (b) Chorioallantoic membrane (CAM) inoculation.

introduction of antibiotics, which greatly reduced the contamination problem; development of an excellent, defined growth medium for cells; and introduction of the enzyme trypsin to free cells from fragments of tissue so they can be grown in single-cell layers.

According to most authorities, the work that ushered in the era of tissue culture was the *in vitro* cultivation of poliomyelitis virus in tissues other than nerve cells. This was achieved in 1949 by J. F. Enders, T. H. Weller, and F. C. Robbins by using human embryonic tissue. Before then, polio virus had been grown only in lower animals and nervous tissue. The destructive action, or *cytopathic effect,* of the virus (Figure 12–27) was clearly demonstrated. The three scientists received the Nobel Prize for their work.

PREPARATION OF ANIMAL TISSUE CULTURES

Although the tissues of plants and cold-blooded animals can be cultivated, we shall concentrate here on the cultivation of mammalian tissue.

In the preparation of animal tissue cultures, cells are removed from animals and maintained under suitable conditions *in vitro*, so that they can serve as hosts for viruses or as sources of nucleic acids. The growth medium must provide ample nutrients to keep the metabolism of the animal tissues functioning well and it must be kept free from contamination by unwanted microorganisms such as mycoplasma and latent viruses. An unexpected problem that confronts tissue culture work is the presence of viruses other than those desired. The animal that is the source of tissue may be harboring a latent viral infection. When these tissues are grown *in vitro*, the viral agent may use its new environment to unleash some destructive effect, thus producing an extremely confusing picture for the virologist.

DETECTION OF VIRAL MULTIPLICATION IN TISSUE CULTURE SYSTEMS

There are several tissue culture indications of viral infection, including cytopathic effects (Figure 12–27) and alterations in cellular metabolic reactions.

Cytopathic Changes. Gross cytopathic changes in virus-infected cultures can readily be seen by standard light microscopy. Although fixation and staining of infected cells is not necessary to detect virus multiplication, they are used for making permanent records of its stages (Color Photographs 54 and 55).

Characteristic cytopathic effects (CPEs) brought about by several viruses include cytoplasmic granulation or vacuolation, formation of giant and multinucleated cells (Figure 12–28), and condensation of nucleic acid and protein material in the nuclear membrane of cells. The particular cytopathic effect produced can sometimes aid in diagnostic virology, the identification of a particular viral group. Certain viruses, however, characteristically do not cause any observable structural change in cells.

Efforts to detect viral infection by observing cytopathic effects are complicated by the fact that newly isolated viruses occasionally must be transferred several times before the characteristic cytopathic effects are produced. Furthermore, changes in the fine structure of cells may be the result of the effects of a temporary lack of nutrients, changes in pH, or other related factors. However, these effects can usually be distinguished from cytopathic effects because they develop within 24 hours and are not neutralized by antiviral substances such as antibodies.

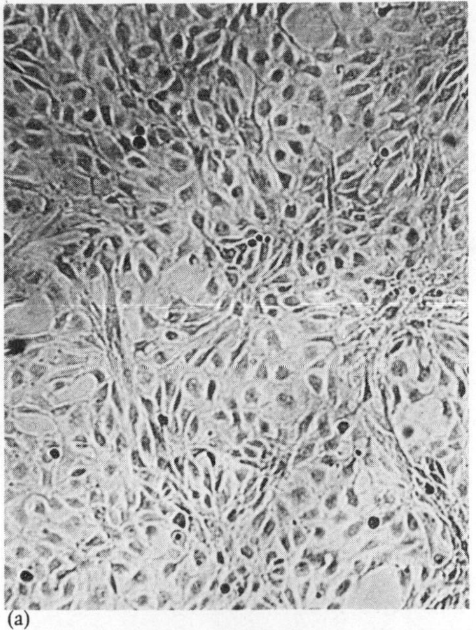

(a)

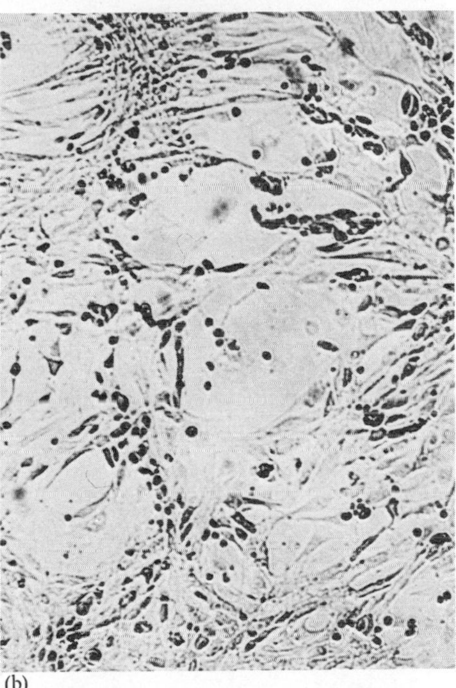

(b)

FIG. 12–27 Demonstration of *in vitro* virus infection. (a) Uninfected tissue culture cells. Note the fairly even distribution of cells. (b) The cytopathic effect (CPE) of viruses is shown here. Cells have a granular appearance and show loss of nuclei and separation from other cells. Higher magnification of cells infected by certain viruses show the presence of inclusion bodies. (See Color Photograph 55.) *Matsunaga, Y., et al.,* Inf. Imm. 18:*495–500 (1977).*

Plaquing Techniques. In the plaquing method, a monolayer tissue culture system is inoculated with a viral suspension. After allowing time for the virus particles to be adsorbed by the tissue cells, the system is overlaid with nutrient agar and incubated at the desired temperature. Viruses that infect the cells multiply within their hosts and produce cellular damage. Because of the agar overlay and the single layer of cells, viruses can spread only along the agar surface, producing clearly defined areas of cellular degeneration (Figure 12–29). Such sites of destruction, called **plaques,** are detected by staining either the remaining living cells (with neutral red) or the dead cells (with typan blue). The characteristics of the plaques, such as their diameter and margin properties, in a particular type of tissue culture system helps in the identification of viruses.

The plaque technique can also be used to obtain pure viral lines. This procedure, called ***plaque purification***, is based on the presumption that a single virus particle produces each plaque just as a single bacterium produces a bacterial colony.

Plaque Assays. Plaque assay is used to determine the number of infectious virus particles in a particular specimen. The measurement of infectivity is accomplished by carrying out the plaque technique with specific dilutions of virus-containing suspensions. The infectivity of the original virus-containing suspension is computed from the number of resultant plaques, each of which is referred to as a *plaque-forming unit* (PFU), together with a correction factor for the specimen dilution employed. Modifications of this technique are necessary at times, depending upon the virus being assayed.

Transformation Assays. Methods have been developed for detecting and measuring the infectivity of viruses that do not cause cell death. One of these is the *transformation assay.* Certain cancer-producing viruses can destroy some cultured cells but can also transform others into malignant systems. Such transformed cells grow in an uninhibited manner to produce a small pile of tumor cells that stands out among the normal cells in a tissue culture. For some viruses, such as the agent of Rous sarcoma, the transformation assay is the basic method for determining viral infectivity.

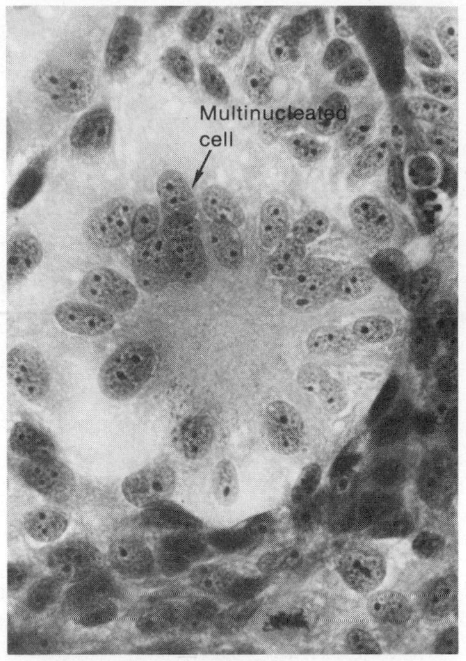

FIG. 12–28 Photograph of measles-virus-induced multinucleated cell formation in monkey kidney cells. *Courtesy of Dr. F. Rapp, Baylor University College of Medicine, Houston.*

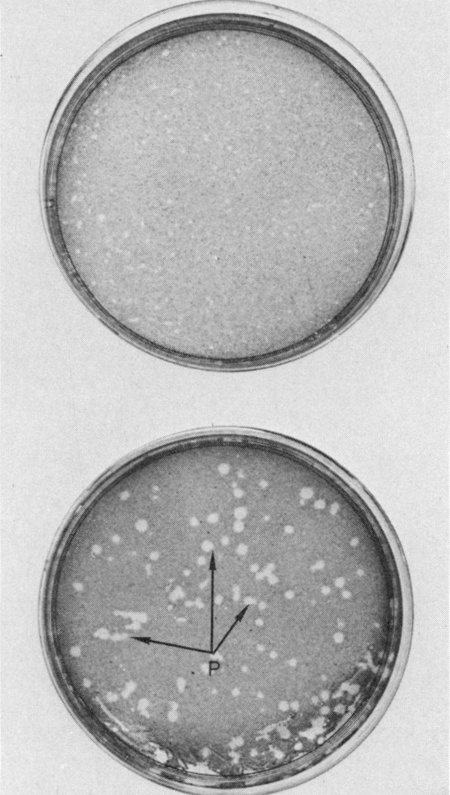

FIG. 12–29 Plaque (P) formation of virulent measles virus in both green monkey kidney (top) and BSC-1 cell (bottom) cultures. *Courtesy of Dr. F. Rapp, Baylor University College of Medicine, Houston.*

Plant Viruses

Virus diseases of plants, although not recognized as such, were known long before the discovery of bacteria. Among the first recorded disease states (in 1576) was a variegation in the color of tulips, which is now called tulip break (Figure 12–30). Since that time over 300 different viruses have been found that affect plants.

Details of ultrastructure, cultivation, symptoms of infections, and demonstration of plant viruses are discussed in the following sections.

Individual plant virions consist of RNA surrounded by a protein capsid. Only one known virus, cauliflower mosaic, contains DNA. The capsomere pattern of virions and the position and orientation of the nucleic acid components to their capsids differ among plant viruses (Figure 12–31).

The shapes of plant virus particles fall into two general categories—polyhedral and helical (Figure 12–32a). The latter group includes rigid rodlike particles, bullet-shaped viruses (Figure 12–32b), and long, flexible threads.

Plant Virus Cultivation

Apart from the need to obtain sufficient material for ultrastructural studies, plant virus cultivation serves many other purposes. These include the study of virus-infected cells, the determination of viral environmental and nutritional requirements, and the evaluation of effects of chemicals and radiation on virus replication and other activities.

Three different procedures are used for cultivation: tissue culture, cell culture, and protoplast culture. In tissue culture, pieces of various plant parts such as roots, stems, and seeds are used. Diseased tissues, including tumors, have also been cultured for virus study. Cell culture techniques use cells isolated from plant tissues. Such cells can be obtained from the vigorous shaking of cut plant parts or from the enzymatic breakdown of the intercellular connecting substances in plant tissues. The methods used to produce protoplast cultures involve the enzymatic digestion of plant cell components.

The presence of viruses in plant cells can be demonstrated in various ways, including staining with fluorescent antibody procedures and electron microscopy.

Plant Virus Infections

Plant viruses apparently have no specific mechanisms to ensure their penetration into host cells. They can enter their hosts through breaks or abrasions in the plant, or they can be introduced by insects, parasitic worms, or other plants such as dodder.

Abnormalities develop in all parts of infected plants. External signs of virus infection include mottling on leaves, with dark green, light green, or yellow areas often accompanied by raised blisterlike spots (Color Photograph 56a); changes in flower color (Color Photograph 56b); formation of unusually small, misshapen, or bumpy fruits; cracked bark; and abnormal growths (tumors) on roots. Of the various internal changes that occur, degeneration of conductive tissues, increase in cell number, and the presence of cellular inclusions are the most common. The cellular inclusions frequently contain virus particles.

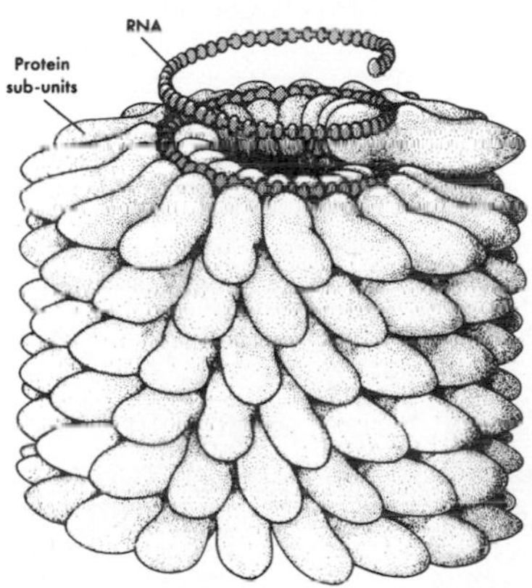

FIG. 12-31 Tobacco mosaic virus. A diagrammatic representation of this virus showing how its RNA chain is arranged within the supporting framework of the capsid. *Caspar, D. L. D., and A. Klug,* Adv. Virus Res. 7*:225 (1960).*

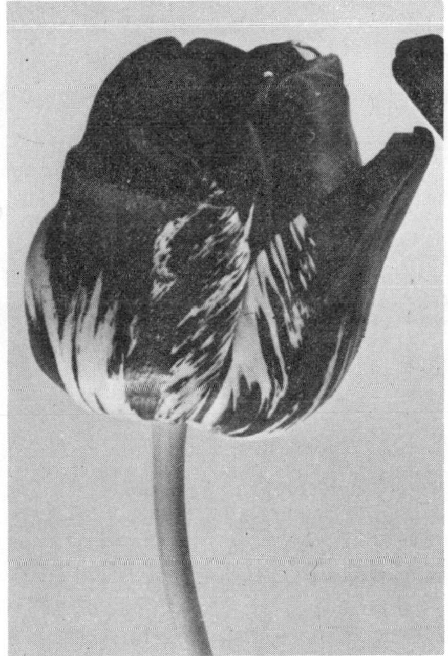

(a)

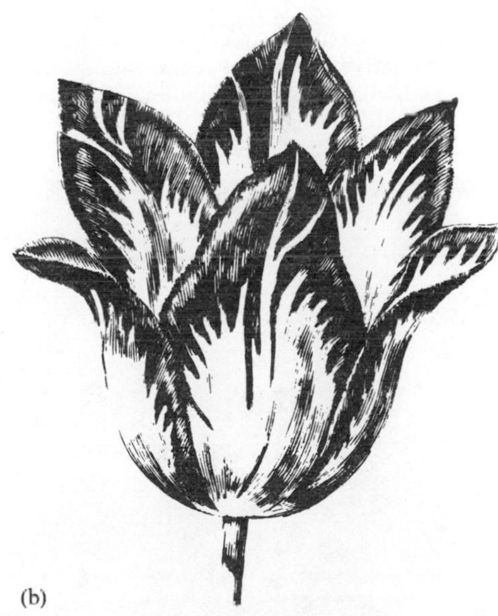

(b)

FIG. 12-30 Virus-caused tulip break. (a) A photo showing the streaking, or "break," of tulips caused by virus infection. (b) A drawing of a similar condition from a book entitled *The Clergy-Man's Recreation,* by J. Lawrence, published in 1714. *Courtesy of Dr. R. Markham, Agricultural Research Council, Cambridge, England.*

Viruses of Eucaryotic Microorganisms

More and more virus associations with eucaryotic microorganisms, including algae, fungi, and protozoa, are being described (Figure 12–33). Such associations take one of two forms. In one type, the eucaryotic microorganism serves as a **vector,** or transmitter, of the virus. This virus-vector relationship appears to be highly specific. At present there is no evidence that any of these viruses multiplies in its eucaryotic microbial vector. Interestingly enough, certain viruses present in these eucaryotes actually may be associated with procaryotic or other eucaryotic microorganisms (endosymbionts) present within the cell (Figure 12–33c). Those eucaryotes that exhibit phagocytosis are likely to acquire viruses of other organisms simply by feeding from a nonsterile environment. Once introduced, such viruses might be kept intact. Various parasitic protozoa have acquired viruses following contact with host cells.

In the second situation, the virus infects the eucaryote, which then functions as a host. Since relatively little is known about virus infections of eucaryotic microbes other than fungi, and since much research has been done on the virus-host association in fungi, we shall concentrate here on these viruses of fungi, or *mycoviruses.*

In 1967 a virus was found in an Ascomycete. Since then, different viruses have been found in over 100 species of fungi, including genera from all the main taxonomic groups of fungi. A number of these mycoviruses have now been characterized *in vitro* (in test tubes or similar containers), and their replication has been demonstrated *in vivo* (in living, whole organisms). In many instances, however, the evidence consists largely of electron micrographs of viruslike particles found in extracts from the fungi.

The viruses studied are primarily nonenveloped, polyhedral particles that contain double-stranded RNA. Recently, an enveloped, double-stranded, herpesvirus-type virus particle was discovered. Transmission of fungal viruses can occur through hyphal connections and through asexual or sexual spores. Although there is sometimes a total absence of harmful effects, these viruses may cause the death of the host or the formation of abnormal mycelial growth activities. From the available evidence, it appears that there is no consistent relationship between the presence or the absence of mycoviruses and the production of antibiotics and mycotoxins such as aflatoxins.

The biological significance of viruses in fungi is still unclear. Under normal conditions, most of these viruses seem to be latent. However, as experience has shown with bacteria and other forms of life, latent infections can be triggered into virulent ones.

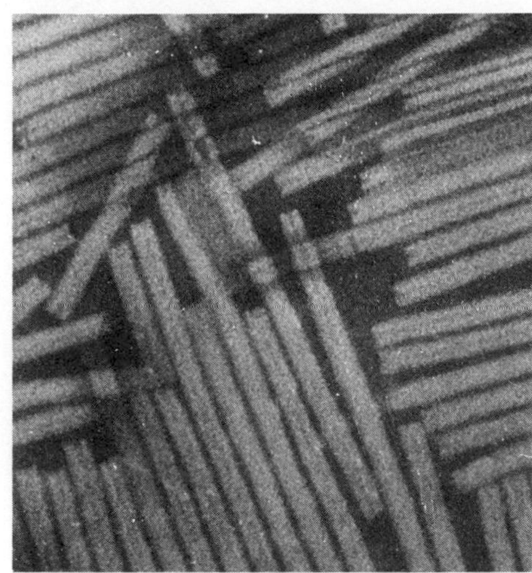

(a)

FIG. 12–32 (a) An electron micrograph of negatively stained tobacco mosaic virus. *Courtesy of Dr. R. Markham, Agricultural Research Council, Cambridge, England.* (b) Negatively stained eggplant mottled dwarf virus. Note the bullet shape and helical nucleocapsid (N). *Russo, M., and G. P. Martelli,* Virology 52:*39–48 (1973).*

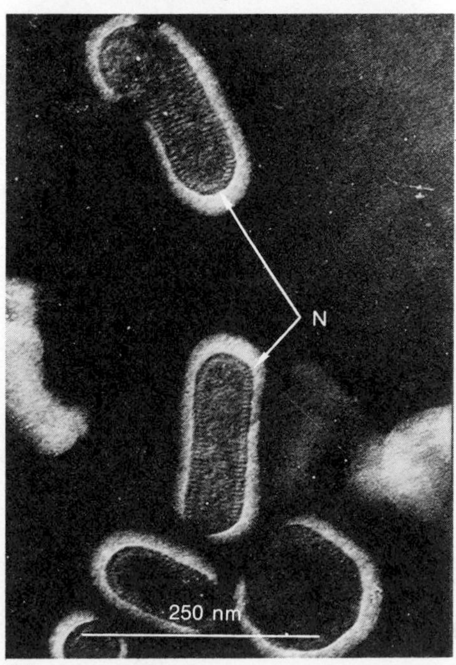

(b)

Viroids

In 1971, T. O. Diener introduced the term **viroid** to represent a newly discovered category of subviral plant pathogen (Color Photograph 57). The first member of this unique class of disease agents was found during research by Diener and W. B. Raymer concerning the agent of potato spindle tuber disease. Two additional plant diseases, chrysanthemum stunt and citrus exocortis, are now recognized as viroid-caused conditions.

All currently known viroids consist of low-molecular-weight (75,000 to 120,000 daltons) RNA, making the viroids about one tenth the size of the smallest known plant virus (Figure 12–34). They are short, with an average length of about 500 Å. Viroids are found primarily in nuclei of infected cells, in close association with cellular chromatin material. There they lead to replication of the viroid RNA and sometimes to disease. Just how viroids produce their effect is not known, although several hypotheses have been offered. It has been suggested that the viroids specifically interfere with host metabolic functions. Such interference could result in cellular malfunction, such as cellular production of faulty proteins. The transmission of agents like the potato spindle tuber viroid can occur through the pollen or ovules (a part of the plant's ovary) of infected plants.

The discovery of viroids poses several important questions for molecular biology, virology, plant pathology, and veterinary and human medicine. This is especially true in the case of medicine, because several low-molecular-weight RNA molecules have been found in association with a number of viral infections.

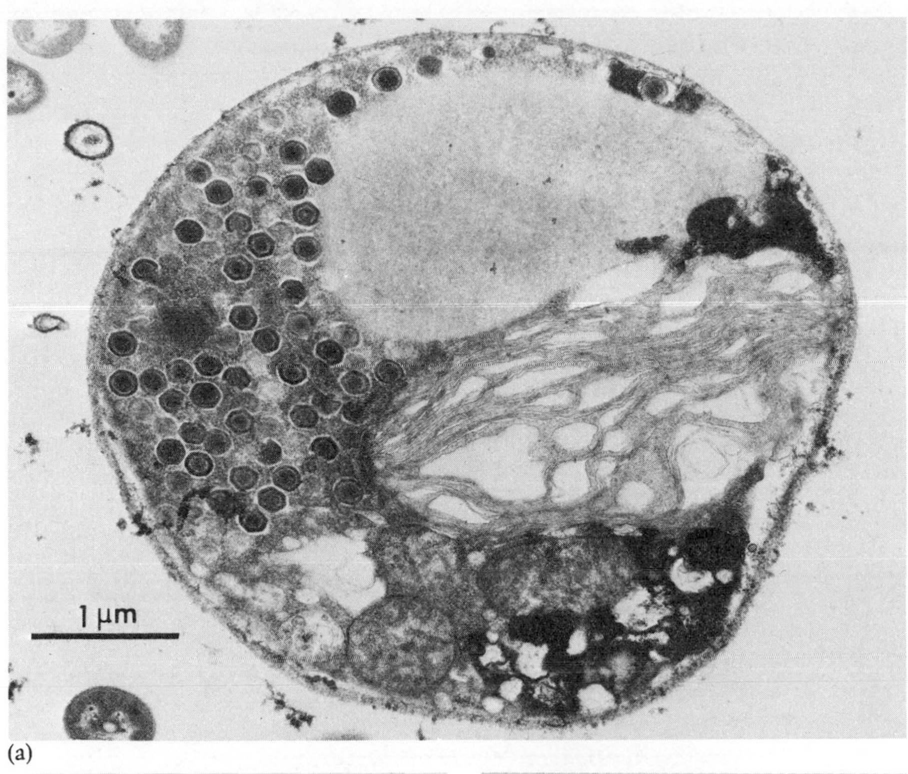

(a)

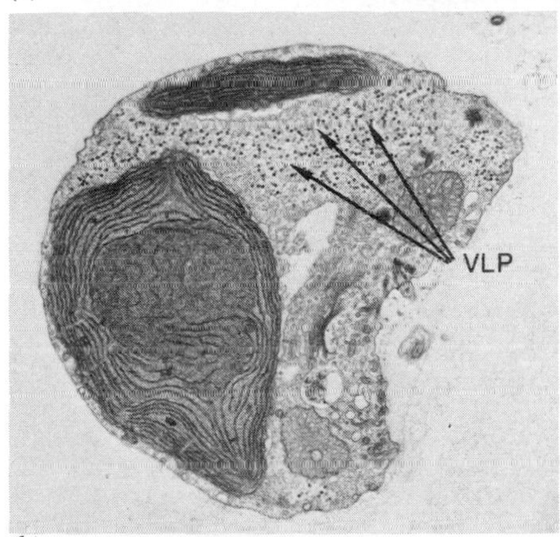

(b)

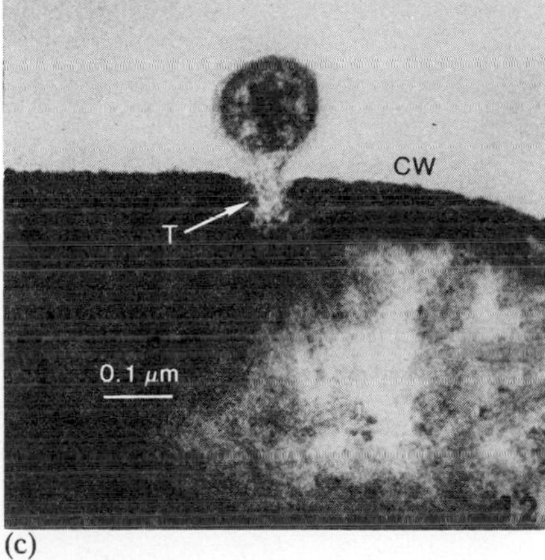

(c)

FIG. 12-33 Viruses of eucaryotic microorganisms. (a) Polyhedral viruslike particles in a spore of the brown alga *Chorda tomentosa*. *Toth, R., and Wilce, R. T.:* J. Phycol. 8:*126–130 (1972)*. (b) Icosahedral, viruslike particles (VLPs) found in green algae. Infection leads to cell destruction. These particles are structurally similar to those that infect other eucaryotic algae. *Reproduced with the permission of the National Research Council of Canada from Hoffman, L. R., and L. H. Staker,* Can. J. Botany 54:*2827–2841 (1976)*. (c) A virus particle invading a green alga through its cell wall. Note the tail-like structure of the invading particle. *Kawakami, H., and N. Kawakami,* J. Protozool. 25:*217–225 (1978)*.

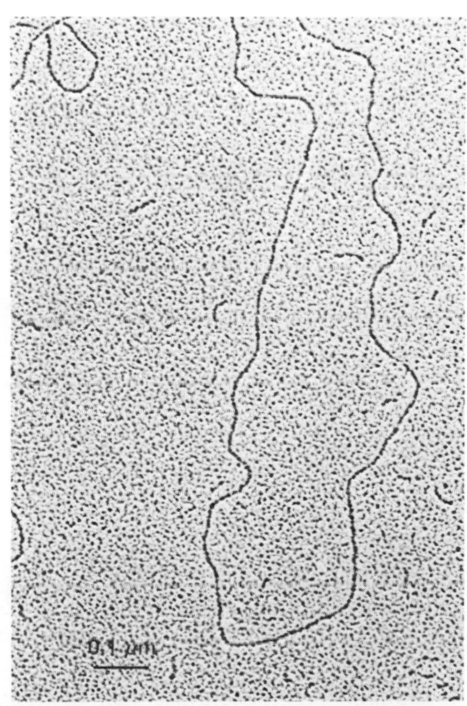

FIG. 12-34 An electron micrograph of the potato spindle tuber viroid (PSTV) in comparison with a conventional viral nucleic acid from bacteriophage T_7. Note the great size difference between the viroids (arrows) and the viral DNA molecule. *Courtesy of T. O. Diener, Research Plant Pathologist, U.S.D.A.*

SUMMARY

Every kind of life can be parasitized by viruses.

What Is A Virus?

A mature virus particle, or *virion,* has several distinguishing properties, including the absence of cellular structures, the possession of either DNA or RNA, viral nucleic acid regulation of new virus production (replication), and a dependence on the host cell and its parts for energy and protein needs.

Basic Structure of Extracellular Viruses

1. A typical viral life cycle consists of both intracellular and extracellular phases. Intracellular phases involve the production of viral parts used in the formation of complete viruses.
2. Most virions exhibit a characteristic structure.
3. A complete virus consists of a nucleic acid core surrounded by a protein *capsid* (coat).

The Nucleic Acid of the Mature Virion

1. The viral nucleic acid, whether DNA or RNA, contains the viral genetic material, or *genome.*
2. The specific type and form of nucleic acid varies according to the virus.
3. Length also varies, but it is constant for a specific virus.

The Nucleocapsid

1. The capsids of viruses consist of subunits known as *capsomeres.*
2. Virus particles can exhibit one of several forms of symmetries. These include *cubic, helical* (springlike), *binal* (a combination of cubic and helical), *bullet-shaped,* and *filamentous.*
3. The *nucleocapsid* consists of the capsid enclosing a viral nucleic acid core.

Enveloped Viruses

1. Viruses which through their intracellular developmental cycle acquire an outer coat, or covering, from the cytoplasmic and/or nuclear membranes of infected host cells are referred to as *enveloped.*
2. The envelopes of some viruses are covered with projecting spikes that may appear as a fringe. Attachment of viruses to cells of various types is associated with these projections.

Shape and Size

Virions vary not only in size, but in shape as well.

Classification

Current classification schemes for viruses are mainly based on capsid organization and nucleic acid chemistry.

Bacteriophages (Bacterial Viruses)

1. Almost all large groups of cultivable bacteria have been found to have viruses.
2. Many bacterial viruses have been useful in identification of bacterial pathogens and in research on the mechanisms of cellular infections.

The Basic Structure of Bacteriophages

1. Bacterial viruses exhibit a great variety of forms.
2. These viruses contain either RNA or DNA.
3. A characteristic feature of some bacteriophages is their tail-like structure, which serves as an attachment device as well as a tube through which viral nucleic acid can be injected into a host cell.

Filamentous Bacteriophages

1. The *filamentous viruses* are among the smallest viruses known to date.
2. Filamentous viruses have focused attention on a form of symbiotic behavior previously unrecognized in bacteria.

The Cultivation of Bacteriophages

1. Actively growing young bacterial cells are used for their cultivation. Either broth or agar cultures are used for this purpose.
2. When agar plates are used, the presence of bacterial viruses is indicated by the development of *plaques.*

Enumeration of Phages

Accurate estimations of the number of virus particles in a sample can be done by several techniques including the plaque count assay and electron microscopy.

Phage Typing

Phage typing is used to identify certain specific bacterial species.

Replication Cycle of Bacteriophages

1. Bacterial viruses that regularly infect and complete their life cycles in bacterial hosts and ultimately produce more virus particles with the accompanying destruction of the host are called *virulent* or *lytic* viruses.
2. Not all virus infections of bacteria end in host cell destruction. Some viruses integrate their DNA into that of the host. Such viruses are said to be *temperate,* and their integrated form is refered to as a *prophage.* The bacterial cell containing a prophage is *lysogenic.*

Lysogeny

1. When a temperate phage infects a host cell, it can either cause the destruction of the host (lytic cycle) or assume a noninfectious state.
2. The presence of a virus in a noninfectious state can result in changes of the host cell, including changes in colonial morphology and toxin production.
3. Bacteria harboring a virus as a prophage are immune to infection by other phages of the same type. This is a form of *resistance.*

The Lytic Cycle

The lytic cycle of bacterial viruses such as the T-even ones includes the stages of adsorption, penetration, replication of new viral DNA, maturation, and new virus particle release.

Growth Curve

A *one-step growth curve* utilizes the events of the lytic cycle to determine the time sequence from injection to the release of mature viruses and the number of virus particles released per cell.

Cyanophages

Cyanophages, viruses of blue-green bacteria, are similar to other bacterial viruses in both structure and infection cycle.

Cyanophage Cultivation and Enumeration

The conditions, media, and procedures used for preparation of suitable hosts for cyanophages are different from those used for bacteriophages.

Animal Viruses

Disease

1. Examples of human diseases include chickenpox, smallpox, and yellow fever.
2. Lower animal diseases include canine distemper, foot-and-mouth disease, and various tumors.
3. The effects of animal viruses can range from mild skin rashes and upper respiratory symptoms to tissue destruction and death.
4. Viruses that attack insects such as honeybees and silkworms can cause severe economic losses.

Animal Virus Replication

Although differences exist among viruses, the general sequence of events involved in replication are attachment to the host cells, penetration, *uncoating* (removal of viral envelope and capsid from the nucleic acid), replication of viral nucleic acid, manufacture of other viral parts, assembly of viral parts to form new virus particles, and release of new viruses.

Animal Virus Cultivation

1. Fertilized eggs are useful for virus cultivation, especially when large numbers of viruses are needed.
2. Egg cultivation of viruses is useful in vaccine production, virus isolation, virus morphology studies, determinations of the effectiveness of drugs on viruses, and in studies dealing with the mechanism of infection.
3. Signs of infection include death of the embryo, demonstration of red blood cell clumping by virus-containing fluids, and the finding of virus particles in embryo material by various types of microscopy.

Tissue Culture Cultivation of Viruses

1. Viruses can be grown in a variety of tissues maintained in various types of containers. This type of cultivation is known as *in vitro*.
2. The destructive effects of viruses in these systems are called *cytopathic effects* (CPEs) and include nuclear changes, formation of multinucleated and giant cells, and vacuole formation. The particular type of cytopathic effect can be used at times for virus identification.
3. Special techniques used in determining the number of virus particles in specimens and in purifying and establishing virus lines include the plaquing method. A *plaque* refers to a clear area in a single tissue culture layer that contains numerous virus particles.
4. Transformation assays are special tissue culture methods used to detect viruses and activities that do not cause cell death.

Plant Viruses

Virus diseases of plants were known long before the discovery of bacteria.

Plant Virus Structure and Shape

1. Most individual plant virus particles consist of RNA surrounded by a protein capsid.
2. The shapes of plant viruses fall into two general categories, polyhedral (many-sided) and helical.

Plant Virus Cultivation

Plant viruses can be cultivated in tissue culture, cell culture, and protoplast culture systems.

Plant Virus Infections

Plant viruses produce both internal and external effects in infected hosts. Abnormalities can be noted on different plant parts including flowers, roots, and bark.

Viruses of Eucaryotic Microorganisms

Viruses may be found in association with eucaryotic microorganisms such as algae, fungi, and protozoa.

Viroids

Viroids represent the smallest infectious agent known and consist only of a low-molecular-weight RNA. They are mainly found in plant disease states.

QUESTIONS FOR REVIEW

1. a. What is a virus?
   b. How does the organization of a virus particle differ from that of a procaryote?
   c. How does the organization of a virus particle differ from that of a eucaryotic microorganism?
2. Explain or define the following terms:
   a. capsomere
   b. virion
   c. capsid
   d. icosahedron
   e. nucleic acid core
   f. envelope
   g. binal arrangement
3. Distinguish between a virion and a viroid.
4. Compare the structural features of:
   a. a typical animal virus
   b. a typical plant virus
   c. a bacteriophage
   d. a cyanophage
5. Do all viruses contain DNA? Explain.
6. Which of the structures shown in the electron micrograph of Figure 12–35 would you *not* expect to find in the following?
   a. bacteriophage
   b. typical green alga
   c. typical flagellated protozoan
   d. a yeast cell

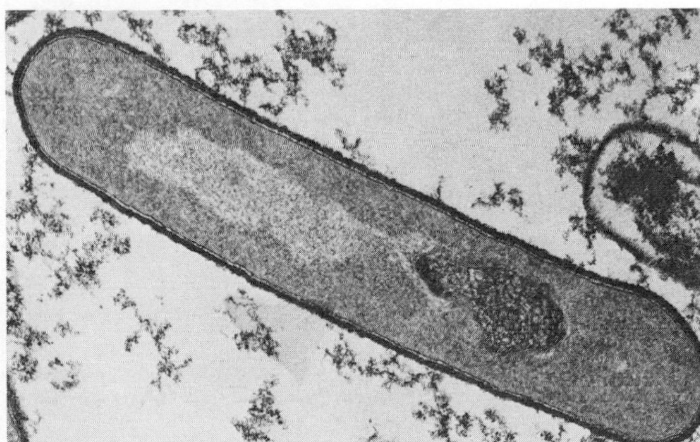

FIG. 12-35 An electron micrograph of an ultrathin section of *Bacillus subtilis. Courtesy of W. Van Iterson, University of Amsterdam, and the North-Holland Publishing Company, Amsterdam.*

7. a. How are viruses classified?
   b. Does virus classification differ from the system used for bacteria? If so, how?

- c. List six properties of viruses used for their classification.

8. a. List three different techniques used for virus cultivation.
   b. How do such techniques differ from the ones used for bacterial cultivation?

9. a. How is the replication of viruses detected in the laboratory?
   b. What does CPE mean?

10. a. Describe, in order, the events that occur in the replication of an enveloped virus.
    b. Describe, in order, the events that occur in the replication of a binal-shaped bacteriophage.

11. What is lysogeny?

12. a. What types of microorganisms harbor viruses?
    b. Do these viruses differ from either animal or plant virus particles? If so, how?

13. Do animal viruses infect plant cells? Explain.

14. What forms of life do not have viruses?

15. List eight specific structures of procaryotes not found in a virus particle.

16. a. Define the statement that viruses are living.
    b. Present arguments against the above statement.
    c. What do you think?

17. The electron micrograph in Figure 12–36 shows the surface of a virus-infected human cell. Emerging enveloped virus particles (arrows) can readily be seen. Briefly outline the events that were necessary for the development of such viruses to occur.

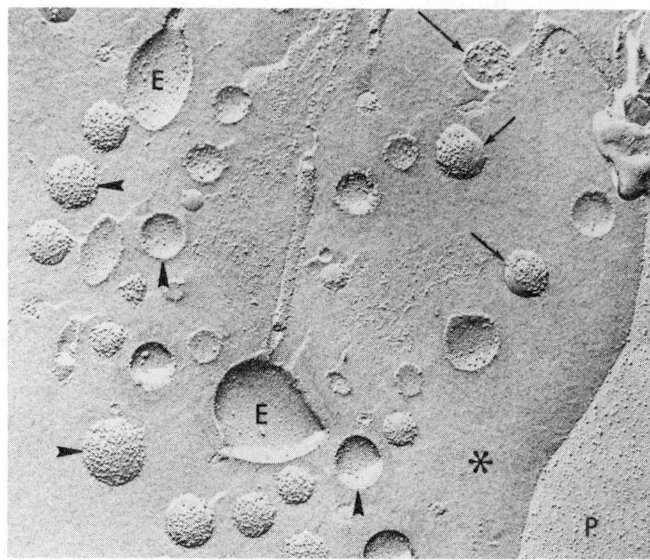

FIG. 12–36 *Rodriguez, M., and M. Dubois-Dalcq,* J. Virol. 26:435–447 *(1978).*

SUGGESTED READINGS

Campbell, A. M., "How Viruses Insert Their DNA into the DNA of the Host Cell," *Sci. Amer.* 237:102 (1976). *Details of the insertion of a virus into the host cell are presented. How viruses can coexist peacefully with host cells without causing cell death is explained.*

Hughes, S. S., *The Virus, A History of the Concept.* New York: Science History Publications, 1977. *This is a good, short book on the history of the virus from the germ theory of infectious disease to concepts of the virus in the twentieth century.*

Lemke, P. A., "Viruses of Eucaryotic Microorganisms," *Ann. Rev. Microbiol.* 30:105–145 (1976). *A review of the ultrastructural, physiochemical, and genetic evidence for the existence of viruses among algae, fungi, and protozoa. The possibility that certain viruses in these microorganisms may actually be associated with procaryotes within algae, fungi, and protozoa is also discussed.*

Lenard, J., "Virus Envelopes and Plasma Membranes," *Ann. Revs. Biophys. Bioeng.* 7:139 (1978). *Enveloped viruses, the origin of viral lipids, the presence of envelope proteins, and the formation of viral envelopes are among the major topics of this review.*

Luria, S. E., J. E. Darnell, Jr., D. Baltimore, and A. Campbell, *General Virology.* 3rd ed. New York: John Wiley & Sons, 1978. *A good, general textbook on virology dealing with subjects such as virion structure, virus-host interactions, the diversity of bacterial, mammalian, insect and plant viruses, and the relationship of viruses to specific diseases and cancer.*

Smith, K. M., *Plant Viruses.* 6th ed. London: Chapman and Hall, 1977. *A concise and readable book that provides a comprehensive, illustrated coverage of plant virology. Chapters dealing with the viruses of algae and fungi and mycoplasma-caused plant diseases are also included.*

Bacterial Growth and Cultivation Techniques

CHAPTER 13

Chapter 13 examines various aspects of bacterial growth, including specific nutritional categories and physical requirements. This chapter also describes the preparation and handling of media; the conditions needed for growth of organisms, with different requirements for oxygen and carbon dioxide; and the phenomenon of growth itself.

After reading this chapter, you should be able to:

1. **Describe the forms of nutrition known as heterotrophy, autotrophy, and hypotrophy.**
2. **Identify microbial categories according to gaseous requirements.**
3. **Describe what is meant by cardinal temperatures and classify bacteria according to temperature requirements.**
4. **Identify the role of pH in bacterial growth and list selected organisms with unusual pH requirements.**
5. **Identify the role and common sources of nitrogen, carbon, vitamins, growth factors, mineral salts, and water in bacteriological media.**
6. **Describe the basic elements of media preparation, the requirements for storage, and selected uses of bacteriological media.**
7. **Identify the role of aseptic technique in bacterial inoculation and transfer procedures.**

8. **Describe the pour-plate and streak-plate techniques and their use in the isolation of pure cultures.**
9. **Explain the need for pure cultures.**
10. **Describe general methods for establishing capneic and anaerobic incubation conditions and the concept of biological indicators.**
11. **Describe what occurs during each phase of the bacterial growth curve.**
12. **Describe differences in how bacteria grow in liquid and solid media.**
13. **Identify the basic aspects and uses of continuous culture techniques.**
14. **Describe techniques used to determine bacterial growth by estimation of cell mass and cell numbers.**

Bacteria are grown for many purposes, including those of medicine, agriculture, industry, and basic research. Each species has particular requirements for its nutrition and other aspects of growth. Because of such precise growth needs, pure cultures must be obtained and verified periodically. This is particularly true when an organism is to be identified, since so many bacteria appear the same morphologically.

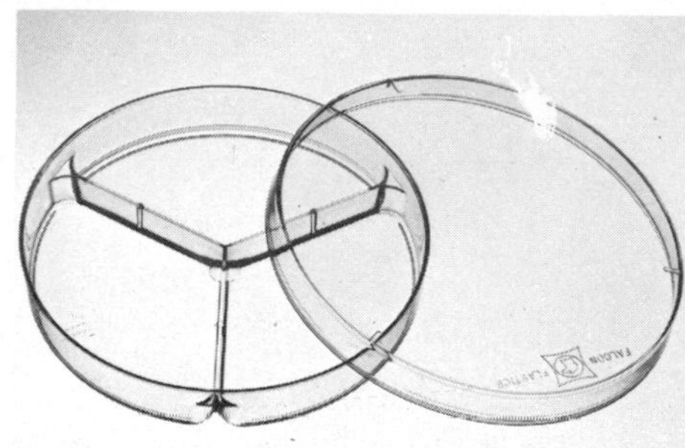

FIG. 13-1 An example of a three-compartment Petri dish. Dishes are also available without compartments or with two or four compartments. Different media or specimens can be introduced into each separate area. *Courtesy of Falcon Plastics, Division of BioQuest, Los Angeles.*

An Introduction to Bacterial Cultivation

A wide variety of procedures and nutrient preparations are used to induce microorganisms to grow and reproduce. Different microbes require different environments and nutrients, called *culture media* (singular, *medium*). Procedures for culturing fungi, for instance, are of little value in inducing viruses to grow.

Microorganisms are cultivated in containers ranging from test tubes, flasks, and Petri dishes (Figure 13-1) to huge steel tanks. The tanks are used commercially to obtain large quantities of the desired organisms or their products, as discussed in Chapter 38. Whatever the actual container material may be, the procedures are referred to as *in vitro*—literally, "in glass," even though such containers are often made of plastic.

Some microorganisms cannot be grown *in vitro*, but only in living animals. Cultivation methods using live animals are called *in vivo* techniques (Color Photograph 53). When animal tissues are removed and used as a culture medium for microbes, the procedure is an *in vitro* one because a culture vessel is used, not the living *(vivo)* animal. Some microbes can be cultured both *in vivo* and *in vitro*.

In order for an organism to cause disease, it must be able not only to survive, but to grow and reproduce in or on the body of its host. These pathogens—as well as nonpathogenic microbes that populate different body regions—carry on their life processes in environments containing different organic and inorganic substances, different oxygen and carbon dioxide concentrations, and different degrees of alkalinity or acidity (pH). Cultivation techniques and media used to provide suitable conditions for the growth of bacteria will be discussed from the viewpoint of these different conditions.

Nutrition and Other Conditions for Growth

Heterotrophy, Autotrophy, and Hypotrophy

The **heterotrophic** organism requires certain preformed organic compounds for its nutrition. These materials may be sources of carbon (sugars), nitrogen (amino acids), vitamins, or other growth factors. The **autotrophic** microorganism, on the other hand, can synthesize all or nearly all of its essential organic materials from inorganic compounds such as carbon dioxide (CO_2). It usually thrives best in soils and bodies of water (Color Photograph 4a); the heterotroph grows well in any environment with a source of organic and other nutrients.

Both heterotrophic and autotrophic organisms are free-living and can, as a rule, be cultivated on artificial media—if the particular nutrients and environmental conditions for growth are known.

A third group of microorganisms, the **hypotrophs,** are obligate intracellular parasites. That is, they will grow only within a living host cell. The hypotrophs include the viruses of animals, plants, and bacteria and most rickettsia.

Gaseous Requirements

In addition to their classification by nutritional requirement, microorganisms are categorized by their response to available gases such as oxygen and carbon dioxide. Oxygen is involved as an electron receptor in metabolism and carbon dioxide is an essential nutrient for some organisms.

Aerobic organisms require oxygen, either at atmosphere levels or at some lower concentration.

Microaerophilic organisms require oxygen at less than the 20 percent concentration found in the atmosphere and surface waters. They do not grow in the upper portions of liquid (broth) cultures where oxygen is abundant. If this avoidance of oxygen is due to a need for more carbon dioxide rather than less oxygen, the microaerophilic organism is called *capneic*. Capneic organisms require an atmosphere with a carbon dioxide level of approximately 3 to 10 percent.

Certain bacteria of medical significance, such as *Neisseria gonorrhoeae*, must be provided with carbon dioxide for growth purposes. With other pathogens, such as *Brucella* spp., causative agents of brucellosis, carbon dioxide is used only for primary isolations. Since many microorganisms of clinical importance grow better in the presence of carbon dioxide, it is likely that capneic incubation will become the preferred technique in the laboratory. Details of conditions of incubation are discussed later in this chapter.

Anaerobes are organisms that have no requirement for free oxygen but that possess varying degrees of oxygen tolerance. *Strict*, or *obligate*, *anaerobes* cannot tolerate any free oxygen in their environment. The human pathogenic agents *Bacteroides* spp. are examples of such organisms. They must be collected from the patient, transported, cultured, and grown under strict anaerobic conditions. The slightest exposure to free oxygen will kill them. *Aerotolerant anaerobes,* on the other hand, can grow in the presence of free oxygen, although it is not used in their metabolism. Streptococci are aerotolerant anaerobes. **Facultative** *anaerobes* will grow in either the presence or absence of oxygen. These organisms usually grow best aerobically. The colon bacterium *Escherichia coli* belongs to this category, as do many yeasts.

One explanation for the sensitivity of obligate anaerobes to an oxygen environment is related to formation of hydrogen peroxide (H_2O_2) during microbial metabolic processes. This product alone can be quite destructive, as shown by the fact that it is commonly used as a disinfectant. Some bacteria produce an enzyme, catalase, that breaks down the peroxide to oxygen (O_2) and water (H_2O). Strict anaerobic bacteria do not produce this enzyme and are therefore poisoned by environments containing peroxide.

An additional explanation for the inability of anaerobes to grow in the presence of oxygen concerns the oxidation-reduction potential of the medium. The oxidation-reduction potential is a concept that indicates the electron-accepting or electron-yielding potentials of substances. When the oxidation-reduction potential of a medium is lowered by the addition of a reducing or oxygen-absorbing compound, such as cysteine or thioglycollic acid, many anaerobes will grow. Because some reducing agents are toxic, they must be selected with care.

Thermal Conditions

As a group, microorganisms have been shown to grow between the temperatures of about freezing and above 90°C. Organisms can be classified as **psychrophiles** (cold-loving, 0° to 20°C), **mesophiles** (moderate-temperature-loving, 20° to 45°C), or **thermophiles** (heat-loving, 45° to above 90°C), based upon their favorable growth temperature range.

An organism, while not actively growing at unfavorable temperatures, may still endure them. For example, many organisms can survive in freezing environments; these forms may be called *psychroduric* or *cryoduric.* Organisms that survive at high temperatures are known as *thermoduric* types. *Bacillus* spp. are good examples of the latter, due to their formation of heat-resistant spores.

The minimum, maximum, and optimum temperatures for an organism are known as its *cardinal temperatures.* The cardinal temperatures for any organism depend upon several factors, including the age of the culture and the supply of nutrients.

Acidity or Alkalinity (pH)

Microorganisms also have certain pH (hydrogen ion concentration) needs, as reflected by their growth responses in various media. The pH is simply the negative logarithm of the hydrogen ion $[H^+]$ concentration. The scale of values representing this property of solutions commonly extends from 0 to 14 (Table 13–1). Aqueous solutions also contain hydroxyl ions $[OH^-]$, which are important in the control of the alkalinity of a solution. A neutral state, in which the concentrations of hydrogen and hydroxyl ions are equal, has a pH of 7. In general, pure water should have this pH. Solutions with pH values from 0 to 6.9 are *acidic,* while those having values from 7.1 to 14 are *basic,* or *alkaline.*

Because of the logarithmic nature of the pH units, a change in one such unit corresponds to a tenfold change in the hydrogen ion concentration. Consider, for example, a preparation with a pH of 0. The $[H^+]$ here is 10^0 or 1 normal (N).

By comparison, a solution having a pH of 1 has a hydrogen concentration represented by 10^{-1} or one tenth normal, that is, N/10 (Table 13–1).

TABLE 13–1 pH Values and Corresponding Hydrogen Ion Concentrations

pH Scale	*pH Value*	*Normal Concentrations*	*Common pH of Substances*	
Highly acid	0	10^0	Human gastric juice	0.9
	1	10^{-1}		
	2	10^{-2}	Orange juice	2.0
	3	10^{-3}		
	4	10^{-4}	Tomato juice	4.2
	5	10^{-5}		
	6	10^{-6}	Media for fungi	5.6
Neutral	7	10^{-7}	Milk	6.6
			Blood (approx.)	7.3
			Bile	7.8
	8	10^{-8}	Some media	8.6
	9	10^{-9}		
	10	10^{-10}		
	11	10^{-11}		
	12	10^{-12}	Lime water	12.3
	13	10^{-13}		
Highly alkaline	14	10^{-14}	A 1-N sodium hydroxide solution	14.0

Various indicators and electronic pH meters are commonly used to measure the hydrogen concentrations of preparations. Examples of indicators incorporated into bacteriological media are bromcresol purple, litmus, and phenol red (Color Photographs 64 and 65).

Some organisms can be found growing in sulfur springs containing sulfuric acid with a pH of less than 2, others in ammoniated solutions at a pH greater than 8. Fungi, as a rule, grow well at an acid pH range of 5.5 or 6. This property is used in the preparation of selective media for these organisms, since many contaminating bacteria cannot grow under these conditions.

Necessary adjustments to obtain the desired pH usually can be made by the careful addition of standard acids, such as hydrochloric acid (HCl), or bases, such as potassium hydroxide (KOH) or sodium hydroxide (NaOH).

The causative agent of Asiatic cholera, *Vibrio cholerae*, can tolerate a pH of 8. This fact can be used in the preparation of isolation media for the organism, since it must be separated from other typical organisms comprising the enteric flora found in feces (Color Photograph 62). As a rule, microorganisms prefer a more neutral pH, between 6 and 7.5. Therefore, acidic and alkaline solutions can exert disinfecting effects on various organisms.

Properties of Bacteriological Media

Combining various substances into nutritive concoctions has long been an integral part of microbiology. Such media are used for the isolation of important organisms from such materials as dairy products, foods, soil, water, and clinical specimens. Most organisms found in these situations are heterotrophic in nature, thus simplifying the task of combining the essential nutrient components into a suitable medium. Some of the important ingredients of media are briefly described below.

Nitrogen Sources

Nitrogen is a component of cellular proteins, nucleic acids, and vitamins. Microorganisms must therefore be supplied with this element in some form. Many can use ammonium salts, for example, ammonium chloride (NH_4Cl), as inorganic nitrogen; others require the breakdown products of proteins, such as peptones (partially hydrolyzed proteins), peptides, and amino acids. Some bacteria (for example, ***Bacillus*** spp.) produce extracellular protein-digesting enzymes (proteases) that break down gelatin and other proteins into the smaller components of peptides and amino acids. These components can then be brought into the cells for further metabolic action. An example of this ability to digest materials in the environment is shown in Figure 13–2. A bacterial culture is shown growing on a nutrient agar that contains the milk protein casein. The presence of the casein causes the agar to appear white. The clear zone around the bacterial growth demonstrates the ability of the bacterial enzymes to digest the protein for use by the cells.

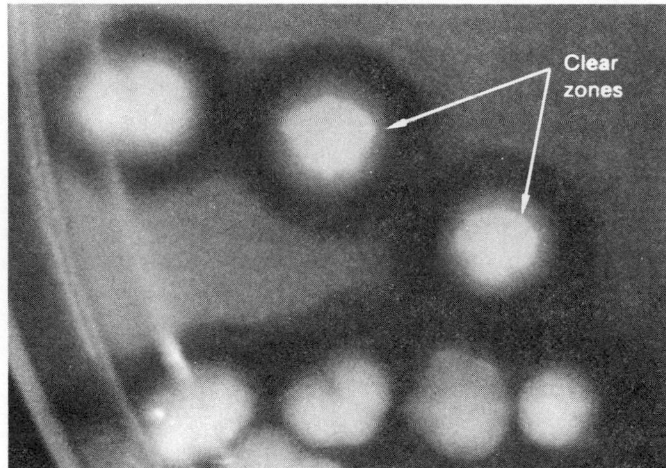

FIG. 13–2 Bacteria growing on casein (milk) agar. The clear zone demonstrates the ability of the bacterial enzymes to digest materials in the environment of the cells.

Carbon and Energy Sources

Carbon is the most basic structural element of all living forms. Organisms obtain it from organic nutrients (carbohydrates, lipids, and proteins) and from carbon dioxide. The ***catabolism*** (metabolic decomposition) of organic compounds produces amino acids, sugar, fatty acids, and other related compounds. Such materials may function in ***anabolism*** (constructive metabolism), thus producing the enzymatic and structural proteins, nucleic acids, carbohydrates, and other biochemical compounds required by the organism. The same compounds may be involved in energy metabolism, producing the impetus for growth and reproduction, or as storage products rich in energy-yielding chemical bonds.

Carbohydrate sources of energy and carbon include starch, glycogen, various pentose (five-carbon) monosaccharides and hexose (six-carbon) monosaccharides, and disaccharides such as lactose, sucrose, and maltose. To utilize the polysaccharides (starch and glycogen), the organism must produce extracellular enzymes to break the complex compound down into smaller molecules that can enter the cell. The enzyme amylase, for example, degrades starch into maltose units, which can then be transported into the cell. Subsequently, the enzyme maltase splits maltose into two glucose units for use in further metabolic activities. This catabolism not only yields building blocks for protein, polysaccharide, lipid, and nucleic acid biosynthesis, but results in the production of energy with which cells can perform anabolic reactions.

Vitamins and Growth Factors

Several of the vitamins important in treatment of human nutritional deficiency diseases are also required by microorganisms. Certain microorganisms are capable of synthesizing their own required vitamins; others must obtain them from their nutrient medium. Vitamin compounds that have been shown effective in microbial nutrition include thiamine chloride, riboflavin, nicotinic acid, pantothenic acid, pyridoxine, biotin, para-amino benzoic acid, folic acid, cyanocobolamine, and inositol.

Vitamins can function as portions of coenzymes or as integral components of other biologically active materials. A **coenzyme** may be thought of as the active portion of an enzyme when it is associated with the protein component of that enzyme.

Various microorganisms require other growth factors as well. These may be vitamin precursors, such as pimelic acid (the precursor of biotin) and beta-alanine (the precursor of pantothenic acid). They may also include purines and pyrimidines for nucleic acid syntheses.

Some microorganisms appear to have peculiar requirements. For example, ***Hemophilus influenzae*** and certain other bacterial species must have a certain component of hemoglobin for growth, in addition to a complete coenzyme—either nicotine adenine dinucleotide (NAD) or its triphosphate (NADP). The interrelationships of the various vitamins and growth factors are more meaningful with a grasp of certain aspects of metabolism presented in Chapter 14.

Essential Mineral Salts

Various inorganic compounds are also essential for microbial nutrition. These include phosphates, which are required in nucleic acid synthesis, and sulfates, which may be needed in the formation of certain amino acids. Potassium, magnesium, manganese, iron, and calcium serve as inorganic cofactors for particular enzymes or may be incorporated into several biochemical reactions. For example, iron is a constituent of cytochromes, which are important in energy metabolism. Calcium is a major component of bacterial spores. Inorganic nutrients required in trace amounts include cobalt, copper, zinc, and molybdenum. Such inorganics are components of special enzymes and are believed to be required by most, if not all, life. Some organisms have special mineral requirements. The diatoms (Color Photograph 4b) require silicon for formation of their cell walls if they are to grow.

Water and Osmotic Pressure

The bacterial cell is approximately 80 percent water and must be in intimate contact with a water supply for its survival, growth, and reproduction. Such contact may involve the presence of a mass of cells on a moist, solid surface or a cell suspension in a liquid medium. When nutrient media are prepared, the various ingredients are dissolved in distilled water, not tap water. Distilled water is used in order to minimize the presence of excess inorganic salts or extraneous organic compounds that may be in tap water. Since tap water may vary in its mineral and dissolved solids composition from day to day, more consistent preparations are obtained with distilled water.

The osmotic pressure (osmolarity) of a suitably prepared medium is comparable to, or at least does not vary greatly from, that found in the microorganism, a condition referred to as *isotonic*. Normal changes in osmotic pressure, caused by the utilization of a medium's components or by partial dehydration of the medium, are not usually sufficient to prevent the growth of the organism.

When cells are taken from an isotonic situation and placed in distilled water at lower osmotic pressure (a *hypotonic* condition), water will enter the cells. This is caused by the greater concentration of dissolved substances within the cell in comparison to the distilled water. Since the dissolved solids cannot distribute themselves because of the microbial membrane, the water molecules are pulled into the cells. In most cases the bacterial cell wall is rigid enough to withstand the increased pressure caused by the incoming water molecules. However, some cells will burst, a condition called **plasmoptysis.** Plasmoptysis occurs more readily in animal cells than in plant or microbial cells, because of the absence of a rigid cell wall. Probably the best example of this reaction is the production of red blood cells *stroma*, or ghosts, caused by introducing whole blood into distilled water. The cell membranes are stretched sufficiently to release most of their cytoplasmic components. Apparently, little holes are temporarily created during this reaction that subsequently close or heal.

When cells are placed into a solution of greater osmolarity or *hypertonicity*, water molecules escape from them, creating a shrinkage known as **plasmolysis.** In this phenomenon, the cytoplasm becomes concentrated and will usually pull away from the cell wall of Gram-negative bacteria but not necessarily of Gram-positive bacteria. In erythrocytes, which have no walls, entire units shrink.

Preparation of Media

Laboratory media have been devised for the cultivation of specific microorganisms to suit their particular growth requirements. As a rule, media of this type can be obtained in dehydrated form from commercial supply companies. Reconstitution is simple. The required weight of the powdered medium is added to distilled water and heated gently to dissolve and mix the ingredients of the preparation. Adjustment in pH may be necessary before the medium is dispensed into smaller vessels. Once this has been done, the medium is sterilized with a high-pressure steam system (autoclaved) according to the directions of the supplier.

Certain components of media, such as serum, plasma, some carbohydrates, and vitamins, are destroyed or inactivated by heat. These components are usually sterilized by filtration and then aseptically introduced into the remaining portion of the medium. It is also possible to filter sterilize the entire medium.

Media Usage and Categories

The cultivation of microorganisms may be necessary for any of the following reasons: the isolation and identification of organisms; the determination of antibiotic sensitivities of pathogens isolated from patients; sterility testing of products destined for human use; food and water analyses; environmental control; antibiotic and vitamin assays; industrial testing; and the preparation of biological products such as materials used for immunizations. The choice of which medium to use for a specific purpose is important and can be a problem. Hundreds of formulations in dehydrated or completed form exist. (Recently, a wide range of sterile, prepackaged, and ready-to-use broth and agar media have become commercially available.) The selection of media can be influenced by such factors as availability and cost, personal habit and experience, preferences of instructors or of chief laboratory personnel, and reported research findings. It should be noted that the most efficient laboratory is not necessarily the one with the greatest variety of media. Efficient performance and results depend on carefully chosen media. The following sections will present the different categories of media used for the cultivation of microorganisms and representative examples of each.

Differential Media

Several combinations of nutrients and pH indicators can be used to produce a visual differentiation of several microorganisms growing on the same medium (Color Photographs 62 and 63). A ***differential medium*** is one that supports the growth of various species while providing an environment that makes it easier to distinguish among different organisms. For example, an ***enriched*** medium such as blood agar can be used to differentiate among many bacterial species belonging to the genus *Streptococcus*. For this group of organisms, approximately 5 to 10 percent sheep blood is added to a base medium (for example, blood-agar base), which is sterilized separately and cooled before the sheep blood is added. Because of the enzymes and other compounds they produce, colonies of different streptococci leave different visual signs on the medium. Based on these effects, a limited classification can be established. A green discoloration of areas around bacterial colonies means alpha (α) hemolysis (hemolysis is the destruction of red blood cells); clear zones surrounding bacterial colonies means beta (β) hemolysis; and no obvious effect means gamma (γ) hemolysis. The typical appearance is shown in Color Photograph 58. (These hemolytic reactions are not limited to streptococci. Other organisms are capable of producing similar effects.)

In addition to different sources of mammalian blood, carbohydrates, proteins, and other nutrients are used for differentiation purposes. The pH indicators may also be included in media. Those most commonly employed are bromothymol blue, neutral red, and phenol red (Color Photographs 64 and 74).

Selective Media

A preparation that can interfere with or prevent the growth of certain microorganisms while permitting the growth of others is a ***selective medium***. Selective media provide a means for isolating a particular species or category of microorganisms. Among the substances that can be used as selective agents are dyes such as crystal violet, eosine Y, methylene blue, and brilliant green, all of which inhibit Gram-positives. Bile salts and high concentrations of sodium chloride may also be used. A medium can be made selective by adjusting its pH to a very high or very low level, thus permitting the growth of some organisms and inhibiting others. A well-known example of a selective medium is Sabouraud's glucose agar with a pH of 5.6, used for fungus cultivation (Color Photographs 34 and 35). The most recent substances employed to make culture media selective are antibiotics such as cycloheximide, kanamycin, neomycin, and vancomycin.

Selective and Differential Media

Many media are both selective and differential. The properties of both types of media are combined for the purpose of identifying and enumerating organisms in one general procedure (Color Photograph 62 and 63).

MACCONKEY AGAR

This medium is used in the selection of Gram-negative enteric bacteria. The bile salts and crystal violet in MacConkey agar (frequently called Mac agar) inhibit the growth of Gram-positive organisms. Bile salts function by reducing surface tension, which apparently is inhibitory to these microorganisms. Crystal violet inhibits a critical step in the synthesis of cell walls of certain Gram-positive bacteria. The carbohydrate lactose serves as the differentiating substance when it is fermented, or broken down.

MANNITOL SALT AGAR

This medium can be used not only to select for a particular bacterial species, but also to differentiate potentially pathogenic organisms from those of a nonpathogenic nature. Mannitol Salt agar is used most often for *Staphylococcus aureus*. In addition to the carbohydrate mannitol, Mannitol Salt agar contains 7.5 percent sodium chloride and the pH indicator phenol red. Potentially pathogenic staphylococci grow on this preparation and ferment mannitol, producing acid. In the presence of acid, the normally light red preparation turns yellow. A typical reaction with a pathogenic *S. aureus* is shown in Color Photograph 74.

The ingredients and applications of many differential, selective, and selective and differential media are discussed in the chapters concerned with particular disease-causing agents. Before leaving this topic, it is important to note that the concentrations of the differentiating and selective components can be critical to achieving desired results. Too little of an ingredient may not accomplish the effect, and an overabundance may inhibit the growth of the microorganism sought.

Other Media

Certain pathogens are today cultured routinely on modified versions of media used many years ago. For example, *Corynebacterium diphtheriae*, the etiologic agent of diphtheria, is routinely cultivated on a modification of the original preparation described by Loeffler in 1887. This medium contains beef blood serum, beef extract, tryptose (peptone), dextrose, sodium chloride, and distilled water. Another organism, *Mycobacterium tuberculosis*, is still grown on the egg-base medium formulated by Lowenstein in 1931 and modified by Jensen in 1932. The medium contains water, eggs, the amino acid asparagine, potassium phosphate, magnesium sulfate, magnesium citrate, potato flour, and malachite green. The last of these is inhibitory for most bacteria other than the mycobacteria found in clinical specimens.

Media for the Cultivation of Anaerobes

Fortunately, most pathogenic anaerobes encountered are heterotrophic and do not require unusual growth factors (are not "fastidious"). Thus, most of these organisms can be cultivated routinely and identified without the use of complicated equipment (Figure 27–4) or complex media. Quite often, the same media may be used for both aerobes and anaerobes, providing that they support adequate growth.

Basically, procedures for cultivation and/or identification of anaerobic bacteria are much like those for aerobes. Many of the specific techniques are identical aside from the incubation atmosphere.

Broth media vary in composition. Some contain a beef extract preparation and partially hydrolyzed proteins (peptones). The beef extract, which is obtained by soaking ground meat in water, usually contains carbohydrates, minerals, peptones, proteins, and vitamins. The peptones provide peptides and amino acids. In other media, a water extract of disrupted yeast may be substituted for the beef extract. The yeast extract usually contains more of the B-complex vitamins. Sodium and various phosphates and chlorides are added. The sodium serves primarily to ensure a suitable osmotic pressure in the medium; the phosophates provide a buffering action against the acids produced by the metabolic activities of cultured organisms. A reducing agent such as sodium thioglycollate may also be incorporated into a medium for the cultivation of microaerophilic and certain anaerobic bacteria.

With a preparation such as thioglycollate medium, anerobic conditions are maintained by two reducing agents, L-cystine and agar, in addition to the thioglycollic acid. Although agar is used as a solidifying agent for many media, its 0.075 percent concentration here is insufficient for this purpose. Here agar functions as an adjunct to the other reducing agents in the medium.

Resazurin serves as an oxidation-reduction indicator. This compound is colorless or nearly colorless in its reduced state, thereby indicating the existence of anaerobic conditions. When oxidized, it turns pink or red, indicating an aerobic state. A sterile tube of this medium suitable for the growth of aerobes, microaerophiles, and several but not all anaerobes will have an upper pink layer and a lower yellow to light brown layer (see Color Photograph 59). Aerobic organisms grow well in the upper region, anaerobes in the lower zone (Figure 13–3).

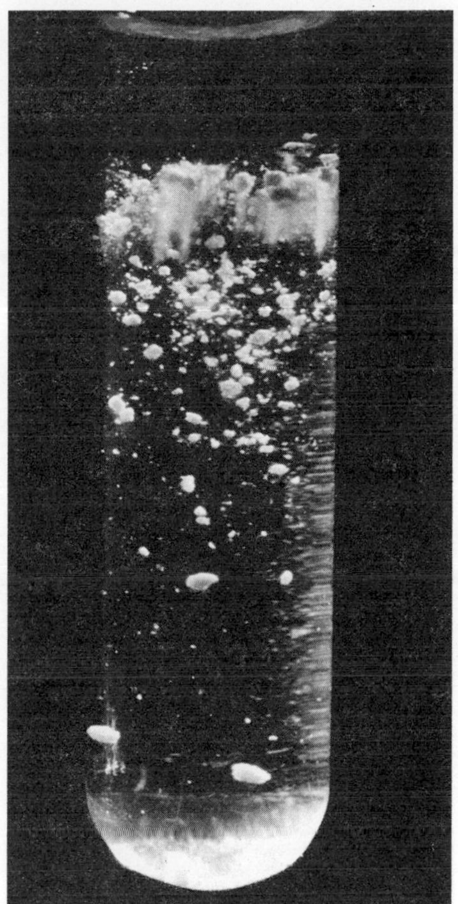

FIG. 13–3 *Arachina propionica.* The appearance of anaerobic growth in fluid thioglycollate medium. Notice the lack of growth near the surface where some oxygen is present. *Gerencser, M. A., and J. M. Slack,* J. Bacteriol. 94:*109–115 (1967).*

Prereduced Anaerobically Sterilized Media

Prereduced anaerobically sterilized media, when used properly, greatly increase the chances of isolating many fastidious anaerobic bacteria. Prereduced anaerobically sterilized media are prepared, dispensed, sterilized, and stoppered in an oxygen-free nitrogen environment, preventing any exposure to oxygen. In order to maintain the exclusion of air during inoculations, a stream of nitrogen or carbon dioxide without any free oxygen is directed into the tube as it is inoculated. Various media of this kind are commercially available.

STORAGE OF MEDIA

Most media can be stored under conditions that prevent dehydration. Media are usually kept refrigerated or in airtight packaging. In either case, the media should first be incubated overnight to determine if sterilization was adequate. All media found to be contaminated should be sterilized and then discarded.

Inoculation and Transfer Techniques

Once the medium is selected and prepared, the next step in culturing a microorganism is inoculation of the medium with the specimen. This is accomplished by use of an inoculating loop (Figure 13–4) or its modified form, the inoculating needle.

The inoculating or transfer tool basically consists of a thin piece of heat-resistant wire, usually platinum or stainless steel, measuring 2 to 3 inches in length, and usually provided with a short handle.

Most types of media, such as broth, agar plates, and slants, may be inoculated with either a transfer loop or a needle. However, the loop is usually used with liquid inocula sources of cultures.

The inoculation and transfer techniques are important to master because they are routinely part of many bacteriological procedures. In addition to inoculation, they may be used for isolation and characterization of pure cultures; transfer of microbial growth from one medium to another; preparation of samples for microscopic examination—smears, hanging-drop, or temporary wet mounts; and maintenance of stock cultures of organisms.

The steps in a typical tube inoculation are shown in Figures 13–4a and b. A tube containing the inoculum and one or more tubes with sterile media are held together in one hand, supported by the three middle fingers. The thumb functions to keep the tubes in proper postion. The inoculating tool, which is in the other hand, is passed through a flame (flamed)—heated to redness to incinerate any organisms on its surface. Next, the plugs of the tubes are grasped by the little and ring fingers of the hand holding the inoculating tool. The mouths of these tubes are passed through the flame. This flaming creates convection currents that prevent air-borne contaminants from falling into the tubes. The heating may also kill some organisms on the glass and prevent them from contaminating any other media or the individual holding the cultures.

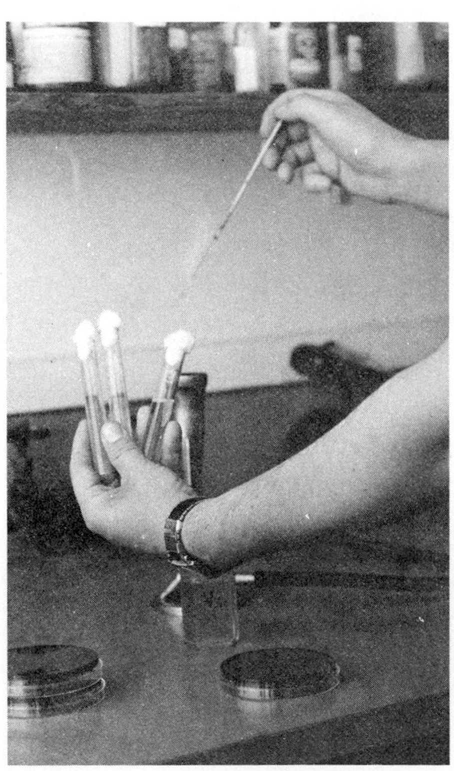
(a)

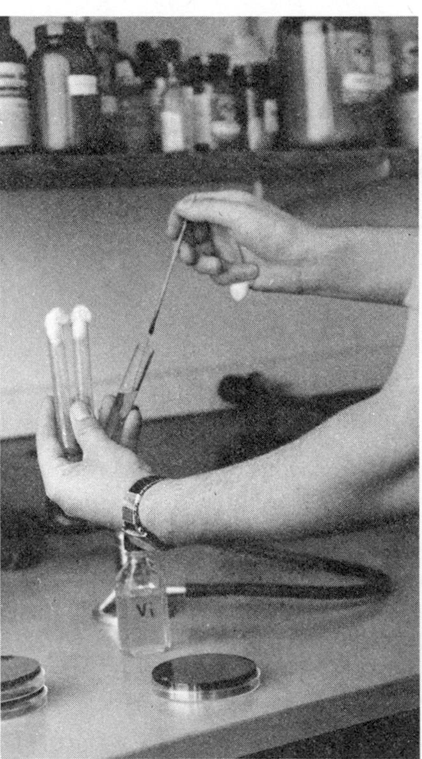
(b)

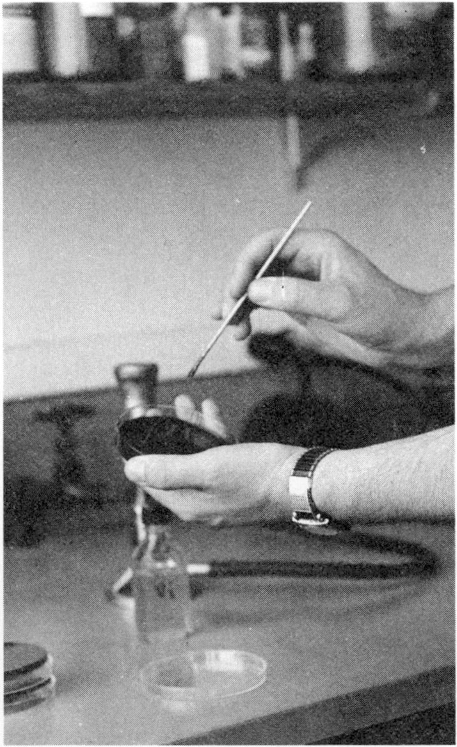
(c)

FIG. 13–4 Inoculation and transfer techniques. (a) Flaming the inoculating tool. Note that the entire wire portion must turn red-hot in order to eliminate undesirable microorganisms. (b) Transferring the inoculum to two sterile tubes of broth. The mouths of both tubes must be flamed before and after the transfer, as must the inoculating tool. Note how the cotton plug is grasped. (c) Streaking an agar plate. This procedure involves spreading an inoculum over the surface of the medium.

When inoculum is obtained and introduced into the proper tubes, the lips of the tubes are again passed through the flame, and each plug is inserted into the same tube from which it was removed. Once again the inoculating loop is flamed to redness.

This technique is carried out to prevent the introduction of contaminating organisms, collectively referred to as *sepsis*. Hence, the term **aseptic technique** is used for procedures of this type.

Other means for the transfer of microorganisms include sterile pipettes, cotton applicator swabs, and syringes. The device used is determined by the needs of the particular situation.

After inoculation, certain cultural characteristics, such as pigmentation, type of growth on agar slants, pellicle formation, and colonial appearance of organisms can be observed (Figures 13–5 and 13–6 and Color Photographs 21 and 22). Such properties are often useful in describing a particular bacterial species.

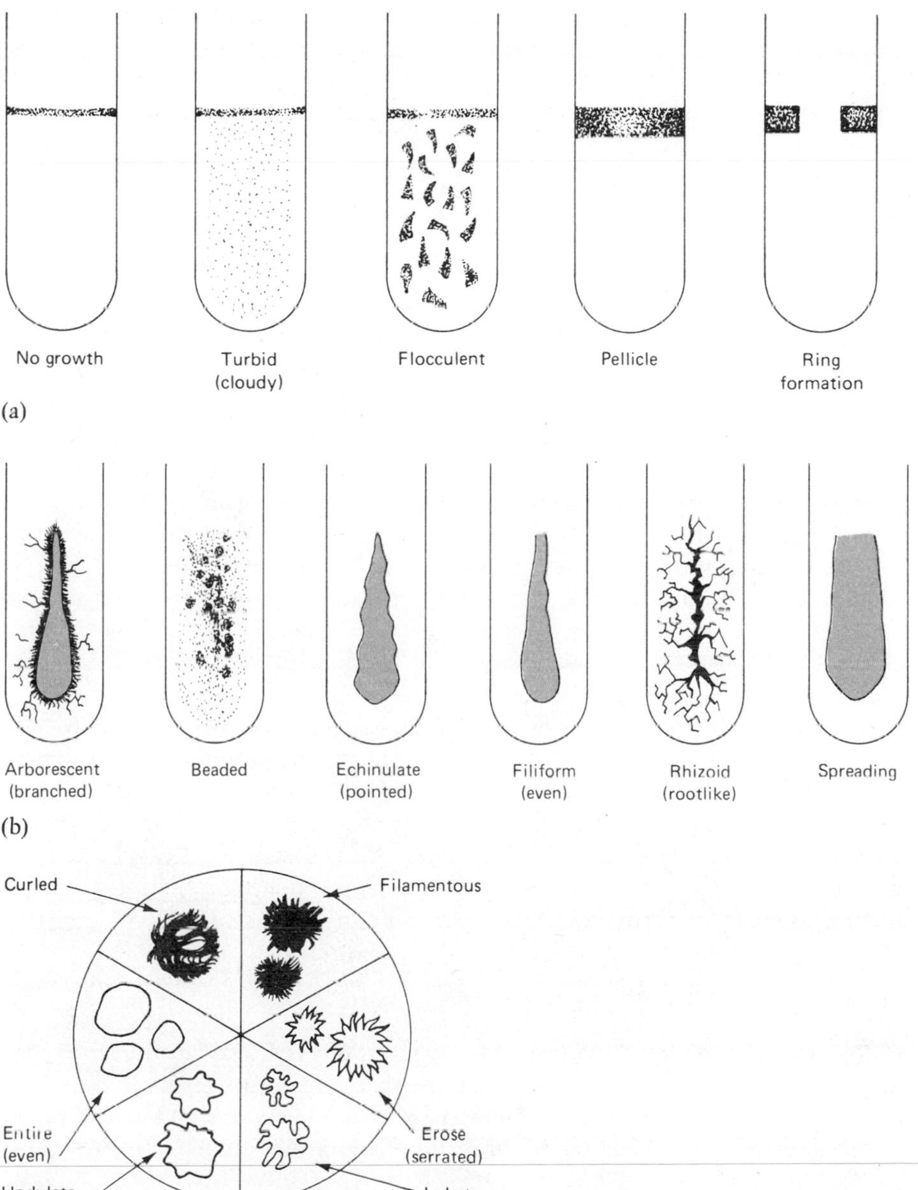

FIG. 13-5 Cultural characteristics of bacteria. (a) Selected features of broth cultures. (b) Agar slant strokes. In this case the inoculum is introduced to the base of the slant and drawn along the surface from this region to the end of the slant. (c) Some margin characteristics of bacterial colonies.

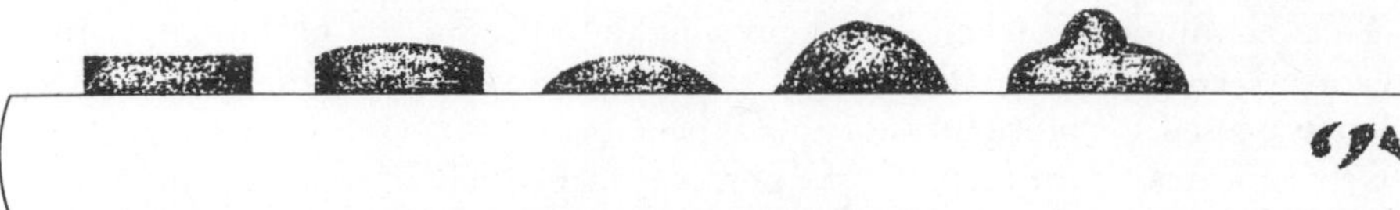

FIG. 13-5 (d) Elevation characteristics of bacterial colonies.

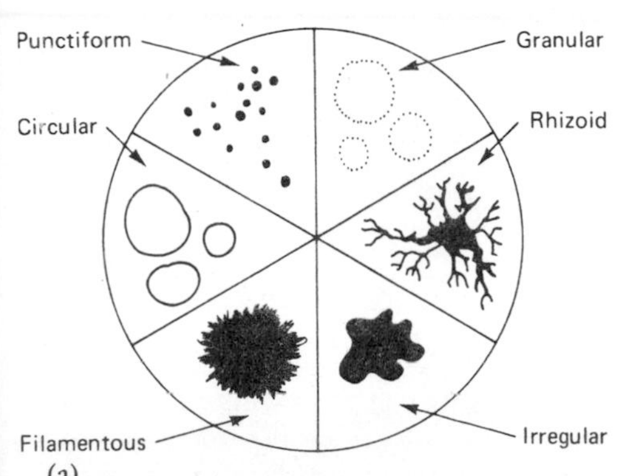

(a)

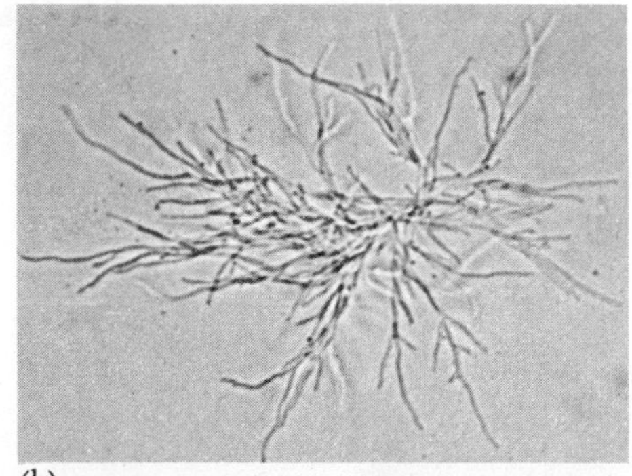
(b)

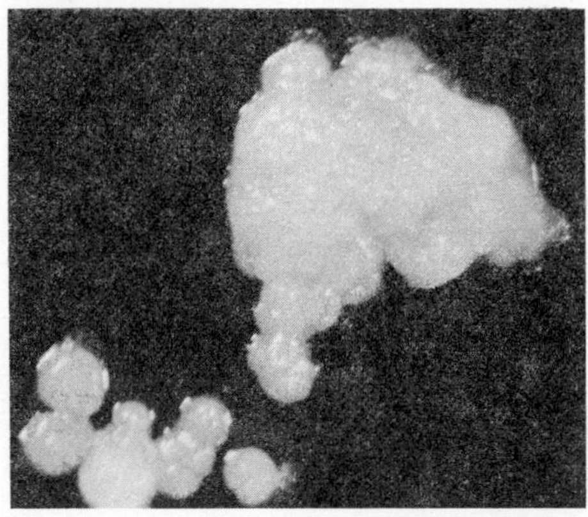
(c)

FIG. 13-6 Selected characteristics of bacterial colonies. (a) Diagrammatic representation of colonial forms of growth. *Gerencser, M. A., and J. M. Slack,* J. Bacteriol. 94:*109 (1967).* (b) A developing microcolony of *Actinomyces propionicus.* Note the filamentous nature of the organism. (c) A "molar" tooth colony of the same organism, shown in its mature form.

Techniques for the Isolation of Pure Bacterial Cultures

The isolation and the subsequent identification of a bacterial species are important facets of microbiology. Many techniques can be effectively used to detect and enumerate different microorganisms present in specimens. Among these procedures, two methods, the ***pour-plate*** and ***streak-plate techniques*** (Color Photographs 60 and 61), have become indispensable to the bacteriologist.

Whichever isolation technique is used, its effectiveness can be greatly increased by using differential or selective culture media, such as Eosin Methylene Blue Agar and Hektoen Enteric media (Color Photographs 62 and 63).

The Pour-plate Technique

The forerunner of the present pour-plate method (Color Photograph 61) was developed in the laboratory of the famous bacteriologist Robert Koch. Today this technique consists of cooling melted agar-containing medium (1.5 percent agar) to approximately 42° to 45°C, inoculating the medium with a specimen, and immediately pouring it into a sterile Petri plate, allowing the freshly poured medium to solidify and incubating the preparation at the desired temperature. When the magnitude of the bacterial population in the specimen is not known beforehand, suitable dilutions must be created in order to ensure that the colonies will be isolated. By means of the pour-plate method, bacteria are distributed throughout the agar and are trapped in position as the medium solidifies. Although the medium restricts bacterial movement from one area to another, it is soft enough to permit growth, which occurs both on the surface and in the depths of the inoculated medium.

In addition to the use of this procedure to isolate and detect bacterial species in a mixed culture, it is also useful in quantitative measurements of bacterial growth. Unfortunately, however, this technique has several drawbacks. Colonies of several species may present a similar appearance in the agar environment, thus making differentiation difficult. Also, certain species of bacteria may not grow under the cultural conditions of the method. And, finally, removing colonies for further study may be difficult.

The Streak-plate Technique

The streak-plate technique (Color Photograph 60) was also developed in the laboratory of Robert Koch—this time by bacteriologists Friedrich Loeffler and Georg Gaffky. The modern method for the preparation of a streak-plate involves spreading a single loopful of material containing microorganisms over the surface of a solidified agar medium. Figure 13-7 shows streaking methods that have been used.

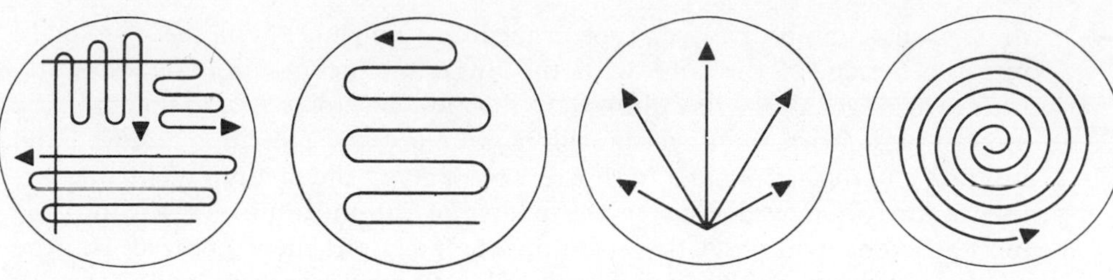

FIG. 13–7 Representative streaking patterns used in the isolation of bacteria.

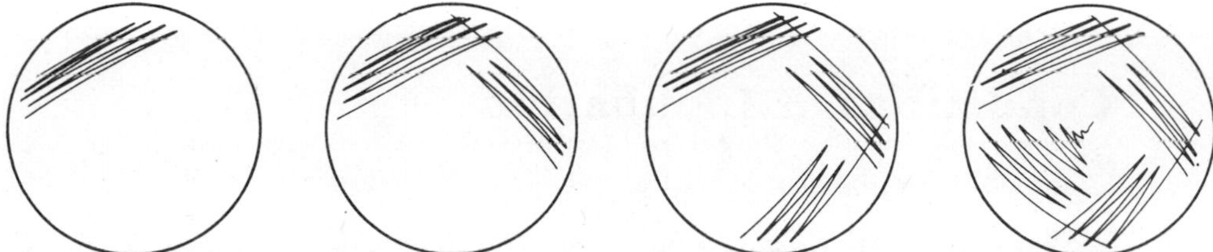

FIG. 13–8 The clock-plate method of streaking.

The clock-plate technique is one of the more common forms of this procedure (Figures 13–8 and 13–9). First the inoculum is spread over a small portion of the medium's surface. Then the inoculating loop is flamed to destroy any residual bacteria, and the plate containing the medium is rotated approximately one quarter of a turn. The flamed loop is next used to make a second set of streaks, thus diluting (spreading) the bacterial population in the original set of streaks. As Figure 13–8 shows, the original surface streaks are crossed only once. Further dilutions of the specimen are carried out by repeating this sequence—flaming the loop, rotating the medium, and making additional streaks.

If this technique is properly performed, well-isolated colonies should grow after incubation at an appropriate temperature (Color Photograph 60). One colony is supposed to develop from a single cell, thereby producing a pure culture. It is customary to "pick" (transfer) a small portion of a desired colony to a tube of medium, such as broth or agar slant, and utilize the culture as a source of organisms for additional studies.

Another technique, the spread-plate procedure, is used in certain types of investigations. Here a bacterial specimen is placed on an agar medium and spread over its surface with the aid of a sterile bent glass rod. The agar plate can be placed on a rotating wheel device to aid the spreading out of the bacterial specimen.

Because of the high concentration of water in agar preparations, condensation forms in most Petri plates. Water of condensation on media surfaces may cause bacterial colonies to run together. Plates are therefore incubated in an inverted position.

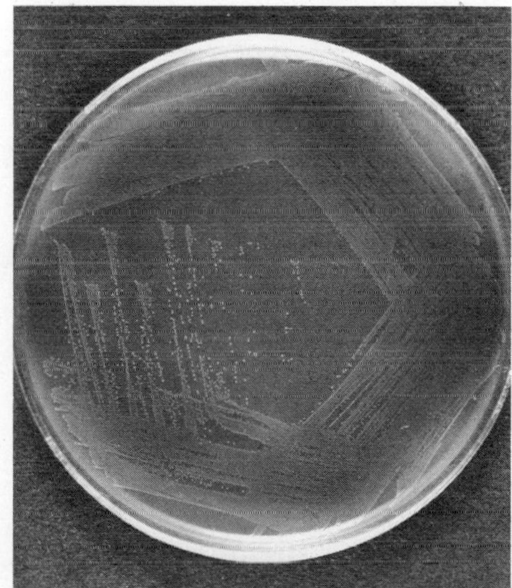

FIG. 13–9 A clear demonstration of the clock-plate technique. Note the isolated colonies of *Moraxella phenylpyruvica*. (See Color Photograph 60.) *Riley, P. S., et al.,* Appl. Microbiol. 28:355 *(1974).*

Anaerobic Transfer

The lack of growth of many clinical isolates may not be due to the oxidation-reduction potential of the properly prepared anaerobic medium, but instead to brief exposure to air during the specimen collection or transportation to the laboratory, or, after growth, during the transfer of organisms to subculture media. In order to prevent inactivation of anaerobes, transfer should be performed under a flowing stream of nitrogen for cultures on solid media or by the use of a pipette for liquid media. For example, in the transfer of cultures from thioglycollate broth to a fresh tube of medium, a pipette should be introduced into the bottom of the tube with the finger on the mouthpiece. Carefully lifting the finger allows inoculum from the most anaerobic area to flow into the pipette. Next, with the finger on the mouthpiece, the pipette is removed and inserted into the bottom of a fresh tube of thioglycollate medium. The finger is then quickly removed, causing the release of the inoculum—again into the most anaerobic portion of the medium. The pipette is then removed, and the newly inoculated preparation is incubated at the desired temperature.

Conditions of Incubation

Aerobic Incubation

Microbial growth, as noted previously, can depend upon suitable levels of oxygen and carbon dioxide. While aerobic organisms may be able to grow under anaerobic conditions, the obligate aerobes must be in intimate contact with air, or approximately 20 percent oxygen. Many organisms have less stringent oxygen requirements and will grow well in the depths of liquid or solid media. Therefore, cultivation of aerobic or facultative anaerobic bacteria is relatively simple under usual laboratory conditions.

Once an appropriate solid or liquid medium has been inoculated and protected from contamination, all that remains to be controlled is the temperature and occasionally the level of humidity. Standard laboratory incubators are usually sufficient to maintain such environmental factors.

With any incubator, it is advisable to employ a maximum-minimum thermometer to determine the temperature range provided by the thermostatic control. The thermometer registers the highest and lowest temperature values in any given time and assures that the incubator is functioning properly.

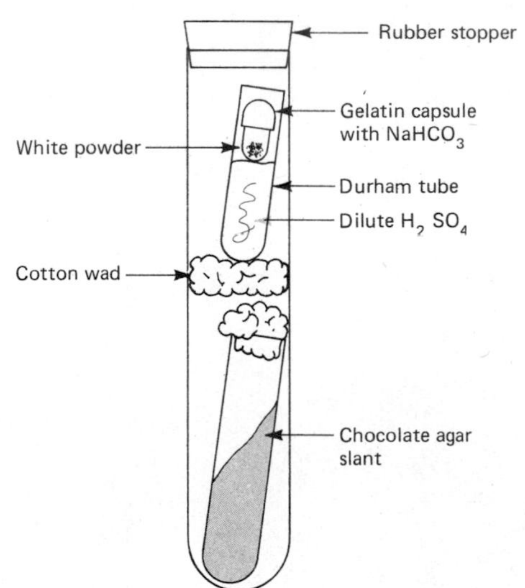

FIG. 13-10 The test tube capneic system. A capsule of sodium bicarbonate ($NaHCO_3$) is added to a small tube of dilute sulfuric acid (H_2SO_4) and the large tube is immediately stoppered. The reaction is the same as that used in fire extinguishers—acidification of bicarbonate to release carbon dioxide (CO_2). The example shown is a chocolate agar slant culture inoculated with *Neisseria gonorrhoeae.*

Capneic Incubation

Air enriched with carbon dioxide is required by some bacteria, including *Neisseria gonorrhoeae, N. meningitidis,* and *Brucella* spp., for primary isolation from clinical specimens. What's more, many other microorganisms, such as *Mycobacterium tuberculosis,* appear to grow better under capneic conditions. An atmosphere enriched with carbon dioxide can be supplied in a variety of ways. The candle jar technique is routinely used for *N. gonorrhoeae* cultivation. With this technique, Petri plates or tubes with inoculated media are placed in a jar with a candle. The lighted candle continues to burn after the lid has been placed on the jar, until the carbon dioxide concentration increases enough to stop combustion, usually around 3 to 5 percent carbon dioxide. This does not represent complete combustion of oxygen, as aerobic organisms will grow and strict anaerobes will not grow in such a candle jar.

To maintain capneic conditions for cultures on slanted media, the test tube capneic system should be considered (Figure 13–10). In this system a capsule of sodium bicarbonate is added to a small tube of dilute sulfuric acid and the large tube is immediately stoppered. The reaction here is the same as that used in fire extinguishers: acidification of bicarbonate to release carbon dioxide.

Anaerobic Incubation

Incubation under anaerobic conditions can be accomplished with vacuum devices. Incubators for this use are usually fitted with gaskets and ports by

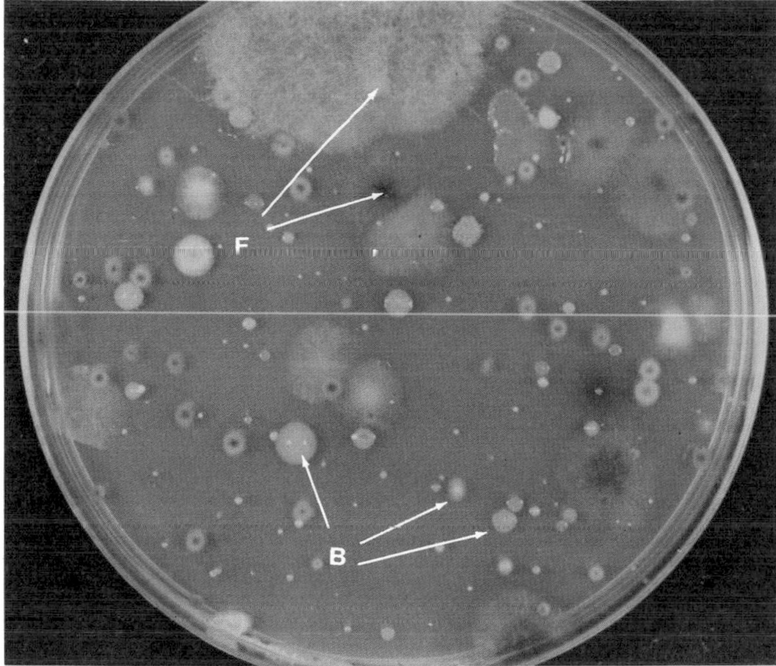

Fig. 1. The appearance of bacterial (b) and fungal (f) growth. After exposing a Petri dish containing a nutrient mixture to room air, colonies of different microorganisms developed within 24 to 48 hours.

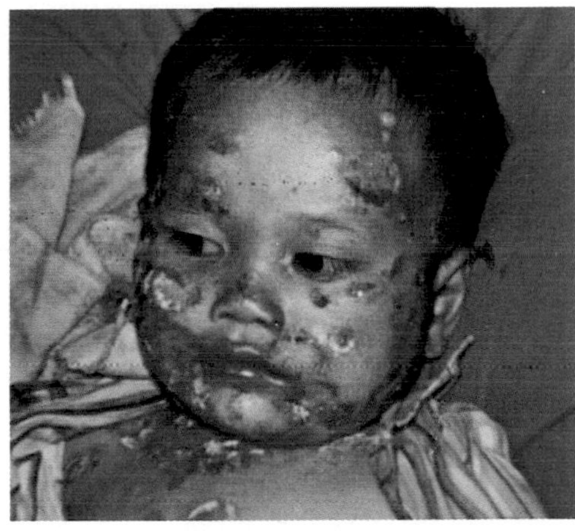

Fig. 2. Impetigo, one of many different types of infection caused by bacteria. *From Allen, A. M., D. Taplin, and L. Twigg,* Arch. Derm., *104:271 (1971).*

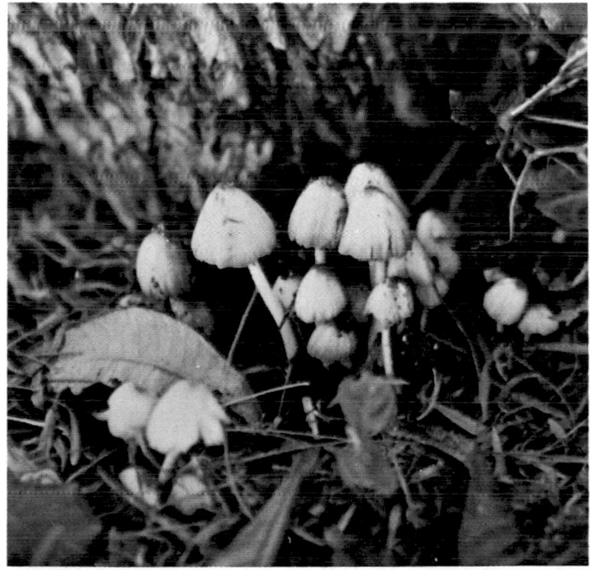

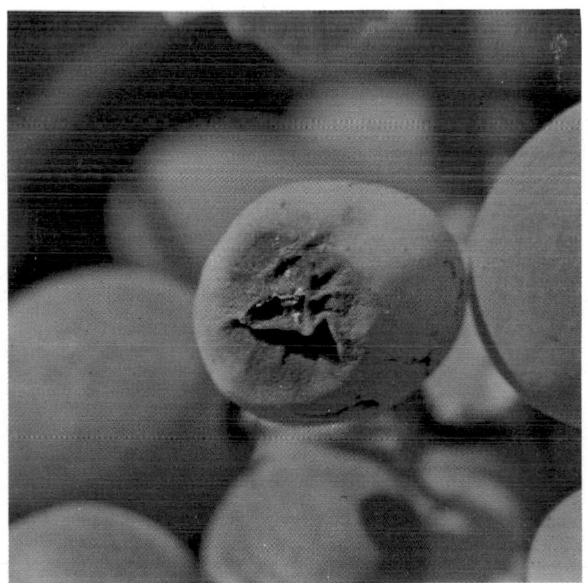

Fig. 3. The many forms of fungi. *(Above) Mycena* species are a common mushroom in areas of rotting and decaying wood and leaves. Over 200 different types of the mycenas are found in North America. *(Right)* An example of the spoilage of agricultural products caused by fungi. On the center Tokay grape, the black, dry fungal growth is obvious.

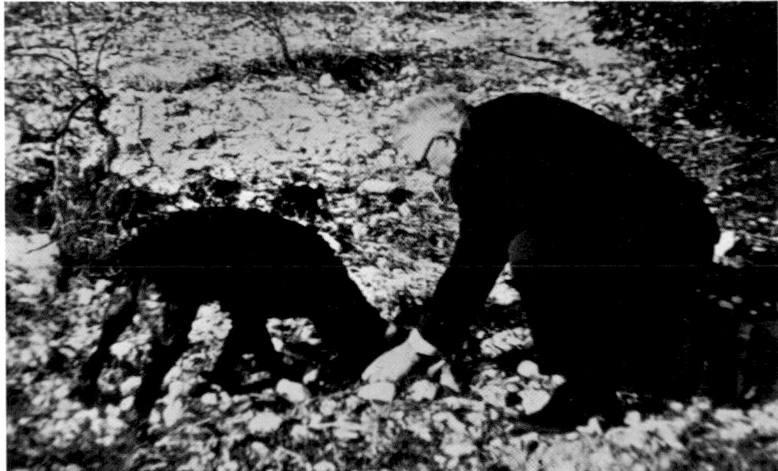

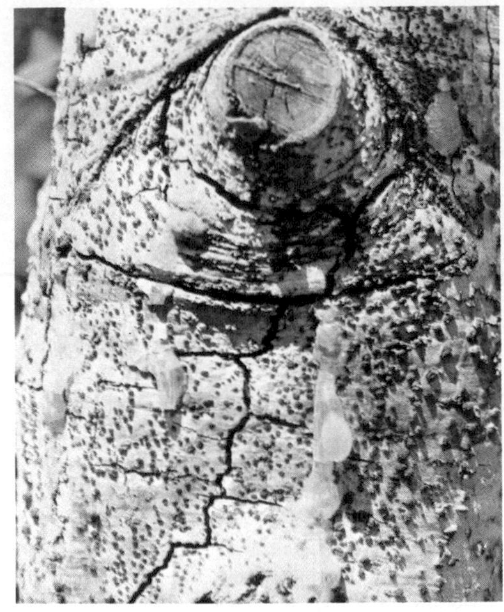

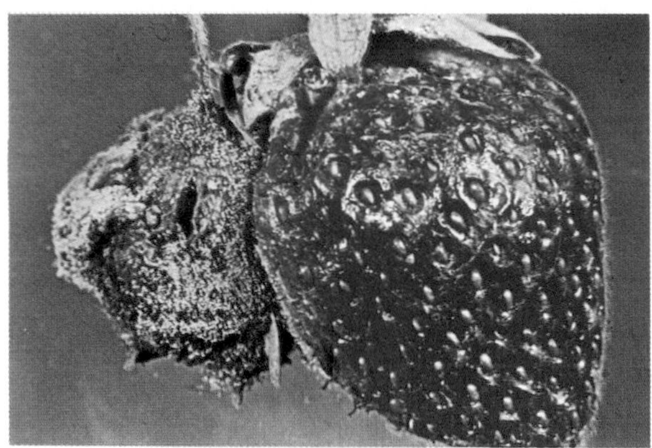

Fig. 37. *(Above left)* A truffle hunt. Trained dogs or pigs are used to search for these particularly edible mushrooms. Most of the desirable truffles are found in France and Italy under oak and beech trees. The truffle grows from 1 to 6 inches below the soil. Although it cannot be seen, the scent can be detected by dogs or pigs. *Courtesy of Food and Wines from France, Inc. Photo by Alain Robert.*

Fig. 38. *(Above right)* Effects of a fungus attack. This Formosan sweet gum tree has a stem canker. Note the gummy resin flow and the orange accumulations of fungal ascospores. *From Snow, G. A., et al., 64:602–605 (1974).*

Fig. 39. *(Left)* Significant losses of fruit and vegetable crops occur yearly. The strawberry on one side has been destroyed by a fungus-caused fruit rot. *Courtesy U.S.D.A.*

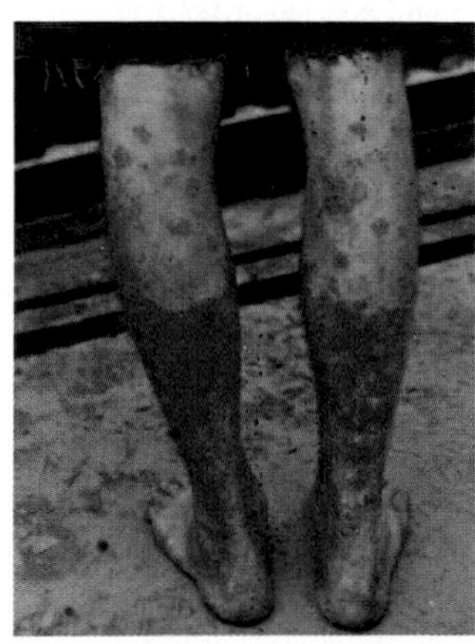

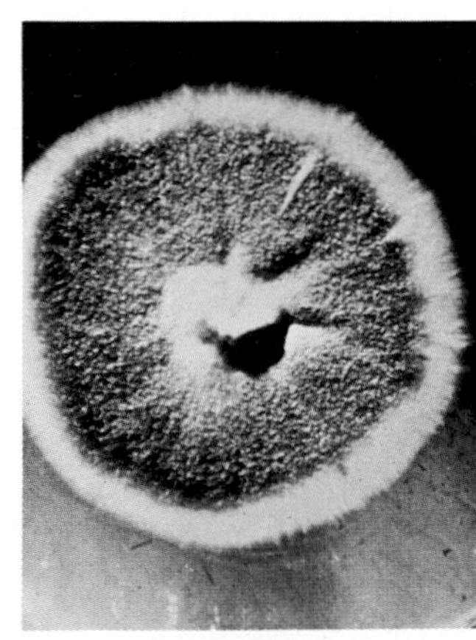

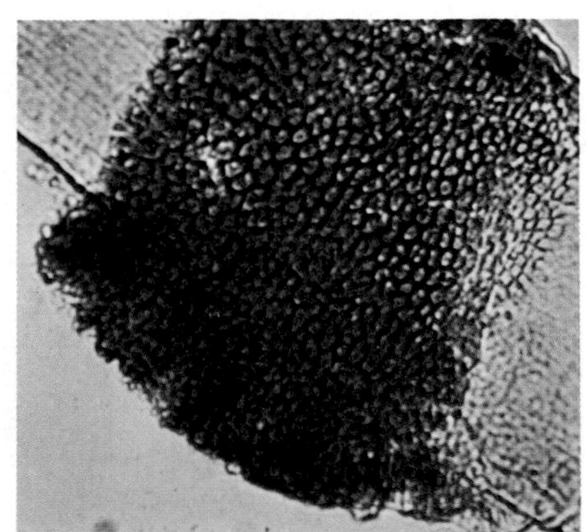

Fig. 40. *(Left)* Disabling ringworm infection on areas of the feet. The patient had been wearing wet boots and socks. This fungus infection, also known as athlete's foot, is a fairly common condition. It generally is much milder in its effects. *From Allen, A. M., and D. Taplin.* JAMA. *226:864 (1973).*

Fig. 41. *(Middle)* The mycelium of *Trichophyton rubrum.* The fungus is a common cause of athlete's foot. *Courtesy of Dr. E. S. Beneke, Department of Botany and Plant Pathology, Michigan State University.*

Fig. 42. *(Right)* The appearance of spores on the surface of a fungus-infected hair. *Courtesy of Dr. E. S. Beneke, Department of Botany and Plant Pathology, Michigan State University.*

which air is removed and inert gases added. One method commonly used involves flushing a specially equipped incubator with 95 percent nitrogen and 5 percent carbon dioxide to remove any oxygen and to introduce carbon dioxide into the system. The latter gas may enhance growth. Hydrogen may also be used for flushing, but it forms an explosive mixture with oxygen. If for some reason anaerobic hydrogen bacteria must be grown in the presence of hydrogen gas, hydrogen should be bubbled through water first; an explosion will not occur with wet hydrogen.

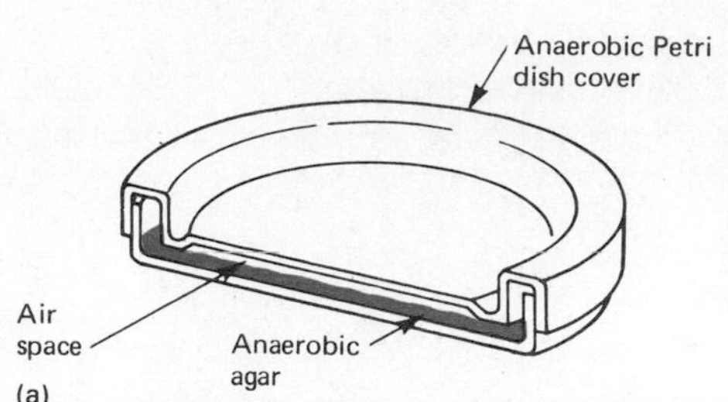

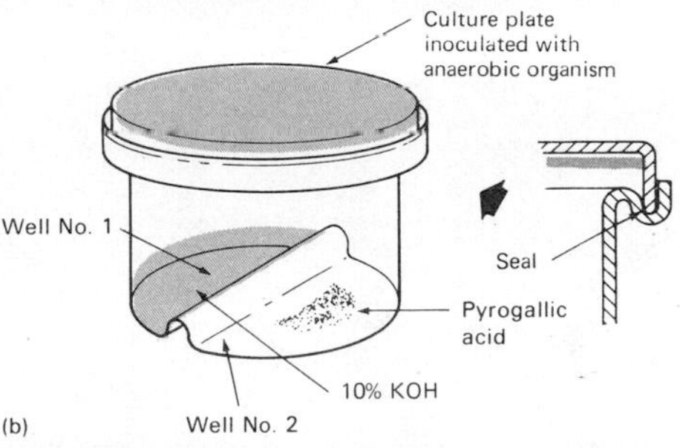

FIG. 13-11 (a) A cut-away drawing of a Brewer Petri dish. (b) Spray dish for anaerobic incubation.

OTHER METHODS OF ANAEROBIC INCUBATION

Before the advent of the anaerobic incubator, two systems for culturing anaerobic bacteria were used. In one system, thioglycollate agar is inoculated and poured into a special Petri dish (Figure 13–11). The cover for this Brewer plate (named for its inventor) forms a seal with the surface of the agar and with the edge of a slight concave opening, to allow a limited surface for organisms to grow on. The trapped oxygen is rapidly reduced by the thioglycollate, thus producing anaerobic conditions.

An alternative to the Brewer plate is the Spray dish (Figure 13–11b). This device consists of a deep, double-well dish and cover. The arrangement of the double wells permits separation of an alkaline solution, such as potassium hydroxide (KOH), from pyrogallic acid. When combined, these chemicals absorb oxygen and produce anaerobic conditions. When this system is used, an inoculated Petri plate is inverted over the bottom dish and sealed into place. The dish is then tipped to mix the chemicals and produce ***anaerobiosis*** (anaerobic conditions).

The Brewer jar was developed to produce a larger incubation system for the anaerobic organisms (Figure 13–12). In this system, the inoculated plates or tubes are placed in the jar, the cover sealed in place, and the container is immediately evacuated and flushed with hydrogen. When a catalyst in the lid (platinum, for example) is heated by an electric current, the hydrogen combines with any remaining oxygen to form water. A slight vacuum is created in the chamber due to the combustion reaction.

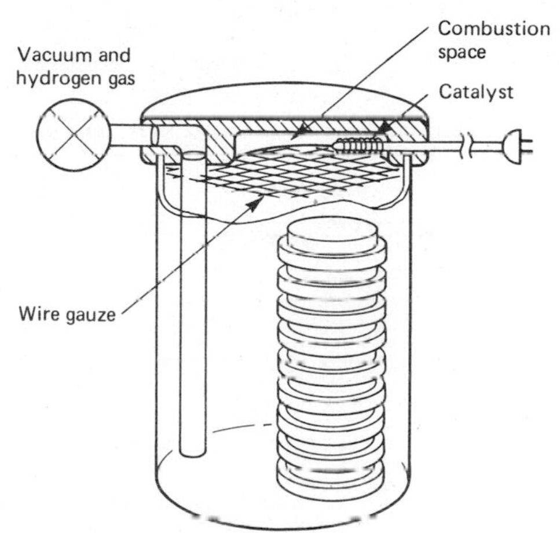

FIG. 13-12 The Brewer anaerobic jar.

A current alternative to the Brewer jar is the Bio Quest disposable Gas Pak. This unit is a self-contained hydrogen-generating and catalyst system, much simpler to use than the Brewer jar. The plates or tubes are placed in the unit with a Gas Pak envelope containing the anaerobic generating system. The envelope is opened, water is added to the reagents, and the self-contained unit is sealed immediately (Figure 13–13). The generation of hydrogen in the presence of air and the catalyst causes reduction of the oxygen to water, which condenses on the side of the unit. This system eliminates the need for hydrogen and nitrogen tanks and vacuum pumps, which greatly enhances the ability of a small clinical laboratory to carry out anaerobic cultivation.

ANAEROBIC INDICATORS

Anaerobic incubation systems should be checked whenever possible to ensure that adequate conditions have been obtained and maintained during incubation. One system used for this purpose incorporates methylene blue as an indicator of oxidation-reduction potential in the medium. It is usually dispensed into small screw-capped vials and autoclaved. This reduces the methylene blue to a colorless state, leucomethylene blue. The procedure for testing involves placing an opened vial of medium in the incubator and initiating the anaerobiosis environment. After a suitable incubation period the vial is removed and examined. If anaerobic conditions were maintained during the

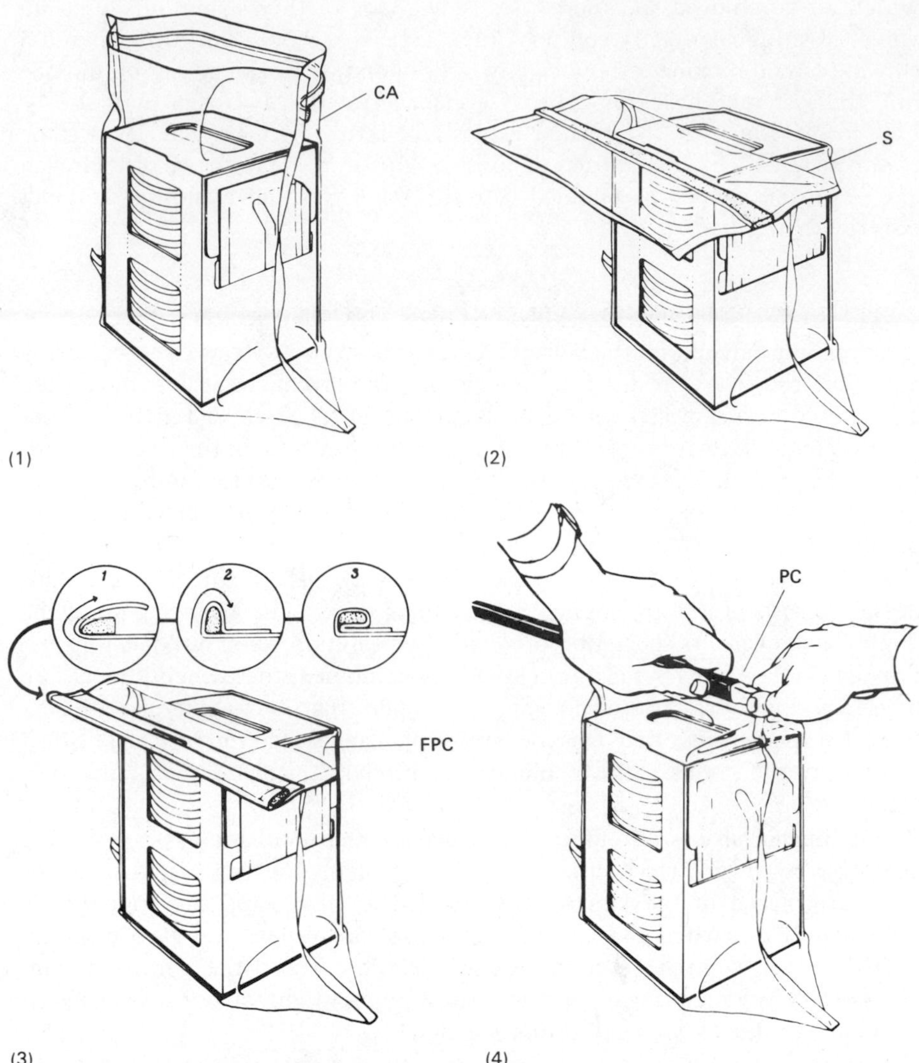

FIG. 13-13 A simple flowchart demonstrating the procedure used for the Gas Pak Disposable Anaerobic System. (1.) Tubes or Petri plates are placed into the carrier. The flaps of the carrier assembly (CA) are closed. (2.) The foil container of a Gas Pak anaerobic indicator is opened (pulled down halfway) and inserted into the slot (S) provided in the carrier assembly. (3.) The incorporation of the hydrogen and carbon dioxide generator envelope and the introduction of water into it is not shown. The entire carrier assembly is placed in the flexible plastic container (FPC), which is folded and pressed flat over the top of the carrier to expel as much air as possible. (4.) The edge of the plastic clamp (PC) is slid along its entire length for clamping purposes. *Courtesy of BioQuest Cockeysville, MD.*

test period, the methylene blue should still be in the colorless reduced state. However, if anaerobiosis was not achieved, the medium will be oxidized and appear blue. (Note that in the first case, the brief exposure to air may cause a slight oxidation of the leucomethylene blue at the surface of the medium.)

Another system for checking an anaerobic incubator involves subculturing an obligate anaerobic bacterium in the same incubator as other specimens. If the indicator organism grows, satisfactory conditions were met. Organisms that may be used for this purpose include certain *Clostridium* and *Bacteroides* spp. However, the use of chemical indicators is recommended because of their simplicity and reliability.

Biological or "Sterility Test" Cabinets

Protection from air-borne contamination is important both for obtaining and maintaining pure cultures and for the safety of those working where microbes are being cultured. Compact cabinets designed for this purpose are shown in Figure 13–14. Such units are valuable in laboratories that handle "biohazardous" substances or that prepare bacteriological media for sterility testing and for inoculation of a variety of media.

Cabinets of this type are equipped with a double transparent viewscreen. Air circulating between the layers creates a "front air barrier" at the opening of the work area (Figure 13–14). This barrier protects both the laboratory personnel and materials from contamination by preventing air-borne particles from leaving or entering the cabinets. Air entering and leaving the working area passes through HEPA (High-Efficiency Particulate Air) filters, which remove particles of 0.3 μm and greater. Although contamination of personnel and materials is prevented in a unit such as this one, workers must still observe aseptic precautions and techniques.

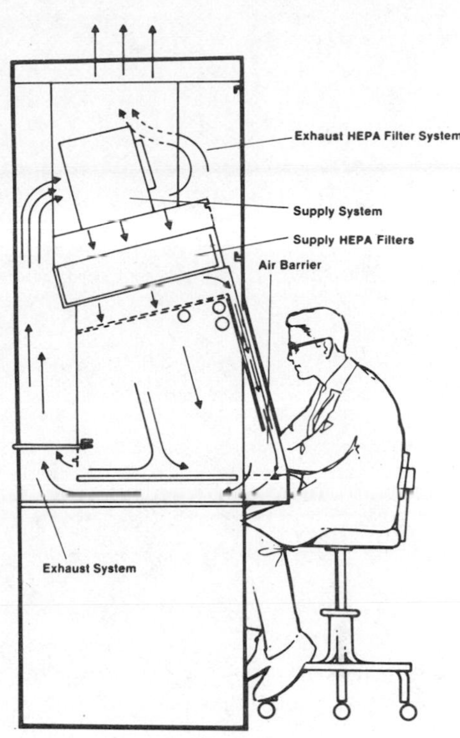

FIG. 13–14 A biological cabinet. The air flow patterns create a barrier to contaminants passing either into or out of the work area. *Courtesy of BioQuest, Cockeysville, MD.*

Bacterial Growth

As a rule, bacteria reproduce by binary fission, the production of two new cells from one parent. This can be seen quite clearly in Figure 13–15. However, some bacterial species, bacterial variants lacking cell walls, and mycoplasma increase their cell numbers asexually by budding. This budding process can be seen quite clearly with the mycoplasma.

Bacterial Growth Curve

When bacteria are transferred to a fresh broth medium without any further changes being made in that medium, subsequent growth follows a typical curve, as shown in Figure 13–16. The actual times and shape of each portion of the curve and the actual numbers of viable organisms obtained will vary between species and different types of media used.

THE LAG PHASE OF GROWTH

The *lag phase* represents what appears to be a transition period on the part of bacteria transferred to new conditions. It is a time in which the bacteria are adjusting to—and at the same time adjusting—their new environment. While there is no increase in cell number, there is a considerable increase in the size of individual cells, with increases in cell protein, DNA, dry weight, and overall metabolic activity. The increased activity appears to be essential to the adjustment process, which may involve altering the pH or oxidation-reduction potential of the medium. These cells are said to be in a state of physiological youth. Although this state of activity is critical to the development of the new culture, it creates conditions potentially detrimental to the cells. During physiological youth, cells are more permeable to materials in their environment and contain a higher percentage of free water. These properties appear to increase the susceptibility of the cells to various toxic chemicals and to heat.

The actual length of the lag phase depends on several factors, including the status of the transferred cells (normal or damaged), the previous environment, and the number of viable organisms in the inoculum. When conditions are

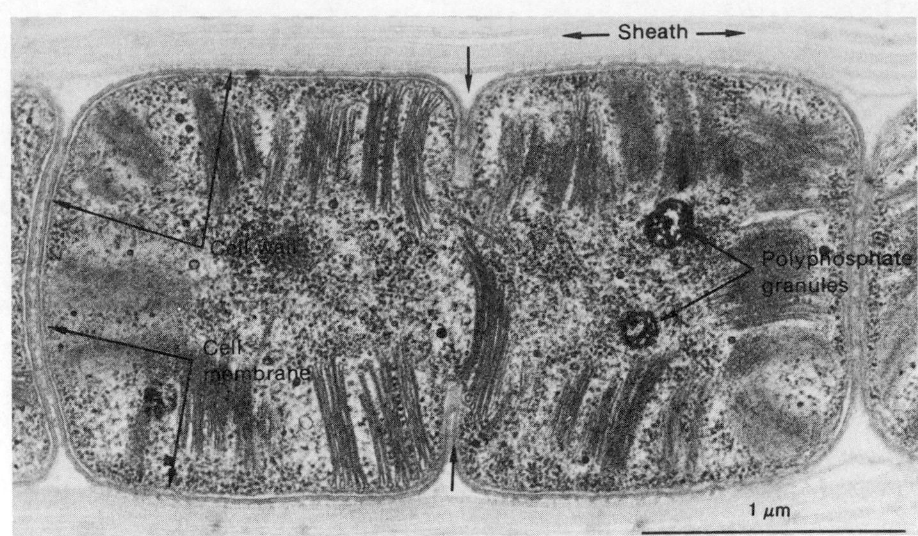

FIG. 13-15 A dividing *Crenothrix* cell. Note the extension of the cell walls into the areas of crosswall, or septum, formation (arrows). The cell walls of the dividing cell are clearly separated from those of its neighbors. *Volker, H., et al.*, J. Bacteriol. *306-313 (1977)*.

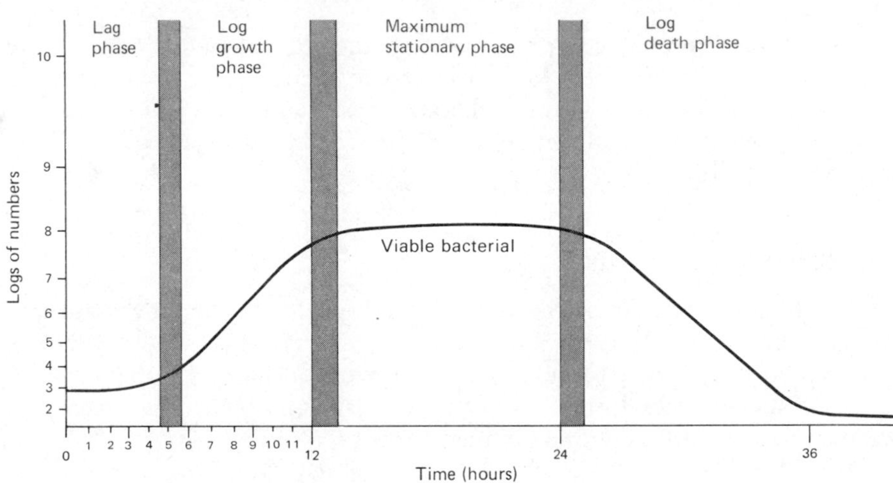

FIG. 13-16 A representation of a generalized bacterial growth curve, showing numbers of bacteria and times of incubation.

suitable, division begins, and after an acceleration in the rate of growth, the cells enter the logarithmic (log) phase.

THE LOGARITHMIC PHASE

During the ***logarithmic (log) phase***, the number of cells increase in a geometrical progression—one splits to make two, two to make four, four to make eight, and so on. Division occurs at a constant and maximum rate. When the number of cells is plotted against time on a logarithmic scale (Figure 13-16), a straight line is obtained. It is from this logarithmic increase in cell number that one is able to calculate the average time for a cell to divide, the ***generation time (g)***. The generation time is equal to the period of time required for the number of cells present to double.

STATIONARY GROWTH PHASE

At some point, the growth rate begins to taper off and the ***stationary phase*** becomes evident. Here the growth and death rates are more nearly identical, and a fairly constant population of viable cells is achieved. In 1929, Bail called this stationary or maximum allowable population for a batch culture the *M concentration*. His experiments showed that no matter how many organisms are used for an inoculum, the same eventual *M concentration* is achieved. When the growth in a tube of medium was removed by centrifuging, introducing a new inoculum into the same medium produced the same M concentration. This procedure could be repeated several times until some essential nutrient was depleted or some by-product toxic for growth accumulated. On the basis of these and other studies, Bail claimed that each living cell required a finite volume or space. He called this property ***lebensraum*** (from the German, meaning "living room").

There are two procedures by which to maximize growth in a liquid medium—a biphasic system and a dialysis bag technique (Figure 13–17).

In the ***biphasic system***, nutrient broth is placed over an agar medium in an appropriate container. The broth is generally the material inoculated. If the liquid surface is large for its volume (that is, for a thin layer of broth), oxygen will not be a limiting growth factor. In systems of this type, some organisms can produce densities that approach a paste consistency.

With the ***dialysis bag technique***, inoculated broth is placed in semipermeable dialysis tubing and suspended in aerated broth that is changed frequently. Very high cell densities are also possible with this method. One advantage of the technique is that the broth surrounding the dialysis tubing need not be sterile, since it is exchanged frequently and contaminating organisms cannot pass through the membrane.

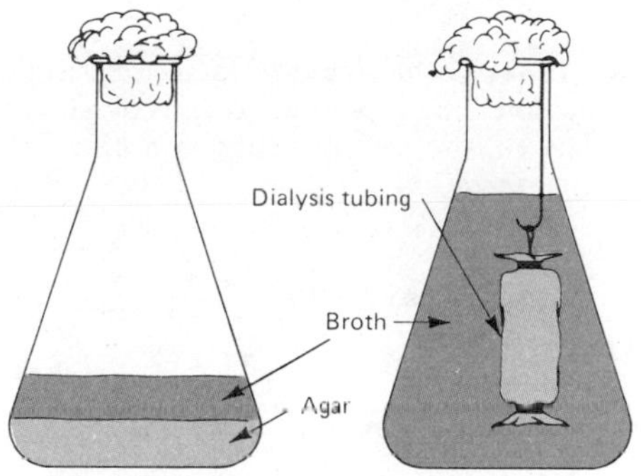

The maximum cell densities of bacterial colonies are also obtainable when organisms are grown on solid media. Here nutrients diffuse to the cells from below, oxygen diffuses into the developing colony, and metabolites released from the cells diffuse into the agar medium.

Dialysis tubing
Broth
Agar

FIG. 13–17 Techniques used to maximize growth in liquid cultures. *Left*, a biphasic system. ***Right***, the dialysis bag procedure.

LOGARITHMIC DEATH RATE

In the stationary, or batch, culture, conditions develop that accelerate the rate of death. These conditions include the accumulation of toxic wastes such as acids and the decreasing concentration of essential nutrients. After a short period, a ***logarithmic death rate*** is observed. During this period, the number of viable cells decrease in a geometrical progression that is the reverse of the one in the log growth phase. This situation will continue until the number of cells is very low and remains almost constant for a time. The culture now has entered the final phase of the growth curve.

Viable cells may persist for some time in this phase. Some may tolerate the ever-increasing accumulation of wastes, and some may even reproduce, although at an extremely long generation time. During this period, dead cells will lyse from naturally occurring ***autolytic enzymes***. Cellular contents and related materials may serve as nutrients. At some point, after days, weeks, even months, conditions will cause even the hardiest organisms to perish. This usually occurs with the drying out of the medium.

Continuous Culture

The batch processes for growing bacteria are often adequate for various biochemical studies and for antibiotic, antigen, and vaccine production. However,

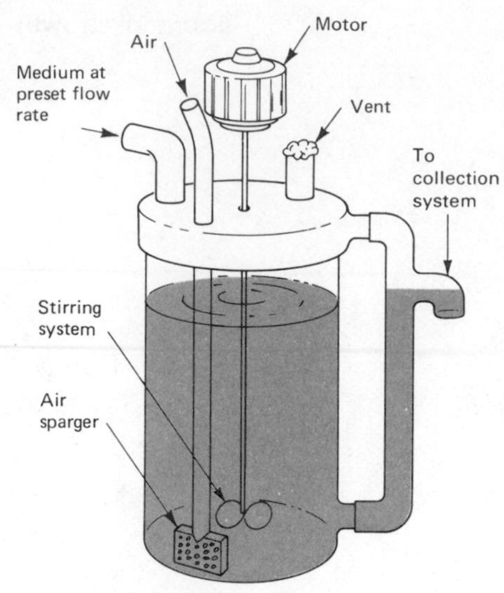

FIG. 13-18 A device for large-scale cell production. The example shown is of a continuous culture system utilizing a growth-limiting medium.

there is usually considerable variation in the ages of the resulting cells and their metabolic activities. Techniques of continuous culture were developed to avoid these variations. Devices like that shown in Figure 13–18 have been used for large-scale cell production and the controlled production of many individual biochemical compounds.

In this system, the rate of growth is controlled by providing a liquid medium with some essential nutrient at a concentration that is less than optimal and with a flow rate less than the growth rate. This ***external control*** keeps all cells in the log phase of growth. For example, in a simple synthetic medium for ***Escherichia coli*** containing glucose, ammonium chloride, and phosphate, the nitrogen source is usually chosen as the ***limiting growth factor***. By keeping the glucose and phosphate at high levels and determining the growth rate or generation time at varying concentrations of ammonium chloride, one is able to determine the suboptimal concentration for the limiting growth factor. With external control, the system is self-stabilizing, continuously providing cells with whatever growth rate is needed to yield the best product.

Growth on Solid Media

Mass culture techniques and biochemical studies usually use either batch or continuous broth cultures. However, colony and slant growth cultures can be extremely useful in evaluating the purity of cultures and in isolating organisms from a mixture and beginning their identification. Common growth patterns and terminology used for their descriptions are given in Figures 13–5 and 13–6. The growth of bacteria into colonies is illustrated by ***Brochothrix (Microbacterium) thermosphactum*** in Figure 13–19.

Measurement of Growth

Microbial growth can be determined by observing an increase in mass or numbers. The selection of techniques for this purpose depends upon the particular organism involved or the requirements of a particular problem. Several different analytical procedures are performed for comparative purposes, taking into account dry weight, protein or nitrogen concentration, and turbidity.

FIG. 13-19 Colony formation in *Brochothrix (Microbacterium) thermosphactum.* *Davidson, C. M., et al.,* J. Appl. Microbiol. 31:*551-559 (1968).*

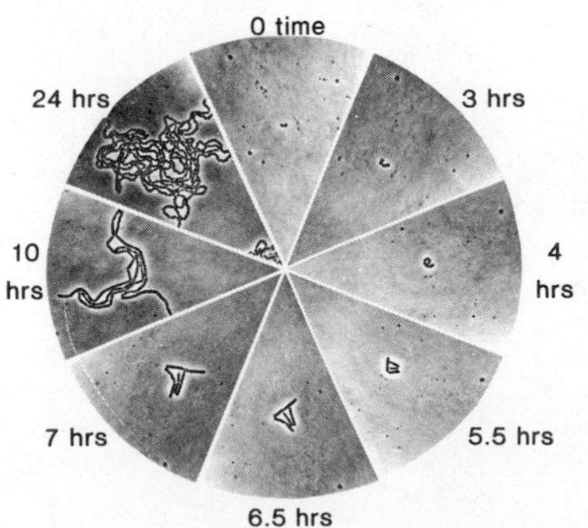

Cell Mass Determination

DRY WEIGHT

Cell mass can be measured from the dry weight of microbial cells in culture. This technique is commonly used to determine the growth of fungi. In this procedure the mycelial mat is removed from the growth medium, possibly washed briefly to remove extraneous solids, placed in a weighing bottle, and dried in a heated dessicator. When the microbial remains appear dry, the contents of the bottle are weighed accurately. Usually this procedure—heating followed by weighing—is repeated until a constant weight is obtained. The weight is used to estimate the fungal mass produced under particular growth conditions. Such data may be used to compare the rates of growth of different antibiotic-producing molds or to determine the relative effects of antifungal agents.

Cell mass values of bacteria can be obtained in essentially the same manner. However, to avoid including growth medium along with the bacteria, it is customary to remove the bacteria by centrifugation from a quantity of the medium, and to then determine the weight of solids present. The weight of a comparable volume of medium treated in the same manner is then subtracted from the total weight of the bacterial suspension to determine the dry weight of the bacterial cells.

Growth can often be differentiated from reproduction in terms of an increase in cell mass rather than in cell numbers. This is not always the case, however, since cellular reserve material may be accumulating without the production of major biological compounds such as nucleic acids or proteins. Thus in some situations an increase in mass is not a reflection of growth. Growth requires the orderly increase in all of an organism's chemical constituents—including nucleic acids and proteins. Growth usually occurs when bacteria are transferred into a growth medium from a different environmental source. The two environments may differ only slightly in their composition, temperature, pH, or osmotic effects.

CHEMICAL ANALYSIS

Mass can also be determined by chemical analyses for protein or nitrogen, since the protein or nitrogen concentration in a growing bacterial culture correlates with the increase in cell mass. In this case, samples of the culture are obtained together with cell-free specimens of the medium for control purposes. In this manner the effect of various nutrients or antimetabolites and related substances upon the protein synthesis of a growing culture can be determined.

TURBIDITY

Dry weight and protein or nitrogen concentrations are not difficult to determine, but a more rapid measure of cell mass is often necessary. One visible characteristic of a growing culture is the increasing cloudiness of the medium. This turbidity can be measured. Changes in turbidity are used in various studies and correlate well with other growth characteristics of a particular organism grown under a particular set of conditions.

Turbidity measurements can be performed with a variety of instruments, including *colorimeters, spectrophotometers,* and *nephelometers.* With the first two instruments, the amount of light beam lost (by absorption or scattering) in passing through the sample is measured. The intensity of the transmitted light is compared with the intensity of light transmitted by the clear medium to give a measure of turbidity called *optical density* (Figure 13–20).

Comparison of the culture medium with the bacteria-free medium, as shown in Figure 13–18, makes it possible to estimate the turbidity produced by organisms even in a medium that is itself colored or slightly cloudy.

Turbidity measurement by light transmission can give readings for solutions that are at least slightly turbid. The sensitivity is not sufficient to monitor suspensions of organisms that do not show some cloudiness. Nephelometry, on the other hand, is most sensitive when microorganisms are in low concentration. The sensitivity of this technique is such that it can detect *Escherichia coli* at 10,000 cells per milliliter. About one million cells per milliliter must be present for light transmission measurements. In nephelometry, the light scattered by the organism is measured, rather than the light transmitted. The mathematics required to prove the greater potential sensitivity of nephelometry is too complex to present here. However, it should be noted that this greater sensitivity is not needed for routine turbidity measurements.

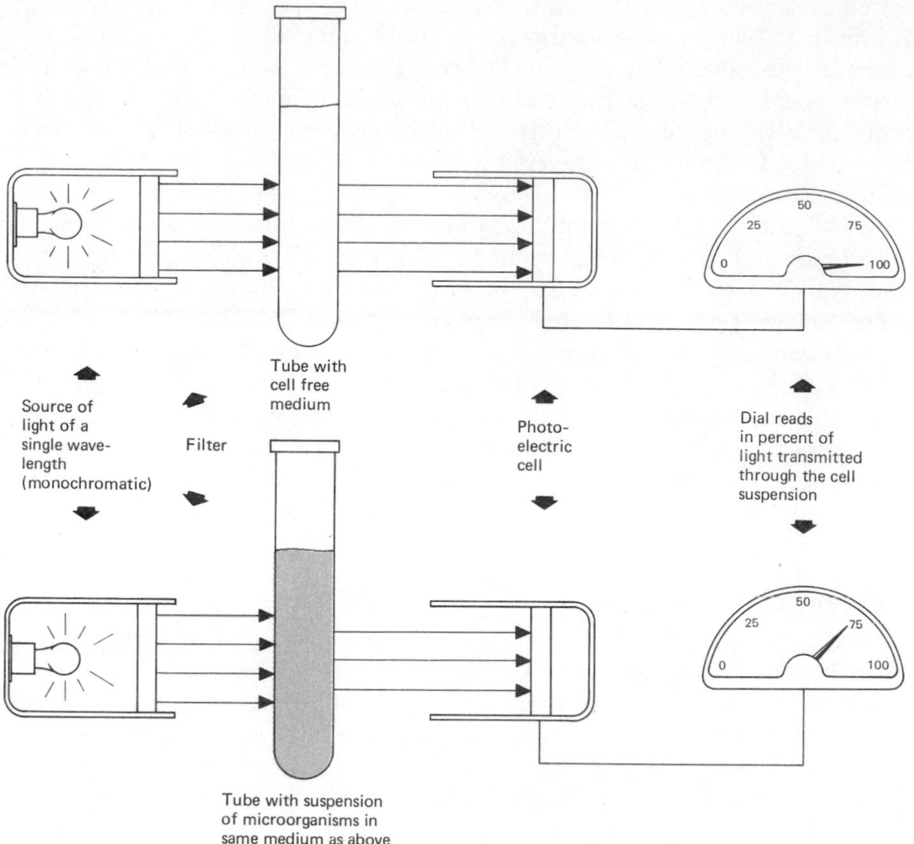

FIG. 13-20 Measurement of turbidity by monitoring of light transmission. (a) A tube with a cell-free medium. (b) A tube with a microbial suspension.

FIG. 13-21 An automatic bacterial colony counter, the Petri-Scan. This device can obtain a colony count from any Petri dish of standard size in one second. The count is flashed on a digital readout visual display (top left-hand corner). *Courtesy of American Instrument Company.*

Viable Counts

Viable counts are carried out to estimate the number of living and/or infective microorganisms in a given material. Cultures of organisms are diluted in a liquid medium and placed in an environment that allows them to produce some type of visual effect. Agar media or membrane filters are used for certain algae, bacteria, and fungi. Tissue cultures are employed for the chlamydia, rickettsia, and viruses. The actual count is of colonies for bacteria (Figure 13-21) and of plaques for viruses. Estimates thus obtained are expressed in *colony-forming* or *plaque-forming units, CFU* and *PFU*, respectively.

To obtain a colony count for bacteria, 1 ml of a well-mixed bacterial suspension (contaminated drinking water in Figure 13-22) is placed in a 99-ml sterile dilution liquid (water blank). This 99 ml of sterile fluid may be nutrient broth, physiological saline, or distilled water. This produces a dilution of 1 to 100. The 1 to 100 dilution can also be expressed as 1/100 or 1×10^{-2}. After the dilution step, one or more 1-ml samples are removed and introduced into separate sterile Petri dishes, followed by the addition of melted and cooled nutrient agar. (This step is not shown in Figure 13-22, and only one Petri dish per dilution is depicted.) The plates are rotated to ensure proper mixing, and the agar is allowed to solidify. The finished plates are then incubated at a desired temperature. After incubation, it can be seen that confluent growth occurred with the 1×10^{-2} dilution (Figure 13-22). This result is represented as being too numerous to count (TNTC). Thus the initial 1/100 dilution was not adequate to obtain the necessary separation of colonies for counting. Unless some additional information is available to give an indication of the expected number of bacte-

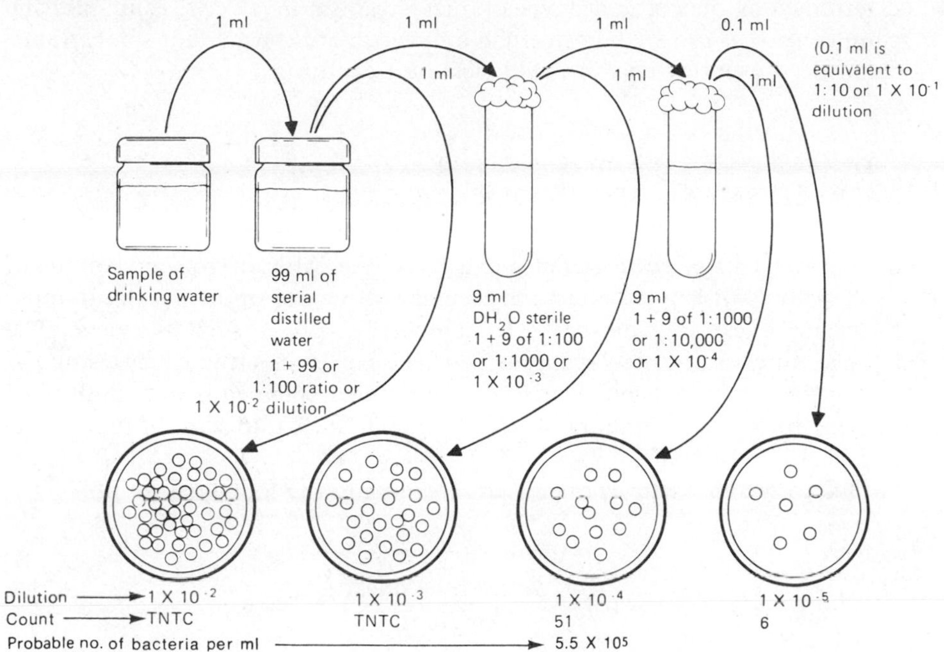

FIG. 13–22 The procedure used to determine the viable population in a bacterial culture. The pour-plate technique is used here.

ria in the original sample, a series of dilutions, must be made. Each of these dilutions must in turn be plated out in a manner similar to the one described.

The remainder of Figure 13–22 illustrates the serial dilution process. A 1-ml sample of the 1/100 dilution is added to a 9-ml dilution blank, which makes a dilution ratio of 1/10 of 1/100, or 1/1000 (also written 10^{-3}). This, too, produces colonies too numerous to count. This procedure is carried still further, to 1/10,000 (or 10^{-4}) and 1/100,000 (or 10^{-5}) dilutions, which are plated, incubated, and counted. Only the 1/10,000 dilution results in separating the organisms sufficiently to yield an easily countable plate. This dilution produced a count of 48 CFU/ml.

A good rule of thumb for accuracy is not to count plates with fewer than 30 or more than 300 colonies. The lower values are likely to be affected by the mixing of the dilution blank, and with the higher figures a large proportion of colonies may be formed by multiple groups of organisms.

To calculate the probable number of bacteria per milliliter in the original sample, it is necessary only to multiply the bacterial colony count by the reciprocals of the dilution and of the volume used. Thus

$$\text{CFU} = \frac{48}{\underset{(10{,}000)}{1 \text{ ml} \times 10^{-4}}} = 48 \times 1 \times 10{,}000$$

$$= 480{,}000 \text{ or } 4.8 \times 10^{5}$$

The result is the estimated number of bacteria in terms of *colony-forming units* (CFU). The latter designation is used rather than absolute numbers, since more than one organism may produce a single colony. This is also true for viral plaques—thus the PFU designation.

Determining Total Counts of Microorganisms

The method used to obtain total counts of microorganisms in specimens is determined by the particular type of microorganism involved. Techniques and equipment that can be used include a direct microscopic count, proportional counting, a counting chamber, and electronic counting.

DIRECT MICROSCOPIC COUNT (BREED SMEAR TECHNIQUE)

A direct microscopic count involves spreading 0.01 ml of a well-mixed specimen over a square centimeter area of a glass slide. After drying, any substance in the sample that might affect the accuracy of the determination (fat in milk, for example) can be removed by an appropriate solvent, such as xylene. The average number of microorganisms per field can be determined by using the high-dry or oil-immersion objectives. The number obtained is then multiplied by a microscope correction factor (MCF), which takes into account the calibration of the instrument.

This correction factor is calculated according to the following formula:

$$\text{MCF} = \frac{\text{Area of the smear}}{\text{Area of the microscopic field}} \times 100$$

Commercially available ocular micrometers are used to measure the diameter of the microscopic field. From this value the area can be calculated according to the formula $A = \pi r^2$, where $\pi = 3.142$ and r is the radius of the field. The dilution factor, which takes into account the volume of material used from the sample and adjusts the number of microorganisms to that found in 1 ml, is represented by 100 in the MCF calculation. In other words, 100 times the number of organisms found in a 0.01-ml sample will give the number of such microbes expected to be present in 1 ml of the sample studied. The final count reported is usually the average of counts on approximately 50 different fields.

Direct microscopic counts have been used in approximating the quality of various grades of raw and pasteurized milk and in computing the growth curves of microorganisms.

Unfortunately, direct microscopic counts are not particularly accurate when few microorganisms are present in a specimen—less than 20,000 to 50,000 per milliliter.

PROPORTIONAL COUNTING

Since the turn of this century, microbiologists have used the technique of proportional counting for estimating microbial populations. In this method a standardized suspension of yeast cells, or of inert particles such as polystyrene latex spheres, is prepared. A measured volume of this suspension is then mixed with a measured volume of the unknown specimen. By examining the mixture, one can determine the relative numbers of specimen organisms and particles or yeast cells present. If the ratio turns out to be 1 to 1, then the original unknown sample contained a number of organisms equal to that in the standardized preparation. This method is used today especially for determining the number of virus particles in suspensions. Ratios are determined with electron microscopy and suitably prepared shadowed specimens.

COUNTING CHAMBER

In a counting chamber, a known volume of sample suspension is placed over a calibrated, etched grid contained in a special chamber. In the Petroff-Hauser device (Figure 13–23), the etched lines can be seen on the central surface. This surface is purposely depressed slightly, so that a space of 0.02 mm is formed when the calibrated region is covered with a special cover glass. The counting chamber consists of regular, partitioned, cubical chambers of known volume.

A bacterial suspension to be examined is introduced into this space with the aid of a calibrated pipette. After the bacteria settle and the liquid currents have quieted down, the microorganisms are counted and their number per unit volume of the suspension is calculated, using an appropriate formula.

Counting chambers can also be used in estimating the total and viable numbers of yeast cells in a suspension. In this case, methylene blue is added to the yeast suspension to act as a *vital dye*, a dye that can distinguish between living and dead cells. Viable yeast cells absorb the dye and reduce it to the leuco or colorless form. Thus living cells are colorless, and dead or dying cells are stained blue. As with the Breed smear, it is essential to have large populations in order to obtain a reasonably accurate count.

This method has not proved practical with bacterial cells. Methylene blue or other oxidation-reduction (redox) indicators are limited in this respect.

ELECTRONIC COUNTING

Electronic counting by a device called a Coulter Counter relies on changes in the electrical conductivity of the medium to signal the presence of a cell. As the suspension passes through a narrow opening, each cell is detected by a fluctuation conductivity across the orifice, and passage of the cell registers on the counter. Counters of this type are used routinely in clinical hematology to count white and red blood cells. Excellent reproducibility and accuracy of results are usually obtained.

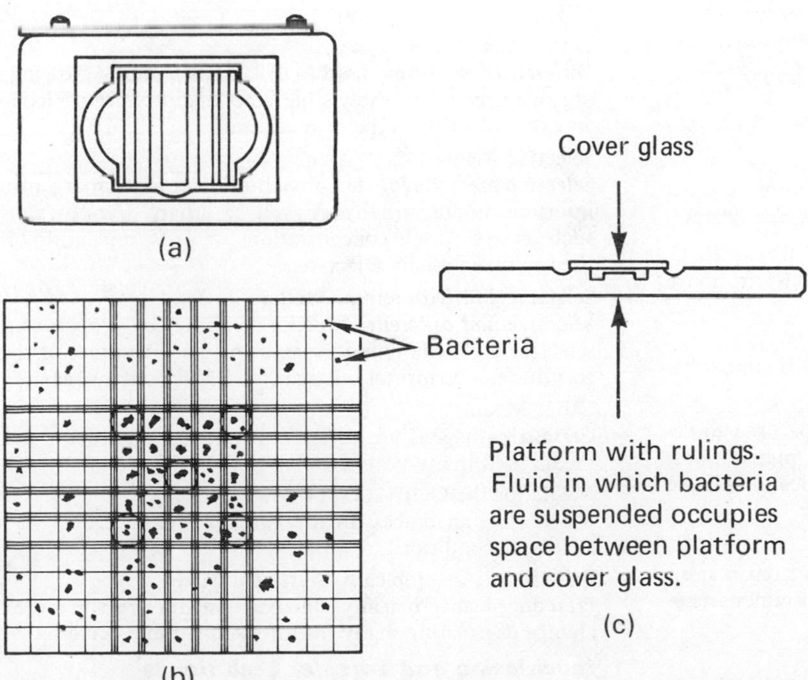

FIG. 13–23 (a) A Petroff-Hauser bacterial counter. *Courtesy of Arthur H. Thomas Co., Philadelphia.* (b) A vertical section view. (c) An enlarged view of the ruled chambers in the center.

SUMMARY

An Introduction to Bacterial Cultivation

1. A wide variety of procedures and nutrient preparations called *culture media* are used for the cultivation of microorganisms.
2. Living animals, plants, and/or their cells are used for those microorganisms that require living cells for growth and reproduction.
3. Procedures using nonliving materials contained in culture vessels are called *in vitro* techniques, while techniques using living cells or entire animals or plants are called *in vivo* techniques.

Nutrition and Other Conditions for Growth

Heterotrophy, Autotrophy, and Hypotrophy

1. *Heterotrophic* organisms need preformed organic compounds for their growth, reproduction, and other activities. Examples of such compounds include amino acids and carbohydrates.
2. *Autotrophic* organisms utilize inorganic compounds such as carbon dioxide and minerals.
3. *Hypotrophs* need living cells for their activities. These forms include viruses and the rickettsia.

Gaseous Requirements

1. Microorganisms can also be grouped by their response to available gases in the environment, such as oxygen and carbon dioxide.
2. Organisms requiring oxygen are called *aerobic*. Those needing low concentrations are *microaerophilic*. Those having no requirement for free oxygen are called *anaerobes*. *Strict*, or *obligate*, anaerobes cannot tolerate any free oxygen in their environment.

Thermal Conditions

1. Microorganisms need specific temperatures for their growth and related activities.
2. The *minimum*, *maximum*, and ideal, or *optimum*, requirements are known as an organism's *cardinal temperatures*.
3. *Psychrophiles* have a temperature range of 0° to 20°C, *mesophiles*, 20° to 45°C, and *thermophiles* 45° to above 90°C.

Acidity or Alkalinity (pH)

1. Microorganisms have certain pH (hydrogen ion concentration) needs for growth.
2. Various indicators and electron devices can be used to determine the hydrogen ion concentrations of preparations. Examples of pH indicators used in bacteriological media are bromcresol purple, litmus, and phenol red.

Properties of Bacteriological Media

Media are used for the isolation of microorganisms from materials such as dairy products, foods, soil, water, and specimens associated with diseases.

Nitrogen Sources

Nitrogen-containing compounds—proteins and their products—are an important ingredient of media.

Carbon and Energy Sources

1. Carbon and energy sources are also important ingredients of media. Organisms obtain carbon from organic nutrients such as carbohydrates, lipids, and proteins, as well as from carbon dioxide.
2. Carbohydrate sources of energy and carbon include starch, glycogen, various pentose monosaccharides and hexose monosaccharides, and various disaccharides.

Vitamins and Growth Factors

Several of the vitamins important in treatment of human nutritional deficiency diseases are also required by microorganisms. Other growth factors may be needed as well.

Essential Mineral Salts

Various inorganic compounds are also essential for microbial nutrition. These include phosphates and sulfates. Potassium, magnesium, manganese, iron, and calcium are also used.

Water and Osmotic Pressure

The bacterial cell is 80 percent water and must be in intimate contact with a water supply for its survival, growth, and reproduction.

Preparation of Media

Many types of media may be obtained in dehydrated (powder) form from commercial establishments. Such preparations are then reconstituted with distilled water, adjusted in pH, dispensed in appropriate containers, and sterilized for use.

Media Usage and Categories

Media can be used for different purposes, such as the isolation and identification of microorganisms, the determination of microbial antibiotic sensitivity, sterility testing of medically important products, analyses of food and water, and the preparation of vaccines.

Differential Media

Differential media are used to distinguish among growing microorganisms based on the visible reactions produced. Blood agar is an example of this type of medium.

Selective Media

Selective media favor the growth of certain microorganisms and interfere or prevent the growth of others. Various substances such as dyes, high concentrations of salts, and antibiotics are used to make media selective.

Selective and Differential Media

Selective and differential media combine the properties of both selective and differential types of media. Examples of this category include mannitol salt agar, and MacConkey agar.

Other Media

Certain pathogens are today cultured on modified versions of media used many years ago.

Media for the Cultivation of Anaerobes

Media for anaerobes incorporate reducing agents to create anaerobic conditions.

Prereduced Anaerobically Sterilized Media

Prereduced anaerobically sterilized media greatly increase the chance of isolating many fastidious anaerobic bacteria.

Inoculation and Transfer Techniques

1. Inoculating instruments, loop or needle, are used for introducing specimens into or onto nutrient media, isolation of pure cultures, culture transfer, and preparation of specimens for microscopic study.

2. Before use, the inoculating instrument must be heated (flamed) to redness to sterilize it. In addition, the lips of tubes from which cultures are removed or into which cultures are introduced must be carefully flamed.

3. *Aseptic technique* refers to the prevention of microbial contamination.

Techniques for the Isolation of Pure Bacterial Cultures

The pour-plate and streak-plate techniques are two of the effective procedures used for the isolation and subsequent identification of bacteria.

The Pour-plate Technique

The pour-plate technique consists of cooling melted agar-containing medium, inoculating the medium with a specimen, and immediately pouring it into a sterile Petri plate, allowing the freshly poured medium to solidify and incubating the preparation at the desired temperature.

The Streak-plate Technique

The streak-plate technique involves spreading a single loopful of material containing microorganisms over the surface of a solidified agar medium.

Anaerobic Transfer

Transfer should be performed under a flowing stream of nitrogen for cultures on solid media or by the use of a pipette for liquid media.

Conditions of Incubation

Aerobic Incubation

Once an appropriate solid or liquid medium has been inoculated and protected from contamination, cultures must be incubated under controlled conditions of temperature and humidity.

Capneic Incubation

Various devices and procedures are used to provide the suitable concentration of carbon dioxide for capneic incubation.

Anaerobic Incubation

Incubation under anaerobic conditions can be accomplished with vacuum devices such as the anaerobic incubator, the Brewer plate, and the Spray dish.

Biological or "Sterility Test" Cabinets

"Sterility test" cabinets protect pure cultures from air-borne contamination, as well as providing for the safety of those working where microbes are being cultured.

Bacterial Growth

Most bacteria reproduce by binary fission, the production of two new cells from one parent cell.

Bacterial Growth Curve

1. Upon transfer of bacteria to a fresh broth medium, and under controlled conditions, a typical growth curve will result.

2. The actual phases and shape of such a curve vary with the species and media used.

3. A bacterial growth curve consists of a *lag phase*, *logarithmic phase*, *stationary growth phase*, and *logarithmic death rate*.

Continuous Culture

Continuous culture techniques were developed to avoid variation in the ages of the bacterial cells that are grown.

Growth on Solid Media

Colony and slant growth cultures can be useful in evaluating the purity of cultures and in isolating organisms from a mixture.

Measurement of Growth

Microbial growth can be determined by observing an increase in mass or numbers.

Cell Mass Determination

Analytical procedures used to determine cell mass include determination of dry weight, chemical analysis for protein or nitrogen concentration, and turbidity, or cloudiness, measurements.

Viable Counts

1. Viable counts are estimates of the numbers of living microorganisms in a given material. For bacteria these estimates can be expressed in *colony-forming units (CFU)*. Only plate counts with 30 to 300 colonies can be used.

2. Colony-forming units can be calculated according to the formula

$$\text{CFU} = \frac{\text{Number of colonies}}{\text{Volume of sample used}} \times \text{dilution used}$$

Determining Total Counts of Microorganisms

Techniques and equipment used to obtain total counts of microorganisms in materials include the direct microscopic count, proportional counting, the counting chamber, and electronic counting devices.

QUESTIONS FOR REVIEW

1. Distinguish between *in vivo* and *in vitro* techniques.
2. What does pH mean? How can the pH of a medium be altered?
3. Compare the nutritional requirements of autotrophic, heterotrophic, and hypotrophic organisms and give examples of each organism.
4. Explain the following terms:
   a. aerobe
   b. microaerophilic
   c. anaerobe
   d. facultative anaerobe
   e. capneic
   f. obligate aerobe
5. What is a hypotroph?
6. Discuss the grouping of microorganisms according to their temperature growth requirements.
7. a. What is a growth medium?
   b. What substances serve as sources of carbon, mineral salts, nitrogen, and vitamins?
   c. Distinguish between broth and agar media and give common examples of each.
8. Discuss anaerobic cultivation methods. Include in your answer a treatment of media and equipment used in general procedures.
9. What is the difference between the Petri dish and the Brewer dish?
10. Describe the pour-plate and streak-plate techniques. What disadvantages does each procedure possess? What advantages?
11. What is aseptic technique?
12. What are synthetic media? Can both bacteria and fungi be grown with them?
13. List three cultural characteristics of bacteria that can be noted from broth cultures. Do the same for agar slant and agar plate cultures.

14. a. Distinguish between selective and differential media.
    b. What is a selective and differential medium?
    c. Give examples of each of these medium categories.
15. Describe three methods by which you can measure growth in microorganisms.
16. Define:
    a. growth
    b. lag phase of growth
    c. reproduction
    d. Breed smear technique
    e. lebensraum
    f. biphasic growth system
    g. proportional counting
    h. continuous cultivation
17. Calculate the colony-forming units of a sample if 1 ml of a 10^{-6} dilution yielded 66 colonies.

SUGGESTED READINGS

Gray, T. R. G., and G. R. Postgate (eds.), *The Survival of Vegetative Microorganisms.* New York: Cambridge University Press, 1976. *This book has several articles dealing with the many ways vegetative microorganisms manage to survive in spite of starvation, cold, heat, osmotic shock, ultraviolet light, and other factors.*

Inniss, W. E., "Interaction of Temperature and Psychrophilic Microorganisms," *Ann. Rev. Microbiol.* 29:445 (1975). *The effects of temperature on psychrophilic microorganisms and their activities, whether in the laboratory or in their natural environments, are discussed.*

Ishikawa, T., Y. Maruyama, and H. Matsumiya (eds.), *Growth and Differentiation in Microorganisms.* Baltimore: University Park Press, 1977. *A collection of papers describing the DNA replication cycle, formation of cell groupings in Gram-positive cocci, synchronization of growth, and bacterial spore formation.*

Pirt, S. J., *Principles of Microbe and Cell Cultivation.* New York: John Wiley & Sons, 1975. *A slightly advanced text describing specific topics associated with methods of cultivation of microorganisms, such as the estimation of biomass and chemostat cultures, as well as the effects of oxygen, temperature, pH, and water on growth.*

Society for General Microbiology, *Microbial Growth.* New York: Cambridge University Press, 1969. *Descriptions of growth of mixed cultures, regulation of enzyme synthesis during growth, differentiation of cells, and development of organelles in lower eucaryotes are found in this publication.*

Microbial Metabolism and Cellular Regulation

CHAPTER 14

Chapter 14 describes the means by which life forms use available biochemicals for energy and for growth and reproduction. Carbohydrate metabolism is discussed briefly to provide a foundation for understanding the interrelationship of carbohydrate, protein, and lipid metabolism. Additional topics to be found in this chapter include: consideration of protein synthesis in the light of recent advances in unraveling the genetic code, brief discussions of methods for measuring metabolism, and various aspects of microbial metabolism. This chapter emphasizes the similarities and differences between metabolic reactions of microbes and other organisms and shows the unity of biochemical activity among life forms.

After reading this chapter, you should be able to:

1. **Discuss, briefly, the concept of metabolism and define anabolism and catabolism in terms of general reactions and energy changes.**
2. **Discuss the involvement of adenosine triphosphate (ATP) in energy production in the cell and the mechanisms for making ATP: photophosphorylation, substrate phosphorylation, and oxidative phosphorylation.**
3. **Outline the general steps in glycolysis in terms of the initial chemical, activation process, and end products.**
4. **Differentiate between the potential energy (numbers of ATP molecules) produced as a result of glycolysis under anaerobic versus aerobic conditions.**

5. **Define fermentation and outline typical reactions that use pyruvic acid.**
6. **Describe the transition reaction, the metabolic step by which pyruvic acid is converted to acetyl CoA.**
7. **Show the general steps in the citric acid cycle by which acetyl CoA is metabolized to CO_2, NADH, $FADH_2$, and ATP.**
8. **Indicate metabolic steps by which proteins and lipids can be utilized for energy in glycolysis and the citric acid cycle.**
9. **Describe general mechanisms for metabolism as exhibited by photosynthetic autotrophs and heterotrophs, and chemosynthetic autotrophs and heterotrophs.**
10. **Discuss what is meant by genetic code, and outline the steps in protein synthesis in terms of transcription and translation, defining "sense strand," complementarity, codon, anticodon, *m*RNA, and *t*RNA.**
11. **Discuss feedback inhibition and inducible and repressible operons as mechanisms for controlling metabolic activities in the cell.**
12. **Describe each of the following as means of studying metabolic reactions: simple fermentation tests, manometry, oxidation-reduction activity, radioisotopes, and chromatography.**

The metabolic activities of microorganisms have been studied for many reasons and have many applications. It is one thing to know that some organisms produce antibiotics, cheeses, or diseases, but it is quite another thing to attempt to understand how these activities occur as normal processes of life.

General Metabolism

Metabolism refers to the entire set of chemical reactions by which cells maintain life. Two general phases of metabolism are **catabolism** and **anabolism.** Catabolic reactions are those by which complex organic nutrients are broken down to simpler organic and inorganic compounds. During these reactions, energy is obtained and stored, usually in the form of adenosine triphosphate (ATP) molecules. This energy is utilized, in part, for the series of reactions that synthesize macromolecules, such as nucleic acids, lipids, polysaccharides, and proteins and the subunits of which these macromolecules are formed. These synthetic processes are called anabolism. In general, then, energy and building blocks for macromolecules are obtained during catabolism and used during anabolism.

Processes Essential to Cellular Growth and Reproduction

The complete breakdown of a carbohydrate, such as that of glucose to carbon dioxide and water, involves a series of enzymatically controlled steps and the release of energy that is associated with reactions in which inorganic phosphate (PO_4^{3-}) is used to form adenosine triphosphate (ATP) from adenosine diphosphate (ADP). The latter type of reactions are known as **phosphorylations.** The important biochemical aspects of glucose degradation will be discussed in terms of *energy metabolism*, *glycolysis*, the *Krebs cycle*, and *electron transport*.

Energy Metabolism

ATP PRODUCTION

The process for making adenosine triphosphate or ATP involves combining adenosine diphosphate (ADP) and inorganic phosphate (Pi).

$$\text{ADP} + \text{Pi} + 7 \text{ to } 8 \text{ Kcal} \longrightarrow \text{ATP}$$

This reaction requires 7 to 8 kilocalories of energy. The energy can be obtained in three different ways. The phosphorylation of ADP is called photosynthetic phosphorylation, substrate phosphorylation, or oxidative phosphorylation, depending upon the source of energy (Figure 14–1).

In *photosynthetic phosphorylation*, the required amount of energy is absorbed by chlorophyll as light. Photosynthesis supplies the blue-green bacteria, the sulfur and nonsulfur photosynthetic bacteria, algae, and plants with the ATP needed for synthesis of all materials, including the polysaccharides used as sources of energy.

The catabolic reactions by which organic compounds such as polysaccharides

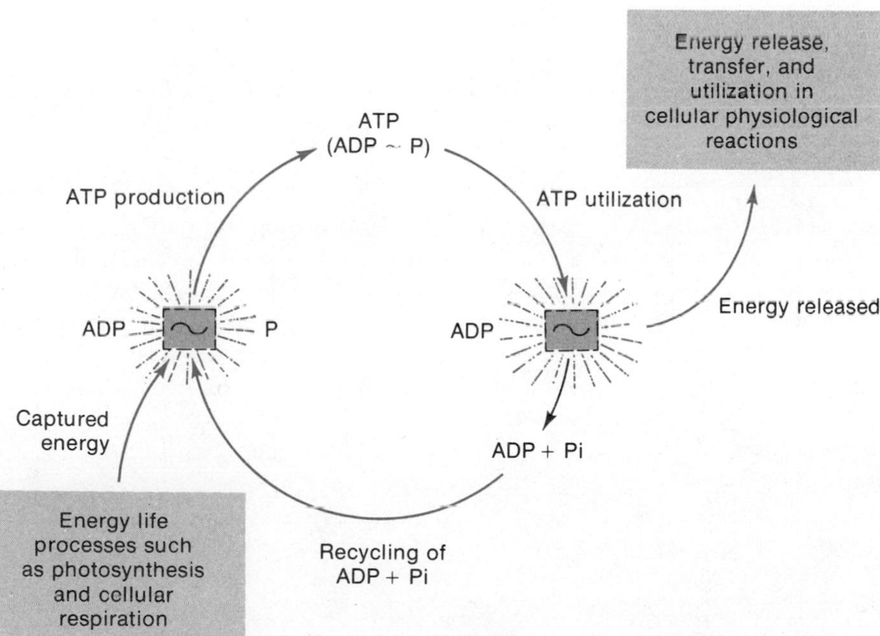

FIG. 14–1 The formation of adenosine triphosphate (ATP), a fuel that serves all living organisms. By means of energy-yielding processes such as photosynthetic phosphorylation and substrate phosphorylation, energy-rich bonds (~) are formed and used to combine ADP and inorganic phosphate (Pi) into ATP. ATP, in turn, is used for various life processes resulting in ADP and released inorganic phosphate. The inorganic phosphate and ADP are used again to continue the cycle.

are converted into other organic compounds are called *substrate reactions.* A substrate is the substance acted upon by an enzyme. During some substrate reactions, energy-rich bonds are formed, and this energy can be used to combine ADP and inorganic phosphate into ATP. These molecules of ATP are formed by *substrate phosphorylation,* which occurs in the cytoplasm of both procaryotes and eucaryotes, as well as in the fluid matrix of eucaryotic mitochondria.

Some enzymes, particularly those that perform oxidation-reduction reactions, require coenzymes for that activity. The most common of these coenyzmes is nicotinamide adenine dinucleotide (NAD), which exists both in an oxidized state (NAD) and in a reduced state, (NADH) (Figure 14–2). Two other coenzymes that participate in oxidation-reduction reactions are nicotinamide adenine dinucleotide phosphate (NADP) and flavin adenine dinucleotide (FAD), which are $NADPH_2$ and $FADH_2$ in their reduced forms. During substrate oxidation reactions, these coenzymes are reduced and can subsequently reduce another substance.

Glycolysis

Literally, the term *glycolysis* means the breakdown of sweets. It refers to the catabolic reactions that convert glucose into pyruvic acid and/or glycerol, and the energy-rich molecules such as adenosine triphosphate (ATP) and reduced nicotinamide adenine dinucleotide (NADH).

Figure 14–3 outlines the general steps in glycolysis. Glucose may be formed in the cell by photosynthesis, or it may be obtained in the form of starch, cellulose, or glycogen, or as glucose and maltose. The first step of glycolysis is *activation* of the sugar molecule by the addition of phosphates. This reaction is

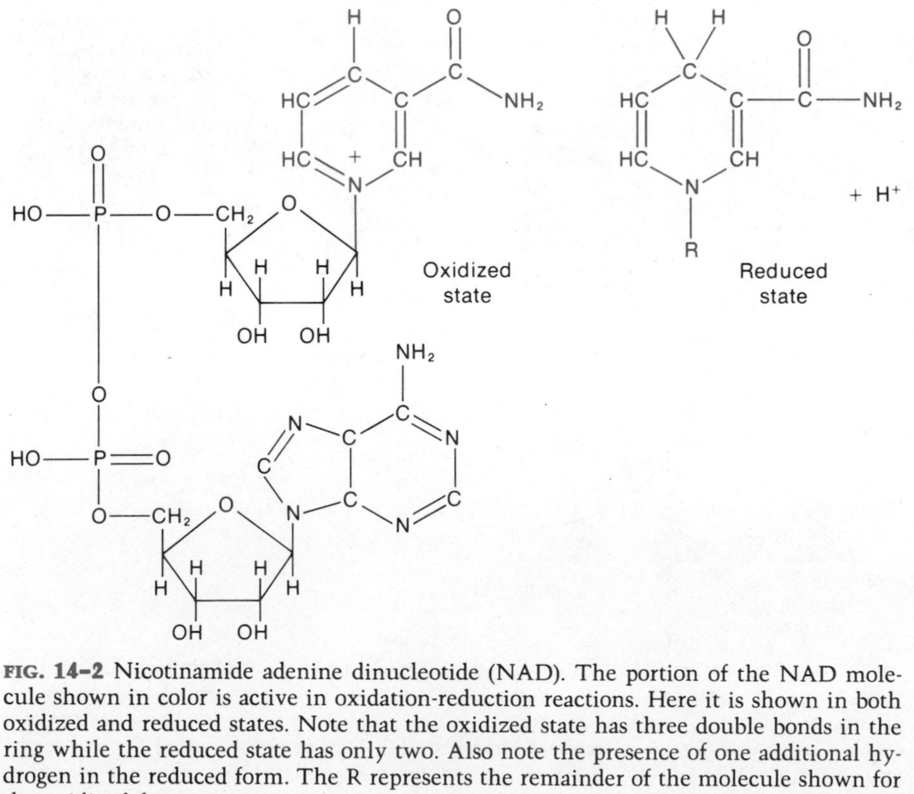

Oxidized state

Reduced state

+ H^+

FIG. 14–2 Nicotinamide adenine dinucleotide (NAD). The portion of the NAD molecule shown in color is active in oxidation-reduction reactions. Here it is shown in both oxidized and reduced states. Note that the oxidized state has three double bonds in the ring while the reduced state has only two. Also note the presence of one additional hydrogen in the reduced form. The R represents the remainder of the molecule shown for the oxidized form.

accomplished using energy released by the hydrolysis of ATP to ADP. The energy released is used for molecular rearrangements; it permits the synthesis of more ATP later, when energy is generated by various oxidation-reduction steps. The molecular rearrangement permits cleavage of a sugar (fructose) diphosphate to form two 3-carbon compounds: glyceraldehyde phosphate and dihydroxyacetone phosphate. As indicated by the double arrows, these trioses can be changed from one to the other. In the more usual pathway to pyruvic acid, two molecules of pyruvic acid are formed for each molecule of glucose metabolized. With microorganisms, under various conditions differing quantities of glycerol and pyruvic acid may be produced. Glycolysis generates a total of four molecules of ATP during substrate reactions converting glucose to pyruvic acid. The ATP molecules are formed after the formation of the two triose phosphate compounds. Two molecules of ATP are required to activate or phosphorylate the glucose yielding fructose diphosphate. Thus, a net gain of two ATP's and two reduced NAD's (NADH) results from glycolysis. These ATP's are available for various cellular activities, such as nucleic acid synthesis and other energy processes necessary for growth and reproduction.

When organisms can perform the glycolytic reactions under aerobic conditions, four times as much energy is released, because energy liberated during metabolism can be utilized more efficiently in aerobic glycolysis. One step following triose phosphate formation is the reduction of a coenyzme, NAD, to NADH. The $NADH_2$ is used to reduce the FAD to $FADH_2$, resulting in the progressive reduction of these coenyzmes and, ultimately, oxygen.

Each pair of electrons going through this electron transport system permits the synthesis of three molecules of ATP. Because two pairs of electrons are generated per glucose molecule during glycolysis, six ATP's are added to the two previously formed, thus producing a total of eight.

Glycolysis is often called anaerobic glucose metabolism because it functions in the absence of oxygen. However, the same reactions occur whether oxygen is present or not. The products are primarily pyruvic acid, $NADH_2$, and ATP. The essential difference between what occurs aerobically and what occurs anaerobically is what happens to the pyruvic acid and the $NADH_2$. Some of the anaerobic processes are called fermentation.

FERMENTATION

Fermentation can be defined as the anaerobic decomposition of organic compounds such as carbohydrates. Organic compounds serve as both ultimate electron donors and acceptors. Thus a fermentable substance such as glucose often yields both oxidizable and reducible metabolites.

During glycolysis, glucose, a 6-carbon sugar, is oxidized to two molecules of pyruvic acid, a 3-carbon compound (Figure 14–4). Some fermenting organisms reduce the pyruvic acid to lactic acid as the sole or primary end product (Figure 14–4). Such organisms are said to be ***homofermentative***. They include species of *Bacillus, Lactobacillus*, and *Streptococcus*. Microorganisms that produce lactic acid, as well as acetic, formic, and other acids, possibly ethanol, other alcohols, and acetone, are referred to as being ***heterofermentative***. This group includes yeasts, other fungi, and bacterial species belonging to the Enterobacteriaceae family, and to the genera of *Clostridium* and *Streptococcus*.

A noncarbohydrate fermentation can occur with amino acids, organic acids, purines, and pyrimidines. A reaction of this type is illustrated by the action of *Clostridium* spp. on amino acids. In one kind of amino acid fermentation, the *Stickland reaction*, two different amino acids participate. One is oxidized, while the other is reduced. The alanine is oxidized and deaminated to yield pyruvic acid and ammonia. The pyruvic acid is further oxidized and decarboxylated to

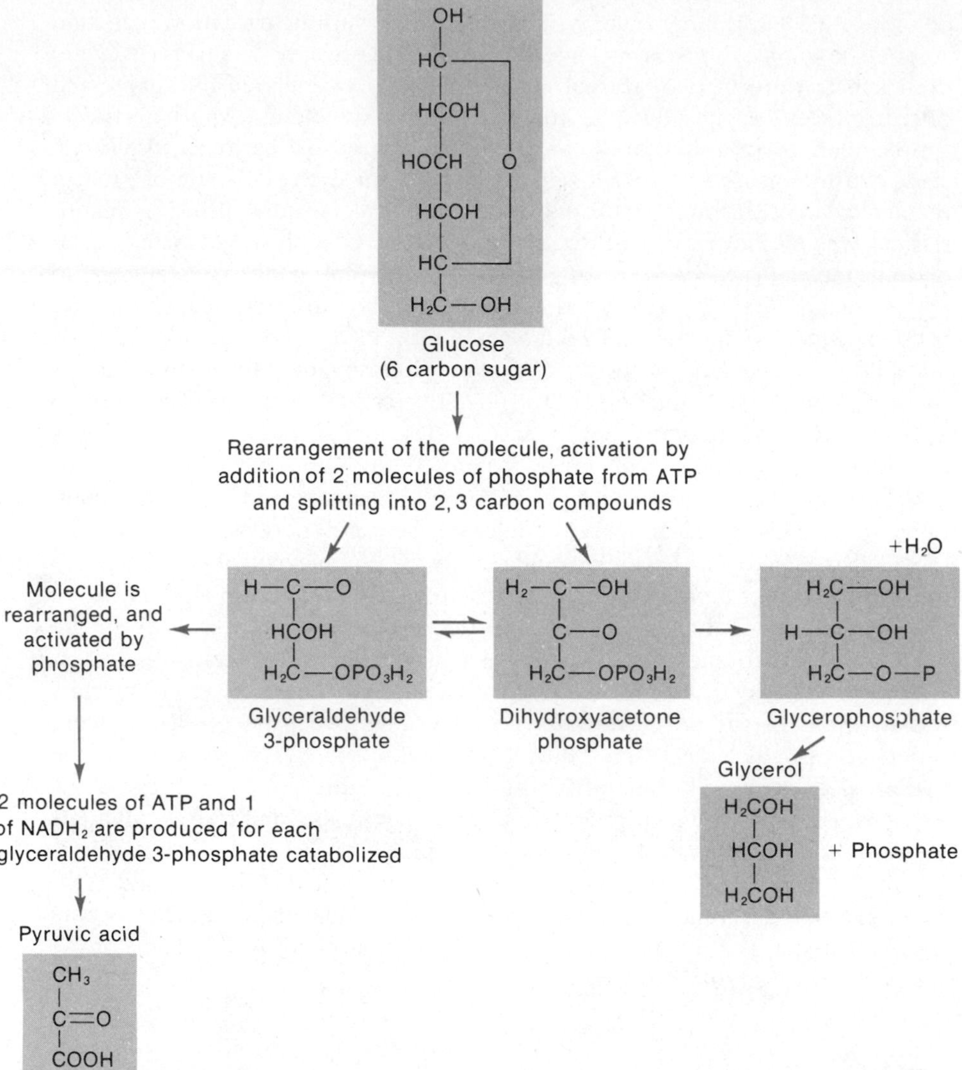

FIG. 14-3 Glycolysis. Refer to Figures 14–4 and 14–10 to see how glycolysis is related to other metabolic processes.

yield acetic acid and carbon dioxide. During this time, glycine is reduced and deaminated to produce acetic acid and ammonia (Figure 14–5).

Krebs (Citric Acid) Cycle

The complete catabolism of glucose to carbon dioxide and water involves three phases. The initial phase is glycolysis, and the second phase is the **Krebs cycle.** The third phase of glucose catabolism is the **electron transport system (ETS),** which can operate with pairs of electrons produced by either the reactions of glycolysis or those of the Krebs cycle.

Another designation for the series of reactions comprising the Krebs cycle is the *citric acid cycle.* This name is an appropriate one because citric acid appears at the beginning of each complete "rotation" of the cyclic series reactions (see Figure 14–6). The cycle is often called "the energy wheel of cellular metabolism" because it is crucial to supplying the energy needs of cells.

When oxygen is available to the cell, the energy in pyruvic acid is released

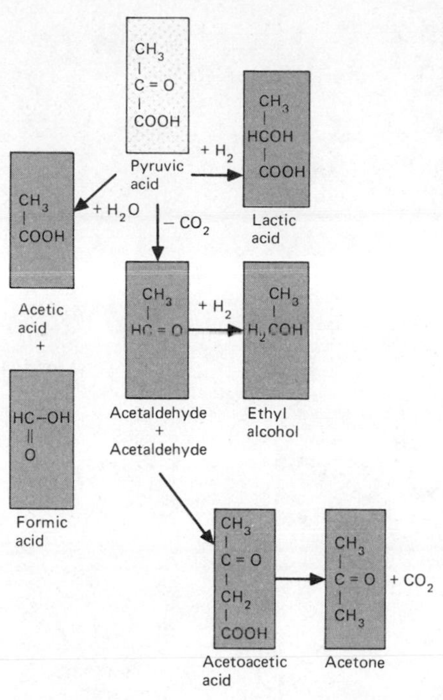

FIG. 14-4 Selected reactions involving pyruvic acid.

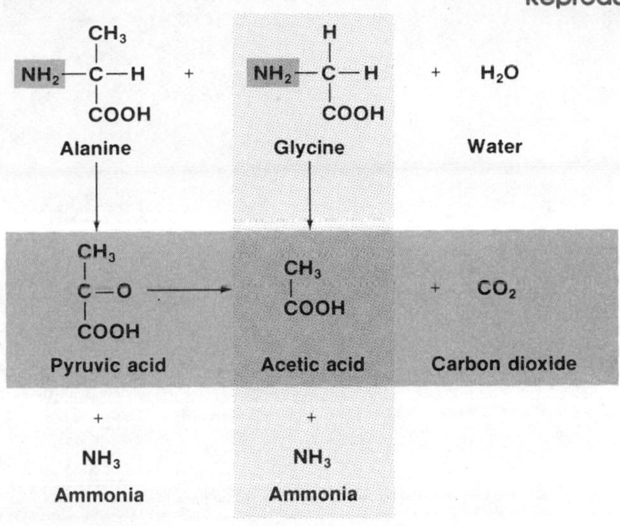

FIG. 14-5 An example of the fermentation of noncarbohydrate compounds. The portions of the amino acids that are deaminated are boxed. Refer to the text for additional details.

through **aerobic respiration.** The first step in this metabolic pathway includes the removal of one of the three carbons in pyruvic acid, the formation of carbon dioxide, and the production of one NADH. The remaining two carbons of the molecule, known as the *acetyl group*, are attached to the compound *coenyzme A* or CoA (Figure 14–6).

In the Krebs cycle, citric acid (6-carbon compound) is converted to oxaloacetic acid (4-carbon compound) through a series of oxidation or decarboxylation reactions. The first step, or the beginning of a new turn of this cycle, involves the addition of acetyl CoA, an activated 2-carbon derivative obtained by the oxidative decarboxylation of pyruvic acid, to the 4-carbon compound oxaloacetic acid. This reaction forms citric acid. Coenyzme A (CoA–SH) has a terminal sulfhydryl group (Figure 14–7). Transfer of the 2-carbon units by CoA–SH produces a high-energy sulfur bond that stores energy from the decarboxylation of pyruvic acid (Figure 14–6). This energy is important in the transfer of activated 2-carbon derivatives into the cycle.

As shown in Figure 14–6, citric acid is decarboxylated twice, once for each acetyl compound. Each of these reactions yields CO_2 and reduced coenyzmes. The citric acid cycle is considered complete and begins again with additional acetyl CoA, as soon as the formation of oxaloacetic acid has occurred. In the course of the cycle, three $NADH_2$'s, one $FADH_2$, and one ATP are produced by substrate phosphorylation. The electrons in $NADH_2$ and $FADH_2$ are degraded to a lower energy level in the cytochrome system, producing additional molecules of ATP in the process. This results in a gradual and controlled release of electron energy, rather than a sudden and explosive reaction that would be extremely harmful for cells.

Each pyruvic acid molecule oxidized via this cycle results in the formation of twleve ATP's. Because each molecule of glucose can result in the formation of two pyruvic acid molecules, a total of twenty-four ATP's can be formed from a single molecule of glucose.

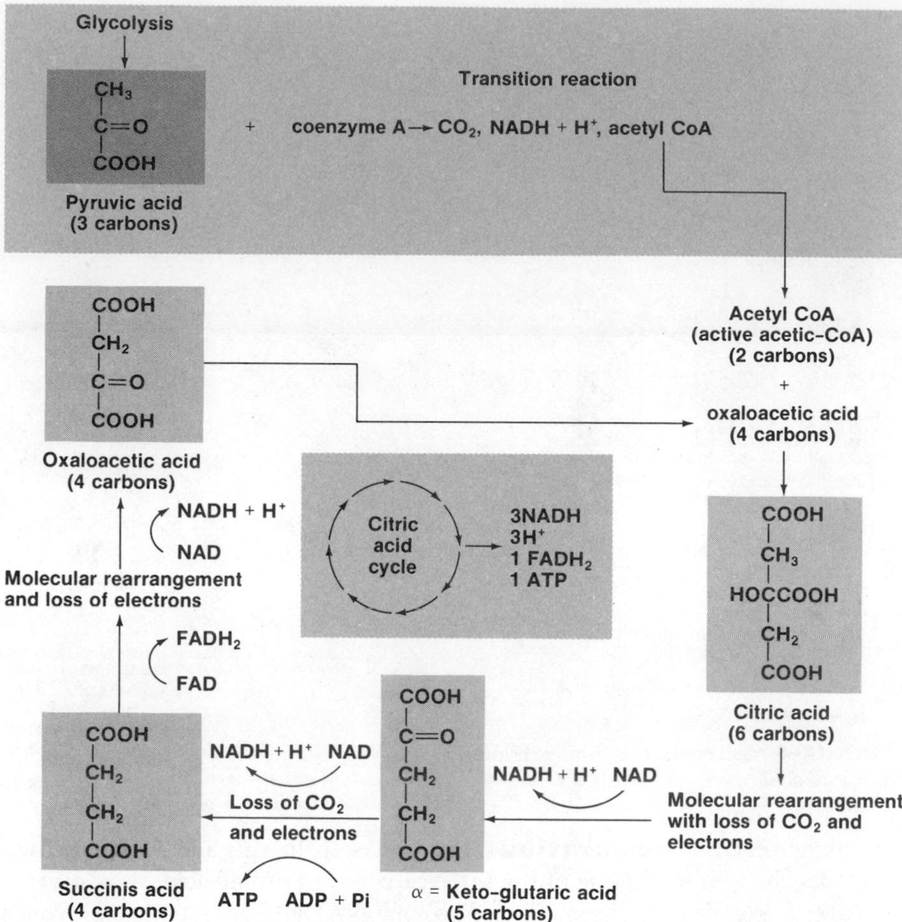

FIG. 14-6 The major steps in the Krebs or citric acid cycle. The number of carbons contained in each compound is shown in parentheses, i.e. (5C), along with major by-products, i.e. CO_2, $NADH_2$, $FADH_2$, ATP.

Electron Transport System

This system, which is also known as the ***respiratory chain***, is a common pathway for the utilization of electrons formed during a variety of metabolic reactions. It is primarily concerned with aerobic metabolism; however, certain components of the system have been identified with anaerobic organisms.

The NADH and $FADH_2$ produced by aerobic respiration and the Krebs cycle are transferred to certain electron carrier molecules which are associated with the lipid components of membranes. The carrier molecules form the ***electron transport system***, which consists of two types of proteins, the flavoproteins and the cytochromes, and the nonprotein carriers, the quinones in the form of coenzyme Q. The cytochromes contain a ferric ion (Fe^{3+}) that can be reduced to a ferrous ion (Fe^{2+}). All members of the system are arranged in precise order (Figure 14–8), and must be capable of being reduced by the reduced form of a previous carrier and oxidized by the oxidized form of a carrier next in line. The sequence of reactions is started by the oxidation of NADH which, in turn, reduces FAD. This process of oxidizing NADH or NADPH and reducing FAD results in the formation of $FADH_2$. What is more significant, it releases enough energy to form ATP as previously described (Figure 14–1). This important step in the system is known as **oxidative phosphorylation.** At the end of the series of oxidations and reductions in this system, electrons freed of their excess energy react with oxygen which then combines with hydrogen ions to form water. Cytochrome oxidase is an enzyme that catalyzes the direct reaction with oxygen.

The flow of electrons through this transport system can be pictured as a series of steps or waterfalls over which electrons pass. With each fall at a particular step, the electron energy that is released is enzymatically captured and used to form ATP molecules from ADP (Figures 14–1 and 14–9). The series of reactions that comprise the electron transport system is shown in Figure 14–8.

Oxidative phosphorylation occurs along the cristae of eucaryotic mitochondria on special stalked particles and on the membranes of mesosomes and related structures of procaryotes.

ANAEROBIC RESPIRATION

The emphasis on oxygen in the electron transport system suggests that corresponding anaerobic systems do not occur. This is not true. The comparable anaerobic system of biological oxidations that does not use oxygen as the final acceptor of electrons is called *anaerobic respiration.* In anaerobic respiration, compounds such as carbonates, nitrates, and sulfates ultimately are reduced. Many facultative anaerobic bacteria can reduce nitrate to nitrite under anaerobic conditions. This type of reaction permits some continued growth when free oxygen is absent, but the accumulation of nitrite, which is produced by the reduction of nitrate, is eventually toxic to the organism. Certain species of *Bacillus* and *Pseudomonas* are able to continue the reduction of nitrite to gaseous nitrogen. This process, called **denitrification,** can occur only when these aerobic organisms are grown under anaerobic conditions. The organisms that reduce sulfate and carbonate are strictly anaerobic. *Desulfovibrio desulfuricans* reduces sulfate to hydrogen sulfide as it oxidizes carbohydrate to acetic acid. *Methanobacterium omelianskii* is able to couple the reduction of carbon dioxide to methane with a similar oxidation of carbohydrate to acetic acid.

The reduction of "bound oxygen" in anaerobic respiration with nitrate, sulfate, and carbonate involves cytochrome-containing electron transport systems comparable to that illustrated for aerobic respiration.

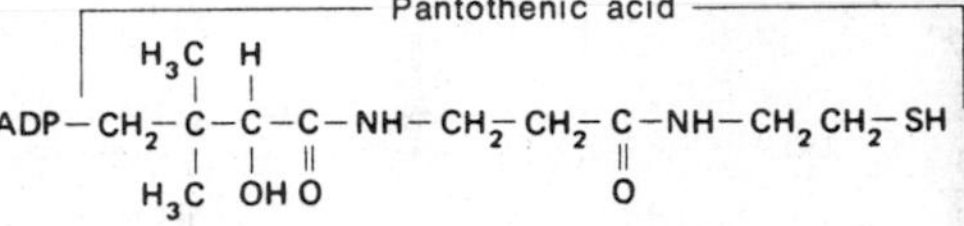

FIG. 14–7 Coenzyme A is a derivative of adenosine diphosphate (ADP). Attached to ADP is a molecule of pantothenic acid which bears a terminal thiol (-SH) group. Coenzyme A also can be symbolized as CoA-SH.

A Summary of Energy Production During Glucose Catabolism

The relationship of ATP production (net gain) to the various pathways in glucose catabolism is shown in Figure 14–9 and can be summed up as follows:

Glycolysis: glucose $\longrightarrow$ 2 pyruvic acids + 2 NADH's + 2 ATP's
Respiration: 2 pyruvic acids $\longrightarrow$ 2 acetyl CoA + 2 CO_2 + 2 NADH's
Krebs Cycle: 2 acetyl CoA's + 2 oxaloacetic acids $\longrightarrow$ 2 oxaloacetic acids + 4 CO_2 + 6 NADH's + 2 $FADH_2$'s + 2 ATP's

Aerobic procaryotic microorganisms can use these reactions to generate a maximum of thirty-eight ATP's from glucose. Glycolysis yields two ATP's by substrate phosphorylation, and subsequently by the same process an additional two ATP's are obtained in Krebs cycle. The total of ten NADH's can yield thirty ATP's, and the two $FADH_2$'s can yield four ATP's, all by oxidative phosphorylation. This totals thirty-eight ATP's.

Aerobic eucaryotic microorganisms, however, can only produce a total of thirty-six ATP's. The transition and citric acid cycle reactions occur within the

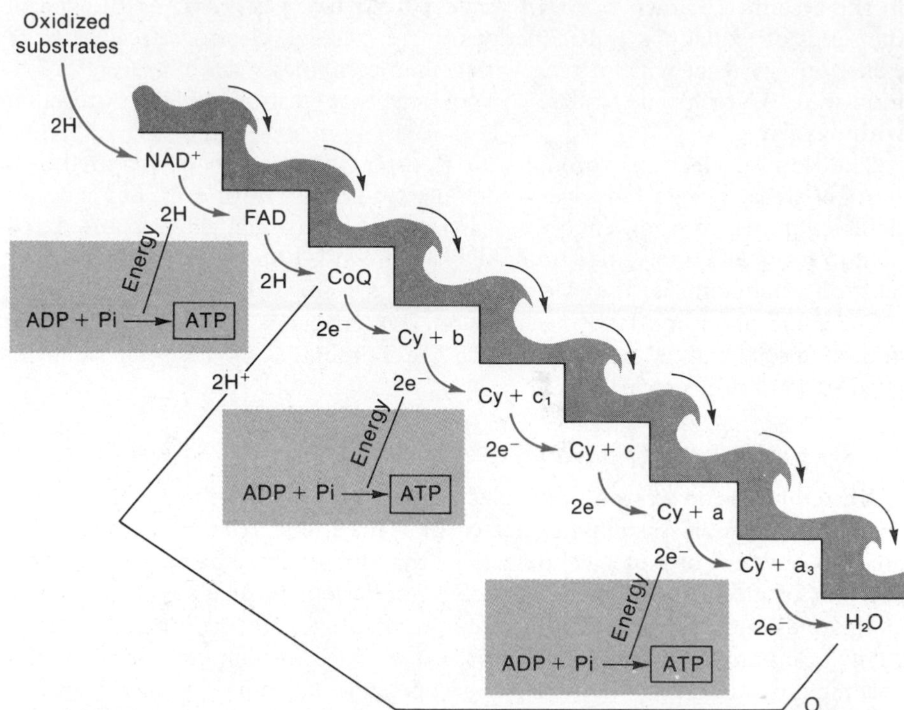

FIG. 14-8 The series of reactions that comprise the electron transport system. The formation of ATP by oxidative phosphorylation is shown in the boxes. Each e^- represents an electron.

fluid matrix of the mitochondria in close proximity to the sites of oxidative phosphorylation activity. However, glycolysis occurs in the cytoplasm, and the two NADH's produced in glycolysis must reduce $FADH_2$'s in the process of entering the mitochondria, thus losing two potential ATP's.

Metabolic Interrelationship of Carbohydrates, Fats, and Proteins

Although the metabolic pathways of carbohydrates, lipids, proteins, and other significant biochemical compounds are often described separately, they are actually closely related. A simplified version of the network formed by these pathways is shown in Figure 14–10.

In the catabolism of glucose to carbon dioxide, water, and energy, acetyl CoA can be produced (Figure 14–7), as previously discussed. Acetyl CoA is also a catabolic product of fat metabolism. Moreover, it is an important precursor in the synthesis of fatty acids. The interrelationship of fatty acid synthesis and glucose catabolism is well illustrated by the dependence of the fatty acid synthesis process on glycerol, an alternate product of glycolysis (Figure 14–4).

Acetyl CoA can also be obtained from proteins. For example, deamination (loss of the $-NH_2$ group) converts the amino acid alanine to pyruvic acid and subsequently acetyl CoA (Figure 14–10).

An additional example of the interrelationship of protein synthesis and glucose catabolism is the conversion of proteins to amino acids and then to pyruvic acid and the citric acid cycle intermediates, α-keto glutaric and oxaloacetic acids. The addition of an amino ($-NH_2$) group converts these compounds into the

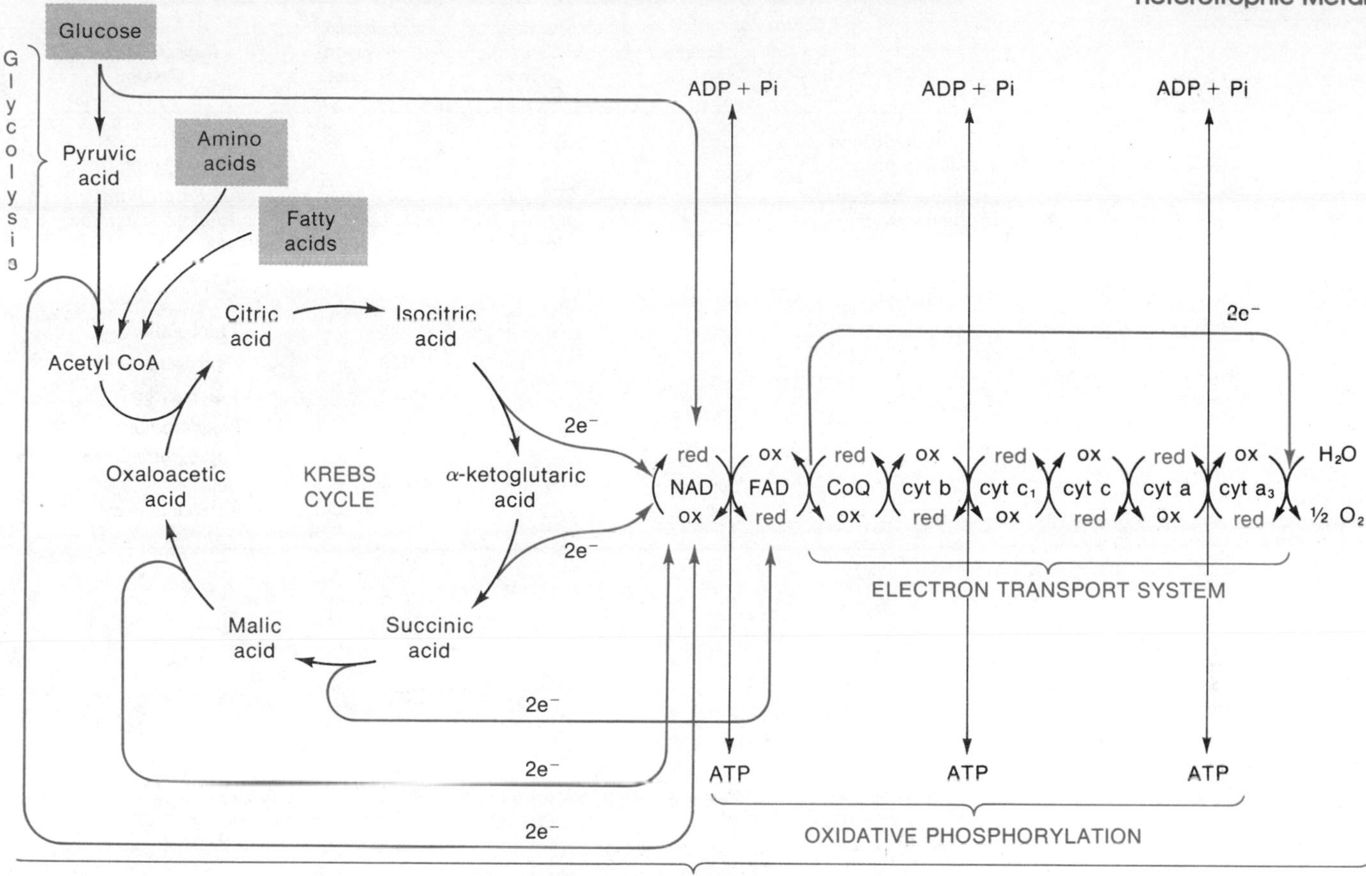

FIG. 14-9 A summary of the pathways by which glucose is oxidized to CO_2 and H_2O and a substantial portion of its energy is captured in the form of ATP. Glycolysis, the Krebs cycle, the electron transport system, and oxidative phosphorylation are shown.

building blocks of protein. Conversely, deamination (loss of $-NH_2$) converts glutamic and aspartic acids to the citric acid cycle intermediates, α-keto glutaric and oxaloacetic acids. Many of the steps in glycolysis are reversible, so that glucose units are available for combination into starch, glycogen, or cellulose. Thus, metabolic intermediates of carbohydrates, lipids, and proteins are used to create energy and building blocks for more carbohydrates, lipids, nucleic acids, and proteins. In this manner, the food digested by living beings becomes distinctively part of them.

Autotrophic and Heterotrophic Metabolism

The differentiation between autotrophic and heterotrophic types of microbial metabolism is based, in part, upon the capacity of organisms to use carbon dioxide as the major carbon source for the synthesis of required biochemical compounds. Autotrophs have this ability, while heterotrophs do not. Both groups are further classified into nutritional types according to the means used to obtain energy for growth and metabolism (Table 14-1).

TABLE 14-1 Classification of Microorganisms by Nutritional Types

Type	*Energy Source*	*Primary Carbon Sources*	*Selected Electron Sources*	*Representative Groups*
Photosynthetic autotroph	Light	CO_2	H_2S	*Chlorobium* *Chromatium*
Photosynthetic heterotroph	Light	CO_2 and organic substances	Organic substances	*Rhodospirillum* *Rhodopseudomonas*
Chemosynthetic autotroph	Oxidation reactions	CO_2	H_2S	*Beggiatoa*
			S^0	*Thiobacillus*
			H_2	*Hydrogenomonas*
			Fe^{++}	*Thiobacillus*
			CH_4	*Pseudomonas*
			CO	*Carboxydomonas*
Chemosynthetic heterotroph	Oxidation reactions	Organic substances	Organic substances	Most microorganisms

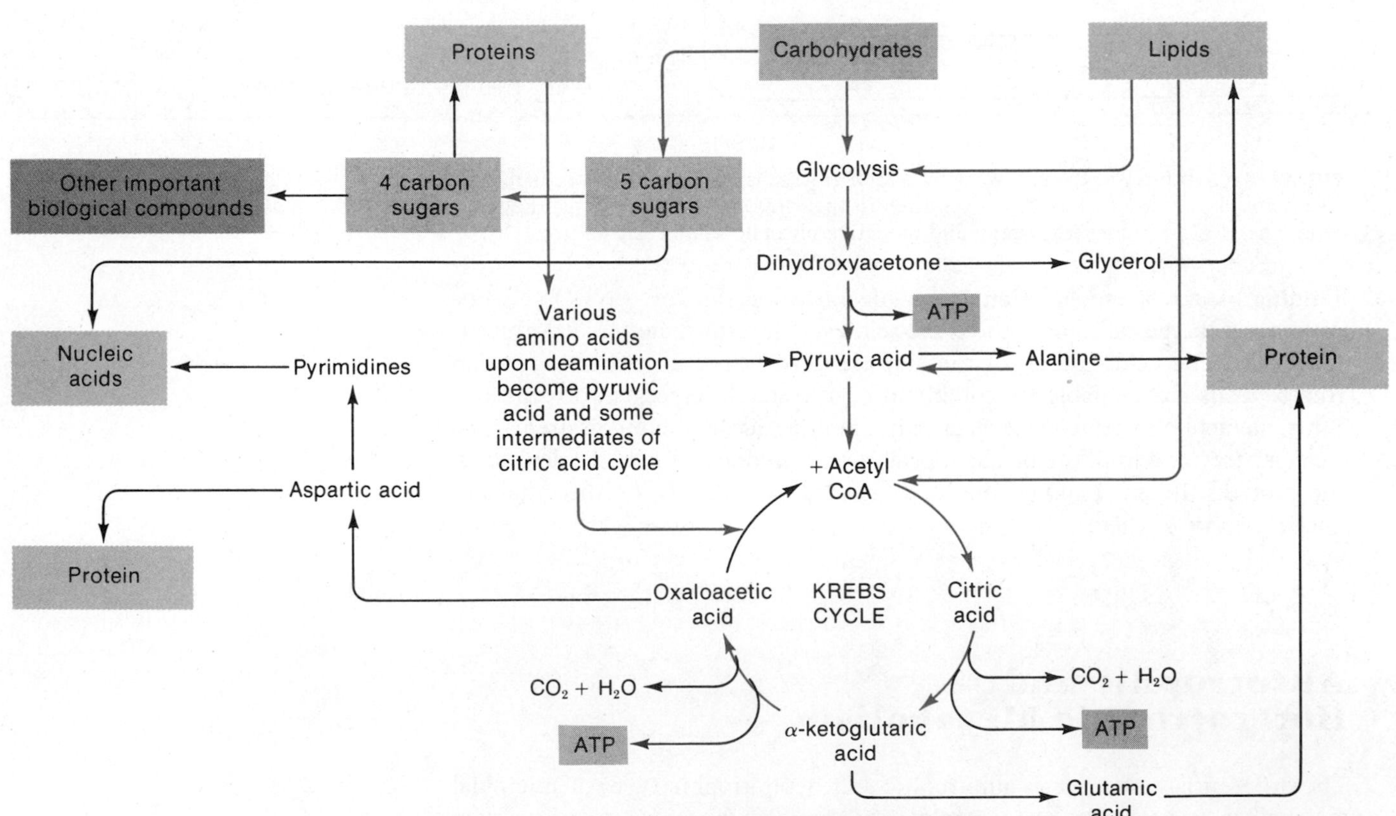

FIG. 14-10 The interrelationship between the metabolic pathways of carbohydrates, lipids, and proteins. Reactions involved with the degradation (breakdown) of compounds (nucleic acids) are indicated by dotted lines, while those reactions leading to the formation of important macromolecules are shown by solid lines.

Autotrophic Microorganisms

PHOTOSYNTHETIC AUTOTROPHS

The photosynthetic bacteria possess chlorophylls chemically similar to those found in plants. Photosynthetic pigments in bacteria are designated ***bacteriochlorophyll-a, -b, -c,*** and ***-d,*** to distinguish them from the plant pigment ***chlorophyll-a.*** In addition to the bacteriochlorophylls, photosynthetic organisms also have various carotenoid pigments, which impart coloration to their colonies. The colors include yellow to orange-brown, red, pink, reddish purple, and violet. Such pigmentation is largely dependent upon the type and concentration of carotenoid present. Green bacteria also contain carotenoids, but these compounds, which are light yellow, do not mask the green bacteriochlorophyll. The carotenoids in photosynthetic bacteria absorb light energy, which is then transferred to the bacteriochlorophyll for use in photosynthesis. Unlike the photosynthesis in cyanobacteria and green plants, photosynthesis by green and purple bacteria does not produce oxygen. In algae, cyanobacteria, and other photosynthetic eucaryotes, the energy absorbed from light by chlorophyll is used to split water molecules, yielding free oxygen and hydrogen ions. The hydrogen serves to reduce NADP to NADPH and is, thereby, made available for reducing additional substrates and for the electron transport system. The light energy thus ultimately causes production of adenosine triphosphate (ATP). Some of the reduced nicotinamide adenine dinucleotide phosphate (NADPH) and ATP are required for fixing carbon dioxide as carbohydrate and cell material. Thus, the energy from light absorption by chlorophyll results in the oxidation of water:

$$2H_2O \rightarrow 4H + O_2 \uparrow$$

and the reduction of CO_2:

$$CO_2 + 2\ NADPH + 3ATP \rightarrow \text{cell material} + H_2O$$

The first step in the fixation of CO_2 is the reaction of this compound and ribulose diphosphate to yield six molecules of phosphoglycerate. The phosphoglycerate is subsequently reduced to glyceraldehyde phosphate, which participates in the reversed glycolysis pathway eventually producing glucose and starch. The newly formed carbohydrate can be used for either energy or growth materials. The photosynthetic cycle is complete when some glyceraldehyde phosphate condenses to generate new ribulose diphosphate that can combine with additional CO_2. These reactions are summarized in Figure 14–11.

Unlike photosynthesis in green plants, noncyanobacterial photosynthesis does not release free oxygen. Because these photosynthetic bacteria do not oxidize water in the preliminary steps of their cycle, they cannot produce oxygen. They must oxidize other electron donor compounds, such as hydrogen sulfide (H_2S) and hydrogen (H_2). These two sets of reactions, which result in the fixation of CO_2, can be shown as follows:

$$CO_2 + 2H_2S \rightarrow \text{cell material} + H_2O + 2S$$

and

$$CO_2 + 2H_2 \rightarrow \text{cell material} + H_2O$$

The sulfide oxidation may result in the accumulation of elemental sulfur (S^o) within or outside the cells. When sulfide is depleted, the sulfur is oxidized to sulfuric acid.

CHEMOSYNTHETIC AUTOTROPHS

These nonphotosynthetic organisms rely on the oxidation of inorganic compounds for the energy necessary to fix CO_2 as the sole carbon source. They may oxidize hydrogen or hydrogen sulfide (like photosynthetic bacteria), ammonia, nitrites, and iron-containing substances. Representative reactions and bacteria capable of performing them are listed in Table 14–2.

TABLE 14–2 Energy Production by the Oxidation of Inorganic Compounds

Representative Bacterial Genera	*Energy-Yielding Reactions*
Hydrogenomonas	$2\,H_2 + O_2 \rightarrow 2\,H_2O$
Nitrobacter	$2\,NO_2^- + O_2 \rightarrow 2\,NO_3^{2-}$
Nitrosomonas	$2\,NH_3 + 3\,O_2 \rightarrow 2\,NO_2^- + 2H^+ + 2\,H_2O$
Thiobacillus	$\begin{cases} 2\,H_2S + O_2 \rightarrow 2S + 2\,H_2O \\ 2S + 3O_2 + 2H_2O \rightarrow 2SO_4{=} + 4H^+ \end{cases}$
	$4\,Fe^{2+} + 4H^+ + O_2 \rightarrow 4\,Fe^{3+} + 2\,H_2O$

Heterotrophic Microorganisms

PHOTOSYNTHETIC HETEROTROPHS

The photosynthetic heterotrophs are adaptable in their oxygen requirements. Anaerobic conditions must be present when the photosynthetic process is being used to obtain energy. This is also true for photosynthetic autotrophs. However,

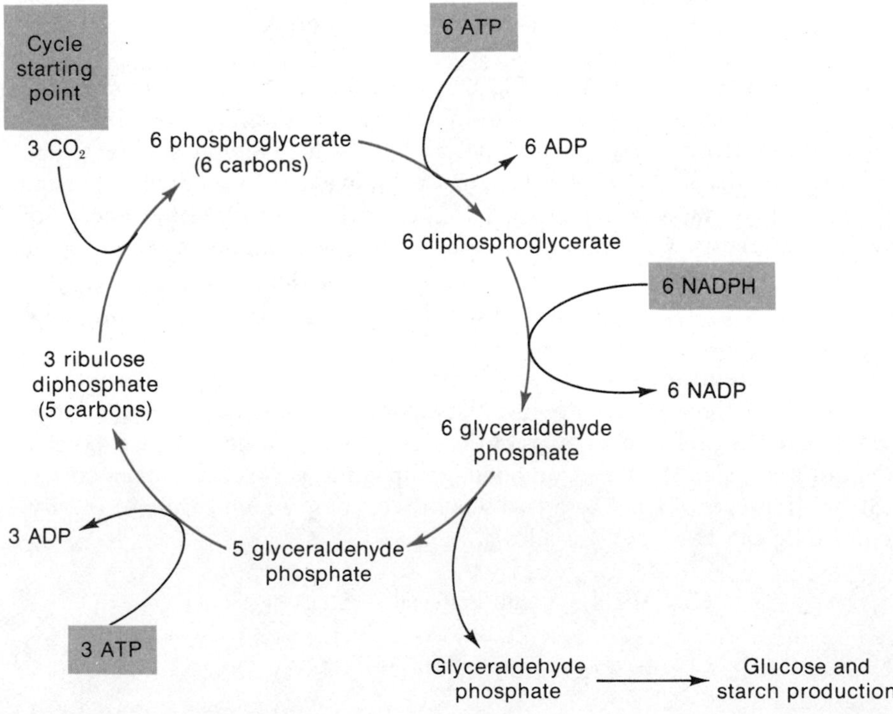

FIG. 14–11 A summary of photosynthetic reactions. The energy that drives the reactions of this cycle is in the form of ATP and reduced NADP. The number of carbon atoms in each compound is indicated.

unlike the autotrophic organisms, the heterotrophs' sources of electrons are alcohols, fatty acids, and other organic acids. Photosynthetic heterotrophs can grow aerobically only in the dark. Under these conditions they are, in essence, the same as chemosynthetic heterotrophs, a class that includes most microorganisms and members of the animal kingdom.

CHEMOSYNTHETIC HETEROTROPHS

These microorganisms are quite varied in their metabolism. However, they all perform the metabolic reactions of carbohydrates, proteins, and lipids described earlier in this chapter. In addition to respiration using molecular oxygen as the ultimate electron acceptor, chemosynthetic heterotrophs also perform the fermentation and anaerobic respiration reactions described above.

Protein Synthesis

Probably one of the greatest scientific accomplishments of the 1960s was the delineation of the steps in protein synthesis. Chief among the critical aspects of this work was the initial breaking of the genetic code, or nucleotide language, reported by Marshall W. Nirenberg in 1961.

Genetic Code

When it had been determined that DNA was, indeed, the genetic substance, the question was posed as to what combinations of the four nucleotides containing the nitrogenous bases guanine (G), adenine (A), cytosine (C) and thymine (T) might code for each of the twenty amino acids found in proteins. The first question to be answered was how many nucleotides were required to specify an amino acid. The four nucleotides could be used to write out only 16 two-letter "code words"—GA, GC, GT, AC, AT, etc.—and could, therefore, specify only sixteen of the twenty amino acids. A code using three nucleotides (GTA, GCA, CTG, etc.) would allow 64 combinations, more than enough to specify all the natural amino acids. Four-letter codes would permit 256 combinations.

The triplet code with its 64 combinations would permit the 20 needed combinations, with 44 extra for alternate combinations to code for certain amino acids and to act as spacers or regulatory areas—punctuation marks of a sort. Nirenberg and others have demonstrated that the triplet code is, indeed, the operating genetic system.

Nirenberg found that synthetic RNA trinucleotides would stimulate the incorporation of specific amino acids onto ribosomes. The first triplets studied, containing uracil (UUU), adenine (AAA), and cytosine (CCC), directed the binding of phenylalanine, lysine, and proline, respectively, in cell-free systems using combinations of ribosomes and messenger (m) RNA, transfer (t) RNA, and DNA. Alternate codes were found for some amino acids.

Examples of representative nucleotide sequences of messenger RNA, reported in 1965 by Bernfeld and Nirenberg, are shown in Figure 14–12. The code specifying a single amino acid may allow for as few as one or as many as four arrangements of nucleotides. The 64 possible combinations allow for an average of 3 combinations per amino acid. The data suggest that most amino acids have two sequences. Three of the 64 combinations do not code for any of the known amino acids. Such codons are referred to as *nonsense* triplets and serve to signal the stopping points of the information for the formation of a particular protein molecule.

The genetic code appears to be universal. Similar code sequences are found in organisms as different as bacteria and mammals. The reason for this universality is not difficult to see if one remembers that all life forms must synthesize many protein molecules with similar functions. Enzymes constitute a good example of such molecules.

One key to understanding protein synthesis is the complementarity discussed earlier. Recall that in DNA the two strands are kept at a specific distance because adenine is always paired by hydrogen bonds with thymine and guanine is always paired with cytosine. We therefore say that, for DNA, the pairs of adenine with thymine, and cytosine with guanine are complementary.

In Figure 14–13, the production of a molecule of messenger RNA (*m*RNA) is shown. This molecule literally carries the code from DNA to the ribosomes in the cytoplasm where the *m*RNA directs synthesis of proteins.

Messenger RNA (*m*RNA) carrying the genetic code for a particular protein is produced in the nucleus or in a plastid such as a mitochondrion or chloroplast. This process is known as **transcription.** The right-hand strand of DNA in Figure 14–13 shows two complete triplets, GCT and CGA, out of dozens or hundreds in the complete code for some protein. Only one DNA strand contains the code for all the possible *m*RNA's that can be produced by transcription from the DNA molecule. This piece of DNA is known as the "sense strand" and serves the role of pattern, or *template.* Each of the triplets GCT and CGA serves as the pattern for complementary code words, or *codons,* in *m*RNA (Figure 14–11), consisting of a nucleotide sequence complementary to the sequence of the DNA strand. In this instance, the codons are CGA and GCU, respectively. (Recall that thymine is not found in RNA: it is replaced by uracil, giving the complementary pair adenine-uracil.) Transcription is under the control of a DNA-dependent enzyme, RNA polymerase. The enzyme appears to bind particularly to specific nucleotide sequences, called *promotor* regions, in the DNA molecule. Such promotors serve as start signals for the transcription of single genes and sometimes for groups or clusters of genes called **operons.** (Operons are discussed later in this chapter.) When the *m*RNA molecule is completed, it passes from its site of formation to the ribosomes, which are nucleoprotein particles.

Decoding the information contained in *m*RNA is referred to as **transla-**

Codon	*Amino Acid*	*Codon*	*Amino Acid*	*Codon*	*Amino Acid*	*Codon*	*Amino Acid*
AAA	lysine	CAC	histidine	GAA	glutamic acid	UAA	nonsense
AAG	lysine	CAU	histidine	GAG	glutamic acid	UAG	nonsense
ACA	threonine	CCC	proline	GCA	alanine	UCA	serine
ACG	threonine	CCU	proline	GCU	alanine	UCG	serine
AGA	arginine	CGA	arginine	GGA	glycine	UGA	nonsense
AGG	arginine	CGU	arginine	GGG	glycine	UGG	tryptophan
AUA	isoleucine	CUC	leucine	GUA	valine	UUA	leucine
AUG	methionine	CUU	leucine	GUG	valine	UUG	leucine

FIG. 14–12 Representative nucleotide sequences of the genetic code. Examples of the RNA nucleotide sequences or *codons* are shown together with the specific amino acids they represent. Two different codons may specify the same amino acid. Nonsense codons, which do not stand for any of the amino acids but serve as punctuation signals in the protein synthesis process, appear in colored boxes. The codons are read from left to right.

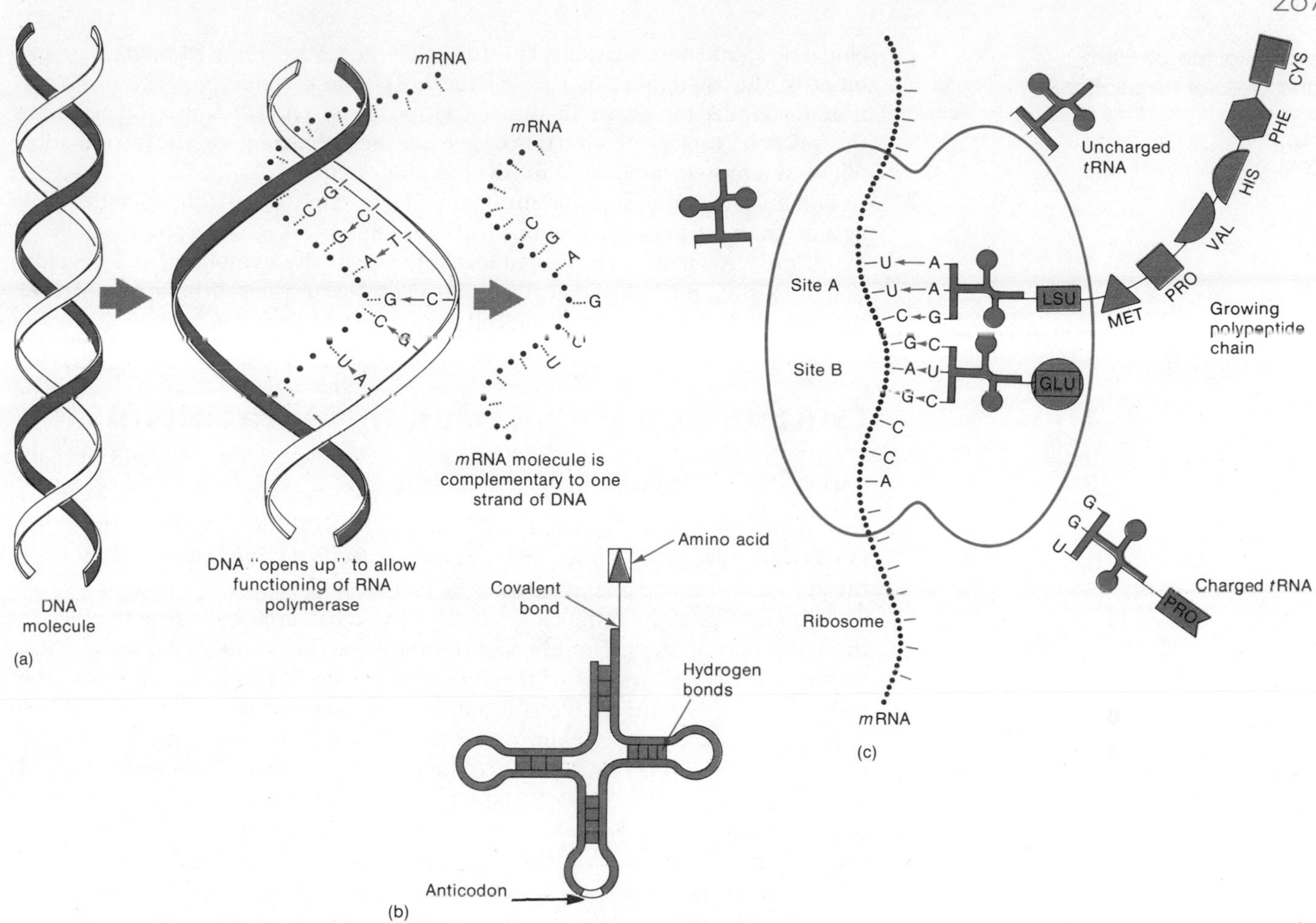

FIG. 14–13 Protein synthesis. (a) Transcription, the formation of a messenger RNA molecule. (b) A transfer RNA molecule. (c) Translation. The processes of decoding and *t*RNA binding are shown.

tion. It consists of two general steps, one of which is ribosome-independent and the other, ribosome-dependent. In the first, free amino acids are activated by enzymatic reactions involving adenosine triphosphate (ATP) and are coupled to transfer RNA (*t*RNA) (Figure 14–13b). For each amino acid there are one or more specific activating enzymes. There are also one or more different *t*RNA molecules. Each *t*RNA molecule contains an ***anticodon***, a sequence of three nucleotide bases that can pair with a complementary codon in an *m*RNA molecule.

During the time that a protein molecule is being synthesized, *t*RNA is continuously released and made available for use by additional amino acids. Once the ATP activation reactions have occurred, the amino acids diffuse to the ribosome and enter the ribosome-dependent phase of the translation process. In the coupling reaction between *t*RNA's and amino acids, specific *t*RNA's recognize and combine with specific amino acids. If the wrong amino acid is attached to the *t*RNA, it may be inserted in an improper position on the protein molecule. A situation of this type could lead to a faulty or nonfunctional protein.

The major function of ribosomes in the second phase of translation is to orient the *m*RNA and the incoming *t*RNA complex (*t*RNA and activated amino acid) so that the information contained in an *m*RNA molecule can be correctly converted into the amino sequence of a protein molecule. The ribosome-dependent process can be divided into the three phases of initiation, elongation, and termination. The initiation phase involves ribosomal attachment to the appropriate portion of the *m*RNA and ribosomal binding to the initiator *t*RNA molecule. In the elongation phase the ribosome travels along the *m*RNA, catalyzing the translation of the molecule. In the termination phase, the protein product is finished and released.

The *m*RNA is unstable and must be replaced fairly often. This liability may be a mechanism to assure that one particular protein is not overproduced. With many *m*RNA's being synthesized and released to the cytoplasm, the degradation of existing *m*RNA makes ribosomes available for the synthesis of whatever structural protein or enzyme the cell may need.

Control and Regulation of Metabolism

Feedback or End-product Inhibition

In many enzymatic reactions, the final product inhibits, or slows, the series of reactions that produced it. This is known as ***feedback inhibition***. Synthesis of the amino acid isoleucine in ***Escherichia coli*** is one such set of reactions. When extra quantities of an amino acid are added to a bacterial culture actively synthesizing that particular amino acid, synthesis of the compound ceases. Thus, by controlling the amount of the isoleucine made available to a culture, the pathway for this compound can be either started or stopped.

As long as isoleucine is required for protein synthesis or for other metabolic reactions, synthesis continues. When the reactions utilizing isoleucine stop and the compound begins to accumulate, it interferes with the particular enzyme responsible for starting the pathway. Studies of this control mechanism using isolated enzymes show that the end product inhibits the activity of the first enzyme involved in the pathway leading to its synthesis (Figure 14–14).

The similarity of molecular structure of the end product (isoleucine) and the substrate of the first enzyme (threonine) in the pathway suggests that these two compounds

```
CH3 — CH2 \
            CH — CH — COOH
          /       |
     CH3          NH2
```

Isoleucine

```
CH3 \
     CH — CH — COOH
    /       |
HO          NH2
```

Threonine

are structurally enough alike to allow isoleucine to fit into the active site of the enzyme and thus block its activity. However, this does not appear to be the mechanism of inhibition.

Evidence indicates that the inhibition is ***allosteric***, or indirect. The isoleucine binds at a site different from the active one. The first enzyme, threonine deaminase, can be partly altered by heat denaturation or mutation in a way that desensitizes the regulatory site. In this case, the pathway functions continuously and isoleucine accumulates beyond normal levels.

Isoleucine synthesis offers one of many examples of regulatory mechanisms

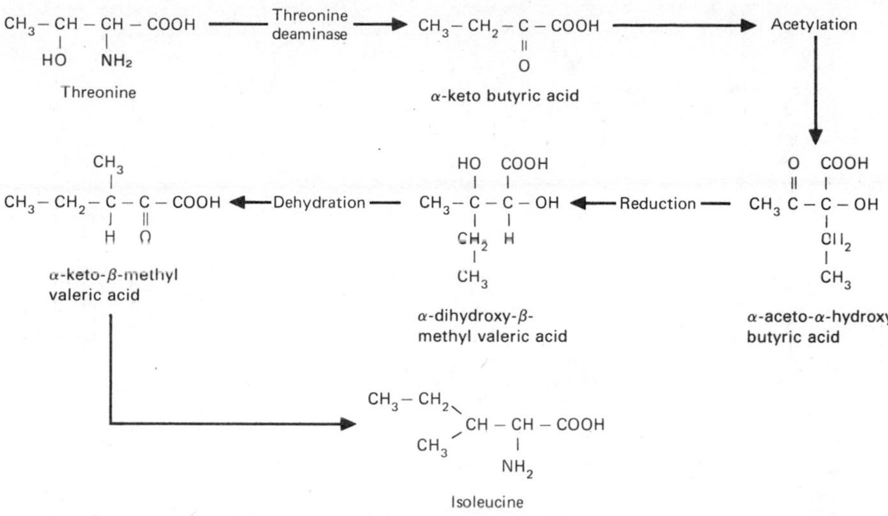

FIG. 14-14 The isoleucine synthetic pathway.

involved in metabolic reactions. The presence of such regulation makes one think of a cell as a finely tuned automated system for the performance of life processes. But the programming for this system can sometimes go awry. Mutations may alter the function of enzymes. The cell can sometimes compensate for this lack or it may simply rely on the environment to provide a particular compound essential to its nutrition. Mutations or biochemical defects can also cause accumulation of certain chemicals that may become toxic to the cell. Such metabolic defects occur in humans as well as in other life forms. One example of this type of situation in humans is phenylketonuria (PKU) in which an enzyme needed for the metabolism of the amino acid phenylalanine is missing.

Operons

Feedback or end-product inhibition depends on control of metabolism at the enzyme level. A given enzyme beginning a pathway is turned off when a particular metabolite accumulates, then turned on when the concentration decreases. This is a clever system, but apparently it does not prevent the synthesis of the enzyme or enzymes involved in the pathway. It might be more efficient for cells to have a means of regulating the synthesis of enzymes they may need at any particular time. Logically, this control would operate at the level of DNA in protein synthesis. Regulatory systems of procaryotes utilize clusters of genes known as **operons** (Figure 14–15).

Operons have been shown to be of two types. One type, the ***repressible*** operons, controls the synthesis of enzymes normally present. The second type, the ***inducible*** operons, controls the synthesis of enzymes normally absent.

The operon consists of structural genes and an operator gene or genes (Figure 14–15). The structural genes contain the information to cause the synthesis of enzymes that perform the steps in the particular metabolic pathway. The operator is a switch that can permit the formulation of *m*RNA from the structural genes (DNA). In addition, there is a control substance produced from one or more regulator genes. In the repressible operon, the operator, or switch, is in the "on" position. An end product of the particular pathway can react with the

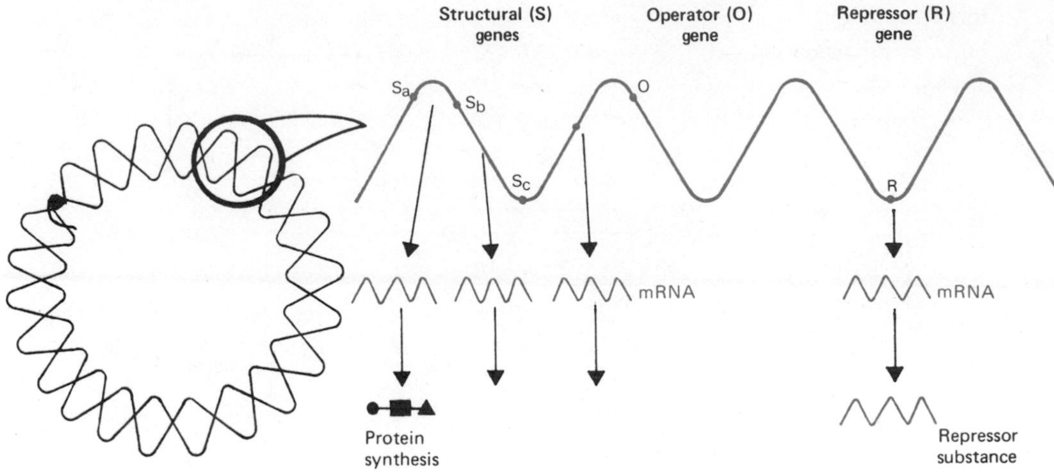

FIG. 14-15 A generalized model of an operon. *Repressible operon:* The end product reacts with a repressor substance, which causes the operator gene(s) to stop formation of *m*RNA for enzyme synthesis. *Inducible operon:* The compound to be metabolized reacts with a repressor substance and causes the operator gene(s) to permit the formation of *m*RNA for enzyme synthesis.

control substance, called the regulator, and turn the operator off. Then no more *m*RNA is produced, and the existing *m*RNA for these enzymes will gradually degrade and stop synthesis of this enzyme. This system is also known as end-product repression. In the inducible operon, the operator is in the "off" position due to the presence of the control substance called the repressor. Apparently a compound to be metabolized reacts with the repressor, allowing the operator to turn on and permit *m*RNA to be made for the synthesis of the required enzymes.

Measurement of Metabolism

Metabolic studies have shown how antibiotics interfere with microbial growth and also how microorganisms can alter their metabolism to become resistant to these drugs. They have also demonstrated some basic differences between pathogenic and nonpathogenic bacteria. The results of such investigations are being used to develop faster methods of identifying clinically important microorganisms. Among the methods used are: (1) simple fermentation tests; (2) manometry; (3) oxidation-reduction activity; (4) the use of radioisotopes; and (5) chromatography.

Simple Fermentation Tests

When an organism has the necessary enzymes to ferment a particular sugar, we are generally able to detect fermentation by the production of organic acids, with or without gas. This can be accomplished either by incorporating some nontoxic pH indicator in the medium, or by adding it after growth. A decrease in pH indicates that a fermentation reaction or the production of organic acids (Color photograph 64) took place. In liquid media, gas production can be observed by the presence of obvious bubbling or by trapping the gas in an inverted small glass tube (Figure 14–16a). This tube, known as a *Durham tube,* is placed upside down in the fermentation medium prior to autoclaving. The formation of gas within the system displaces the liquid in the inverted vial.

Generally, the Durham tube indicates only the presence or absence of gas. The *Smith fermentation tube* (Figure 14–16b) can be used to measure the relative proportions of different gases produced. Because microorganisms often produce more gas than the Durham tube is capable of holding, the Smith tube is preferable for obtaining a reasonably accurate measurement of the volume of gas produced. This can be accomplished by measuring the portion of tube containing gas before (Figure 14–16b) and after (Figure 14–16c) the addition of alkali to absorb CO_2. Thus one can determine the relative amounts of CO_2 produced. Because the remaining gas is primarily H_2, the measurements indicate the ratio of H_2 to CO_2 formed.

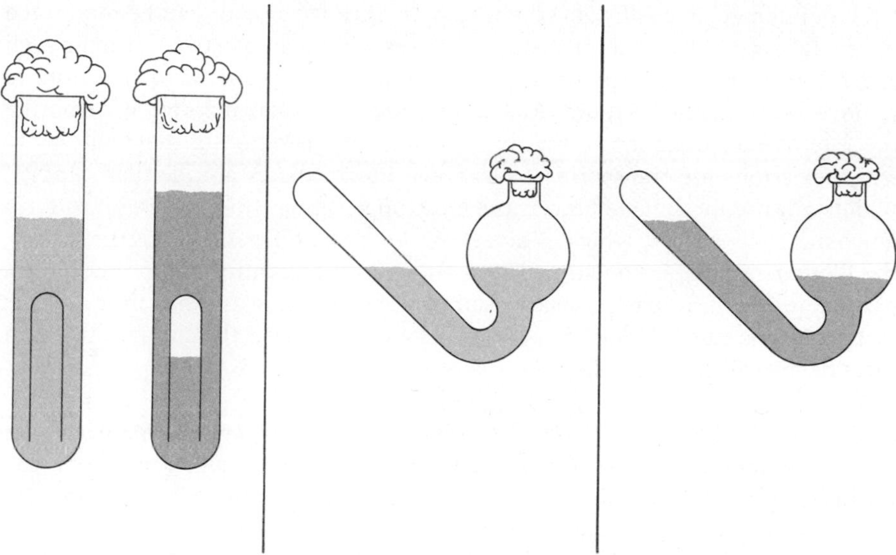

FIG. 14–16 Comparison of gas production from sugar fermentations. (a) Uninoculated Durham fermentation tube and the results of active fermentation. Note the displacement of the fluid from the inverted vial. (b) A Smith tube before the addition of an alkali compound. (c) The results after addition of an alkali compound.

Manometry

Manometry, or differential gas pressure measurement, can be used in any closed system where gas is either consumed or evolved. The Warburg apparatus (Figure 14–17), which can be used to make such determinations, consists of several manometer-flask systems. The flasks are submerged in a constant-temperature water bath and agitated to mix the reactants and speed diffusion of gas into and out of the reaction mixture.

To demonstrate how measurements are made, let us assume that the following conditions have been carried out: A resting (nonmultiplying) suspension of *Escherichia coli* is placed in the flask around the raised central well (Figure 14–17b). Alkali is introduced into the well for the purpose of absorbing CO_2, and a solution of some organic acid is placed in the side arm so that it is not in direct contact with the *E. coli*.

To examine the rate of hydrogen production under anaerobic conditions, the system is assembled, flushed with sterile nitrogen gas, and allowed to reach temperature and gas pressure equilibrium in the water bath. After a certain period, during which time any changes in pressure have been recorded on the manometer, the flask is tipped to cause the organic acid to mix with the test

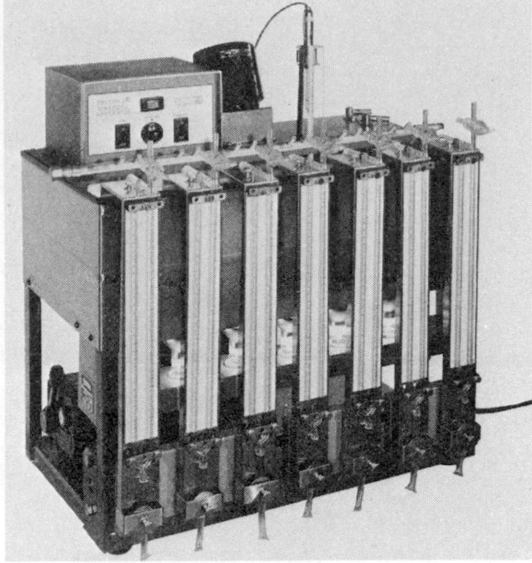

(a)

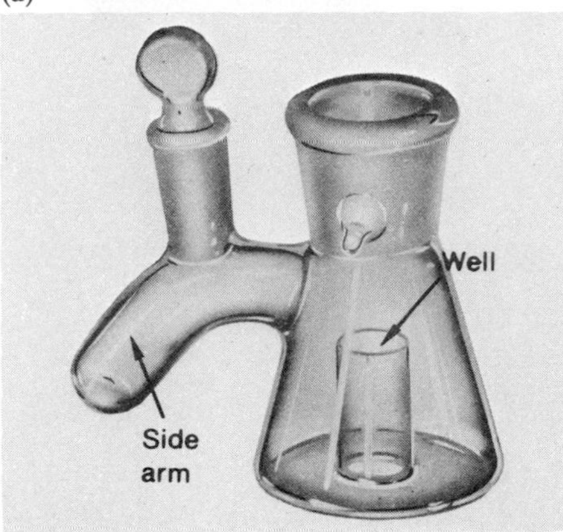

(b)

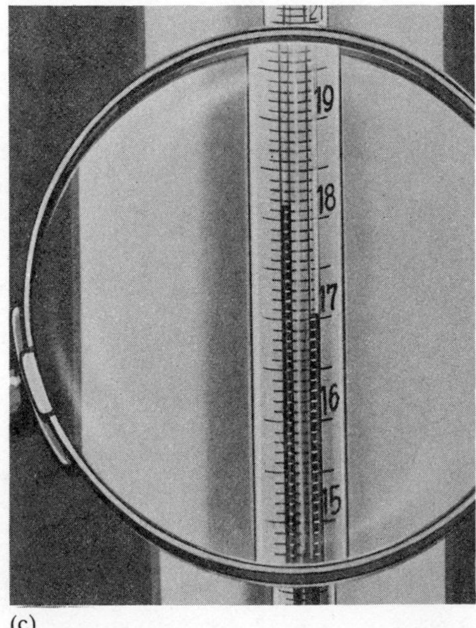

(c)

FIG. 14-17 (a) A Warburg apparatus for manometric measurement. *Courtesy of Precision Scientific Co.* (b) A Warburg reaction flask. The locations of materials used in measurements are indicated. *Courtesy of Precision Scientific Co.* (c) A Warburg manometer. *Courtesy of Bronwill Scientific Inc.*

organisms. Because CO_2 is absorbed in the center well by the alkali, any other gas produced (presumably H_2) by the test organism acting on the organic acid will increase the system's pressure and be evident on the manometer. By regularly recording the increasing pressure, the information necessary to calculate the rate of gas production under these particular conditions is collected.

Similar experiments can be performed with other materials, including cell-free extracts, tissue homogenates, and fractionated extracts of homogenates. Thus, one can determine the effect of atmospheric composition, added cofactors, or various metabolites on any biochemical system capable of consuming or producing gas.

Oxidation-Reduction Activity

Under anaerobic conditions, the metabolic activity of cells can be monitored in several ways. One such procedure involves adding an electron acceptor such as methylene blue to a resting suspension and then exposing it to a vacuum to remove air from the medium. Metabolic activity is then monitored by noting the rate of decolorization of the dye. During the operation of metabolic pathways, electrons are transported by various intermediates and dehydrogenases, which can use methylene blue as the electron acceptor, thus causing it to form leuco-methylene blue, which is colorless. A device for performing these tests, the ***Thunberg tube***, is shown in Figure 14–18. To determine the presence of a particular dehydrogenase, a specific substrate is placed in the side arm and the system is evacuated. Then the tube is sealed by turning the top portion with the side arm (Figure 14–18b).

A common source of electrons in biological systems is the Krebs cycle intermediate, succinic acid. If succinic acid dehydrogenase is present in a particular unknown system, the resting suspension will remove electrons from the substrate to methylene blue with some intermediate steps. The loss of color indicates the presence of that dehydrogenase. Using properly controlled studies, one can determine: (1) possible metabolic pathways; (2) the effect of various respiratory inhibitors; and (3) blocks in metabolic pathways.

Radioisotopes

Some of the elements that make up biochemical compounds, such as carbon, nitrogen, oxygen, and phosphorus, exist in several forms, called ***isotopes***. Isotopes of an element have the same atomic number but different atomic masses. Certain isotopes are unstable; as they deteriorate, they release various radioactive particles—alpha, beta, and gamma rays. These can be detected by radiation counters or by their effect on photographic emulsions. Table 14–3 lists some of the common isotopes used in biochemical research and their respective ***half-lives*** (the time required to lose half of their radioactivity).

TABLE 14–3 Common Isotopes Used in Biochemistry

Element	*Radioisotope*	*Half-Life*
Carbon (^{12}C)	^{14}C	5,570 years
Hydrogen (^{1}H)	^{3}H	12.2 years
Sulfur (^{32}S)	^{35}S	87.1 days
Iron ($^{55.8}Fe$)	^{59}Fe	45 days
Phosphorus ($^{30.9}P$)	^{32}P	14.3 days
Iodine ($^{126.9}I$)	^{131}I	8 days

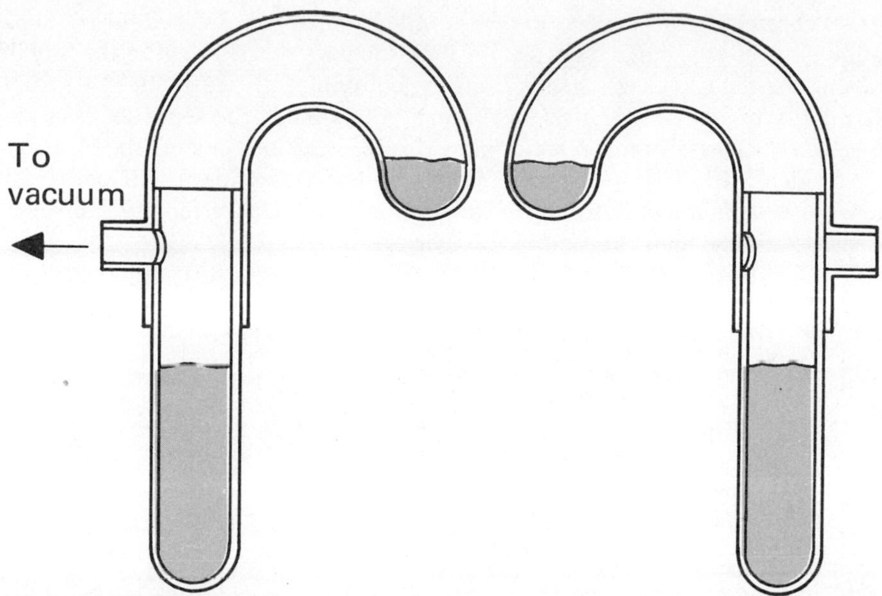

FIG. 14–18 The Thunberg tube. On the left, the tube is being prepared for the test determination. On the right, the system is ready for testing.

METABOLIC STUDIES OF MICROBES USING RADIOISOTOPES

Melvin Calvin began a study on the pathway of carbon in photosynthesis in 1946, using radioactive carbon dioxide $^{14}CO_2$. $^{14}CO_2$ was introduced into the atmosphere of growing algae organisms. Periodically the photosynthetic process was interrupted briefly to remove small samples of compounds formed. The various carbon compounds of the algae were isolated and tested for radioactivity, an indication of carbon-14. In this manner the pathway of carbon in the photosynthesis cycle could be traced step by step through the presence of C-14 in successive metabolic products.

Tritium (^3H) labeled thymidine was used by John Cairns to obtain an autoradiograph (photographic record) of the ***genome*** of *E. coli*. Cairns first fed the nucleic acid precursor to *E. coli* and later lysed the bacteria cell and very carefully transferred the bacterial DNA to photographic plates. After a two-month exposure, the autoradiograph shown in Figure 14–19 was obtained. It shows the circular nature and mode of replication of the bacterial chromosome.

Chromatography

The term ***chromatography*** refers to procedures that separate the components of a mixture by causing the mixture to migrate through a solid matrix such as filter paper carried by two or more solvents. Under these conditions one solvent is adsorbed to the matrix and the remaining solvents remain mobile. As the solvents seep through the matrix, different conditions for adsorption of the mixture's components occur, and the components separate.

The first major study involving chromatography was made by Michael Tswett in 1906. By running an ether solution of chlorophyll through a column of calcium carbonate, he was able to separate the various colored pigments.

Chromatography can be performed with various solvent mixtures on filter paper, silica, or cellulose-coated glass, or in columns containing various solid matrices such as powdered calcium carbonate or alumina.

Gas chromatography is a form of column chromatography used for the separation of gases or vaporized chemicals, with some inert carrier gas as the mobile solvent. As the carrier gas passes from the column, it enters a detector, which commonly uses the differences in thermal properties of the separated material to detect it. Generally the detector plots this information on a graph. Materials can be identified by comparing their times of detection under particular conditions with tabulations of times for known materials. Gas chromatography has been used in the identification of microorganisms.

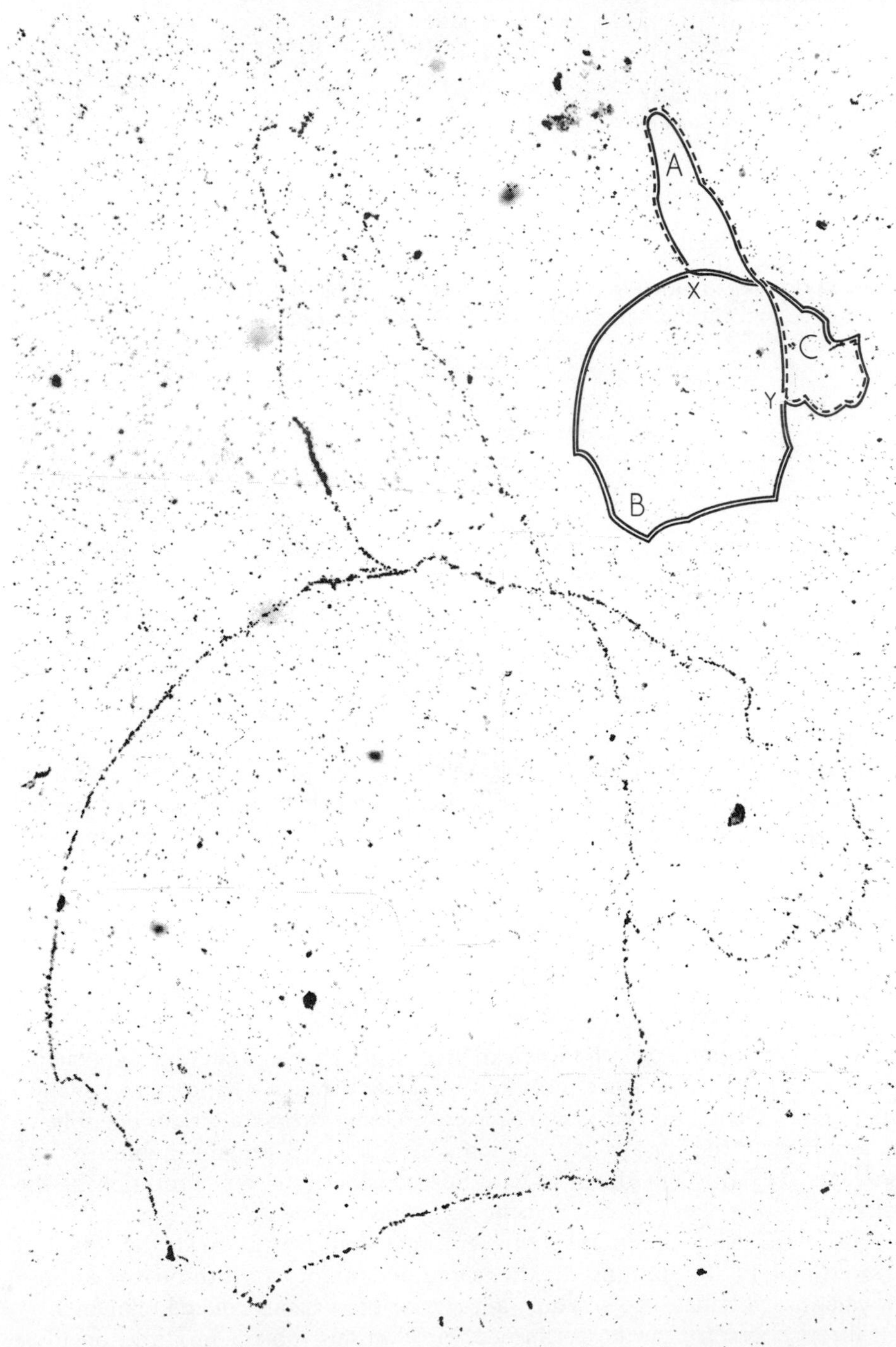

FIG. 14-19 An autoradiograph of *Escherichia coli* DNA. *Cairns, J.:* Cold Spring Harbor Symp. Quant. Biol. 28:*43–46 (1963).*

SUMMARY

General Metabolism

1. Metabolism refers to the entire set of chemical reactions by which a cell produces and forms the various macromolecules it needs to maintain itself. The two general categories of metabolism are *catabolism* and *anabolism*.
2. Catabolic reactions through which complex compounds are broken down with the release of energy are linked to anabolic reactions which result in the formation of important macromolecules.

Processes Essential to Cellular Growth and Reproduction

Energy Metabolism

1. The basic process for producing adenosine triphosphate (ATP) involves combining adenosine diphosphate (ADP) with inorganic phosphate (Pi). This reaction requires energy, which can be obtained through *photosynthetic phosphorylation*, *substrate phosphorylation*, or *oxidative phosphorylation*.
2. In photosynthetic phosphorylation, the required energy is obtained from the absorption of light by chlorophyll.
3. During substrate phosphorylation reactions, energy is released from substances (substrates) acted upon by enzymes. This energy can be used to form ATP.

Glycolysis

1. Glycolysis refers to the catabolic reactions that convert glucose into pyruvic acid and/or glycerol, and molecules such as ATP and NADH.
2. Glycolysis can occur under both aerobic and anaerobic conditions. Some of the anaerobic processes are called fermentation.

Krebs (Citric Acid) Cycle

1. The complete breakdown of glucose involves three phases: glycolysis (anaerobic), the Krebs cycle, and the electron transport system (ETS, aerobic). Energy in the form of ATP results from the reactions associated with these phases.
2. The Krebs cycle includes the conversion of the 6-carbon compound, citric acid, to the 4-carbon compound, oxaloacetic acid.
3. Acetyl CoA is a major intermediate compound involved in the Krebs cycle.

Electron Transport System

1. Oxidative phosphorylation requires coenzymes such as nicotinamide adenine dinucleotide (NAD), adenine dinucleotide phosphate (NADP), and flavin adenine dinucleotide (FAD). During a series of oxidation and reduction reactions, enough energy is produced to form ATP. This series of reactions constitutes the *electron transport system*.
2. Oxidative phosphorylation occurs along the cristae of eucaryotic mitochondria and mesosome membranes of procaryotes.

A Summary of Energy Production During Glucose Catabolism

By means of substrate phosphorylation and oxidative phosphorylation, a total of thirty-eight ATP's are produced from the breakdown of one glucose molecule.

Metabolic Interrelationship of Carbohydrates, Fats, and Proteins

1. Several aspects of the metabolism of carbohydrates, lipids, proteins, and other compounds are interrelated.
2. Various metabolic intermediate compounds of these pathways are used for energy and the construction of other macromolecules.

Autotrophic and Heterotrophic Metabolism

Autotrophs can use carbon dioxide as their major carbon source for the formation of essential biochemical compounds. Heterotrophs do not have this capacity.

Autotrophic Microorganisms

1. The bacteriochlorophylls found among photosynthetic autotrophic bacteria include *a*, *b*, *c*, and *d*. Such chlorophylls are different from those found in plants.
2. The photosynthetic process carried out by green or purple bacteria does not result in the formation of oxygen. Cyanobacterial photosynthesis does produce oxygen.
3. Photosynthetic bacteria combine carbon dioxide with ribulose diphosphate to form other macromolecules, which can be used for energy and growth.
4. Nonphotosynthetic organisms such as the *chemosynthetic autotrophs* rely on the oxidation of inorganic compounds, including hydrogen or hydrogen sulfide, for the energy to fix carbon dioxide.

Heterotrophic Microorganisms

1. Heterotrophic organisms that are capable of photosynthesis can adjust to varying levels of oxygen.
2. Chemosynthetic heterotrophs perform metabolic reactions involving carbohydrates, proteins, and lipids similar to those performed by other organisms.

Protein Synthesis

1. Deoxyribonucleic acid (DNA) directs the formation of proteins with the aid of different types of ribonucleic acid (RNA) molecules.
2. The DNA molecule involved in protein synthesis unwinds and serves as a pattern or mold for the formation of messenger RNA. *Transcription* is the process by means of which the specific information necessary for the formation of a protein molecule is incorporated into the newly formed molecule.
3. The messenger RNA travels to a site within the cell where ribosomes decode the information contained within the molecule. This process is called *translation*.
4. After activation of specific amino acids, these building blocks of proteins are carried to the site of protein production by transfer RNA.
5. Finished proteins are used by cells for enzymes or structures.

Control and Regulation of Metabolism

Feedback or End-product Inhibition

1. Feedback inhibition is one of several metabolic regulatory mechanisms found in cells.

2. It refers to the control of a series of enzymatic reactions by the end product of a specific metabolic pathway.

Operons

1. An **operon** represents a mechanism for the regulation of enzyme production.
2. Two types of operons are recognized, ***repressible*** and ***inducible***. Repressible operons consist of a cluster of genes that control the formation of normally present enzymes. Inducible ones control the formation of enzymes normally absent.
3. An operon consists of structural and operator genes. Structural genes are associated with the synthesis of metabolically important enzymes, while operator genes control the activities of the structural genes.

Measurement of Metabolism

1. Metabolic studies have shown how antibiotics may interfere with microbial growth and cause changes in metabolic activities of microorganisms.
2. Specific methods used to study microbial metabolism include simple fermentation tests, manometry, oxidation-reduction activity, radioisotopes, and chromatography.

QUESTIONS FOR REVIEW

1. Differentiate between catabolic and anabolic reactions in a cell's metabolism.
2. Describe, briefly, the basic differences between each of three mechanisms for making ATP during catabolism.
3. Outline the general steps in glycolysis and indicate the primary end products of this process.
4. Compare the total numbers of ATP molecules that can be formed by glycolysis in terms of substrate and oxidative phosphorylation, under anaerobic and aerobic conditions.
5. What is meant by fermentation? List typical products that may be produced by bacteria from pyruvic acid under anaerobic conditions.
6. What is anaerobic respiration?
7. What occurs during the transition reaction between glycolysis and the citric acid cycle in aerobic metabolism?
8. Outline the general process known as the citric acid cycle, indicating the starting materials and products of each reaction.
9. Summarize aerobic catabolism in terms of each major phase and the numbers of ATP's possible from substrate and oxidative phosphorylation.
10. Indicate how proteins and lipids can be catabolized and utilized to make ATP's in aerobic metabolism.
11. Differentiate between the general mechanisms of metabolisms of photosynthetic autotrophs and heterotrophs and chemosynthetic autotrophs and heterotrophs.
12. Define transcription, translation, sense strand, complementary pairing, codon, anticodon, *m*RNA, and *t*RNA.
13. Outline the process of protein synthesis, indicating for the following triplet of the "sense strand" of DNA, AAA, the corresponding codon in *m*RNA and its corresponding anticodon on a *t*RNA.
14. Discuss three mechanisms by which enzyme activity in the cell is regulated.

SUGGESTED READINGS

Doelle, H. W. (ed.), *Microbial Metabolism*, Stroudsburg, Penn.: Dowden, Hutchinson, and Ross, Inc., 1974. *A collection of papers covering topics such as carbohydrate metabolism, metabolism of inorganic compounds such as nitrogen and sulfur, aromatic carbon metabolism, and anaerobic fermentation.*

Glenn, A. R., "Production of Extracellular Proteins by Bacteria," *Ann. Rev. Microbiol.*, 30:41, 1976. *This review deals with the fascinating biological problem of how bacterial cells synthesize and secrete often vast amounts of potentially lethal enzymes.*

Lascelles, J. (ed.), *Microbial Photosynthesis*, Stroudsburg, Penn.: Dowden, Hutchinson, and Ross, Inc., 1973. *Basically a collection of noteworthy papers on bacterial photosynthesis, the organisms involved, and the photosynthetic mechanism.*

Nierlich, D. P., "Regulation of Bacterial Growth, RNA and Protein Synthesis," *Ann. Rev. Microbiol.*, 32:393, 1978. *This article discusses the growth of bacteria as measured by their ability to make protein and the genetic elements involved in protein synthesis.*

Microbial Genetics

CHAPTER **15**

Two of the longest-standing basic questions in biology have dealt with the ability of changes to occur in populations as a part of evolution, and with the apparent paradox that populations tend to show little change. How change and stability both have been studied in microorganisms constitutes a major portion of this chapter. We shall deal mostly with the genetics of microorganisms that reproduce asexually and with their role as test systems for understanding heredity at the molecular level. Consideration also will be given to some applications of microbial genetics, including the use of microorganisms as "guinea pigs" in genetic engineering.

After reading this chapter, you should be able to:

1. **Explain how experiments performed by Hershey and Chase helped to prove that DNA is the genetic material.**
2. **Describe what is meant by mutation, how mutation can occur biochemically, and how specific agents cause mutation.**
3. **Define the terms minimal medium, prototroph, and auxotroph.**
4. **Explain the one-gene, one-enzyme hypothesis.**
5. **Describe Lederberg's indirect selection procedure for proving the spontaneous nature of mutations in microorganisms.**
6. **Distinguish between transformation, conjugation, and transduction as means of recombination in asexual organisms.**
7. **Explain what is meant by sexduction and lysogenic conversion.**

8. **Describe the use of conjugation as one means of mapping the bacterial chromosome.**
9. **Differentiate between autonomous and semiautonomous cytoplasmic inheritance.**
10. **Define and/or describe plasmids, episomes, bacteriocins, resistance transfer actors (RTF), and metabolic plasmids.**
11. **Explain how a scientist might develop a biological assay for a particular amino acid.**
12. **Explain how genetic studies can be used to determine taxonomic relationships between asexual organisms.**
13. **Explain what is meant by gene manipulation. Contrast potential benefits and hazards, and describe one technique for gene manipulation with *Escherichia coli*.**

Microorganisms are serving as unique test "animals" for the science of genetics. Research with bacteria such as *Streptococcus pneumoniae* and *Escherichia coli* raised, and essentially resolved, the modern dilemma of the chemical nature of the genetic material and of mutations. Study of *Neurospora crassa*, a common bread mold, lead to the careful mapping of metabolic pathways and of genetic fine structure. Techniques now being developed will enable genes from a totally unrelated cell to be transplanted into a bacterium so that the progeny of that cell can make medically important drugs, such as human insulin.

Evolution and Inheritance

Any consideration of the basis of genetics and the mechanisms of inheritance must begin with the viewpoint of Jean Baptiste de Lamarck (1744–1829). The concept of *evolution* was first introduced by Lamarck, who defined it as a continual process of gradual changes in plant and animal species in response to environmental conditions. Thus, according to Lamarck, exposure to the sun accounted for the difference between the white and black races. The protective coloration of birds and animals, especially insects, was caused by their prolonged exposure to the natural conditions that they came to resemble. Giraffes became long-necked by continually stretching to reach the leaves on high branches of trees. According to this theory of acquired characteristics, the properties that an individual develops in response to the environment become a part of the individual's genetic makeup.

An opposing theory was developed by the nineteenth-century naturalist, Charles Darwin, who wrote in *The Origin of Species* that evolution of new species occurred because of natural selection. Darwin argued that natural differences or variations appear spontaneously among individuals of a species. The conditions of the environment exert selective pressures on these varying individuals, and the resulting struggle for existence in the environment determines which individuals survive to pass on their characteristics to future generations. Thus a dark-colored bird had a greater chance of survival than his lighter relative because he was better able to hide from hawks. Any creature that could fight better, run faster, take better care of its young, or could utilize more sources of food had a survival advantage; its characteristics would tend to continue by natural selection and thereby implement evolution.

Modern biology recognizes that changes in cells and organisms are the result of permanent genetic changes, or **mutations.** Microorganisms have been used extensively to study mutation, and evidence presented in this chapter will show that these organisms seem to follow the Darwinian concept of natural variation.

How does modern biology explain the apparent stability of populations, that is, of members of the same species, in the face of evolution? The key to stability in populations is associated with sexual reproduction, which permits the mixing of hereditary units or genes throughout a breeding population, that is, throughout a species. This flow of genes tends to keep changes due to mutation at low levels in the *gene pool,* the total of all the genes of all the individuals in a population. Sexual reproduction thus inhibits the expression of mutations.

This explanation of population stability is satisfactory for those eucaryotic microorganisms that reproduce sexually, but what about the asexual procaryotes and eucaryotes? **Recombination,** or the mixing of genetic material from two organisms, has been investigated in bacteria since 1908. The accumulation of evidence showing that procaryotes have their own form of sexuality allowing population stability is described later in the chapter. Before dealing with these important issues in microbial genetics, we shall discuss the chemistry of genetics and mutation.

The Chemistry of Genetics

DNA and Chromosomes

The basic genetic material was first isolated by Frederick Miescher in 1868. His isolate, which he called *nuclein* because it came from the nuclei of white blood cells, had interesting chemical composition: 14 percent nitrogen and 2.5 percent phosphorus. We now know that Miescher's nuclein was mainly deoxyribonucleic acid (DNA).

In 1881, nuclein was shown to be associated somehow with chromosomes. Findings of this kind suggested to some biologists that nuclein was responsible for the transmission of hereditary characteristics. Until the mid twentieth century, the predominant view, however, was that the protein of the nucleus was the material responsible for heredity. It was argued that nuclein could not be the genetic substance because the amount of nuclein appeared to vary during asexual cell division or mitosis. Protein, on the other hand, appeared to be more constant. The belief that nuclear protein was the basis of heredity remained widespread until 1949 when quantitative chemical analyses of DNA from cell nuclei proved that DNA, not protein, remained constant throughout the mitotic cycle of cell division. This finding suggested that DNA was probably the critical substance in chromosomes.

Meanwhile, a series of experiments on the biological role of DNA that began in the 1920s finally yielded decisive results in 1952. In that year, A. D. Hershey and M. Chase reported evidence from bacteriophage research demonstrating the genetic role of DNA. Their viruses, which consisted of protein and DNA, were used to learn whether both biochemicals entered the bacterial cells during infection. Using two radioactive isotopes, sulfur-35 to label protein and phosphorus-32 to label the DNA, they were able to show that all of the DNA and very little of the protein entered the cells. Because only the radioactive phosphorus appeared in the new virions produced in infected bacteria, Hershey and Chase concluded that the DNA must be the genetic material.

The Chemistry of Mutations

DNA consists of a linear chain of nitrogen bases known as the purines (adenine and guanine) and the pyrimidines (thymine and cytosine). These compounds are linked by sugar-phosphate components. The DNA of most forms of life is double-stranded and complementary: adenine in one strand is always opposite thymine in the other and guanine is always paired with cytosine.

The apparent simplicity of DNA originally caused many scientists to disregard it as the genetic substance. Since then, however, its purines and pyrimidines have been shown to form combinations that allow for a sufficiently complex formulation. Three bases are normally necessary to code for a particular amino acid. Permanent hereditary changes—mutations—result from changes in a triplet codon.

Mutations may develop as a consequence of natural or spontaneous events, or may be induced by various physical or chemical agents. The result of a mutation depends upon the change it causes in the transcription of the DNA code into RNA, messenger RNA, and protein synthesis.

The change in one base would cause the substitution of a complementary base in *m*RNA. The resulting codon would be read by a different transfer RNA, thereby causing the placement of an amino acid in the forming protein molecule different from the one specified by the code.

The effect of this change depends upon the location of that amino acid. Most of the amino acids in a particular enzyme form its structural framework; other amino acids in a specific sequence function in the enzyme's active sites, the particular areas of the enzyme that are involved in enzymatic activity. Most changes in the genetic code associated with the structural aspects of enzymes probably would not affect activity; however, changes in amino acids that are involved in determining shape could cause the enzyme to bind with a substrate in a manner that would still permit maximum activity. Other changes—those affecting the active portion of the protein—could eliminate activity. Research on ***Escherichia coli*** demonstrated that certain mutations that deactivated a particular enzyme did permit the synthesis of a protein that was practically identical in all other characteristics. Changes of one or more amino acids in hemoglobin have been shown to cause sickle cell anemia and other blood abnormalities.

A mutation involving deletion of one or more purine or pyrimidine bases or their abnormal placement in a DNA molecule will cause complete misreading of the genetic code (Figure 15-1). These events are called "reading-frame shifts." A mutation of this type will cause the synthesis of a nonfunctional protein.

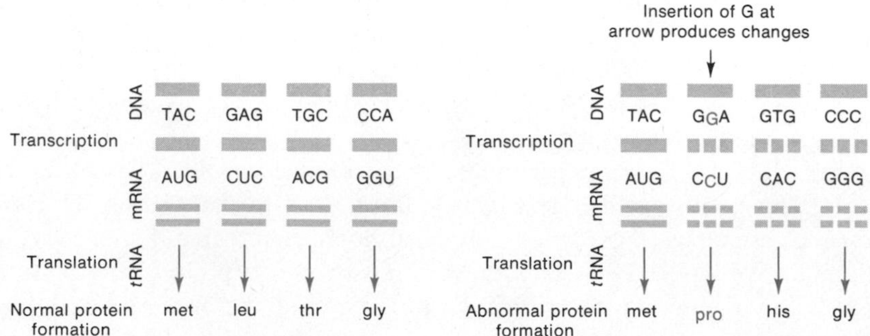

FIG. 15-1 The effects of alterations in a chromosome. A normal triple sequence in a DNA molecule is shown at the top with the corresponding messenger RNA (*m*RNA) molecule directly beneath it. The insertion of one new base G (arrow) changes the reading of the genetic code at every point beyond the site of mutation. The altered DNA and *m*RNA molecules are respectively underlined with broken lines.

Mutations can also be caused by the rearrangement of chromosome pieces on the same or separate chromosomes. Situations of this nature are referred to as being a *translocation* form of chromosomal aberration.

MUTAGENIC AGENTS

Early work on mutations with *Drosophila* was performed with x-ray irradiation because x rays cause chromosomal breakage. One of the first chemical mutagens studied, mustard gas, was chosen because it acts in a way similar to that of x rays. Mustard gas represents a group of mutagenic chemicals known as *alkylating agents*, which replace a hydrogen with another group, for example, methyl ($-CH_3$) or ethyl ($-CH_2CH_3$) on a molecule such as guanine. The substituted guanine appears to cause defects by pairing with a thymine molecule rather than with cytosine. Thus, in the next generation of DNA, the original guanine is replaced by adenine, which will pair with the incorrect thymine. Alkylating agents also produce deletions and chromosome rearrangements.

Many other chemical and physical agents have been tested for mutagenic activity. Ultraviolet rays appear to act as a mutagen because UV wavelengths are strongly absorbed by DNA. Some of the chemicals studied include molecules of similar structure to the components of DNA. These base analogs are purines and pyrimidines not normally found in DNA. Their incorporation into DNA, during nucleic acid synthesis, results in incorrect pairing during the replication process. For example, 5-bromouracil can be incorporated into DNA in place of thymine. Because of stereochemical differences, 5-bromouracil pairs with thymine rather than adenine, thus changing the code.

Another group of chemical mutagens, the acridines, appear to penetrate the DNA in a way that separates the bases. This separation might lead to the unnatural insertion or deletion of a base, which causes reading-frame shifts. The mutagen nitrous acid was originally tested because of its known interaction with proteins, which were thought to be the genetic material. However, experiments have shown that nitrous acid does cause mutations by removing an amino group (NH_2) found in adenine, guanine, and cytosine. When these bases are **deaminated** by removal of the amino group, they are converted to hypoxanthine, xanthine, and uracil, respectively. The new compounds will not pair with the appropriate purine or pyrimidine, thus creating spot changes in the genetic code.

Mutations in Microorganisms

The theory that mutations are actually defects in enzymes preventing specific metabolic activities has been tested, primarily with microorganisms. The first significant work in this area was reported by George W. Beadle and Edward L. Tatum in 1941. Their research organism was *Neurospora crassa*, an ascomycete fungus often found as a pink-red mold on bread. The important feature of the microorganism was that it grew on a simple, defined medium called *minimal medium*. This means that the primary, or parent, culture did not have complex nutritional requirements. For example, the minimal medium for *N. crassa* would include ammonium chloride for nitrogen, glucose for energy and carbon, a few mineral salts, one or more vitamins, water, and agar (when used for solid media). The parent culture was called *wild type*, meaning the form usually found in nature. After irradiation, mutants of *N. crassa* were found that could not grow on the minimal medium but would grow on a complex medium containing added malt and yeast extracts. Beadle and Tatum found that each mutant had one particular nutritional requirement rather than a general requirement for different nutrients. These growth requirements were for a specific amino acid, vitamin, purine, or pyrimidine, and each mutant would grow on the minimal medium supplemented with its particular requirement. Such mutants are called **auxotrophs** in contrast to the parent or wild type culture referred to as a **prototroph.** (An auxotroph is defined as a mutant having additional nutritional requirements from its parental culture.) The fact that each mutant tended to have a specific nutritional requirement served as the basis for the *one-gene, one-enzyme* hypothesis proposed by Beadle and Tatum, that is, that each gene is responsible for the production of a single enzyme. These scientists were able to correlate the development of the nutritional requirement with the absence of a particular enzyme. This hypothesis has proven particularly helpful in determining metabolic pathways in both procaryotic and eucaryotic cells. Since the early 1940s, mutational research has included most if not all microorganisms, a favorite being *Escherichia coli* and its viruses.

Microbial Experiments and the Nature of Mutation

The controversy between proponents of the theories advanced by Lamarck and Darwin, discussed in the introduction to this chapter, has carried over into microbiology. The idea that changes are caused by adaptation to conditions is certainly logical. An excellent example involves the development of resistance to antibiotics by microorganisms.

Consider a penicillin-sensitive *Staphylococcus aureus* culture obtained from a patient. Administration of penicillin should greatly reduce if not eliminate the infection. However, the patient may subsequently return to the hospital with a severe uncontrolled infection, and the staphylococcus culture obtained this time is found to be penicillin-resistant. According to the Lamarckian adaptation theory, some of the bacteria that were in contact with the antibiotic managed to survive by adaptation. On the other hand, proponents of modern Darwinism would theorize that those bacteria that happened to be resistant to the antibiotic were the only survivors. In either case, the time between apparent recovery and relapse is the time required for the resistant bacteria to increase to sufficient numbers. The question that remains is to differentiate between adaptation and random variation.

In 1943, S. E. Luria and M. Delbrück reported an indirect approach to finding the nature of microbial mutation. The procedure used was a "fluctuation test," designed to determine statistically whether mutation to bacterial virus resistance in *E. coli* was random or directed. Their data presented strong evidence for the spontaneous, random nature of mutation.

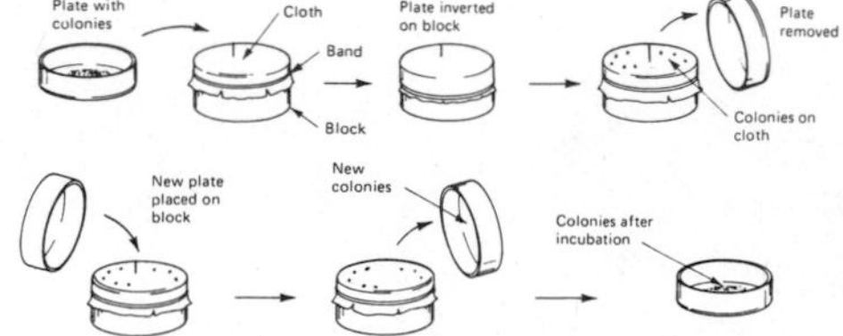

FIG. 15–2 The replica-plating technique. Among other applications, this procedure can be used to demonstrate that spontaneous mutations arise in microorganisms.

The Lederbergs' Indirect Selection Procedure

After the demonstrations by Luria and Delbrück and others that mutation is spontaneous in microorganisms, J. and E. W. Lederberg developed a relatively simple method by which virus-resistant mutants could be isolated without any exposure to the bacterial virus. In this replica-plating technique (Figure 15–2), a velveteen nap was used to transfer bacteria from colonies on one plate to several other plates containing fresh media. When this is properly done, the transferred bacteria develop into colonies at locations on the new plates corresponding to those occupied by the same colonies on the original inoculum plate (Figure 15–3). The relative locations of such colonies on all plates inoculated with the same velveteen pad should be the same. Using the bacterial colonies on one nutrient agar plate (1) as their inoculum sources, the Lederbergs introduced these organisms onto one with nutrient agar and one plate with nutrient agar plus a bacterial virus (2) that could infect and kill the bacteria, thus preventing colonies from developing.

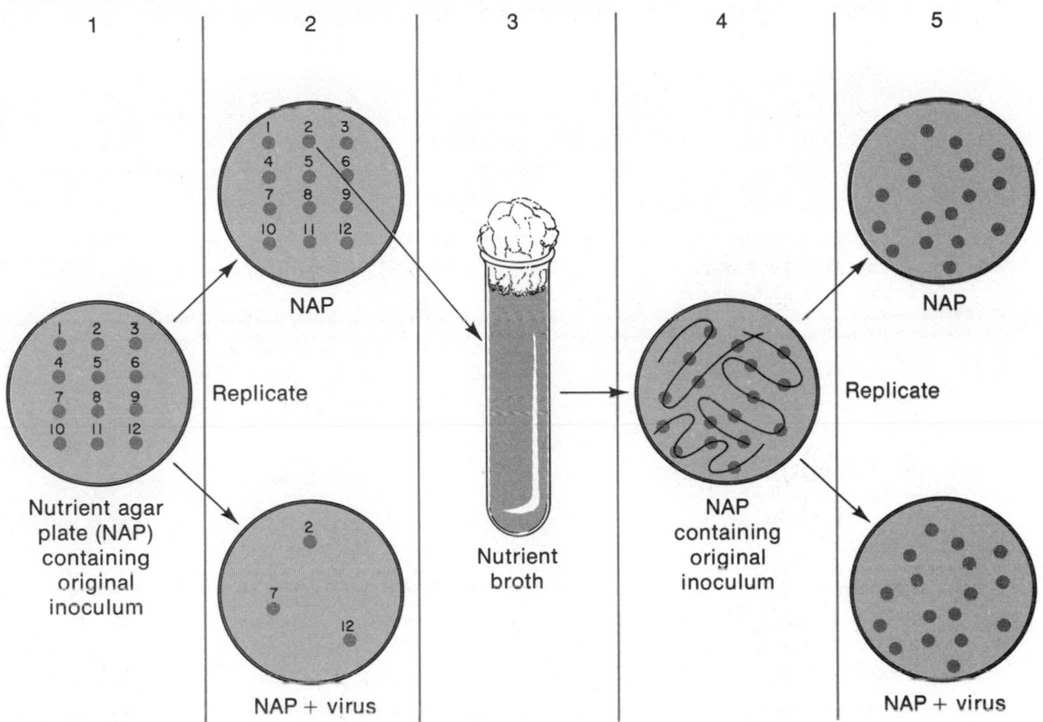

FIG. 15–3 Spontaneous mutation in bacteria as shown through replica plating. The selective agent here is a virus to which the bacteria used are sensitive.

The sequence diagrammed in Figure 15–3 has been greatly simplified for clarity and brevity. Only three colonies of the original twelve—numbers 2, 7, and 12—were resistant to virus and developed on the medium containing the virus. Because the two plates were oriented in the same way as the original one, colonies that appeared on the medium without virus could be identified and related by position to those found to be virus resistant. Colony number 2 from the plate without virus was moved by an inoculating needle from the nutrient agar plate to nutrient broth and allowed to grow (3). When growth from the nutrient broth was streaked on a nutrient agar plate, twelve colonies developed (4) and were used as the original inoculum to repeat the replication technique as before. This time, the resultant colonies appeared on both types of media (5). We would not have known that virus-resistant bacteria had arisen and were present unless such colonies had been identified by replicating onto the second plate containing the virus. This procedure clearly leaves no doubt that the virus-resistant cells were there on the first plate used before any exposure to virus had been made.

The techniques developed by Luria and Delbrück and by the Lederbergs have been used to study mutations of a wide variety of characteristics with many different microorganisms, including antibiotic resistance in *Staphylococcus aureus, Escherichia coli, Pseudomonas aeruginosa, Shigella* spp., and *Salmonella typhi.*

Recombination in Procaryotes

The generally accepted view that the hybridization produced by sexual cross-breeding is important to the survival of a species (hybrid vigor) does not seem to apply to bacteria because they are haploid. That is, they contain a single set of unpaired chromosomes. Although plant and animal species are classified according to their ability to combine gametes with a resultant diploid (paired-chromosome) cell, microbial species are classified primarily by common structural and biochemical characteristics, usually independent of genetic relatedness. Bacteria have exchanged genetic material between genera and between species.

The process by which new combinations of genes are obtained from two different types of cells is called *genetic recombination.* On a molecular level, a new chromosome is formed from the DNA contributed by the two different parental cells. In bacteria, four processes by which such recombinant chromosomes can form are **transformation, conjugation, sexduction,** and **transduction.** Genetic material is transferred from a donor cell to a recipient and does not involve cell fusion, which is a common feature of the sexual process as it occurs with eucaryotes.

Transformation

The way in which the haploid bacterial cell solves this apparent genetic problem became clear in 1928, when F. J. Griffith observed some startling results while investigating the destructive effects of pneumococci in mice. The ability of a pneumococcus to produce disease is largely dependent upon the polysaccharide capsule that prevents its destruction by phagocytes (white blood cells) in the host. These encapsulated organisms can mutate to unencapsulated forms which are *avirulent,* unable to produce disease. If the virulent pneumococcus culture was heat killed and then injected into mice, virulence was lost, as you might expect (Figure 15–4). Griffith inoculated mice with a mixture of live, unencapsulated, avirulent bacteria and heat-killed encapsulated pneumococci of a virulent type. To his surprise, some of the mice died (Figure 15–4). Analyzing his results, Griffith concluded that neither the avirulent live bacteria nor the heat-killed virulent ones could have killed the mice, because neither had that effect when injected alone. He isolated living pneumococci from the dead mice and identified them as encapsulated organisms of the type represented by the heat-killed bacteria. It therefore appeared that either the dead bacteria were rejuvenated by the living avirulent ones, or the dead bacteria somehow transformed the avirulent organisms into virulent ones.

In 1933, J. L. Alloway reported the next major step in explaining this transformation phenomenon. He performed *in vitro* the same type of experiment that Griffith had performed *in vivo.* In place of the killed cells, these studies used a sterile, cell-free extract of the virulent pneumococci. This extract did not cause the death of mice when injected alone, but when mixed with avirulent bacteria of a different type, the result was the production of virulent pneumococci, indistinguishable from the ones that were used to make the extract. A substance called a *transforming principle (TP)* had been prepared in crude form. During the 1940s it was proved absolutely that Alloway's TP was DNA.

Thus began the era of intensive investigations into the molecular basis of genetics and of life itself. The crude extracts of TP were separated into protein, lipid, polysaccharides, RNA, and DNA, and it was shown that only the DNA

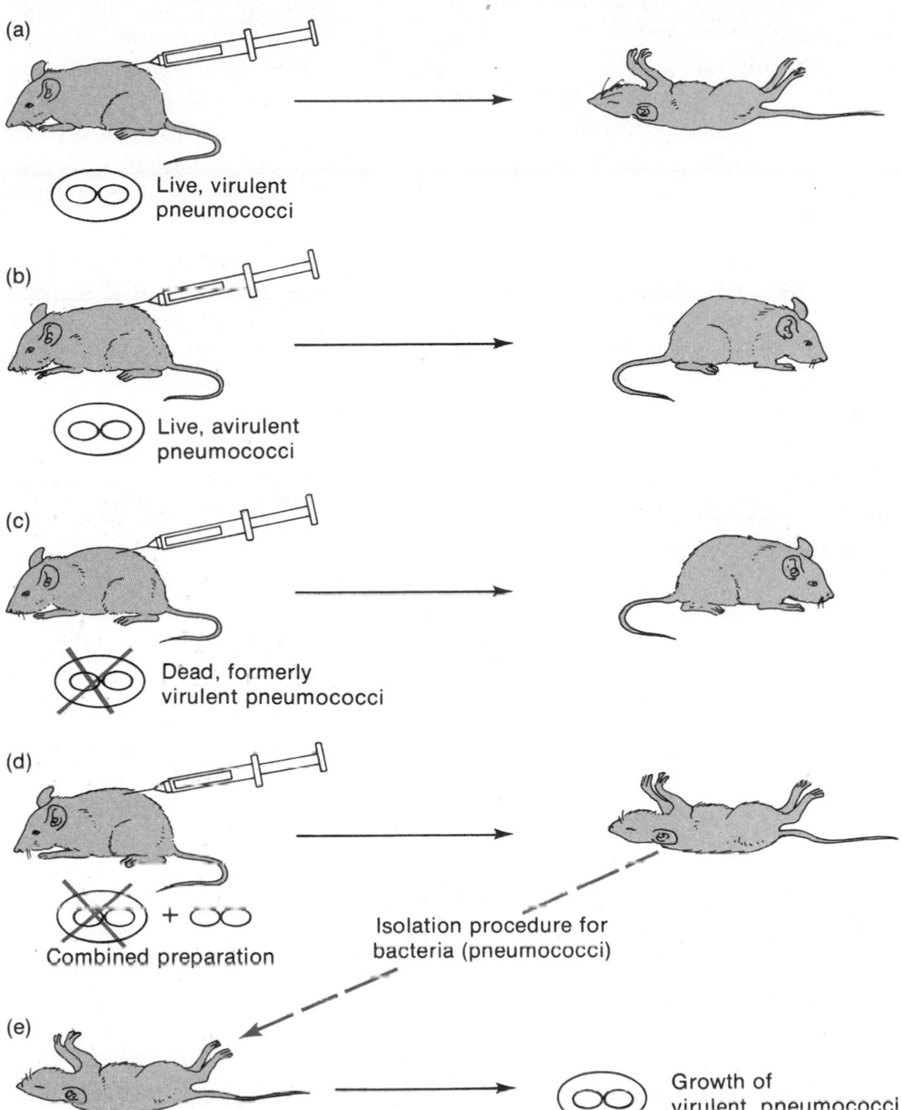

FIG. 15-4 Griffith's experiment contributed greatly to the understanding of transformation and the nature of DNA.

fraction caused transformation. The identity of DNA was proved by a wide variety of established chemical and physical analytical techniques.

Then, in 1948, it was shown that the active DNA had to be highly polymerized and that only certain of the avirulent pneumococci could be transformed by the DNA. A recipient cell that is able to absorb donor DNA and subsequently undergo transformation is a *competent cell.* Competence appears to develop as a function of population density: when the cell concentration of a culture reaches a critical level, most cells exhibit competence. (However, loss of this property can occur abruptly.) As competence appears in a culture, a protein is produced that can change incompetent cells into competent ones. Although the exact mechanism involved is not known, it is believed that this *competence factor* influences some change in cell surfaces that causes development of receptor sites or increases permeability to DNA molecules.

Since Griffith's pioneering work with *Streptococcus pneumoniae,* transformation has been demonstrated with many genera, including *Hemophilus, Bacillus, Rhizobium, Neisseria, Acinetobacter,* and *Escherichia.* The research with the pneumococci and *Hemophilus* was complicated by their complex nutritional requirements, making it difficult to study more than a few characteristics at any one time. Recall that the study of mutation with *Neurospora crassa* was facilitated by that organism's relatively simple nutritional needs. This property allowed careful study of metabolic pathways and the formulation of the one-gene, one-enzyme hypothesis. The discovery of transformation in *Bacillus subtilis* in 1961 made such studies in transformation possible, because *B. subtilis* has relatively simple nutritional requirements.

An exciting study in transformation with *B. subtilis* showed that DNA extracted from an animal virus such as vaccinia (cowpox) could be used in transformation to lead to the development of animal viruses in infected *B. subtilis.* This process is called *transfection.* One can, therefore, speculate that potentially pathogenic human viruses may use normally present bacteria as a reservoir; these bacteria may serve as "carriers" until some later time when the virus becomes active and causes the disease for no readily apparent reason.

Transformation experiments can yield much information on the transfer of genetic information per se and the location of genes on the chromosomes or genomes of several bacterial species.

Bacterial Conjugation

Conjugation is the transfer of genetic material between two living bacteria that are in physical contact. Conjugation, or recombination, the major means of genetic exchange and variability in sexually reproducing higher organisms, had been investigated with bacteria as early as 1908. However, bacterial conjugation was not proven until Lederberg and Tatum obtained multiple mutants *(polyauxotrophs)* of *Escherichia coli* in 1946.

The bacterial strains used were biochemically deficient mutants. Each had two or more different genetic defects. One parent organism had defects that caused it to require the vitamin biotin (B) and the amino acid methionine (M) for survival; the other parent strain required the amino acids threonine (T) and leucine (L) but not biotin or methionine. These parent strains were symbolized as $B^-M^-T^+L^+$ and $B^+M^+T^-L^-$, respectively. The minus signs represented a requirement for the particular biochemical substance for growth on minimal medium, and the positive signs indicated no deficiency requirement. Neither strain was able to grow on minimal medium. Only a transfer of B^+M^+ to one parent or T^+L^+ to the other would permit growth on the minimal medium of the test conditions (Figure 15–5).

When the two strains were mixed and placed on minimal medium, some bacteria were able to survive and grow. These organisms represented the natural type of genetic makeup, $B^+M^+T^+L^+$. The statistical probability of the double spontaneous mutations yielding the same result would be of the order of one chance in 10^{14}. The number of resulting colonies obtained was far greater than this. These findings suggested that recombination by crossing over was occurring, indicating a linear arrangement of genes *(linkage)* in bacteria, as in higher organisms. The crossing over of the T^+L^+ portion of a chromosome would produce a wild type *E. coli.* This phenomenon can be represented as follows:

$$\begin{array}{c} \underline{B^+M^+T^-L^-} \\ \diagdown\!\underline{\quad\quad} \\ B^-M^-T^+L^+ \end{array} = \underline{B^+M^+T^+L^+}$$

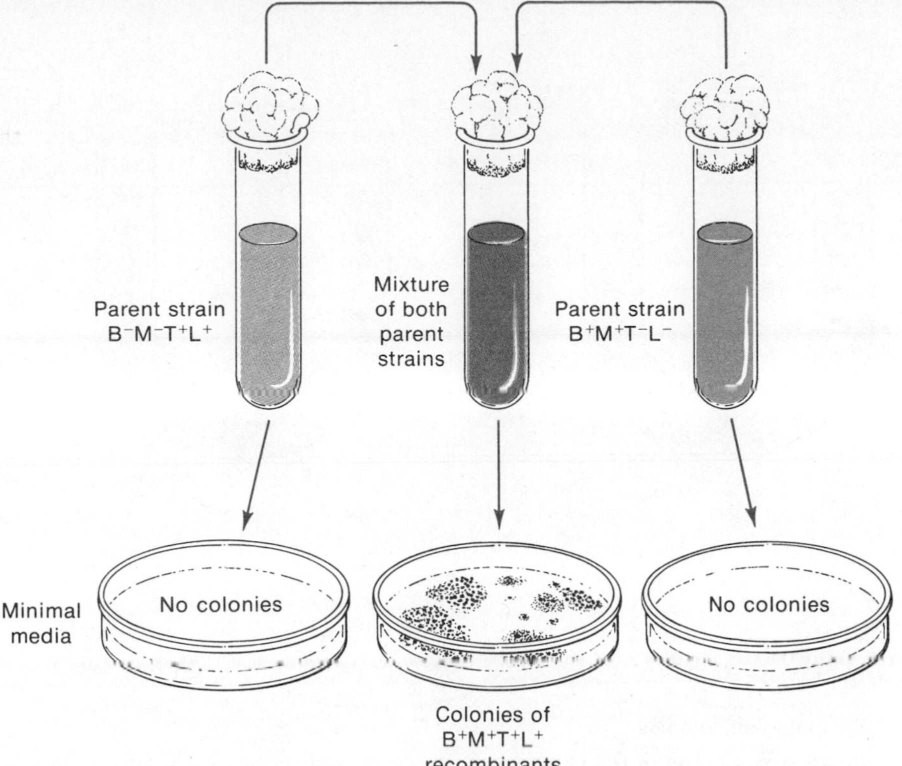

FIG. 15–5 Lederberg and Tatum's original conjugation experiment. The parent strains, $B^-M^-T^+L^+$ (left) and $B^+M^+T^-L^-$ (right), were unable to grow when plated on minimal media. However, when these strains were mixed, allowed to conjugate, and then plated, colonies developed on minimal media which represented the presence of $B^+M^+T^+L^+$ recombinants.

To eliminate the possibility that transformation, transfer of DNA without contact between cells, might be taking place, B. Davis in 1950 carried out a series of experiments using a U-tube device (Figure 15–6). The U-tube was constructed with two arms, (A) and (B), separated by a porous glass filter (C) which would prevent passage of bacteria between the arms but would not block DNA. When two biochemically deficient parental strains such as $B^+M^+T^-L^-$ and $B^-M^-T^+L^+$ were placed in the same arm, recombinants were obtained at expected frequencies. However, if one mutant strain was placed in (A), the other in (B), and the medium flushed between the arms, no recombinants were obtained. Thus transformation was eliminated as an explanation of this phenomenon, and the need for intimate contact between bacteria was firmly established.

Sexduction

F^+ AND F^- PARTICLES

Through subsequent research in this area, sexuality in bacteria was discovered. In addition certain strains were shown to be donors of genetic material and others, recipients, in any bacterial population in which conjugation occurs. Donor (male) cells are designated $\mathbf{F^+}$, while recipient (female) cells are indicated as $\mathbf{F^-}$. Only donor cells contain extra pieces of DNA, known as F (fertility) particles, which are not a part of the chromosomes of such cells (Figure 15–7).

Upon the mixing of F^+ and F^- bacteria, the F^+ cells attach to the recipient F^- cells by sex pili and, within minutes, F particles are transferred. F^- cells become F^+ cells through this process. Bacterial chromosomes, however, are not

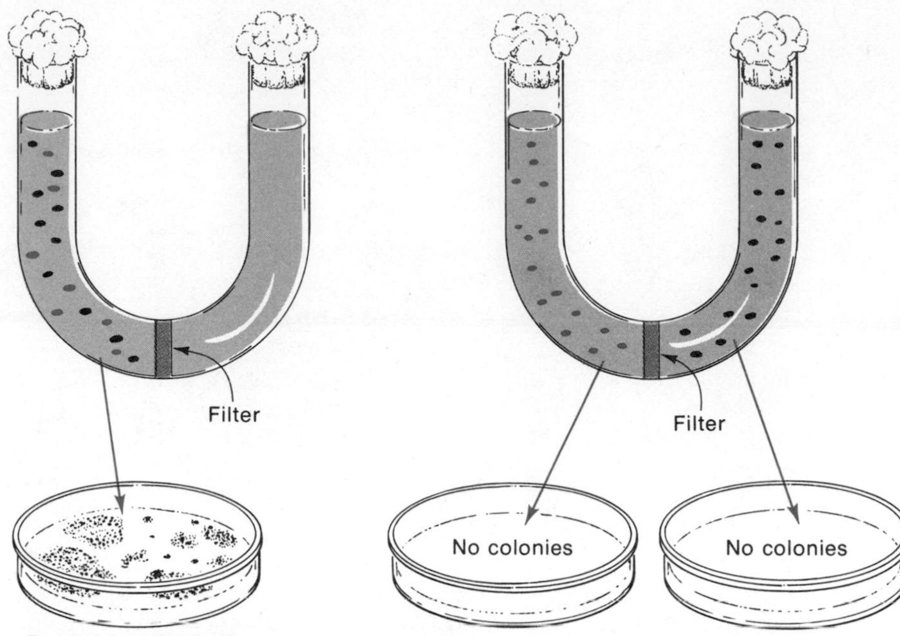

FIG. 15-6 A diagram of the U-tube experiments performed by Davis. In the system on the left, two biochemically deficient parent strains such as $B^+M^+T^-L^-$ and $B^-M^-T^+L^+$ are placed in the same arm. Upon plating a sample, recombinants develop. When the individual strains are placed in different arms and separated by a filter, as in the system on the right, no recombinants develop upon plating.

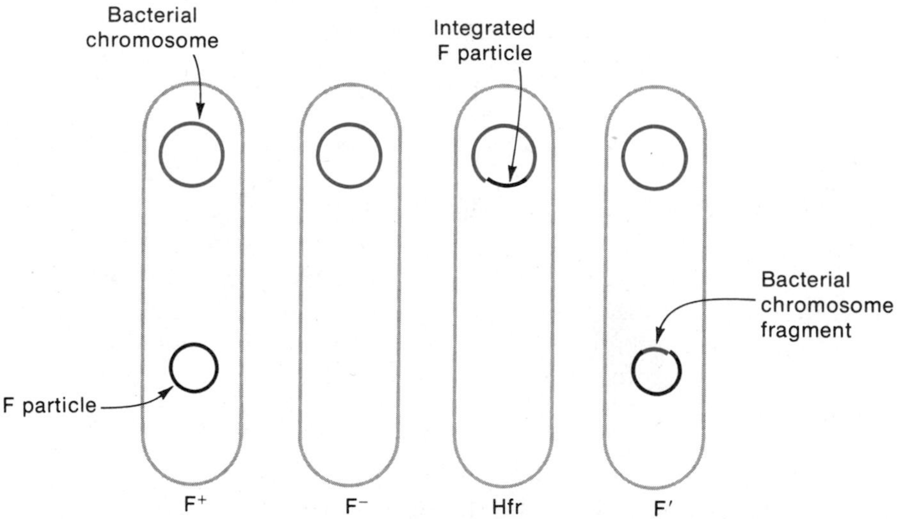

FIG. 15-7 The structure of F^+, F^-, Hfr, and F′ bacterial cells. The diagram shows the possible relationships between the bacterial chromosome and F particle.

transferred, so recombinants do not develop.

The F particle is an extrachromosomal genetic complex composed of circular DNA that possesses genes for the following: (1) the regulation of its own replication; (2) the synthesis of sex or F pili (Figure 15-7) necessary for conjugation so that donor DNA can pass to a recipient cell; and (3) the formation of a particular surface component that may serve to lower negative electrical surface charges of donor cells, so that intimate contact with recipient cells can occur after random collision.

Hfr CELLS

Bacterial chromosomes are transferred to F^- cells by a cell type known as Hfr, an abbreviation for ***high frequency of recombination*** (Figure 15-8). Such cells arise from the integration of the F particle into the donor cell chromosome (Figure 15-7). This F particle integration appears to mobilize donor chromosomes for the transfer process.

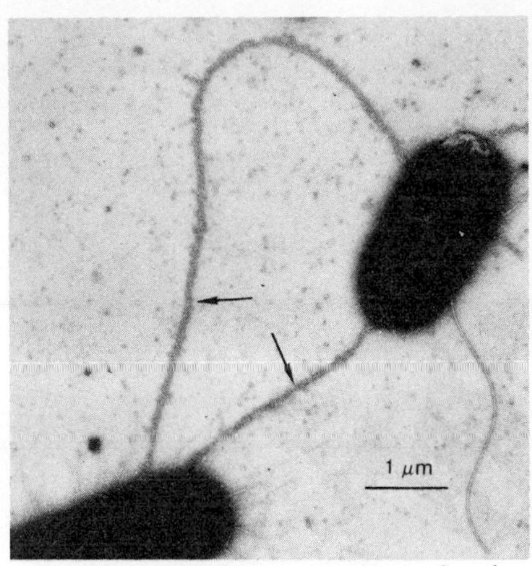

FIG. 15-8 An electron micrograph of a presumed specific pairing between an Hfr cell (bottom) and an F^- cell. The sex pili (S) can be clearly differentiated from other pili (P). *Curtiss, R., III, et al.,* J. Bacteriol. 100:*1091-1104 (1969).*

THE F-PRIME (F′) PARTICLE

There is another type of extrachromosomal particle which some bacterial strains are capable of transferring. Such particles carry several chromosomal genes of a donor cell (Figure 15-7). F particles can change their extrachromosomal status by integrating into a bacterial cell chromosome. They also can, in rare situations, detach themselves. However, when such detachment occurs, several bacterial chromosome genes remain attached to the particle. The resulting F particle carrying bacterial genes is referred to as an ***F-prime*** (F′) ***particle.*** It behaves in a manner similar to an F^+ particle. As a consequence of an $F' \times F^-$ mating, the recipient bacterial cell acquires the additional genes carried by the F′ particle upon integration into the recipient's chromosomes.

Transduction

When Lederberg extended his recombination research to *Salmonella* species, the unidirectional transfer of genetic material occurred. This phenomenon resembled conjugation as observed with *E. coli;* but when performing these studies in a Davis U-tube, Lederberg observed that physical contact was not required. This, then, appeared similar to the observed transformation as with pneumococci, *Hemophilus* spp. and *B. subtilis.* To confirm the transformation in *Salmonella,* DNAase, the enzyme that breaks down free DNA, was added to the culture to prevent the genetic transfer of free DNA. Contrary to expectation, the DNAase did not prevent the transfer of genetic information. This surprising result spurred research into the transduction phenomenon.

In 1952, N. D. Zinder and J. Lederberg reported finding bacterial genetic transfer via a filterable agent identified as a bacterial virus. Certain bacteriophages are able to infect a bacterial cell and, through the process of lysogeny, become an integral part of the bacterial genome. In this condition the viral DNA has actually become part of the bacterial chromosome. However, the virus is eventually activated, either spontaneously or by ultraviolet light, replicates at the expense of the cell, and eventually causes the host cell to disintegrate. Thus, many viruses can be released into the culture to infect other bacteria. Some of these may carry one or more bacterial genes, small pieces of the bacterial DNA that remained with the maturing bacteriophage (prophage) as it broke loose from the host cell chromosome. It is these small pieces of genetic material that are transferred to other bacterial cells by bacterial viruses in ***transduction.***

Compared with bacterial conjugation, transduction permits the transfer of relatively small segments of DNA because of limited space within the virus. Usually this transfer consists of the virus DNA (prophage) and a segment of DNA taken from its attachment site on the bacterial chromosome.

Two forms of transduction are recognized, ***generalized*** and ***specialized.*** In the generalized type, virtually any gene (genetic marker) of the host bacterium can be transferred and does not require lysogeny. In specialized transduction situations, only genes near the attachment site of the virus on the chromosome of host cell are involved. This phenomenon has been used to study the fine structure of the bacterial DNA according to short linkage patterns.

Lysogenic Conversion

During the 1950s an event more medically significant was discovered, namely, *lysogenic,* or *viral, conversion.* In lysogenic conversion, unlike transduction, a particular genetic change occurs in all infected microorganisms, as a consequence of lysogeny. Such conversions, which are recognized as physical changes, include the development of smooth colonial types in mycobacteria and alterations of the antigenic types of salmonellae, and are of clinical significance.

Probably the most significant alteration of a microbial characteristic by lysogeny was reported by V. J. Freeman in 1951. This investigation showed that the bacteria causing diphtheria, *Corynebacterium diphtheriae,* could produce toxin only when infected by a specific bacteriophage. There are other requirements as well, primarily the presence of a certain concentration of iron, but if the phage is absent, lysogenic state toxin production does not occur.

Toxin production as a consequence of lysogeny can be demonstrated by a relatively simple procedure. The presence or absence of toxin can be observed by its reaction with antitoxin to form a precipitate. A strip of filter paper impregnated with antitoxin is placed on the surface of a sterile serum agar medium. Cultures of *C. diphtheriae* exposed to bacteriophage or suspected of being toxigenic are then streaked across the plate as shown in Figure 15–9. When the streak cultures grow to a reasonable size, the presence of toxin is shown by zones of precipitation in the agar where the streaks cross the impregnated filter paper strip.

These zones of precipitation are formed when the toxin diffusing from the bacterial cultures and the antitoxin diffusing from the filter paper meet at the proper concentrations. This phenomenon, a form of *immunodiffusion,* is used widely as a standard immunological technique.

Plasmids

In addition to F particles, various small, extrachromosomal DNA particles capable of independent replication have been found in bacteria. These genetic elements are called **plasmids.** They occur in the cell's cytoplasm and *do not* become integrated into the cell's chromosome. Those extrachromosomal units that can replicate either autonomously or as part of the host (usually a bacterial cell) chromosome and are capable of shifting between these two modes of replication are referred to as episomes. All others are called plasmids.

Plasmids have been studied in a variety of bacteria, including the members of the bacterial genera *Vibrio, Pasteurella, Staphylococcus,* and *Bacillus.* These DNA-containing structures are categorized as nongenetic factors. They concern nonessential properties that can be transferred between bacteria by conjugation, transduction, and possibly transformation. The following have been found to be plasmid in nature: the F particle, the production of *bacteriocins,* resistance transfer factors (RTF), and metabolic plasmids.

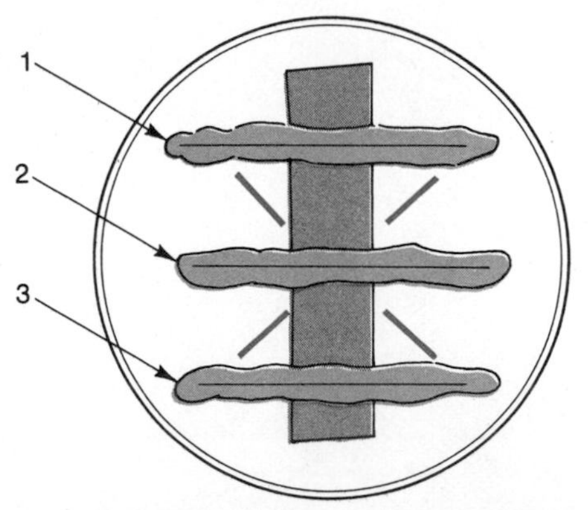

FIG. 15–9 Demonstration of toxin production by lysogenic culture of *Corynebacterium diphtheriae.* (1) and (3) are nonlysogenic, (2) is lysogenic. Note the absence of lines of precipitation at the top and bottom of the plate. Lines of precipitation (color) form where the optimum concentration of toxin from the bacterial culture has reacted with the optimum concentration of antitoxin from the filter paper.

BACTERIOCINS

The bacteriocins were first described in 1932 as antibiotic-like material, from *Escherichia coli.* Bacteriocins are a diverse group of substances, usually proteins, that inhibit or kill sensitive members of strains closely related to the one that produced the material. Colicins, bacteriocins produced by *E. coli,* act by adsorbing to specific molecular groupings, or receptors, on the surfaces of sensitive organisms, causing modification or loss of these receptor sites.

Antibiotic-like substances similar to those from *E. coli* have been found in

Pseudomonas (pyocin) and *Bacillus megaterium* (megacin). Collectively, these substances are ***bacteriocins***. The ability to form bacteriocins requires a bacteriocinogenic plasmid. Chemically, bacteriocins may be simple proteins, proteins and carbohydrates, or comparable to incomplete bacteriophage particles (phage tails). The mode of action differs among bacteriocins: some appear to damage the cell membrane of susceptible hosts; others interfere with the synthesis of nucleic acid or protein.

RESISTANCE TRANSFER FACTOR (RTF)

The resistance transfer factor (RTF) was first described as an episomal element in *Staphylococcus aureus*, which is a standard test organism for bacterial resistance studies. As many as six different antibiotic-resistance characteristics may be associated with episomes in *S. aureus*. This is particularly significant because autonomous episomes are destroyed by treatment with the antiseptic chemical acriflavine. Loss of resistance to these antibiotics can be demonstrated by acriflavine treatment *in vitro*. We may speculate on the potential use for it in the treatment of patients with severe staphylococcal infections. Such *in vivo* use could combine one or more antibiotic with acriflavine.

Transfer of multiple drug resistance requires cell contact and generally involves conjugation, although RTFs can also be transferred from cell to cell by transduction. The agents responsible for the drug resistance, R factors, consist of two distinguishable parts, the basic resistance transfer factor (RTF) and a variable genetic determinant for antibiotic resistance (*r* determinant), which contains the genes for drug resistance (R genes). The genetic *(r)* determinants cannot be transferred unless they fuse with a transfer factor.

METABOLIC PLASMIDS

Pseudomonas spp., commonly found in soil, have unique metabolic activities. They can break down xylene, hexane, phenol, and camphor. The complete set of enzymes in each catabolic pathway is synthesized under the control of genes on a plasmid. These plasmids may be transferred by conjugation, transduction, or along with the sex factor plasmid. When they are transferred to a recipient cell, that cell acquires an entire metabolic pathway.

TRANSPOSONS

Small pieces of plasmids known as **transposons** can migrate between molecules of DNA of significantly different base composition. Thus, certain genes can move from one plasmid to another in the same cell, as well as migrating from a plasmid to the cell's chromosome. Genes which determine antibiotic resistance, R genes, are examples of transposons.

Cytoplasmic Inheritance in Eucaryotes

The genetic characteristics of eucaryotic animal and plant cells are not entirely regulated from within a nucleus or nucleus-type organelle. Several observations indicate that certain hereditary characteristics are under cytoplasmic control. Chloroplasts and mitochondria of certain animal, plant, and microbial cells can self-duplicate and are apparently independent of the nucleus. These plasmids contain DNA in addition to the biochemical materials, such as enzymes, required for their particular functions within the cell. An example of such regulatory influences is the "petite colony" mutant of yeast. This mutation appears to be a defect in the mitochondria that produces both a respiratory deficiency and small cell size. The expression of these cytoplasmic or extranuclear elements may be due to autonomous (independent) units without strict chromosomal control, may be self-duplicating and yet under chromosomal direction (semiautonomous), or may be due to episomes or extrachromosomal DNA that are integrated into the cell's chromosome.

Treatment with the chemical acriflavine destroys the elements of cytoplasmic inheritance. When in the autonomous state, episomes are inactivated by such compounds. This characteristic is used to determine whether a cytoplasmic inheritance unit is episomal.

THE KILLER SYSTEM AND KAPPA PARTICLES

The killer system of *Paramecium aurelia,* shown to be a genetic system by Sonneborn in 1943, is the classic example of cytoplasmic inheritance in eucaryotes. Certain strains of *P. aurelia,* which are known as killers, have been observed to contain ***kappa particles.*** These kappa-particle-containing protozoans produce a toxin that kills paramecia that do not have the particles. The particles can be transmitted only by cytoplasmic mixing (Figure 15–10).

Kappa particles present in the cytoplasm of "killer" strains are self-duplicating, and under the control of a dominant gene, K, located in the nucleus. They are 0.2 to 0.8 μm in diameter and contain DNA. Sensitive, nonkiller strains lack either kappa particles or the dominant K gene. Those nonkiller strains without the dominant K gene would have two recessive kk genes (Figure 15–10). Both elements are necessary to maintain the killer system.

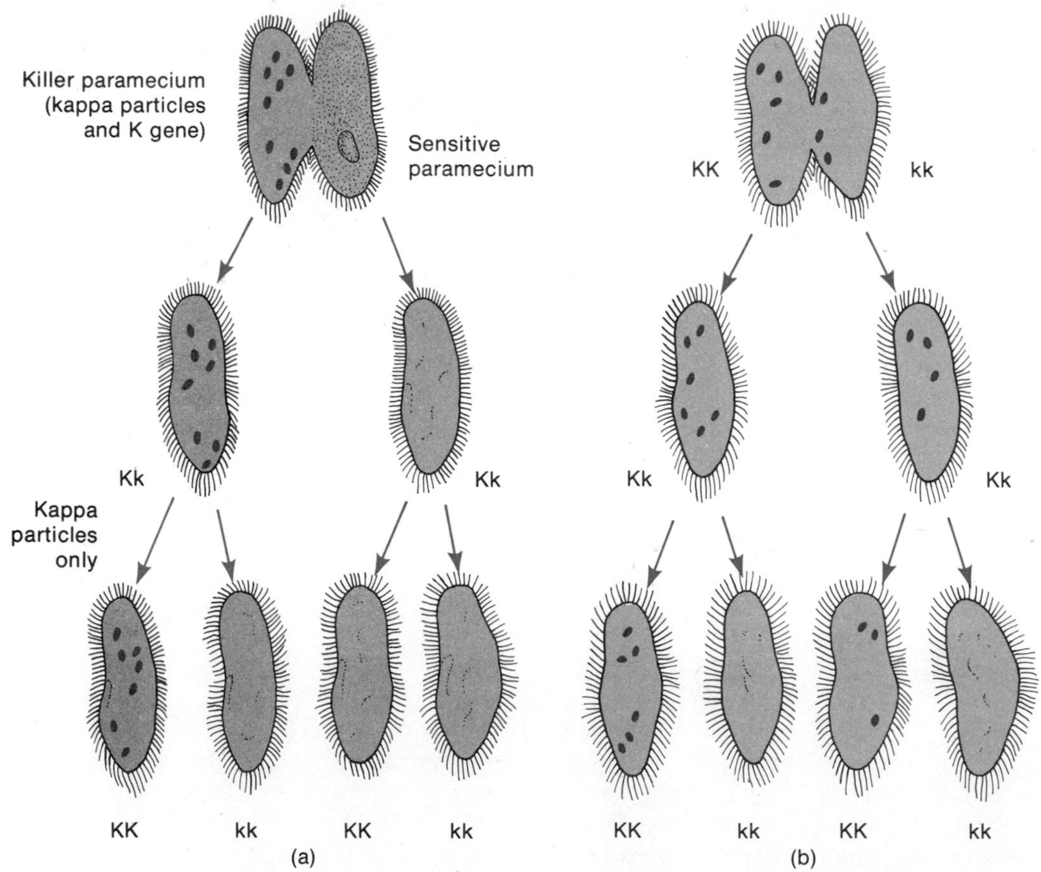

FIG. 15–10 (a) Mating between a killer paramecium with *kappa* particles and a sensitive organism without cytoplasmic exchange. The nuclear *K* gene is transferred, but the kappa particles are not. (b) Mating betwen a killer paramecium (KK with *kappa* particles) and a sensitive organism (kk) with cytoplasmic exchange.

Recent studies have shown kappa particles to be bacterial in nature. Particles found in other paramecia have been cultured outside their protozoan hosts and identified as Gram-negative bacteria.

Mapping the Bacterial Genome

Transformation, transduction, and conjugation techniques are all used to determine the location of individual genes on the bacterial chromosome. The characteristics transferred by transformation or transduction are usually very small linkage groups. Many very complex analyses of recombinant cells are, therefore, necessary to piece together enough information to map the genes. Although the process of mapping by conjugation is probably equally complex, it is much more easily described.

Linear transfer of DNA between the F^+ and F^- bacteria yielded information on genetic mapping in *E. coli*. Before extensive work was begun, it was known that, with a particular F^+ strain, rates of recombination of the order of one in a million occurred. Unfortunately, this was not often enough to permit large-scale studies of conjugation. However, during these studies, mutants of F^+ strains, the Hfrs, were found that recombined at a rate of approximately one in a hundred. As indicated earlier, investigations with these mutant strains have shown that fertility in *E. coli* depends upon the presence of the F particle in the bacterium. In F^+ cells, the sex particle is present as an individual cytoplasmic unit. When an F^+ cell is mated with an F^-, the F^- cell receives this F particle at a high rate without the bacterial genome. Only in the case of Hfr is this F particle integrated with the genome, allowing other genes to be transferred to the recipient (Figure 15–7). Thus, it was found that the small rate of recombination observed in F^+ populations was caused by the presence of a small number of Hfr mutants in the population.

In 1955 a relatively simple procedure for genetic mapping analyses in *E. coli* was reported. After Hfr and F^- strains were mixed, conjugation could be interrupted by whirling the bacteria in a kitchen blender. Analysis of recombinants in the F^- bacteria indicated that the genome was indeed linear. This was demonstrated by breaking the mating pairs after different intervals and observing that, after certain intervals, additional genetic characteristics were expressed by the original F^- bacteria.

Figure 15–11 summarizes the conjugation process in *E. coli*. In the hypothetical experiment presented, Hfr and F^- strains of *E. coli* are mixed, and samples of the mixture are removed to a blender after selected time intervals. After blending to rupture the conjugation tube, the recombinants are cultured on media suitable for analyzing nutritional characteristics and characteristics of antibiotic and bacterial virus resistance. These genetic traits, or ***markers***, are indicated in Figure 15–11 by numbers 1 through 9. The sexuality factor or F is always the last marker transferred. When it is transferred, the former F^- cell becomes either an Hfr cell or an F^+ cell.

The time intervals at which the mating bacteria were separated can be used to locate the genes on the chromosome. Suppose, for example, that in a hypothetical experiment using interrupted mating, one additional characteristic was transferred to the recipient cell during each 5 minutes of mating. By the end of the experiment, the F^- cells contained all the characteristics under study. The order of transfer would indicate the order in which the characteristics are located along the length of the chromosome.

Actual research has shown that the entire chromosome of over 450 genes in

E. coli is transferred in 90 minutes. Resistance to penicillin, for example, is transferred at 83 minutes; resistance to streptomycin, at two points, 7 and 64 minutes; and formation of pili, at 88 minutes.

This and other types of analysis have proved that the bacterial chromosome is truly one strand and is circular. This circular strand of genetic information, which controls the destiny of *E. coli*, always breaks at the point of F particle integration.

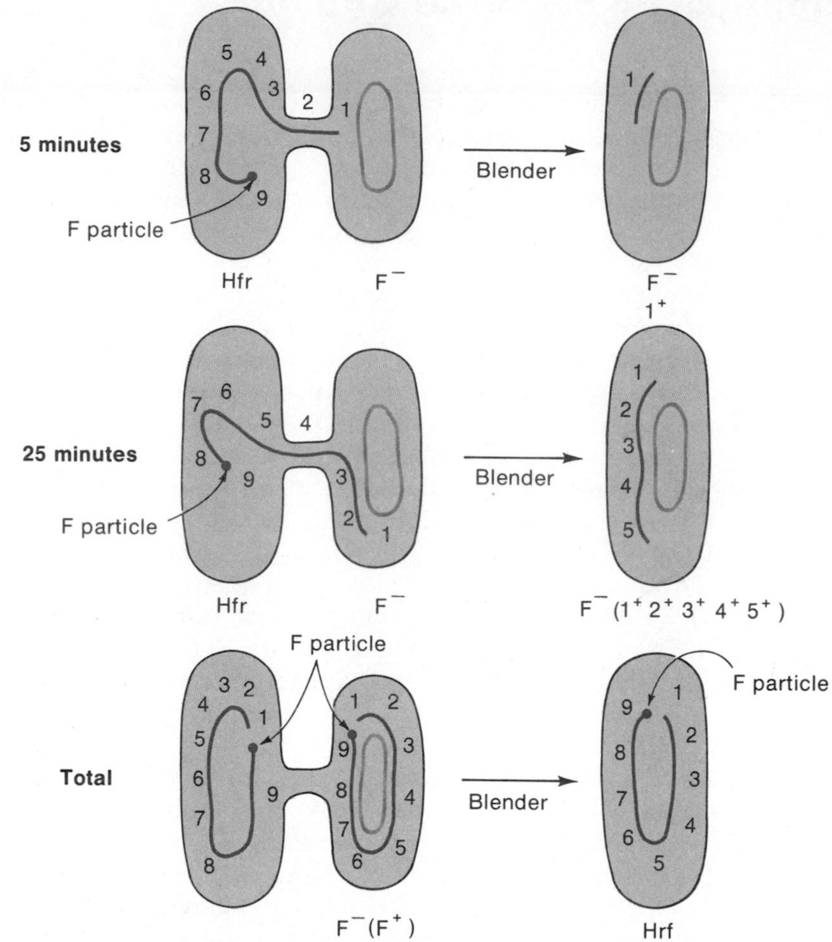

FIG. 15-11 Conjugation in *Escherichia coli.*

Applications of Microbial Genetics

Use of mutations to determine metabolic pathways and to map the bacterial chromosome are two important applications of microbial genetics. Similar processes have been used to map the DNA in bacterial viruses. Biological assays, determination of taxonomic relationships between microorganisms, and gene manipulation also use techniques of genetic research. Microbial testing for carcinogens, another application, is described in Chapter 36.

Biological Assays

As described earlier with *Neurospora crassa,* it is possible to increase the rate of microbial mutations. Many of these genetic changes involve specific nutritional requirements. An auxotroph with the requirement for the vitamin biotin can be used to determine the amount of biotin in a food, for example. First the growth response of the auxotroph is measured as increasing quantities of the vitamin are added to the minimal medium. Figure 15–12 shows that the organism grows to an optical density of 0.5 when given 4 micrograms per milliliter of biotin and to 1.0 with 8 mg/ml. If an extract of some particular food allowed the organism to grow to a density of 0.6, the graph (Figure 15–12) would indicate that the food probably provides 5 mg/ml biotin.

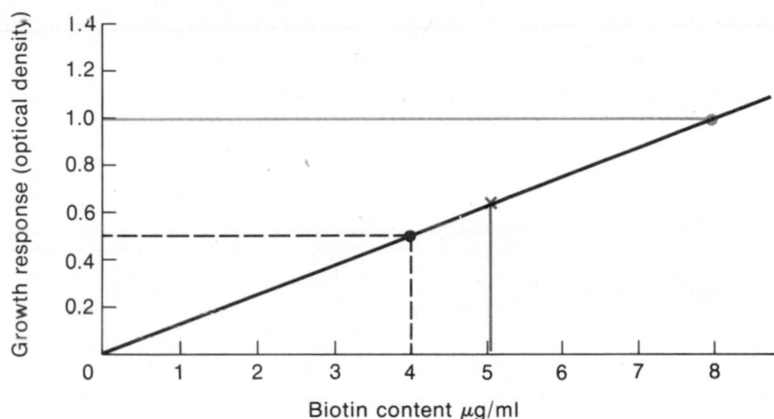

FIG. 15–12 Growth response of an auxotroph requiring biotin.

Genetics and Taxonomy

PERCENT G + C COMPARISON

One means of studying the relationship between genetics and taxonomy involves determining the percent of guanine and cytosine, % (G + C), in the DNA of an organism, as compared to the total base composition, of adenine, thymine, guanine, and cytosine. Organisms with similar values of % (G + C) have been shown to be related genetically and very similar in terms of numerical taxonomy. Selected bacteria and their % (G + C) values are presented in Table 15–1.

TABLE 15–1 Selected Bacterial Genera and Their Percent Guanine and Cytosine (G + C) Ratios

Percent (G + C)	*Representative Genera*
30–36	*Bacillus, Clostridium, Fusobacterium, Staphylococcus, Streptococcus*
38–44	*Bacillus, Coxiella, Hemophilus, Lactobacillus, Neisseria, Proteus, Streptococcus*
46–52	*Clostridium, Corynebacterium, Enterobacter, Escherichia, Klebsiella, Neisseria, Pasteurella, Proteus, Salmonella, Vibrio*
54–60	*Alcaligenes, Corynebacterium, Enterobacter, Klebsiella, Lactobacillus, Pseudomonas, Serratia, Spirillum*
62–68	*Bacillus, Micrococcus, Mycobacterium, Pseudomonas, Rhizobium, Vibrio*
70–80	*Mycobacterium, Nocardia, Sarcina, Streptomyces*

In many instances, genera are well grouped by their % (G + C) value. However, certain significant discrepancies exist, either because of incomplete data or because of true unrelatedness.

DNA HYBRIDIZATION

When the DNA double-stranded helix is heated, the hydrogen bonds holding the base pairs together are weakened and the strands can separate. Upon cooling, the strands reassociate and the DNA appears to be identical to the original. As would be expected, when DNA from *Escherichia coli*, for example, is studied in this manner, there is complete reassociation with more DNA from *E. coli*. When two different strains, or species, are mixed and heated, the degree of relatedness of the two organisms can be measured by determining the ability of their respective DNAs to reassociate to form a "hybrid" DNA molecule. This tendency to reassociate can be measured in a variety of ways, including enzymatic cleavage of single-stranded DNA and radioisotopic tagging of one source of DNA. When such studies compared *E. coli* with *Salmonella typhimurium* and with *Pseudomonas aeruginosa*, relationships of 71 percent and 1 percent, respectively, were obtained.

Gene Manipulation

Transformation, transduction, and conjugation are natural means by which asexual organisms produce DNA recombinations similar to that of sexual organisms. When these processes are performed in the laboratory rather than in nature, they are examples of ***gene manipulation***. This section will deal primarily with processes geared to produce recombinant DNA situations that might be called unnatural, such as producing microorganisms with DNA of entirely unrelated microorganisms or of higher forms of life incorporated in their genetic makeup, most commonly as plasmids.

Potential Benefits

Among the many potential benefits of controlled gene manipulation are development of simple processes for synthesizing human insulin by bacteria. Others might be improving sources of antibiotics; incorporating nitrogen-fixing capabilities in more soil organisms; making animal proteins for food by fermentation; improving palatability and digestibility and removing toxicity associated with some sources of single-cell protein; adding photosynthetic enzymes to more kinds of microorganisms; producing hormones more simply; and creating biological pesticides of broader usefulness than the currently available microorganisms.

Potential Hazards

On the other hand, a number of potential hazards have been suggested. For example, it is feared that mixing genes between widely separated species of life forms might create some deadly monster. Recombinant organisms are called ***chimeras*** after the fire-breathing mythological monster with the head of a lion, body of a goat, and the tail of a dragon. It might be possible to create a chimera that produces toxins and has a greater potential for spreading disease than the original bacterium. Let us assume that an irresponsible scientist were to create an *Escherichia coli* chimera with the capability of making botulism toxin. Normally, *Clostridium botulinum*, an anaerobic soil organism, finds only occasional access to conditions where its toxin can be produced, ingested, and ultimately cause food poisoning. However, a strain of *E. coli* with that capability normally living in the human intestine might more easily find access to a suitable environment and might produce an epidemic. Some concern has also been voiced over creating bacterial chimeras with antibiotic resistance patterns not found in nature and chimeras of tumor or other animal viruses and bacteria. Imagine *E. coli* with the genetic information to cause cancer, rabies, viral encephalitis, or even severe birth defects such as those caused by the virus of German measles.

The concern over such potential hazards led to the development of strict research guidelines in 1976 by the National Institute of Health Recombinant DNA Molecule Program Advisory Committee. The guidelines include handling all bacterial chimeras as highly virulent pathogens with appropriate pro tective clothing and laboratory isolation procedures.

Techniques

There are four essential elements in gene manipulation:

1. breaking and joining DNA from different sources,
2. obtaining a suitable gene carrier that can replicate with foreign DNA attached,
3. introducing the composite DNA into a bacterium, and
4. selecting the chimera produced from the large number of bacterial cells exposed to the gene carriers.

Two key biochemicals found in *E. coli* allow the process to occur with relative ease. They are an enzyme called ***restriction endonuclease*** and the ***RTF plasmids*** described earlier.

RESTRICTION ENDONUCLEASE

A restriction endonuclease is a unique DNAase that not only breaks DNA at particular points but, in doing so, creates a condition that permits attaching portions of foreign DNA cleaved by the same enzyme. The enzyme produces regions of unpaired bases at the ends of the DNA strands ("sticky ends") as shown in Figure 15–13a. The *E. coli* restriction endonuclease called ***EcoRI*** is capable of splitting the DNA complementary sequences

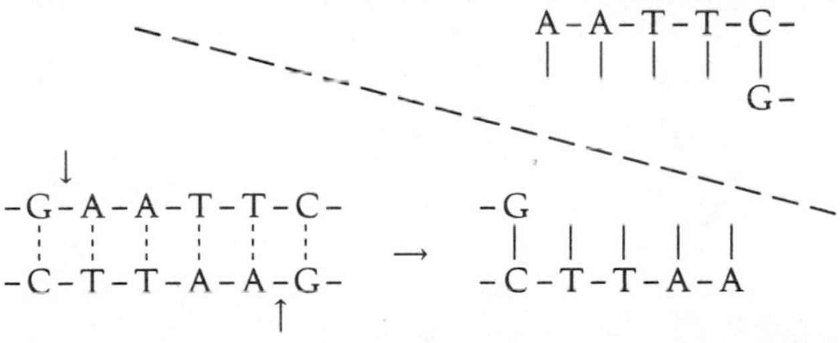

```
                                    A-A-T-T-C-
                                    | | | | |
                                            G-
   ↓
-G-A-A-T-T-C-          -G
 : : : : : :    →       | | | | |
-C-T-T-A-A-G-          -C-T-T-A-A
           ↑
```

at the G–A and A–G bonds, thereby creating the "sticky ends." The restriction endonuclease apparently functions by recognizing the A-A-T-T / T-T-A-A pattern, which has been called a palindrome. By definition, a palindrome is a word, verse, or sentence that is the same when read backward or forward.

The enzyme does not distinguish between different species in which that sequence is found and therefore produces the complementary single strands wherever the sequence is present (Figure 15–13b). This technique, or a similar one, has been used to produce composite DNA structures between *E. coli* and

Staphylococcus aureus, as well as between *E. coli* and DNA from the frog, *Xenopus laevis.* When the pieces of foreign DNA are mixed with the opened plasmid, complementarity rules, and the appropriate single-stranded ends are joined to form the composite DNA, Figure 15–13c.

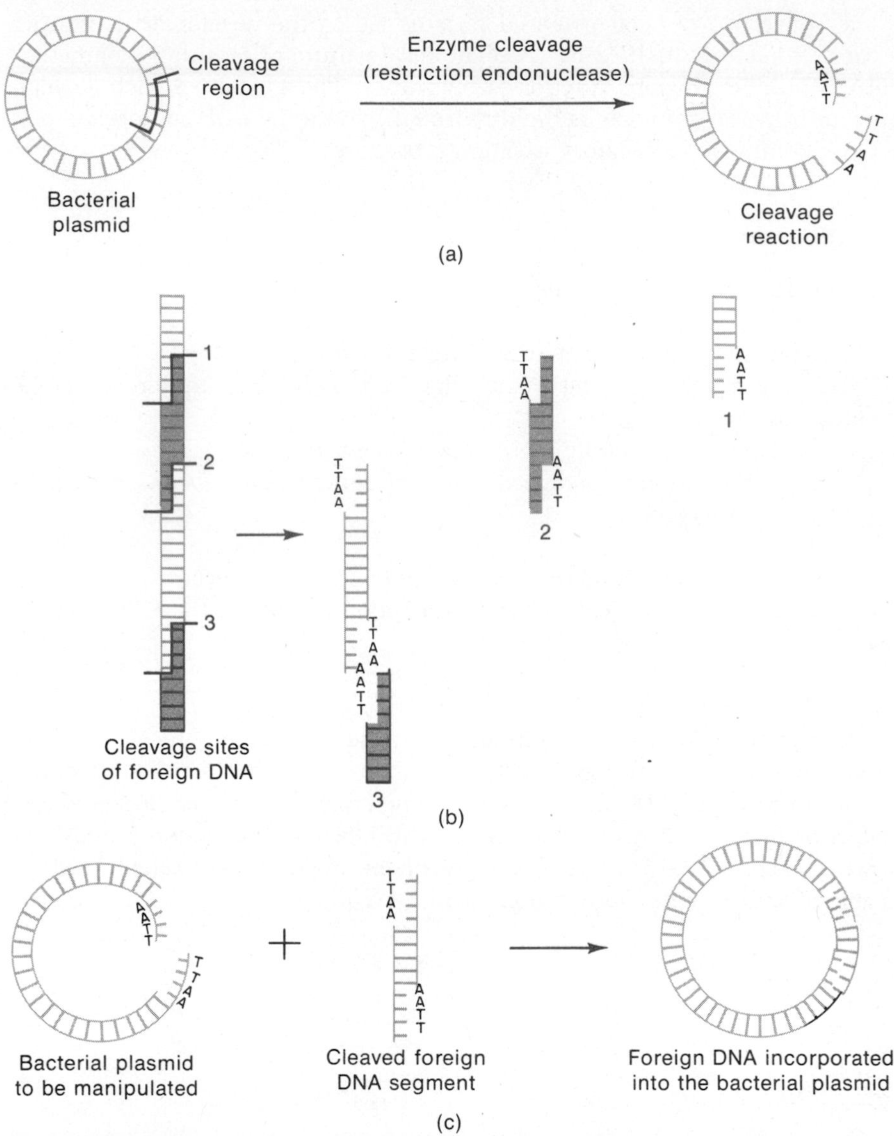

FIG. 15–13 How foreign DNA segments can be incorporated into a bacterial plasmid. This is an example of gene manipulation.

RTF PLASMIDS

The second key biochemical from *E. coli* are the plasmids carrying genetic information for resistance to antibiotics. The RTF plasmids can replicate in an appropriate host bacteria, thereby making more copies of the foreign gene or genes. Some strains of bacteria may produce as many as twenty copies of the plasmid or composite plasmid and make twenty times as much gene product.

This has been called ***gene amplification***. Another significant property of the RTF plasmid is that the antibiotic resistance it conveys to the host cell enables the investigator to recognize and isolate the chimera easily. For example, plasmid pSc101 has the gene for resistance to tetracycline. The host bacterium that gains this trait will grow in the presence of that antibiotic. Because all the many bacteria that do not have this resistance will not grow under these conditions, the chimera can be found easily.

So far we have discussed first, second, and fourth elements of gene manipulation. The remaining one deals with introducing the composite plasmid made in test tubes into the recipient bacterial cells. With *E. coli* this process is sufficiently difficult that many believe it cannot occur in nature. The actual process is a form of transformation, as shown in Figure 15–14. The difficulties include making the cells receptive by treating them with calcium chloride and incubating for several hours at 0° C in the presence of calcium chloride.

E. coli has been used to produce clones of foreign DNA from *S. aureus* and the frog *Xenopus laevis*, as mentioned earlier. In addition it has been the recipient of sea urchin, *Drosophila melanogaster* (fruit fly), mouse mitochondria, and yeast. This transformation capability is not limited to *E. coli*. It has been reported that plasmids from *E. coli* have been inserted into cowpea protoplasts where they were later found to be stable extranuclear particles. A very exciting experiment showed that the fungus *Pseudosaccharomycete* Tc-1176 could be transformed with extracted DNA from pancreatic beta cells and that these fungi were able to synthesize the biologically active insulin normally made by the beta cells. The scientists, Thinumalachar, Narasimhan, and Anderson, were awarded a patent in 1978 to make insulin by this process.

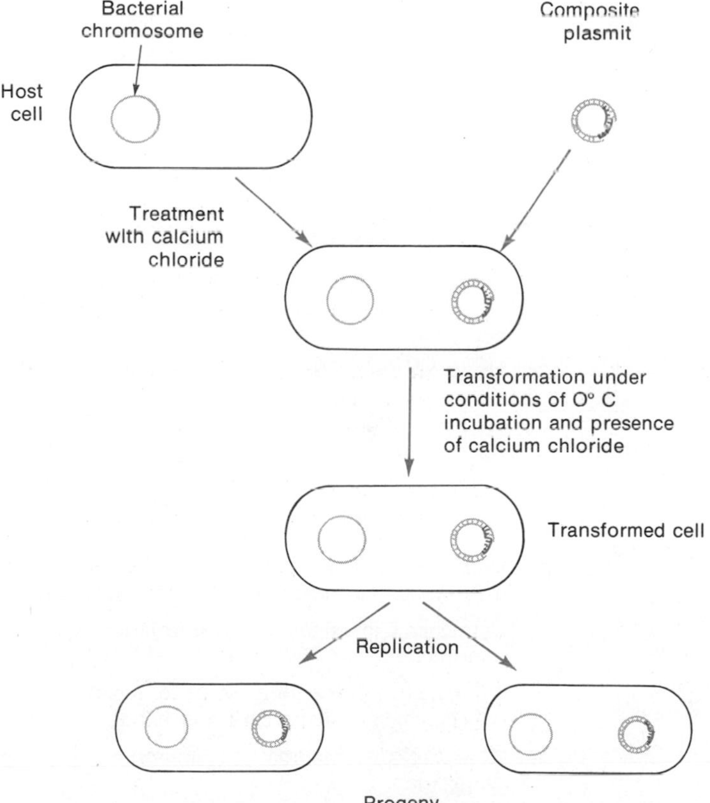

FIG. 15–14 Transformation process for gene manipulation in *Escherichia coli*. Here a plasmid (foreign DNA) is introduced into a receptive host cell. The newly received DNA is replicated along with the host cell's chromosome and is passed on to future offspring.

SUMMARY

Evolution and Inheritance

1. The concept of evolution introduced by Lamarck during the early 1800s was defined as a continual process of gradual changes of animals and plants in response to environmental conditions.
2. Darwin argued that spontaneously occurring variations and natural selection were the causes of evolutionary change.
3. Modern biology recognizes that changes in cells and organisms are the result of permanent genetic changes known as *mutations.*

The Chemistry of Genetics

1. Deoxyribonucleic acid (DNA) has been proven conclusively to be the genetic substance of cells.
2. DNA consists of a double strand or linear chains of nitrogen bases, the purines (adenine and guanine) and the pyrimidines (thymine and cytosine), linked together by means of sugar-phosphate molecules.
3. Mutations result from changes in the sequences of purines and pyrimidines in DNA strands.
4. Various chemical and physical factors can cause mutations. Such mutagenic agents include mustard gas, nitrous acid, and ultraviolet light.

Mutations in Microorganisms

1. Mutations are expressed as defects in enzymes that prevent specific normal metabolic activities from occurring.
2. Experiments involving bacterial resistance to viruses have provided strong evidence for the spontaneous, random nature of mutation and the Darwinian theory of natural selection.

Recombination in Procaryotes

1. Genetic material can be exchanged between members of different bacterial genera and species. Such exchanges can occur by means of transformation, bacterial conjugation, sexduction (F-duction), and transduction.
2. Transformation results in a genetic change caused by soluble extracts of DNA.
3. Bacterial conjugation refers to the transfer of genetic material between two living bacteria that are in intimate physical contact.
4. Sexduction, or F-duction, is a process whereby genetic material is transferred by an extrachromosomal genetic particle, or F particle, to a cell lacking this particle.
5. Transduction is a process in which genetic material transfer is accomplished by a bacterial virus.
6. Notable changes occur in microorganisms as the result of virus infection. Such *lysogenic,* or *viral, conversions* are of medical importance and include toxin production and antigenic changes.
7. Plasmids are small extrachromosomal DNA particles capable of independent replication. Plasmids control nonessential properties of bacteria, including antibiotic resistance, the synthesis of bacteria-killing substances called bacteriocins, and certain metabolic activities.
8. The killer system of the protozoan *Paramecium aurelia* is a classic example of cytoplasmic inheritance in eucaryotic microorganisms. The killer trait is associated with cytoplasmic particles known as *kappa particles* which are controlled by a dominant gene in the cell nucleus.

Mapping the Bacterial Genome

Transformation, transduction, and conjugation techniques can be used to determine the location of individual genes on the bacterial chromosome.

Applications of Microbial Genetics

Applications of microbial genetics include mapping metabolic pathways, performing biological assays for vitamins and other materials in foods, determining the specific genetic relatedness between microorganisms, and testing substances of various types for cancer-producing activity.

Gene Manipulation

1. Laboratory controlled DNA recombination of bacteria is *gene manipulation.*
2. The possible benefits of gene manipulation include the potential for improving sources of antibiotics, producing important hormones, and making animal protein for food by fermentation. One possible hazard is that of creating uncontrollable or difficult-to-control disease agents.
3. Current techniques to incorporate strands of DNA in existing bacterial chromosomes utilize a unique enzyme called restriction endonuclease.

QUESTIONS FOR REVIEW

1. What was the basis of the Hershey and Chase experiment with bacterial viruses that showed that DNA was the genetic material?
2. Using the chemistry involved in transcription and translation, describe how ultraviolet light and nitrous acid can cause mutations.
3. What is the one-gene, one-enzyme hypothesis of Beadle and Tatum?
4. Define: minimal medium, prototroph, auxotroph.
5. Explain Lederbergs' indirect selection procedure for proving the spontaneous nature of mutation in microorganisms.
6. Define and distinguish: transformation, conjugation, and transduction.
7. Compare transformation with conjugation, and compare lysogenic conversion with transduction.
8. How can the bacterial chromosome be mapped using conjugation?
9. What is meant by autonomous and semiautonomous cytoplasmic inheritance?
10. Define: plasmid, episome, bacteriocin, RTF, and metabolic plasmid.

11. You want to develop a biological assay for the amino acid histidine in milk and milk products. How would you attempt to do so?
12. Describe the use of % (G + C) and DNA hybridization studies in classifying organisms.
13. What is the function of a restriction endonuclease in gene manipulation?
14. Discuss the potential benefits and hazards of gene manipulation.

SUGGESTED READINGS

Carlberg, D. M., *Essentials of Bacterial and Viral Genetics.* Springfield, Ill.: Charles C. Thomas, 1976. *A general, well-written textbook covering such topics as history of the discovery of genetic material, protein synthesis, mutations, recombination, bacterial viruses and plasmids.*

Curtiss, Roy, III, "Genetic Manipulation of Microorganisms: Potential Benefits and Biohazards," *Ann. Rev. Microbiol.* 30:507–533 (1976). *A clear look at the current state of technology associated with genetically altering microorganisms, together with benefits and unsolved problems.*

Fox, M. S., "Some Features of Genetic Recombination in Procaryotes," *Ann. Rev. Genet.* 12:47 (1978). *A discussion of the events that result in the formation of genetic recombinants in bacterial transformation and conjugation. Generalized transduction and bacteriophage recombination also are given attention.*

:kson, D. A., and S. P. Stich (eds.), *The Recombinant DNA Debate.* Englewood Cliffs, N.J.: Prentice-Hall International, Inc., 1979. *A thorough presentation of recombinant DNA debate. Sufficient background of the issues and concepts are provided for the reader to intelligently evaluate the new and powerful methodology in the area of genetic research.*

King, R. C. (ed.), *Handbook of Genetics,* vol. 1. New York: Plenum Press, 1974. *A collection of short papers on the genetics of various genera and species of bacteria, fungi and bacteriophages of importance.*

Maniatis, T. and M. Ptashne, "A DNA Operator-repressor System." *Sci. Amer.* 234:64 (January 1976). *The working of an operator-repressor system is the subject of this article.*

Starlinger, P., "DNA Rearrangements in Procaryotes," *Ann. Rev. Genet.* 11:103 (1977). *The interactions of bacterial, plasmid, and phage chromosomes with each other and chromosomal rearrangements occurring in their vicinity and spontaneous aberrations also are discussed.*

Watson, J. D., *Molecular Biology of the Gene,* 3rd ed. New York: W. A. Benjamin, 1976. *A masterful and understandable summary of general and biochemical genetics based on experiments with bacteria and viruses.*

CHAPTER 16 Microbial Ecology

The soils and waters of the planet earth abound with microorganisms. The influence of the environment on these organisms and on the relationships among microbes and other life forms is critical to the survival of life as we know it. The vast majority of microorganisms do not cause spoilage or disease, but they do perform a variety of natural processes that affect the well-being of life on this planet. This chapter describes many of these microorganisms, their environments and their interaction with different life forms.

After reading this chapter, you should be able to:

1. **Define the term *ecosystem*.**
2. **Distinguish between the abiotic and biotic factors of an ecosystem.**
3. **Describe the types of natural habitats in which microbes are found.**
4. **List representative microbial types found in specific natural habitats.**
5. **Define *symbiosis*.**
6. **List, explain, and give examples of three different types of symbiotic associations.**
7. **Define or explain the following terms:**
   - **a. lichen**
   - **b. biosphere**
   - **c. autotroph**
   - **d. heterotroph**
   - **e. population**
   - **f. community**
   - **g. habitat**
   - **h. niche**
8. **Explain the role of producers, consumers, and decomposers in an ecosystem.**

9. **Discuss what is meant by the following types of coaction, giving examples for each type: syntrophism, competition, and predation.**
10. **Describe and discuss examples of commensalism, parasitism, and mutualism as types of symbiosis.**

The word *ecology* was coined by Ernst Haekel in 1869. He wrote: "By ecology we mean the body of knowledge concerning the economy of nature—the investigation of the total relations of the animal both to its inorganic and its organic environment."* Haekel's use of the word "economy" in the definition is very apt, for "economy" is derived from two Greek words, *oikos* and *nemain*, meaning "to manage a home." Thus ecology is the study of the relationships among different forms of life and their interactions with their physical environment. It includes all the activities and relationships by which living and nonliving components of the environment manage to sustain life on this planet.

Basic Ecological Principles

Life and the physical environment go together, for the environment supplies both the nutrients and the conditions for the existence of life. This combination of living things and the environment in which life exists is the **biosphere.** The biosphere extends up into the atmosphere to more than 10,000 meters, down into the ocean to a depth of approximately 8000 meters, and more than 250 meters below land surfaces.

Most forms of life are adapted to a particular environment that is restricted in general living conditions and food resources. Moreover, the nutrition of any species must be in balance with the biosphere as a whole. Thus the biosphere is a global biological system based on a continuous, or cyclic, flow of energy and nutrients.

Despite their small size, microorganisms have important roles in many natural processes that contribute to the survival of animals, plants, and microbes.

The purpose of this chapter is to survey environmental microbiology, including descriptions of representative microorganisms in their natural environments and discussions of microbial nutrition as related to the requirements of other forms of life.

The Organization of the Biosphere

At the present time, earth, among all the planets of our solar system, is the most favorable for the production and survival of life. Its distance from the sun, neither too close nor too far, creates an environment that permits the various biochemical and biophysical reactions on which life as we know it depends. Environment includes all factors external to the organism that in some way affect it.

The biosphere is made up of ecological units called **ecosystems.** Groups of individuals having similar properties and living in the same area are called **populations.** When various populations interact with one another, they

*Quoted in R. Brewer, *Principles of Ecology* (Philadelphia: W. B. Saunders Company, 1979).

form a **community** (Figure 16–1). The interactions of such a community and its physical environment constitute an *ecosystem*. An ecosystem, then, refers to the organisms in the system and to the physical environment that supports their life.

The living members of an ecosystem are divided into three categories, depending on their role in maintaining the stable ecosystem: *producers, consumers*, and *decomposers* (Figures 16–2 and 16–3).

Photosynthesizers, such as the cyanobacteria and purple and green bacteria, microscopic algae, and large plants, function as the producers of organic compounds from inorganic materials. Such forms of life, as noted in Chapter 13, are called autotrophs. The consumer category is made up of heterotrophs, species that cannot produce organic substances from inorganic ones. Microbial consumers are mostly protozoans (Figure 16–2). The microbial decomposers are various bacteria and fungi that break down complex organic products such as the remains of animals, plants, and other microbes into smaller compounds, or into inorganic materials that can be used by plants for their producer activity. In short, these microorganisms are microscopic "recycling centers." It would be difficult for life to continue normally without them.

Decomposers function in the ecosystem by using rotting organic matter as nutrients. Like consumers, these saprophytic organisms are heterotrophic. They secrete a variety of extracellular enzymes such as proteases, carbohydrates, and lipases, which render the waste materials on which they act soluble, so that they and other organisms can utilize them for food. Subsequent metabolic activities by these and other organisms further decompose the wastes and return their essential elements to forms that can be used in the nutrition of plants and other organisms.

The activities of producers, consumers, and decomposers together constitute members of **food chains.** These are circular processes that promote the exchange of nutrients and energy flow in the ecosystem.

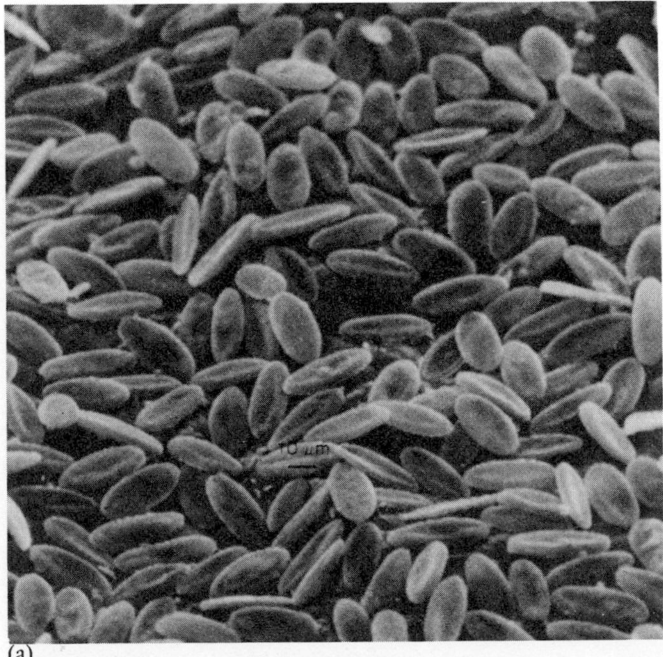

(a)

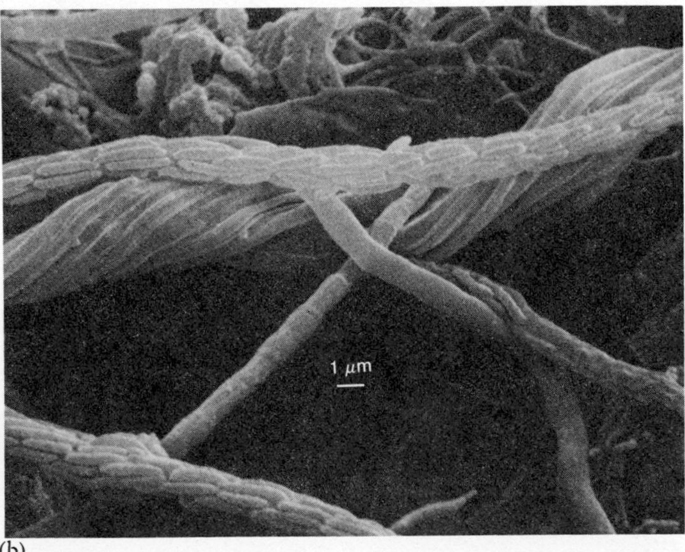

(b)

FIG. 16–1 Some microbial members of the biosphere. (a) An impressive number of the diatom *Cocroneis scutellum* forming an algal community. *McN. Sieburth, J., and C. D. Thomas,* J. Phycol. *9:46–50 (1973)*. (b) Microbial communities in the intestinal tract of a termite. What bacterial shapes are present? *Boyle, P. T., and R. Mitchell,* Science *200:1157–1159 (1978)*.

TABLE 16-1 Three Abiotic Factors and Selected Microorganisms That Grow Under Extreme Conditions in Nature

Abiotic Factor	*Microorganism*	*Conditions for Growth*
Temperature	Blue-green bacterium	73°C
	Thermoactinomyces spp.	68°C
	Rhodotorula sp.[a]	14°C
	Flavobacterium spp.	4°C
	Bacillus globisporus	−10°C
pH	*Agrobacterium* sp.	12.0
	Vibrio cholerae	9.0
	Bacillus pasteurii	8.5
	Sulfolobus sp.	0.5
	Thiobacillus thiooxidams	0
Osmotic Pressure	*Candida* spp.[a]	60% sugar[c]
	Hansenula spp.[a]	60% sugar[c]
	Saccharomyces spp.[a]	60% sugar[c]
	Halobacterium salinarum	27–30% NaCl[b]
	Sarcina morrhuae	27–30% NaCl
	Pseudomonas cepacia	Distilled water

[a]These organisms are yeasts, all others are bacteria.
[b]This concentration of NaCl can be found in Great Salt Lake, Utah, and the Dead Sea.
[c]Honey is one example of such a high sugar concentration in nature.

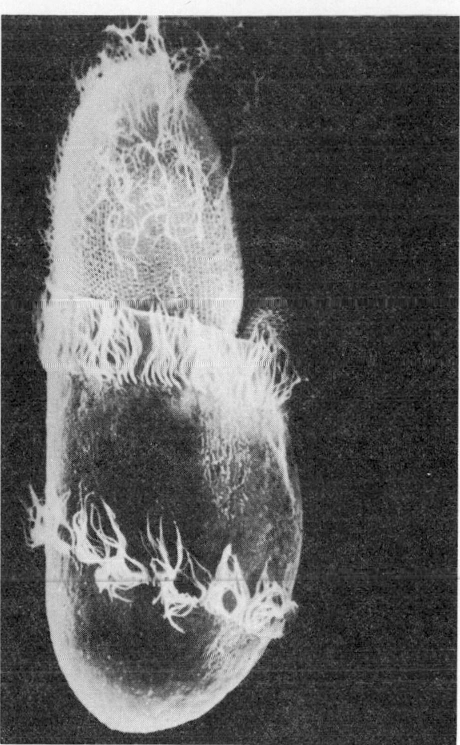

FIG. 16–2 The ingestion of the protozoan *Paramecium* by another ciliated form, *Didinium*. The half-swallowed *Paramecium* is shown in the feeding apparatus of *Didinium*. *Wessenberg, H., and G. Antipa.* J. Protozool. 17:*250–270 (1970).*

The Components of an Ecosystem

The activities and reactions of living and nonliving components in a natural physical location form a stable, self-nourishing system. The specific location or place of residence of an organism is called its **habitat;** its specific role or function in a community is referred to as its **niche.** The concept of niche is often difficult to define, since it includes an organism's habits, relationships to other forms of life, food-related reactions, and ability to change or be changed by its environment. No two species can occupy the same niche at the same time. Thus, certain plants produce food for a community, while other forms of life have the role of decomposer and, at times, predator. An invasion of an organism's niche by another form of life results in *competition* and ends in one species being eliminated.

Ecosystems include lakes, forests, ponds, or even smaller regions such as a fish bowl or a handful of soil. The human body is also an excellent example of an ecosystem.

BIOTIC AND ABIOTIC FACTORS

The possible habitats for any living organism are limited by both *biotic* (living) and *abiotic* (nonliving) factors in the biosphere. Biotic factors include other animals, plants, and microbes that may compete or otherwise interfere with essential processes. Examples of abiotic components are hydrostatic pressure, osmotic pressure, pH, light, and temperature. The nonliving components also include a variety of inorganic substances such as water, carbon dioxide, oxygen, and minerals, as well as organic substances.

Abiotic factors include those physical and chemical conditions in the environment that are not necessarily due to life forms. For example, a low pH can be a result of mining wastes or the oxidation of sulfur by microorganisms. A high temperature may be due to volcanic activity or to microbial catabolism.

Table 16–1 presents selected microorganisms and the extreme conditions under which they grow.

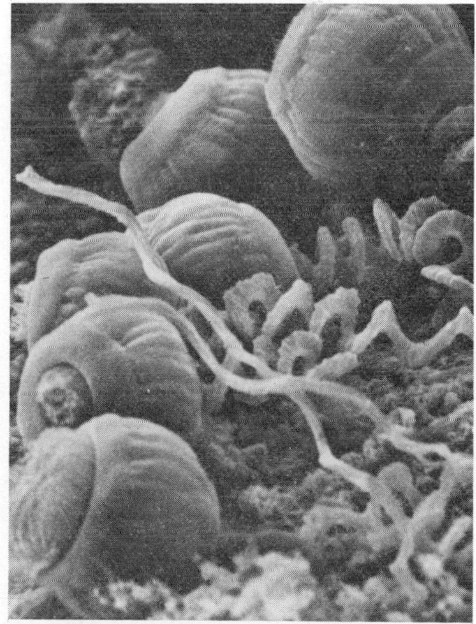

FIG. 16–3 Protozoa on leaf litter from a stream. *Suberkropp, K. F., and M. J. Klug,* Microbial Ecol. 1:*96–103 (1974).*

Temperature. Microorganisms have been observed growing in extremes of −10° to 92°C in their natural habitats. *Psychrophilic* ("cold-loving") yeasts have been isolated from glacial ice and soil from Antarctica. A ***Flavobacterium*** sp. isolated from the Great Lakes demonstrated higher respiration rates at 4°C than at 20°C. Since this organism grows best at 4°C, it is considered an obligate psychrophile. Other genera that contain psychrophiles are ***Achromobacter, Alkaligenes, Bacillus, Pseudomonas, Vibrio,*** and ***Xanthomonas.*** Psychrophilic yeasts are found in the genera of *Candida* and *Rhodotorula*. Psychrophiles that grow and metabolize optimally at 4°C or less play a crucial role as decomposers. They also perform other functions in the cold ecosystems, particularly in deep ocean waters, 90 percent of which are at these temperatures.

Thermophilic ("heat-loving") microorganisms grow in volcanic soils and heated water ecosystems, as well as in ***compost.*** Compost is the natural decomposition product of microbial activity in mixtures of vegetation supplemented with manure. This decomposition of cellulosic and animal wastes is usually an anaerobic process, but it can be made aerobic by frequent mixing of the materials. Heat generated by composting can reach 80°C, which is usually adequate to disinfect the compost. The final product is used for soil enrichment. ***Thermoactinomyces*** spp. have been observed growing optimally at 65° to 68°C and have been isolated with other thermophilic bacteria from compost piles.

Probably the most remarkable organisms are the blue-green bacteria isolated from hot sulfur springs, where the water may be 92°C or higher.

pH. Land (terrestrial) and aquatic habitats vary in acidity and alkalinity. The pH of such environments is determined by the types and amounts of various minerals and microbial activities. For example, bacteria can oxidize sulfur to sulfuric acid, creating aquatic environments with pH values as low as 0 to 2.0. A pH of 0 means that the acidity is equivalent to a 1 N solution of a strong acid, which is a great amount of acid for a living creature to tolerate. Bacteria are also known to decompose urea and proteins to produce large quantities of ammonia. This compound forms ammonium hydroxide in both water and soil and in these areas produces pH values as high as 12.0.

Acidophilic ("acid-loving") microorganisms include ***Thiobacillus thiooxidanas,*** a sulfur oxidizer that will grow at pH 0, although its optimum pH for growth is 2.0 to 3.5. ***T. ferrooxidans,*** an iron oxidizer, has been isolated from acid soils such as peat bogs and from acid mine waters. Some sulfur-containing waters of volcanic habitats are also hot, and as indicated earlier, the bacterium ***Sulfolobus*** sp. has been isolated and shown to be thermophilic as well as acidophilic. Fungi in general prefer a somewhat acid environment of pH 5.0 to 5.5.

Alkaliphilic ("alkaline-loving") microorganisms include ***Bacillus pasteurii,*** which will grow at pH levels of 8.5 and higher; Vibrio cholerae at 9.0; and ***Agrobacterium*** sp. at 12.0.

Osmotic Pressure. As the amount of dissolved materials increases in the immediate environment of living cells, a condition of hypertonicity results and water tends to escape from the cells. This drying out of cells with hypertonic solutions is used in meat and fish preservation, since common spoilage microorganisms cannot tolerate pickling brines of 30 percent sodium chloride. It is also used in the preparation and preservation of fruits by the addition of 40 to 60 percent sugar to make jams, jellies, preserves, and syrups.

Such conditions also occur in nature. The Dead Sea and Great Salt Lake in Utah have salt concentrations of 27 percent. Some areas can be found with concentrations as high as 30 percent salt. Halophilic ("salt-loving") microorganisms such as ***Halobacterum salinarum*** and ***Sarcinia morrhuae*** will grow in 36 percent salt. As a rule, these organisms will not grow in salt concentrations of less than 12 to 15 percent. Although species of ***Spirillum*** and ***Vibrio*** can be found as protoplasts or L-forms in marine environments with less than 12 percent, active growth will only occur when the salt concentration increases, usually by evaporation. Obligate halophilic bacteria require the sodium and magnesium ions in the saline solutions to maintain the integrity of their cell envelope, since their cell walls have little or no rigid layer. They require the high osmotic pressure for the same purpose. One halophile, *Pediococcus halophilus,* has been reported to grow in the range of 0 to 20 percent salt and thus has a different mechanism operating in its halophilic existence.

Saccharophilic ("sugar-loving") microorganisms can be found naturally in honey and other high-sugar-content materials. These microorganisms are primarily fungi. Saccharophilic yeasts include species of *Candida, Hansenula, Pickia, Saccharomyces,* and *Torulopsis.* Species of the molds *Rhizopus* and *Neurospora* may also be saccharophilic.

At the other extreme of osmotic environments we find three strains of *Pseudomonas cepacia* capable of growing in distilled water. Organisms such as this one can achieve a population density of 10^6 to 10^7 with only the trace amounts of volatile organic materials, salts, and metal ions usually present in distilled water. Under these conditions the organism is able to grow within a wider temperature range and exhibits a very small cell size. Certain microorganisms can survive for up to five years in distilled water. Examples of such organisms include bacteria such as *Nocardia* spp., species of yeasts belonging to the genera *Candida, Cryptococcus,* and *Geotrichum* and species of molds, such as *Alternaria* and *Aspergillus.*

Hydrostatic Pressure. Organisms that live at great depths in the ocean are called barophiles (Figure 16–4). For every 10 meters of depth, the hydrostatic pressure increases by 1 atmosphere, that is, 15 pounds per square inch (psi). Microorganisms exist that require pressures of as much as 1000 atmospheres. This level of pressure is obtained at 10,000 meters, or 10 kilometers, a little more than 6 miles deep. A pressure of 15,000 psi can denature proteins in nonbarophilic microorganisms. Research into the growth characteristics and metabolic activities of barophilic microorganisms requires special equipment to maintain the *in situ* pressure while the water samples are brought to the surface and studied.

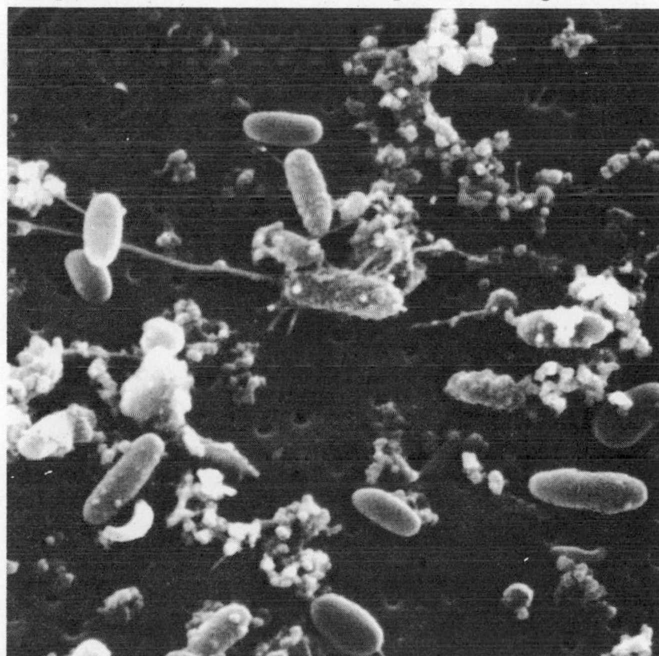

FIG. 16–4 A scanning micrograph of bacteria from material collected on a membrane filter at an ocean depth of 4400 meters and fixed prior to decompression. *Courtesy of Dr. H. W. Jannasch, Woods Hole Oceanographic Institution.*

THE EFFECTS OF POLLUTANTS

If either a biotic or abiotic factor changes abruptly, the balance of the system is jeopardized, and the entire ecosystem may be disrupted. Chemical pollutants pose such dangers. Although some chemicals can be utilized as new nutrients in an ecosystem, others may be toxic to the organisms of a food chain. A particularly striking effect of such toxicity on the protozoan *Tetrahymena pyriformis* is shown in Figure 16–5. Normal cells have the typical pear shape and obvious cilia. Exposure to an environmental chemical pollutant, phenol, sometimes used as a disinfectant, produces the damaging effects shown in Figures 16–5b and c.

The Natural Habitats of Microorganisms

Our planet can be divided into three zones. These are the ***atmosphere,*** the gaseous region surrounding the earth; the ***hydrosphere,*** or aquatic environments such as lakes, rivers, and oceans; and the ***lithosphere,*** the solid portions of the earth consisting of rock and soil.

While the earth provides many suitable habitats for a variety of organisms (Color Photographs 33, 47, and 66), the same type of life is not found everywhere. In fact, every environment, no matter how slightly it differs from others, supports a community of organisms that is somewhat different from that found in similar habitats.

Terrestrial Habitats

The great variety of terrestrial (land) habitats extends from the rocky slopes of mountains to the lush tropical jungles, to the hot desert sands. All terrestrial environments are composed of either rock or rock materials. Disintegrating rock material forms gravel, sand, silt, and clay, in order of decreasing particle size. These particles also form the basis for the loose surface material that covers the earth's crust, the ***soil.*** Particles of soil often bear a film made of moisture, organic materials, and associated microbes. It is estimated that fertile soils commonly contain as many as 100,000 to 500,000 organisms per gram of soil.

Aquatic Habitats

Over 70 percent of the earth's surface is water. The aquatic habitats that this water represents fall into two general categories: ***fresh water*** and ***marine water.*** Freshwater habitats, which make up about 2 percent of the hydrosphere, include ponds, streams, lakes, and rivers. Marine habitats contain salt concentrations of 3.5 percent and higher and include the oceans, seas, and certain inland lakes such as the Great Salt Lake in Utah. ***Estuaries,*** coastal regions where sea water mixes with fresh water, are frequently found associated with marine environments.

Two unique features make water habitats suitable for microorganisms: (1) there is less temperature variation in bodies of water than in terrestrial environments, and (2) sunlight penetrates the water, allowing photosynthetic activities well below the surface. Like terrestrial habitats, aquatic environments are rich in nutrients in the form of waste organic material.

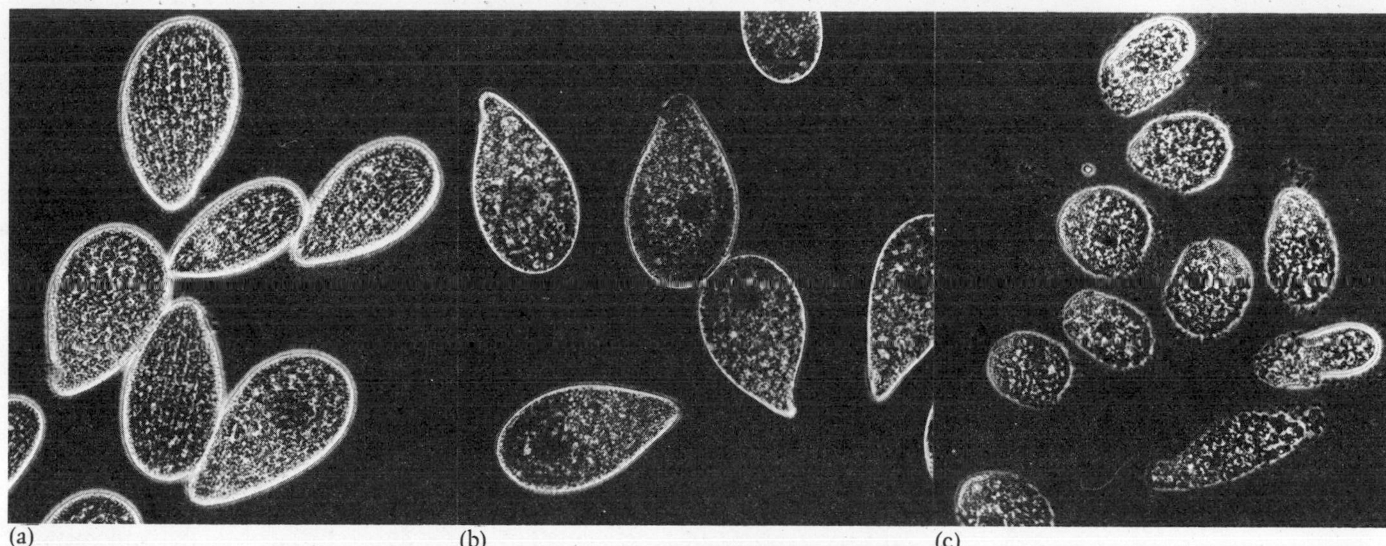

FIG. 16-5 Dangerous environmental pollutants resulting from various industrial processes are being discovered. One of these is phenol. This series of micrographs shows the effect of this organic pollutant on ciliated protozoa, which are important links in the food chain and occur world-wide in a variety of fresh-water habitats. (a) *Tetrahymena pyriformis,* control organisms. (b) After three-minute exposure to phenol (100 mg/liter). (c) After sixty-minute exposure. *Schultz, T. W., and J. N. Dumont,* J. Protozool. 24:*164–172 (1977).*

Microhabitats

The habitats of interest in microbiology are often much smaller than a forest or lake. These small, inhabited regions are called ***microhabitats.*** Every environment consists of many different microhabitats. A decaying piece of wood, the moist undersurface of a fallen leaf, and the carcass of a fish or bird are just a few of the microhabitats to be found in a forest. Just these few examples represent a wide range of conditions in terms of pH, temperature, and gaseous oxygen and moisture content. Each is dynamic in that conditions change constantly due to abiotic factors and the microbial activities of various producers, consumers, and decomposers.

The human body contains a variety of microhabitats. Many microorganisms normally share our bodies and form various ecosystems on the skin and in the upper respiratory tract, mouth, lower gastrointestinal tract, and various body openings. These habitats and niches are discussed in later chapters in terms of potential microbial benefits and hazards.

Microbial Habitats

Microorganisms have been found in nearly all regions of the earth. In many cases the organisms are only transients in the environment, but some are definitely native, or ***indigenous,*** microorganisms. These indigenous microorganisms are able to grow during those climatic periods when environmental conditions are appropriate and to survive during periods when conditions for growth are unsuitable. Survival in some cases is due to the formation of bacterial endospores, cysts and conidia, blue-green bacterial heterocysts and akinetes, and protozoan cysts.

Microbial Interactions

The pioneer American ecologist F. E. Clements has classified the activities in ecosystems as one of three kinds: *action, reaction,* or *coaction.* Action deals with the way abiotic forces affect organisms. Reaction deals with the biological activities in the ecosystem: how organisms react to the environment and perform their functions in shaping the environment. Coaction is concerned with the effect organisms have upon one another. The remainder of this chapter will describe coaction involving microorganisms, plants, and animals. The four kinds of coactional relationships, **syntrophism, competition, predation,** and **symbiosis,** will be presented.

Syntrophism

Organisms exhibiting syntrophism are not intimately associated with one another, but benefit from one another. For example, a major activity found in soil is the decomposition of the polysaccharide cellulose in decaying plant matter. This involves bacteria from the genera *Cytophaga* and *Spirillum* and a number of fungi, all of which produce the cellulose-digesting enzyme cellulase. The digestion produces the disaccharide cellobiose, which is used not only by the microorganisms that help produce it but also by others in the general area. Cellobiose is subsequently degraded to glucose, which is used by many organisms in the immediate environment. Thus several different organisms feed together. Other examples of this basic activity include processes involved with yogurt production, waste digestion in sewage disposal and the actions of different microorganisms in the digestive tracts of various animals.

Competition

Ecologists define competition as the interaction between organisms resulting from a demand for nutrients and energy that exceeds the immediate supply in a habitat. Some organisms compete by secreting toxic substances into the environment. Molds such as *Penicillium* and other antibiotic-producing organisms in the soil may be able to compete by controlling the growth of bacteria sensitive to their secretions. Microorganisms produce various substances that have an inhibitory effect on other organisms (Figure 16–6).

Predation

Predation plays an important role in controlling the populations of higher forms of life, as well as those of microorganisms. The *predator* is the species that ingests other species, the *prey*. The paths of two different forms of life cross and interact to the betterment of one and to the detriment of the other. The predator is usually larger than the prey, but as Figure 16–2 shows, the smaller protozoan, *Didinium*, is able to ingest the larger *Paramecium* with little trouble. Microbial predators may show little or no preference for one prey or another.

Symbiosis

In symbiosis two different forms of life coexist in an intimate ecological relationship. This relationship, which may be of long or short duration, requires close physical contact (Figure 16–6). Symbiotic associations in which one partner is actually inside a cell or tissue of the other partner are called **endosymbiotic;** those in which one member is external to the other are

ectosymbiotic. The participants in these associations are called *endosymbionts* and *ectosymbionts,* respectively.

Symbiosis is classified as of one of three forms, depending on the benefits it provides the symbionts. In **mutualism,** both members benefit from the association; in **commensalism,** only one organism benefits, while the other partner neither benefits nor is harmed; and in **parasitism,** one organism benefits at the expense of the other.

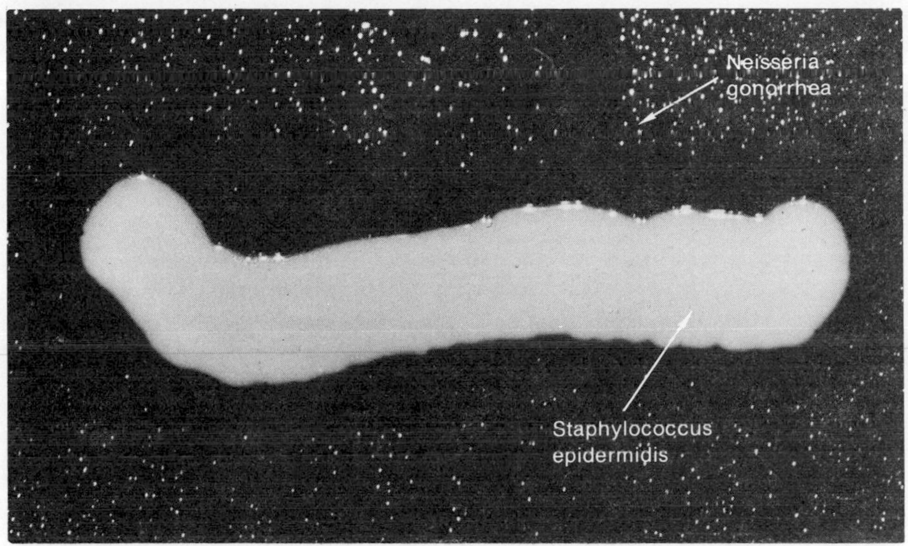

FIG. 16–6 Bacterial interference. Various bacteria produce substances that can inhibit the growth of other bacteria in their vicinity. Here the growth of *Niesseria gonorrheae* is inhibited by another bacterium, *Staphylococcus epidermidis. Reproduced with the permission of the National Research Council of Canada, from Shtibel, R.,* Can. J. Microbiol. 22:*1430–1436 (1976).*

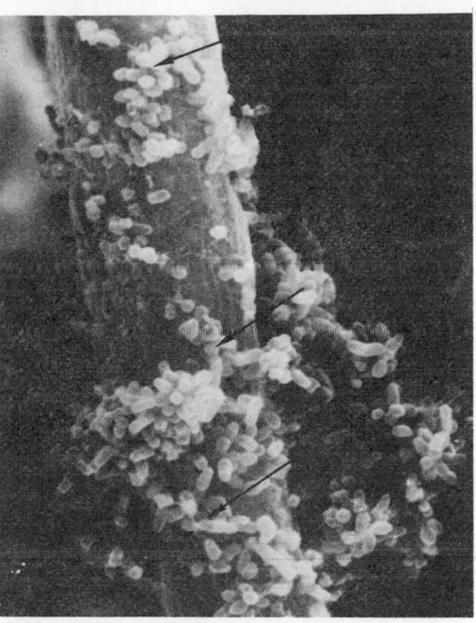

FIG. 16–7 Symbiotic relationships require close contact. In the ectosymbiotic association shown, physical attachment of the bacteria (arrows) to the plant part (P) is essential for the microorganisms to infect and cause developmental changes. *Spiess, L. D., et al.,* Amer. J. Bot. 64:*1200–1208 (1977).*

Mutualism, like the other forms of symbiosis, occurs widely among most of the principal groups of animals, plants, and microorganisms and includes an amazing range of physiological and behavioral adjustments. Mutualism is usually essential to the survival of the organisms involved because of the dependence they have developed for one another. In many situations, one partner cannot survive without the other.

Intermicrobial Mutualism. Among microorganisms, the lichens represent the ultimate mutualistic association. Lichens consist of highly specialized fungi that house green algae or cyanobacteria among their hyphae. The fungus absorbs moisture, minerals, and carbon dioxide from the environment. The algae or cyanobacteria then perform photosynthesis and supply themselves and the partner fungus with organic nutrients and oxygen (Color Photographs 51 and 52).

Microbe-Plant Mutualism. Some of the most advanced and ecologically important examples of mutualism exist among plants. Nitrogen fixation, described more fully in Chapter 17, is conversion of gaseous nitrogen (N_2) into a form that can be used by plants or other soil or water organisms. In nature this is usually accomplished by microorganisms. Nitrogen-fixing bacteria of the genus *Rhizobium* live in specially formed nodules in the roots of legumes such as alfalfa, clover, and soybeans (Figure 16–8). Here, in exchange for the protection and a constant environment provided by the plant, these bacteria provide the legume with substantial amounts of nitrates essential to its growth (Figure 16–9).

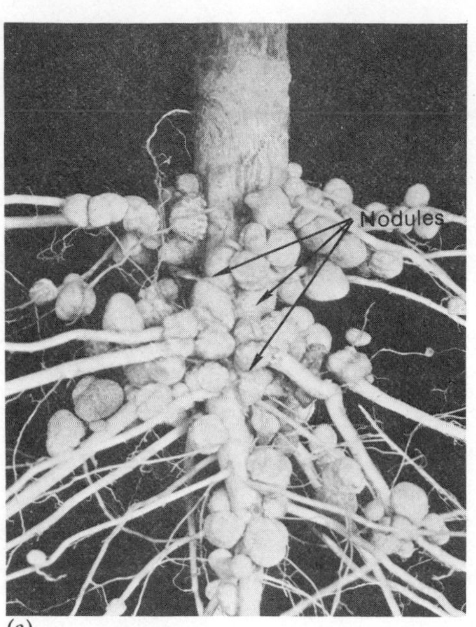

(a)

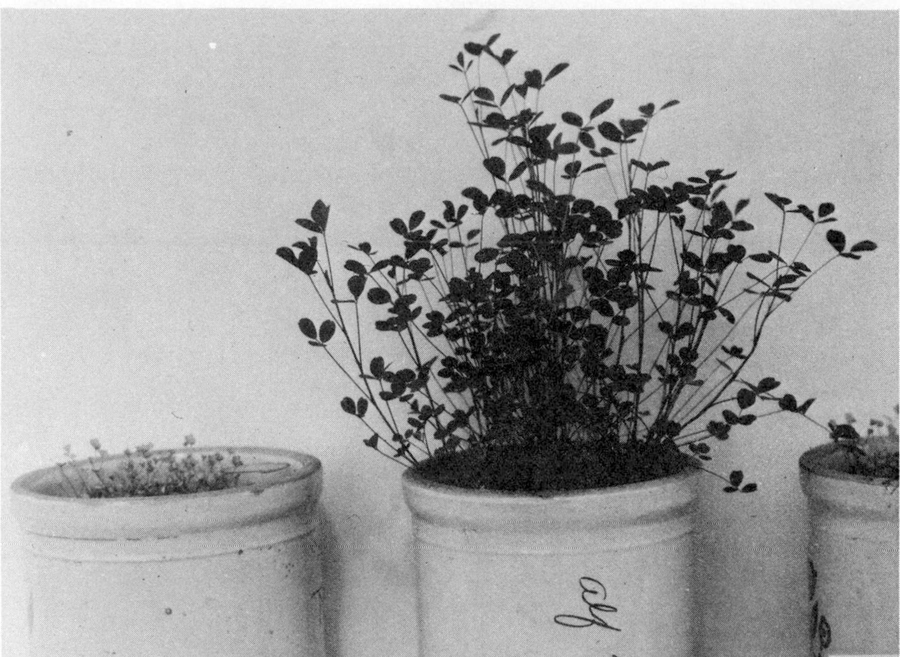

FIG. 16–9 The effects of symbiotic nitrogen fixation. The alfalfa plant on the left does not have nodules and is growing in nitrogen-poor soil. The plant on the right is nodulated and is flourishing despite the nitrogen-poor soil. *Courtesy Nitagin Company.*

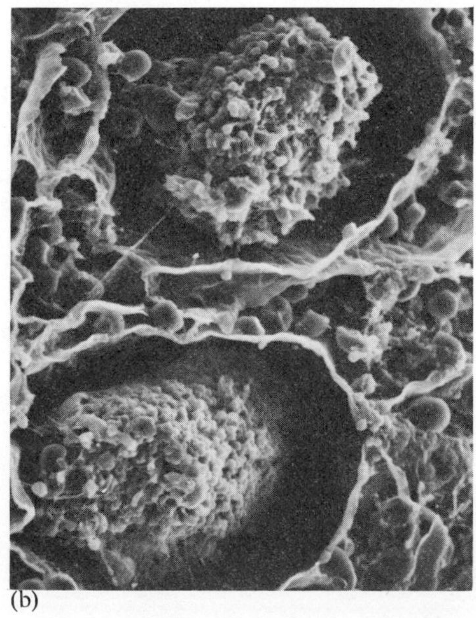
(b)

FIG. 16–8 Nitrogen fixation. (a) Nodules (small tumors) that house nitrogen-fixing bacteria. *Courtesy USDA.* (b) A view through a nodule showing the bacterial endosymbionts within large cells of the nodule. *Kummerow, J., et al.,* Amer. J. Bot. *65:63–69 (1978).*

Microbe-Animal Mutualism. Mutualistic partnerships between microorganisms and animals are quite common. One of the most famous pairs is the termite and its intestinal protozoan populations, discussed in an earlier chapter. Another interesting and unusual example is the fungus-garden-cultivating ant (Figure 16–10). Several ant species have mutually beneficial relationships with fungi that parallel those between humans and crop plants. Depending on the ant species, the fungi are provided with bits of fresh leaves, plant debris (mulch), or ant excrement as nourishment. Workers among the ants tend the fungus beds inside the ant colony and remove certain fungi that the colony does not eat (that is, the weeds). The fungi may be carried to a new ant colony by the young queen, sometimes in a special body pouch and usually as fungus (hyphal) fragments. The participating fungi that have been identified are mostly mushrooms (or related forms) and yeast. The arrangement is clearly beneficial to both parties. The hyphae or spores provide food for the ants, while the fungi receive nutrients and are freed from fungal competitors. The growing fungi also function to keep a constant level of moisture in the colony.

Other insects, such as termites and beetles, are also known to cultivate particular fungi as foods. The insects involved usually construct their nests in decaying plant materials, which are invariably inhabited by fungi. Probably the insects originally fed indiscriminately on fungi, but the nutritional advantages of utilizing certain fungi resulted in the evolution of lines that fed on and maintained only one kind of fungus.

Another interesting mutualistic relationship is the one between species of luminescent bacteria such as *Photobacterium fischeri* (Figure 16–11c) and various ocean fish. Much of the light in ocean depths originates in bacteria specially nurtured in fish structures called light organs. For example, the flashlight fish (Figure 16–11a and b) swims above reefs in the Indian Ocean and Red Sea shining its beam of light much like a car on a dark country road. These luminous organs are used by fish to attract and capture prey, as well as to communicate with other members of its species.

Why this type of mutualistic relationship comes into being is unknown. Some investigators believe that it is a matter of nutrient exchange. The bacteria obtain glucose from the fish; the fish utilize pyruvic acid excreted by the luminous bacteria. What *is* known is that the light organs are surprisingly specific as to what bacteria they will host. The light-producing reaction in these bacteria (Color Photograph 67) is similar to that in fireflies. An enzyme called luciferase combines hydrogen from a component in the electron transport system of the bacteria with oxygen to make water and transform an aldehyde compound into an acid. The energy released by this reaction is given off as light.

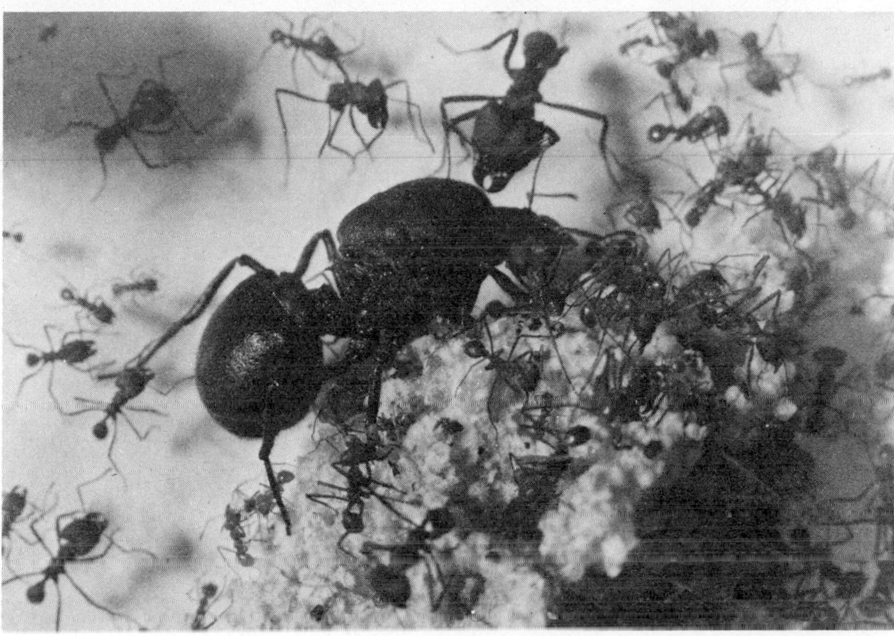

FIG. 16–10 Fungus-gardening cultivating ants. The queen ant of a young *Atta sexdens* colony on her fungus garden. The smaller workers that constitute the queen's brood are also evident. *Weber, N. A.,* Science 153*:587–604 (1966).*

Rumen Symbiosis. Rumen symbiosis is a mutualistic relationship that involves a higher form of animal life. The ruminants are a group of plant-eating mammals including cows, goats, camels, and sheep that have a special structure known as the *rumen* in their digestive tracts (Figure 16–12). Within this structure, microbial digestion of cellulose and other plant polysaccharides takes place. Like other mammals, ruminants are incapable of manufacturing the enzymes necessary to digest cellulose. The rumen, which actually comprises the first two of four stomachs, serves as large incubation chambers in which anaerobic bacteria and protozoa break down cellulose. The types of reactions associated with a typical ruminant are shown in Figure 16–12. The ingested grasses and leafy plant material are mixed with large amounts of saliva and then moved into the rumen. There cellulolytic bacteria such as *Bacteroides, Butyrvibrio fibrisolvens, Clostridium lochheadii,* and *Ruminococcus albus* and ciliated protozoans hydrolyze cellulose to the disaccharide cellobiose and the monosaccharide glucose. Microbial fermentation of these sugars by various bacterial species produces acetic, butyric, and propionic acids, as well as the gases carbon dioxide and methane. The ruminant absorbs and uses these organic acids as its main source of energy.

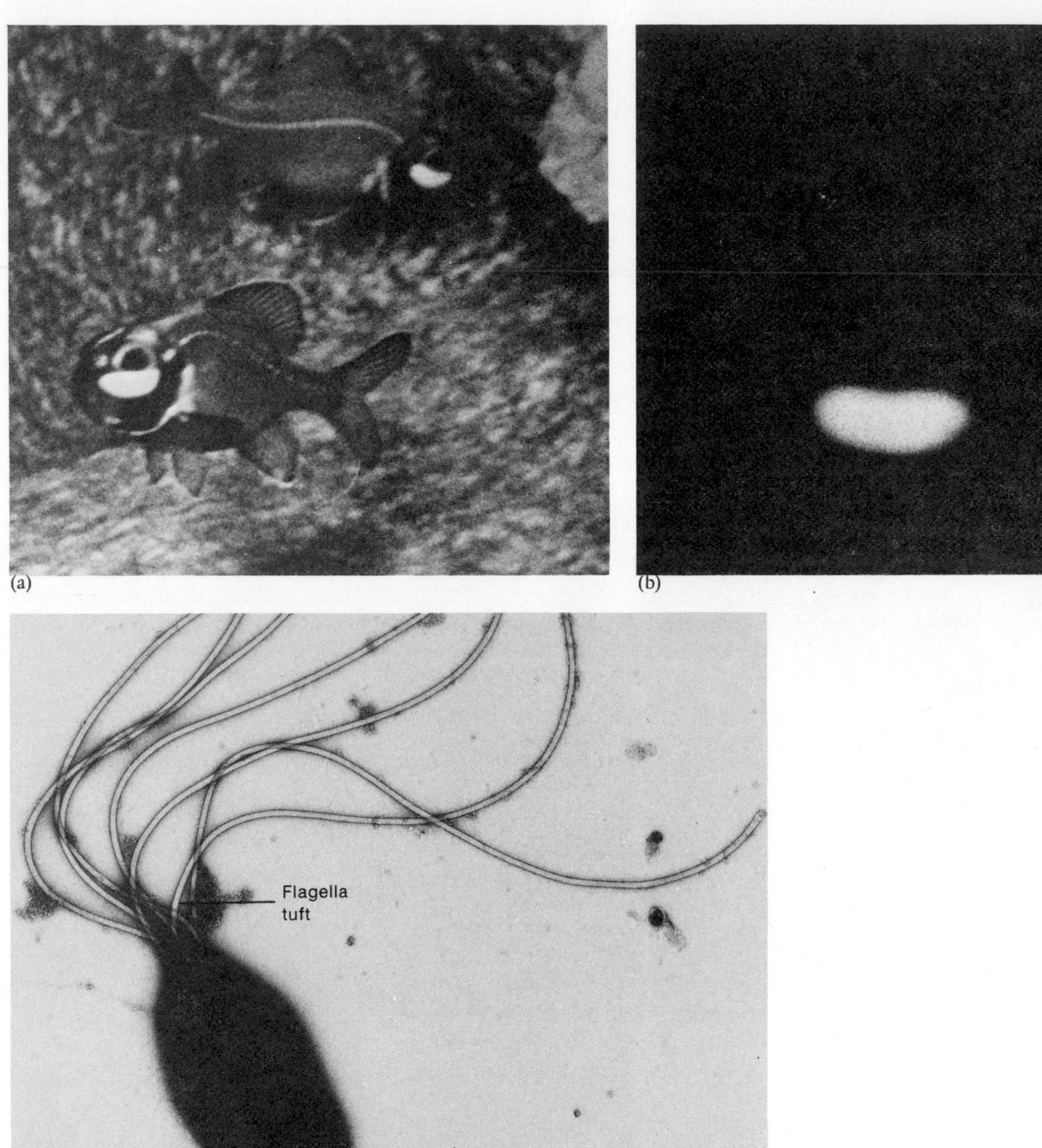

FIG. 16–11 Luminous bacteria and the flashlight fish, an interesting symbiotic association. The flashlight fish, *Photoblepharon palpebratus* has a microbiological light-generating organ that can be used for several functions. It can frighten off a would-be predator or assist the flashlight fish in capturing prey and communicating with members of its own species. (a) The location of the luminous region. (b) The light emitted by the fish's luminous organ at night. *Morin, J. G., et al.,* Science 190:74–76 *(1975)*. (c) *Photobacterium fischeri*, one of several species known to colonize the luminous organs of fish and other aquatic life. Note the tuft of flagella. (Refer to Color Photograph 67 for a demonstration of the light emitted by these bacteria in culture.) *Reichelt, J. L., and P. Bauman,* Arch. Microbiol. 94:*283 (1973)*.

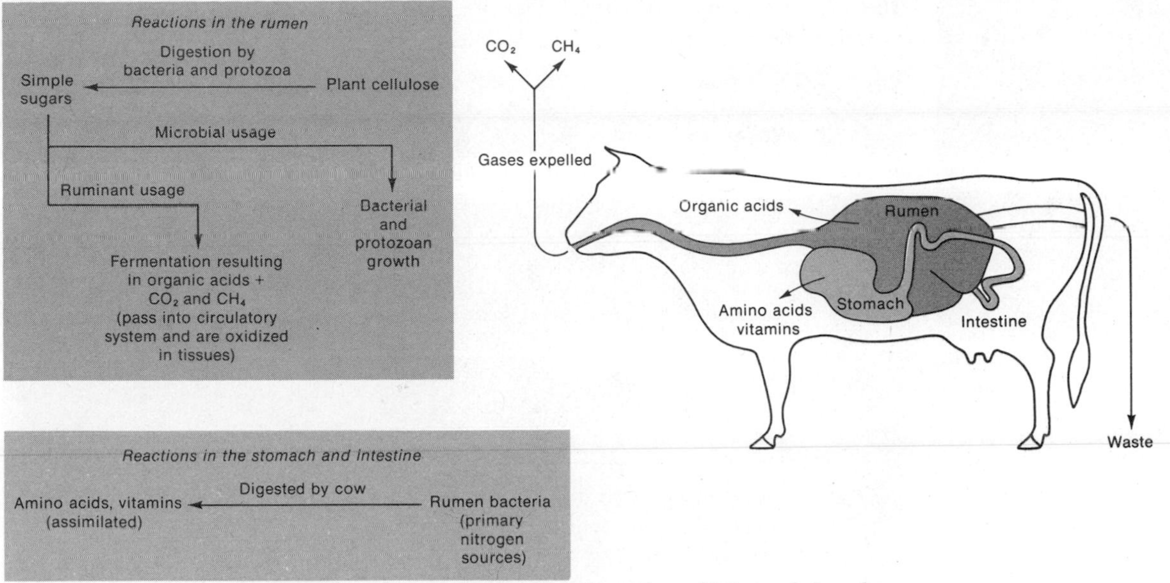

FIG. 16-12 Ruminants, like other mammals, cannot digest the cellulose of the plants they ingest because of their inability to make cellulases. With the mutalistic relationship they have with microorganisms, ruminants, such as cows, can eat and make use of cellulose, their major source of carbon. The digestive tract of a typical ruminant and the microbial reactions and processes that occur in specific locations are shown in this diagram.

The microorganisms in the rumen also provide other specific functions, such as the synthesis of amino acids and vitamins. Some microorganisms leave the rumen and are digested in other parts of the gastrointestinal system to serve as a major supply of proteins and vitamins for the ruminant. This is particuarly important for the nutrition of ruminants because grasses are deficient in protein.

The biochemical reactions occurring among the participants in the rumen are complex and involve vast numbers and varieties of microorganisms. While we have emphasized the bacteria, the protozoans in the rumen are also important. They, too, serve as sources of protein and appear to control the bacterial populations within the system.

COMMENSALISM

The literal meaning of ***commensalism*** is "eating at the same table." Commensalism is an association between two organisms in which one partner is benefited and the other is neither benefited nor harmed. Many intestinal bacteria such as *Escherichia coli* are normally commensals, as are many intestinal protozoa such as *Entamoeba coli* and trichomonads. It is not always easy to distinguish between a commensal organism and a parasite. This is because many commensals living harmlessly on or in body surfaces also have a capacity for disease production.

PARASITISM

Parasitism is an association between two specifically distinct organisms in which one, the **parasite,** lives on or within the other in order to obtain essential nutrients. The organism that harbors a parasite is called the **host.**

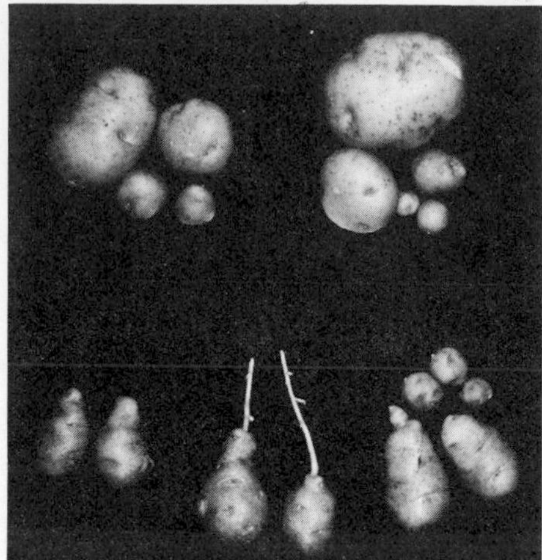

FIG. 16-13 Potato spindle tuber disease, one effect of viroid infection. Healthy potatoes are shown at the top, and diseased specimens at the bottom. *Semancik, J. S., et al.,* Virology 52:*292-294 (1973).*

One of the more familiar parasites is the tapeworm, but parasitism is not limited to multicellular animals. Parasites may also be plants, such as mistletoe and dodder, or microorganisms (Color Photograph 68). All disease-producing agents can be considered parasites. This category includes viroids (Figure 16-13), viruses, bacteria, fungi (Figure 16-14), and protozoa. Later chapters will describe their effects.

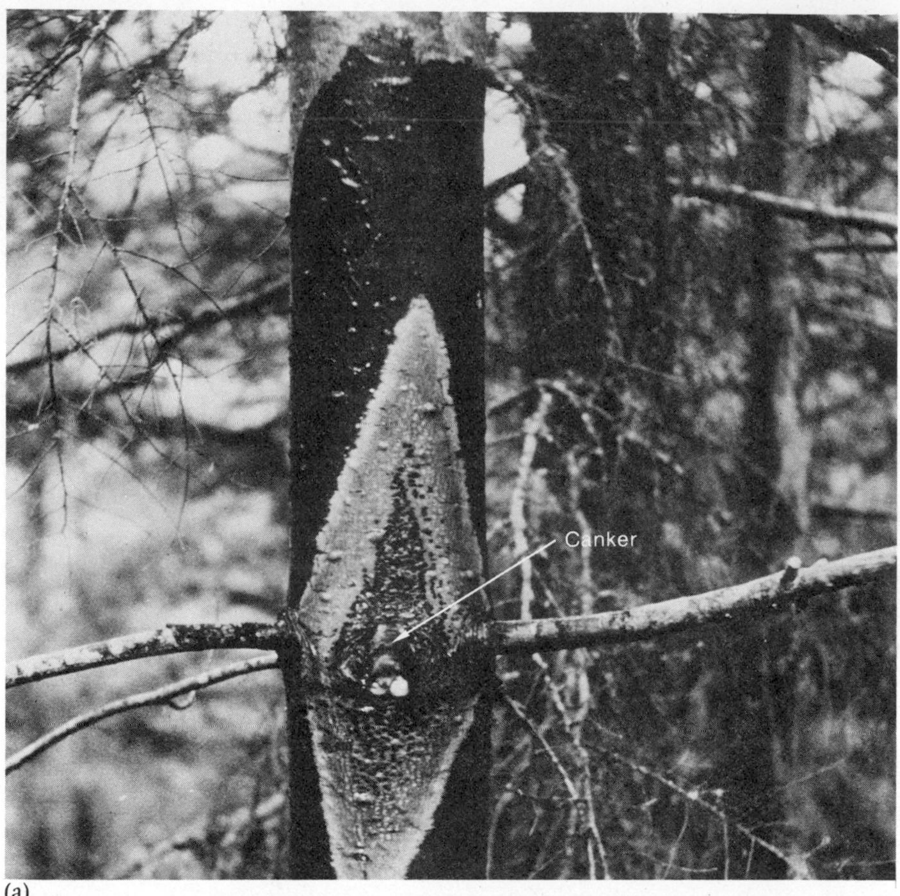

(a)

FIG. 16-14 Parasitism in plants. (a) A fungus-caused canker on the bark of a pine tree. (b) Plant (parenchyma) cells, showing the presence of the fungal components (arrows) that cause the canker. *Welch, B. L., and N. E. Martin,* Phytopathology 64:*1541 (1974).*

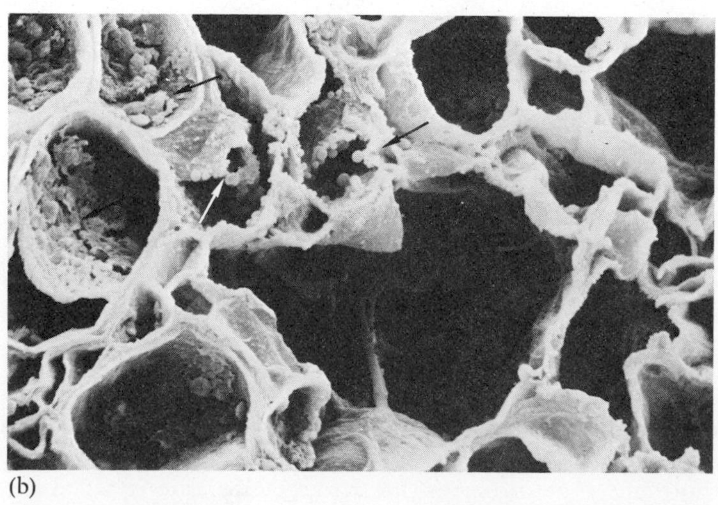

(b)

SUMMARY

The influence of the environment on all forms of life and the various relationships among organisms is critical to their survival.

Basic Ecological Principles

1. The *biosphere* includes the general environment of all living things. It extends up into the atmosphere to more than 10,000 meters, down into the ocean to about 8000 meters, and more than 250 meters below land surfaces.
2. The biosphere is a global biological system based on a continuous, or cyclic, flow of energy and nutrients.

The Organization of the Biosphere

1. *Ecosystems* are ecological units of the biosphere.
2. Groups of individuals having similar properties and living in the same area are called *populations.*
3. The different forms of life of an ecosystem fall into three categories: *producers, consumers,* and *decomposers.* These organisms are responsible for maintaining the stability of the system.
4. Producers, which include photosynthesizing algae, bacteria, and plants, form organic compounds from inorganic materials.
5. Consumers utilize these organic compounds for their essential activities.
6. Decomposers break down complex decaying organic matter, which can then be used by plants and other organisms for their producer activities.
7. Producers, consumers, and decomposers together constitute circular processes that promote the exchange of nutrients and energy flow in the ecosystem.

The Components of an Ecosystem

1. The specific location or place of residence of an organism is called its *habitat;* its specific role in a community is its *niche.*
2. Habitats for any living organism are limited by both *biotic* (living) and *abiotic* (nonliving) factors.
3. Biotic factors include other animals, plants, and microbes, while examples of abiotic components are hydrostatic pressure, light, moisture, minerals, osmotic pressure, pH, temperature, and chemical pollutants. The balance of an ecosystem can be disrupted by disturbing a factor of either type.

The Natural Habitats of Microorganisms

1. The earth can be divided into three zones: the *atmosphere* (gaseous regions), the *hydrosphere* (aquatic environments), and the *lithosphere* (solid portions).
2. Most habitats are *terrestrial* (land settings) and *aquatic* environments.
3. *Terrestrial habitats* include the rocky slopes of mountains, the lush tropical jungle, and the hot desert sands.
4. *Aquatic* environments fall into two general categories: fresh water and marine water.
5. *Estuaries* are coastal regions where sea water mixes with fresh water.

Microbial Interactions

1. The activities in ecosystems can be one of three types: *action, reaction,* or *coaction.*
2. Action deals with how abiotic factors affect organisms.
3. Reaction is concerned with the biological activities in an ecosystem.
4. Coaction deals with the interactions among organisms.
5. Four types of coactional relationships are recognized: *syntrophism, competition, predation,* and *symbiosis.*

Syntrophism

1. While organisms are not intimately associated with one another in syntrophism they benefit from one another's activities.
2. Examples of syntrophism include the feeding of organisms in soil where the digestion of decaying plant material occurs; yogurt production; and waste digestion in sewage disposal.

Competition

1. Competition is the interaction between organisms resulting from a demand for nutrients and energy that exceeds the immediate supply.
2. Some microbes compete by secreting toxic substances.

Predation

Predation plays an important role by controlling various populations of life. The *predator* ingests other species, called the *prey.*

Symbiosis

1. In symbiosis two different forms of life coexist in an intimate ecological relationship. This type of relationship requires close physical contact.
2. *Endosymbiotic* relationships refer to situations in which one partner is actually inside a cell or tissue of the other partner; in *ectosymbiotic* relationships, one member is external to the other.
3. Symbiosis can take one of three basic forms: in *mutualism* both members benefit from the association; in *commensalism,* only one organism benefits from the association, while the other partner neither benefits nor is harmed; in *parasitism,* one organism benefits at the expense of the other.
4. Mutualism can be found between microorganisms (lichens), between microorganisms and plants (nitrogen-fixing legumes), and between microorganisms and animals (termites, fungus-cultivating ants, fish with luminous organs, and ruminants).
5. An example of commensalism is the relationship between higher forms of animal life and their intestinal microorganisms.
6. In parasitism, the organism living on or within the other partner is called the *parasite,* while the supplier of nutrients is the *host.* Parasites can be animal, plant, or any disease-producing microorganism.

QUESTIONS FOR REVIEW

1. a. What is the biosphere?
   b. How is it organized?
   c. What is the difference between a population and a community?
2. Describe the functions and importance of producers, consumers, and decomposers in an ecosystem.
3. a. Distinguish between abiotic and biotic factors in the biosphere.
   b. How do these factors affect one another?
4. a. What is an ecosystem?
   b. Give two examples.
5. Distinguish between a habitat and a niche.
6. Give the major features of terrestrial and aquatic habitats.
7. In what types of habitats are microorganisms found?
8. Define each of the following relationships and give at least one example of each type of association involving microorganisms:
   a. syntrophism
   b. predation
   c. mutualism
   d. commensalism
   e. competition
   f. parasitism
9. What is a barophile?
10. Of what value is nitrogen fixation?
11. Define or explain each of the following terms:
    a. lichen
    b. autotroph
    c. ectosymbiont
    d. host
    e. prey
    f. rumen
    g. nodule
    h. viroid

SUGGESTED READINGS

Brill, W. J. "Biological Nitrogen Fixation." *Sci. Amer.* 236:68–81 (1977). *Describes the relationships between plants and bacteria. Bacteria free in nature and how these organisms form ammonia from atmospheric nitrogen are also discussed.*

Cooke, R. *The Biology of Symbiotic Fungi.* New York: John Wiley & Sons, 1977. *Attempts to outline all major symbiotic relationships that exist between fungi and either animals or plants, describing how these various associations function.*

Frederickson, A. G. "Behavior of Mixed Cultures of Microorganisms." *Ann. Rev. Microbiol.* 31:63 (1977). *This review describes the behavior of mixed populations of microorganisms in which the organisms are known and the composition of the medium is also known.*

Hale, M. E., Jr. *The Biology of Lichens.* 2nd ed. London: Arnold: 1974. *A modern treatment of all aspects of lichens.*

Hungate, R. E. "The Rumen Microbial Ecosystem." *Ann. Rev. Ecology and Systematics* 1:639 (1975). *Describes the bacteria and protozoa associated with the rumen.*

Jannasch, H. W., and C. O. Wirsen. "Microbial Life in the Deep Sea." *Sci. Amer.* 236:42 (1977). *Includes a discussion of how the microbes in the sea are affected by the high pressures and low temperatures of the deep-sea environment.*

Luria, S. E.; J. E. Darnell, Jr.; D. Baltimore; and A. Campbell. *General Virology.* 3rd ed. New York: John Wiley & Sons, 1978. *A good, general textbook on virology, including topics such as the structure of virions, virus-host interactions, bacteriophages, molecular biology of viruses, and animal viruses.*

The Environmental Activities of Microorganisms

CHAPTER **17**

Chapter 17 discusses ways that microorganisms react to the environment. These reactions produce many important materials, including carbon, nitrogen, sulfur, and oxygen compounds, available for use and reuse by all life forms on this planet. On the other hand, microorganisms may harm the environment by the bioconcentration of certain toxic wastes, such as pesticides and radioisotopes.

After reading this chapter, you should be able to:

1. **Define and discuss reaction as an ecological concept in microbiology.**
2. **Describe the carbon, nitrogen, sulfur, and oxygen cycles in terms of their significance in ecology.**
3. **Interrelate the carbon, nitrogen, and sulfur cycles with the oxygen cycle to show that these cycles are not independent events.**
4. **Explain the phrase "microbial infallibility."**
5. **Discuss the role of bioconversion in nature in association with methanogenesis, petroleum degradation, pesticides, and mercury.**
6. **Discuss the role of bioconcentration in nature as it relates to manganese deposits and the toxic accumulations of pesticides and radioisotopes.**
7. **Define or explain:**

a.	**biogeochemistry**	**e.**	**nitrogen fixation**
b.	**photosynthesis**	**f.**	**nitrification**
c.	**chemosynthesis**	**g.**	**denitrification**
d.	**respiration**	**h.**	**oxidase**

The various types of microbial, animal, and plant life on this planet have used and reused inorganic materials since life began. For an estimated 3.5 billion years, water, carbon, oxygen, nitrogen, phosphorus, sulfur, iron, manganese, and many more materials have been cycled through the biosphere. Oxidized and reduced inorganic and organic forms are used repeatedly to make energy and cell substance. Some metabolic reactions cause insoluble, stored compounds to go into solution and become available. The reverse process stores excess materials to prevent their loss from the immediate environment. The participation of organisms in this recycling is one aspect of ***reaction***, the response of organisms to abiotic factors and their function in shaping nature. The reactions that cycle critical materials are often called collectively ***biogeochemistry***. This term simply refers to the important role of life ***(bio)*** in the chemistry of the earth ***(geo)***. In this chapter we shall discuss the role of microorganisms in biogeochemistry and in ***bioconversion*** and ***bioconcentration***.

The Life-supporting Biogeochemical Cycles

The earth's colorful and diverse appearance is mainly the result of microbial, plant, and animal activities, which endlessly change inanimate rocks and gases into an immense variety of organic substances.

The various elements that are vital to the structures and activities of living systems, including carbon, hydrogen, nitrogen, oxygen, phosphorus, and sulfur, are drawn from the environment, incorporated into the cells, and eventually returned to the environment to be used over again. The earth does not receive any substantial quantities of matter from other portions of the universe, nor does it lose any matter to outer space. Interrelated series of natural biogeochemical cycles ensure the flow of essential elements between the living and nonliving parts of ecosystems. In these cyclic transformations of chemicals from one form to another, microbes such as bacteria, fungi, and protozoa are intricately associated with animals and plants (Figures 17–1 through 17–7). It is important to emphasize here that no one cycle can function in the absence of the others. Moreover, all cycles are working at the same time.

The Carbon Cycle

Carbon is one of the most common and important of the elements involved with living systems. It circulates among a large number of biosphere components by means of the **carbon cycle** (Figure 17–1). This cycle is of particular importance because it is the route by which useful energy from the sun is stored in the biosphere. Through photosynthesis, carbon dioxide is first absorbed by many different plant and microbial producers to form cellular substances; later it is released to the atmosphere by consumers. Most photosynthetic organisms use the energy from the sun to generate oxygen, energy-rich organic molecules, and some heat. The consumers, which are mainly animals, utilize the organic molecules and, by respiration, generate heat and return some of the carbon dioxide to the air or water. A small amount of carbon dioxide dissolves in water where it can be trapped into ice caps and groundwater or may form bicarbonate ions. Bicarbonate ions react with calcium ions to form limestone (calcium carbonate). The carbon in this substance may not be returned to the atmosphere for millions of years. Carbonates formed by living organisms as shells or other protective structures of animals and protozoans can also accumulate on lake and sea bottoms and eventually form limestone.

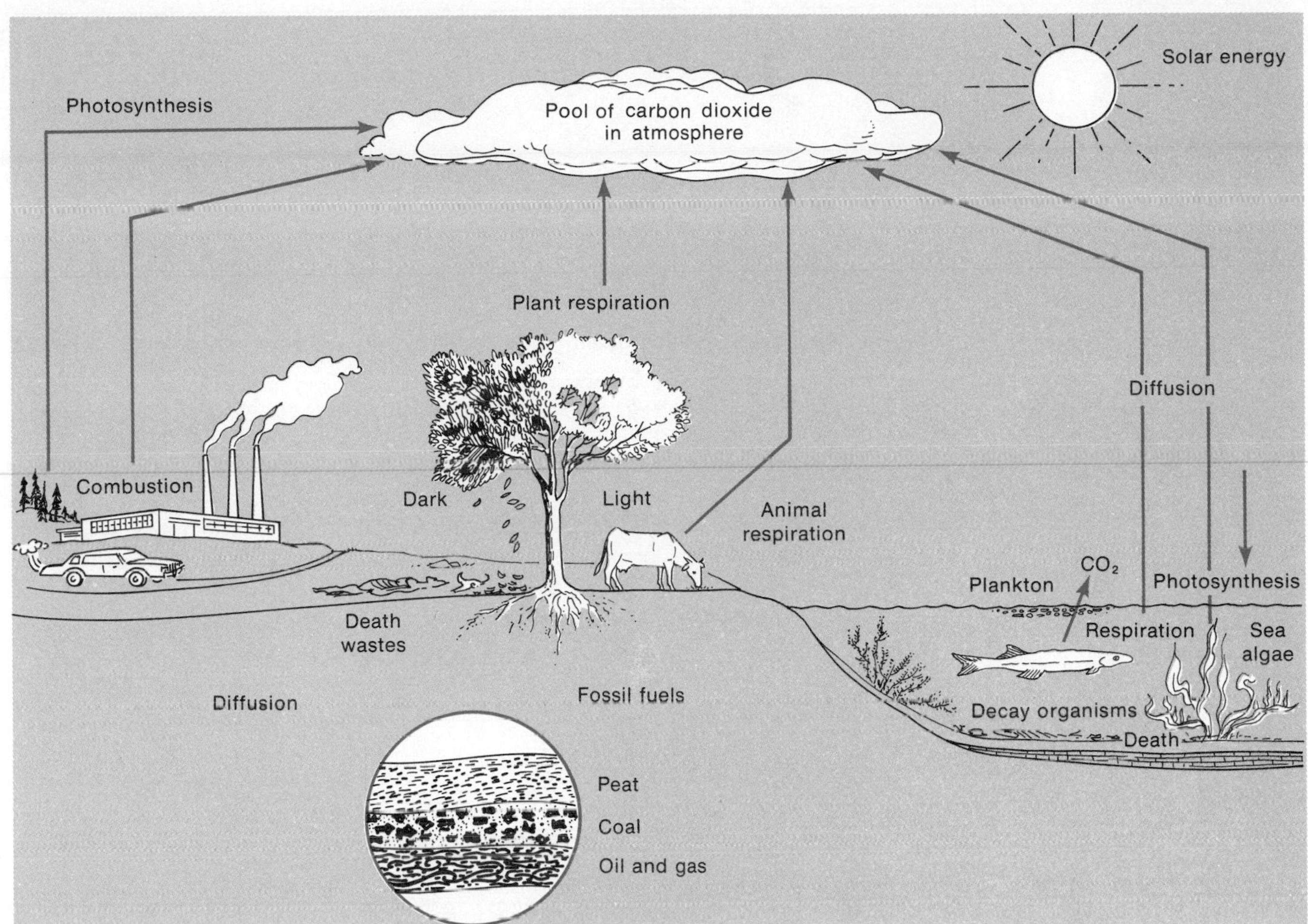

FIG. 17-1 The biogeochemical cycle of carbon involves a chemical element needed by all forms of life to synthesize a full range of organic compounds and cellular components. Energy from the sun is used by higher plant life, algae, and various microorganisms to convert carbon dioxide and water into organic compounds. Eventually these compounds are decomposed to again form carbon dioxide and release it into the atmosphere. A variety of microorganisms are involved in this decomposition phase of the cycle.

When burned, wood and fossil fuels yield large quantities of carbon dioxide to the atmosphere. Under conditions of limited oxygen, incomplete combustion occurs, resulting in carbon monoxide (CO). Interestingly, certain bacteria metabolize this toxic gas, converting it to carbon dioxide and energy.

Under anaerobic conditions, carbon dioxide is reduced to methane (CH_4) by many microorganisms. This metabolic activity is discussed later in this chapter because of its significance as a means of producing fuel. Other anaerobic organisms such as *Methylococcus* spp. are able to oxidize methane as a source of energy and produce carbon dioxide.

Ultimately, various decomposer microorganisms, mainly bacteria, oxidize animal and plant remains with the production of additional heat and the return of carbon dioxide to the environment. The bulk of plant materials is made up of cellulose and lignin, the structural polymers of vascular plants. They usually decompose slowly. Some cellulose decomposition occurs in digestion by ruminants. Lignin digestion is performed by the bacterial thermophile *Thermonospora fusca* and the fungi *Polysporus versicolor, Phanerochaete chrysosporium,* and *Coriolis versicolor.* These organisms apparently require cellulose as an energy source in order to digest lignin. Under certain conditions, such as those that exist in acid soils and bogs, lignin and cellulosic wastes do not degrade and may be converted to peat. This type of process appears to be the origin of most, if not all, of our fossil fuels.

The Nitrogen Cycle

Organisms need nitrogen to synthesize essential compounds such as amino acids, proteins, and nucleic acids. Although 79 percent of the atmosphere is nitrogen gas (N_2), this elemental form of nitrogen is useless to most organisms. Producer organisms such as plants must obtain their nitrogen from the soil in the form of inorganic nitrogen compounds, the *nitrates.* Animals secure their nitrogen from the compounds produced by plants. By means of the **nitrogen cycle** (Figure 17–2), the essential compounds are converted from one type to another by various organisms, often with the release of energy that is captured during metabolic activity. The cycle consists of three phases: *nitrogen fixation, nitrogen assimilation,* and *nitrogen recovery.*

NITROGEN FIXATION

Nitrogen fixation is the reduction of atmospheric molecular nitrogen to ammonia (NH_3) and other biologically essential nitrogen-containing compounds. Under natural conditions, nitrogen fixation can occur in two ways: (1) by inorganic chemical processes in the atmosphere, such as photochemical and electrical (lightning) reactions, and (2) by biological processes involving fungi, cyanobacteria, and various other bacterial species.

Certain microorganisms can reduce nitrogen symbiotically or nonsymbiotically and produce intracellular ammonia. Nitrogen fixation reaction requires a bacterial enzyme, nitrogenase, and adenosine triphosphate (ATP). The active component of the enzyme is formed from two protein molecules and iron and molybdenum. The nitrogenase binds the nitrogen (N_2) and reacts with a special electron carrier protein, oxidizing the carrier and picking up 6 hydrogen ions (H^+) to form two molecules of ammonia. The overall process can be pictured as follows:

$$\underset{\text{atmospheric nitrogen}}{N_2} + \underset{\text{hydrogen}}{6\,H^+} + \underset{\text{electrons}}{6\,e^-} + \underset{\text{adenosine triphosphate}}{12\,ATP} \xrightarrow{\text{nitrogenase}} \underset{\text{ammonia}}{2\,NH_3} + \underset{\text{adenosine diphosphate}}{12\,ADP} + \underset{\text{inorganic phosphate}}{12\,P\,(i)}$$

The combined nitrogen compound (NH_3) is incorporated by the producer of the system in amino acids and proteins. These nitrogen-containing compounds circulate from the primary fixers through consumer organisms. When consumers eat plants, the plant proteins are converted to animal proteins. Ultimately, such proteins or related compounds become available to decomposers and are converted into progressively simpler compounds.

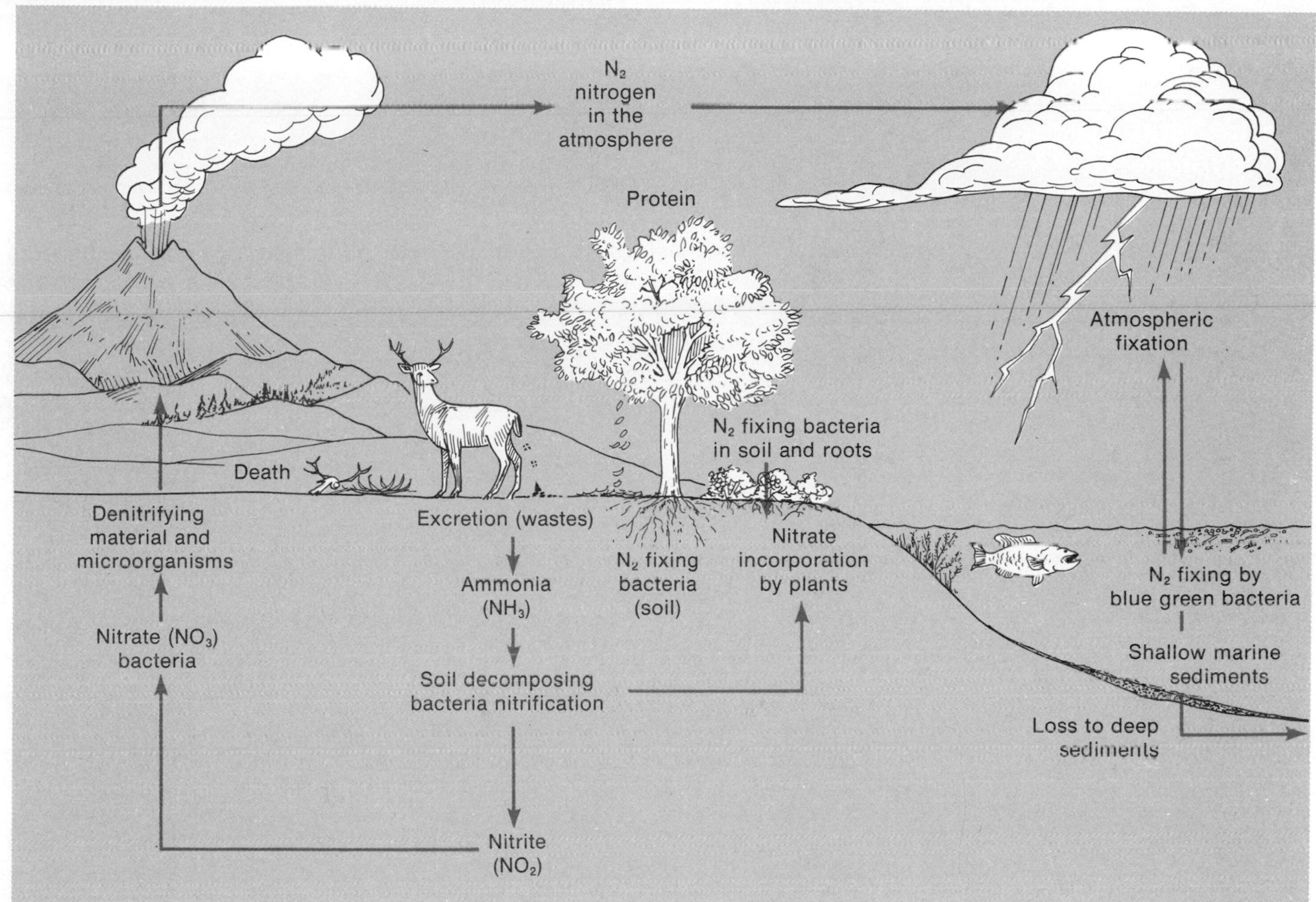

FIG. 17–2 The nitrogen cycle. One of the most important microbial processes in the nitrogen cycle is nitrogen fixation, the conversion of nitrogen gas, N_2, into nitrogen compounds. As this diagram shows, the process is carried out by microorganisms. Higher plants are dependent on microorganisms and this process for their nitrogen requirements. By far the most important nitrogen-fixing organisms in soils are those that are symbiotic.

Nitrogen-fixing organisms can usually be grouped in three categories: (1) free-living bacteria; (2) cyanobacteria; and (3) leguminous plants and their symbiotic bacteria. However, nitrogen fixation also occurs with some non-leguminous root-nodule plants, plants with leaf nodules, and lichens.

Nonsymbiotic nitrogen fixation. Many free-living cyanobacteria and other bacteria that exist both in soil and water habitats are known for their nonsymbiotic nitrogen fixation. These microorganisms can be found in environments as extreme as the soil and rocks of Antarctica and the Hot Springs of Yellowstone National Park. Representatives of this group are listed in Table 17–1.

TABLE 17-1 Genera of Nonsymbiotic, or Free-living, Microorganisms Capable of Nitrogen Fixation

Free-living Bacteria	*Cyanobacteria*	*Yeast*
Azotobacter	*Anabaena*	*Pullularia*
Azotomonas	*Aphanizomenon*	*Rhodotorula*
Bacillus	*Chlorogloea*	
Clostridium	*Nostoc*	
Desulfovibrio	*Stigonema*	
Klebsiella	*Trichodesmium*	
Nocardia		
Pseudomonas		
Rhodospirillum		

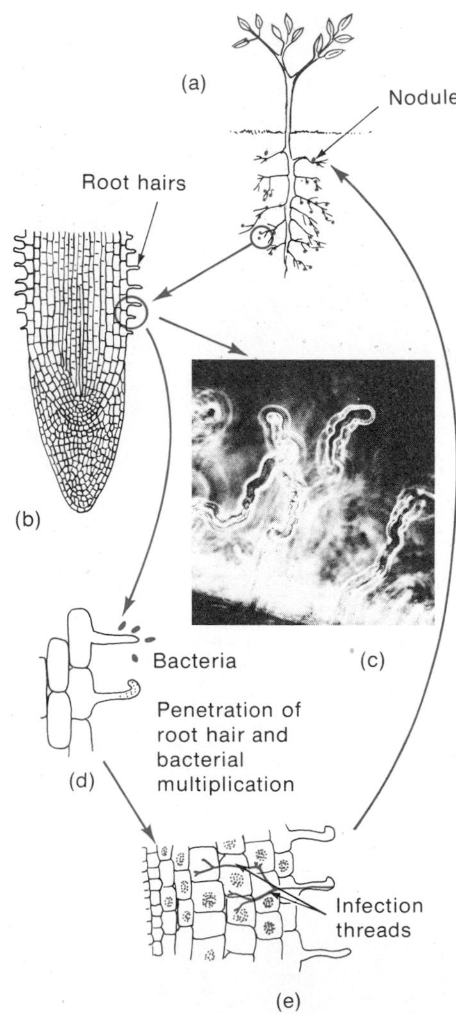

FIG. 17-3 Formation of a root nodule in a legume infected by species of *Rhizobium*. (a) The appearance and location of root nodules. (b) Root hairs, extensions of specialized surface root cells. (c) Close-up of root hairs on a clover plant. (d) Penetration and multiplication of bacteria. (e) Infection thread formation and the spreading of infection thread to nearby cells leading to nodule formation. *Dazzo, F. B., and D. H. Hubbell,* Appl. Microbiol. *30:1017–1033 (1975).*

Symbiotic nitrogen fixation. Most of what is known today about nitrogen fixation has been learned from studies of the mutualistic relationship between certain bacteria and leguminous plants that are members of the pea family. The bacteria in this association are all species of the genus *Rhizobium* and are specific to each host plant in which they occur (Table 17-2). These nitrogen-fixing microorganisms normally live in the soil, where they have the opportunity to invade and infect the roots of the legumes (Figure 17-3). After the invading organisms establish themselves through a series of complex interactions with the plant host, additional plant cells in the interior of the root become infected and eventually enlarge to form localized swellings, or nodules. Free nitrogen picked up by these nodule systems from the soil is converted into ammonia. Although various other nitrogen-fixing systems exist (Figure 17-2), the microbe-legume association is extremely efficient in trapping nitrogen and is thought to be the most important source of nitrogen fixation.

TABLE 17-2 Selected Symbiotic Nitrogen-fixing Systems

Mutualistic Microorganisms	*Host Plant or Animal*
Anabaena azollae[a]	Water fern *(Azolla)*
Frankia alni	Alder tree
Frankia ceanothi	Chaparral shrub *(Ceanothus)*
Klebsiella sp.	Termite
Nostoc Muscorum[a]	Tropical herb *(Gunnera)*
Rhizobium japonicum	Soybean
Rhizobium meliloti	Alfalfa
Rhizobium trifolii	Clover
Spirillum lipoferum	Tropical grass *(Digitaria)*

[a]cyanobacterium

NITROGEN ASSIMILATION AND RECOVERY

The proteins produced by plants are consumed and eventually returned to the environment, mainly in excretions. Through the enzymatic activities of the microorganisms associated with decay, the organic nitrogen molecules in such excretions and in decaying matter are broken down to ammonia (Table 17-3). Ammonia or ammonium ion (NH_4^+) formation is known as ***ammonification.*** Most of the ammonia produced through decay is converted into nitrates (NO_3^-) in two steps. Chemosynthetic bacteria belonging to the genus *Nitrosomonas* oxidize NH_3 to nitrites (NO_2^-). Nitrites, in turn, are oxidized to

TABLE 17-3 Selected Nitrifying and Denitryfying Microorganisms

Nitrification Step 1: $NH_3 \rightarrow NO_2$ *Bacteria*	Step 2: $NO_2 \rightarrow NO_3$ *Bacteria*	*Denitrification* $NO_3 \rightarrow NO_2 \rightarrow NH_3 \rightarrow N_2$ *Bacteria*
Halobacterium	*Nitrobacter*	*Alcaligenes*
Nitrococcus	*Nitrococcus*	*Bacillus*
Nitrosococcus	*Nitrospina*	*Corynebacterium*
Nitrosolobus		*Flavobacterium*
Nitrosomonas	Molds	*Halobacterium*
Nitrosospira	*Aspergillus*	*Pseudomonas*
Nocardia	*Cephalosporium*	
Streptomyces	*Penicillium*	
Molds		
Aspergillus		
Cephalorium		
Penicillium		

nitrates (NO_3^-) by bacteria of the genus *Nitrobacter.* The end products of these reactions are not only made readily available to plants through their roots, but are also used by other members of the microbial community (Table 17-4). Some bacteria, such as *Pseudomonas,* and a few fungi use nitrate as an oxygen source in poorly aerated soil. This results in the loss of nitrate from the biological cycle as gaseous N_2.

TABLE 17-4 Microorganisms That Can Assimilate Nitrate

Bacteria	*Molds*	*Yeasts*
Aeromonas	*Alternaria*	*Candida*
Bacillus	*Aspergillus*	*Hansenula*
Clostridium	*Fusarium*	*Rhodotorula*
Nocardia	*Penicillium*	*Trichospora*

Denitrification completes the nitrogen cycle. By means of certain reactions, nitrates are converted to nitrogen gas, which reenters the atmosphere or water. Once again, microorganisms in terrestrial and aquatic environments are the agents involved (Table 17-3). The major steps in the nitrogen cycle are shown in Figure 17-4.

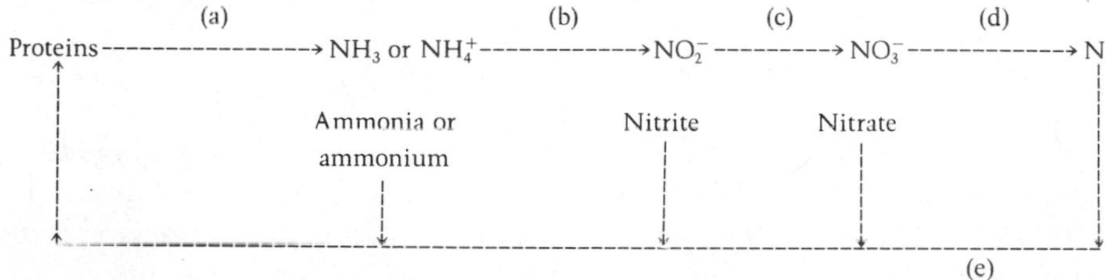

FIG. 17-4 The major steps in the nitrogen cycle. (a) Ammonification. (b, c) The two steps of nitrification. (d) Denitrification. (e) Nitrogen fixation.

The Phosphorus Cycle

Phosphorus is essential for the growth and development of all forms of life. Without phosphorus there could be no organic phosphorus-containing compounds such as adenosine triphosphate (ATP), deoxyribonucleic acid (DNA), and ribonucleic acid (RNA).

See Chapter 5 for descriptions of these compounds.

Producer organisms acquire phosphorus in the form of inorganic phosphate (PO_4^{3-}) and convert it into organic phosphates important in the metabolism of carbohydrates, fats, and nucleic acids. Lower animals obtain their phosphorus as inorganic phosphate in water or as inorganic and organic phosphate compounds in the food they consume.

The **phosphorus cycle** (Figure 17–5) is not as completely balanced as the others described. As water runs over rocks, gradually wearing away their surfaces, various minerals, including phosphates, are carried as sediments to the bottom of the sea faster than they can be returned to land. Sea birds have an important role in this process, since they return phosphorus to the cycle in the form of phosphate-rich droppings. Fish also recover phosphates from the sea and thereby serve as a source of the mineral.

Under natural conditions, much less phosphorus than nitrogen is available to organisms. However, various human activities have substantially increased the concentration of this mineral. Phosphates in fertilizers, detergents, and sewage are being added to ocean sediments faster than phosphates can be recycled in the aquatic ecosystem. One outcome of this has been a dramatic increase in algal and cyanobacterial populations (Color Photograph 69), for which phosphorus had been a limiting nutrient. This proliferation of microorganisms, in turn, has brought about other changes in the ecology of aquatic environments.

The Sulfur Cycle

Sulfur is another essential component of proteins and is therefore required by all life forms. In nature, sulfur exists in the form of elemental sulfur (S^o) and in oxidation states including hydrogen sulfide (H_2S), sulfites (SO_2^{2-}), and sulfates (SO_4^{2-}). Natural deposits of elemental sulfur are due to volcanic action and microbial activity.

The **sulfur cycle** (Figure 17–6) includes the following sequence of events. Animal or plant protein is first broken down through a series of enzymatic reactions to yield amino acids. Three specific amino acids contain sulfur: cysteine, cystine, and methionine. The sulfur from these compounds is completely reduced and removed as the toxic product hydrogen sulfide (H_2S). This breakdown process is anaerobic and occurs in sewage, polluted waters, fresh and marine water and muds, and in the rumen of ruminants. The conversion reactions are performed by sulfate-reducing bacteria. The most widespread organisms of this group belong to the genera of *Desulfovibrio* and *Desulfotomaculum.*

Hydrogen sulfide can also be produced by decomposition of protein by a wide variety of other microorganisms. Species of *Salmonella* and *Proteus* are noted for this ability, and it is used in their identification.

Before elemental sulfur can be taken up by plants and utilized as a primary nutrient, it must be oxidized to sulfate (SO_4^{2-}). Various strictly autotrophic bacteria are responsible for this process. Among them are species of *Beggiatoa, Thiobacillus, Thiobacterium, Thiospira,* and *Thiotrix.* This process occurs in fresh and marine water and muds, sewage, bogs, coal-mine drainage, sulfur springs, and bodies of stagnant water. The oxidized sulfur is assimilated by most forms of life and incorporated into the sulfur-containing amino acids.

The Oxygen Cycle

The atmosphere of our planet is a reservoir of molecular oxygen. Some microorganisms and all higher forms of life require oxygen for cellular respiration and the generation of energy by the electron transport system. The oxygen pool serves the needs of all terrestrial respiring organisms, and since atmospheric

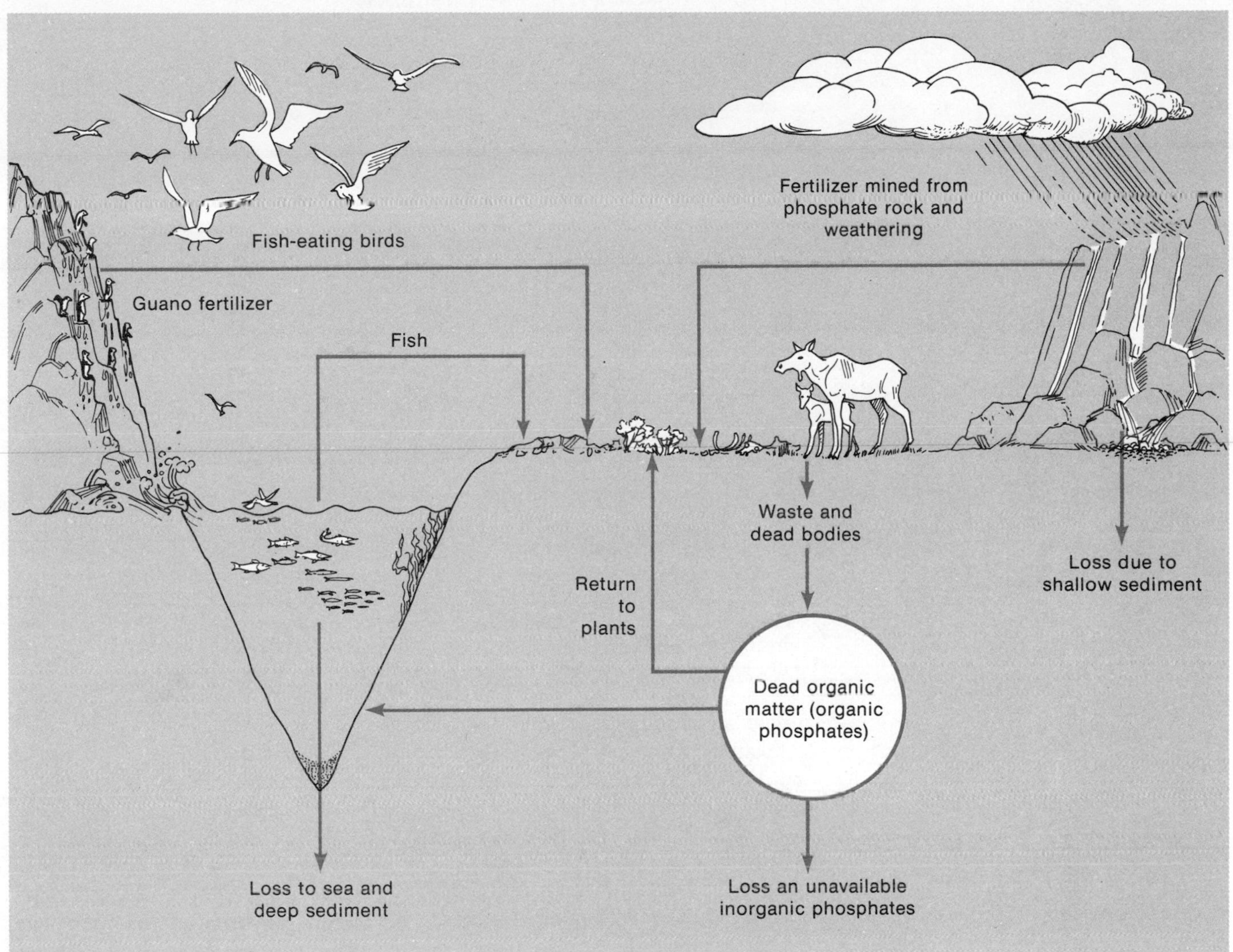

FIG. 17–5 A simplified version of the phosphorus cycle.

oxygen dissolves in water, the needs of aquatic organisms as well. In the respiration process, oxygen functions as the final acceptor of electrons removed from the carbon atoms of food. The enzyme oxidase catalyzes this reaction and the product formed is water. The **oxygen cycle** is completed in the photosynthetic process as light energy is utilized to remove electrons from the atoms of oxygen in water. These electrons reduce the carbon atoms of carbon dioxide to form carbohydrates. Molecular oxygen is left over in its free form as a gas, and the cycle is complete. The oxygen cycle is shown in Figure 17–7.

Reactions of Ecological Concern

There is a common belief among microbiologists that given sufficient time, soil microorganisms can decompose any organic molecule. This has been called

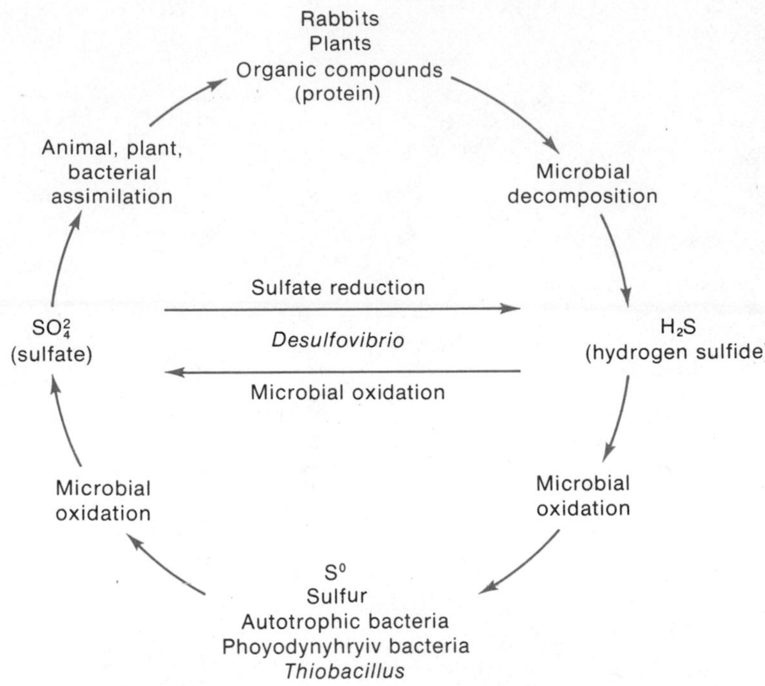

FIG. 17-6 Sulfur cycle. Several forms of sulfur exist in nature; the three forms that are of practical significance are ***sulfate*** (SO_4^{2-}), ***sulfide*** (S^{2-}) and elemental sulfur S^0. Only the biological aspects of the cycle are shown. The burning of fossil fuels and other industrial processes have added substantially to the concentration of gaseous sulfur compounds in the atmosphere.

microbial infallibility by the noted soil microbiologist Martin Alexander. Alexander admits, however, that certain materials are quite resistant to decomposition. These include certain pesticides, unique detergents, various plastics, and lignin.

Most metabolic reactions in terrestrial and aquatic environments are beneficial in that they recycle important materials for general use. The natural metabolic cycles for carbon, nitrogen, sulfur, and oxygen are only a few examples. These types of reactions can be called **bioconversion,** the enzymatic modification of chemicals. During natural cycles, some reactions lead to storage deposits of particular materials, for example, limestone storage of carbon, sulfur deposits in or near bacterial cells, and rare nitrate deposits probably produced by nitrification. These types of reactions can be called **bioconcentration.**

The remainder of this chapter will describe additional examples of bioconversion and bioconcentration, indicating both beneficial and harmful reactions of ecological concern.

Bioconversion

As used here, bioconversion refers to the biological or enzymatic production of a useful product, such as methane; the degradation of petroleum products as pollutants; and the detoxification of organophosphate pesticides.

METHANOGENESIS

Methane production occurs as a normal part of the carbon and oxygen cycles. The worldwide concern over dwindling petroleum reserves has focused attention on methane as an important fuel. Methane is especially interesting because it is, in essence, a recyclable commodity. Various plant and animal wastes and vegetation forms have been investigated as raw materials for commercial methane production. For example, an important by-product of sewage treatment is methane. A 1975 research report detailed a process of cattle waste digestion that yields nearly twenty times the methane produced during normal sewage treatment.

Methanogenesis is an anaerobic process in which methanol, organic acids, or carbon dioxide are reduced to methane. This occurs in aquatic sediments, black muds, marshes, swamps, and in the rumen of appropriate animals. The methane-producing bacteria depend upon the syntrophic production of the necessary substrates, including hydrogen, in these habitats. In freshwater sediments, acetate is a major substrate, and nearly pure methane has been collected at a slow but consistent rate in Lake Erie. In salt marshes along the southeastern coast of the United States, hydrogen and formic acid were found to stimulate methanogenesis. Ruminants are also known to have a system in which carbon dioxide and hydrogen are the important substrates in methanogenesis, since the organic acids produced by fermentation in the rumen are absorbed by the animal for its own nutrition.

Typical methanogenic bacteria are *Methanococcus* spp. in rumens, *Methanosarcinia thermoautotrophicum* and *Methanospirillum hungatii* in sewage sludge, and *Methanobacterium arbophilum* in the wet wood of a living tree.

PETROLEUM, OR HYDROCARBON, DEGRADATION

The degradation of crude oil materials is a major ecological concern. It was estimated in 1971 that 12 million metric tons of petroleum pollute marine environments each year as a result of spills by tankers or wells or as a result of the cleaning of tankers while they return to load more cargo. Crude oil is a complex mixture of hydrocarbons containing paraffins, kerosene, octane, petroleum oils, and many other components. The fact that oil spills eventually disappear from waters, soil around refineries, leaky pipelines, and polluted beaches is clear evidence that microorganisms can decompose these hydrocarbons.

A species of *Corynebacterium* has been isolated that can oxidize paraffin in a manner comparable to fatty acid catabolism to acetyl CoA. *Pseudomonas putida* strains from terrestrial and aquatic habitats have been shown to oxidize benzene, toluene, ethylbenzene, octane, naphthalene, camphor, and salicylates as sole sources of carbon. Metabolic plasmids control many of the hydrocarbon-degrading enzymes in these organisms.

Petroleum-degrading microorganisms adsorb to oil droplets. The smaller the droplets, the greater the ability of the organisms to oxidize the substrates and reproduce. These organisms also have the ability to produce emulsifying agents that help form small droplets (Figure 17–8). Yeasts (Figure 17–8) such as *Candida tropicalis* produce cell wall material of mannan and fatty acid, which assists in droplet formation. Most organisms excrete some form of extracellular material for this process.

Although oil-degrading microorganisms have been found in varied habitats, including arctic coastal water, their use to inoculate oil spills has proven ineffective. The major problem appears to be the low levels of nitrogen and phosphorus compounds in sea water. One solution that has been tried is to treat urea and octyl phosphate with paraffin to produce a slow-release fertilizer. This material, distributed with the organisms in powder form, appears to promote microbial action.

Although the prospects for using microorganisms to clean up oil spills is

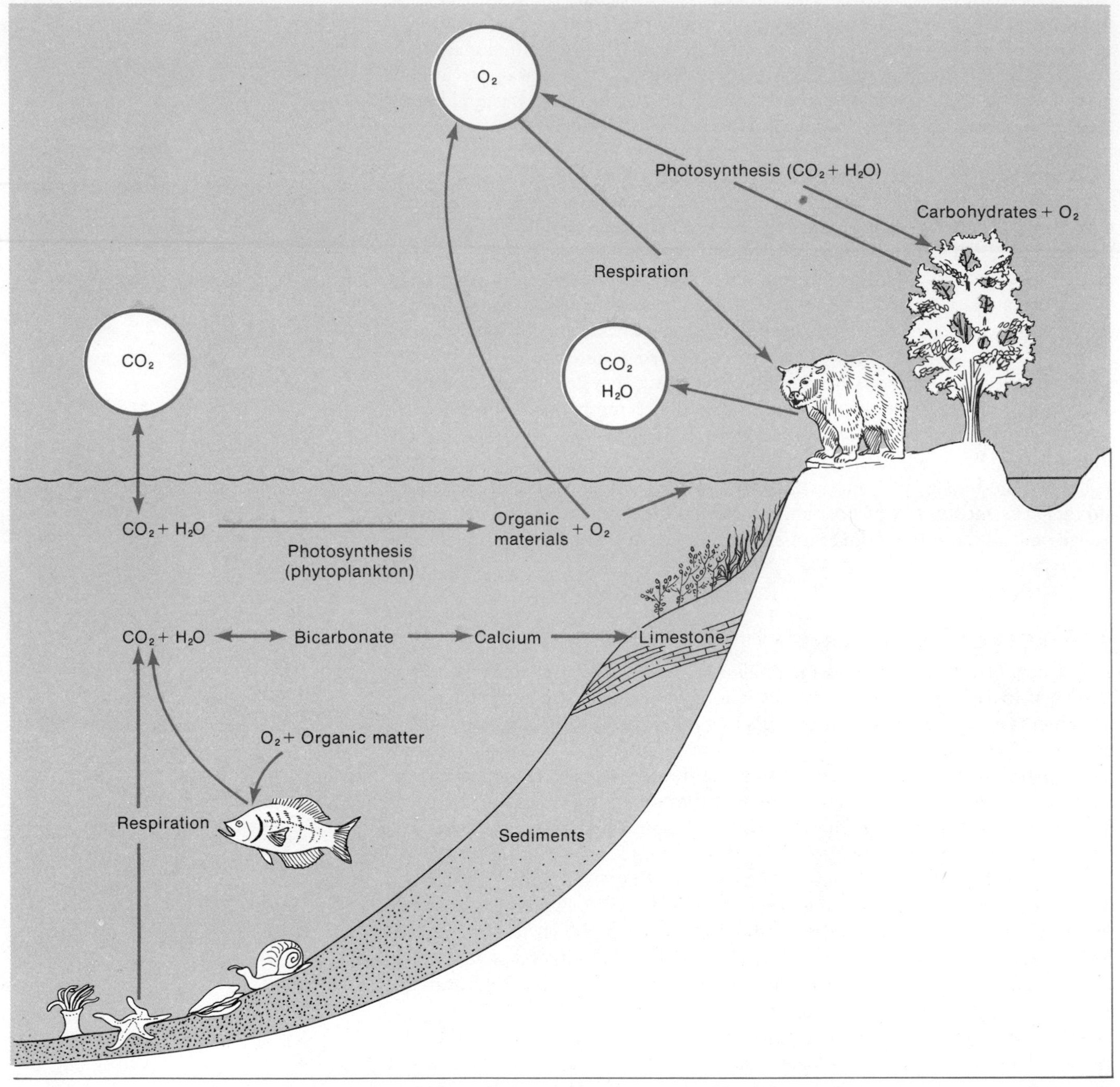

FIG. 17–7 The oxygen cycle. Oxygen occurs in the organic molecules of all forms of life and in water, in carbon dioxide, and in the atmosphere. Virtually all of the molecular oxygen present in the atmosphere was provided by photosynthesizing microscopic algae and higher plant life.

encouraging, it must be kept in mind that microorganisms can also cause spoilage and deterioration of petroleum products. Species from the bacterial genera *Pseudomonas, Chromobacterium, Alcaligenes, Mycobacterium,* and *Sarcina,* as well as certain fungal species of *Aspergillus* and *Monilia,* can decompose gasoline. In addition, the deterioration of asphalt highways and pipe coatings has been caused by species of *Mycobacterium* and *Nocardia.*

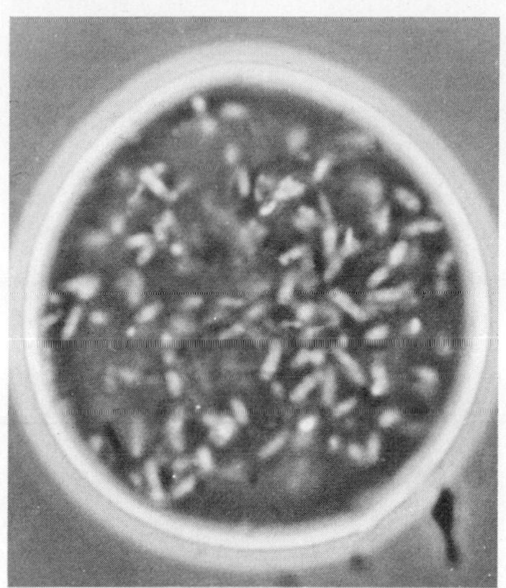
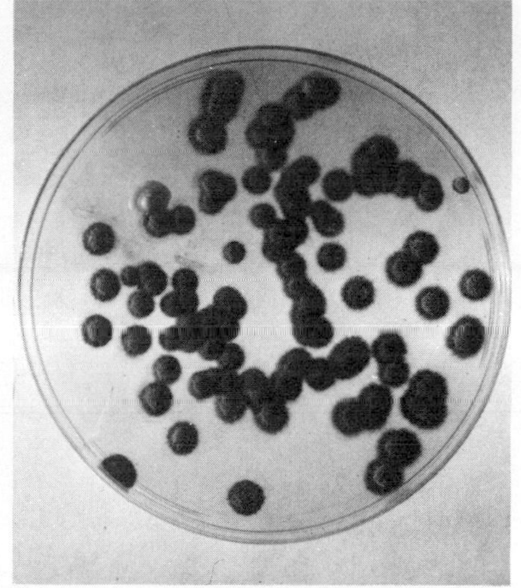

(a) (b)

FIG. 17–8 Petroleum-degrading microorganisms. (a) Bacteria in an oil globule from an Eastern Bay sediment. (b) Petroleum degrading yeasts. *Walker, J.D., and R. R. Colwell,* Microbial Ecol. 1:*63–95 (1974).*

PESTICIDES AND MERCURY

The pesticide parathion belongs to a large group of chemicals known as organophosphates. These compounds are extremely toxic to insects and all other animals because they prevent nerve cell conduction across synapses. They are so effective that they have been tested extensively for use as nerve gas. In a study relating to the concept of microbial infallibility, various soil and sewage microorganisms were tested for their ability to detoxify parathion. Mixed bacterial cultures were found to be effective in preliminary studies. Some of the organisms involved were species of *Brevibacterium, Pseudomonas,* and *Azotomonas.*

Unfortunately, the experience with another group of pesticides has not been so promising. The chlorinated hydrocarbons, which include DDT, aldrin, DDD, lindane, and endrin, can be "degraded" under anaerobic conditions by various facultative anaerobic bacteria and yeast, but the end products are still extremely toxic. In one study, it was observed that DDT (dichloro-diphenyl trichloroethane) was dechlorinated to form DDD (dichloro-diphenyl dichloroethane), another very toxic pesticide. The problems associated with the buildup of chlorinated hydrocarbons in various aquatic and terrestrial environments appears to be related to their relative invulnerability to attack by microorganisms.

Another problem pollutant in terrestrial and aquatic environments is mercury. Mercury is toxic to humans and other life forms, as demonstrated by the mercury poisoning tragedy that occurred in Minamata Bay, Japan, where industrial pollution produced exceptionally high mercury levels in their fish. The form of mercury in the fish was methyl mercury, which is 50 to 100 times more toxic than inorganic mercury compounds. This methylation of mercury can occur abiotically, but considerable evidence points to a significant role of many bacteria and fungi in this reaction. Some organisms, such as *Clostridium cochlearium,* introduce a methyl group on the molecule cobalamin by using vitamin B_{12} and cystine. Subsequently, the methyl group can be transferred to mercury nonenzymatically. *C. cochlearium* is anaerobic, performing the methylation in aquatic bottom sediments and sludge. The ability to methylate mercury has also been shown to exist in indigenous microorganisms such as species of *Pseudomonas* on the gills and in the intestines of fish. Aerobic methylation also occurs. Soil organisms with this capacity include a species of the bacterial genus *Pseudomonas* and the yeast *Neurospora crassa*. One source of mercury in soils has been the application of organomercurial fungicides. Research in Sweden since the introduction of these fungicides has shown considerable increases of methyl mercury in plant and animal tissues.

Bioconcentration

Bioconcentration is the ability of microorganisms to store materials in the environment. The storage may be within cells, as in the case of sulfur, or outside the cells, as in the case of nitrate or sulfur. The metabolic activities of sulfur oxidizers have been used to concentrate low-grade mineral ores. Sulfur oxidizers, such as *Thiobacillus*, can grow in slag from copper mines, the material remaining after ore is roasted to remove most of the copper. The sulfuric acid produced by the growth of *Thiobacillus* dissolves the copper, and copper sulfate accumulates at the base of the slag pile. A similar process is used to concentrate uranium from ores in the form of uranyl sulfate.

Bioconcentration has caused the formation of commercially attractive deposits of manganese but also hazardous accumulations of pesticides and radioisotopes in nature.

MANGANESE DEPOSITS

Manganese, an important trace element in plant nutrition, is found widely distributed in terrestrial and aquatic environments. It is commercially important in alloys of iron, aluminum, and copper. In the soil, bacteria such as *Leptothrix (Sphaerotilus) discophorus* oxidize manganese compounds and accumulate manganese dioxide (MnO_2) in their cells. This oxidation may be a primary energy source for these organisms. The accumulation depletes the manganese available to plants until reducer organisms render MnO_2 deposits soluble and available once more.

In the oceans, both of these reactions have also been noted. A species of *Arthrobacter* has been found associated with ferromanganese nodules. These nodules contain as much as 63 percent MnO_2 deposited by the oxidative capacity of the bacteria. A species of *Bacillus* isolated from nodules and deep-sea sediments can reduce MnO_2 as a stage of its electron transport system. The reduction process must be significantly slower than that of oxidation or the nodules would not have formed to the extent that has been observed. International discussions have been held on cooperative ventures for the mining of these nodules.

PESTICIDES AND RADIOISOTOPES

In 1976 the United States Council on Environmental Quality reported an incident involving the chlorinated hydrocarbon kepone. A Virginia company had been making kepone for sixteen months and cases of poisoning in their personnel had been linked to kepone. When the United States Cancer Institute reported animal studies showing kepone to be carcinogenic, the company was required to stop making the pesticide. Evaluation of the environment, including the James River, showed that water and shellfish contained traces of the chemical as far away as 40 miles. It is suspected that the kepone accumulated in microorganisms upon which the shellfish feed.

More definitive examples of the accumulation of toxic substances have been reported for radioisotopes, which have also been shown to be carcinogenic. In "The Myth of the Peaceful Atom," by Curtis and Hogan, two pertinent examples are presented.* The Savannah River Nuclear Power Plant in Aiken, South

*R. Curtis and E. Hogan, "The Myth of the Peaceful Atom," in C. E. Johnson, *Eco-crisis* (New York: John Wiley & Sons, 1970).

Carolina, released "insignificant" amounts of radioactivity in its cooling water. An examination of algae in the water, however, showed a concentration up to 6000 times the level in the water itself. These algae serve as food for the bluegill fish; the bones of this fish had a concentration 8200 times that in the water.

The Hanford Nuclear Power Plant in Hanford, Washington, used the Columbia River for cooling water. As suspected, the water there, too, had "insignificant" levels of radioactivity and was considered "safe." Algae and other microorganisms in the water concentrated this safe level of radioactivity as much as 2000 times. Fish who fed on the plankton had levels of 15,000 times that in the water. Ducks that fed on vegetation in the water had levels of 40,000 times that in the water, while their egg yolks had concentrations of one million times that of the safe water. Clearly one aftermath of the failure of the Three Mile Island Power Plant in 1979 that will be closely followed is the bioconcentration of radioactivity in the plant and animal life in and around the Susquehanna River.

These few examples of bioconversion and bioconcentration of toxic materials in nature should serve not only to render the concept of microbial infallibility suspect, but also to stop our reliance on aquatic and terrestrial habitats for the dumping of waste materials.

SUMMARY

The processes by which microorganisms are involved in natural cycles for the use and reuse of critical elements are collectively called *biogeochemistry*.

The Life-supporting Biogeochemical Cycles

1. Biologically important elements such as carbon, hydrogen, oxygen, nitrogen, phosphorus, and sulfur are removed from the environment, incorporated into cellular structures, and eventually returned to the environment to be used over again.
2. The natural biogeochemical cycles are interrelated to ensure the flow of essential chemical elements between the living and nonliving parts of ecosystems. No one cycle can function without the others.

The Carbon Cycle

1. Carbon is one of the most common and important of the elements involved with living systems.
2. The *carbon cycle* is the route by which useful solar energy enters the biosphere through the photosynthesis process.

The Nitrogen Cycle

1. Organisms need nitrogen to synthesize amino acids, proteins, and nucleic acids.
2. The *nitrogen cycle* serves to convert essential compounds from one type to another, often with the release of energy that is captured during metabolic activity.
3. The cycle consists of three phases, *nitrogen fixation, nitrogen assimilation*, and *nitrogen recovery*.
4. Nitrogen fixation is the reduction of atmospheric molecular nitrogen to ammonia (NH_3) and other biologically essential nitrogen-containing compounds. The process involves cyanobacteria and other bacteria.
5. Nitrogen fixation can occur symbiotically between legumes and bacteria of the genus *Rhizobium*, and nonsymbiotically by some cyanobacteria and various other bacteria, or nonleguminous root-nodule plants.
6. In nitrogen fixation, the enzyme *nitrogenase* binds N_2 and the following reaction occurs:

$$N_2 + 6\,H^+ + 6\,e^- + 12\text{ ATP} \rightarrow 2\,NH_3 + 12\text{ ADP} + 12\text{ P (i)}$$

7. Microbial enzymatic activities involving decaying organic matter break down organic nitrogen molecules to ammonia (NH_3). The process is known as *ammonification*.
8. Chemosynthetic bacteria of the genus *Nitrosomonas* oxidize NH_3 to nitrites (NO_2^-), which in turn are oxidized to nitrates (NO_3^-) by *Nitrobacter* species.
9. Denitrification completes the nitrogen cycle and results in the conversion of nitrates into nitrogen gas.

The Phosphorus Cycle

1. Without phosphorus, compounds such as ATP, DNA, and RNA would not be formed.
2. Through the *phosphorus cycle*, producer organisms convert inorganic phosphate (PO_4^{3-}) into organic phosphates.

The Sulfur Cycle

1. Sulfur is another essential component of proteins.
2. Through the *sulfur cycle*, oxidized sulfur is obtained and assimilated by living organisms into sulfur-containing amino acids, cysteine, cystine, and methionine.

The Oxygen Cycle

By means of the *oxygen cycle*, an oxygen pool is generated to meet the needs of all land and aquatic respiring organisms.

Reactions of Ecological Concern

Most metabolic and recycling reactions in terrestrial and aquatic environments are beneficial.

Bioconversion

1. The biological or enzymatic formation of a useful product is referred to as a *bioconversion.*
2. Examples include methane production, degradation of polluting petroleum products, and the detoxification of certain pesticides.

Bioconcentration

Bioconcentration refers to the ability of microorganisms to store materials in the environment. Such materials include sulfur, manganese deposits, pesticides and radioactive materials.

QUESTIONS FOR REVIEW

1. What is meant by the term *reaction* as an ecological concept?
2. Briefly outline the carbon, nitrogen, sulfur, and oxygen cycles.
3. Of what biological value is phosphorus to living systems?
4. Explain or define each of the following terms:
   a. photosynthesis
   b. chemosynthesis
   c. nitrogen fixation
   d. legume
   e. nitrification
   f. denitrification
   g. oxidase
5. Define and discuss *microbial infallibility.*
6. Discuss methanogenesis as a bioconversion process of considerable importance.
7. What is the involvement of microorganisms in the degradation of petroleum in nature?
8. Relate microbial activities to the detoxification of organophosphate pesticides and to their role in modifying chlorinated hydrocarbons and inorganic mercury.
9. What is the involvement of microorganisms in the bioconcentration of manganese in the oceans?
10. Relate microbial activities to the toxic accumulation of chlorinated hydrocarbons and radioisotopes in aquatic and terrestrial habitats.

SUGGESTED READINGS

Brill, W. J. "Biological Nitrogen Fixation." *Sci. Amer.* 236:68, 1977. *A nicely illustrated article on the few bacteria and algae that can "fix" atmospheric nitrogen into ammonia.*

Davis, J. B. *Petroleum Microbiology.* New York: Elsevier Publishing Co., 1967. *The actions of microbes, both in the formation and degradation of petroleum and petroleum products, are discussed in detail.*

Gutnick, D. L., and E. Rosenberg. "Oil Tankers and Pollution: A Microbiological Approach." *Ann. Rev. Microbiol.* 31:379, 1977. *The review stresses the special character of hydrocarbon-utilizing bacteria and the use of these organisms in some of the problems arising from oil tanker operations.*

Han, Y. W. "Microbial Utilization of Straw." *Adv. in Applied Microbiol.* 23:119, 1978. *This review discusses some of the problems of using cellulosic agricultural wastes as feed and also some of the microbiological processes considered for converting such waste into useful materials.*

Mah, R. A.; D. M. Ward; L. Baresi; and T. L. Glass. "Biogenesis of Methane." *Ann. Rev. Microbiol.* 31:309, 1977. *The methane bacteria are discussed as regards their role in interspecies hydrogen transfer, methane from carbohydrates, acetate, and the bacteria isolated and grown in pure culture thus far.*

Weinberg, E. D. (ed.). *Microorganisms and Minerals.* New York: Marcel Dekker, Inc., 1977. *Describes the way microbial cells acquire and store selected mineral elements and the function of Mg, Ca, Mn, and Fe in microbial cells. Microbial roles in cycling of mineral elements and antimicrobial action of mineral elements are also discussed.*

PART THREE

The Control of Microorganisms

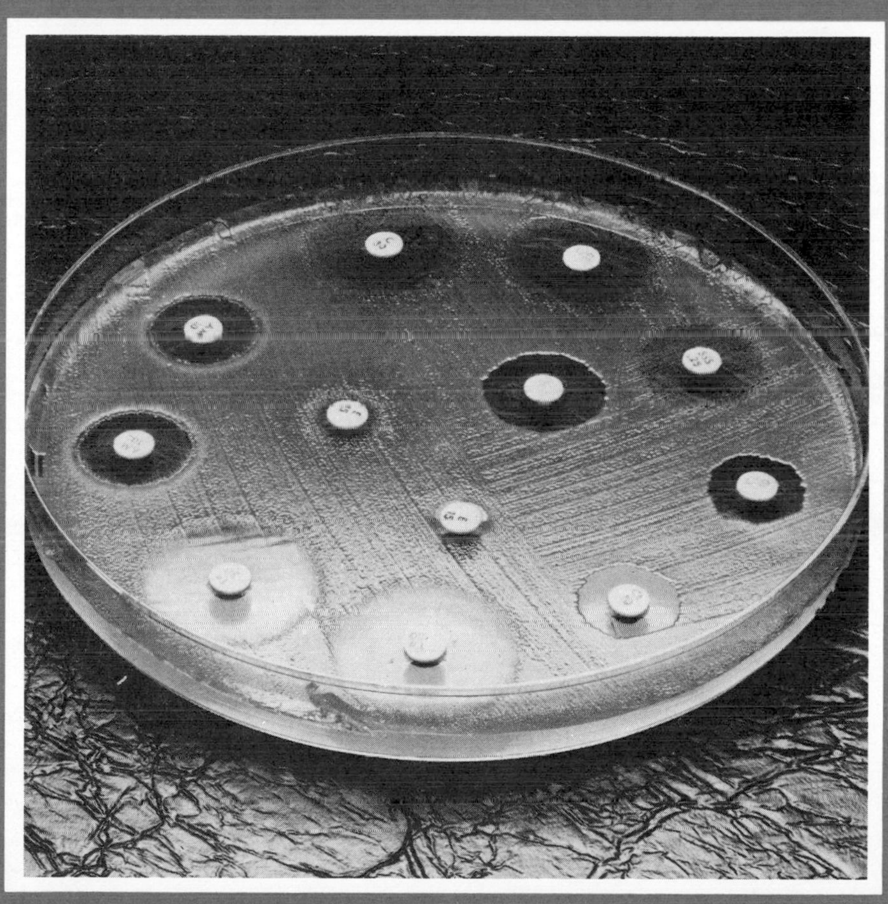

CHAPTER 18

The Use of Chemicals in Disinfection and Sterilization

Many chemicals are available for use in the control of microorganisms. Chapter 18 presents basic concepts in chemical control, discussions of selected chemicals, and the means by which they can be tested and compared.

After reading this chapter, you should be able to:

1. **Define the following terms: disinfection, antisepsis, sterilization, disinfectant, antiseptic, bactericidal, bacteriostatic, and sanitizer.**
2. **Identify the contributions of Paré, Semmelweis, Lister, Koch, Neuber, and Krönig and Paul.**
3. **List and describe seven general directions for using a chemical in antisepsis and disinfection.**
4. **Discuss representative chemical agents from each of the following groups in terms of mechanism of killing microorganisms, general effectiveness, and advantages and disadvantages: halogens, alcohols, phenols, peroxides, detergents, heavy metals, aldehydes, and gaseous sterilants.**
5. **Describe the phenol coefficient test for comparison of chemicals as antiseptics or disinfectants.**
6. **Describe the use-dilution method for testing chemicals.**
7. **Describe a testing procedure to determine if a chemical is bacteriostatic or bactericidal.**

8. Discuss the significance of the toxicity index as a means of comparing chemicals used in disinfection and antisepsis.

The problem of controlling disease-causing microorganisms has troubled scientists for as long as the origin of disease has been known. Many substances have been tested in attempts to find the perfect one to eliminate microbial contamination of living and nonliving surfaces. In the process, many different chemicals and disease control concepts have come about.

The antimicrobial agents developed have a wide range of effectiveness and are appropriate to use in many different circumstances. The terms by which they are described reflect these differences. An **antiseptic** and a **disinfectant,** for example, differ mainly in the way they are used—an antiseptic is applied to living tissue, a disinfectant for contaminated inanimate objects (fomites). Table 18–1 lists and defines the most important terms in chemical and physical control of microorganisms.

Historical Background

The Arabs learned several hundred years ago that *cauterization* of a wound with hot metal prevented infection. This was a common procedure, despite the fact that the patient would be scarred for life. Even though cauterization was traumatic, it gave victims more of a fighting chance to overcome the effects of disease agents. In 1537, the French surgeon Ambroise Paré treated gunshot wounds with bandages soaked in egg yolk, turpentine, and other materials. The turpentine caused a kind of chemical cauterization, and the egg material supplied the antibacterial enzyme lysozyme.

The concept of antisepsis was introduced largely by Ignatz Semmelweis (1816–1865) and Joseph Lister (1827–1912).

TABLE 18-1 Important Terms in Chemical Disinfection and Sterilization

Term	*Explanation*
Antisepsis	Prevention of the growth or activity of microorganisms either by inhibition or killing; applies to the use of chemicals on living tissue.
Antiseptic	A chemical agent used for the purpose of antisepsis.
Disinfection	The killing of pathogenic organisms, but not usually bacterial spores, by chemical or physical means; applies to use directly on inanimate objects.
Disinfectant	An agent, usually chemical, used for the purpose of disinfection.
Sanitizer	Any agent that reduces the numbers of microbial contaminants to acceptable levels; applies to use of agents on inanimate objects and is usually associated with the cleaning of eating and drinking utensils and the cleaning operations for dairy equipment.
Sterilization	Any process, chemical or physical, that kills or removes *all* forms of life, especially microorganisms.
-cide	Suffix used to denote agents, usually chemical, that kill. Commonly used terms are *bactericide, fungicide, virucide,* and *algicide.* The term *germicide* is used if the agent kills pathogens but not necessarily spores. An agent that kills bacterial spores is a *sporocide.*
-static	Suffix used to denote agents, usually chemical, that prevent growth but do not necessarily kill the organism or bacterial spores. Commonly used terms include *bacteriostatic* and *fungistatic.*

Ignatz Semmelweis

Ignatz Semmelweis, a Hungarian physician working in Vienna, observed that the incidence of childbed fever, otherwise known as puerperal fever, was much higher in the obstetrics ward run by physicians in the Vienna General Hospital than in a similar ward run by midwives. In comparing the procedures in both locations, Semmelweis observed that the midwives washed their hands frequently, whereas the physicians came directly from performing autopsies to treat patients, without changing their blood-splattered clothes or washing their hands. Semmelweis guessed that these procedures were important factors accounting for the difference in infection rates between the two wards. To lower the rate of infection in his maternity clinics, he required the attendants to wash their hands with chlorinated lime. The infection rate dropped significantly. Unfortunately, Semmelweis's efforts to persuade other physicians of the necessity for cleanliness and disinfection ended in failure, and he was dismissed from the hospital staff.

In the early nineteenth century, infections were still believed to be caused by some magical power in the air or by an imbalance of body fluids. Certainly contaminated hands were not involved. It took the incredible tenacity of Pasteur to show the world that microorganisms could not only ferment fruit juice to wine but could also cause spoilage of the wine, before the idea that microorganisms could cause disease could evolve.

Surgical Antisepsis

Aware of Pasteur's work, Joseph Lister in England sought to prevent surgical infections. His efforts with carbolic acid (phenol) clearly established modern surgical procedures.

In 1881, Koch and his associates evaluated seventy different chemicals for use in disinfection and antisepsis. Among these chemicals were various phenols and mercuric chloride ($HgCl_2$). In 1886, Neuber applied the latter compound as a surgical antiseptic as well as for the disinfection of operating rooms. He also insisted that patients wear clean gowns and that surgeons wear clean apparel in the operating room.

In 1897, Krönig and Paul published standardized procedures for the evaluation and comparison of chemical disinfectants. Their reports specified the concentrations of chemical compounds, specific test bacteria used, viable plate counts, the temperatures at which the tests were performed, and the culture media used. Effectiveness was reported in terms of the number of surviving bacteria as related to the period of exposure.

The Use of Antiseptics and Disinfectants

Today an almost limitless number of chemical agents are used for controlling microorganisms, and new ones appear on the market regularly. A common problem confronting those who use disinfectants or antiseptics is which one to select and how to use it. Since there is no "ideal" or "all-purpose" agent, the compound to choose is the one that will kill the organisms present in the shortest time, without any damage to the contaminated material.

General Directions for Chemical Disinfection

All surfaces of the contaminated material that are to be treated must be exposed to the chemical agent. Therefore, before chemical treatment is begun, the material must be thoroughly cleaned. Furthermore, there must be enough space left between items so that all surfaces of each item are fully exposed to the solution.

If possible, the cleaning agent should be germicidal, so that microorganisms will not remain in the solution and perhaps contaminate floors or attendants by splashing.

The time at which a particular article is immersed in solution and the time for its removal should be noted. This prevents others from interrupting the process before it is completed.

As solutions used to kill spores are highly volatile, the room in which they are used should be well ventilated.

Certain chemicals alter the composition of the materials to be treated. Usually the labels of containers with such compounds indicate the materials on which they should not be used. Never use a chemical without first checking the label.

Disinfectants should always be diluted in the proportions suggested by the manufacturer.

Solutions should be changed often, especially if cloudiness or sedimentation appears.

It is generally a good practice to have hand lotions in the vicinity for proper hand care after using disinfectants.

Chemical Antiseptics

Antiseptics are usually applied and allowed to evaporate, as in the case of alcohol. Some are rinsed off with alcohol after drying, as in the case of iodine-alcohol; or rinsed off with sterile water for surgical preparations, as in the case of iodophors; or rinsed with water, leaving an active residue, as with hexachlorophene preparations.

In general, 70 to 90 percent isopropyl alcohol is the least expensive, yet a very effective, antiseptic. The addition of iodine to alcohol greatly increases its disinfecting properties. With or without iodine, isopropyl alcohol solutions are not active against spores. The least expensive and best sporicidal formulation appears to be the combination of formaldehyde and alcohol, but this solution is too toxic for antiseptic use. Since disinfectant solutions or gases do not have to come into contact with human skin or mucous membranes, greater toxicity is acceptable, making them more generally applicable as antimicrobial agents.

The choice of antiseptic depends largely upon the needs of the particular operation and the desired effects. Consideration should be given to the fact that some compounds are extremely irritating, and skin sensitivity varies greatly.

Selected Disinfecting and Sterilizing Chemicals

Chemical disinfectants and sterilants are used in what are often termed "cold sterilization" methods. Choosing among the many agents available involves considering the conditions under which the material will be used. Then the product or formulation (combination of substances) that best suits the particular requirements should be selected. Table 18–2 summarizes many of the factors that enter into making the right choice.

THE HALOGENS

The halogens include the compounds of chlorine and iodine, both organic and inorganic. Most of the inorganic halogen compounds are deadly to living

TABLE 18-2 Selected Compounds for Chemical Control of Microorganisms

Procedure	*Effectiveness*	*Advantages*	*Disadvantages*	*Preferred Use*	*Recommended Exposure Time*
Halogens: 1. Chlorine	Kills most vegetative cells, some viruses and fungi; spores usually resistant	Excellent deodorant	Activity reduced by organic material and some metallic catalysts; irritating odor and residue; solutions are somewhat unstable	Purification of drinking water	Immediate effect (from seconds to minutes, depending upon compound and concentration)
2. Iodine	Kills vegetative cells, some spores and viruses when used in high concentration	Extremely useful as a skin disinfectant; can be used over wide pH range	Irritating odor and residue, except with iodophors	Wound dressing, preoperative preparation	At least 60 seconds to kill vegetative bacterial cells
Alcohols	Kills vegetative cells and many viruses; spores unaffected	Unaffected by organic compounds; no residue left; stable and easily handled	No outstanding disadvantages as a disinfectant	Skin and surfaces	10 to 15 minutes in 70% to 80% solutions
Phenols and related compounds	Kills vegetative cells and some fungi; only moderately effective against spores	Stable to heating and drying; unaffected by organic compounds	Pure phenol is harmful to tissues and has disagreeable odor	In combination with halogens and detergents, they make excellent disinfectants	Effect is immediate
Detergents, quaternary ammonium compounds	Kills bacteria (including staphylococci and some viruses; tuberculosis (TB) and spores unaffected	Stable in the presence of organic compounds; easy to handle; no irritating residue left	Hard water, detergents, and fibrous materials interfere with activity; can rust metals	Small metal instruments	Depends upon type and concentration, generally 10 to 30 minutes
Heavy metals	Kills some vegetative cells and viruses; TB and spores unaffected	Fast and inexpensive; no special equipment required	Inactivated by organic compounds and chemical antagonists	Rarely used except as preservatives and in fungal and protozoan infections	Effective as long as in contact
Aldehydes	Kills staphyloccocci, TB[a], and viruses readily; spores killed only upon prolonged exposure	Glutaraldehyde is nontoxic and nonirritating to tissue	Prolonged exposure required	Instrument disinfection	A 2% solution for 3 to 18 hours
Ethylene oxide	100% effective if properly managed	Can treat critical items that would be destroyed by other techniques	Slow; equipment is expensive; leaves irritating residue; materials must be aired before use	Plastics, rubber, and instruments that are sensitive to heat or chemicals	1 to 2 hours at 60°C for small loads; 10 to 12 hours necessary for large loads

[a]Recent evidence suggests that aldehydes may not be as effective against *Mycobacterium tuberculosis* as once thought.

cells. They kill cells by oxidizing protein and thus disrupting membranes and inactivating enzymes.

Iodine. Iodine solution, either in water or alcohol, is highly antiseptic and has been used for years as a preoperative preparation of the skin, usually applied to the skin's surface immediately before a surgical procedure. It is also effective against many protozoans, such as the amoeba that causes dysentery. In proper concentration, iodine does not seriously harm human tissues. However, the clinical use of tincture (alcohol solution) of iodine stains tissue and may cause local skin irritation and occasional allergic reactions. Preparations of iodine compounded with nonionic detergents and polymers such as polyvinylpyrolidone have been developed for disinfection and antiseptic uses, respectively. The iodine binds loosely with the organic compound and is released slowly to produce effective disinfection. Antiseptic iodophors are used routinely for preoperative skin cleansing and disinfection.

Chlorine. Free chlorine, like free iodine, has a characteristic color (green) and a pungent odor. Chlorine in any of its various forms has long been recognized as an excellent deodorant and disinfectant. It is a standard treatment for drinking water in all communities. Unfortunately, most compounds of chlorine are inactivated in the presence of organic material and some metallic catalysts.

Hypochlorite solutions are those most commonly used in disinfecting and deodorizing procedures, as they are relatively harmless to human tissues, easy to handle, colorless, and nonstaining, although they do bleach. They are widely employed in hospitals to disinfect rooms, surfaces, and nonsurgical instruments. They tend to leave a residue that can be irritating to skin and tissues.

Several organic chlorine derivatives are also used to disinfect water. This is particularly useful for campers and others who must use water that is likely to be contaminated. The most common of the compounds employed is halazone, or parasulfone dichloramidobenzoic acid (Figure 18–1a). A halazone concentration of 4 to 8 milligrams per liter safely disinfects even fairly hard water containing typhoid bacilli in approximately 30 minutes. Another compound used for the same purpose is succinchlorimide (Figure 18–1b). A concentration of 11.6 mg will disinfect a liter of water in 20 minutes. These organic chlorides are quite stable in tablet form, becoming active when placed in the water.

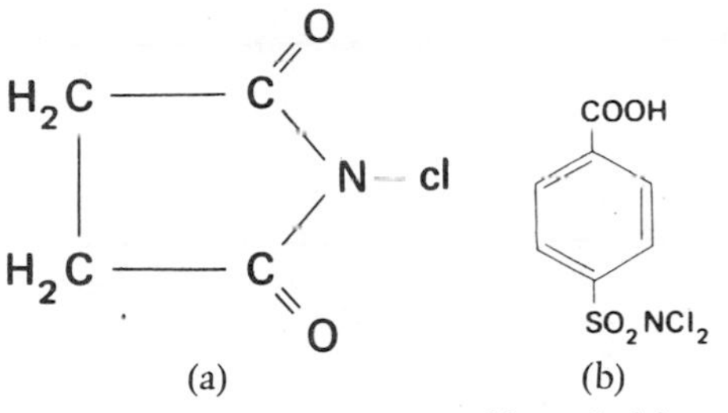

FIG. 18–1 (a) Halazone (parasulfone dichloramidobenzoic acid). (b) Succinchlorimide.

THE ALCOHOLS

Alcohols are among the most effective and heavily relied upon agents for sterilization and disinfection. Alcohols denature proteins, possibly by dehydration, and also act as solvents for lipids. Thus, membranes are likely to be disrupted and enzymes inactivated in the presence of alcohols. Three alcohols are used: methanol, CH_3OH; ethanol, CH_3CH_2OH; and isopropanol $(CH_3)_2CHOH$. As a general rule, the bactericidal value increases as the molecular weight increases; isopropyl alcohol is therefore the most widely used of the three. In practice, a solution of 70 to 80 percent alcohol in water is employed. Percentages above 90 and below 50 are usually less effective, except for isopropyl alcohol, which is effective up to solutions of 99 percent.

Although alcohols are somewhat affected by organic material, they leave no residue on surfaces. Large pieces of office equipment and furniture are commonly wiped with alcohol. A 10-minute exposure is sufficient to kill vegetative cells but not spores.

The alcohols, alone or in combination, are often used as skin disinfectants. A quick wipe is not really enough to sterilize, but only to cut down the population and thus reduce the chance of infection. It has been common practice to dip instruments into alcohol and then flame them. The effectiveness of this procedure is questionable, and it should not be substituted for better sterilization methods.

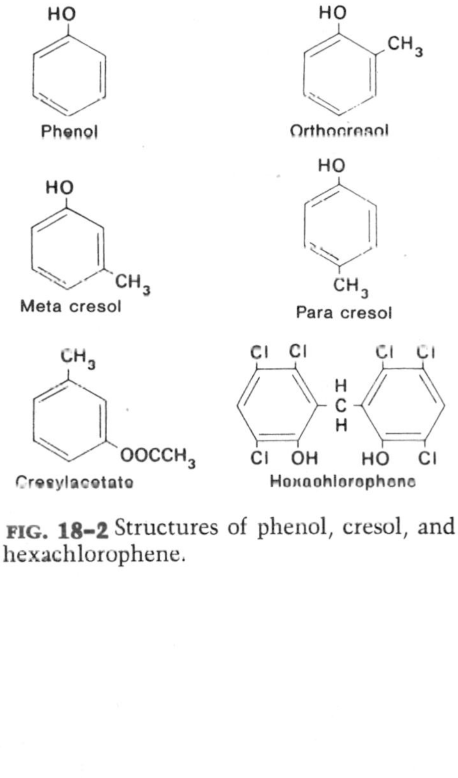

FIG. 18–2 Structures of phenol, cresol, and hexachlorophene.

THE PHENOLS

Phenol (carbolic acid) is probably the oldest recognized disinfectant. It was used by Lister in 1867 as a germicide in the operating room. In low concentration, its deadly effect is due to the fact that it precipitates proteins actively. Like the alcohols, the phenols denature protein. In addition, they disrupt membranes by lowering surface tension. Phenol is the standard of comparison for determining the activities of other disinfectants. Phenol and cresol (methylated phenol) (Figure 18–2) have a typical odor and are corrosive to tissues. However, they are very stable to heating and drying and retain activity in the presence of organic material. Unfortunately, they are only moderately effective against bacterial spores. The addition of a halogen such as chlorine or a short chain organic compound enhances the activity of the phenols.

Hexachlorophene is one of the most useful of the phenol derivatives. Combined with a soap, it is a commonly used, highly effective skin disinfectant, although slow acting. Unlike most phenolic compounds, hexachlorophene has no irritating odor and has a high residual action. It is also a good deodorant, a property put to extensive use by commercial deodorant and soap makers before such widespread use in over-the-counter preparations was banned by the FDA.

An interesting feature of phenol and the cresols is their pain-killing properties. They can only be used externally because they are highly toxic. Slight modification of cresol yields cresylacetate (Figure 18–2), which has been used in spray form for antisepsis and as an analgesic on the mucous membranes of the ear, nose, and throat.

THE PEROXIDES

Hydrogen peroxide (H_2O_2) is an effective and nontoxic antiseptic. The molecule is unstable, and when warmed, degrades into water and oxygen:

$$2\,H_2O_2 \longrightarrow 2\,H_2O + O_2\uparrow$$

During the generation of oxygen gas, the superoxide radical (O_2^-) is formed in the presence of metal ions usually present in the cytoplasm. This highly reactive species reacts with negatively charged groups in proteins and leads to inactivation of vital enzyme systems.

At concentrations of 0.3 to 6.0 percent, H_2O_2 is used in disinfection, and concentrations of 6.0 to 25.0 percent have been used in sterilization. It is particularly recommended for materials such as surgical implants and hydrophilic soft contact lenses, as it leaves no residual toxicity after a few minutes of exposure. A concentration of 0.1 percent H_2O_2 in milk at a temperature of 54°C for 30 minutes results in a 99.999 percent reduction of total bacteria and significant disinfection. There is good evidence that H_2O_2 at 10 percent is actively virucidal and sporocidal. A 3-percent solution is often used to cleanse and disinfect wounds, since anaerobic bacteria are particularly sensitive to oxygen. Sodium peroxide (Na_2O_2) paste has been used for the treatment of acne. Zinc peroxide (ZnO_2) is used medically in a creamy suspension with zinc oxide (ZnO) and zinc hydroxide [$Zn(OH_2)$] for skin infections caused by microaerophilic and anaerobic organisms.

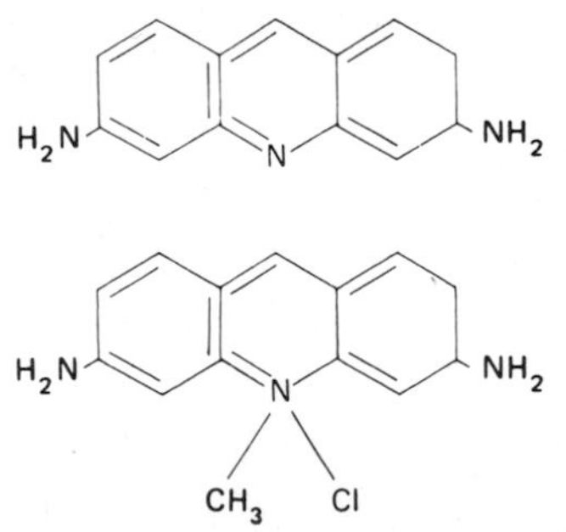

H_2N NH$_2$ N

H_2N NH$_2$ N CH_3 Cl

FIG. 18–3 Diaminoacridine (top) and diamino-methyl-acridinium-chloride (bottom).

THE ANTISEPTIC DYES

There are a variety of dyes that have a growth-inhibiting, or **bacteriostatic,** activity. We shall present two of these varieties, the *acridine* derivatives and *rosaniline* dyes. *Acriflavine*, a mixture of an acridine derivative and another compound (Figure 18–3), has low toxicity and is relatively free from skin-sensitizing properties. It has a broad spectrum of activity and has been used for treatment of urinary tract infections. The mechanism of action appears to be due to the ability of acridines to react with DNA.

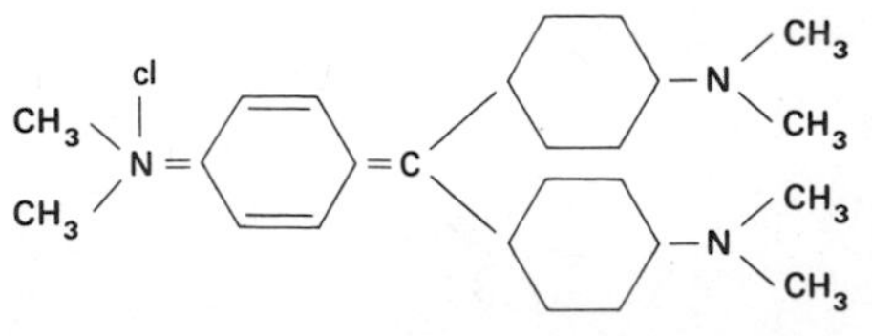

One methyl derivative of a rosaniline dye, *crystal violet*, is a potent bacteriostatic agent for Gram-positive bacteria, besides being the primary stain in the Gram reaction (Figure 18–4). Crystal violet has been used for the treatment of candidiasis and *Trichomonas*-caused vaginitis. *Candida albicans* is particularly sensitive to the dye. The mechanism of action of this compound against Gram-positive bacteria appears to be very similar to that of penicillin, blockage of a final step in the synthesis of cell wall material.

cl CH_3 N= CH_3 =C N CH_3 CH_3 N CH_3 CH_3

FIG. 18–4 Crystal violet (hexamethylpararosaniline).

THE DETERGENTS

Detergents are organic compounds which, because of their structure, bond both to water and to nonpolar organic molecules. The molecules of a detergent have one ***hydrophilic*** end, which mixes well with water, and one ***hydrophobic*** end, which does not. Therefore, the detergent molecules orient themselves on the surfaces of organic material with their hydrophilic ends toward the water (Figure 18–5).

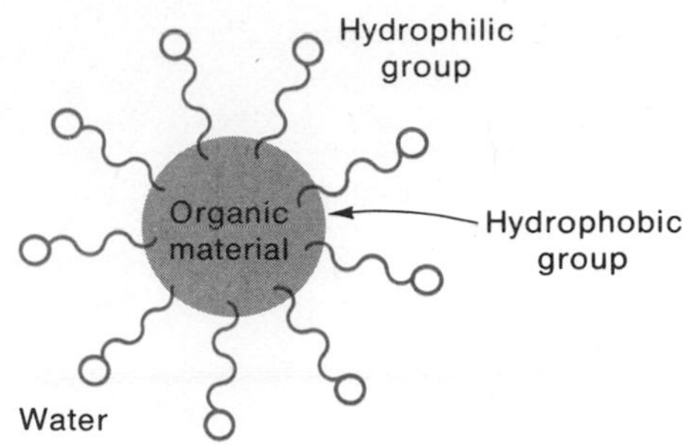

FIG. 18–5 Detergent molecules bond both to nonpolar material and to water.

Detergents may or may not be ionic (electrically charged) (Figure 18–6). The nonionic ones do not usually qualify as good disinfectants and may in some cases even support the growth of bacteria and fungi. Of the ionic surface active agents, the *anionic*, or negatively charged, ones are only mildly **bactericidal.** The *cationic*, or positively charged, detergents are extremely bactericidal, especially for *Staphylococcus* and some viruses, although they do not affect spores.

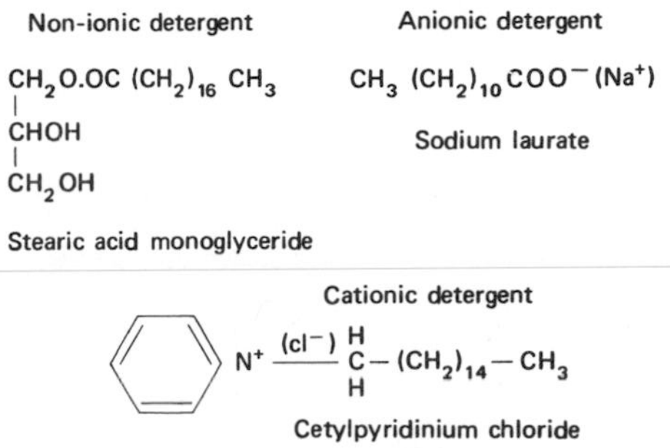

The most widely used cationic detergents are quaternary ammonium compounds, which contain four organic groups bonded to a nitrogen atom. It is thought that they act by dissolving the fatlike substances or lipids on or in cell walls or membranes. Unfortunately, there are a few problems with cationic detergents. They are absorbed by porous or fibrous materials, which may lessen their efficiency in the presence of this type of substance. Hard water, containing calcium or magnesium ions, interferes with their action. Also, they rust metal objects unless an antirust agent, such as nitrite, is added. Even with these drawbacks, cationic detergents are among the most widely used disinfecting chemicals, as they are easily handled and are not irritating to tissues in the concentrations ordinarily used.

Non-ionic detergent

$CH_2O.OC\ (CH_2)_{16}\ CH_3$
$CHOH$
CH_2OH

Stearic acid monoglyceride

Anionic detergent

$CH_3\ (CH_2)_{10}COO^-\ (Na^+)$

Sodium laurate

Cationic detergent

$C_5H_5N^+\ (Cl^-)\ CH_2-(CH_2)_{14}-CH_3$

Cetylpyridinium chloride

FIG. 18–6 Structures of various detergent-disinfectant molecules.

HEAVY METALS

Heavy metals in antimicrobials usually act by precipitating enzymes or other essential proteins of the cell. The most commonly used heavy metals are mercury, silver, arsenic, zinc, and copper.

Mercury. Mercuric bichloride ($HgCl_2$), once a popular disinfectant, is largely deactivated by the presence of organic material and is now considered obsolete. Organic mercury compounds are effective in the treatment of minor wounds and as a preservative in serums and vaccines.

Silver. At a 1-percent concentration, silver nitrate (Argyrol) is used to prevent possible gonococcal and other infections of the eyes of newborns. The chemical is placed in the eyes of the infant immediately after birth, because if the pathogens are present in the birth canal, the resulting infection might cause blindness. For a number of years, penicillin was used instead of silver nitrate. However, with increase in penicillin resistance among these bacteria, the heavy metal has been brought back into more common use.

Arsenic. Arsenic achieved fame as the first known treatment for syphilis and is still used in the treatment of protozoan infections.

Zinc. A mixture of a long-chained fatty acid and the zinc salt of the acid is commonly used as an antifungal powder or ointment. It is particularly effective for the treatment of athlete's foot. The zinc salt also acts as an astringent and aids in healing any superficial lesions, as does zinc oxide paste, which is commonly recommended for treating diaper rash and concurrent bacterial or fungal infections.

THE ALDEHYDES

The aldehydes, too, kill cells by protein denaturation. A 20-percent solution of formaldehyde (Figure 18–7) in 65 to 70 percent alcohol makes an excellent sterilizing bath if instruments are suspended in it for 18 hours. However, because of the residue it leaves, the instruments must be rinsed before use. A related compound, glutaraldehyde (Figure 18–7), in solution is as effective as formaldehyde, especially if the pH is 7.5 or more. Staphylococci and other vegetative cells are killed within 5 minutes, *Mycobacterium tuberculosis* and viruses in 10 minutes, and spores sometimes in 3 hours, although as much as 12 hours may be required. The solution is nontoxic and practically nonirritating to patients.

GASEOUS METHODS

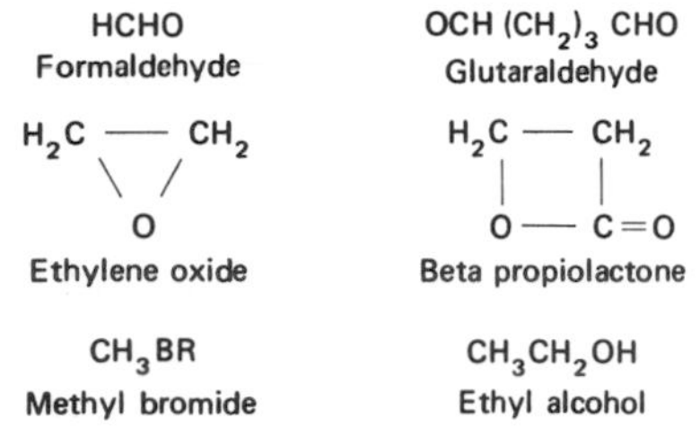

HCHO Formaldehyde	OCH $(CH_2)_3$ CHO Glutaraldehyde
H_2C — CH_2 \ / O Ethylene oxide	H_2C — CH_2 | | O — C=O Beta propiolactone
CH_3BR Methyl bromide	CH_3CH_2OH Ethyl alcohol

FIG. 18–7 Chemical structures of aldehyde disinfectants and gaseous sterilants.

Ethylene oxide. Perhaps the best-known and most often used sterilizing gas is ethylene oxide (Figure 18–7). Ethylene oxide (EtO) kills cells by acting as an alkylating agent. This means that the $CH_2CH_2O^-$ portion of the gas molecule replaces —H of proteins, nucleic acids, and probably other biochemicals. This addition of the ethylene oxide molecule is called alkylation and results in the blocking of reactive groups. In the case of proteins, this causes denaturation.

Introduced in 1940, EtO is a highly explosive gas that is soluble in water. A special autoclave-type sterilizer is available for use with EtO (Figure 18–7). chamber should be humidified for at least one hour before the actual sterilizing for highest EtO activity. To ensure sterility of critical objects, an overnight exposure to 12 percent EtO at 60°C is recommended. Because the gas is explosive in air, it must be used with caution. EtO is often diluted with carbon dioxide, freon (another inert gas), or, more rarely, methyl bromide.

The maximum allowable concentration for prolonged human exposure to EtO has been set at 50 mg/liter. One particular study showed that acute human exposure resulted in nausea, vomiting, and mental disorientation. No deaths were reported in that study. Due to the significant toxicity of EtO, recommendations have been made to license or to certify personnel who must operate EtO sterilizers as part of their job.

Unfortunately, EtO leaves a residue that is irritating to tissue, and all exposed items must be well aired before use. The procedure is slow and time consuming, and the equipment is expensive. The true advantage of EtO lies in the ease with which it penetrates plastic to sterilize contents of wrapped or sealed packages. Materials that are heat- or moisture-sensitive and *not damaged by EtO* are readily sterilized. These materials include optical equipment, catheters, heart-lung machine components, artificial heart valves, respiratory therapy equipment, and often difficult-to-decontaminate items such as pillows, mattresses, and shoes. Other chemicals used in gaseous disinfection and sterilization include formaldehyde, beta-propiolactone, methyl bromide, and ethyl alcohol.

Formaldehyde vapor. We have discussed the usefulness of formaldehyde in liquid disinfection. It can also be very useful as a gas. When formalin (37 percent aqueous formaldehyde) or paraformaldehyde (polymerized HCHO) is warmed, it releases formaldehyde vapor, an extremely effective disinfectant for instruments and various materials that have been contaminated with spores or *Mycobacterium tuberculosis.* Formalin and paraformaldehyde are not without disadvantages. The vapor has poor penetration, reacts with extraneous organic materials, and has a tendency to polymerize as a thin white film on the surface of the objects being treated.

Beta-propiolactone. Beta-propiolactone (BPL) (Figure 18–7) is stable at temperatures below freezing, but when vaporized in a humid environment at room temperature, it becomes a powerful sterilant. BPL is also a powerful alkylating agent. In this case the active group would be $-CH_2CH_2COO^-$. As a liquid, BPL has been used to sterilize vaccines, tissues, sera, and surgical ligatures. BPL decomposes rapidly on exposure to moisture and within a few hours, none is left. When used properly as a vapor, it can be relatively nontoxic. However, liquid BPL has been shown to be carcinogenic (cancer causing).

Methyl bromide vapor. Methyl bromide vapor requires humidity for activity. Although it penetrates well, its microbicidal activity, which is by alkylation, is weak. It has been used primarily as a disinfectant for fungi and non-spore-forming bacteria.

Methyl bromide in combination with ethylene oxide has reportedly been used to sterilize Russian spacecraft. The mixture is said to be synergistic, supposedly generating better penetration and kill then either chemical alone.

Ethyl alcohol. When a piece of apparatus is to be used in intimate contact with an individual over some period of time, it is often advisable to disinfect it gently and periodically if this can be done safely. In one such case, aerosolized, warmed 70 percent ethyl alcohol was used to disinfect the hoses and filter traps in a space suit testing program. Additional items, such as the heat exchanger for condensation of moisture from the air, were sterilized with 6 percent hydrogen peroxide. This combination of disinfectants was used primarily because neither left any residue that might have interfered with the testing program or posed any toxicity hazard to test subjects.

Testing Methods for Antiseptics and Disinfectants

The same standards of effectiveness are applied to antimicrobials whether they are intended as disinfectants or antiseptics. Until the early 1950s, the only accepted procedure for proving sterilizing power was the ***phenol coefficient test.***

Phenol Coefficient Test

The phenol coefficient test compares the activity of a given product with the killing power of phenol under the same test conditions. Various dilutions of phenol and the test product are mixed with a specified volume of a broth culture of *Staphylococcus aureus* or of a certain species of *Salmonella.*

At intervals of 5, 10, and 15 minutes, a specified volume of each diluent tube is removed, added to a nutrient broth medium, and incubated for at least two days. The broth medium is selected to suit the product being tested. For example, oxidizing chemicals or mercurials must be tested with fluid thioglycollate medium, while a broth made up of nutrient ingredients plus lecithin and sorbitan monooleate ("Tween 80") is necessary for testing phenolics and quaternary ammonium compounds. If the product is bacteriostatic rather than bactericidal, it may be necessary to incubate the system for as long as ten to fourteen days to determine the agent's effectiveness.

After the incubation period, the broth subcultures from the disinfectant dilutions are examined for visible evidence of growth. The ***phenol coefficient*** is defined as the ratio of the highest dilution of a test germicide that shows kill in 10 minutes but not in 5 minutes to the dilution of phenol that has the same effect. However, this value does not indicate the relative effectiveness of the product for use in disinfection of floors or walls. For example, if the greatest dilution of a test disinfectant producing a killing effect was 1:200, and the greatest dilution of phenol showing the same result was 1:90, the phenol coefficient value would be 2.2. The value is calculated by dividing the phenol dilution into the dilution of the test substance used: 200/90 = phenol coefficient.

The Use-dilution Test

Certain questions are often raised concerning products for floor and wall disinfection. What concentration should be used for disinfecting surfaces? Is a given disinfectant compatible with soaps and detergents or might it be deactivated by them? Is the disinfectant active in hard water or at low or high pH levels? What is the spectrum of activity against various microorganisms? Until the development of standard ***use-dilution*** methods by the Association of Official Analytical Chemists (AOAC), the "appropriate" dilution of a germicide was computed by multiplying the phenol coefficient by 20. While this practice appeared reasonable for some products, its applicability was not universal.

The AOAC use-dilution method has now been adopted to establish appropriate dilutions of a germicide for actual conditions. In this procedure, three bacterial species are tested against the product: *Staphylococcus aureus* (ATCC 6538); *Salmonella cholerasuis* (ATCC 10708); and *Pseudomonas aeruginosa* (ATCC 15442). (The ATCC designation refers to the catalog number for the particular organism at the American Type Culture Collection in Rockville, Maryland. Cultures of these bacterial species can be obtained from this agency.) The cultures and dilutions of disinfectant are prepared according to the specific instructions of the AOAC. The bacterial species are used to contaminate small stainless steel cylinders, which are dried briefly and then placed in specified volumes of the test product. The cylinders are exposed for 10 minutes, allowed to drain on the side of the test product tube, transferred to appropriate subculture media, and incubated for two days. The results are read simply as "growth" or "no growth," using at least ten replicates of each organism at the test dilution of the product. A satisfactory use-dilution is one that kills all test organisms, producing at least a 95 percent level of confidence. Occasionally it may be necessary to perform a 30- or even 60-cylinder test per organism in order to achieve this level of effectiveness.

The AOAC use-dilution method, although superior to the phenol coefficient procedure, should not be considered infallible. It is essential that each institution modify this AOAC procedure to take into account the use conditions and pathogens of that particular locale.

Bacteriostatic-Bactericidal Test

Many compounds may be either bacteriostatic or bactericidal, depending on the concentration at which they are used. This point can be tested by inoculating serially diluted disinfectant solutions in growth media. After a two-day incubation period, the dilutions that show no growth are subcultured to fresh media. If the growth was prevented by bacteriostatic, rather than bactericidal, action, the organisms will grow on subculture. In this manner, the concentration of a particular product that is bacteriostatic can be compared with results of the bactericidal tests discussed previously.

Tissue Toxicity Test

One approach to comparing antiseptics has been the *tissue toxicity test*. Germicides were tested for their killing effect with bacteria and their toxicity for chick-heart tissue cells. A *toxicity index* was formulated, defined as the ratio of the greatest dilution of the product that can kill the animal cells in 10 minutes to the dilution that can kill the bacterial cells in the same period of time and under identical conditions. For example, a tincture of iodine solution was found to be toxic for chick-heart tissue at a 1:4000 dilution and bactericidal for *Staphylococcus aureus* at a 1:20,000 dilution, giving a toxicity index of 1/5 or 0.2. In contrast, a tincture of merthiolate solution was found to have a toxicity index of 3.3, and tincture of metaphen an index of 10.0. Theoretically, an antiseptic should have an index less than 1.0, indicating a greater toxicity to bacteria than to tissue cells. But it is difficult to assess exactly how an index based upon toxicity to chick heart *in vitro* relates to human skin *in vivo*.

Virus Disinfection

Disinfection of objects contaminated with viruses poses a difficult problem. While some viruses, such as influenza, are as sensitive as vegetative bacteria, others, such as enteroviruses (for example, polio, ECHO, and coxsackie), are more resistant and therefore comparable to *Mycobacterium tuberculosis*. The true resistance of hepatitis viruses is as yet unknown. If hepatitis viruses are suspected, heat sterilization is the preferred method, even if it degrades the contaminated material. Cases of hepatitis virus infection have resulted because chemicals, rather than heat, were relied upon to disinfect dental tools.

SUMMARY

Historical Background

1. Preventing the growth or activity of microorganisms by inhibition or killing by means of chemicals applied to living tissues is known as *antisepsis*.
2. The concept of antisepsis was introduced in the mid-1800s by Ignatz Semmelweis and Lister.

The Use of Antiseptics and Disinfectants

An ideal disinfectant is a chemical that kills pathogens rapidly without damaging the contaminated material.

General Directions for Chemical Disinfection

1. All surfaces of contaminated material to be disinfected must be exposed to the chemical agent.
2. For efficiency and safety, all procedures should (a) be timed; (b) use properly diluted, fresh disinfectant solution, and (c) be performed in well-ventilated rooms.
3. The choice of antiseptic depends largely upon the demands of the particular operation. Consideration should be given to the fact that some compounds are irritating.

Selected Disinfecting and Sterilizing Chemicals

1. Chemical disinfectants and sterilants are used in "cold sterilization" methods.
2. A large number of such agents are used and include:
   a. *halogens:* compounds of chlorine and iodine that disrupt membranes and inactivate enzymes by the oxidation of protein.
   b. *alcohols:* three types of alcohols, ethanol, methanol, and isopropanol, which disrupt membranes and inactivate enzymes by denaturizing proteins and by removal of lipids.
   c. *phenols:* cresol and other phenolic derivatives, which disrupt membranes, usually by protein denaturation.

d. *peroxides:* hydrogen peroxide and related compounds generate oxygen gas, which inactivates essential enzyme systems.
e. *antiseptic dyes:* acriflavine and crystal violet, which react with DNA and interfere with cell wall formation, respectively.
f. *detergents:* molecules with nonpolar and polar regions, which generally act by dissolving the fatlike substances or lipids on or in cell walls or membranes.
g. *heavy metals:* compounds containing mercury, silver, arsenic, zinc, and copper inactivate and/or disrupt the functions of enzymes and cellular parts by precipitating proteins.
h. *aldehydes:* formaldehyde and glutaraldehyde kill cells by protein denaturation.
i. *gases:* ethylene oxide, beta-propiolactone, and vapors of formaldehyde, methyl bromide, and ethyl alcohol denature proteins.

Testing Methods for Antiseptics and Disinfectants

Phenol Coefficient Test

1. The *phenol coefficient test* is a standard accepted procedure for determining the antimicrobial activity of various compounds.
2. This test compares the relative activity of a given product with the killing power of phenol under the same conditions.

The Use-Dilution Test

1. Developed by the Association of Official Analytical Chemists (AOAC), the *use-dilution method* is an accepted procedure to establish appropriate germicide dilutions to use for disinfection.
2. A satisfactory use-dilution is one that kills all test organisms, producing at least a 95 percent level of confidence.

Bacteriostatic-Bactericidal Test

Many compounds may be either *bacteriostatic* or *bactericidal*, depending on the concentration used.

Tissue Toxicity Test

The toxicity of antiseptics can be determined by exposing tissue culture systems to different dilutions of the test solution.

Virus Disinfection

Disinfection of objects contaminated with viruses poses a difficult problem because of the resistance of some species.

QUESTIONS FOR REVIEW

1. Define disinfection, antisepsis, sterilization, disinfectant, antiseptic, bactericidal, bacteriostatic, and sanitizer.
2. Describe the contributions of the following scientists: Paré, Semmelweis, Lister, Koch, Neuber, and Krönig and Paul.
3. List and describe seven general directions for using a chemical as a disinfectant or antiseptic.
4. Describe each of the following chemicals in terms of the mechanism by which it kills microorganisms, its general effectiveness, and its advantages and disadvantages: chlorine, isopropyl alcohol, hexachlorophene, hydrogen peroxide, quaternary ammonium compounds, silver nitrate, glutaraldehyde, and ethylene oxide.
5. How is the phenol coefficient test performed and interpreted?
6. How is the use-dilution method performed and interpreted?
7. A chemical has been shown to prevent growth of *Staphylococcus aureus*. How can you tell if that chemical is bactericidal or bacteriostatic?
8. What is the purpose of the toxicity index and how is it interpreted?
9. Which disinfectant or particular method might be considered in each of the following cases?
   a. oral thermometer for use with tuberculous patients
   b. blood pressure cuff
   c. a child's rectal thermometer
   d. disposable needles and syringes
   e. kitchen floor
   f. dishes from an individual with the flu

SUGGESTED READINGS

American Society of Civil Engineers, Proceedings of the National Specialty Conference on Disinfection. New York: Amer. Society of Civil Engineers, 1970. *Several methods of chemical disinfection are discussed, including disinfection with halogens, ozone, and other gases.*

Block, S. S. (ed.), *Disinfection, Sterilization, and Preservation.* Philadelphia: Lea and Febiger, 1977. *An all-encompassing book on methods of testing disinfectants, sterilization, applications to medicine, and the mode of action of antimicrobial preservatives and protectants. Numerous references are also included.*

Borick, P. M., *Chemical Sterilization.* Stroudsburg, Pa.: Dowden, Hutchinson, and Ross, Inc., 1973. *Various methods of chemical sterilization are described, including antibacterial agents, ethylene oxide, formaldehyde, and detergents.*

Johnson, J. D. (ed.), *Disinfection of Water and Wastewater.* Ann Arbor, Mich.: Ann Arbor Science Publishers, Inc., 1975. *The details of the chemical and microbiological basis of the treatment of drinking, swimming, and wastewater with chlorine, bromine, iodine, and ozone are presented.*

Physical Methods of Microbial Control

CHAPTER 19

Physical agents as well as chemical ones are used to control microorganisms. Chapter 19 concentrates on sterilization through heat, radiation, and filtration.

After reading this chapter, you should be able to:

1. **Discuss general principles for preparation of materials for heat sterilization.**
2. **Define thermal death point, thermal death time, *D* value, and *Z* value.**
3. **Explain the use of *D* and *Z* values in microbiology.**
4. **Explain the mechanism by which moist heat, dry heat, and radiation kill microorganisms.**
5. **Discuss the monitoring of heat sterilization procedures and give examples of physical, chemical, and biological devices for accomplishing it.**
6. **Discuss the essential points in using an autoclave properly, and list the autoclaving pressure-temperature-time relationships for the following pounds per square inch of steam: 15, 20, and 30.**
7. **Differentiate between boiling and pasteurization as means of heat disinfection.**
8. **List hot-air sterilization time-temperature relationships for the following temperatures: 121°C, 140°C, 160°C, and 170°C.**
9. **Describe heat transfer methods that do not use air as the sterilization medium.**

10. Explain the processes of photoreactivation and dark reactivation in protecting microorganisms against ultraviolet light.

11. Discuss what is meant by the target theory in the effectiveness of ionizing radiation to kill microorganisms.

12. Explain how filters can sterilize fluids and give several examples of materials used for filtration.

In biblical times, the clothes and other belongings of lepers were burned because it was believed that purification by fire was the only way to prevent contamination. The use of heat to sterilize and disinfect is still important in public health. However, during this past century, other physical means have been developed to cleanse and sterilize. Table 19–1 summarizes the commonly used methods of physical control with the advantages, disadvantages, and applications of each.

Preparing Materials for Physical Sterilization

With all sterilization procedures, it is absolutely essential that everything to be sterilized be scrupulously clean. This means the complete removal of all debris, particularly organic material such as blood or serum. Cutting down a bacterial population through the physical action of wiping organisms off surfaces aided by the bactericidal effect of a good detergent enhances the effect of any sterilizing technique. Instruments and other metal objects should be placed in hot sodium triphosphate solution to remove organic debris before being disinfected or sterilized.

TABLE 19–1 Selected Physical Control Methods

Procedure	*Effectiveness*	*Disadvantages*	*Preferred Use*	*Recommended Exposure Time*
Autoclaving	Liquids can be sterilized; good penetration; 100% effective	Equipment is expensive; dampens fabrics; corrodes metals; new high-pressure autoclaves improved but costly	All critical materials that can withstand temperature and pressure	Generally 15 to 30 minutes at 121°C and 15 pounds pressure
Dry heat, oven	Easily handled; 100% effective	May char fabric and melt rubber; poor penetration, so procedure is slow	Glassware, wax, oils, powders	1 to 2 hours at 160°C and 170°C, respectively
Dry heat, heat transfer	Can disinfect complex mechanical equipment that cannot be handled by other methods	Items must be dried after treatment; residue left; effective only with small items	Dental handpieces and small instruments	Oils and beads: 125°C for 20 to 30 minutes; spores: 160°C for 1 hour
Ultraviolet radiation	Kills bacteria, some viruses, and some fungi; leaves no residue	Poor penetration (surface disinfection only); effects may be reversible; may cause burns to human tissue	Air and surface disinfectant	Prolonged exposure
Filtration	100% effective for bacteria and larger organisms; may be used for removal of viruses (ultrafiltration)	Some filter media are adsorptive, fragile, or electrically charged	For thermolabile liquids, for example, enzymes, some sugars, and certain antibiotics	Not applicable

For items that must be wrapped before sterilization, either paper or muslin is recommended. A loosely woven material such as muslin allows for better penetration and circulation of heat than more tightly woven fabrics. Items should be wrapped with several thicknesses and then sealed with a heat-sensitive tape. Hinged instruments should be wrapped in open position to ensure proper sterilization. The date must be written on wrapped packs when they are sterilized, since they must be resterilized if not used within four weeks.

Danger of Hepatitis Infection

In a physician's office, the greatest potential danger to the patient, excluding obvious disease, lies in the use of contaminated needles and the transmittance of serum hepatitis. Infected patients often carry the living virus in their bloodstreams for several weeks before symptoms arise, and for several years after recovery from the disease. In either case, the organism is highly infective and can cause severe illness and even death. Its transmission has been traced directly to the injection of the virus by the use of contaminated needles and syringes. Hepatitis virus is extremely stable and resistant to considerable heating, drying, and most chemicals. For this reason, any items that come into contact with serum or blood must be processed rigorously to ensure sterilization. Perhaps the easiest and surest way to protect a patient is to use the many disposable presterilized products available commercially.

Heat Killing of Microorganisms

Thermal procedures are usually simple, reliable, and relatively inexpensive. Much of the knowledge concerning the heat destruction ("thermal kill") of microorganisms comes from studies by the food processing industry.

Terminology of Thermal Kill

Although this chapter does not compare various procedures in depth, four important terms concerning the thermal kill of microorganisms should be introduced and defined:

1. ***Thermal death point:*** That temperature at which a suspension of organisms is sterilized after a 10-minute exposure.
2. ***Thermal death time:*** The length of time required for a particular temperature to sterilize a suspension of organisms.
3. ***D value:*** The time required to kill 90 percent of the organisms in a suspension at a specified temperature. The temperature is generally expressed as a subscript, as in $D_{100°C}$ or $D_{59°F}$.
4. ***Z value:*** The number of degrees of temperature increase needed to reduce the *D* value to one tenth its original value.

The thermal death point and the thermal death time take into consideration the interaction of time and temperature without any particular guidelines. The *D* value is the actual number of minutes required to reduce the viable count of microbes according to certain established guidelines. Lastly, the *Z* value relates

D values. The following example shows the relationship between these terms.

Bacillus megaterium spores have a reported $D_{100°C} = 1$ min. If the same spores had $D_{95°C} = 10$ min, then the Z value is obviously 5, the temperature increase that decreases the D value by a factor of ten. The Z value could also be calculated according to the following formulas:

$$Z = \frac{T_1 - T_2}{\log D_2 - \log D_1}$$

where $T_1 = 100$, $D_1 = 1$, $\log D_1 = 0$, $T_2 = 95$, $D_2 = 10$, and $\log D_2 = 1$. Therefore,

$$Z = \frac{100 - 95}{1 - 0} = \frac{5}{1} = 5$$

This hypothetical experiment shows that for ***B. megaterium***, a change of 5°C can cause a tenfold change in D, the time required to kill 90 percent of the organisms. With this information, we could then predict that $D_{105°C}$ would be 6 seconds and $D_{110°C}$, 600 milliseconds. Assuming that a suspension of these spores contained one billion spores per milliliter, it would take approximately 7 seconds at 110°C to reduce the viable count to less than one per milliliter. Thus, by knowing a few simple concepts and the heat stability of the material to be disinfected or sterilized, we can calculate the appropriate temperature and time duration for sterilization.

How Heat Works

Moist heat appears to kill by denaturing proteins, chiefly enzymes and cell membranes. Another theory of the killing action of moist heat involves a change in the physical state of cell lipids. This view is supported by the observation that ***Clostridium botulinum*** spores are more heat-resistant when grown in the presence of higher-molecular-weight fatty acids, which would liquify at a higher temperature. When grown in lipid-free media, the spores exhibited less heat resistance. There are probably several factors involved in the effects of moist heat.

Bacterial death caused by dry heat appears to be due largely to the oxidation of the cell components. Studies have shown that the drier the preparation, the greater the heat resistance. If dried organisms are heated in a vacuum or under nitrogen, the killing effect is slower and the organisms appear to be more resistant. Lyophilized pellets of ***Escherichia coli*** prepared by rapidly freezing and dehydrating cell suspensions in a vacuum have shown levels of resistance to dry heat close to those of spore-forming bacteria. If, however, pellets are dropped in boiling water, the *E. coli* cells are killed rapidly. Thus, the rapid denaturation of proteins and possibly the physical change in lipids appear to occur more rapidly in moist heat sterilization than oxidative effects alone.

Monitoring Sterilization

Sterilization necessarily requires the killing or removal of ***all*** forms of life, especially microorganisms. Tables 19–1, 19–2, and 19–3 summarize the conditions of time and temperature needed to ensure sterilization. Should these conditions not be met at any time, the items being treated will probably not be sterile.

It is imperative that some means of monitoring sterilizers be used. There are physical, chemical, and biological approaches to following the sterilization procedure. With either moist or dry heat, a thermometer is very important to indicate whether adequate heat has been applied to the materials. A recording thermometer is particularly helpful, since an actual record can be filed for future reference. With the pressurized steam sterilizer ***(autoclave)***, the use of a pressure gauge is also useful. It should be used with the thermometer, not in place of it, as we shall explain later.

Chemicals that darken on exposure to specified heat treatments are also used to monitor moist- and dry-heat sterilization. These substances are often impregnated in paper strips or wrapping tape in such a way that heating causes the chemical to spell out STERILE. This is useful both in identifying sterilized materials and in monitoring the sterilizing device.

Biological indicators offer the surest means of monitoring sterilizers. Two bacterial spore-formers have been selected for use (Figure 19–1). ***Bacillus stearothermophilus*** spores are extremely resistant to steam; ***Bacillus subtilis*** var. ***niger*** spores are more resistant to dry heat. After undergoing the sterilization procedure, the control spore materials are incubated at an appropriate temperature. Growth after 24 to 48 hours constitutes a failure of the sterilizer.

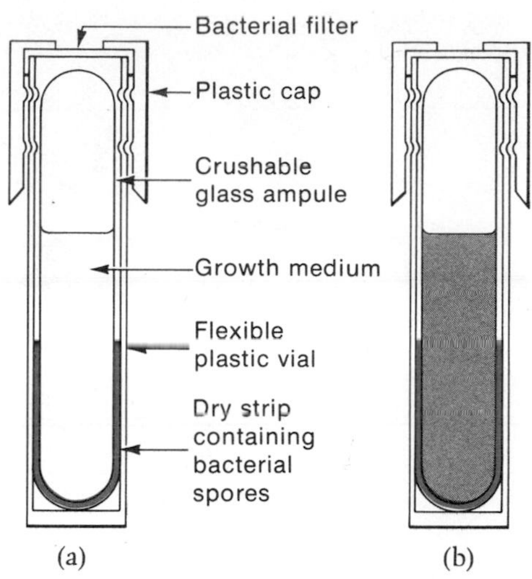

FIG. 19–1 (a) A diagram of one type of biological monitoring system (the Attest Indicator) that can be used to test the effectiveness of either steam or gas sterilizers. After the sterilizing period, the indicator system is removed and allowed to cool; the ampule is crushed between the thumb and forefinger, thereby mixing the broth medium with the dry spore strip. The preparation is then incubated. (b) If growth appears after incubation, as indicated by a cloudiness of the medium, the sterilizing procedure and/or sterilizer were not effective.

Moist Heat

AUTOCLAVING

The surest and preferred technique for sterilization is the application of steam under pressure, or ***autoclaving***. The autoclave (Figure 19–2a) consists of a steel chamber capable of withstanding more than one atmosphere, or 15 pounds per square inch (psi), of pressure. Items to be sterilized are placed in the autoclave. As steam vapor enters the chamber, the air inside is forced out a vent. When the temperature inside the chamber reaches 100°C, or boiling, and all the air is removed, the vents are closed, but the steam continues to enter. This causes an increase in the internal pressure to 15 psi above atmospheric pressure. Most autoclaves have a control valve that can be set for any desired pressure. A temperature of 121.5°C at a pressure of 15 psi must be maintained for 15 minutes for sterilization. In theory, all living material, including bacteria, fungi, spores, and viruses, is destroyed in 10 to 12 minutes. The extra time is a margin of safety. Thick packs or large liquid volumes may be held for a longer time—up to 30 minutes—to ensure that adequate sterilizing temperatures have been reached at their centers. The various components of an autoclave and the path of proper gas flow for sterilization are shown in Figure 19–2b.

In an autoclave the moist heat does the sterilizing, ***not*** the pressure. It is essential that ***all air in the autoclave be forced out*** by the steam in order to achieve the appropriate temperature. Residual air will contribute to the pressure in the system, but it will effectively lower the maximum attainable temperature. Adequate ***circulation of steam*** within the chamber is also essential. Improper loading of items can create "dead spaces" that are not heated to temperature. This, of course, may cause conditions within the chamber that prevent sterilization. When the chamber is being loaded, vessels or beakers must be arranged so that all the air may be freely replaced with steam. Packs or wrapped goods must be positioned so that the steam can reach the center of each. This usually means that these items must be tipped or laid on their sides and dry goods set far enough apart so that steam can circulate between them.

Condensation of the steam on cooler items causes the release of the latent heat from the water to that item's surface, raising its temperature to a level incompatible with life. Unfortunately, the collection of water upon cooler surfaces during autoclaving dampens fibrous materials, dulls the edges of instru-

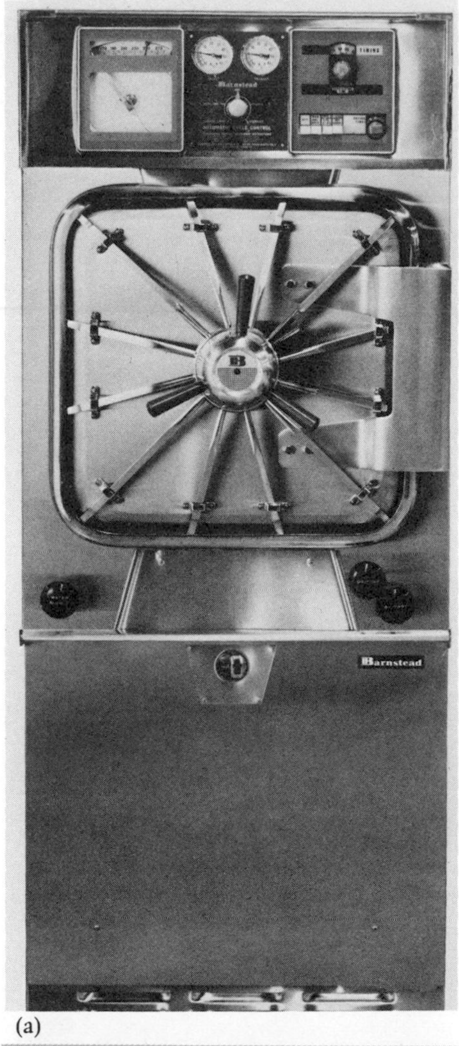

(a)

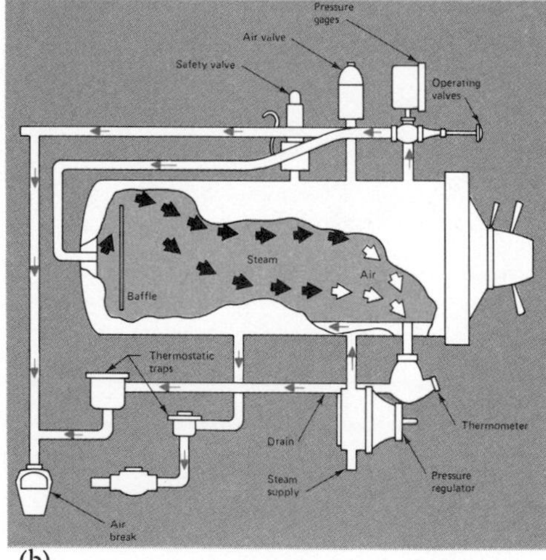

(b)

FIG. 19–2 (a) A modern automatic autoclave. *Courtesy of Barnstead Still and Sterilizer Company, Boston.* (b) A diagram of a downward displacement (gravity) sterilizer, showing various components and the path of air flow (light arrows) and steam flow (dark arrows). Safety valves are not shown.

ments, and causes metals to rust. It is recommended that a *corrosion inhibitor* such as sodium benzoate or other commercially available products be used to protect metallic items before autoclaving.

Materials can be dried in the autoclave by turning off the steam to the chamber and opening the evacuation valve. The excess pressure dissipates immediately, and as the chamber cools, moisture is removed from the sterilized equipment by evaporation.

If operating instructions are followed accurately, and the loading of the chamber is done correctly, the use of the autoclave for sterilization is foolproof. Unfortunately, the equipment is expensive and requires special installation.

Faster autoclaves are commercially available, and others are being developed. These instruments operate at higher temperatures, produced by steam at higher pressures. Table 19–2 presents steam pressures, temperatures, and suggested sterilization times that are possible with various kinds of autoclaves. It is essential to repeat that *the temperature is the critical variable and is dependent upon the proper displacement of the air.*

STERILIZING SOFT ITEMS

Surgical packs, dressings, linen, and various cloth, paper, and other materials usually require drying after exposure to the steam condensate during autoclaving. This can be accomplished by evacuation of the chamber. For sterilizing software, the standard gravity autoclave is being replaced by high-vacuum systems. Reasons for this change include shortening of overall exposure to heat, more complete drying, and shortening of the overall process time.

In a high-vacuum system, the load is subjected to a prevacuum of 15 mm Hg absolute pressure for a few minutes prior to the entrance of steam. This allows the steam to penetrate all parts of the load more rapidly than would be possible otherwise. The load is then processed at 121.5°C for 15 minutes, or at 135°C for 3 minutes. The steam is removed until the pressure comes down to about 40 mm Hg absolute pressure to remove excess heat and moisture. Then sterile air is let in to bring the internal pressure to 760 mm Hg (15 psi). This procedure produces a dry, sterile load.

BOILING

The least expensive and most readily available disinfection technique is boiling. The recommended time for this procedure is 15 minutes once the water has reached a rolling boil. Vegetative cells are killed with 5 to 10 minutes exposure. However, most spores and viruses can survive many hours of this treatment. The addition of certain substances and chemicals to the boiling bath may add to the killing power of this method. However, for critical items, a better and more reliable technique is advised.

PASTEURIZATION

Pasteurization is a method of heat disinfection commonly applied to milk, wine, and cider. The process prolongs the shelf life of such products by decreasing the number of organisms that may cause spoilage. Although this was the original intent of pasteurization, the process has attained greater significance as a means of preventing milk-borne diseases such as tuberculosis, brucellosis (undulant fever), Q fever, certain streptococcal infections, staphylococcal food poisoning, salmonellosis, shigellosis, and diphtheria. Pathogens may gain access to milk from infected cows or handlers or by contamination of the product before pasteurization. Adequate sanitation is uppermost in preventing contamination after pasteurization.

TABLE 19-2 Autoclaving Pressure-Temperature-Time Relationships

Steam Pressure in Pounds Per Square Inch (psi)	Temperature °C	°F	Sterilization Time (min.)
15	121	250	15
20	126	259	10
30	135	273	3
50[a]	146	298	1

[a]For experimental autoclave.

The microorganisms that cause the milk-borne diseases are killed by exposure to 62.9°C for 30 minutes or 71.6°C for 15 seconds. The causative agents of tuberculosis, *Mycobacterium tuberculosis* and *M. bovis,* were once thought to be the most heat-resistant of the pathogenic microorganisms encountered in milk. Consequently, they were used to test the pasteurization method for its general applicability in controlling milk-borne disease. However, as improved techniques for studying rickettsia were developed, it was found that *Coxiella burnetti,* the causative agent of Q fever, could survive pasteurization under certain conditions that the TB organisms could not. During the batch process most commonly used for pasteurization, milk is placed in kettles and heated at 62.9°C for 30 minutes with some mixing (Figure 19-3). This method does not produce the desired temperature at the surface of the dairy product—an inadequacy that became apparent only after the development of several Q fever cases traced to pasteurized milk. With improvement in mixing, the danger of contracting Q fever was eliminated.

The ***high temperature short time*** (HTST) or ***flash pasteurization method*** (71.6°C for 15 seconds) is conducted in coiled tubing or with thin sheets of milk flowing between metal plates. Proper mixing is not a problem, but adequate disinfection depends upon the cleanliness of the milk, as dirt and debris protect organisms, resulting in failure of the pasteurization process.

Milk that has been properly pasteurized has good flavor and sufficient food

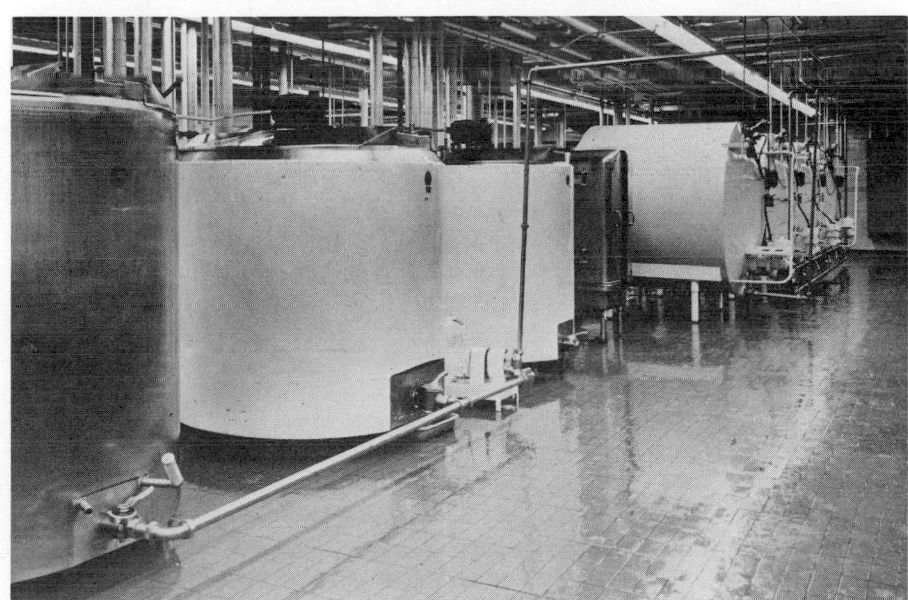

FIG. 19-3 Batch pasteurization of milk. *Courtesy of Borden, Inc., N.Y.*

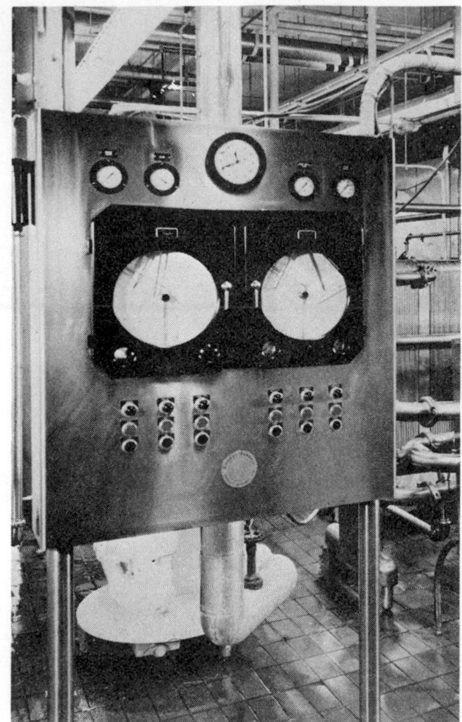

FIG. 19–4 Flash pasteurization of milk. The control panel and related equipment are shown. The central large recording devices function as visible records of temperatures used in the process. *Courtesy of Borden, Inc., N.Y.*

value. However, excessive heating causes a flavor change objectionable to some people. Moreover, the vitamin content may be substantially reduced.

The temperatures used for pasteurization are adequate to control what appear to be the significant disease agents (Figure 19–4), but they do not inactivate staphylococcal enterotoxin, a bacterial product that causes severe gastroenteritis. The organisms present in milk from cows with infected udders (mastitis) are killed by pasteurization; however, their toxic product is not inactivated. For this reason, dairy herds are frequently inspected for the presence of infected cows.

Dry Heat

DIRECT FLAMING OR INCINERATION

One of the simplest sterilization procedures is direct flaming. No special equipment, other than a hot flame, is needed, and the method is 100 percent effective. It merely requires that the material to be sterilized be heated to a red glow. No known living organism can withstand such treatment. As a practical means of sterilization, however, direct flaming has little application. Obviously, it cannot be used on flammable materials such as cloth, rubber, and plastic, nor on liquids. Moreover, instruments and other metal objects can not withstand repeated exposure to the high temperature. Nevertheless, the bacteriologist finds this technique of great value in the flaming of wire transfer loops for the inoculation of sterile tubes and flasks.

HOT-AIR STERILIZATION

Items to be sterilized by hot-air sterilization are placed in an ovenlike apparatus capable of temperatures of 160° to 170°C. Materials are placed well inside the oven to allow good circulation. Hot-air sterilization procedures require a 2-hour exposure at 160°C or 1 hour at 170°C. Because dry heat has less power of penetration than moist heat, a longer exposure time is necessary to kill all forms of life (see Table 19–3).

This method offers two advantages over autoclaving. First, there is no water present to dampen materials or to corrode instruments. Second, the hot-air equipment is relatively economical. Little installation is necessary and hot-air ovens are easy to use.

There are, however, several disadvantages. Many smaller offices cannot afford to have equipment tied up with procedures of washing, sterilizing in dry heat, and cooling. The entire sterilization process may require a total of several hours. Another limitation is that not all items can be sterilized by this method. Fibrous materials are often scorched or charred at the prolonged high temperatures necessary for sterilization. Plastics and rubber, unless they are the more expensive heat-resistant varieties, do not fare well in dry heat. Even certain kinds of solder will melt at 170°C.

But for the sterilization of glassware such as Petri dishes and pipettes, dry heat is the method to use. After Petri plates have been sterilized by this means, the oven is often used as a convenient storage facility. Dry-heat sterilization is also the method of choice for powders, waxes, mineral oil, vaseline, and other materials that must be kept dry or that do not allow moisture to penetrate.

A newer technique for dry-heat sterilization of instruments using 200°C has been proposed. Stainless steel and metal items have been sterilized in 38 minutes, including a 10-minute cooling time. Because of the higher heat necessary, this type of procedure may be of only limited use.

TABLE 19–3 Hot-air Sterilization Time-Temperature Relationships

Temperature (°C)	(°F)	*Time* (*min.*)
121	250	1080–1440 (18–24 hrs.)
140	285	180
150	300	150
160	320	120
170	340	60

HEAT TRANSFER

HEATING IN OIL OR SILICONE FLUID

One method of "dry"—nonsteam—heat sterilization uses hot oils or silicone fluids. Items to be sterilized are thoroughly cleaned and dried. They are then placed in an oil or silicone bath and heated at 150°C for 15 minutes, or 125°C for 20 to 30 minutes.

After sterilization, the instruments must be dried and the residual oils wiped off, usually with carbon tetrachloride. This type of action may cause recontamination, thus making this type of sterilization procedure unacceptable for critical items.

Obviously this procedure is useful only on nonfibrous materials. It has been used primarily for the sterilization of dental handpieces and small instruments. It must never be used on syringes or needles because of the danger of introducing an oil embolism.

This technique has other limitations. For example, oil has poor penetrating powers. Bacterial spores are unaffected unless the bath is heated to at least 160°C and the instruments treated for an hour.

GRANULAR HEATING MEDIA

Sand, glass beads, and stainless steel beads of small diameter have been tried as a replacement for liquids in sterilizing systems. These materials have the advantage of allowing other, nonmetallic materials to be sterilized. The steps in these procedures are about the same as those described earlier. They also have the same major disadvantage, namely, that the temperature may vary considerably from the center to the edges of the "bath." Moreover, large instruments should not be placed in this type of sterilizing unit, because they will cause a drastic drop in the temperature and sterilization will not occur.

Some present applications of dry heat sterilization will probably be replaced by the use of high vacuum steam sterilization, which incorporates exposure of the items to low moisture levels for shorter periods of time at lower temperatures.

Radiation

Ultraviolet Radiation

Microorganisms in the air are killed by exposure to ultraviolet light (UV). The wavelengths for killing microorganisms are found in the range of 290 to 220 nm; the most effective radiation is 253.7 nm. Compounds such as purines and pyrimidines absorb UV at approximately 260 nm. The aromatic amino acids, such as tryptophan, phenylalanine, and tyrosine, absorb UV at 280 nm.

It appears that absorption of UV radiation produces chemical modifications of the nucleoproteins, creating cross-linkages between pairs of thymine molecules. These abnormal linkages may cause a misreading of the genetic code, resulting in mutations that impair vital functions of the organism and consequently cause its death.

Ultraviolet radiation has been applied with some success to air and water sterilization. However, the poor penetration of the rays is a limiting factor. Material to be sterilized, whether liquid, gas, or aerosol, must be passed over or under the surface of a suitable lamp in thin layers if the treatment is to be effective. Persons working at or near a UV source must wear glasses to protect their corneas from severe irritation or possible permanent damage.

Commercial UV units have been developed for use in water systems where chlorination is to be avoided. Such units may have a capacity of up to 20,000 gallons per hour and have been used with wells, swimming pools, aquarium systems, shipboard drinking water, and in the treatment of sea water for shellfish aquaculture. In the latter case, chlorine was found to inhibit the feeding of oysters. Water UV systems have been shown to kill coliforms, three types of polio virus, several types of ECHO virus, several coxsackie viruses, and some reoviruses. Similar UV units have been used in the preparation of vaccines and in combination with beta propiolactone to sterilize plasma.

The potential of ultraviolet radiation as a relatively inexpensive treatment of raw water is receiving considerable study. The findings suggest that UV irradiation may be an effective tool in the disinfection of sewage effluent in estuaries. Such treatment may protect shellfish and their consumers from contamination and infection.

REACTIVATION OF ULTRAVIOLET-TREATED ORGANISMS

In experiments on ultraviolet killing of *Escherichia coli*, certain suspensions, although treated in the same manner as others, were observed to exhibit a lower incidence of mutation or death. Further investigation showed that the length of exposure to visible light to which the suspensions were subjected after UV exposure but prior to their placement in the dark incubators correlated well with the decrease in mutation or kill efficiency. This ***photoreactivation*** was found to be caused by an enzyme active in the presence of visible light (540 to 420 nm) but not in a dark environment. The enzyme involved in photoreactivation is capable of breaking the thymine cross-linkages formed in DNA by ultraviolet exposure. It thus repairs the UV-induced defect.

Dark reactivation may also occur by a mechanism that appears to be quite different from photoreactivation. The thymine-thymine linkage is not simply broken, but removed. The defect is then corrected by a DNA polymerase that replaces the thymines, using the complementary DNA strand for the necessary information.

To avoid dark reactivation, the irradiated suspension must be stored cold or in an inadequate growth medium prior to the completion of the experiment.

Ionizing Radiation

Ionizing electromagnetic radiation includes alpha, beta, gamma, and x rays, cathode rays, and high-energy protons and neutrons. On absorbing such radiation, an atom emits high-energy electrons, thus ionizing its molecule. The ejected electron is absorbed by another atom, creating a chain of ionizations, or an ionization path, in the irradiated substance. This activity excites chemical groups in DNA, causing the production of highly reactive, short-lived chemical radicals. Such radicals may alter chemical groups in DNA or actually break DNA strands, causing mutations.

According to the ***target theory***, a cell will be killed when an ionization path occurs in a significant portion of its "sensitive volume." It is safe to assume that the target, or sensitive volume, is none other than DNA. When one wades through the complicated mathematics of the target theory concerning the relative sensitivities of different organisms to ionizing radiation, it becomes evident that such cells are sensitive inversely to the size of their DNA volume. Thus the smallest cells with the smallest targets are the most resistant.

In general, bacterial spores are the most resistant and Gram-negative bacteria the most sensitive to ionizing radiation. Yeasts and molds tend to be intermediate in their resistance. One conspicuous exception is the extremely radiation-resistant Gram-positive coccus *Micrococcus radiodurans*.

Organisms can be protected to some degree against ionizing radiation by reducing agents such as sulfhydryl-containing compounds and various chemicals that bind metal ions.

Ionizing rays have been considered for disinfection and sterilization procedures. However, expense has been a consideration. The main industrial application of ionizing radiation is for the sterilization of plastic hypodermic syringes and sutures. High levels of radiation have also been used to prevent spoilage in packaged meats, without causing significant changes in the appearance, taste, texture, or nutritive value of the product. Ionizing radiation has been used for the "radiopasteurization" of fruits, sea food, eggs, and poultry products, as an adjunct to refrigeration, thus increasing the market life of these foods. Ionizing radiation has also been used to sterilize insect pests in stored grain. Since 1963, the U.S. Food and Drug Administration (FDA) has permitted unrestricted public consumption of fresh bacon "radiosterilized" with cobalt 60.

Radiation sterilization can be used to produce vaccines. A 1970 report of Reitman and his associates indicates that gamma irradiation was used to produce an effective vaccine against Venezuelan equine encephalitis virus infection. The vaccine that was formed appeared to be superior to both the live and the formalin-inactivated vaccines.

Filtration

Filtration simply involves the passage of a liquid or gas through a screenlike material having pores small enough to retain microorganisms of a certain size. The screen or filter medium becomes contaminated while the liquid or gas that passes through it is sterilized. Certain filters also utilize materials that adsorb microorganisms. Most commonly used filters do not remove viruses.

Filtration is used for sterilizing substances that are sensitive to heat. Included in this group are enzyme solutions, bacterial toxins, cell extracts, and some sugars.

Liquid Filtration

Liquids can be filtered through any of a variety of materials, such as clay, paper, asbestos, glass, diatomaceous earth, and cellulose acetate. The earliest filters of this type, developed by Chamberland in Pasteur's laboratory, were made of unglazed porcelain. A cylinder of unglazed porcelain, closed at one end, was made of hydrous aluminum silicate, or kaolin (china clay) and quartz. This was heated just enough to bind the particles in the mixture but not to glaze the porcelain formed. Varying the proportions of the ingredients produced cylinders of varying porosities. A filter arrangement with the Chamberland device is shown in Figure 19–5.

DIATOMACEOUS EARTH FILTERS

Berkefield and Mandler filters are cylinder types made of a white powder composed primarily of diatomaceous earth, the silicon residue of diatoms, and water, asbestos, and organic matter or plaster of paris. The cylinders are made of the wet claylike material, formed, dried, and baked to bind the constituents. With this type of filter, the centrally situated filter cylinder or candle is held in a mantle or funnel connected by means of a clamp or nut (Figure 19–6).

FRITTED GLASS FILTERS

Fritted glass filters are made by placing finely ground glass particles in a suitable disk mold and heating them enough to cause some melting and cohesion of the particles. The porosity of this filter disk can be controlled by the fineness of the ground particles and the fusion temperature used. Once formed, the disk is usually fused into a funnel (Figure 19–7). The device can be used with negative or positive pressure in a suitable flask.

ASBESTOS AND PAPER

Pads of compressed paper or asbestos can be used in disk form when held firmly in a two-part funnel holder. A commonly employed filter, the Seitz filter, uses asbestos pads. The two compartments of the filter are clamped together to hold the pad in place between them. This is comparable to the fritted glass disk arrangement described above.

CELLULOSE ACETATE MEMBRANE

Membrane filters of cellulose acetate are also made in disk form. However, the filter pad is usually much thinner than those mentioned previously. Membrane filters are 0.1 mm thick, compared to thicknesses of approximately 5 mm for the Seitz and fritted glass filters. The membrane is held in place on a supporting screen by a suitable holder (Figure 19–8).

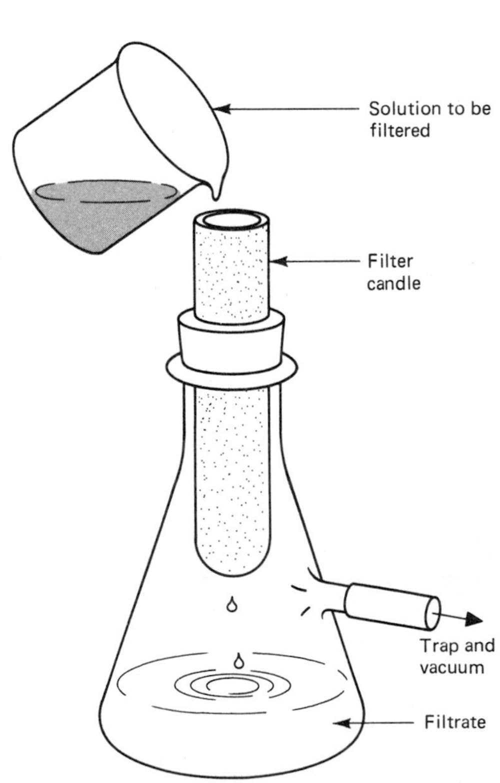

FIG. 19–5 The Chamberland porcelain filter.

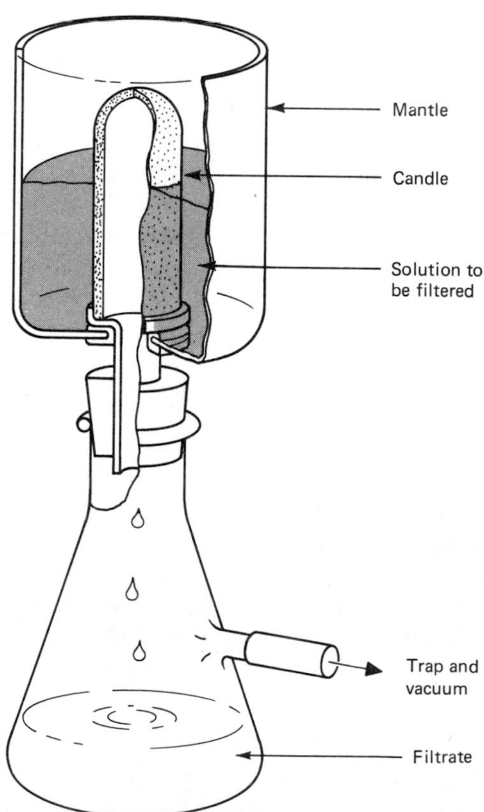

FIG. 19–6 Diatomaceous earth filtration.

All the other filters described above combine sieving with adsorption based on opposite charge effects. Thus, filtration of various organic compounds through porcelain, diatomaceous earth, glass, or asbestos devices may yield a filtrate of lower concentration than the original liquid. In addition to charge effects, the adsorptive nature of such filters removes certain components from solutions. The cellulose acetate filter, on the other hand, truly works by sieve action alone. This disposable membrane filter is being used more frequently because of its nonadsorptive nature. Applications include the processing of various pharmaceutical products and certain alcoholic beverages such as beer and wine.

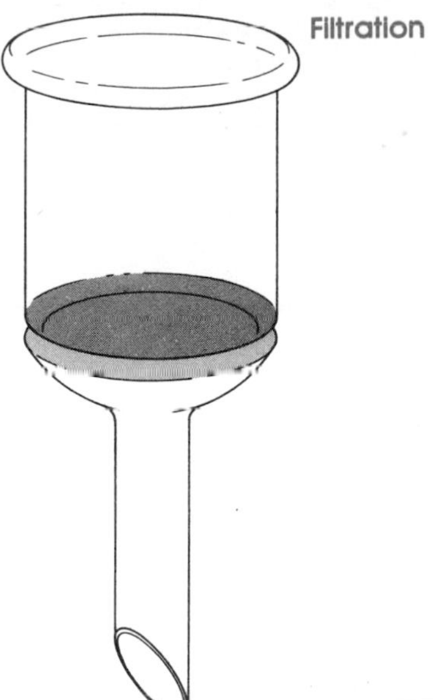

A fritted glass filter.

Air Filtration

Filtering air to reduce microbial contaminants has found significant application in hospital operating rooms and in assembly rooms for space vehicles, among other uses. Air filtration has been practiced by microbiologists for nearly

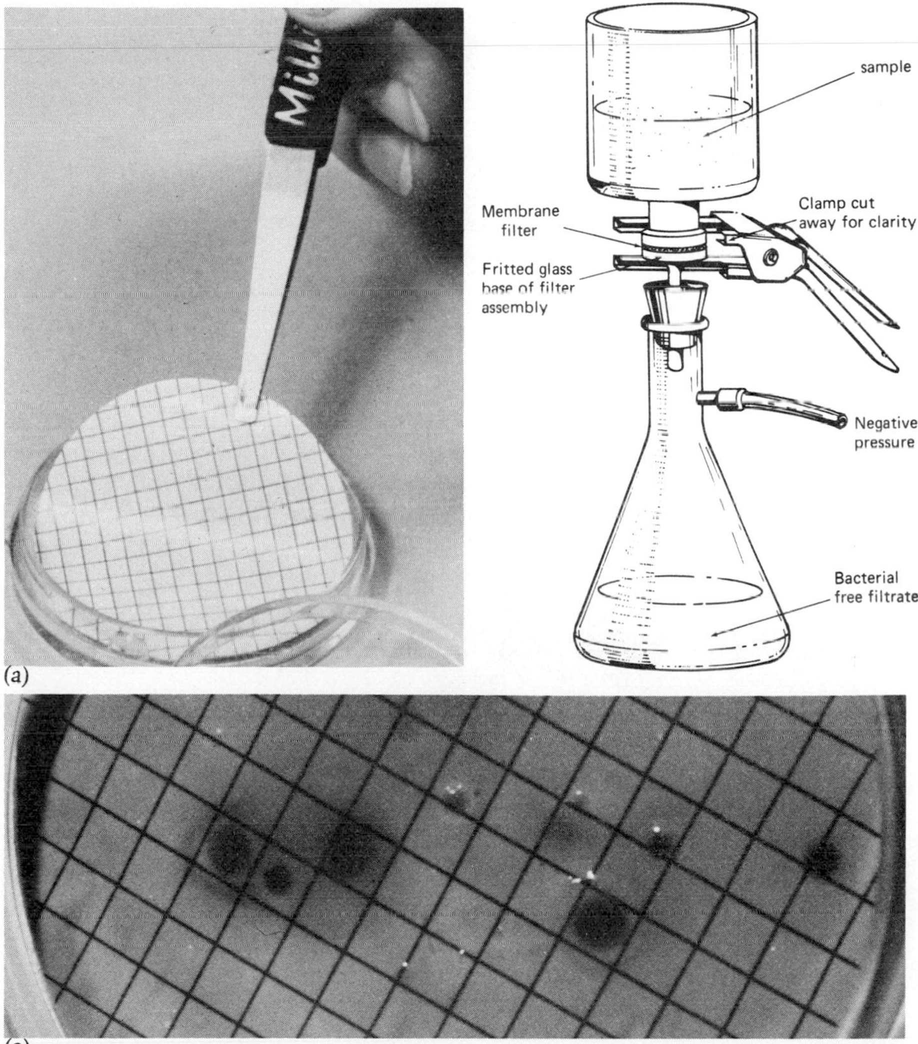

FIG. 19-8 Membrane filtration. (a) After filtration of a sample, the membrane can be placed directly on a selective and differential medium. After incubation, distinct colonial types, which can be counted and identified, form on the membrane filter's surface. (b) The basic features of a membrane filter apparatus. The sample is pulled through the membrane filter by negative pressure. Bacteria and related organisms unable to pass through the membrane's pores remain on its surface. (c) Bacterial colonies on a membrane filter. *Courtesy Millipore Corporation, Bedford, Massachusetts.*

a century to prevent contamination of culture media. Sterile nonabsorptive cotton is one of the oldest known materials used for this purpose. When it is properly inserted to plug a test tube or flask of medium (Figure 19–9), the sterilized contents will remain sterile unless the cotton becomes charred or moistened. A wet cotton plug allows bacteria to penetrate.

Surgical masks, which are made of cloth, paper, or fiberglass, behave in a similar manner. Because bacteria penetrate wet masks, masks must not be worn longer than 20 to 30 minutes and should be changed more often if necessary.

The access of bacteria to culture media can also be prevented by the use of plastic or stainless steel caps, which fit over the mouth of the tube or flask (Figure 19–9). The enclosure forces the air stream to reverse its direction to enter the tube. Solid particles continue in the original direction because of velocity and gravity. This was the basic principle used by Pasteur to disprove the idea that air contained some vital force responsible for the spontaneous generation of life. The Pasteur flask is shown in Figure 2–7.

ENZYME-COATED FILTERS

In the mid-1970s, Enright and his associates coated filter materials with enzymes to improve removal and inactivation of microorganisms. The data indicate that microorganisms probably move through filter media slowly before being blown out the other side. Given sufficient contact time (0.5 to 2 seconds) and moisture in the air stream, the microorganisms are inactivated by the enzymes. Lysozyme was found useful against *Escherichia coli* and *Micrococcus* sp.; trypsin was useful against herpes simplex and *Coxsackie* viruses, but not against two types of influenza viruses. Nucleases were found generally effective with viruses, especially RNAase for RNA viruses and DNAase for DNA viruses. Enzyme coating may significantly enhance the use of high-efficiency particulate air filter systems, described next.

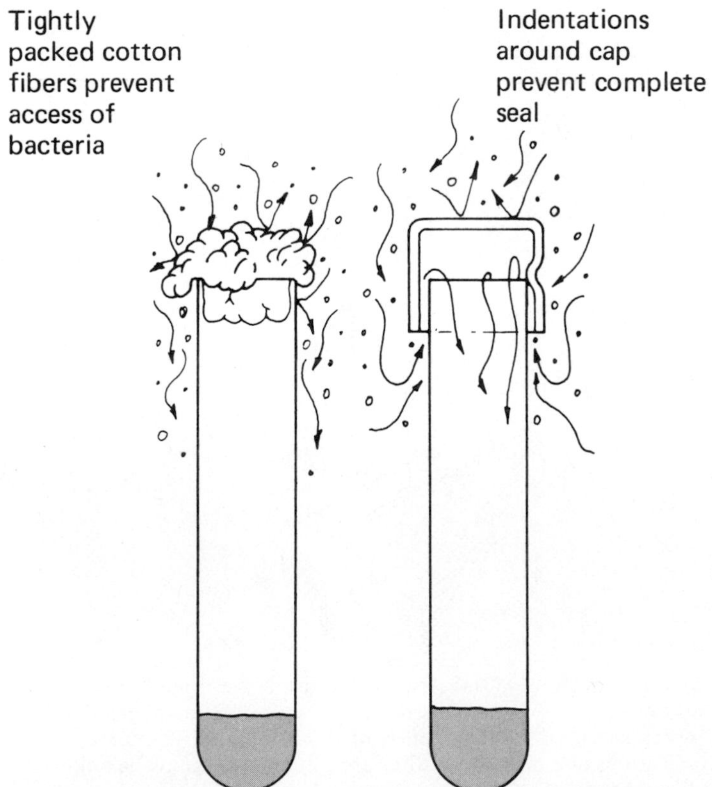

FIG. 19–9 Air filtration by means of a cotton plug and metal cap.

HIGH-EFFICIENCY PARTICULATE AIR (HEPA) FILTERS

Commercial air filtration systems for air conditioning perform with a wide range of efficiency. The application of such devices to the extensive decontamination of air requires the use of high-efficiency particulate air (HEPA) filters. These systems have an efficiency of 99.97 percent for the removal of 0.3-μm diameter particles.

HEPA filters are constructed of cellulose acetate pleated around aluminum foil and are manufactured in various sizes for different applications. One such application is the formation of nonturbulent, or laminar, flow for maximum contamination control in a given area. This use of HEPA filters is shown in Figure 19-10.

One problem commonly encountered when pouring media into culture vessels is contamination by air-borne microorganisms. To prevent such contamination, some HEPA filter systems have been designed with one entire wall consisting of banks of filters. The opposite wall is used for the air exhaust. In this system, any particles in the room that might become aerosolized (suspended in air) are removed by the average air velocity of 50 to 100 feet per minute.

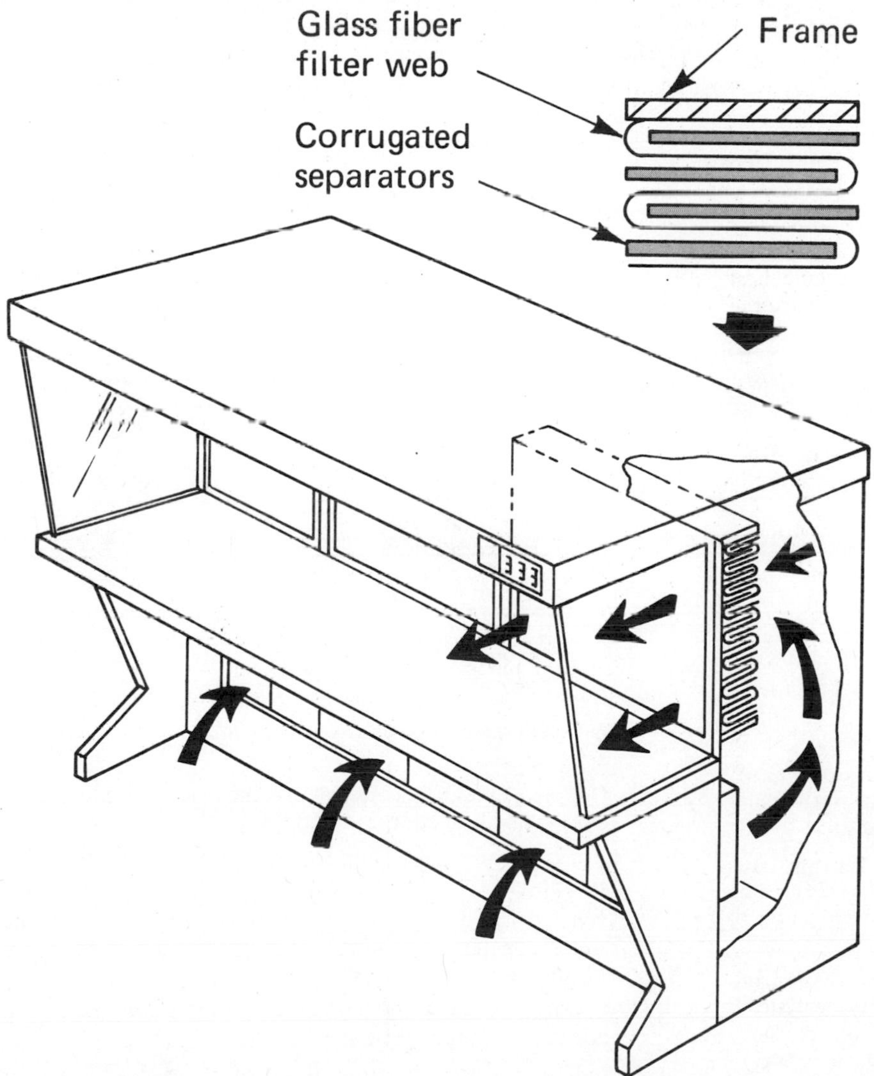

FIG. 19-10 A laminar air flow bench for the prevention of sterile media contamination.

SUMMARY

Preparing Materials for Physical Sterilization

1. Sterilization refers to any act or process that kills or removes all forms of life, especially microorganisms.
2. Items to be sterilized must be cleaned to remove all organic material such as blood or serum.
3. Wrapped sterilized materials should be labeled with the date of sterilization.

Danger of Hepatitis Infection

1. Hepatitis viruses are extremely stable and resist considerable heating, drying, and most chemicals.
2. The use of disposable, presterilized instruments has reduced the potential transmission of such diseases by contaminated needles and syringes.

Heat Killing of Microorganisms

1. Sterilization by heat is usually simple, reliable, and relatively inexpensive.
2. Moist heat kills by causing the denaturation of proteins in cell membranes and enzymes.
3. Dry heat causes the oxidation of cell parts.

Monitoring Sterilization

1. Several different devices and materials are used to determine whether sterilization is effective.
2. Examples of such sterilizing monitors include recording thermometers, paper strips or wrapping tape impregnated with chemicals that darken on exposure to specific heat treatments, and biological indicators containing bacterial spores.

Moist Heat

1. The most effective sterilization technique is the application of steam under pressure, or *autoclaving.*
2. A temperature of 121.5°C at a pressure of 15 pounds per square inch (psi) maintained for 15 minutes is commonly used in this technique.
3. *Boiling* is the least expensive and most readily available disinfection technique. Fifteen minutes after the water has reached a rolling boil is generally effective.
4. *Pasteurization* decreases the number of spoilage-causing organisms and pathogens that gain access to certain products. Temperatures of 62.9°C for 30 minutes or 71.6°C for 15 seconds are used for the procedure.

Dry Heat

1. One of the simplest means of sterilization is direct flaming, or incineration. The technique is of great value in the flaming of transfer tools during inoculation procedures.
2. Hot-air sterilization is carried out in an ovenlike apparatus capable of temperatures ranging from 160° to 170°C. The technique is the method of choice for the sterilization of various types of glassware.
3. Nonfibrous materials can be sterilized by heating in oil, silicone fluid, and low-fusion solder. Such dry-heat sterilization procedures have limited applications.

Radiation

Ultraviolet Radiation

1. The most effective wavelength for killing microorganisms is 253.7 nm.
2. Absorption of UV radiation produces chemical changes in the nucleoproteins of cells, creating cross-linkages between pairs of the pyrimidine thymine. Such abnormal linkages may cause mutations.
3. Commercial UV light units are used in vaccine preparation and water treatment procedures.

Ionizing Radiation

1. Ionizing electromagnetic radiations include alpha, beta, gamma, and x rays, cathode rays, and high-energy protons and neutrons.
2. Application of ionizing radiation causes changes in DNA molecules and leads to mutations.
3. Industrially, ionizing radiation is used for the sterilization of plastic items and the preservation of certain food products.

Filtration

1. Filtration involves passing liquids or gases through porous material having pores small enough to retain microorganisms of certain sizes.
2. Filtration is used for sterilizing substances that are sensitive to heat.
3. Some materials used as filters are diatomaceous earth, ground glass, asbestos, and cellulose acetate.

QUESTIONS FOR REVIEW

1. How would you prepare to sterilize a surgical device that must be wrapped?
2. Define:
   a. thermal death point
   b. thermal death time
   c. *D* value
   d. *Z* value
3. A bacterium has a $D_{100°C}$ value of 10 minutes and a *Z* value of 10. Explain what calculations can be made with these data.
4. Differentiate between the mechanism of kill for moist and dry heat.
5. How can physical, chemical, and biological monitoring be used to test heat sterilizers?
6. What are the key points to remember when using an autoclave?
7. What are the required time of exposure for sterilization and the expected temperature for pressurized steam at 20 psi?
8. Explain why boiling and pasteurization are means of disinfection rather than sterilization.
9. Indicate the required times of exposure for sterilization at the following hot-air temperatures: 121°C and 160°C.

10. Explain how solder and oil can be used to sterilize small instruments.
11. What is meant by photoreactivation and dark reactivation in terms of ultraviolet radiation treatment of microorganisms?
12. Explain the target theory.
13. What types of materials are used for filtration?
14. Do filters sterilize fluids? Explain.

SUGGESTED READINGS

Block, S. S. (ed.), *Disinfection, Sterilization, and Preservation.* Philadelphia: Lea and Febiger, 1977. *An all-encompassing book on methods of testing disinfectants, sterilization, applications to medicine, and modes of action of antimicrobial preservatives and protectants. A large number of references are also included.*

Brock, P. M. (ed.), *Chemical Sterilization.* Stroudsburg, Pa.: Dowden, Hutchinson and Ross, Inc., 1973. *A basic text dealing with various chemical and physical methods of sterilization, including ethylene oxide, heat, radiation, and quaternary ammonium compounds.*

Perkins, J. J., *Principles and Methods of Sterilization in Health Sciences.* Springfield, Ill.: Charles C. Thomas, 1969. *Short history of sterilization, with definitions and detailed descriptions of the methods of sterilization, explaining why they control microorganisms.*

Phillips, G. B., and W. S. Miller, *Industrial Sterilization.* Durham, N.C.: Duke University Press, 1973. *The results of a symposium dealing with various sterilization methods such as ethylene oxide, radiation, formaldehyde, heat. When these methods should be used and their applications to industry are also discussed.*

Stumbo, C. R., *Thermobacteriology in Food Processing.* New York: Academic Press, 1973. *How and where foods may be contaminated and how to control the contamination with various heating methods are the major topics presented in this publication.*

CHAPTER **20**

Antimicrobial Chemotherapy

Antibiotics represent one approach to the treatment and control of many diseases caused by microorganisms. What is an antibiotic? How do such drugs work? Do they pose any problems? These and several other topics are the subject of Chapter 20.

After reading this chapter, you should be able to:

1. **Define antibiotic and chemotherapy.**
2. **List and describe six factors influencing drug selection.**
3. **Distinguish between bacteriostatic and bactericidal antibiotics.**
4. **List at least six commonly used antibiotic drugs and indicate their respective ranges of effectiveness.**
5. **Describe the general mechanisms of antibiotic action.**
6. **Define minimal inhibitory concentration (MIC).**
7. **Outline drug sensitivity testing methods for bacteria and viruses.**
8. **Discuss the importance and basis of microbial drug resistance.**
9. **Summarize problems and limitations of drugs used in the treatment of fungus, protozoan, and viral diseases.**

Antibiotics are among the most frequently prescribed drugs for treatment and control of microbial infections. In recent years, however, problems that threaten the effectiveness of antibiotics have appeared with increasing frequency. These include antibiotic-resistant bacteria, the transfer of drug resistance among organisms, the multiple effects of the host environment on antibiotic action, and drug toxicity. Knowledge of the mechanisms and effectiveness range of antibiotics is critical to dealing with such problems.

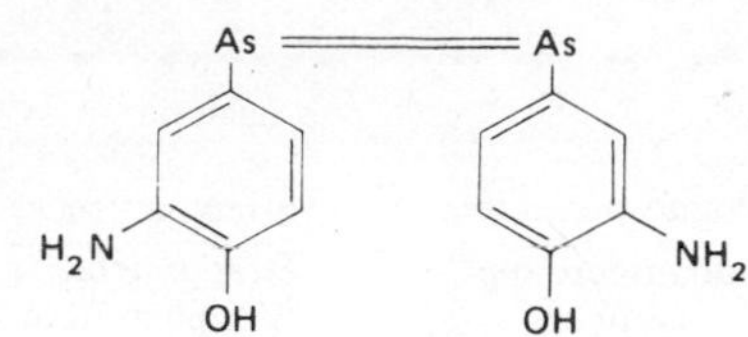

FIG. 20-1 Salvarsan, Ehrlich's 'magic bullet.' This arsenic-containing compound was useful in the treatment of a form of sleeping sickness caused by trypanosomes in horses, as well as for treatment of syphilis.

Historical Background

The discoveries of Salvarsan by Ehrlich in 1909, sulfa drugs by Domagk in 1935, and penicillin by Fleming in 1929 ushered in the modern era of chemotherapy as a means of controlling infectious diseases. Various drugs for the treatment of such diseases have been in use since ancient times. However, they were largely in the form of extracts of plants and their parts. During the sixteenth century, for example, extracts of cinchona bark (quinine) were used to treat malaria, and extracts of ipecacuanha roots (emetine) were used in the treatment of amoebic dysentery. Until Paul Ehrlich (Figure 2–11a) developed the "magic bullet," Salvarsan (Figure 20–1), for the treatment of syphilis, the selection and study of synthetic compounds or natural extracts for therapeutic purposes was largely haphazard. Ehrlich's approach to chemotherapy laid the groundwork for all modern drug development. He stressed that the effectiveness of a chemotherapeutic drug was dependent on the degree of its *selective toxicity.* Thus a functional drug would kill or inhibit the growth of a parasite without causing serious damage to the host.

Chemotherapeutic Agents

All chemotherapeutic agents originate in one of two ways: (1) as natural products of microorganisms or (2) as antimicrobial substances or agents synthesized in the laboratory. The term **antibiotic** originally referred only to chemicals produced by one microorganism that could kill or inhibit the growth of other microbial forms. Today, the term is applied to a variety of antimicrobial drugs including the totally synthesized laboratory products and the chemically modified (semisynthetic) forms of natural antibiotics.

After Sir Alexander Fleming's discovery that microorganisms produce substances that inhibit or kill other microorganisms, the search for antibiotics blossomed. Table 20–1 lists the microbial sources of over twenty antibiotics. Several of these drugs are antibacterial, antifungal, antiprotozoan, and antiviral in nature. The organisms producing them are largely soil and water species that must constantly compete for food and room to live. Thus, the production of antibiotics, which is a natural means of controlling competing microbe populations *in situ,* has been put to many uses in addition to the treatment of human infections. In recent years, attention has been given to agricultural uses of antibiotics, such as for feed additives to protect plants and livestock against infectious diseases and to accelerate their growth. They have also been used as food additives to retain product freshness for an extended period.

Antibiotics are also of great interest in research. They offer remarkable experimental devices for biochemistry—novel biochemical tools that can make a significant contribution to progress in this and related fields.

Today the continuing search for synthetic antimicrobial agents involves efforts to isolate new natural antibiotics from microorganisms as well as synthetic research. Antimicrobial activity is occasionally discovered under rather un-

TABLE 20-1 Common Microbial Sources of Some Antimicrobial Drugs

Bacteria			Fungi		
			Deuteromyces (Fungi Imperfecti)		
			Moniliaceae[a]		
Micromonosporaceae[a]	Streptomycetaceae[a]	Bacillaceae[a]			
Micromonospora spp.	*Streptomyces* spp.	*Bacillus* spp.	*Cephalosporium* spp.	*Penicillium* spp.	*Aspergillus* sp.
Gentamicin	Amphotericin B[b]	Bacitracin	Cephalosporins	Griseofulvin[b]	Fumigillin[c]
	Chloramphenicol	Colistin		Penicillin	
	Erythromycin	Polymyxins		Statalon[d]	
	Kanamycin				
	Lincomycin				
	Neomycin				
	Mystatin[b]				
	Rifampin				
	Streptomycin				
	Tetracyclines				

Note: Drugs are primarily antibacterial unless otherwise designated.
[a]Family taxonomic rank.
[b]Antifungal drugs; have also been used against certain protozoan pathogens.
[c]Antiamoebic drug.
[d]Antiviral drug.

usual circumstances, such as those reported by Schmidt and Rosenkranz in 1970. They found that local anesthetics used in obtaining lung specimens for culture were in some cases preventing the growth of the pathogens being tested. They discovered that these anesthetics were antibacterial and antifungal for several organisms.

Principles of Chemotherapy

When a pathogenic microorganism has been isolated from a patient, its sensitivity to a variety of antimicrobial agents is checked. With the results of such tests, a physician can choose the drug best suited for the patient. The administration of an antibiotic depends upon several factors, including the patient's general physical condition, existence of drug allergies, the pathogen, and the site of infection. The site of infection is particularly important. For example, certain orally administered drugs may reach high levels in urine and fair levels in blood. However, they may fail to cross the blood-brain barrier or may not penetrate well into the tissue that contains the organisms causing the particular problem.

Another factor to consider is the dosage of the antibiotic to be given. When the laboratory performs drug-susceptibility tests and reports that a certain organism is sensitive to a particular antibiotic, the result should mean that the organism is sensitive to the level of drug that can be achieved in the body. Unfortunately, it is not always possible to correlate laboratory findings with results in the body. Part of the problem is the selective concentration of chemotherapeutic agents in certain tissues, which produces drug concentrations either greater or lower than those used in laboratory testing. It is important, therefore, that the achievable levels of the drug in the various parts of the body be known, as well as the relative sensitivities of the pathogen. This relative sensitivity is called the **minimal inhibitory concentration** (MIC), meaning the lowest concentration of a drug that will prevent growth of a standardized suspension of the organism. Additional discussion dealing with antibiotic testing methods is presented later in this chapter.

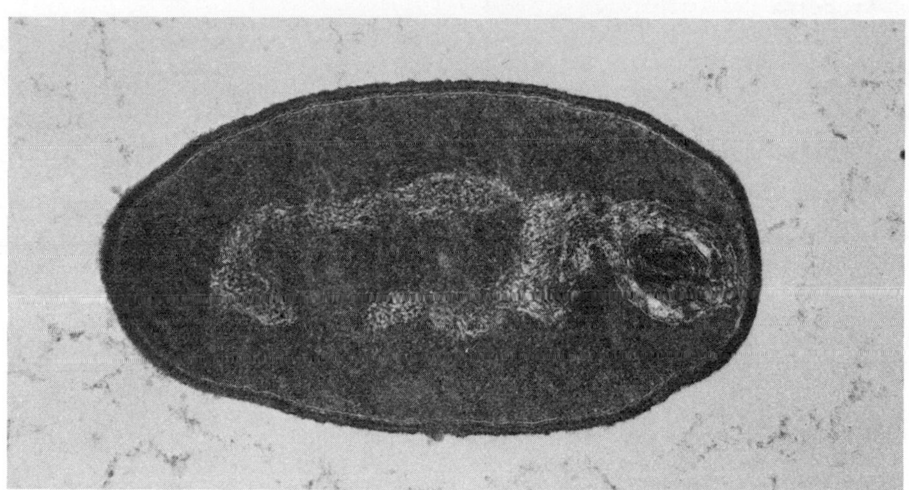

FIG. 20–2 Certain drugs can cause dramatic changes in the organization of nuclear material. In this cell the nuclear fibrils have uncoiled in expanded strands through the cytoplasm. *Van Iterson, W., and J. A. Aten,* Antonie van Leeuwenhoek *42:365–386 (1976).*

Minimal Antibacterial (Active) Concentration (MAC)

Minute amounts of antibacterial agents have been shown to produce morphological changes in bacteria and to inhibit growth of bacteria (Figure 20–2). The effects and the significance associated with the use of sublethal or minimal active concentrations (MACs) of drugs are of great importance to successful treatment of disease states and to determining the mechanism of antibiotic action.

Properties of an Effective Antibiotic

Before any chemotherapeutic agent can be considered for use, it must meet two important criteria. First, the drug must be shown to be relatively nontoxic to the host. Second, it must exhibit antimicrobial activity at low concentrations when introduced into the body of an infected individual.

Physicians frequently are faced with the problem of balancing the usefulness of a chemotherapeutic agent for a particular pathogen against its potential undesirable side effects, which may include nerve damage; irritations of the gastrointestinal tract or kidneys; interference with natural defense mechanisms of the host, such as phagocytosis; elimination of the host's normal microbial flora (this may create an imbalance of microbial populations within the body that can lead to unchecked growth and reproduction of pathogenic microorganisms); and the development of a sensitivity or allergy to the drug itself. Table 20–2 lists a broad range of antibiotics and other preparations used to treat various infectious diseases, as well as their possible side effects. Most of the drugs listed are routinely used. The association of a single drug with a particular microorganism should not be considered an endorsement. Furthermore, it should be noted that under certain conditions, some medications may not be effective.

Mechanisms of Action of Antimicrobial Agents

The use of several chemotherapeutic agents leads to irreversible injury of susceptible microorganisms and ultimately cell death. Effects of this type are referred to as *cidal.* A drug that causes the death of bacteria is termed **bacteri-**

TABLE 20-2 Chemotherapy of Selected Bacteria

Microorganism	*Disease*	*Drug of Choice or Multiple Therapy*	*Primary Effects*	*Possible Side Effects*
Gram-positive				
Bacillus anthracis	Anthrax	Penicillin	Bactericidal	Allergy
Clostridium tetani	Tetanus	Penicillin	Bactericidal	Allergy
Streptococcus pneumoniae	Pneumonia, meningitis, etc.	Penicillin	Bactericidal	Allergy
		Clindamycin	Bactericidal	Diarrhea, nausea
Staphylococcus aureus	Wound infection, boils, pneumonia, meningitis, etc.	Methicillin	Bactericidal	Allergy, renal toxicity, neutropenia (a reduction in the number of neutrophils).
		Clindamycin	Bactericidal	Diarrhea, nausea
		Rifampin	Bactericidal	Some disturbance of liver activity
Streptococcus hemolyticus	Strep throat, skin infections, meningitis, etc.	Penicillin	Bactericidal	Allergy, hemolytic anemia
Gram-negative				
Bacteroides fragilis	Wound infections, lung abcesses, etc.	Tetracyclines	Bacteriostatic	Nausea, vomiting, diarrhea, skin irritation (dermatitis), vaginitis, allergy
Bordetella pertussis	Whooping cough	Clindamycin	Bacteriostatic	Diarrhea, nausea
		Ampicillin	Bactericidal	Allergy, bone marrow depression, diarrhea, yeast infection (candidiasis)
Brucella abortus	Brucellosis	Tetracyclines	Bacteriostatic	Nausea, vomiting, diarrhea, dermatitis, vaginitis, allergy
Escherichia coli	Urinary tract and wound infections	Ampicillin	Bactericidal	Allergy, bone marrow depression, diarrhea, candidiasis
Hemophilus influenzae	Pneumonia, meningitis	Tetracyclines	Bacteriostatic	Nausea, vomiting, diarrhea, dermatitis, vaginitis, allergy
		Rifampin	Bacteriostatic	
Neisseria gonorrhoeae	Gonorrhea	Penicillin	Bactericidal	Allergy
		Rifampin	Bactericidal	
Yersinia pestis	Plague	Streptomycin	Bacteriostatic	Dermatitis, fever, kidney damage, nerve injury, hearing loss
		Tetracyclines	Bacteriostatic	Nausea, vomiting, diarrhea, dermatitis, vaginitis, allergy
Proteus mirabilis	Urinary tract and wound infections	Kanamycin	Bacteriostatic	Kidney damage, hearing loss
Pseudomonas aeruginosa	Urinary tract infection, infected burns, pneumonia	Gentamicin, carbenicillin (alone or in combination with gentamicin)	Bacteriostatic	Kidney damage, hearing loss
Salmonella typhi	Food poisoning, gastroenteritis	Chloramphenicol	Bacteriostatic	Drug-associated fever, interference with blood cell formation
Shigella dysenteriae	Dysentery	Ampicillin	Bactericidal	Allergy, interference with blood cell formation, diarrhea, candidiasis
Acid-fast or Partially Acid-fast Microorganisms				
Actinomyces israeli	Actinomycosis	Sulfonamides	Bacteriostatic	Vertigo, malaise, headache, fever, dermatitis, blood in the urine (hematuria)
Mycobacterium leprae	Leprosy	Diamino diphenyl sulphone (DDS or dapsone)	Probably bacteriostatic	Vertigo, malaise, headache, fever, reduction in white blood cells, hematuria
Mycobacterium tuberculosis	Tuberculosis	Isonicotinic hydrazide	Bacteriostatic	Renal toxicity, constipation, gastritis, nerve injury, drowsiness
		Para-amino-salicylate	Bacteriostatic	
		Streptomycin	Bactericidal	Dermatitis, fever, kidney damage, and nerve injury
		Rifampin	Bactericidal	Some disturbance of liver function
Nocardia asteroides	Nocardiosis	Sulfonamides	Bacteriostatic	Vertigo, malaise, headache, fever, dermatitis, hematuria

TABLE 20-2 Chemotherapy of Selected Bacteria (Continued)

Microorganism	Disease	Drug of Choice or Multiple Therapy	Primary Effects	Possible Side Effects
Other Bacterial Species				
Chlamydia trachomatis	Trachoma	Tetracyclines	Bacteriostatic	Nausea, vomiting, diarrhea, dermatitis, vaginitis, allergy
Coxiella burnetti	Q fever	Tetracyclines	Bacteriostatic	Nausea, vomiting, diarrhea, dermatitis, vaginitis, allergy
Chlamydia psittaci	Psittacosis	Tetracyclines	Bacteriostatic	Nausea, vomiting, diarrhea, dermatitis, vaginitis, allergy
Mycoplasma pneumoniae	Primary atypical pneumonia	Tetracyclines	Bacteriostatic	Nausea, vomiting, diarrhea, dermatitis, vaginitis, allergy
Rickettsia rickettsii	Rocky Mountain spotted fever	Tetracyclines	Bacteriostatic	Nausea, vomiting, diarrhea, dermatitis, vaginitis, allergy
Treponema pallidum	Syphilis	Penicillin	Bactericidal	Allergy

cidal. Those chemotherapeutic agents that do not cause cell death but inhibit growth produce a *static* effect. Dilution or removal of such drugs enables microorganisms to resume growth and reproductive activities. A chemotherapeutic agent that inhibits bacteria is referred to as **bacteriostatic.**

Antibiotics that inhibit a single bacterial group or only a few species are considered to have a narrow, or limited, spectrum of activity. Other drugs active against several Gram-positive and Gram-negative bacteria are said to have a *broad spectrum*.

Whether a drug exerts a static or cidal effect can be an important factor on the outcome of certain diseases. Static chemotherapeutic agents are dependent on the host's immune mechanisms for the eventual elimination of pathogenic microorganisms. If such mechanisms are ineffective, relapses or a worsening of the host's condition can result. Cidal drugs usually are independent in their actions and cause their effects directly on disease agents.

Specific Mechanisms of Action

There are several major mechanisms of action by which antimicrobial agents can inhibit or kill microorganisms (Table 20–3). These include (1) inhibition of the formation of a specific product of metabolism (metabolite); (2) inhibition of cell wall formation (Figure 20–6); (3) inhibition of protein synthesis; (4) irreversible damage to the cell membrane; and (5) inhibition of nucleic acid synthesis (Figure 20–2). The following sections will describe the specific effects of some commonly used antimicrobial drugs.

Some Commonly Used Antimicrobial Drugs

Sulfa Drugs

Gerhard Domagk reported in 1935 that a red dye compound, prontosil, was chemotherapeutic for streptococcal infections in mice. This drug was not active *in vitro* and supported Ehrlich's assumption that a chemotherapeutic agent must be modified in the body in order to be effective. By 1936, scientists at the Pasteur Institute in Paris had discovered that prontosil was converted to sulfanilamide (Figure 20–3), which was active both *in vitro* and *in vivo*.

TABLE 20-3 Summary of Mechanisms of Action for Some Commonly Used Antibiotics

Antibiotic	*Process Affected*
Bacitracin Cephalosporin Cycloserine Penicillin Vancomycin	Cell wall synthesis
Aminoglycosides Chloramphenicol Lincomycin Puromycin Tetracyclines	Protein synthesis
Mitomycins	DNA synthesis
Actinomycin Rifamycins	RNA synthesis

Sulfanilamide is but one of many types of sulfa drugs. Each of these compounds has certain peculiarities related to their solubilities and relative toxicities.

RANGE OF ACTIVITY

Sulfa drugs are used for treatment of *Escherichia coli* urinary tract infections, meningococcal infections, certain protozoan diseases, chancroid, trachoma, and infections caused by *Nocardia* spp. They are not particularly effective in the presence of dead tissue or pus and therefore are used only for mild to moderate infections.

MECHANISM OF ACTION

Sulfa drugs are bacteriostatic, acting upon bacteria that are growing and actively metabolizing. Their mechanism of action depends upon the similarity of their structure to para-aminobenzoic acid (PABA), which is a part of the essential coenzyme and growth factor folic acid (Figure 20–3a).

Thus, a sulfonamide may enter a metabolic reaction in place of the PABA and interfere with the synthesis of folic acid. A lack of this coenzyme will disrupt normal cellular activities. Sulfonamides are active against bacteria that synthesize their own folic acid, and cannot differentiate between these compounds and PABA. The mechanism here is an example of competitive inhibition of enzymes. Sulfa drugs do not usually inhibit growth of cells that require preformed folic acid (Figure 20–3b). The level of sensitivity of the sulfa drugs varies widely from one bacterial species to another.

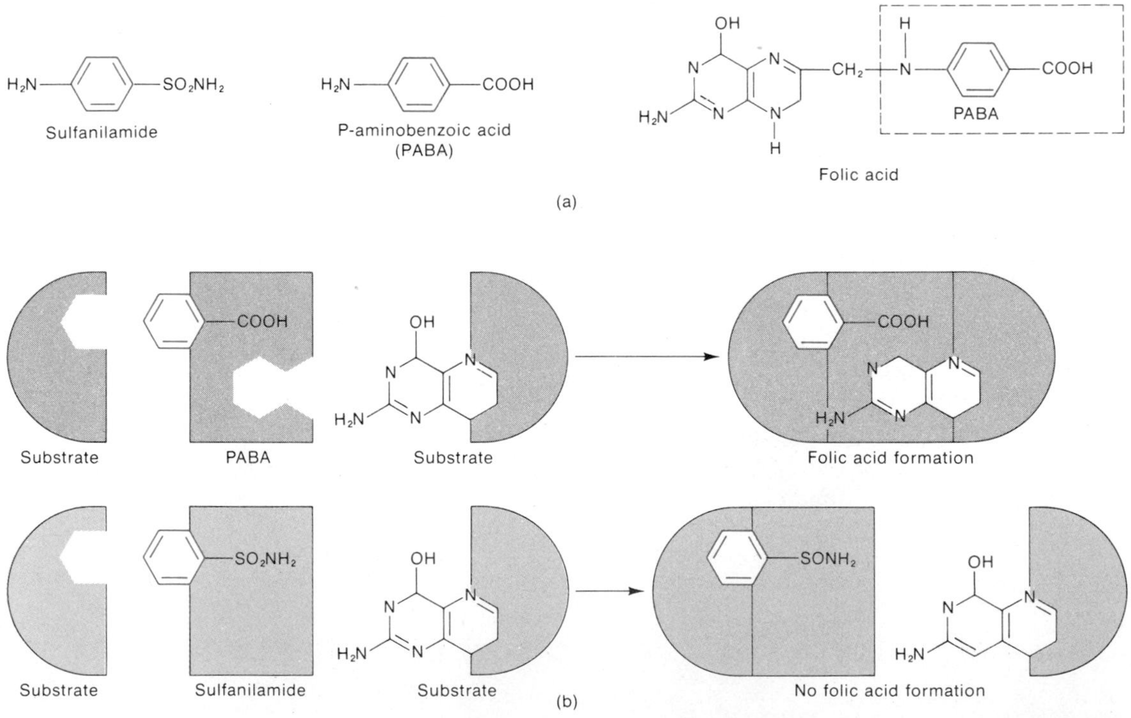

FIG. 20–3 Sulfa drugs and their mode of action. (a) The formulas of the simplest sulfa drug, sulfanilamide, and para-aminobenzoic acid (PABA), an important compound needed by many bacteria for the formation of the essential growth factor, or coenzyme, folic acid. Note the position of PABA in folic acid. (b) Para-aminobenzoic acid normally combines with other reacting molecules (substrates) to form the pure product folic acid (top). Sulfonamides inhibit the growth of susceptible organisms by replacing or competing with PABA in this type of reaction, thus preventing the formation of folic acid (bottom).

Penicillins

Penicillin, the first widely used antibiotic, was introduced to clinical use for the general public in 1945. Figure 20–4 shows the basic structure of penicillin as it appears in (1) the natural product, Penicillin G; (2) a semisynthetic penicillin, ampicillin; (3) another semisynthetic penicillin, carbenicillin; and (4) cephalosporin N, one of a new group of natural and semisynthetic "penicillins" called cephalosporins.

The cephalosporin antibiotics are included with penicillin because of the extreme similarities in basic structure. The portions of the molecules shown in color in Figure 20–4 differ from the natural Penicillin G, while those portions to the right are identical.

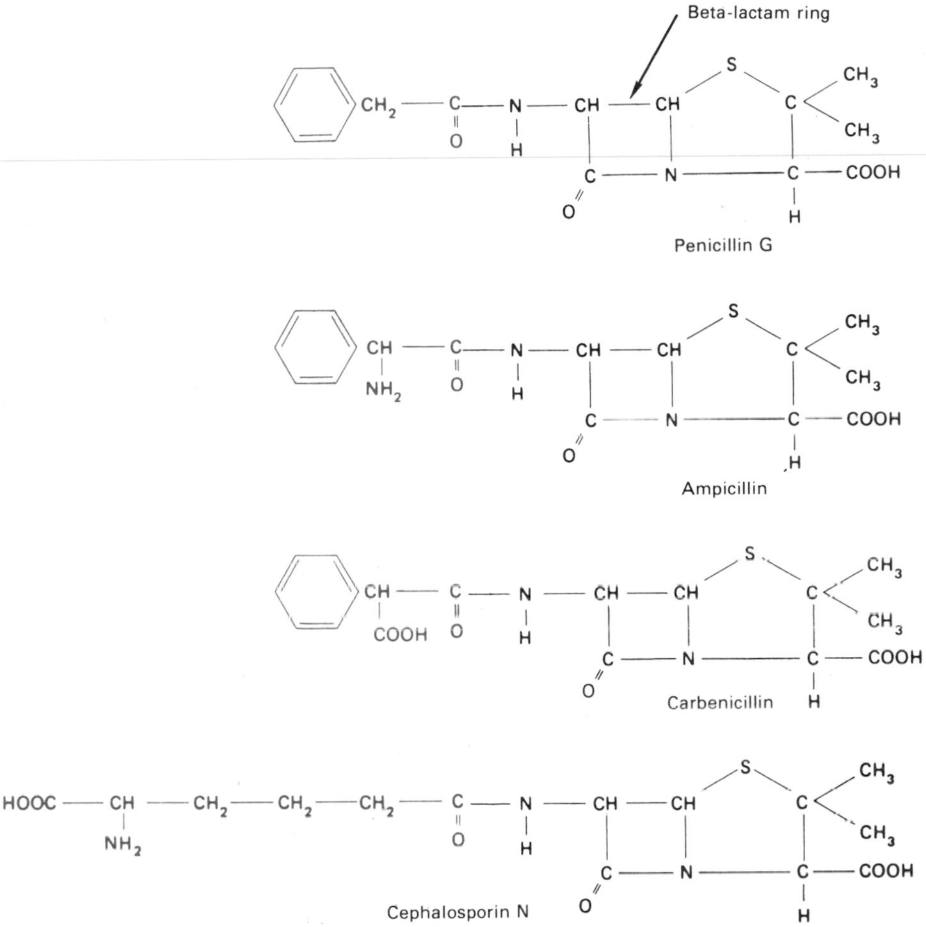

Beta-lactam ring

Penicillin G

Ampicillin

Carbenicillin

Cephalosporin N

FIG. 20–4 Four antibiotics of the penicillin family. The penicillin core is shown on one side for each of the antibiotics. The beta-lactam ring is also indicated.

Ampicillin was developed in an effort to obtain improved drugs. The slight modifications of the molecule by the addition of an amino (NH_2) group converted penicillin into a broader-spectrum chemotherapeutic agent.

Disodium carbenicillin was the first semisynthetic penicillin to attain extensive clinical use specifically because of its pronounced activity against selected Gram-negative organisms, primarily *Pseudomonas* and certain strains of *Proteus.* The main application of this antibiotic, alone or in combination with gentamicin, has been for serious *Pseudomonas* infections such as severe burns and infections of the pulmonary and urinary systems. Microbial resistance to carbenicillin appears to develop primarily through inappropriate use of the drug.

The original cephalosporin-producing molds, *Cephalosporium* spp., were isolated from salt water by Brotzu in 1945. As with penicillin, additional work showed that other antibiotics obtained from these molds were more effective than the original. By making chemical changes in their basic formula, several new broad-spectrum antibiotics were developed. Among those currently available for use are cephalothin, cephalexin, cefazolin, and cephaloridine.

RANGE OF ACTIVITY

Penicillin G and closely related drugs are highly active against sensitive strains of Gram-positive and Gram-negative cocci, Gram-positive bacilli, and Gram-positive and Gram-negative anaerobic bacteria. At high concentrations, which can be produced in the urinary tract, penicillin is known to be effective against *E. coli* and *Proteus mirabilis*. However, ampicillin is the drug preferred because it can be used in smaller concentrations against *E. coli*, *P. mirabilis*, *Hemophilus influenzae*, *Salmonella*, and *Shigella* spp., as well as the other organisms that respond to penicillin. The spectrum of the cephalosporins is similar to that of ampicillin, but they are active also against pneumococci, *H. influenzae*, and most anaerobic bacteria. Unlike penicillin and ampicillin, cephalosporins are not inactivated by penicillinase, an enzyme produced by penicillin-resistant staphylococci, but they are susceptible to cephalosporinases produced by various bacteria.

MECHANISM OF ACTION

All four of these chemotherapeutic agents are bactericidal, and all act by interfering with cell wall synthesis. The portion of their structure associated with the four-member lactam ring is comparable to a region of the dipeptide alanylalanine (Figure 20–5).

Apparently the penicillins are incorporated in cell walls in place of this compound. Penicillin is effective only during the growth stages of sensitive organisms, since fully formed cell walls are not sensitive to its action. Sensitive bacterial cells grown in the presence of penicillin or modified forms of the antibiotic have unusual shapes and abnormal internal organization (Figure 20–6).

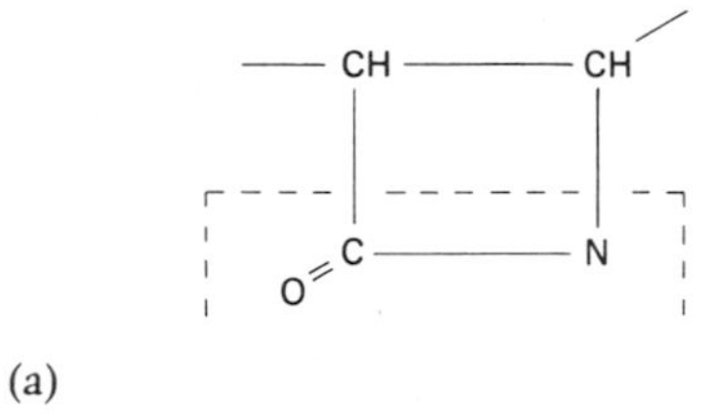

(a)

(b)

FIG. 20–5 The portion of the lactam ring of penicillin (a) that is comparable to a region of the dipeptide (alanylalanine) (b) it prevents from being incorporated into the developing bacterial cell wall.

Clindamycin: A Useful Alternative to Penicillin-cephalosporin Antibiotics

Clindamycin is a semisynthetic antibiotic active mainly against Gram-positive bacteria. The antibiotic inhibits pneumococci, streptococci, and most *Staphylococcus aureus* isolates. It is not active against the commonly encountered Gram-negative rods. Clindamycin acts by inhibiting protein synthesis in the bacterial cell.

Chloramphenicol and the Tetracyclines

Chloramphenicol and one naturally occurring tetracycline, chlortetracycline (Figure 20–7), are both produced by species of *Streptomyces*. These compounds are bacteriostatic, broad-spectrum antimicrobials having the same mechanism of action. Both are thought to disrupt protein synthesis by blocking the transfer of activated amino acids from transfer RNA to the growing polypeptide chain. Two new synthetic tetracyclines, doxycycline and minocycline, which have become available in recent years, differ only in minor respects from other tetracyclines.

RANGE OF ACTIVITY

Chloramphenicol is particularly useful for infections caused by many Gram-positive and Gram-negative bacteria, rickettsia, and chlamydia. It is the drug of choice for typhoid fever. However, because of its highly toxic effect on blood-cell-forming tissues, chloramphenicol must be reserved for cases resistant to other forms of treatment.

Chlortetracycline is also active against a variety of Gram-positive and Gram-negative bacteria, as well as the rickettsia and chlamydia. It is much less toxic than chloramphenicol and can be used more freely. However, it is inferior to chloramphenicol for *Salmonella* infections.

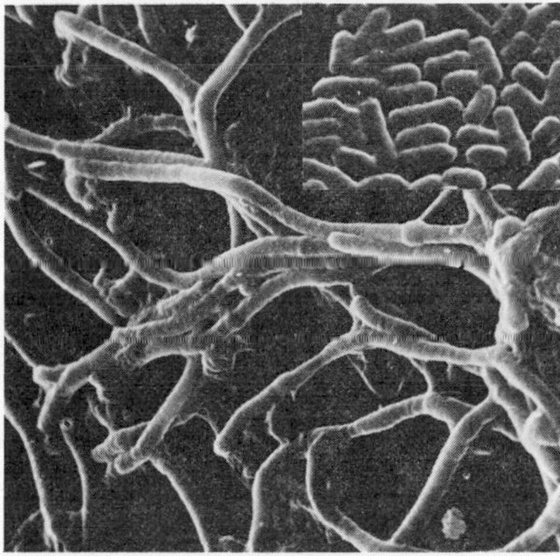

(a)

(b)

FIG. 20–6 The effects of penicillin and its modified forms on bacteria. Even small amounts of these antibiotics are associated with changes in morphology and/or growth inhibition. (a) Antibiotic treatment with ampicillin converts *Salmonella typhimurium* from the form shown in the inset to long filaments. (b) The formation of several crosswalls in *Staphylococcus aureus* after exposure to a sublethal inhibitory concentration of penicillin. *Lorian, V., et al.*, Proceedings of the 10th International Congress of Chemotherapy, *American Society for Microbiology, pp. 72–78 (1978).*

Aminoglycosides (Streptomycins)

The aminoglycosides include streptomycin, kanamycin, and gentamicin (Figure 20–8).

The name of this group of antibiotics is derived from the complex structure, which includes the connection of two or three components by glycosidic bonds (Figure 20–8). Streptomycin was discovered by Waksman and Schatz in 1944 as a product of *Streptomyces griseus.* Kanamycin was isolated from *Streptomyces kanamyceticus.* Gentamicin is produced by species of *Micromonospora,* which are closely related to the *Streptomyces.*

RANGE OF ACTIVITY

Streptomycin's primary activity is against Gram-negative bacteria, enterococci, and *M. tuberculosis.* Since organisms rapidly develop resistance to this drug, it must be used in combined therapy. When combined with penicillin or ampicillin, it is particularly effective against enterococcus infections, especially endocarditis. In the treatment of tuberculosis, it can be combined with isonicotinic hydrazide (INH) and para-aminosalicylic acid (PAS).

Kanamycin is active against a wide variety of Gram-positive and Gram-negative bacteria and *M. tuberculosis.* It is not particularly effective against *Pseudomonas* spp., various streptococci, or anaerobes.

Although gentamicin is a broad-spectrum drug, it is primarily active against infections from Gram-negative bacteria and is a drug of choice for *Pseudomonas* infections. It is effective against most *Proteus* spp., but kanamycin is usually the more effective drug.

All three aminoglycosides may be toxic to kidneys and auditory nerves.

MECHANISM OF ACTION

These aminoglycosides, although somewhat different in spectrum, are all bactericidal and interfere with protein synthesis. They appear to act by combining with a subunit of the ribosome, causing a misreading of the genetic code.

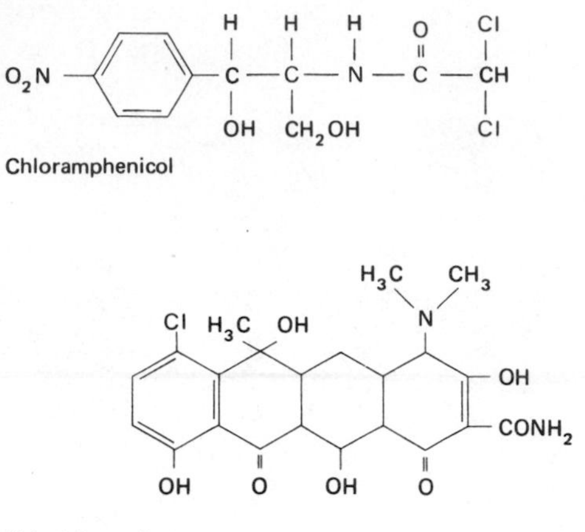

Chloramphenicol

Chlortetracycline

FIG. 20-7 Chloramphenicol and Chlortetracycline.

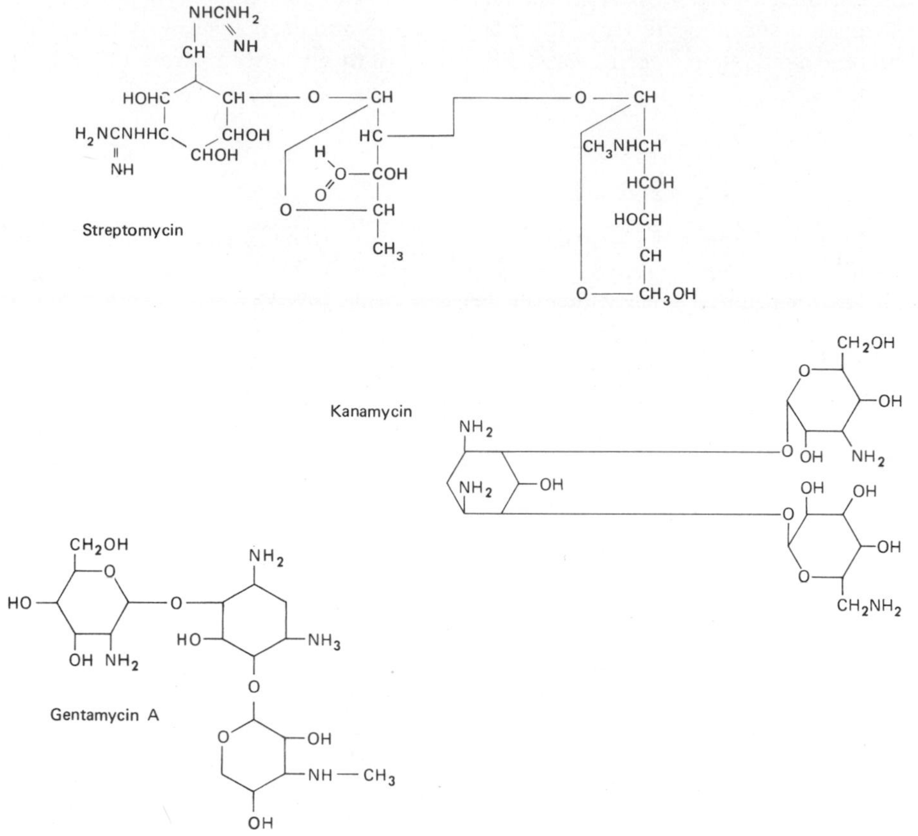

Streptomycin

Kanamycin

Gentamycin A

FIG. 20-8 Representative antibiotics of the aminoglycoside group. The parts of these and other antibiotics are connected by glycosidic bonds, which are links between the hydroxyl (OH^-) group of one molecule and the aldehyde group ($\overset{O}{\underset{C}{\|}}$— H) of another molecule. These glycosidic linkages are indicated for these antibiotics.

Polypeptides

Two of the more common drugs in this group are polymyxin B and colistin (polymyxin E). The members of this group can be isolated from ***Bacillus polymyxa***. Colistin was also found in a ***Bacillus colistinus*** culture from Japanese soil.

RANGE OF ACTIVITY

These drugs are effective against most Gram-negative bacteria, with the exception of ***Proteus*** spp. They are used with gentamicin for ***Pseudomonas*** infections.

MECHANISM OF ACTION

Polymyxin B and colistin act as detergents on the microbial membranes, causing leakage of essential cytoplasmic components. They may be bacteriostatic or bactericidal, depending upon the dosage used and the relative number of organisms to be treated. Both compounds are somewhat toxic. However, kidney damage and nerve injury are usually reversible.

Antimycobacterial Drugs

Two drugs commonly used in combination with streptomycin are isonicotinic hydrazide (INH) and para-aminosalicylic acid (PAS) (Figure 20–9).

RANGE OF ACTIVITY

After the discovery that the activity of sulfa drugs is based on competition with PABA in microbial metabolism, investigators set out to apply this type of mechanism to other organisms. Salicylic acid was found to stimulate the metabolism of *Mycobacterium tuberculosis*. On the basis of this finding, para-aminosalicylic acid was shown active against bovine tuberculosis in 1946.

In acting against tuberculosis, INH penetrates into the tissues so well that it can act against bacilli located in tubercles and inside phagocytes—unlike streptomycin and PAS. Isonicotinic hydrazide is relatively nontoxic, but it may cause renal (kidney) complications, particularly in patients with renal tuberculosis.

(a) O, C—NHNH$_2$, N

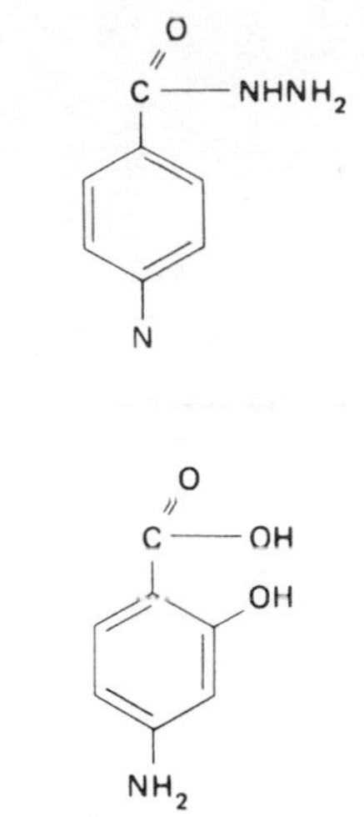

(b) O, C—OH, OH, NH$_2$

FIG. 20–9 Two antimycobacterial drugs. (a) Isonicotinic hydrazide. (b) Para-aminosalicylic acid.

MECHANISM OF ACTION

Isonicotinic hydrazide is bacteriostatic initially, becoming bactericidal later. The activity appears to be due to its incorporation into nicotinamide adenine dinucleotide (NAD) or nicotinamide adenine dinucleotide phosphate (NADP), both of which are coenzymes. Isonicotinic hydrazide also resembles vitamin B and probably interferes with those enzymes that incorporate vitamin B_6 into a coenzyme molecule. Thus, INH appears to act by blocking essential enzyme activity due to its incorporation into coenzymes. PAS acts as sulfa drugs do, by interference with PABA metabolism (Figure 20–3b). PAS is a relatively ineffective bacteriostatic drug. The prime value of this antitubercular agent is its activity in delaying the emergence of resistance to streptomycin and INH. The usual side effects of PAS are nausea and vomiting, which are commonly prevented by the simultaneous administration of an antacid compound.

Rifampin

Rifampin is a relatively new semisynthetic derivation of rifamycin B produced by *Streptomyces mediterranei*. This is a broad-spectrum drug that is chemically unrelated to other antibiotics. It is active against Gram-positive and Gram-negative organisms and is highly effective in the treatment of tuberculosis. The development of rifampin is a major advance in antituberculosis chemotherapy, since it is of great value in patients with drug-resistant organisms. Microbial resistance to rifampin can also develop, however. Therefore, in antituberculosis therapy it is used in combination with other drugs. Rifampin interferes with nucleic acid synthesis.

Mechanisms of Drug Resistance

When a great many antimicrobial agents became available for chemotherapy in the early 1950s, these "wonder drugs" were thought to be the final answer to the control of infections. Penicillin, in particular, was added to items such as chewing gum, mouthwash, and toothpaste. In addition to this indiscriminate use of drugs, many physicians routinely prescribed them for minor infections. Partly as a result of drug misuse, microorganisms such as *Staphylococcus aureus* became resistant to these agents and consequently became more difficult to eliminate. Even with the development of more and more specific and broad-spectrum drugs, resistance remains a problem that requires constant consideration.

Some mechanisms by which organisms develop resistance to antimicrobial agents include (1) an enzymatic alteration of the drug, (2) a change in the selective permeability of the cell walls and membranes of organisms, (3) a change in the sensitivity of affected enzymes, and (4) an increased production of a competitive substrate. One example of antibiotic inactivation is the production of the enzyme penicillinase by *Staphylococcus aureus*. Since the portion of the penicillin molecule attacked by the enzyme is a beta lactam ring (Figure 20–4), the enzyme is more correctly known as penicillin-beta lactamase. The pharmaceutical industry has attacked this particular problem of penicillin resistance by modifying the structure of the drug. As a result, the drugs methicillin, oxacillin (Figure 20–10), and nafcillin have been produced. These compounds are effective against penicillinase-producing staphylococci.

One example of drug resistance due to changes in cellular permeability and sensitivity involves streptomycin. Apparently streptomycin interferes with translation of genetic information involving mRNA and ribosomes. Resistance here can occur by the development of a decreased sensitivity of the enzymes concerned with attaching mRNA to ribosomes. Streptomycin also appears to affect cell membrane permeability. Resistance, therefore, can occur because of changes in the selective permeability of the cell.

Sulfonamides also seem to act both at an enzymic level (the pathway from para-aminobenzoic acid to folic acid) and at membrane sites. Resistance to sulfonamides may therefore be due to changes in enzyme sensitivity and/or selective permeability. With sulfonamides, the bacterium can also develop resistance by overproducing PABA, as occurs in *S. aureus*.

The Dangers of Antibiotic Abuse

As more antibiotics become known, both medical and nonmedical uses increase. Very few of these compounds have become obsolete or have been withdrawn from the market. Currently, however, it appears that several of these antibiotics are overused and overprescribed. For example, market research data show that almost two thirds of the prescriptions given to patients for the common cold are for antibiotics, yet most colds and sore throats are caused by viruses, microorganisms that are not affected by most currently available antibiotics or antimicrobials. Increased unnecessary exposure to these drugs has produced a significant increase in antibiotic-resistant organisms. Furthermore, as many as 1.5 million people are hospitalized annually in the United States for adverse drug reactions, and approximately 130,000 die from reactions associated with antibiotics and antimicrobials.

Transferable Antibiotic Resistance

Since the discovery of transferable antibiotic resistance in 1959, a fairly clear picture of the process as it occurs in the laboratory has emerged. Furthermore, it is well known that in most cases the introduction of a new antibiotic, effective against bacteria such as *Staphylococcus aureus*, for example, has been followed by the appearance of strains resistant to that antibiotic. During the 1940s and 1950s, antibiotic resistance in bacteria was generally thought to arise by mutation and selection. However, since 1960, evidence has accrued to show that most antibiotic resistance in organisms belonging to the Enterobacteriaceae, such as *Escherichia coli, Citrobacter freundii,* and *S. aureus,* is determined and controlled by extrachromosomal particles called ***plasmids.*** At times, such plasmids are physically distinct from a bacterium's chromosome, and depending on the bacterium, can be transferred from one organism to another by several means, including bacterial viruses. It should be noted that certain cases of antibiotic resistance are chromosome-mediated.

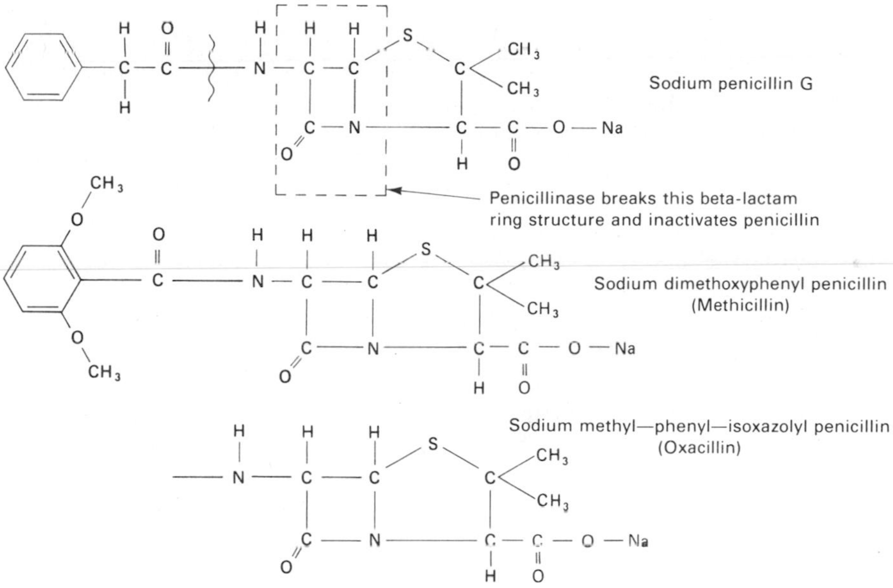

Sodium penicillin G

Penicillinase breaks this beta-lactam ring structure and inactivates penicillin

Sodium dimethoxyphenyl penicillin (Methicillin)

Sodium methyl—phenyl—isoxazolyl penicillin (Oxacillin)

FIG. 20-10 Comparison of penicillin G and several penicillinase-resistant penicillins. The portion of the penicillin molecule susceptible to attack is shown with the sodium penicillin G molecule.

The overall impact of the plasmid on a population of bacterial cells is that it provides a means for greater flexibility to survive under a variety of environmental factors. Several studies have shown that penicillinase production is plasmid-determined in the great majority of penicillin-resistant strains. Thus under natural or laboratory conditions, this antibiotic resistance could be imparted to antibiotic-sensitive organisms through cell transfer mechanisms. With such transfer, the usefulness of an antibiotic can be greatly decreased. Although this may be a valuable evolutionary weapon for organisms, it obviously poses a serious threat to the effectiveness of antibiotic therapy and to the control of infectious disease. The use of antibiotics has undoubtedly increased the number of plasmid-containing bacteria. Future application of chemotherapeutic agents must be directed toward reducing the incidence of such plasmid carriers if the usefulness of antibiotics is to be not only retained but also improved.

Antibiotic Sensitivity Testing Methods

Minimum Inhibitory Concentration Determination

The best methods for determining the antibiotic susceptibility of microorganisms involve careful estimation of an antimicrobial agent's minimum inhibitory concentrations (MICs). This is the lowest concentration of an antimicrobial agent capable of preventing growth. The determinations can be performed in either liquid or solid media.

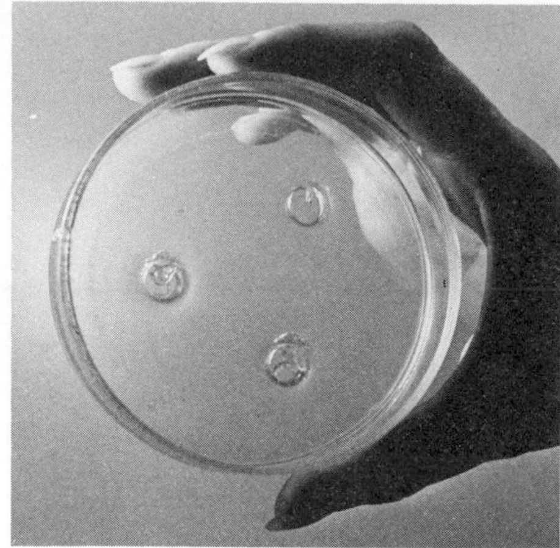
(a)

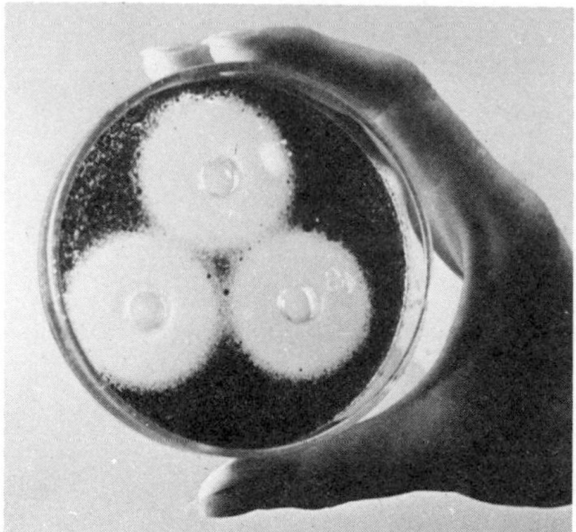
(b)

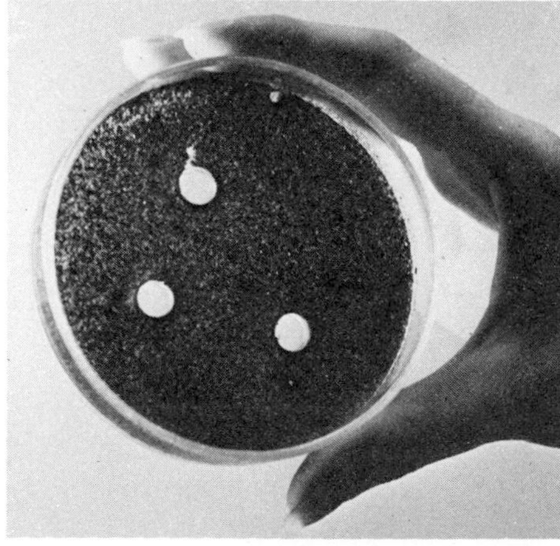
(c)

FIG. 20–11 (a) A Petri dish containing a medium seeded with a test organism. Three wells have been cut for the placement of an experimental drug. (b) The results of a test in which the test organisms are sensitive to the drug. (c) Drug resistance on the part of the test organisms. *Courtesy of Lederle Laboratories, Pearl River, N.Y.*

Drug Diffusion Methods

CYLINDER AND WELL METHODS

The screening of large numbers of bacteria with various antibiotics requires simple techniques that can be used with several samples at the same time. For example, small cylinders can be placed into the agar plates or wells can be cut into the agar for the purpose of holding a specified quantity of a particular antimicrobial agent. This type of procedure is shown in Figure 20–11a. The Petri dish here contains an agar medium seeded with a test organism. The three wells have been cut out and filled with solutions of a drug. If the antimicrobial agent is effective against the test organism, three zones of inhibition will develop (Figure 20–11b). However, if the drug is ineffective, then the results shown in Figure 20–11c are found.

FILTER-PAPER DISK

Because the well method is still a bit awkward to perform as a routine laboratory procedure, ***impregnated paper disks*** have received wide acceptance (Figure 20–12). A. Bondi in 1947 reported using filter paper disks containing specified concentrations of antibiotics (Color Photograph 76). The standardization of variables to minimize difficulties in interpretation was a critical aspect of this work.

Several factors can affect the size of the zone of antibacterial activity. These include (1) the depth of the medium used, (2) the choice of medium, (3) the size of the inoculum, and (4) the diffusion rate of a particular antibiotic. The last factor, in particular, has resulted in unfortunate misinterpretations of results.

Until recently, most laboratories used single- or double-disk methods. The single-disk methods use one disk of either a high or low antibiotic concentration. Determining the relative sensitivity of the organism to the drug requires interpretation of zone sizes. With the double-disk method, the interpretation is simpler. Here both high- and low-strength disks are applied for each antibiotic to be tested. The organism is reported as being sensitive if a clear zone appears around both disks. If a zone appears around the high-concentration disk alone, the organism is called ***moderately susceptible***. If zones are lacking in both disks, the organism is considered resistant to the drug. Although interpretation is simpler here, the accuracy of the double-disk method does not approach that of the Kirby-Bauer procedure.

KIRBY-BAUER (K-B) STANDARDIZED SINGLE-DISK METHOD

First reported in 1966, the Kirby-Bauer method uses a single high-strength antibiotic disk with Mueller-Hinton agar dispensed in 150×15 millimeter (mm) Petri plates. The depth of the medium is 5 to 6 mm (approximately 80 ml of medium). Standardization of the test organisms is accomplished by (1) introducing the growth from 5 isolated colonies into 4 ml of brain-heart infusion broth; (2) incubating the preparation for 2 to 5 hours in a water bath or thermal block, or until adequate turbidity is evident; and (3) adjusting the turbidity of the bacterial suspension according to a standard made from barium sulfate

(McFarland Standard 0.5).

A sample is taken by means of a sterile cotton swab. Excess fluid is removed by rolling the swab against the side of the tube containing the bacterial suspension.

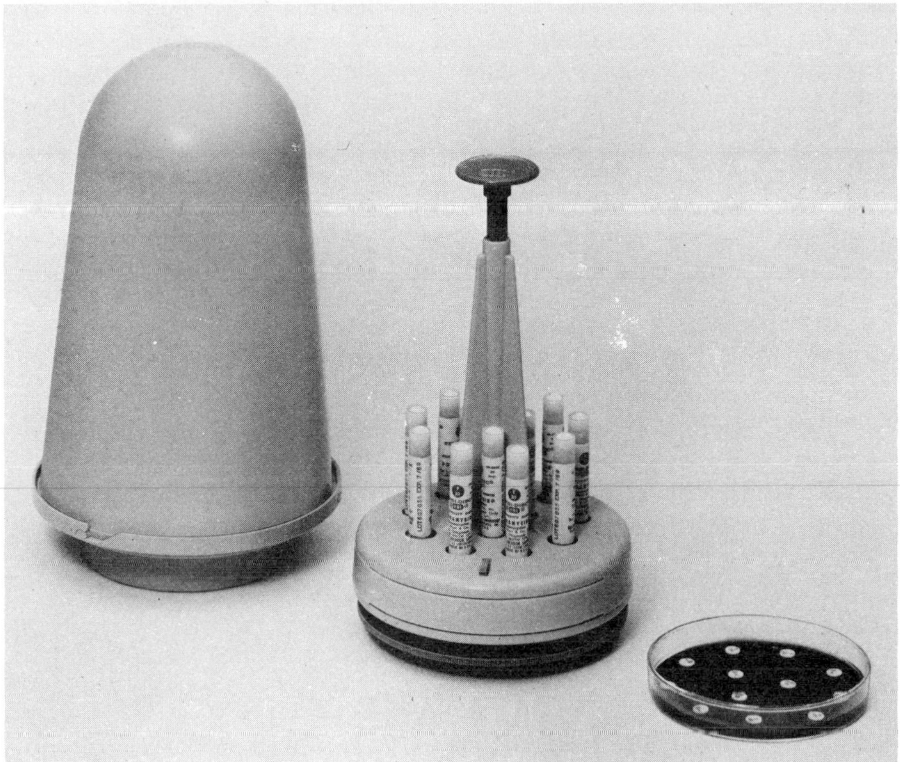

FIG. 20–12 Commercially available paper disks can be obtained in cartridges and applied to the medium in a Petri plate. This is usually done with a multiple applicator device of the types shown. *Courtesy of BioQuest, Division of Becton, Dickinson and Company, Cockeysville, MD.*

Then it is used to spread the organisms onto the surface of the agar medium. After a few minutes wait for the surface moisture to be absorbed by the agar, disks are applied. This procedure may be done with the large-size applicator like the one shown in Figure 20–12. After incubation, the sizes of zones can be measured with the aid of calipers, or they can be compared against a template consisting of various zones, the sizes of which are based on the data published by Ryan and his associates in 1970.

The zone sizes for selected drugs are presented in Table 20–4. These were evaluated according to MICs for pathogens and obtainable levels of antimicrobial agents in the human body. With this system, when an organism is reported to be sensitive (S) or resistant (R), the level of confidence in such a report is very high. An intermediate (I) classification indicates that the organism is probably resistant to obtainable body levels of the drug in question. The drug should not be used without first performing a tube dilution test confirming the MIC obtained. In practice, the I designation is considered the same as an R rating—meaning the drug is not effective. The drug is not used if the microorganism has been found to be sensitive to several other drugs.

The K-B method and the agar-overlay modification techniques presented next are suitable only for rapidly growing pathogenic bacteria, such as staphylococci and *Pseudomonas* spp. Fortunately, most pathogens are in this category. The other single- or double-disk procedures can be used with most bacterial species. However, without some form of standardization, the accuracy of the results is questionable.

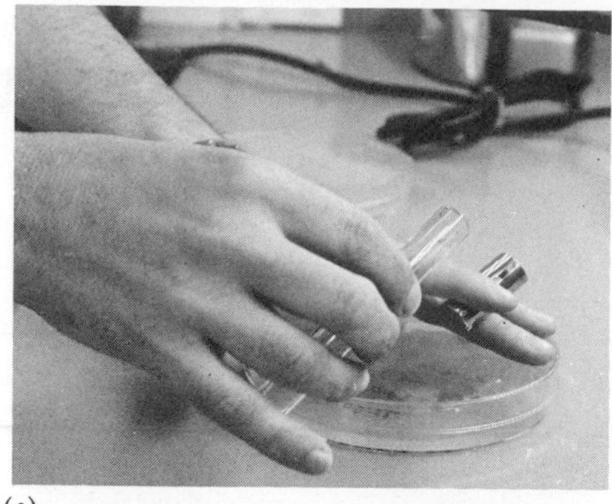
(a)

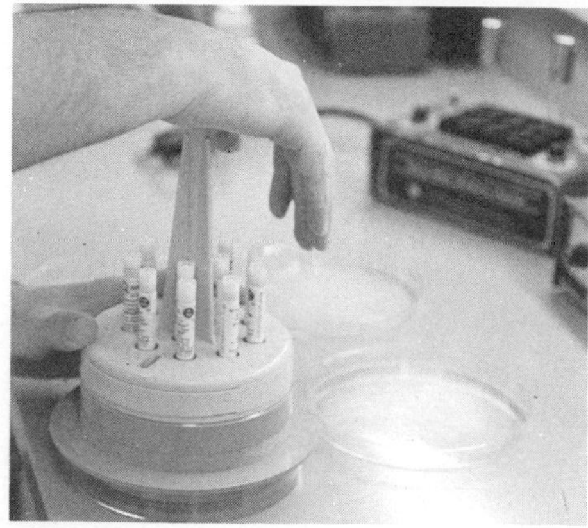
(b)

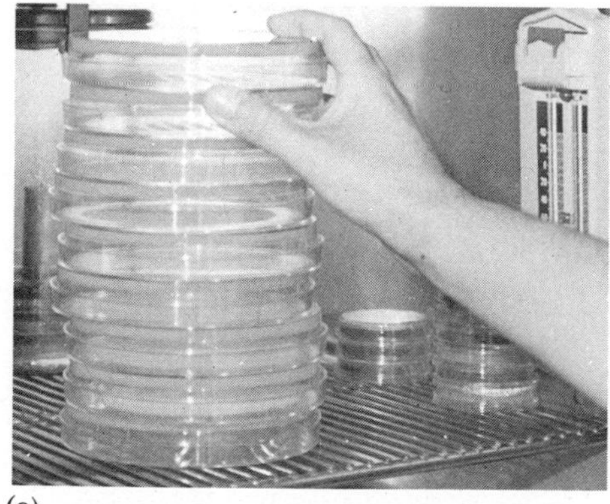
(c)

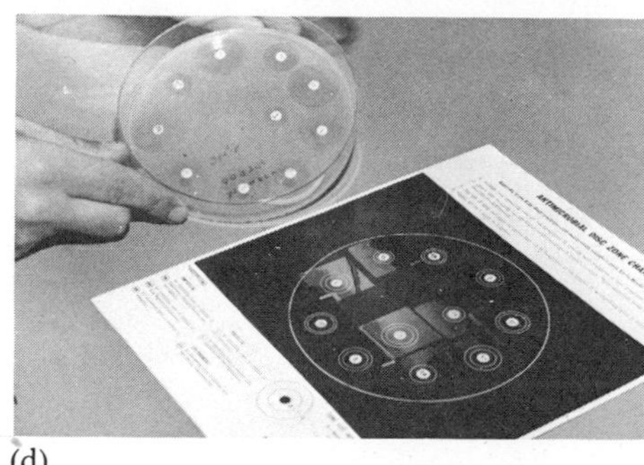
(d)

FIG. 20–13 Agar-overlay modification of the Kirby-Bauer standardized antiobiotic disk sensitivity test. *Courtesy of St. Mary's Long Beach Hospital, Long Beach, California.*

THE AGAR-OVERLAY METHOD

The agar-overlay modification of Barry, Garcia, and Thrupp (1970) has greatly simplified the Kirby-Bauer procedure without affecting the interpretation of zone sizes. Figure 20–13 shows some of the steps involved in this test.

In this procedure, 0.5 ml of brain-heart infusion broth is inoculated with the test colonies to make the solution slightly cloudy. The tube is then held at 37°C for four to eight hours. During this incubation period, tubes containing 8 ml of melted 1.5 percent agar are placed in a constant temperature bath or block maintained at approximately 52°C.

After the incubation period, 0.001 ml of the broth culture is introduced by means of a calibrated loop into a tube of melted agar. The contents of the tube are mixed and then poured onto the surface of 70 ml of solidified Mueller-Hinton agar in 150 × 15 mm plastic Petri plates (Figure 20–13a). It is imperative that the plates be warmed to at least room temperature before attempting this last step. Tilting and/or rotating the plate is usually necessary to produce a uniform layer of the seeded agar. The colder the plate, the more difficult this step is to perform.

TABLE 20–4 Zone Size Comparison of Selected Chemotherapeutic Drugs

Chemotherapeutic Drug	*Concentration in Disk*	*Inhibition Zone Diameter (mm)* R[a] *less than*	I *between*	S *more than*
Ampicillin[b]	10 μgm	21	21–28	28
Chloramphenicol	30 μgm	13	13–17	17
Colistin	10 μgm	9	9–10	10
Kanamycin	30 μgm	14	14–17	17
Penicillin[b]	10 units	21	21–28	28
Sulfonamides	300 μgm	13	13–16	16
Tetracyclines	30 μgm	15	15–18	18

[a]R = resistant, I = intermediate resistance, S = sensitivity. See text for additional information concerning the differences between R and I and reasons for the various zone sizes for different drugs.
[b]Interpretation of zone sizes with ampicillin and penicillin varies with different organisms. These values are primarily for staphylococci.

The required antibiotic disks are applied three to five minutes after the agar layer has solidified (Figure 20–13b). These disks are placed firmly on the agar surface. Then the Petri plate cover is replaced and the entire system is incubated overnight at 35°C (Figure 20–13c). The zones of inhibition that develop are compared with standards to determine relative sensitivities (Figure 20–13d).

Blood Levels of Antimicrobial Agents

Antimicrobial therapy is becoming increasingly complex as more resistant organisms emerge as important pathogens. *In vitro* susceptibility tests performed in most laboratories indicate whether an infection caused by the organism tested is likely to respond to the antibiotic concentration recommended for treatment (Color Photograph 76). In cases of life-threatening diseases, proper treatment often requires close monitoring of blood levels of antibiotics in the patient.

A number of tests are available to perform such serum assays, but they have not been standardized to the same extent as the better known bacterial susceptibility methods. In these tests, specimens are obtained from patients who have received the drug for at least 24 hours. The blood is usually drawn just before administration of the antibiotic (trough level) and also at the time the highest concentration of antibiotic is expected in the bloodstream (peak level). Biological or enzymatic methods are then used to measure antibiotic concentrations.

In biologic assays, the concentration of antibiotic in the patient's bloodstream is measured by comparing growth inhibition of a test organism by the patient's serum to inhibition of the same organism by a known amount of the antibiotic administered. A disk diffusion procedure is widely used for this purpose (Figure 20–14).

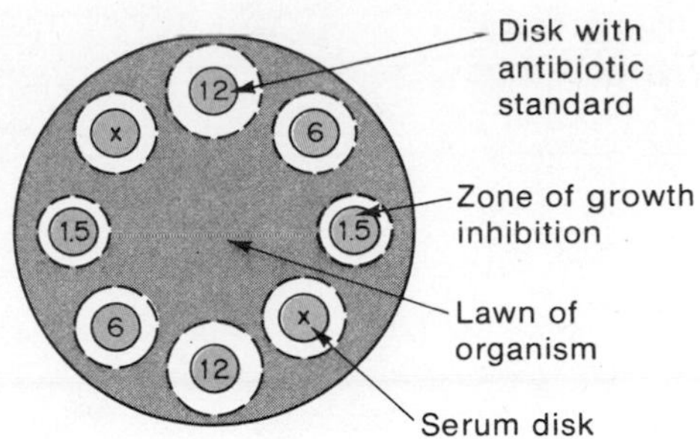

FIG. 20–14 A diagram of the disk diffusion assay plate and its components.

Two plates are normally used for each assay. Specified amounts of the patient's serum and of three standard concentrations of antibiotic are incorporated onto one-quarter-inch filter-paper disks. Two sets of disks are placed clockwise on each agar plate, with the disk containing the most concentrated antibiotic standard first and the serum disk last. After two to three hours of incubation at 35° to 37°C, the zones of inhibition caused by the antibiotic and by the patient's serum are measured, compared, and used to calculate the inhibitory concentrations of the antibiotic being monitored.

Enzymatic assay is more rapid, accurate, and specific than biologic assays. The test uses radioactive material and an appropriate counter to detect levels of radioactivity of reaction mixtures.

Antimycotic Agents

Unlike chemotherapy for bacterial infections, treatment of fungus infections or mycoses by chemical agents is still quite limited. There are several reasons for this situation. Infections caused by fungi are much less common than those produced by bacteria or other microorganisms, and the most frequent mycotic infections, such as the various ringworm conditions (Color Photographs 40 and 42), are not life threatening and in most cases are trivial. Also, it has proven especially difficult to develop antifungal agents that have a specificity for fungal cellular structures and for cellular macromolecular synthetic processes such as protein and ribonucleic acid (RNA) synthesis.

The most important antifungal agents are those that affect cell membranes. Of these, the polyene antibiotics (Figure 20–15) are the most important and most useful in the treatment of clinical infections. These antibiotics interact with the membranes of susceptible cells and distort their selective permeability. This results in the leakage of potassium and magnesium ions followed by decreased protein and RNA synthesis. All organisms susceptible to polyenes contain sterols. These include algae, flatworms, mammalian cells, protozoans, and yeasts. Because of their effect on membrane permeability, some polyenes have been found to increase the effectiveness of other drugs. Some problems have been encountered with the polyenes, however, especially with respect to absorption, solubility, stability, and toxicity.

Other important antifungal, or antimycotic, agents are 5-fluorocytosine, which affects RNA synthesis, and griseofluvin, which inhibits cell division in a variety of different types of cells. Both of these agents are taken orally. The characteristics of several traditional as well as new antimycotic agents are given in Table 20–5.

The Treatment of Protozoan Diseases

At the present time, control of most of the protozoan diseases of humans and domestic animals relies largely on drugs. Even though several medications have been developed for most of these disease states, they are not always readily available. Chemotherapeutic agents used for protozoan diseases have other limitations. Some preparations, especially those containing arsenic or antimony, are highly toxic. Others are not effective against all stages of the parasite. Resistance to certain drugs is also becoming a greater problem.

Antiprotozoan drugs are thought to exert their antimicrobial action by several mechanisms. These include interference with energy metabolism (Figure 20–16); disruption of membrane function; and interference with nucleic acid production, protein synthesis, or other biosynthetic reactions of the parasite. Later chapters will discuss specific drugs for treatment of protozoan diseases.

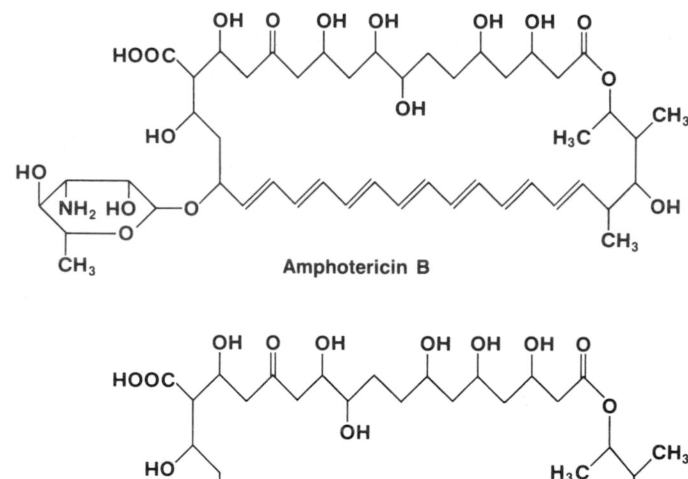

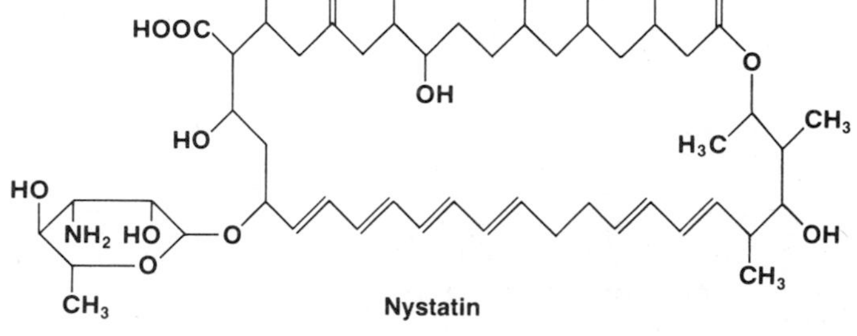

FIG. 20–15 The chemical structures of selected antifunal agents. Two polyene antibiotics are shown, amphotericin B and nystatin. Interactions between these antibiotics and the membranes of susceptible cells causes leakage of potassium and magnesium ions followed by decreased protein and ribonucleic acid synthesis.

(a)

20 μm

(b)

FIG. 20–16 The dramatic effect of chemotherapeutic agents. (a) The protozoan *Trypanosoma brucei*, one of the causative agents of African sleeping sickness, before treatment. (b) After treatment with salicyl hydroxamic acid and glycerol. Note the absence of trypanosomes and the remaining two flagella (arrows). *Clarkson, A. B., Jr., and F. H. Brohr,* Science *194: 204–206 (1976).*

Antiviral Agents

Until quite recently, chemotherapy of true virus diseases had been virtually nonexistent. Considerable prophylactic and therapeutic success had been achieved with a large number of viral agents through the use of vaccines, but no success had been obtained with chemotherapeutic drugs. During the last few years, several promising antiviral drugs have been developed. Examples of these include amantadine, 5-iodo-2′-deoxyuridine (IDU), methisazone, interferon inducers, and cytosine arabinoside (cytarabin). Table 20–6 provides a comparative summary of these antiviral agents, and Figure 20–17 shows their chemical structures.

TABLE 20-5 Characteristics of Antimycotic Drugs

Drug	*Fungus Diseases Affected*	*Side Effects*
Amphotericin B (Fungizone)	Superficial candidiasis	Essentially none
	Systemic candidiasis, not involving the heart (endocarditis)	Kidney damage, convulsions, hypotension, nausea, vomiting, abdominal pain, metallic taste, cardiac arrest, and anemia[a]
	Deep-seated fungus infections, including aspergillosis, coccioidomycosis, histomycosis, systematic sporothricosis, blastomycosis, and cryptococcosis	Same as for systemic candidiasis
Clotrimazole	Ringworm of the skin	Generally none
Fluorocytosina (Ancobon)	Systemic candidiasis, not involving the heart, and cryptococcosis	Gastrointestinal distress and reduction of white blood cells (leukopenia)
Griseofulvin (Fulvicin, Grifulvin, Grisactin)	Dermatophytoses (ringworm of the hair, nails, and/or skin)	Fatigue, skin eruptions, nausea, vomiting, and diarrhea
Haloprigin	Ringworm of the skin	None
Miconazole	Dermatophytoses (ringworm of the hair, nails, and/or skin), candidiasis, candidal vulvovaginitis, and deep-seated fungus infections such as aspergillosis and coccidioidomycosis	Bleeding and ulcerations at sites where the drug is introduced
Nystatin (Mycostatin)	Intestinal candidiasis	Basically none
Tolnaflate	Dermatophytoses of hair and nails	None

[a]The side effects listed occur more readily with the rapid introduction of the drug

Antiviral Agent Sensitivity Testing

With the recent unraveling of many of the biochemical, biological, and biophysical properties of disease-causing viruses has come great anticipation of an era of effective viral chemotherapy. Despite the wealth of knowledge that has been gathered, there remain many serious problems peculiar to the field of viral chemotherapy. Among these obstacles is the fact that chemical agents effective against viruses are often also toxic to mammalian cells. Furthermore, antiviral agents are affected by a multiplicity effect. An agent may be effective against viruses in low concentration but ineffective against high concentrations

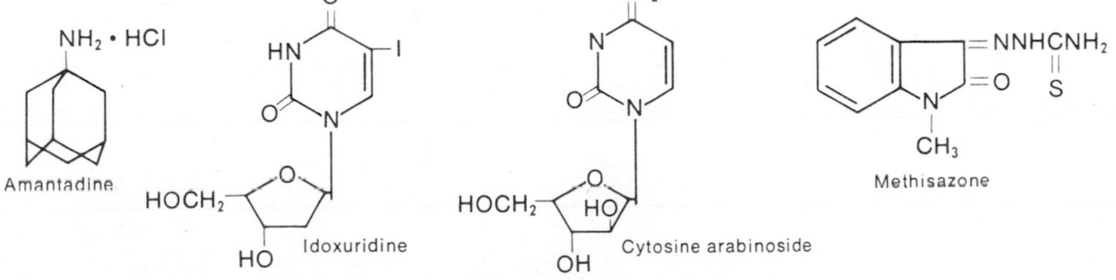

FIG. 20-17 The chemical structures of antiviral agents.

TABLE 20–6 A Comparative Summary of Antiviral Drugs

Drug	*Representative Viral Disease(s) Affected*	*Possible Side Effects*	*Mechanism of Action*
Amantadine	Influenza A_2 (Asia)	General irritability, insomnia, confusion, hallucinations, inability to concentrate	Prevents penetration of certain viruses into host cells
5-Iodo-2′-deoxyuridine	Severe *Herpesvirus hominis* (herpes simplex) infection	Nausea, vomiting, hair and fingernail loss, lowering of white blood cells (leukopenia) and platelets (thrombocytopenia)	Blocks synthesis of nucleic acids
Cytosine arabinoside	Progressive varicella (chickenpox) and zoster (shingles) infections	Nausea, vomiting, loss of appetite, chromosomal changes, lowering of white blood cells and platelets, anemia	Inhibits DNA synthesis
Methisazone	Progressive vaccinia	Nausea, vomiting, loss of appetite, liver toxicity (hepatotoxicity)	Interferes with protein synthesis at the level of translation

of viruses. Demonstrating the clinical effectiveness of antiviral agents is difficult, and drug-resistant viral strains may well emerge.

Of all these important problems, the evaluation of clinical effectiveness is especially critical, because a drug must be thoroughly tested before it can be made available for general use. The clinical value of a few antiviral drugs has been established (Table 20–7). Before the clinical effectiveness of an antiviral agent can be determined, the drug in question must be evaluated for antiviral activity and toxicity both in cell culture and in animal models. In the second phase of drug evaluation, human experimentation is performed with the objective of determining tolerable dosages and general effects of the antiviral agent on the body. The third phase is the formal therapeutic trial, which is directed toward determining the true clinical effect of the drug on actual cases of virus infections. Certain preparations satisfy some of these drug-evaluation requirements but for various reasons fall short of satisfying all of them. Clearly, the problems peculiar to viral chemotherapy must be overcome before a proven treatment for viral diseases will be at hand.

TABLE 20–7 Current Clinical Status of Antiviral Agents

	Type of Application			
	Topical		*Systemic*	
Agent	*Prophylaxis (preventative measure)*	*Therapy*	*Prophylaxis*	*Therapy*
Amantadine	–	+	+	–
Cytosine arabinoside (AraC)	–	–	–	–
Idoxuridine (IDU)	–	+	–	–
Interferon	+[a]	–	–	–
Methisazone	–	–	+	–

[a]Refer to Chapter 21 for a discussion of interferon.

SUMMARY

1. Antibiotics are among the most frequently prescribed drugs for treatment and control of microbial infections.
2. Certain problems have appeared which can limit their effectiveness. These include antibiotic resistant microorganisms, transfer of drug resistance among organisms, and the effects of the host on antibiotic action.

Historical Background

The discoveries of Salvarsan by Ehrlich in 1909, sulfa drugs by Domagk in 1935, and penicillin by Fleming in 1929 ushered in the modern era of chemotherapy.

Chemotherapeutic Agents

1. Chemotherapeutic agents are either natural products of microorganisms or antimicrobial agents produced in the laboratory. Today the term *antibiotic* applies to both categories of substances.
2. Antibiotics can be used as feed additives to protect plants and livestock against infectious diseases as well as to keep agricultural products fresh for extended periods.

Principles of Chemotherapy

1. The administration of an antibiotic depends on several factors, including the physical condition of the recipient, the existence of drug allergies, the pathogen, the site of infection, and the dosage of the antibiotic to be given.
2. Laboratory findings of effective antibiotic levels do not always correlate with similar levels in the body.
3. Laboratory testing is used to determine the lowest concentration of a drug that will prevent the growth of a standardized microbial suspension. This relative sensitivity is expressed as *minimal inhibitory concentration* (MIC).

Minimal Antibacterial (Active) Concentration (MAC)

Minute amounts of antibacterial agents can produce morphological changes as well as inhibition of growth.

Properties of An Effective Antibiotic

An effective chemotherapeutic agent must be relatively nontoxic to the host and exhibit antimicrobial activity at low concentrations in the body of an infected individual.

Mechanisms of Action of Antimicrobial Agents

1. Chemotherapeutic agents causing irreversible damage or death to microbial cells are called *cidal* drugs. These preparations are independent in their actions on microorganisms.
2. Drugs inhibiting growth and reproduction of microbial cells exert a *static* effect. Static drugs are dependent on the host's immune system for the elimination of pathogens.
3. Drugs active against several Gram-positive and Gram-negative bacteria are called *broad spectrum*. Those active against a single group or only a few species have a narrow, or limited, spectrum of activity.

Specific Mechanisms of Action

Major mechanisms by which antimicrobial agents can inhibit growth or kill microorganisms include (1) inhibition of cell wall formation; (2) inhibition of protein synthesis; (3) irreversible damage to the cell membrane; (4) inhibition of nucleic acid synthesis; and (5) inhibition of specific products of metabolism.

Some Commonly Used Antimicrobial Drugs

Sulfa Drugs

1. Sulfa drugs are bacteriostatic and act upon growing and metabolizing cells.
2. The mechanism of action is an example of competitive inhibition of enzymes, which interferes with cellular metabolism.

Penicillins

1. Penicillins are bactericidal and act by interfering with cell wall formation.
2. The penicillins are effective only during the growth stages of sensitive organisms.

Cylindamycin, A Useful Alternative to Penicillin-cephalosporin Antibiotics

This semisynthetic antibiotic inhibits protein synthesis.

Chloramphenicol and the Tetracyclines

1. These agents are bacteriostatic, broad-spectrum antibiotics.
2. Both antibiotics inhibit protein synthesis.

Aminoglycosides (Streptomycins)

The aminoglycosides are all bactericidal and interfere with protein synthesis.

Polypeptides

These antibiotics include polymyxin B and colistin and cause a leakage of essential cytoplasmic parts.

Antimycobacterial Drugs

Drugs commonly used against tuberculosis include isonicotinic hydrazide (INH) and para-aminosalicylic acid (PAS).

Rifampin

Rifampin is a broad-spectrum drug used against tuberculosis.

Mechanisms of Drug Resistance

Mechanisms by which organisms develop resistance to antimicrobial agents include enzymatic alteration of the drug; changes in selective permeability of cell walls and membranes; changes in the sensitivity of affected enzymes; and increased production of a competitive substrate.

The Dangers of Antibiotic Abuse

Increased unnecessary exposure to antibiotics has resulted in a significant increase in antibiotic-resistant organisms.

Transferable Antibiotic Resistance

1. Antibiotic resistance in certain bacteria is determined and controlled by extrachromosomal particles called *plasmids.*
2. The ability of organisms to transfer resistance limits the effectiveness of antibiotics.

Antibiotic Sensitivity Testing Methods

Methods for determining the antibiotic susceptibility of microorganisms include drug diffusion techniques, performed with cylinders and filter paper disks, and tests monitoring blood levels of antibiotics in patients.

Blood Levels of Antimicrobial Agents

With life-threatening diseases, it is often necessary to monitor blood levels of antibiotics in the patient.

Antimycotic Agents

1. Fewer agents exist for the treatment of fungus infections

than for bacterial diseases.

2. Antifungal drugs affect both cell membrane permeability and RNA synthesis and inhibit cell division.

The Treatment of Protozoan Diseases

1. Chemotherapeutic agents for protozoan diseases are toxic and not always readily available.
2. Their antimicrobial action is similar to those of drugs used against other microbes.

Antiviral Agents

1. Some promising antiviral agents have been developed.
2. Before such drugs can be used, they must be shown to have antiviral activity and be nontoxic.

QUESTIONS FOR REVIEW

1. a. What are antibiotics?
   b. Of what value are such chemicals?
   c. What are the sources of antibiotics?
2. Differentiate between bacteriostatic and bactericidal drugs.
3. List the properties of a functional antibiotic.
4. a. List and explain four ways in which antimicrobial drugs interfere with microbial cells and/or activities.
   b. Give an example of one antibiotic that acts by each mechanism listed in 4a.
5. What is a broad-spectrum antibiotic?
6. Why are antibiotics such as penicillin and streptomycin ineffective against viruses?
7. a. What is an *in vitro* antibiotic sensitivity test?
   b. What factors affect the accuracy of such procedures?
8. a. Of what value is the determination of the blood or serum levels of an antibiotic in the treatment of a disease?
   b. What methods are used for this type of determination?
9. a. Explain microbial drug resistance.
   b. How is such resistance transferred among bacteria?
   c. What mechanisms are responsible for drug resistance?
   d. Is such resistance increasing or decreasing? Explain.
10. What is the value of semisynthetic or synthetic antibiotics?
11. Why are antibiotics, which are effective against bacterial pathogens, given to individuals with viral infections?
12. a. How do antimycotics function?
    b. List three antimycotic agents.
13. a. How are antiviral agents tested and selected?
    b. Are there any limitations to the use of such agents?
14. Does the host of an infectious agent exert any influence on the effectiveness of an antibiotic?
15. Define or explain the following:
    a. MIC
    b. *Streptomyces*
    c. competitive inhibition
    d. plasmid

SUGGESTED READINGS

Ainsworth, G. C., *Introduction to the History of Mycology.* Cambridge: Cambridge University Press, 1976. *An interesting and scholarly work containing many anecdotes associated with various 'breakthroughs' in microbiology. The account of Sir Alexander Fleming's discovery of penicillin and how it revolutionized the practice of contemporary medicine is particularly worthwhile.*

Davies, J., and D. I. Smith, "Plasmid-determined Resistance to Antimicrobial Agents," *Ann. Rev. Microbiol.* 32:469–518 (1978). *A review organized along the lines of possible biochemical mechanisms for antibiotic resistance in microorganisms.*

Garrod, L. P., H. P. Lambert, and F. O'. Grady (eds.), *Antibiotics and Chemotherapy.* 4th ed. Edinburgh: Churchill Livingstone, 1973. *An excellent presentation of the modes of action of antibiotics and other chemotherapeutic agents. Emphasis is placed on antibiotic usage in the treatment of infectious diseases, although sulfonamides and synthetic drugs are covered.*

Glasby, J. S., *Encyclopaedia of Antibiotics.* A Wiley-Interscience Publication. New York: John Wiley & Sons, 1976. *An encyclopedic listing of antibiotics together with their properties, including formula, structure, microbial source, abbreviated methods of preparation and purification toxicity, and those microorganisms against which the substances are effective.*

Hopwood, D. A., "Extrachromosomally Determined Antibiotic Production," *Ann. Rev. Microbiol.* 32:373–392 (1978). *An up-to-date review of the involvement of plasmids (extrachromosomal material) in antibiotic production.*

Kobayashi, G. S., and G. Medoff, "Antifungal Agents: Recent Developments," *Ann. Rev. Microbiol.* 31:291–308 (1977). *This is a comprehensive review of what is known about the most important antifungal agents used in clinical infections.*

Stuart-Harris, C. H., and L. Dickinson, *The Background in Chemotherapy of Virus Diseases.* Springfield, Ill.: Charles C. Thomas, 1964. *This book describes the problems scientists have encountered in attempts to make an antiviral drug.*

Whitley, R. J., and C. A. Alford, "Developmental Aspects of Selected Antiviral Chemotherapeutic Agents," *Ann. Rev. Microbiol.* 32:285–300 (1978). *The difficulties encountered in developing an antiviral chemotherapeutic agent are discussed. Some of the newest antiviral agents are described.*

PART FOUR

Principles of Immunology

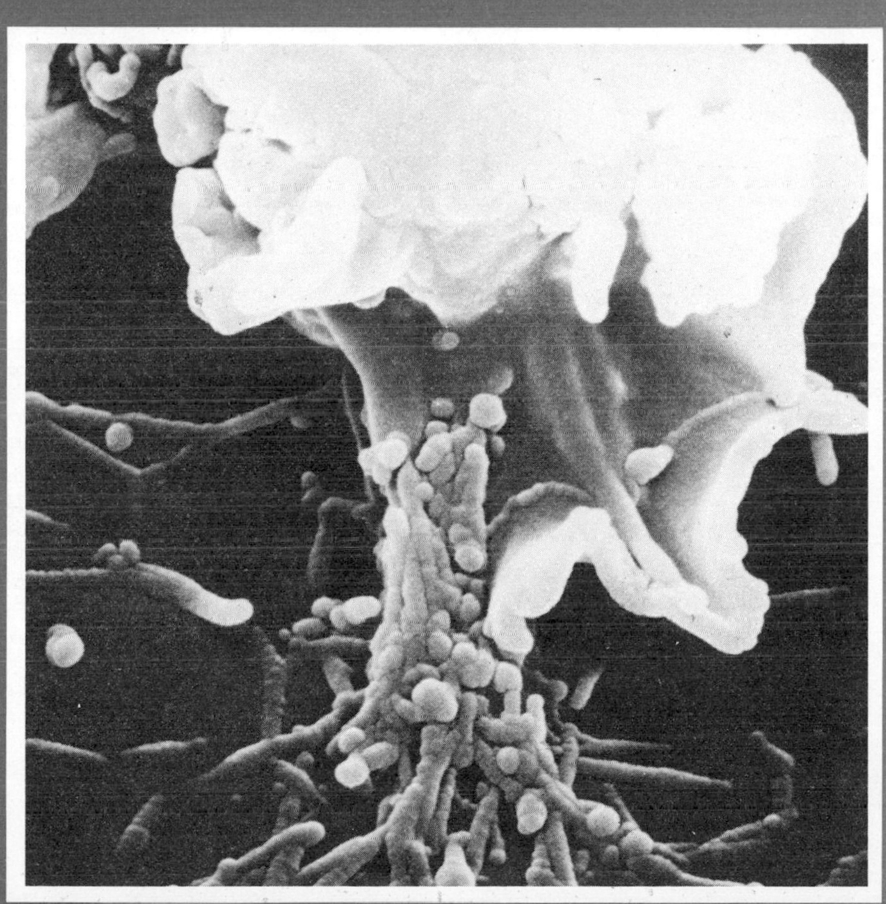

CHAPTER **21**

Resistance in Host-Parasite Interactions

Chapter 21 deals with the various means and mechanisms by which the body normally combats infectious disease agents. We shall also see what happens when such protection fails and what various factors and conditions lower an individual's resistance to microbial attack.

After reading this chapter, you should be able to:

1. **List and explain the roles of five body components important to the defense against disease agents.**
2. **Explain the benefits of indigenous microbes to resistance.**
3. **Differentiate among the various cellular components of blood and their respective roles in health and disease.**
4. **Describe the stages of phagocytosis and the cell types involved in the process.**
5. **Identify the significant factors and conditions that lower host resistance.**
6. **List and describe the antimicrobial substances produced in the human body.**
7. **Explain the functions and importance of phagocytosis, inflammation, and fever in host resistance.**
8. **List and describe the events and signs of inflammation.**

Humans and other vertebrates are protected in varying degrees from disease-causing microorganisms and cancer cells by a surveillance mechanism, referred to as the *immune system*. Collectively, the various components of the system provide protection by imposing barriers to invasion by microorganisms and other disease agents or by selectively eliminating foreign invaders that do find their way into the body.

Among the body's defense mechanisms are some that provide *specific immunity* against particular microorganisms and their products. Other defense mechanisms are general, used against any and all disease-causing agents. This form of immunity is called *nonspecific resistance*. Some contributing factors in nonspecific resistance are species or racial factors, mechanical and chemical barriers, phagocytosis, inflammation, and various antimicrobial chemical products of the body.

Species or Racial Resistance

It is well known that some animal species are normally nonsusceptible to diseases that can have disastrous effects on other animals. Humans exhibit such *nonsusceptibility* toward a variety of infectious diseases of other animals, including canine distemper, cattle plague, chicken cholera, and hog cholera. On the other hand, lower animal species are similarly resistant to human-associated bacterial infections such as dysentery, gonorrhea, typhoid fever, and whooping cough, and to viral diseases such as measles and mumps. This kind of nonsusceptibility, or *species resistance*, is determined by physiologic and anatomic properties of the particular animal species and is inheritable. Demonstrable antibodies (protective protein molecules) are not associated with this state of resistance.

Changes in body temperature, diet, and stress can affect species resistance, as is shown by several classic experiments. Chickens and frogs normally are not susceptible to the bacterial disease anthrax. However, the cold-blooded frog will succumb to inoculation with the infectious agent if its temperature is artificially raised to approximately 35° C, and the warm-blooded chicken will succumb if its body temperature is lowered to that level. The multiplication of various pathogens depends upon the availability of growth factors in usable form. Some disease agents depend on the food of their host. For example, dogs are normally resistant to anthrax; however, when meat is omitted from their diets, they become susceptible to the infection.

Species or racial resistance depends on the interplay of many factors, not all of which are known.

Mechanical and Chemical Barriers: The Body's First Line of Defense

Several systems of the body are barriers to potential disease-causing agents. Their effectiveness depends on the physiologic or pathologic state of the host. Conditions such as alcoholism, poor nutrition, and the debilitating effects of aging, fatigue, and prolonged exposure to extreme temperatures and to immunosuppressive therapy contribute to establishment of a disease process. Chapters in the next division contain general descriptions of the various body defense systems. Some pathogenic agents seem to initiate their infectious process only when they gain access through a particular portal of entry, each of which has its own defense barriers.

Intact Skin

Unbroken skin serves as an excellent mechanical barrier which most microorganisms cannot penetrate. In addition, certain bactericidal secretions are formed by glands associated with the skin layers. Injuries to the skin, such as abrasions, lacerations, or burns, provide the opportunity for microorganisms to pass this first line of defense. However, the mere penetration of the skin does not establish an infection. Once organisms enter the body by this means, they may or may not encounter conditions favorable for their growth and multiplication; nevertheless, accidental injuries, regardless of how minor they appear to be, should not be neglected. Given the right set of circumstances, any type of wound can result in a serious infection.

Mucous Membranes

The respiratory system is protected by several mechanisms. In addition to the presence of nasal hairs that trap particles in the air, the mucous membranes of this region are covered with a thick, slimy secretion known as mucus, which serves to entrap dust, foreign particles, and various microorganisms. Parts of the respiratory passages are also lined with cilia, which beat rhythmically in such a way as to move particles trapped by mucus upward toward the back of the throat where they are swallowed. These barriers, plus the coughing and sneezing reflexes, help to eliminate foreign particles. If microorganisms evade them, certain white blood cells, or leukocytes, operating in the body are called forth to stop them.

Genitourinary System

The mucous membranes of the female genitourinary tract are afforded protection against several pathogens by a thick secretion that tends to trap certain invading organisms. In addition, the acidity of the vaginal environment discourages some infectious agents. The outward flow of urine and its acidity contribute to the defense of the urinary tract; however, various pathogens, including those causing gonorrhea and syphilis, are able to invade the body by this portal.

Eyes

Several factors function to prevent disease agents from entering and attacking the inner lining of the eyelid (the conjunctivae). These include the mechanical motion of the eyelids, the eyelashes, and eyebrows and the washing effects of tears, which contain the bactericidal substance ***lysozyme***, discussed later.

Gastrointestinal System

The composition and acidity of gastric juice provides considerable protection to the stomach; however, some organisms are shielded by the presence of food.

In the small intestine, mucus, certain enzymes, bile, and the process of phagocytosis are important factors contributing to the body's defense. The large intestine usually harbors many microorganisms (indigenous flora) that are important in maintaining a "normal" balance.

Indigenous or Normal Flora

The flora and fauna indigenous to humans are often referred to simply as *normal flora.* In this context, "flora" denotes all microscopic life forms and "normal" becomes a statistical term. The reader must not equate normal with nonpathogenic, for many organisms found on and in the body can pose problems under conditions such as the following:

1. Deterioration of the host's defense mechanisms.
2. Relocation of microorganisms, as when an organism finds its way to an area of the body previously uninhabited by it.
3. A disturbance of the balance of the "normal flora."

Normal flora are commonly referred to as **amphibionts,** ranging from beneficial commensals to pathogens. The amphibionts are obligately parasitic for humans or other animals but are not necessarily pathogenic. They are found at least as often in the absence of disease as in its presence. The indigenous microorganisms may flourish in the general region of tissue damage and contribute to the disease state as **opportunists,** rather than primary etiological agents. That is, they take advantage of a host's weakened defenses to cause disease.

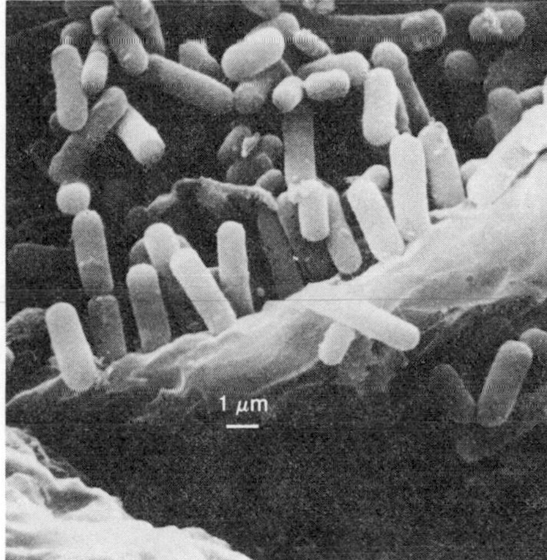

FIG. 21-1 Attachment of short, rod-shaped bacteria to the epithelial surface of an adult mouse's gastrointestinal system. *Savage, D. C., and R. V. H. Blumershine:* Infect. Immun. *10:240–250 (1974).*

Amphibiont Sites

As a rule, few or no microorganisms are found in the following anatomical locations: blood, larynx, trachea, nasal sinuses, bronchi, esophagus, stomach, upper intestinal tract, upper urinary tract (including the posterior urethra), and posterior genital tract (passage above cervix included).

The major habitats for indigenous microorganisms include the skin and contiguous mucous membranes (Figure 21–1), conjunctivae, portions of the upper respiratory tract, the mouth, lower intestine, and several of the external and internal parts of the reproductive system. It will become apparent later that certain characteristics of each region allow a different range of microorganisms to thrive. These differences can be categorized into the following three types of environment:

1. Extremely high levels of both moisture and nutrients, as in the lower intestines and the mouth.
2. A high level of moisture and a low level of nutrients, as with mucous membranes.
3. A low level of moisture and a moderate level of nutrients, as on the skin.

Other variables include availability of oxygen, pH, temperature, and relative exposures to contaminants and ventilation.

Development

Because the infant is bathed during gestation in a sterile amniotic fluid, development of the indigenous flora begins with the normal birth process. As the baby passes through the birth canal, it picks up organisms, many of which may remain with it throughout its lifetime. Additional microorganisms are acquired by contact with the air, with hospital personnel, and with the mother. Such organisms may be transient (temporary) in nature, or may become permanent members of the flora. Cultures from the mouths of infants 6 to 10 hours old show appreciable numbers of bacteria. Bacteria appear in the feces 10 to 20 hours after birth.

Because each anatomical area varies in pH, oxygen content, nutrients, moisture, and bactericidal factors, different organisms will predominate. While the amphibionts persist in their respective locations, saprophytic organisms and many parasitic microorganisms are destroyed or excreted. Conditions in these locations can change as a result of maturation of the individual, alteration in dietary habits, or chemotherapy. Thus, microorganisms may be of a temporary or permanent nature, depending upon the conditions that exist in the body.

The microorganisms listed in Table 21-1 are considered representative of the normal flora of the human adult; each appears to exist in at least 5 percent of the adult population. Clearly, many potential pathogens are present in various habitats in the absence of disease. A slight imbalance of the host's defense mechanisms or ecological shifts as a consequence of chemotherapy or other factors could result in disease.

TABLE 21-1 The Variety of Indigenous Microorganisms

Bacteria	*Fungi*	*Protozoa*
Actinomyces spp.	*Candida* spp.[a]	*Chilomastix mesnili*
Bacteroides spp.	*Epidermophyton floccosum*	*Dientamoeba fragilis*
clostridia	*Pityrosporum*	*Endolimax nana*
Corynebacterium spp.	*Torulopsis glabrata*[a]	*Entamoeba* spp.
Escherichia coli	*Trichophyton* spp.	*Enteromonas hominis*
fusobacteria		*Giardia intestinalis*
Hemophilus spp.		*Iodamoeba butschlii*
Leptotrichia		*Retortomonas intestinalis*
Micrococcus spp.		*Trichomonas* spp.
Moraxella spp.		
mycobacteria		
Mycoplasma spp. and L-forms[b]		
Pseudomonas spp.		
spirilla and spirochetes		
staphylococci		
streptococci		
Veillonella		

[a]Yeast.
[b]These microorganisms can be found in all body habitats of humans and other animals. They appear routinely in the mouth, upper respiratory, intestinal, and genitourinary tracts.

Benefits

Probably the main benefit derived by humans from their microbial inhabitants is protection from disease. This may seem contradictory because we have noted that the amphibionts can cause disease under certain circumstances. The key phrase is *under certain circumstances.* As a rule, the normal flora occupy their own niches and thus inhibit foreign organisms invading from other portions of the body or from the external environment. Such inhibition is brought about by competition for food, by the production of antibiotics or other inhibitory substances, or by changes in environmental conditions, such as oxygen content or pH.

This ecological balance apparently prevents indigenous pathogens, such as the yeast *Candida albicans* and the bacteria *Streptococcus pneumoniae*, *Hemophilus influenzae*, and *Staphylococcus aureus*, from causing severe disease. When the balance is upset by chemotherapy, for example, one or more pathogens may grow unchecked. A frequent sequel of antibiotic therapy is the appearance of *Candida albicans* infections. These infections may occur in the mouth or in the perianal region. Untreated candidiasis can result in serious involvement of the lungs, meningitis, and septicemia. Indigenous microorganisms that have been shown to inhibit the growth of *C. albicans* include *Enterobacter aerogenes*, *Escherichia coli*, *Pseudomonas aeruginosa*, and streptococci.

Another significant role played by indigenous organisms is helping to maintain mechanisms for antibody production. Studies with germ-free animals show that such animals generally have very low levels of immunoglobulins, the protective proteins formed by the body in response to various foreign substances. Because indigenous flora are lacking and their immune responses are weak, these animals are particularly susceptible to infection. The available evidence indicates that the amphibionts act as a constant source of antigens or irritants to the antibody-producing systems of the body and thereby permit a more rapid immunological response when it is needed.

There is some concern that prolonged space travel may lead to weakening of immunological responses. Investigations have shown that under isolation humans develop a condition of reduced normal flora that might lead to some deterioration of antibody-producing systems. In the lower animals studied, deterioration of this nature has occurred. Because of this potential danger, some space scientists have advocated adding *Lactobacillus* pills to the diet of astronauts. Lactobacilli are noted for their ability to stabilize the intestinal flora. For the same reason, pediatricians sometimes prescribe their use in cases of diarrhea.

The role of amphibionts in nutrition is the subject of considerable research. Some of these organisms synthesize a variety of vitamins in excess of their own needs, which are thus made available for the host. These vitamins include biotin, pyridoxin, pantothenic acid, and vitamins K and B_{12}. This function of the amphibionts must be of a supplementary rather than indispensable nature. If not, certain vitamin deficiency diseases would not have been so readily discovered. However, it is likely that some individuals with deficient diets are benefited by this function. One interesting side effect of chemotherapy is the occasional development of symptoms of vitamin B_{12} deficiency, perhaps as the result of a reduction in the population of normal flora.

The Immune System

The invasion of the body by foreign microorganisms or chemical agents may pose a threat to health. Defending against the effects of such foreign invaders or antigens is the function of the various components of the *immune system*, a series of protective mechanisms, specialized cells and molecules operating in the body. The immune system has several means of coping with disease agents. Among these mechanisms are (1) removing them from the body; (2) neutralizing infectious organisms and biologically active molecules; and (3) destroying foreign cells. Some of the components of this important system and their associated activities are described in the following sections.

The Components of Normal Blood and Their Roles in Health and Disease

Blood is the body's transportation system and the means of intercommunication between the various tissue cells of the body. It transports food and hormones, removes cellular waste products, assists in the regulation of body temperature, and aids in the removal and, in certain situations, the destruction of foreign substances and invading microorganisms. As several of the following chapters will show, blood can play an important role in the transmission, production, diagnosis, cure, and prevention of many conditions caused by microorganisms.

As a liquid, blood is a somewhat atypical form of connective tissue. It consists of cellular elements in a fluid substance called **plasma** (Figure 21–2). The structural components of mammalian blood are not all considered true cells. They are often referred to as the *formed elements.* These include ***erythrocytes*** (red cells), ***leukocytes*** (white cells), and ***platelets*** (Figure 21–3). *Chylomicrons,* which are visible minute fat globules, are also suspended in the plasma portion of blood. The cellular elements comprise approximately 45 percent of the blood, and plasma constitutes the remaining portion. A special type of calibrated tube called a ***hematocrit*** can be used to determine the proportions of cells and liquid portion or plasma in a blood sample.

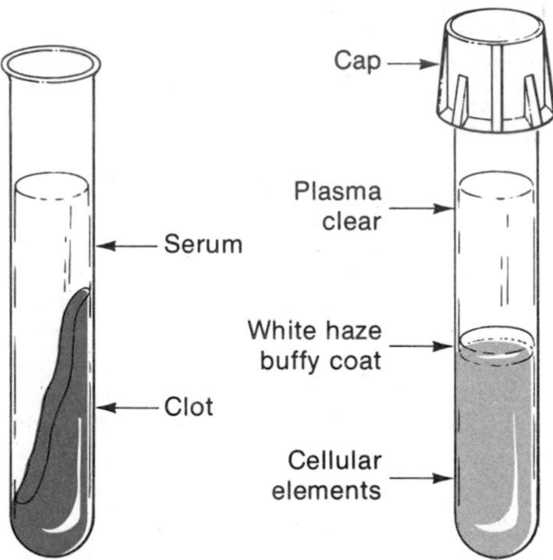

FIG. 21–2 The distinction between serum (left) and plasma (right). Serum does not contain fibrinogen.

PLASMA AND SERUM

When blood is removed from the body by means of a sterile syringe and needle and introduced into a test tube, the specimen normally clots within 2 to 6 minutes. The complex mechanism of clotting is shown in Figure 21–4. The soluble protein substance *fibrinogen,* which normally circulates in the plasma, is converted into the insoluble protein called *fibrin,* which forms the fiber framework of the clot. Most of the blood cells in the specimen become enmeshed in the fibrin. Within a few hours, the clot shrinks and expels a clear, yellow fluid called *serum* (Figure 21–2). The serum contains several types of proteins, including albumin and normal and immune globulins. *Normal globulins* are proteins important to the maintenance of adequate cellular nutrition and a normal osmotic pressure. *Immune globulins* or immunoglobulins are the so-called antibodies that are produced by the body in response to: (1) infectious agents, (2) vaccine preparations of killed, weakened, or attenuated organisms, or their products; or (3) other foreign protein substances, such as pollens.

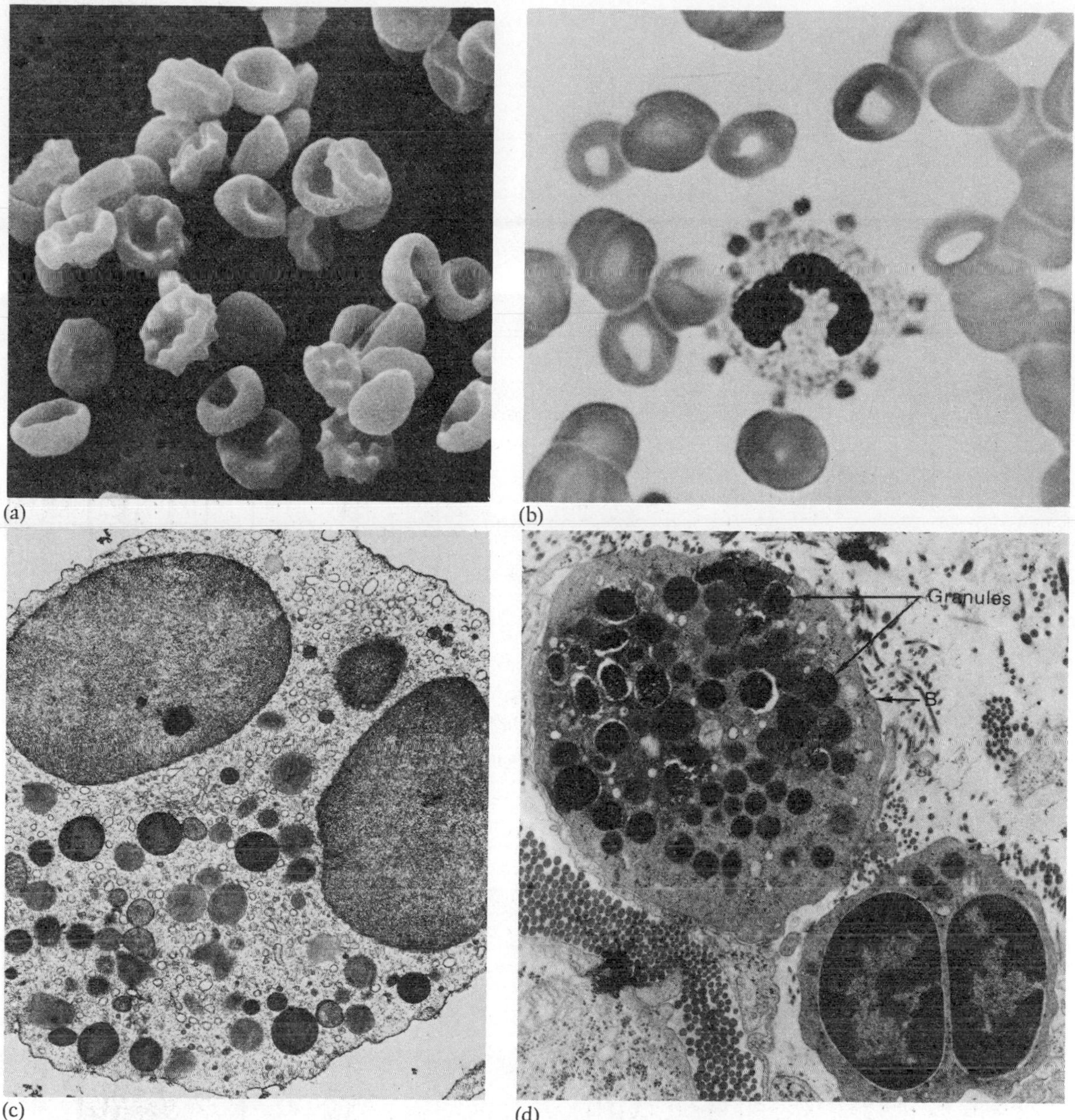

FIG. 21-3 Components of normal blood of humans and other vertebrates. (a) Red blood cells (erythrocytes) are manufactured in the bone marrow. During maturation they lose their nuclei and become disk-shaped, with slight concavities on each side. *Sheetz, M. P., R. G. Painter, and S. J. Singer:* J. Cell Biol. *70:193–203 (1976).* (b) A light micrograph showing a neutrophil surrounded by a number of smaller platelets. Platelets are the smallest formed components in the blood. They are produced by very large cells, known as megakaryocytes, in the bone marrow. *Courtesy of L. F. Skinnider.* (c) A human eosinphil. This electron micrograph shows the presence of crystalline structure within the granules of this cell. *Burns, C. P. and J. C. Huak:* J. Ultrastruct. Res. *50:143–149 (1975).* (d) An electron micrograph of a basophil. Note the characteristic granules of this white blood cell type. *Clark, J. M., G. Altman, and F. B. Fromowitz:* Inf. Imm. *15:305–312 (1977).*

In the laboratory, plasma is obtained by mixing a blood sample with an anticoagulant such as potassium, sodium oxalate, or heparin. These substances interfere with the formation of ***thrombin*** (Figure 21–4). The cellular elements will settle to the bottom of the tube containing the specimen, either on standing or centrifugation. The clear fluid left above is called ***plasma***. Thus, plasma is blood without cells but with fibrinogen; serum is ***defibrinated*** plasma.

Plasma is a complex mixture of substances, including carbohydrates, lipids, proteins, gases, inorganic salts, hormones, and water. The pH of plasma normally is slightly alkaline, approximately 7.4.

ERYTHROCYTES

Red cells, or erythrocytes, are formed in the bone marrow and measure about 7.5 to 7.7 μm in diameter and 1.9 to 2 μm in thickness. In mammals, they are not nucleated when mature and appear as biconcave disks (Color Photograph 17). The red cells are composed of a membrane which is in close association with the iron-containing protein compound ***hemoglobin***. Hemoglobin has great attraction for oxygen, and the red cell is specialized for the transport of this gas. In addition, these cells possess the major, minor, and Rh blood factors. An erythrocyte's life-span generally ranges from 100 to 120 days. Production of insufficient or hemoglobin-deficient red cells by the body is known as ***anemia***.

LEUKOCYTES

White cells, or leukocytes, are classified into two groups based upon: (1) the presence and type of cytoplasmic granules, (2) the shape of the nucleus, (3) the appearance of the cytoplasm, and (4) the size. The groups are called **granulocytes** and **agranulocytes.** Granulocytes contain distinct cytoplasmic granules and have irregular and multilobed nuclei. Like erythrocytes, they are formed in the bone marrow. The life-span of these cells is no longer than two weeks. Upon staining (as in the case of blood-smear preparations), these

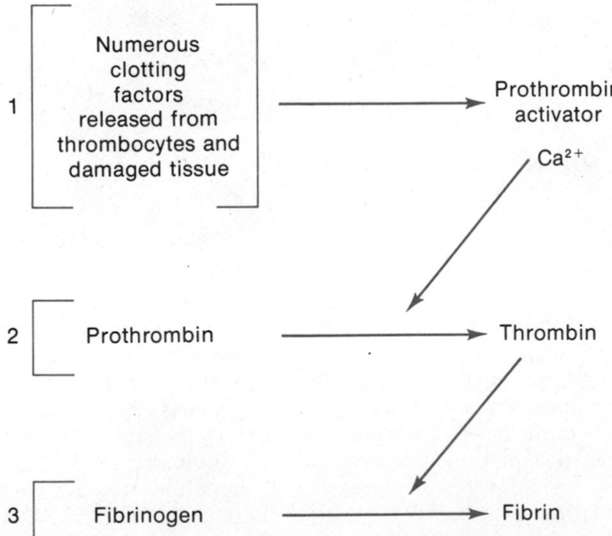

FIG. 21–4 The three stages of blood clotting (fibrin formation). Many clotting factors are necessary to react with a prothrombin activator to convert prothrombin, in the presence of calcium (Ca^{2+}), to thrombin. Thrombin in turn, converts the soluble circulating fibrogen into an insoluble meshwork of fibrin strands. Free blood cells become enmeshed in the fibrin framework.

cytoplasmic components react with dyes to yield characteristic colors. Based upon the resulting chemical reaction, three types of granulocytes are defined (Color Photograph 17): (1) *Eosinophils* containing granules that react with acid dyes and become red. They help combat certain parasitic worm infections. Eosinophils are present in greatest number in individuals with parasitic infections or allergies. (2) *Basophils* with granules that react with basic dyes and become blue. Basophils are phagocytic, capable of engulfing and digesting invading foreign particles. They are also known to play a role in immunity to virus infection and in rejection of grafts. These cells also contain chemical substances that have powerful effects on the body's blood vessels and pulmonary system. (3) *Neutrophils* or *polymorphonuclear leukocytes* (PMNLs) containing granules that react with neutral dyes or acid and basic dye mixtures, and become neutral or orange-colored. Neutrophils are also phagocytic. The number of neutrophils in the blood increases rapidly in the early stages of bacterial infection.

The *agranulocytes* do not possess granules, and their nuclei are rounded rather than lobed. The two general cell types of this group are the *lymphocyte* and the *monocyte* (Color Photograph 17).

Lymphocytes have individual rounded nuclei that occupy most of the cell. Some lymphocytes survive for as long as 200 days. Lymphocytes are principally produced in the appendix, lymph nodes, spleen, thymus, and other lymphoid tissues. Monocytes are larger than lymphocytes, and their nuclei are generally kidney-shaped. They are formed in the bone marrow. As to function, certain lymphocytes and monocytes are involved with specific antibody formation. When in tissues, monocytes also participate in phagocytosis.

Disease states can cause changes in the proportions of the different types of leukocytes. Also, certain pathogens produce an increase of white cells, called *leukocytosis*. These include *Streptococcus pneumoniae* (which causes lobar pneumonia), *Neisseria gonorrhoeae* (the cause of gonorrhea), and *Staphylococcus aureus* (the cause of boils, carbuncles, pneumonia, etc.). Other microorganisms cause a reduction in the number of leukocytes, *leukopenia*. The etiologic agents of influenza, measles, tuberculosis, and typhoid fever are included in this group.

Differential count. A *differential count* is performed to determine the proportions of the various white cells. This count is made from a stained blood smear. The normal values, based on an approximate total of 100 cells, are as follows:

Cell type	Count
Granulocytes	
Basophils	0–1
Eosinophils	1–4
Neutrophils	60–70
Agranulocytes	
Large lymphocytes	0–3
Small lymphocytes	25–30
Monocytes	4–8
	90–116

The Lymphatic System

The cells and molecules of the immune system are carried to most tissue by the blood stream. They enter the tissues by penetrating the walls of the capillaries (Figure 21–5). These cells eventually make their way to a return vascular system of their own, the *lymphatic system*. Components of this system include lymphatic vessels, lymph fluid, lymph nodes, and lymphocytes. The lymphatic vessels exist throughout most of the body (Figure 21–6). They pass through lymph nodes, which are nodular accumulations of lymphocytes and macrophages. Macrophages are derived from circulating blood monocytes. They are capable of several immunologically related functions, including clearing and degrading foreign substances within the body (phagocytosis) and preparing foreign substances in the antibody formation process. In addition to being of particular value in the transport of fatty acids, proteins, and white blood cells, the lymphatics are also important during times of infection or other tissue injury. This system serves to remove material that accumulates at the site of tissue damage, such as foreign cells and their products, white cells, and tissue debris. Pathogens and their products are carried by the lymphatics to the lymph nodes, where the immune responses by the host's macrophages and lymphocytes are initiated. During times of infection, lymphatic vessels may become inflamed and involved lymph nodes, considerably enlarged.

THE RETICULOENDOTHELIAL SYSTEM

The reticuloendothelial system (RES) consists of a variety of cells that ingest and digest foreign and host substances. Such phagocytic activity is carried out by cells called macrophages that may be either attached to tissue or free to wander into tissues. The fixed cells are found in the body's network of loose connective tissue (reticulum), lining the capillaries and the sinuses, and in regions such as the liver (Figure 21–7), spleen, bone marrow, and lymph nodes. The wandering phagocytes are found in air sacs of the lungs (Figure 21–8a), blood, and cavity holding portions of the digestive system.

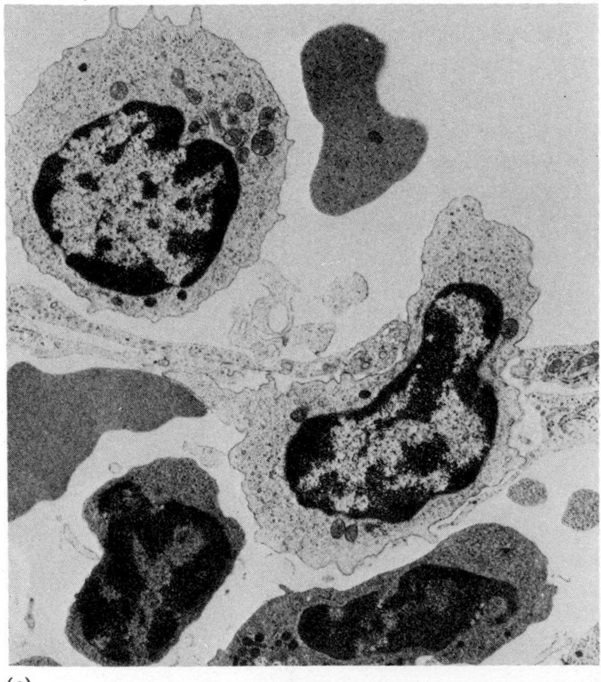

(a)

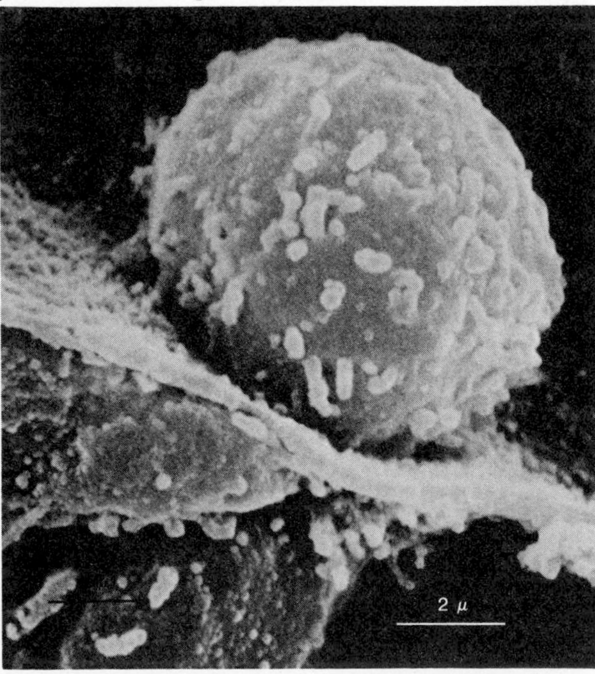

(b)

FIG. 21–5 A granulocyte in transit. (a) This transmission electron micrograph shows the white blood cell passing through the capillary wall. (b) A similar cell shown by scanning electron microscopy. *Chamberlain, J. K., P. F. Leblond, and R. I. Weed:* Blood Cells *1:655–674 (1975).*

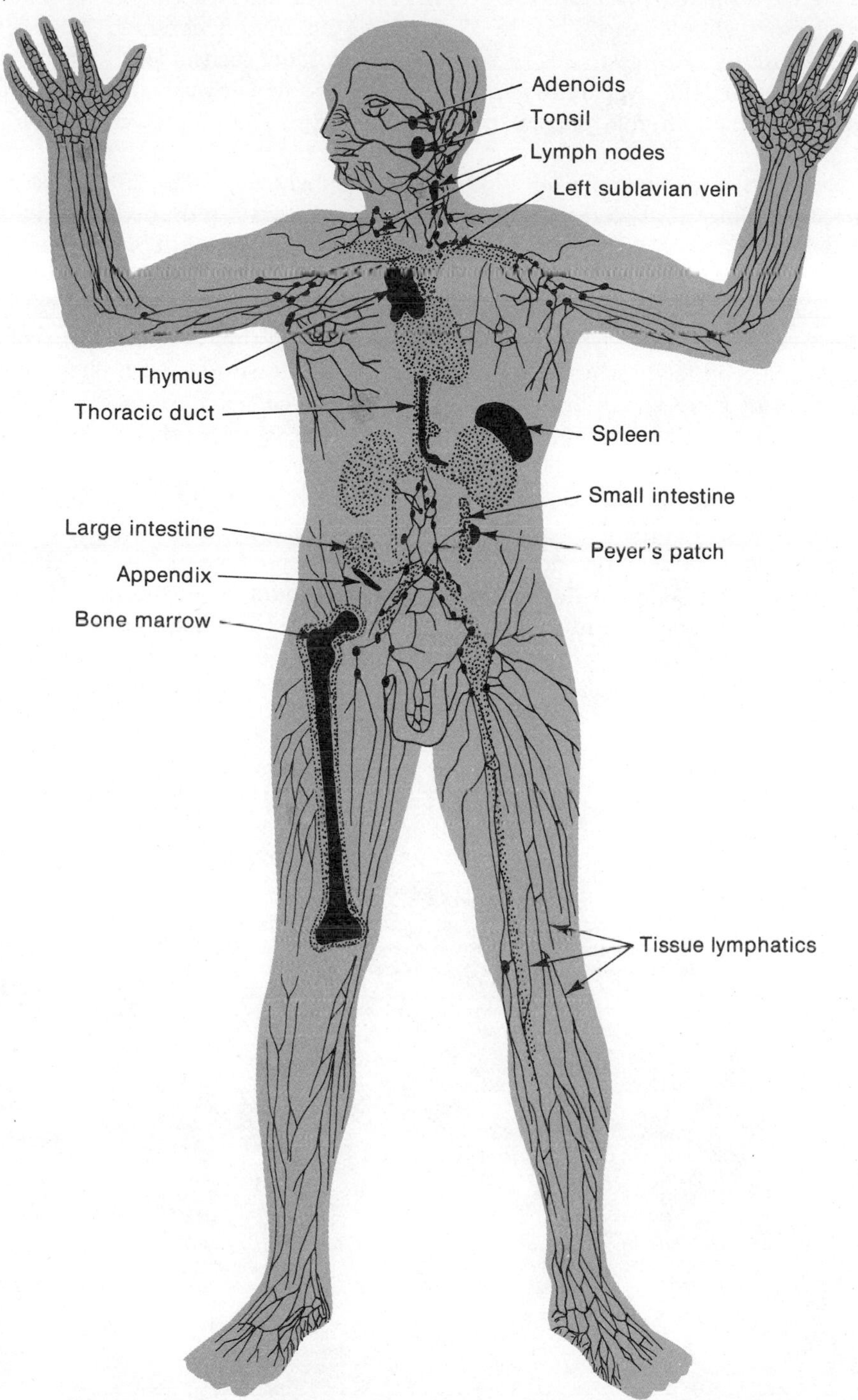

FIG. 21-6 The human lymphatic system. Components are shown in a darker color.

Phagocytosis

After the mechanical barriers provided by the skin and mucous membranes, phagocytosis is one of the organism's most important defenses against invading matter. **Phagocytosis** is the ingestion and subsequent digestion of particles by single cells. This process is carried out by circulating granulocytes (Figure

21–5) and by fixed macrophages. Foreign matter is ingested by extensions of phagocytic cells (Figure 21–8). In 1882, Elie Metchnikoff observed "ameboid cells" (leukocytes) ingest cells of the yeast *Monospora bicuspidata* within the water flea *Daphnia*. Apparently he was among the first investigators to recognize the important role played by leukocytic ingestion in protecting a host from disease.

Noncellular components of blood have been shown to be important in phagocytic ingestion. By the early twentieth century, immune serum was known to enhance active phagocytosis. When a specific antibody combines with microbial cells in the presence of a complex group of proteins known as complement, cells are made susceptible to phagocytosis. This process is called **opsonization.** Opsonizing antibodies combine with the surface antigens of a cell (antigen-antibody complex) and prepare it for ingestion by the phagocyte. Ingestion of bacteria can occur in the absence of detectable antibody. In this phenomenon, called *nonimmune* or *surface phagocytosis,* the pathogen is trapped against tissue surfaces.

If phagocytosis of the invading organism is complete, the disease state is either averted or cured. However, in the event that pathogens manage to escape ingestion and intracellular destruction, they can reproduce and cause serious infections. This tends to happen with *Mycobacterium tuberculosis, Neisseria gonorrhoeae, N. meningitidis,* and pathogenic staphylococci. Exposure to certain anesthetics, significant increases or reductions of body temperature, and various drugs can depress phagocytic activity, thus seriously lowering an individual's resistance.

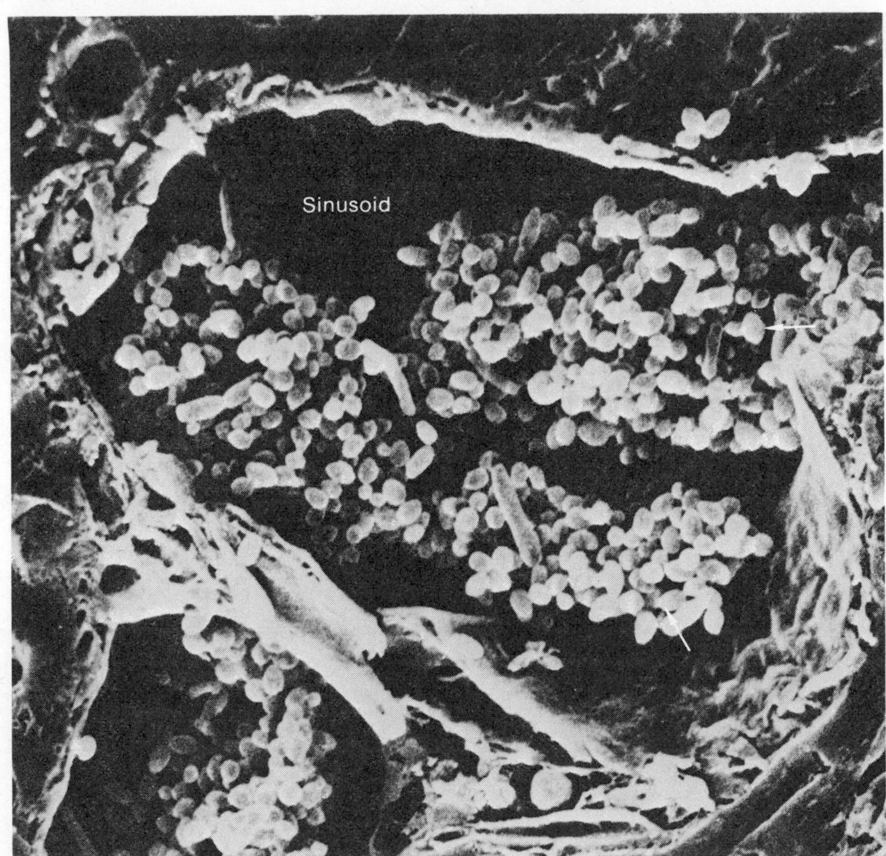

FIG. 21–7 The removal of the yeast *Candida albicans* from the bloodstream by the liver. This organ, part of the reticuloendothelial system, helps remove foreign microorganisms by trapping cells (arrows) in its spaces (sinusoids). *Sawyer, R. T., R. J. Moon, and E. S. Beneke:* Inf. Imm. *14:1348–1355 (1976).*

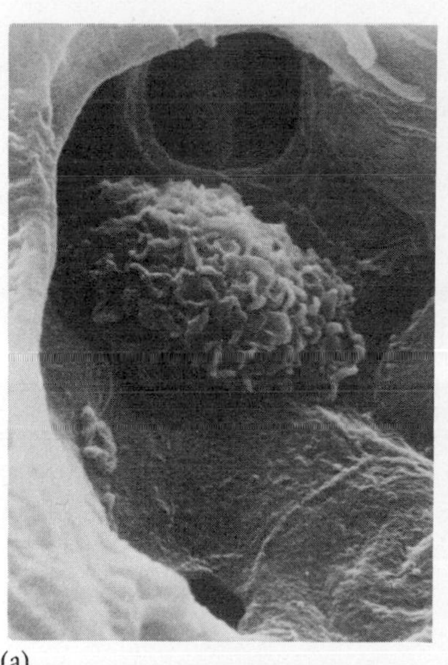
(a)

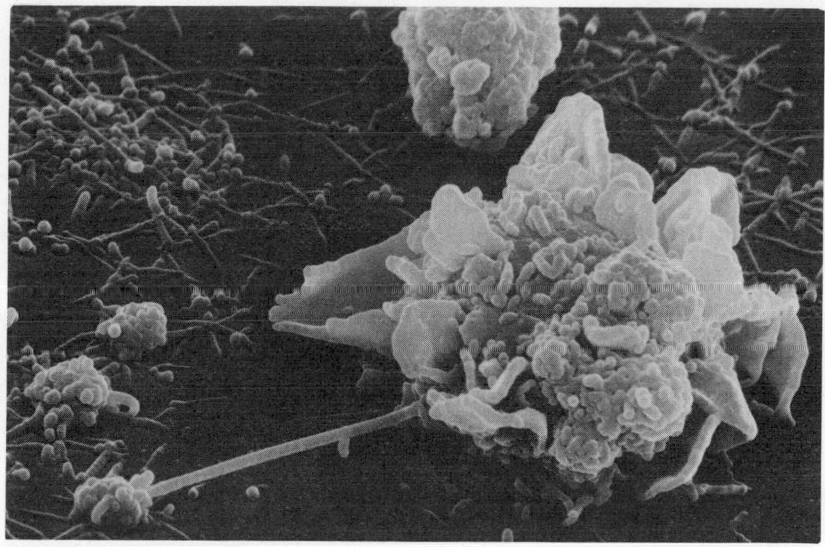
(b)

FIG. 21-8 Phagocytic cells in action. (a) A wandering macrophage on the surface of an air sac lying just beneath the entrance to the lung. *Greenwood, M. F., and P. Holland,* Lab. Invest. *27:296 (1972).* (b) Phagocytosis of bacteria. Note the cellular extension. *Powell, D. A., and K. A. Muse,* Lab. Invest. *37:535 (1977).*

Phagocytic Cell Types

It was Metchnikoff who first distinguished two major kinds of cells having phagocytic capabilities. He named them ***microphages*** and ***macrophages.*** The microphage category includes polymorphonuclear leukocytes (PMNLs), of which neutrophils appear to have the most pronounced phagocytic activity. PMNLs are the principal cells involved in the inflammatory response to invading microorganisms. Inflammation, as described later, is the result of a complex series of reactions that are coordinated to isolate and destroy harmful agents and to prepare the damaged area for healing and repair.

The ***fixed macrophages*** of the RES function in disposing of old and fragmented red blood cells. The ***wandering*** type of macrophage, which includes monocytes, also aids in the disposal of various blood cells. This is especially true of macrophages that have passed through and out of blood vessels. In addition, these macrophages assist in the repair of tissue damage by destroying and absorbing cellular debris.

Stages in Phagocytosis

Destruction of microorganisms by phagocytosis occurs in three stages: (1) contact between the phagocyte and the particle to be ingested; (2) ingestion; and (3) intracellular killing and destruction (digestion).

CONTACT

This stage may be either random or directed. Random contact depends upon chance collision between ingesting cells and particles to be ingested. In the more specific response, phagocytic cells migrate toward bacteria or particulate matter, drawn by ***chemotaxis,*** reaction to chemical stimuli. Several bacterial extracts or whole organisms have been reported to attract leukocytes ***(positive chemotaxis).*** The exact mechanism of chemotactic responses is unknown.

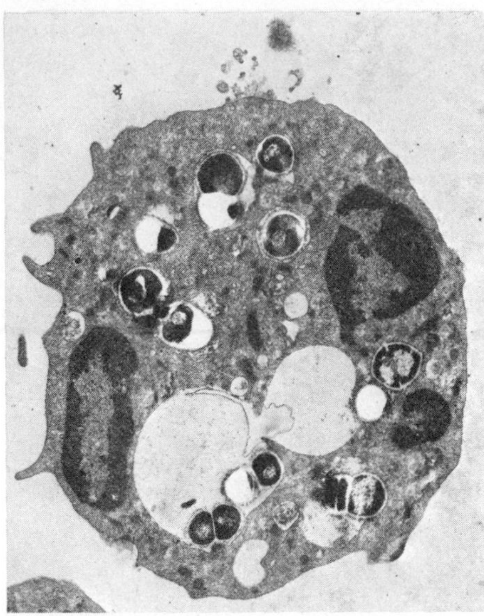

(a)

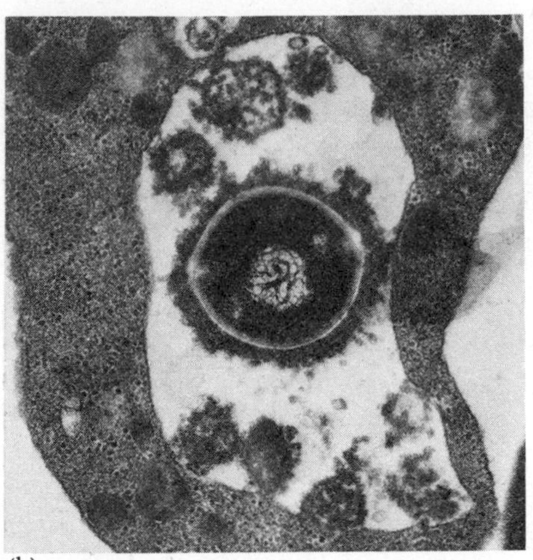

(b)

FIG. 21–9 Intraphagocytic degradation of group A streptococci as shown by electron microscopy. (a) Streptococci contained within polymorphonuclear leukocytes (PMNLs) 45 minuts after *in vitro* phagocytosis. Early evidence of degradation can be seen with certain bacteria (arrows). (b) A streptococcal cell undergoing the initial process of intro-phagocytic degradation in the vacuole (V). Changes in the cell wall (CW) and internal regions are evident at this point. *Ayoub, E. M., and J. G. White:* J. Bacteriol. *98:728–736 (1969).*

INGESTION

This stage of phagocytosis is similar to food intake by amoeba. Bacteria are ingested through an invagination of a leukocyte's cytoplasmic membrane. In general, bacteria or particles coated, or opsonized, with antibody molecules are more readily ingested. In the ingestion process, a phagocytic vacuole (Figure 21–9) forms, engulfing the bacterial cell. This activity requires the expenditure of energy by the leukocyte, energy derived for the most part from glucose metabolism. The vacuole migrates into the cytoplasm. There it collides with lysosome-like granules, which explosively discharge their antibacterial contents into the bacterium-containing vacuole. The membranes of the vacuole and granule fuse, forming a digestive vacuole, or ***phagolysosome.***

The granules of phagocytic cells appear to decrease in number as the organisms or particles are ingested. This event is called the ***degranulation phenomenon*** and is directly related to the number of particles ingested. Chemical analysis has shown the granules to contain ***phagocytin,*** as well as a large number of degradative enzymes.

INTRACELLULAR DESTRUCTION

Both lysosomal components and metabolic products contribute to the bactericidal activity in the phagocyte. As a result of the burst of metabolic activity following ingestion, lactic acid (which lowers the pH in the vacuole) and the strong oxidizing agent hydrogen peroxide are produced. These, together with histones, lysozyme, phagocytin, and various digestive enzymes released from lysosome granules, degrade the dead bacterium. Several of these antimicrobial agents are discussed in more detail elsewhere in this chapter.

Two types of lysosome granules are formed as neutrophils mature: primary and secondary granules (Figure 21–10). The first to form is the primary granule, which contains typical lysosomal enzymes. The secondary granule is the predominant granule in a mature cell and contains various bactericidal substances. Both can discharge their contents into phagocytic vacuoles.

Failure of intracellular destruction. Once ingested by phagocytes, several Gram-positive cocci are killed and degraded. This set of events is well documented for pneumococci and streptococci. However, toxin-producing staphylococci are apparently not killed after ingestion. Tubercle bacilli are readily ingested, but they remain intact inside the phagocyte because of their resistance to digestion. Such tubercle bacilli are provided not only with an environment in which to multiply, but a means for spreading to other regions and establishing new infections.

Several types of phagocytic dysfunction are known. Many of them are genetic disease states. One currently under study is the rare genetic disease Chediak-Higashi syndrome (C-HS). This condition has been found in cattle, humans, mice, and killer whales. Its characteristics include increased susceptibility to bacterial infections and the presence of large, abnormal granules (C-HS granules) in several different cell types. Large primary granules that fail to degranulate after phagocytic ingestion appear to be a major factor in the increased susceptibility to infection (Figure 21–10). In humans this change in granule activity is accompanied by impaired capacity to kill certain Gram-negative and Gram-positive bacteria, although the ingestion of organisms generally is normal.

Inflammation

Inflammation is the body's second line of defense against infection. Inflammation can be produced by infectious disease agents and by irritants such as chemicals, heat, and mechanical injury.

Signs

The characteristic or *cardinal signs* of inflammation are heat, pain, redness, swelling, and loss of function. The redness is the result of increased blood in the involved area. The dilation of local blood vessels causes a slowing of blood flow. This dilation of blood vessels is accompanied by an increased permeability which causes a swelling, ***edema,*** as tissue fluid accumulates in the spaces surrounding tissue cells. The increased diameter of the blood vessels increases the flow of warm blood to the injured area, thereby raising the temperature. Clots can form in small vessels in the general area of injury, which may prevent infectious agents or their products from entering the circulatory system. The pain experienced in an inflammatory reaction is believed to be caused by the pressure accumulating tissue fluid exerts on sensory nerves. The blood dilating substances also may irritate those nerve endings. The loss of function is associated with the pain.

As the inflammation response develops, a noticeable change occurs in the behavior of granulocytic cells. These cells first attach themselves to the inner lining of small blood vessels, the capillaries, and then push their way between the cells of these blood vessels into the areas of tissue injury at a rate faster than normal. In the later stages, these granulocytes are replaced by monocytes.

Pus formation may also be associated with inflammation. After the phagocytes have destroyed the microbial cells and engulfed the tissue debris, they become degranulated and die. In the involved area, a central mass of fluid is formed by the remains of damaged tissue cells, dead phagocytes, and microbial casualties. This fluid is pus.

Mechanism

Inflammation is a complex mechanism. Its characteristic symptoms are thought to be caused by substances released from damaged cells. Included in this group of suspected factors are the compounds ***histamine*** and ***serotonin.***

Inflammatory Exudate

The process of inflammation brings several mechanisms of the host's defense into play. With the increased blood flow to the injured area, the concentration of white blood cells and various antimicrobial factors in the fluid or exudate associated with the inflammatory reaction are greatly increased. The injuries and the increasing number of dead host cells cause the release of still more antimicrobial substances, which make the involved area increasingly unfavorable for the several types of microorganisms.

The exudate associated with inflammation also contains the elements needed for blood coagulation. These may wall off the site of activity, preventing its spread to other areas. A closed region or sac of this type, containing pus and microorganisms, is referred to as an **abscess.** Pimple, boil, and furuncle are common terms for this kind of lesion. Abscesses that are not isolated but intercommunicating are known as ***carbuncles.***

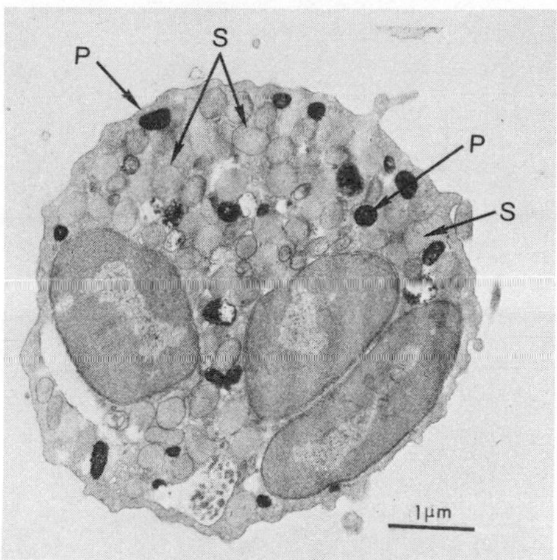

(a)

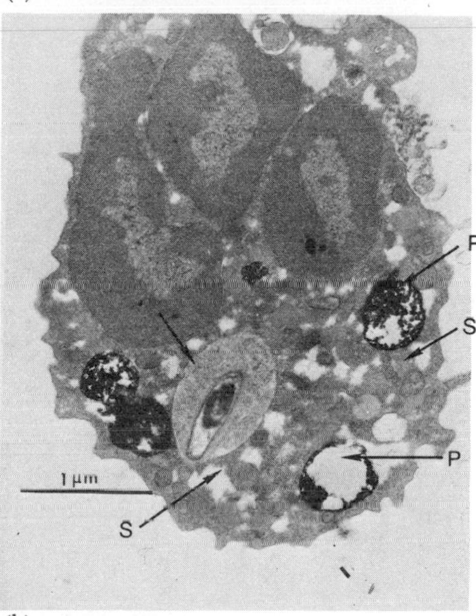

(b)

FIG. 21-10 Leukocyte dysfunction in Chediak-Higashi syndrome (C-HS). (a) An electron micrograph of a normal PMNL incubated without bacteria. The cell contains primary (P) and secondary (S) granules characteristic of mature cells of this type. (b) A C-HS polymorphonuclear leukocyte incubated in the presence of ***Bacillus subtilis.*** Phagocytic vacuole formation has occurred with an intact, apparently undigested bacterium (arrow). However, the appearance of the cell indicates that the degranulation of primary granules (P) was delayed. *Renshaw, H. W., W. C. Davis, H. H. Fudenberg, and G. A. Padgett,* Infect. Imm. *10:928–937 (1974).*

Fever

Fever is an elevation of body temperature above normal. It is a frequently treated symptom of many disease states. Attempts to lower body temperature during a febrile (feverish) episode are based on the assumption that fever is a harmful by-product of infection. Although the effects of fever may be disagreeable, they are beneficial, if the body temperature does not rise too high. Temperatures of 38 5 to 39.0° C speed the destruction of disease agents by increasing immunoglobulin production and phagocytic activity. Fever is thought to be caused by the action of toxic substances, known as ***pyrogens***, entering the bloodstream. These pyrogens are products of the disintegration of microorganisms or other cells in an injured area of the body.

Antimicrobial Substances

Chemical substances capable of *in vitro* antimicrobial activity have been isolated from various animal fluids and tissues. The full extent of their *in vivo* effectiveness is not known. Several antimicrobial substances and the types of microorganisms affected by them are listed in Table 21–2. The better known of these are discussed more fully below.

TABLE 21–2 Representative Antibacterial Substances in Animal Tissues and/or Fluids

Substance	*Common Sources*	*General Chemical Composition*	*Types of Microorganisms Affected*
Complement	Sera of most warmblooded animals	Believed to be a protein-carbohydrate-lipoprotein complex	Gram-negatives
Histone	Components of the lymphatic system	Protein	Gram-positives
Interferon	Virus-infected cells	Protein	Various viruses and certain protozoa
Leukin	Leukocytes	Basic peptides (protein-like)	Gram-positives
Lysozyme	Include leukocytes, saliva, perspiration, tears, egg whites	Protein	Mainly Gram-positives
Phagocytin	Leukocytes	Protein	Gram-negatives
Properdin	Serum	Protein	Gram-negatives and certain viruses
Protamine	Spermatozoa	Protein	Gram-positives
Spermidine, spermine	Prostate and pancreas	Basic polyamines	Gram-positives
Tissue polypeptides	Components of the lymphatic system	Basic peptides	Gram-positives

Source: Adapted from Carpenter, P. L.: *Immunology and Serology.* Philadelphia: W. B. Saunders Company, 1965.

Complement

The bactericidal property of serum, as well as of whole blood, has been recognized since approximately 1888. These antibacterial substances were found to be inactivated by heating to 56° C for 30 minutes and to function as bactericides only in the presence of specific antibody. P. Ehrlich discovered that antibody was also required for other activities, such as the lysis of red blood cells (hemolysis) by this thermolabile (heat-sensitive) component of serum which he named **complement.** Unlike the immunoglobulins and other serum factors, complement concentrations do not rise in response to immunization.

Complement, commonly designated C′, is a complex group of at least eleven major proteins normally present in the sera of most vertebrates. Some of these proteins are themselves complexes. For example, the first component of complement, C′l, is a macromolecule that consists of three subunits, C′lq, C′lr, and C′ls. When complement participates in a reaction, these protein components activate one another sequentially. Although all eleven components are necessary to produce a destructive (lytic) antigen antibody reaction, other immunobiologic activities of complement require the sequential participation of only some of the protein fractions.

Only limited information exists on the synthesis of complement components. Macrophages have been shown to manufacture C′4 and C′2. C′l synthesis has been associated with epithelial cells of the gastrointestinal mucous membranes, and the liver has been suggested as the site for the formation of other components.

Complement is well known for its ability to react with a wide variety of antigen-antibody combinations to produce important physiological results. Included in this group of reactions are: (1) the destruction of erythrocytes as well as other tissue cells; (2) the initiation of inflammatory changes; (3) the lysis of certain bacterial cells; and (4) enhancement of phagocytosis involving some opsonized particles. The cytotoxic effect of complement has been put to use in the diagnosis of several infectious diseases as in the complement-fixation test (Chapter 23).

Leukins

In 1891, Hankin prepared an extract from the lymph nodes of both cats and dogs that had bactericidal activity against ***Bacillus anthracis***. Some years later, Schneider obtained active substances from leukocytes which he called ***leukins***. Other studies yielded leukins and leukin-like compounds from various mammals including man. The substance from rabbit white blood cells was found to be heat-stable and to contain a large quantity of the basic amino acid arginine.

Lysozyme

Lysozyme, a thermostable enzyme, is present in several body fluids and tissues, including leukocytes, perspiration, saliva, and tears. Its bactericidal action is associated with the hydrolysis of bacterial cell walls, especially where repeating units of N-acetylglucosamine and N-acetylmuramic acid are exposed. Lysozyme is effective against Gram-positive bacteria and, under certain conditions, against several Gram-negative species. Recent studies have shown lysozyme's effectiveness against several microorganisms to be increased by the presence of very low antibody concentrations.

Phagocytin

Phagocytin is a protein extracted from leukocytes that is active against Gram-negative organisms and against staphylococci and some streptococci. Approximately 70 to 80 percent of the phagocytin of man, rabbits, and guinea pigs is contained in the granules of PMNLs. The substance is believed to function in conjunction with other tissue and fluid products, such as lysozyme and histones.

Properdin

Properdin was first reported in 1954 as a relatively heat-sensitive protein found in normal serum. The substance was described as having bactericidal activity against Gram-negative bacteria in the presence of magnesium ions (Mg^{2+}) and complement. Recent studies indicate that properdin is a system consisting of at least four protein factors. These factors unite to activate certain complement components.

In addition to its bactericidal action, properdin has been reported to cause the inactivation of various viruses, produce hemolysis, to provide protection against total body irradiation, and to participate in activities, such as opsonization, that promote phagocytosis.

Spermine

In 1953, Dubos and Hirsh isolated a basic peptide that is active *in vitro* against tubercle bacilli. This substance, called *spermine,* is known to be present in human tissues and those of various other animal species. The effectiveness of the peptide in these tissues is unknown. Chemically, spermine is low in the amino acid lysine but high in arginine. Its *in vitro* activity against tubercle bacilli depends upon activation by the enzyme spermine oxidase. Dubos found that tissue containing this enzyme was more resistant to tubercle bacilli than those tissues apparently lacking spermine oxidase.

Interferon

Several studies have demonstrated the production of a protein called **interferon** by certain virus-infected cells. Interferon, which is secreted into the extracellular environment, exerts an antiviral action before specific antibody levels are high enough to be effective. Interferons are synthesized by cells of different animal species and appear to be host specific: the interferon produced by a given species is the same regardless of the viral agent that causes its formation. They differ, however, among animal species with respect to antigenicity and molecular weight.

Many reports suggest that interferon is an important antiviral factor in host resistance. This can be demonstrated by removing interferon from virus-infected tissue cultures and introducing it into other systems to protect uninfected cells from viral challenge.

Many other microorganisms, particularly those with an intracellular phase in their growth cycle, also bring about the synthesis of interferon. Included in this group are the causative agents of malaria, the rickettsia, and other bacteria, such as *Brucella abortus* and *Francisella tularensis.* Many pure chemical substances will also induce interferon. These include bacterial endotoxins, double-stranded ribonucleic acid, synthetic ribonucleic acid, and complex polysaccharides and *mitogens,* proteins that stimulate cell division in lymphocytes.

Most mitogen-stimulated production of interferon takes place in T lymphocytes, the cells responsible for rejection of foreign tissue grafts and for the strong skin reaction in the tuberculosis skin test. Because of this type of activity, the mitogen-stimulated interferon has been called *immune interferon.* It differs from the virus-induced form in several properties, including molecular structure. Its actions, properties, and potential for controlling disease and manipulating the immune response are currently being studied.

PROPERTIES

In addition to the properties mentioned earlier, interferons exhibit unusual stability at low pH and a general resistance to temperatures of 50° C and slightly higher in certain instances. They are susceptible to various protein-digesting enzymes. Interferon has low toxicity for host cells but acts against several viruses, to varying degrees.

ACTION

When interferons are produced by cells infected with virions, the quantity of interferon formed by cells varies considerably, usually depending on the virus concentration. It can be altered by inactivating the virus with heat or ultraviolet light. Interferon production is dependent on viral nucleic acid. Studies have shown that empty virus cores do not induce its formation. Other sources of nucleic acids (e.g., laboratory synthesized) can stimulate synthesis of interferon. Thus, it appears that the cells producing these protein substances are reacting to the presence of foreign nucleic acids.

The importance of interferon in host resistance lies in its potential as an inhibitor of viral synthesis. Depending on interferon concentrations, various cellular activities involved in viral replication can be inhibited. As inhibition becomes more complete, the quantities of viral DNA and viruses synthesized are greatly reduced (Figure 21–11).

One currently held concept of interferon action is that it interferes with the translation of viral *m*RNA by ribosomes without inhibiting normal-cell *m*RNA translation. Thus, interferon interferes with the synthesis of viral proteins. Interferon does not inhibit all viruses equally. Several viruses, including arboviruses, influenza, and vaccinia, are quite sensitive, while adenoviruses and Newcastle disease virus are relatively resistant.

THERAPEUTIC VALUE

Because of its range of activity and its low toxicity for host cells, interferon appears to have great potential as a therapeutic agent against viruses. Progress in this direction is hindered by difficulty in obtaining large quantities of interferon, the lack of an effect on viral synthesis already in progress, and the short duration of activity. If a means can be found to maintain high and effective levels of interferon, the control of several virus-caused diseases can be achieved.

Conditions That Lower Host Resistance to Disease Agents

Preceding sections of this chapter have emphasized the importance of various factors and mechanisms to host resistance. Some consideration should be given to circumstances that can lower host resistance to infectious disease agents. A representative number of conditions are listed in Table 21–3. In most cases of infection, more than one of these conditions is involved. The frequency of

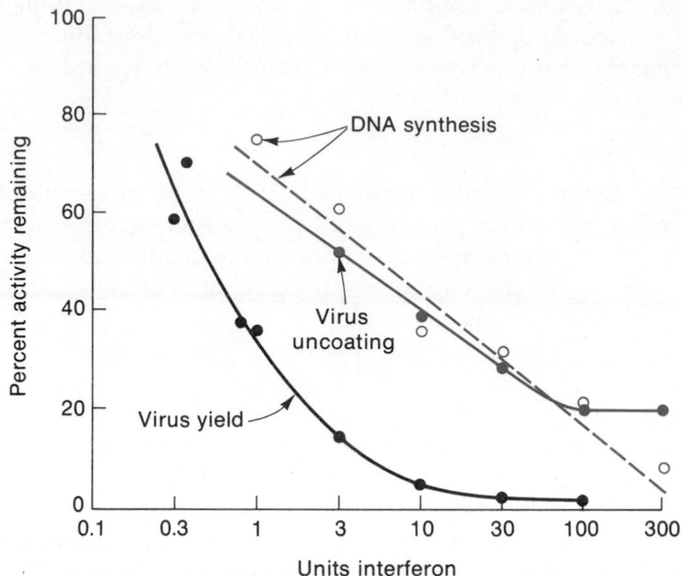

FIG. 21-11 Results of studies showing the effect of interferon concentrations on vaccina-virus uncoating, DNA synthesis, and new particle formation in a chick embryo tissue culture system. Such studies show the dramatic reduction of virus particle uncoating (colored line), viral DNA synthesis (dotted line), and new viral particle production (black line) with increasing interferon concentrations. The dots represent actual observed data; the curves are generalizations from the observed data. *Magee, W. L., and S. Levine:* Ann. N. Y. Acad. Sci., *173:362–378 (1970). The New York Academy of Sciences (1970). Reprinted by permission.*

these conditions as direct or indirect causes varies with different segments of the population and with the nature of health care services provided. Developmental and genetic defects are also important.

TABLE 21-3 Conditions or Factors that Lower Host Resistance to Infectious Disease Agents

Condition or Factor	*Selected Effects*
Acute radiation injury	Alteration of the cellular defenses of the host.
Age	Decreased efficiency of antibody synthesis and cell-mediated immunity at extremes of age; decreased levels of certain complement components during first 3 months of gestation.
Agranulocytosis	Reduction or absence of phagocytosis by neutrophils.
Alcoholism	Nutritional deficiencies; possible depression of the inflammatory response to bacterial infection.
Altered lysosomes	Extensive or limited inability of macrophages and neutrophils to destroy ingested microorganisms.
Atmospheric pollutants	Depressed immunological function of polymorphonuclear leukocytes.
Circulatory disturbances	Localized destruction of tissues; congestion; accumulation of fluid in tissue.
Complement deficiencies and/or defects	Limited or extensive inability to inactivate and/or destroy certain infectious disease agents.
Excessive or indiscriminate use of antibiotics	Elimination of natural flora that provide protection; overgrowth of resistant microbial forms; interference with digestive process and vitamin utilization.
Immunological deficiency	Interference with immunoglobulin production and/or cell-mediated immunity.
Immunosuppression	Impairment of cell-mediated immunity mechanisms.

Condition or Factor	Selected Effects
Mechanical obstruction of body drainage systems (urinary, tear, and respiratory mechanisms or systems)	Interference with the mobilization and functioning of phagocytic cells.
Nutritional deficiencies	Interference with and/or changes in several immune mechanisms, including antibody production; phagocytic activity; and integrity of mucous membranes and skin.
Traumatic injury	Direct access to body tissues for opportunists and pathogens; possible interference with immunity mechanisms; possible obstruction of body drainage systems.

SUMMARY

1. The immune system provides varying degrees of protection from or resistance to disease-causing microorganisms and cancer cells.
2. This system may impose barriers to invasion by microorganisms or selectively eliminate foreign invaders that do get into the body.
3. Specific immunity mechanisms provide protection against particular microorganisms and their products, while nonspecific resistance mechanisms are used against any and all disease-causing agents. Factors contributing to nonspecific resistance include species or racial factors, mechanical and chemical barriers, phagocytosis, inflammation, and various chemical products of the body.

Species or Racial Resistance

1. Species or racial resistance to disease agents is determined by the interplay of many factors, including physiologic and anatomic properties of a particular animal species. This type of resistance is inheritable.
2. Changes in body temperature, diet, and stress can affect this kind of nonsusceptibility.

Mechanical and Chemical Barriers: The Body's First Line of Defense

1. The effectiveness of the body's barriers to potential disease-causing agents depends on the general health of the host.
2. Mechanical and chemical barriers include unbroken skin, mucous membranes of the respiratory and genitourinary systems, nasal hairs, coughing and sneezing reflexes, tears and their associated washing action, eyelashes, and the various secretions and microbial contents of the different portions of the gastrointestinal system.
3. The effectiveness of these barriers against disease can be reduced by conditions such as alcoholism, poor nutrition, the debilitating effects of aging, fatigue, and prolonged exposure to extreme temperatures and to immunosuppressive therapy.

Indigenous or Normal Flora

1. The normal flora of the human include all microscopic forms of life normally found in or on the body and are referred to as ***amphibionts.***
2. Such normal inhabitants may, under certain conditions, cause disease or pose other problems. Microorganisms that take advantage of a host's weakened defenses to cause disease are known as ***opportunists.***
3. The major habitats for indigenous microorganisms include the skin, mucous membranes, portions of the upper respiratory tract, mouth, lower intestine, and the external and internal parts of the reproductive system. Different anatomic regions provide characteristic environments favoring a different range of microorganisms.
4. Development of the indigenous flora begins with the normal birth process and changes with subsequent exposures to other environments throughout the lifetime of the individual.
5. Benefits provided by indigenous microorganisms include inhibiting foreign microorganisms, stimulating the production of antibodies and protective proteins, and synthesizing vitamins.

The Immune System

The Components of Normal Blood and Their Roles in Health and Disease

1. Depending on the circumstances, blood can play an important role in the transmission, production, diagnosis, cure, and prevention of many conditions caused by microbes.
2. In the body, blood consists of red blood cells, white blood cells (leukocytes), and platelets in a fluid called *plasma.*
3. When blood is removed from the body, the plasma can be separated from the cellular elements with the use of an anticoagulant. If the blood clots, the clear fluid formed is called *serum.*
4. Erythrocytes, or red blood cells, are nonnucleated; formed in the bone marrow; contain major, minor, and Rh blood factors; and appear as biconcave disks.
5. Leukocytes, or white blood cells, are nucleated and can be

classified into two groups: *granulocytes*, which contain distinct cytoplasmic granules, and the *agranulocytes*, which lack such granules.

6. Based on staining reactions, three types of granulocytes are found in blood smears: eosinophils (red granules); basophils (blue granules); and neutrophils or polymorphonuclear leukocytes, or PMNLs (orange granules).
7. Agranulocytes consists of two general types, the lymphocyte with a rounded nucleus and the larger monocytes with a kidney-shaped nucleus.
8. Disease states can cause changes in the proportions of different types of leukocytes.

The Lymphatic System

1. The lymphatic system consists of lymphatic vessels, lymph fluid, lymph nodes, and lymphocytes.
2. The system participates in the transport of fatty acids, proteins, and white blood cells, and in the removal of foreign cells and their products, white blood cells, and tissue debris that accumulate at sites of infection and injury.
3. The reticuloendothelial system (RES) consists of a variety of cells that ingest and digest foreign and host substances.

Phagocytosis

1. Phagocytosis is one of the most important defenses against invading matter. It is the ingestion and subsequent digestion of foreign matter by circulating granulocytes, monocytes, and fixed macrophages.
2. Some disease agents can escape the ingestion and intracellular destruction of phagocytosis.

Inflammation

1. Inflammation is another defense mechanism of the body. It can be produced by infectious disease agents and by irritants such as chemicals, heat, and mechanical injury.
2. The characteristic or cardinal signs of inflammation are heat, pain, redness, swelling, and loss of function.
3. Pus formation may also be associated with inflammation. Pus is fluid formed by the remains of damaged tissue cells and dead phagocytes and microorganisms.
4. Fever is an elevation of body temperature above normal.
5. Fever is a frequently treated symptom of many disease states; however, temperatures of 38.5 to 39° C are known to speed the destruction of disease agents by increasing immunoglobulin production and phagocytic activity.

Antimicrobial Substances

1. Chemical substances capable of *in vitro* antimicrobial activity have been found in various animal fluids and tissue. These include complement, interferon, lysozyme, phagocytin, and spermine.
2. One of these substances, complement (C′), is a complex group of proteins. It is well known for its ability to react with a variety of antigent-antibody combinations to produce important physiological reactions, including the destruction of various tissue cells, the destruction of bacterial cells, and the enhancement of phagocytosis.
3. Interferon, a protein normally produced in response to certain virus infections, has great potential for the treatment of virus infections. It interferes with the formation of viral proteins.

Conditions That Lower Host Resistance to Disease Agents

Radiation injury, aging, alcoholism, atmospheric pollutants, circulatory disturbances, and complement deficiencies may lower host resistance to infectious disease agents.

QUESTIONS FOR REVIEW

1. a. What significant role do the normal body flora play in the control of infectious disease agents?
   b. Are pathogens encountered as normal flora? If so, list several representative microorganisms in this category.
   c. Are all types of microorganisms found as normal flora members? Explain.
2. What parts or regions of the human body act as mechanical barriers to microorganisms? Explain how each functions in this capacity.
3. Compare the composition of whole blood and plasma, and of plasma and serum.
4. Differentiate among the various types of formed elements in blood with regard to their morphological features and functions.
5. Explain the roles played by the following cells and processes in maintaining the defense mechanisms of the body:
   a. lymphocyte
   b. interferon
   c. monocyte
   d. phagocytosis
   e. eosinophil
   f. neutrophil
   g. complement
   h. inflammation
   i. properdin
   j. lysozyme
6. What is a differential count? What is its significance?
7. Describe the stages of phagocytosis.
8. What is phagocytic dysfunction? Describe one type of phagocytic dysfunction.
9. What are interferon inducers?
10. List and describe at least six factors that lower host resistance to pathogens.

SUGGESTED READINGS

Anderson, R. E., and N. L. Warner, "Ionizing Radiation and the Immune Response," *Adv. Immunol.* New York: Academic Press, 1976. *This review describes the effect of irradiation on normal lymphoid tissues, lymphocytes, antibody production and tolerance.*

Burke, D. C., "The Status of Interferon," *Sci. Amer.* 236:42 (1977). *This article includes a discussion of interferon and how it helps defend cells against virus infection, how it has been purified and characterized, and its promises for the future in combating viral diseases.*

Burnet, F. M. (ed.), *Reading from Scientific American: Immunology.* San Francisco: W. H. Freeman, 1976. *A collection of articles dealing with such topics as the immune response, cells associated with immunological reactions, and immune deficiency, transplantation immunity and infectious disease, and auto-immunity. Articles are written on a general level.*

Katz, D. H., *Lymphocyte Differentiation, Recognition, and Regulation.* New York: Academic Press, 1977. *A comprehensive and up-to-date description of cellular interactions and the cells involved in immunological reactions and responses.*

Mayer, M., "The Complement System," *Sci. Amer.* 229:54 (1973). *The components and reactions involving the complement system are presented in an understandable and well-illustrated fashion.*

Miller, M. E., *Host Defenses in the Human Neonate.* New York: Grune and Stratton, 1978. *A current publication dealing with the general concept of the susceptibility of newborn infects to infectious diseases. Other topics covered include the immune response of the neonate, phagocytic cells, and immune disorders.*

Pauling, L., *Vitamin C and the Common Cold.* San Francisco: W. H. Freeman, 1970. *A controversial study of the relationship between the common cold, general balanced health, and the use of vitamin C.*

Spiegelberg, H. L., "Biological Activities of Immunoglobulins of Different Classes and Subclasses," *Adv. Immunol.* 259:19 (1974). *A descriptive article dealing with the nature of immunoglobulins and the mechanisms triggered by the combination of antibodies with specific antigens.*

CHAPTER **22**

Microbial Virulence

How does a microorganism gain a foothold in the body and set up a disease process? Chapter 22 begins with a look at the bacterial structures and products that assist disease agents in entering a host. Attention is then focused on the various types of microbial toxins and their effects. Finally, viruses and their destructive activities are also discussed.

After reading this chapter, you should be able to:

1. **Discuss virulence and list the virulence factors involved with the causation of an infectious disease.**
2. **Identify and describe the surface components of bacteria that contribute to their invasiveness.**
3. **Describe how bacterial components interfere with host defense mechanisms.**
4. **Distinguish between endotoxins and exotoxins.**
5. **Describe the properties of algal toxins, mycotoxins, and bacterial phytotoxins and their impact on human well-being.**
6. **Discuss the pathological effects of viruses.**
7. **Explain the properties and importance of slow virus infections.**
8. **Describe the relationship of viruses to toxin-producing bacteria.**
9. **List at least three factors that contribute to opportunistic infections.**
10. **Discuss the use of the Limulus test and other techniques for detecting microbial toxins.**

Infectious Disease and Virulence

Only a small percentage of the tens of thousands of known microorganisms are capable of overcoming the defense mechanisms of a host to cause disease.

Moreover, a large number of these disease-producing agents, or pathogens, can maintain themselves only within the systems of the animals and plants they invade. In short, their existence is dependent on the availability of a suitable host, a type of *obligatory parasitism.*

To cause disease, a pathogen must: (1) attach to the surface of and gain entrance into a susceptible host (Figure 22–1); (2) multiply in host tissues; (3) resist, or not stimulate, host defenses; and (4) damage the host, often by the secretion of *toxins,* or poisons. An organism's capacity to establish a disease process in a specific animal or plant host depends on the means and mechanisms by which it carries out these steps.

An *infectious disease* may be described as an interference with the normal functioning of a host's physiochemical process caused by the activities of another organism living within its tissues or on its surfaces.

Apparently most microorganisms have disease-producing potential, given suitable environmental conditions and host. Table 22–1 lists mechanisms of action of several pathogens. Portions of this chapter and the following one describe these mechanisms and the pathogens exhibiting them.

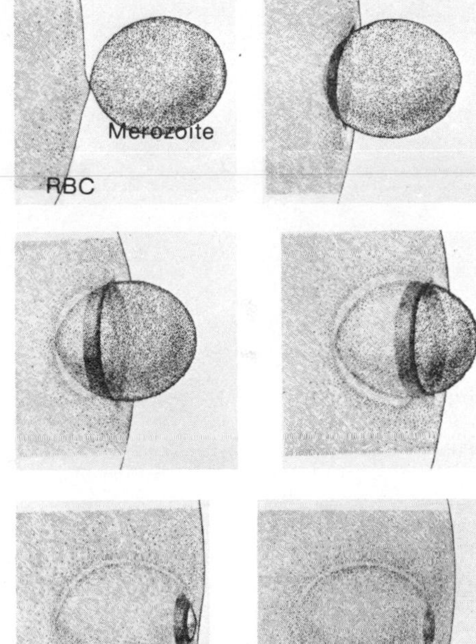

(a)

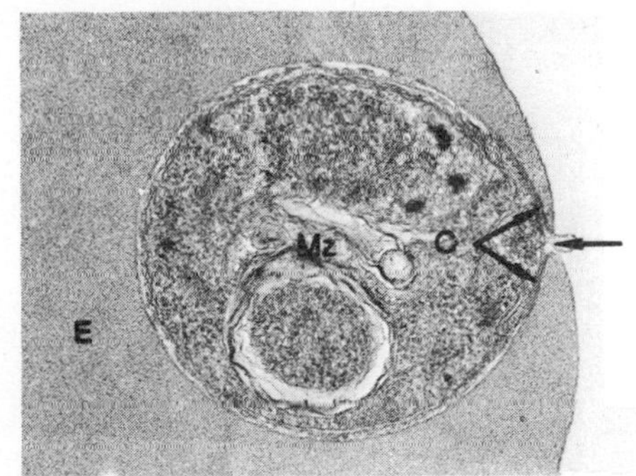

(b)

FIG. 22–1 Adherence, penetration, and growth. (a) The sequence of steps in the invasion of a susceptible cell by a malarial parasite (merozoite). (b) An electron micrograph of the parasite (Mz) beginning its growth and development. Note its point of entry (arrow). *Aikawa, M., L. H. Miller, J. Johnson and J. Rabbege,* J. Cell Biol. 77: 72–82 *(1978).*

TABLE 22–1 Some Mechanisms of Action Exhibited by Infectious Disease Agents[a]

Mechanism	*Some Disease States and/or Pathogens Exhibiting the Mechanism*
Allergic reactions (e.g., delayed hypersensitivity)	Deep-seated fungus infections, dermatomycosis (fungus skin diseases), helminthic diseases, leprosy, protozoan infections, syphilis, and tuberculosis
Blood loss and/or utilization of vitamin B_{12}	Hookworm and fish tapeworm
Fusion of cellular and viral membranes; includes the formation of giant cells known as syncytia	Viruses including herpes simplex or *Herpesvirus hominis,* measles, parainfluenza, respiratory syncytial disease, and varicella-zoster agent
Genetic integration (incorporation of nucleic acid of a virus into that of the host)	Botulism, diphtheria, and cancerous states induced by oncogenic viruses
Immunodepression (interference with a host's immune responses)	Lepromatous leprosy, measles, syphilis, tuberculosis, and virus-induced cancer
Interference with essential body functions	Anthrax, botulism, cholera, diphtheria, plague, rickettsial infections, salmonellosis, and shigellosis
Interference with phagocytosis	Infections with bacterial pathogens such as anthrax bacilli, menigococci, pneumococci, and group A streptococci, yeasts such as cryptococci, and influenza viruses
Interference with phagocytic killing	Bacterial diseases, including brucellosis, gonorrhea, leprosy, meningococcal meningitis, tuberculosis, and typhoid fever; fungus diseases, including histoplasmosis; and protozoan infections, such as leishmaniasis, pneumocystis pneumonia, and trypanosomiasis
Intracellular growth and cellular destruction	Bacterial diseases, such as brucellosis, leprosy, salmonellosis, shigellosis, tuberculosis, and rickettsial infections; most viral infections
Mechanical blockage of organs and/or associated vessels	Helminth diseases, including ascariasis, filariasis, and schistosomiasis; fungus diseases, such as aspergillosis and candidiasis; the bacterial disease lymphogranuloma venereum (LGV); and the protozoan disease malaria
Migration through body tissues and/or organs	Helminth diseases including ascariasis, fasciolopsiasis, hookworm, strongyloidiasis, trichinosis

[a]These include microorganisms as well as helminths (worms). The helminths are discussed in Chapter 37. The other disease states mentioned here are discussed in Chapters 29 and 31–36 (see the Index for exact page numbers).

Microbial Virulence

The capacity of a given pathogen to produce disease is called **virulence,** or **pathogenicity.** Virulence generally depends on features of the organism including its invasiveness, its ability to survive and reproduce in the face of the host's defensive mechanisms, and its production of *toxins* harmful to the host. Some pathogens may be both invasive and toxogenic. Experimentally, the virulence of a particular disease agent is measured by the numbers of such organisms required to kill a particular host under standardized conditions within a specified time. Naturally, the resistance of the host is an important factor. The relationship of virulence *(V)*, numbers of pathogens or dosage *(D)*, and the resistant state *(RS)* of the host to the establishment of an infectious disease can be shown by the frequently quoted formula:

$$\text{Infectious disease} = \frac{V \times D}{RS}$$

Invasiveness

Unfortunately, the terms used to express the invasiveness of disease agents with respect to the bloodstream are sometimes applied loosely, leading to misunderstanding. Here we shall use these terms with the following definitions: The presence of bacteria in blood as detected either by means of bacteriological culture or microscopic examination is referred to as *bacteremia*. This type of finding does not imply that the organisms are pathogenic, since blood may, from time to time, contain temporary invaders. The presence of organisms in the blood and their association with the toxic or septic symptoms of a host is referred to as *septicemia*. A disease state in which pathogens produce localized collections of pus in the tissues of the host is called *pyemia*.

Relatively Nontoxic Bacterial Structures and Products Contributing to Invasiveness

Invasiveness refers to the ability of a parasite not only to survive, but to establish itself in the tissues of the host. Thus, from a microorganism's point of view, several obstacles must be overcome as it penetrates deeper into the tissues of the host. This group of barriers includes phagocytosis, the lytic action of serum in the case of Gram-negative organisms, and the difficulty of spreading through tissues.

CAPSULES

Because phagocytic and other antimicrobial activities of the host involve the surfaces of invading organisms, it is not unusual to find bacterial and yeast pathogens equipped with certain protective substances. Early studies clearly described the presence of a halo-like area surrounding various pathogenic bacteria (Color Photograph 13). These regions, which later came to be known as *capsules,* are an extremely important class of surface components. Representative bacterial species with capsules include the anthrax bacillus, *Hemophilus influenzae, Klebsiella pneumoniae,* meningococci of groups A and C, the pneumococci, and certain strains of staphylococci. Loss of the ability to form capsules lowers the organism's virulence because it lowers resistance to phagocytosis.

COAGULASE

Most pathogenic staphylococci are noted for their production of the extracellular enzyme *coagulase* or *staphylocoagulase*. Human or rabbit blood treated with citrate or oxalate to prevent its normal coagulation will be caused to clot by coagulase (Color Photograph 75). In order for the reaction to occur an accessory factor, coagulase-reacting factor (CRF), must be present in the host's plasma. This serum substance is heat-labile, inactivated by heating to 56° C, and reacts slowly with the inactive coagulase to form the active enzyme. The CRF is believed to be protein. Once activated, coagulase converts fibrinogen to fibrin, and a clot forms. Staphylocoagulase has antigenic properties. At least seven distinct varieties have been reported.

HYALURONIDASE

The ability of pathogens to spread among the tissues of their host has long been a subject for study. The existence of so-called spreading factors was suggested early in such investigations. One of the substances implicated was the enzyme ***hyaluronidase,*** which is produced by various organisms, including clostridia, pneumococci, and streptococci. Several parasitic worms, or ***helminths,*** also produce hyaluronidase. This enzyme hydrolyzes hyaluronic acid, a thick, high-molecular-weight polysaccharide that is an essential component of the intracellular ground substances of several tissues, and of clotted material that accumulates in host inflammation. The effect is to greatly increase tissue permeability.

STREPTOKINASE

Several Gram-positive bacteria produce this enzyme, which dissolves fibrin clots. Included in this group of organisms are gas gangrene bacteria, hemolytic streptococci, and staphylococci. Streptokinases have a marked specificity. For example, the kinases produced by human strains of streptococci dissolve only human fibrin, and those produced by canine strains of the microorganism liquefy only the fibrin of dogs. Purified streptokinase can be used therapeutically to dissolve clots.

Microbial Toxin Production

Bacterial Toxins

Several normal components or products associated with bacterial cells are known to be toxic for higher forms of life. The toxins of bacteria are categorized as either ***endotoxins*** or ***exotoxins.*** Endotoxins are substances that are liberated only after the organism disintegrates by ***autolysis.*** Exotoxins are products generally released during the lifetime of an organism and, at times, by autolysis. Occasionally, enzymes released from cells also are considered exotoxins. Hyaluronidases and coagulase are two such enzymes. Others include fibrinolysins, such as streptokinases, which dissolve fibrin clots; proteinases, which dissolve proteins; and lecithinase, which decomposes lipids. Representative toxins and substances that aid microorganisms in their invasion of a host are discussed in the following sections.

ENDOTOXINS

Endotoxins are formed in the cell walls of Gram-negative bacteria. Chemically, they are lipopolysaccharide-protein complexes. When the two components are separated, the lipopolysaccharide (LPS) fraction is toxic and pyrogenic ***(fever causing),*** while the protein portion imparts antigenic properties to the

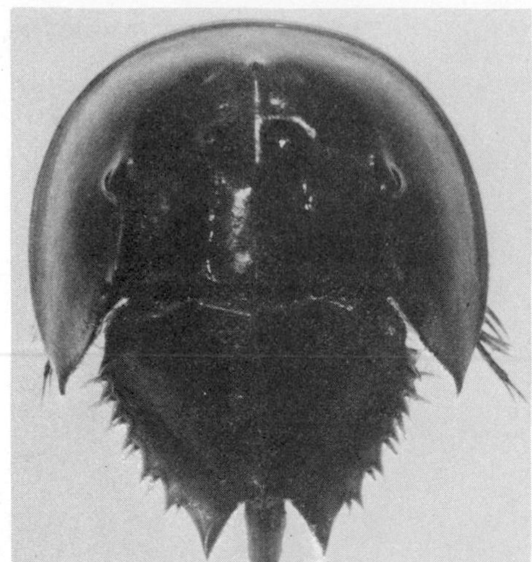
(a)

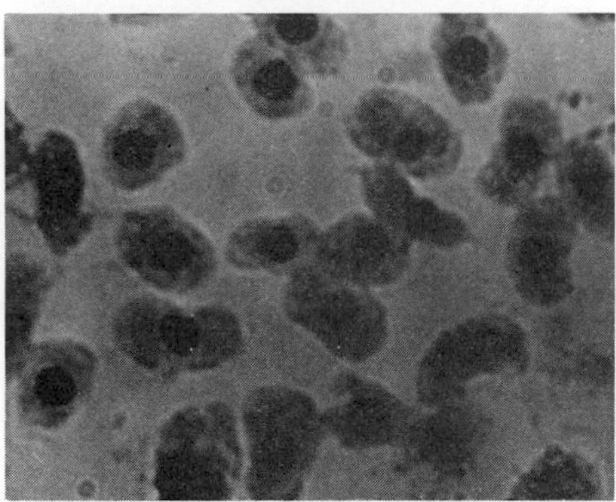
(b)

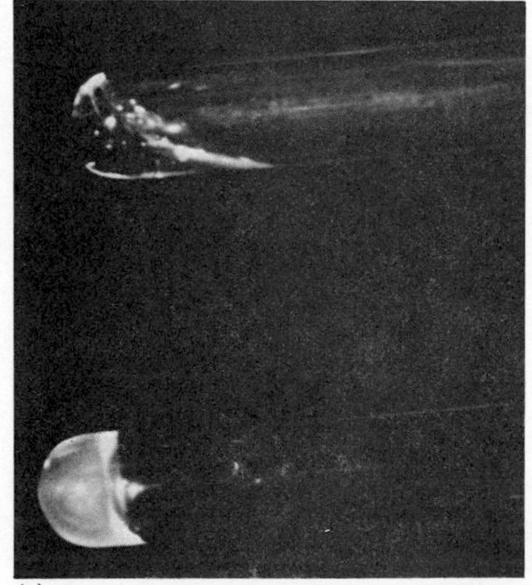
(c)

FIG. 22-2 The Limulus test. (a) The horseshoe crab. *Photographs courtesy of Dr. James H. Jorgensen, University of Texas Health Science Center at San Antonio, Texas.* (b) A microscopic view of the cells of the horseshoe crab, amoebocytes, involved with the test. *Jorgensen, J. H., and R. F. Smith,* Appl. Microbiol. 26:43, 1973. (c) A close-up view of a negative result (top tube) and a strongly positive result (bottom tube).

entire complex identical to the cell wall or somatic (O) antigens of the intact bacterium.

Endotoxins from several pathogenic and nonpathogenic Gram-negative organisms have been isolated and studied, including species of *Escherichia, Neisseria,* rickettsiae, *Salmonella, Serratia, Shigella,* and *Veillonella.* Several of the characteristics that distinguish endotoxins from exotoxins are listed in Table 22-2.

TABLE 22-2 A Comparison of Selected Characteristics of Endotoxins and Exotoxins

Characteristic	*Endotoxin*	*Exotoxin*
Chemical composition	Lipopolysaccharide-protein complex	Protein
Source	Cell walls of Gram-negative bacteria; released only on autolysis or artificial disruption of cells	Mostly from Gram-positive bacteria; excretion products of growing cells, or in some cases, substances released upon autolysis and death
Effects on host	Nonspecific	Generally affects specific tissues
Thermostability	Relatively heat-stable (may resist 120° C for 1 hour)	Heat-labile; most are inactivated at 60° to 80° C
Toxoid[a] preparation for immunization possible	No	Yes

[a]Modified protein toxin that is not toxic but still causes the production of antibodies.

MODES OF ENDOTOXIN ACTION

Endotoxins are clearly involved in disease states caused by Gram-negative bacteria, but their exact role is not understood. Various studies have shown their effects to be nonspecific. Apparently they cause the release of a fever-inducing substance from PNMLs and other cells which in turn interferes with the temperature regulatory centers in the brain. Endotoxins also cause blood clotting disorders and shock.

ENDOTOXIN DETECTION

Even minute concentrations of endotoxins can be detected by the Limulus test. The test is based on the fact that an aqueous extract of amoebocytes (lysate) from the blood of the horseshoe crab (Figure 22-2) forms a gel in the presence of very small amounts of endotoxin.

The Limulus assay is performed by adding dilutions of specimen samples to equal volumes of Limulus lysate in glass test tubes. The reaction mixtures are incubated for 60 minutes at 37° C. After incubation, the presence of a solid gel or a marked increase in viscosity (Figure 22-2c) represents a positive test. Since its initial description in 1968, the lysate procedure has been used for the detection of bacteriuria (bacteria in the urine), for the diagnosis of Gram-negative spinal meningitis, and for the detection of pyrogens (fever-causing agents) in radiopharmaceuticals and biologicals. Because of its extreme sensitivity, it is quite possible that the test can be used routinely to determine pollution in natural bodies of water, such as lakes and streams, and to detect Gram-negative bacterial contamination in various food products. The assay is unique in that it can be used to detect endotoxin in concentrations of as little as 5×10^{-4} μg/ml.

EXOTOXINS

Exotoxins may be secreted during the growth of bacteria, or, as certain recent studies have shown, they may be released on the death and autolysis of cells. They are responsible for many of the disease symptoms and for the eventual disease of the organism in many disease states. These poisonous substances are distinguished from endotoxins by several properties (Table 22–2). Chief among these are their protein nature and specificity of action. Several bacterial species produce a wide variety of exotoxins (Table 22–3).

TABLE 22-3 Selected Representative Exotoxins Produced by Bacterial Pathogens

Bacterial Species	*Gram Reaction*[a]	*Disease*	*Toxin Designation*	*Type of Toxin Action*
Bordetella pertussis	−	Whooping cough	Pertussis (whooping cough toxin)	Necrotizing (tissue destructive)
Clostridium botulinum	+	Botulism	Six type-specific toxins[b]	Paralytic (blocks acetylcholine release)
Clostridium novyi[c]	+	Gas gangrene	Alpha (α) toxin	Necrotizing
			Beta (β) toxin	Hemolytic lecithinase, necrotizing
			Delta (δ) toxin	Hemolytic
Clostridium perfringens[c]	+	Gas gangrene	Alpha toxin	Hemolytic lecithinase, necrotizing
			Theta (θ) toxin	Hemolytic cardiotoxin (heart tissue destructive)
			Lambda (λ) toxin	Proteolytic (protein digesting)
Clostridium tetani	+	Tetanus	Tetanolysin	Hemolytic cardiotoxin
			Tetanospasmin	Spasm-causing
Corynebacterium diphtheriae	+	Diphtheria	Diphtheritic toxin	Necrotizing
Yersinia pestis	−	Plague	Plague toxin	Probably necrotizing
Shigella dysenteriae	−	Bacillary dysentery	Neurotoxin	Hemorrhagic, paralytic
Staphylococcus aureus	+	Food poisoning	Enterotoxin	Vomiting
		Pyogenic infections	Alpha toxin	Hemolytic, leucocidic, necrotizing
			Beta toxin	Hemolytic
			Delta toxin	Skin destructive, dermonecrotic, hemolytic, leucolytic
			Leucocidin	Leucocidic
Streptococcus pyogenes	+	Pyogenic infections and scarlet fever	Alpha toxin	Hemolytic
			Erythrogenic toxin	Scarlet fever rash
			Streptolysin O	Cytotoxin, hemolytic
			Streptolysin S	Smooth muscle contraction, hemolysin

Source: Modified from B. Davis, R. Dulbecco, H. Eisen, H. Ginsberg, and W. Wood: *Microbiology*. New York: Harper & Row Publishers, Inc., 1968.
[a]− = Gram-negative; + = Gram-positive.
[b]Two of these toxins, C and D, affect lower animals.
[c]Only a few of the several toxins produced by this species are given.

An interesting aspect of exotoxin production is its association in certain cases with particular bacterial viruses. For example, diphtheria bacilli produce an exotoxin only when they are harboring a particular temperate bacteriophage. Only those bacteria infected by such specific viruses form the toxin. A similar situation exists with cells of *Clostridium botulinum* and *Streptococcus pyogenes*, which produce the erythrogenic toxin associated with scarlet fever only under the influence of certain temperate viruses.

TABLE 22-4 Conditions and/or Factors Involved in Bacterial Opportunistic Infections

Predisposing Condition and/or Factor	Bacteria	Infection or Disease State
Abdominal and other forms of surgery	*Bacteroides fragilis*	Blood poisoning (septicemia)
	Streptococcus spp.	Blood poisoning and lung disease
Alcoholism	*Haemophilus* spp.	Infection of brain coverings (meningitis)
	Klebsiella pneumoniae	Lung disease (pneumonia)
	Mycobacterium tuberculosis	Tuberculosis
Antimicrobial therapy	*Escherichia coli*, *Proteus vulgaris*, *Serratia marcescens*	Urinary tract infection
	Staphylococcus aureus	Blood poisoning (septicemia)
Breaks in skin, wounds, burns, etc.	*Acinetobacter calcoaceticus*, *Bacteroides*, *Clostridium* spp.	Blood poisoning
	Pseudomonas spp., *Staphylococcus aureus*, *Streptococcus* spp.	Blood poisoning, lung infection
Diabetes mellitus	Anaerobes	Foot ulcers
	Haemophilus spp.	Infection of brain coverings
	Nocardia spp., *Streptococcus pneumoniae*	Lung infection
Immunosuppression	*Corynebacterium* spp.	Lung infection
	Escherichia coli	Urinary tract infection
	Staphylococcus aureus	Blood poisoning
Malnutrition	*Mycobacterium tuberculosis*	Tuberculosis
Malignancies (various types of cancer)	*Aeromonas hydrophilia*, *Clostridium perfringens* and other clostridia, *Citrobacter* spp., *Escherichia coli*, and *Pseudomonas* spp.	Blood poisoning and lung infections
Sickle cell disease	*Haemophilus* and *Yersinia* spp.	Blood poisoning
Transplants	*Arizona* spp.	Blood poisoning
	Mycobacterium spp.	Lung infection
	Mycobacterium tuberculosis	Tuberculosis

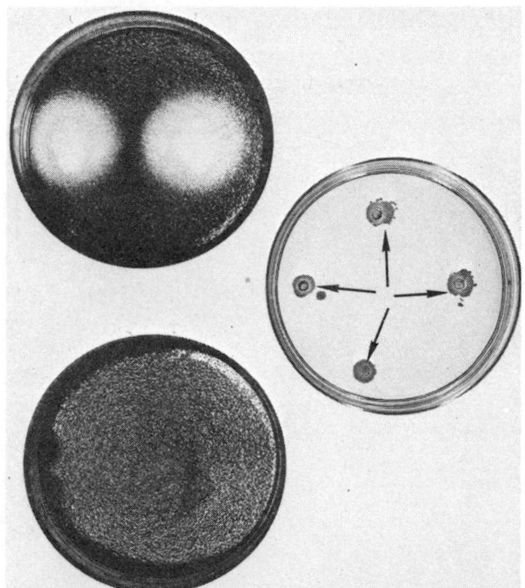

FIG. 22-3 The colony overlay test (COT), a method for detecting toxin production (toxicogenicity) by *Corynebacterium diphtheriae* strains in tissue culture. The plate on the right shows growth of bacterial cultures 18 hours after inoculation. The cultures located at 3 and 9 o'clock are toxin producers, whereas the remaining two are not. This is evident in the top tissue culture plate where toxin from two toxin-producing strains has destroyed a monolayer of tissue culture cells. The lower plate, a control, shows no tissue destruction.

MODES OF EXOTOXIN ACTION

The mechanisms and sites of action have been studied in several of the classic exotoxins, including botulism, diphtheria, and tetanus. In general, exotoxins function by destroying specific components of cells, or by inhibiting certain cellular activities. Some of these substances work only on specific cell types. Further details will be discussed in the chapters dealing with these toxin-producing agents.

EXOTOXINS OF MAJOR CLINICAL SIGNIFICANCE

Botulism. The exotoxin of *Clostridium botulinum*, the causative agent of fatal food poisoning, affects only nerve tissues; that is, it is a *neurotoxin*. This poisonous substance interferes with the mechanisms involved in the transmission of stimuli to muscles by blocking the release of acetylcholine.

Diphtheria. The diphtheria exotoxin appears to inhibit protein synthesis. It is also noted for general destructive effects on various types of tissues (Figure 22–3).

Gas gangrene. Several members of the genus *Clostridium* may be associated with this disease state. One of them, *C. perfringens,* is known to produce an alpha (α) toxin that can destroy cell membranes.

Tetanus. The exotoxin formed by *Clostridium tetani,* the causative agent of lockjaw, is also a neurotoxin. It exerts its destructive effects mainly on the anterior horn cells of the central nervous system.

OTHER EXOTOXINS OF CLINICAL SIGNIFICANCE

Several exotoxins normally play a lesser role in clinical disease states, either because, under normal conditions, they are produced in small quantities or because they are not extremely toxic. However, under certain conditions, these exotoxins may cause serious illness. Examples of these exotoxins include dysentery bacillus neurotoxin, scarlet fever erythrogenic toxin, staphylococcal enterotoxin, and streptolysins O and S.

The erythrogenic toxin of scarlet fever. A small number of the strains belonging to beta hemolytic group A streptococci are capable of producing this "minor" toxin. These streptococci belong to one of the several immunological groups differentiated on the basis of their antigenic composition. Three toxins are recognized, labeled A, B, and C. The first of these toxins occurs with the greatest frequency. Erythrogenic toxins have a selective action on the skin and are neutralized by scarlet fever antitoxin. No effects are suffered by the streptococci multiplying at the time.

Staphylococcal enterotoxins. Many coagulase-positive strains of *Staphylococcus aureus* produce enterotoxins. These toxins are: (1) protein in nature, (2) poor antigens, (3) resistant to boiling temperatures for approximately 30 minutes, and (4) not neutralized by antitoxins prepared against other toxins produced by staphylococci. Humans and monkeys appear to be the only naturally susceptible victims for this enterotoxin. Affected individuals generally experience nausea and vomiting within a few hours after the toxin's ingestion. Fatalities are rare.

Streptolysin O. Certain streptococci produce two distinct soluble hemolysins, enzymes that destroy red blood cells. One of these bacterial products is called *O lysin* because of its sensitivity to oxygen. The other hemolysin, designated *S lysin,* in addition to other properties, is noted for its extreme sensitivity to heat. Certain streptococci produce only O lysin, while others secrete only S lysin. Most members of group A produce both.

Streptolysin O is elaborated by most streptococci in group A, those organisms of human habitation in group C, and certain members of group G. This streptolysin can be inactivated by heating at 37° C for 2 hours. It is a protein and is antigenic, as is evident during infections caused by streptococci. Streptolysin O is noted for its toxic action on red blood cells and various other types of cells, including frog heart and mammalian kidney and heart (Figure 22–4). Several studies indicate that it may play a significant role in rheumatic heart disease.

Streptolysin S. This exotoxin is produced by most strains of group A streptococci and probably by members of other groups. Because streptolysin S

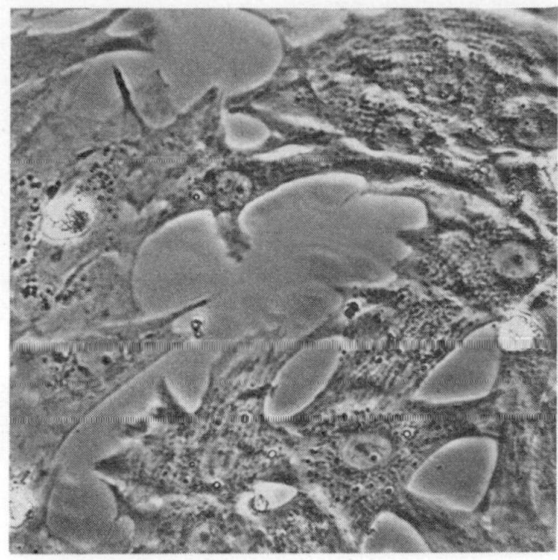

(a)

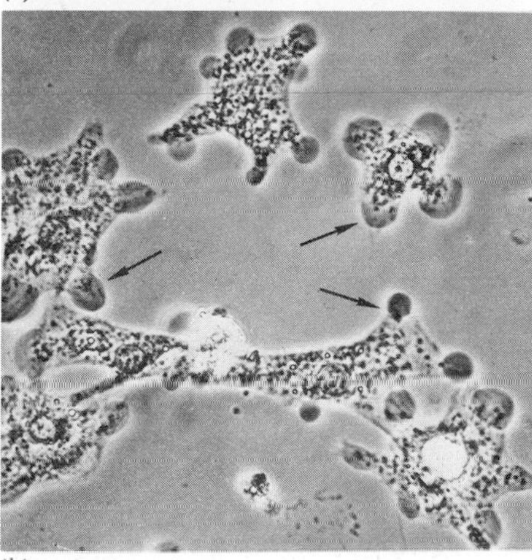

(b)

FIG. 22–4 The toxic effect of streptolysin O or beating mammalian heart cells in tissue culture, as observed by phase contrast microscopy. (a) The appearance of normal rat heart ventricle cells after two days of growth. Before exposure the myocardial cells on the right exhibited striations and were beating vigorously. (b) The same cells three minutes after exposure to group C streptolysin O. Note the granulation and numerous plasma membrane blebs (arrows) associated with killed myocardial cells. *Thompson, A., S. P. Halbert, and U. Smith,* J. Exp. Med. *131:745–763 (1970).*

has resisted attempts at purification, its chemical makeup remains in doubt. It is believed to be either polysaccharide or protein in nature.

The toxin is not antigenic in the generally accepted sense upon injection into laboratory animals. It is, however, noted for a pronounced toxicity on the tissues of laboratory animals. The hemolysis that develops around surface-located colonies on blood agar plates is caused by streptolysin S.

Shigella dysenteriae **exotoxin.** This simple protein substance is noted for its neurologic effects in man and various laboratory animals. Its toxicity is comparable to that of the tetanus and botulism neurotoxins. Fortunately, the quantities produced per cell in cultures of *S. dysenteriae* are quite low.

Bacterial Phytotoxins

Humans are virtually dependent for survival on certain food crops. Among them are barley, cassava, corn, oats, potato, rice, soybean, sweet potato, sugarcane, and wheat. Unfortunately, all of these plants are hosts for pathogenic bacteria, many of which are known to produce toxins. Such **phytotoxins** (plant poisons) can cause plants to wilt or to lose their coloration, or they may bring about extensive destruction of leaves, stems, or flower parts. Species of *Corynebacterium, Erwinia, Pseudomonas,* and *Xanthomonas* are known to produce one or more phytotoxins. Chemically, these toxins are polysaccharides, peptides, and related compounds.

Toxins of Blue-green Bacteria

Poisoning of lower animals and even of humans by blue-green bacterial blooms is well documented. Toxic blooms have occurred in the lakes, ponds (Color Photograph 4A), and reservoirs of Africa, Asia, Australia, Europe, and North and South America. Toxic freshwater blue-green bacteria are becoming an important factor in water quality, especially as more marginal water supplies are coming into public use. Unlike freshwater species, most marine cyanobacteria have not presented serious health or economic problems. However, swimmers in tropical waters have experienced rashes and blisters of the skin, lips, and genitals after exposure to disrupted blue-green bacteria.

Algal Toxins

Algal toxins contribute a wide variety of poisonous substances to aquatic environments. Thus far, many algal toxins, which become poisonous to fish, waterfowl, mussels, and clams and subsequently to humans who eat shellfish, have been studied in crude form only. One of the few that has been isolated in pure form is produced by the dinoflagellates associated with the toxic red tides. The toxin is a highly potent poison: it causes death in experimental animals in less than 30 minutes, and it produces paralysis and death in humans.

Toxin-producing algae pose a serious threat to human well-being. Many algal species that may represent a potential food supply produce toxins, and the poisonous substances produced by marine algae threaten edible marine organisms. The problem could become more acute as the world becomes more dependent upon food from aquatic sources.

Mycotoxins

Mycotoxicoses are disease states caused by the ingestion of foodstuffs contaminated with fungus toxins. This is to be distinguished from another fungus disease category, **mycosis,** which involves a general invasion of living tissue by actively growing fungi. Mold-induced deterioration of foods and feeds causes economic losses and poses a serious health hazard. Ergotism, the effect of the mycotoxin ergot, has been known for years, and isolated other mycotoxicoses in animals have been reported. There is an increasing awareness of mycotoxins as potential natural environmental contaminants.

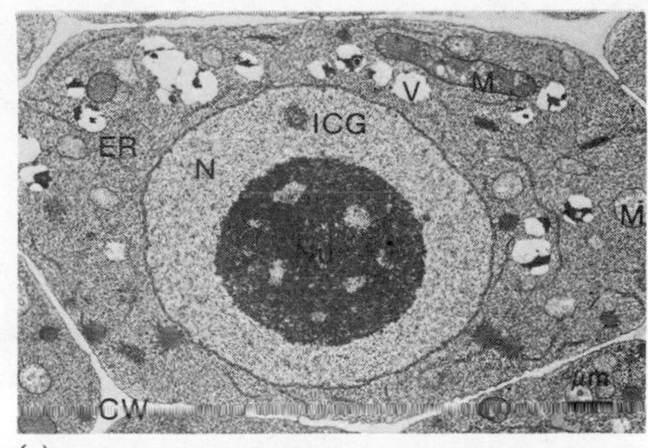

(a)

(b)

FIG. 22-5 The effects of a fungal toxin (specifically, aflatoxin) on plants. Cellular changes after exposure to aflatoxin are obvious in the electron micrographs of root cells. (a) Control cells. (b) The effects of treatment with aflatoxin. (*Abbreviations:* CW, cell wall; ER, endoplasmic reticulum; ICG, interchromatin granules; L, lipid bodies; M, mitochondria; N, nucleolus; V, vacuole; and arrow, light nucleolar cap.) *Crisan, E. V.,* Appl. Microbiol. *12:991–1000 (1973).*

The distinctive characteristics of a mycotoxicosis include the following: (1) the disease is not transmissible; (2) drug or antibiotic treatments have little or no effect on the disease; (3) outbreaks in the field are often seasonal because certain climatic conditions affect mold development; (4) the outbreak is usually associated with a specific feed or foodstuff; and (5) examination of the suspected food or feed reveals signs of fungal activity.

Of the mycotoxins studied, those produced by species of *Aspergillus,* the *aflatoxins,* are the best known. These poisons are a unique group of low-molecular-weight compounds. Aflatoxins have been found in a wide array of edible commodities, including beans, cereals, coconuts, milk, peanuts, sweet potatoes, and commercially prepared animal feeds.

In addition to their intoxication effects, aflatoxins have been found to have carcinogenic properties. This finding has reinforced, but not confirmed, the concept that naturally occurring mycotoxins may be a cause of human cancer on a broad basis. Studies during the 1960s demonstrated the involvement of aflatoxins with liver damage in several birds, fish, and mammals and with tumor formation in ducklings, ferrets, rats, and trout. Specific toxicological and biochemical studies with experimental animals have shown that mycotoxins cause such effects as ultrastructural alterations; changes in the synthesis of DNA, RNA, and protein; and mitochondrial activity. Despite the vast number of these studies, the precise mode of action of aflatoxin is not known. Like many carcinogens, aflatoxins act as nonspecific cell poisons that exert multiple effects on the structures and biochemistry of susceptible cells. Because most of these changes may be secondary to carcinogenic activity, they must be identified as such if the primary mode of action is to be defined.

Some mycotoxins also show antibacterial, antifungal, antiprotozoan, and antitumor effects. Plants are also susceptible, but although a great amount of data has been accumulated, few studies have been conducted on the *in vivo* effects of aflatoxin on plants. In these hosts, aflatoxin has been found to inhibit seed germination, growth, and chlorophyll development, and to induce chromosomal abnormalities and changes in cellular structures (Figure 2–5).

Other mycotoxins also exhibit a number of carcinogenic, mutagenic, and developmental, or teratogenic, (Figure 22–6) effects in both procaryotic and eucaryotic systems. In animal systems, the biological action of mycotoxins is affected by the sex and species of the animal, environmental factors, and nutritional status. Thus, the biological effects of mycotoxins are as varied as their chemical structures.

Viral Pathogenicity

Many microbial pathogens are intracellular parasites. Some viruses enter the tissues of a host directly through some injury or insect bite. Most viral infections, however, start on the mucous membranes of the respiratory or gastrointestinal tract. To start an infectious process, *virions* must first survive on these mucous membranes in the presence of other microorganisms (including normal flora). To replicate, they must enter susceptible host cells, either in the mucous membrane or in tissues distant from the point of entry. Replication of the virus that invades the mucous membrane can produce disease effects directly, as in the case of respiratory infections. Sometimes, however, it sets the stage for damaging replication in another part of the host. Poliovirus is a good example of this situation. The virus replicates first in alimentary-tract cells and ultimately in specific sites in the central nervous system. Knowledge of the factors that affect the early stages of viral infections is incomplete.

Viruses break through host defenses to cause disease. As with bacteria, this process depends not only on the strength of the defenses and on the microorganism's capacity to counteract them, but also on the number of invaders. A sufficiently large infecting dose can overwhelm the initial defenses of a susceptible host and cause irreparable injury before adequate defenses can be brought into action.

Natural disease states and most laboratory experiments involve small infecting doses of viruses. Before a disease state is reached, viral numbers must be built to a population large enough to damage the activities of host defense mechanisms.

The Pathological Effects of Viruses

In studies on the effects and mechanisms of viral pathogenicity, two important questions arise: Which pathological effects are specific to virus attack, rather than being the host's nonspecific responses to general injury? How are the pathological effects produced? Our discussion will concern itself with the second question.

Cellular damage of animal tissues by virus attack has been recognized for many years. For example, brain cells are damaged by Newcastle disease virus, and respiratory epithelium is changed and injured by a variety of respiratory viruses (Figure 22–7).

LATENT INFECTIONS

Electron microscopy and immunofluorescent techniques have shown that viral replication can occur in cells without significant damage. Clearly, not all viral infections result in the death of the host cell. A good example of this situation is given by the *Herpesvirus* that causes cold sores or fever blisters. This virus can remain dormant or silent for months, years, or even decades. The virus lies latent within nerve cells of ganglia, producing no disease symptoms until stresses such as fever, exposure to extreme cold, emotional problems, or sunburn trigger the virus, causing small skin eruptions to develop. Yet between outbreaks the herpesvirus apparently does not destroy the nerve cells in which it continues to exist.

SLOW VIRUS INFECTIONS

In recent years it has also become apparent that some slowly developing, persistent diseases that superficially do not appear to be infectious can be caused or triggered by unusual "slow" viruses. Strong evidence has accumulated that several severe neurological diseases are caused by the agents. There is also preliminary evidence, as yet inconclusive, that several common degenerative diseases, such as diabetes, leukemia, multiple sclerosis, and rheumatoid arthritis, may actually be the result of slowly developing viral infection.

CYTOPATHIC EFFECT

For many years it was thought that virus-induced cell damage was only a side effect of virus replication: excessive production of virus or viral components might deplete cellular components essential for cell life or for the repair of mechanical injury. There is increasing evidence that viruses are more actively responsible for cell damage. One process by which this damage occurs is virus cytotoxic activity. There are two levels at which pathologically important cytotoxic activity can operate, namely, biochemical damage without morphological damage and biochemical damage with morphological damage (cell lysis, fusion, or death). Morphological damage is usually referred to as a cytopathic effect.

Further research will undoubtedly uncover other mechanisms by which viruses can establish infections. Such information will add to the understanding of microbial virulence and may provide a basis for developing effective means of treatment and control.

Opportunists and True Pathogens

True pathogens are the relatively small fraction of those organisms harbored by most forms of animal and plant life that can directly invade tissues and cause obvious infections. *Opportunists* are organisms that have the potential to produce infections if they accidentally gain access to the tissues of the host under special circumstances. An opportunistic microorganism takes advantage of weakened defense mechanisms to cause damage to a "compromised" host. Such microorganisms may or may not be members of a host's normal resident flora, and they may or may not be pathogenic to a normal host.

Knowledge of the mechanisms that open the way for invasion by opportunistic microbes is incomplete. Several situations have been identified as contributing to opportunistic infections. Such factors include genetic defects, the use of antibiotics, and immunosuppressive therapy to limit the activity of the immune system, as in cases of cancer or of tissue transplantation. Table 22-4 lists several of these factors and the bacteria to which they predispose the host.

The distinction between an opportunist and a true pathogen can be difficult to make. This is because, in a clinical setting, it is difficult to decide whether a patient's weakened defenses were or were not a necessary precondition for a given disease.

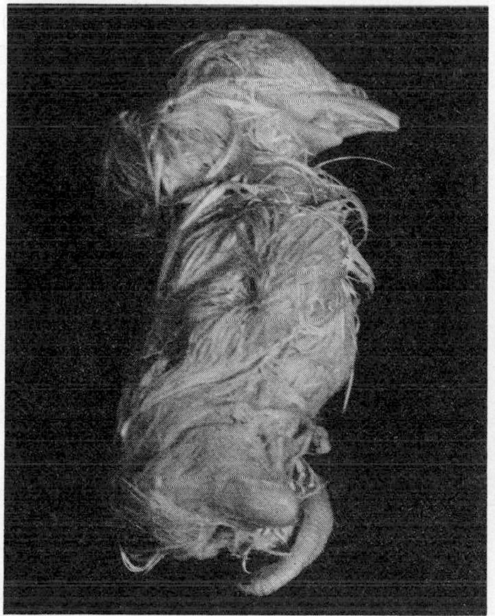

(a)

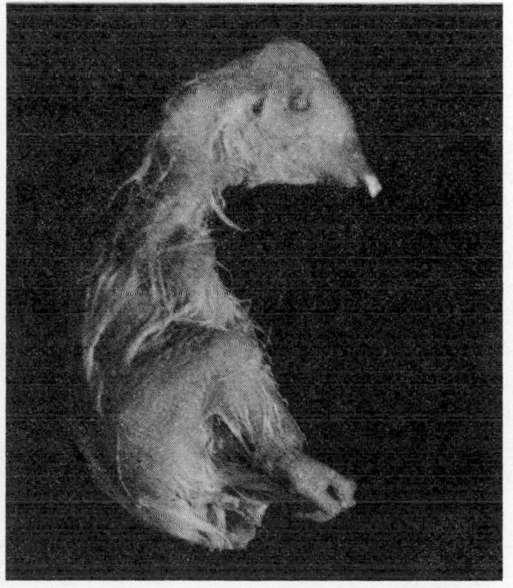

(b)

FIG. 22-6 Certain mycotoxins can interfere with the development of chicken embryos. (a) Control. (b) Embryo exposed to the mycotoxin citrinin. Note the twisted head. *Ciegler, A., R. F. Vesonder, and L. K. Jackson,* Appl. Environ. Microbiol. *33:1004–1006 (1977).*

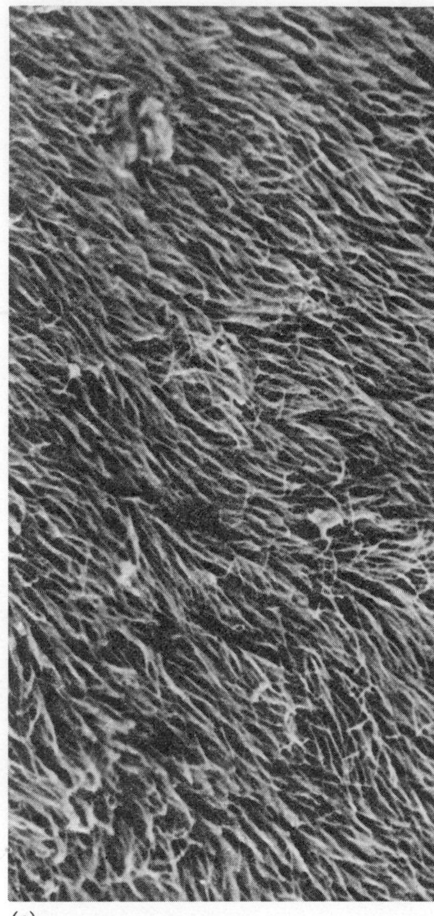
(a)

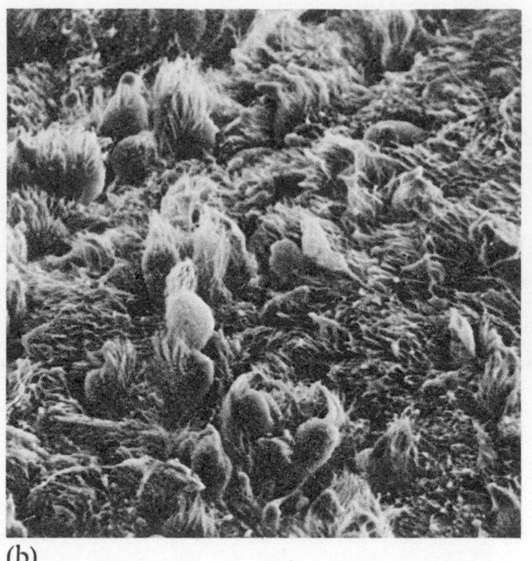
(b)

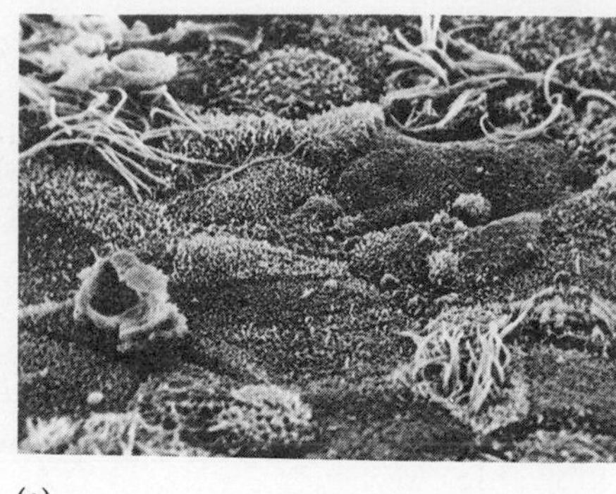
(c)

FIG. 22-7 The destructive effects of respiratory viruses. (a) A scanning electron micrograph showing the appearance of normal tracheal tissue culture cells taken from a calf. Note the number of cilia. (b) The rapid destructive effects of a rhinovirus on the ciliated epithelium, six days after inoculation of ths tissue culture system. (c) Similar destruction by a parainfluenza virus, eleven days after inoculation. *Reed, S. E., and A. Boyde:* Infec. Immun. 6:68–76 *(1972).*

SUMMARY

Infectious Disease and Virulence

1. Only a small percentage of microorganisms cause disease.
2. To cause disease a pathogen must be able to: (1) attach to and gain entrance into a susceptible host; (2) multiply in host tissues; (3) resist or not provoke host defenses; and (4) damage the host, often by the secretion of toxins.
3. An infectious disease interferes with the normal function of a host's physiochemical process, because another organism is living within or attached to the host's tissues.
4. Given suitable environmental conditions and a susceptible host, most organisms will exhibit disease-producing potential.
5. *Virulence* refers to a pathogen's capacity to cause disease. It depends on properties of the organism such as invasiveness, ability to survive and reproduce in the presence of the host's defense mechanisms, and toxin production.

Invasiveness

Three terms used to express the invasiveness of pathogens with respect to the bloodstream are: *bacteremia,* the laboratory demonstration of bacteria in blood samples; *septicemia,* the presence of organisms in the blood and their association with toxic symptoms of the host; and *pyemia,* the production by pathogens of localized collections of pus in host tissues.

Relatively Nontoxic Bacterial Structures and Products Contributing to Invasiveness

1. *Invasiveness* refers to an organism's abilities to survive and to establish itself in host tissues.
2. Obstacles faced by pathogens include phagocytosis, the destructive action of serum upon Gram-negative bacteria, and difficulty in spreading through tissues.
3. Bacterial structures and products which can help pathogens to overcome host obstacles include capsules and enzymes such as coagulase, hyaluronidase, and streptokinase.

Microbial Toxin Production

Bacterial Toxins

1. Bacterial toxins are categorized as either *endotoxins* or *exotoxins.*
2. Endotoxins are associated with the cell walls of Gram-negative bacteria. They are lipopolysaccharide-protein complexes involved with certain disease states caused by Gram-negative organisms.
3. Minute amounts of endotoxins can be detected by means of the Limulus test, which uses cells from the horseshoe crab.
4. Exotoxins may be secreted during the growth of bacteria or

upon the autolysis of cells. They are protein in nature and function by destroying specific parts of cells, or by inhibiting certain cellular activities. Some exotoxins are produced under the direction of bacterial viruses.

5. Exotoxins of clinical significance are associated with diseases such as botulism, diphtheria, gas gangrene, scarlet fever, staphylococcal food poisoning, and tetanus.
6. Certain bacterial species, called phytotoxins, also produce toxins which affect important food crops.
7. Blue-green bacteria are also sources of potentially dangerous toxins.

Algal Toxins

Many algal toxins have been found to be poisonous to fish, waterfowl, mussels, and clams.

Mycotoxins

1. Ingestion of foods contaminated with fungus toxins can cause disease states called *mycotoxicoses.*
2. Distinctive properties of mycotoxicoses include non-transmissibility, ineffectiveness of drug or antibiotic treatment, seasonality of outbreaks, association of outbreaks with a specific food item, and demonstrated fungal activity in the suspected food.
3. Mycotoxins produced by *Aspergillus* species, the *aflatoxins,* are the best known.
4. Some mycotoxins also show antibacterial, antifungal, antiprotozoan, and antitumor effects. Some also are carcinogenic.
5. In animal systems, the biological action of mycotoxins is affected by host and environmental factors.

Viral Pathogenicity

1. Many microbial pathogens are intracellular parasites.
2. The establishment of a virus disease process depends not only on the host's defenses, but on the pathogen's ability to counteract them and on the number of invading organisms.

The Pathological Effects of Viruses

1. Cellular damage of animal tissues by virus attack has been known for many years.
2. Viral replication can occur in cells without significant damage. Not all virus infections result in cell death. An example of this type of situation is found with cold sores and fever blisters.
3. Some slowly developing, persistent diseases that do not appear to be infectious can be caused or triggered by unusual "slow" viruses. Certain severe neurological diseases may be caused by such agents.
4. Viruses' cytotoxic activity can operate at two levels: biochemical injury without cellular damage and biochemical injury with cellular damage (e.g., cell destruction, fusion, or death). Cellular damage is usually referred to as a *cytopathic effect.*

Opportunists and True Pathogens

1. Opportunists are organisms that have the potential to produce infections, but do not have the capacity to directly invade the tissues of a host.
2. Opportunists may or may not be members of a host's normal resident flora.
3. Several situations may contribute to the establishment of infections caused by opportunists. These include genetic host defects, use of antibiotics, and immunosuppressive therapy.

QUESTIONS FOR REVIEW

1. Distinguish between the following:
   a. virulence and pathogenicity
   b. opportunist and pathogen
   c. endotoxins and exotoxins
   d. aflatoxin and carcinogen
   e. mycotoxin and algal toxin
   f. mycotoxicoses and mycosis
2. What microbial factors can influence the course of infection?
3. List any microbial structures or activities that contribute to virulence.
4. List at least four bacterial species that can produce powerful exotoxins, together with the diseases each causes.
5. a. What factor or factors may cause a decrease in a pathogen's virulence?
   b. How might virulence be increased?
6. What mechanisms are involved in viral pathogenicity?
7. How important are algal toxins to human welfare?
8. Are all microorganisms pathogenic? Explain your answer.
9. a. What is the Limulus test?
   b. What other methods are available to detect microbial toxins?
10. What effects do toxins cause in the human or other animals?
11. What factors or conditions contribute to opportunistic infections? List five.

SUGGESTED READINGS

Benenson, A. S. (ed.), *Control of Communicable Diseases in Man.* 12th ed. Washington, D.C.: The American Public Health Association, 1975. *Among the topics presented in this publication are the control, causative agents, occurrence, and mode of transmission of many diseases listed by the disease agent that causes them.*

Brander, G. C. and P. R. Ellis, *The Control of Disease.* London: Bailliere Tindal, 1977. *This book discusses the challenges humans must face in the 1970s in the control of disease.*

Burke, J. F. and G. Y. Heldick-Smith, *The Infection-Prone Hospital Patient.* Boston: Little, Brown and Company, 1978. *A short book containing a sufficient amount of information and references to serve as an introduction to the increasing problems of infection-susceptible patients.*

Docherty, J. J. and M. Chopan, "The Latent Herpes Simplex Virus," *Bacteriol. Revs.* 38:337–355, 1974. *An interesting article describing one of the most interesting concepts in the study of host-pathogen relationships.*

von Graevinitz, A., "The Role of Opportunistic Bacteria in Human Disease," *Ann. Rev. Microbiol.* 31:447–471, 1977. *More and more attention has turned to infections that occur in individuals having generalized or local defects in the immune defense system. This article concerns itself with bacteria taking advantage of such weakened or compromised hosts.*

Wogan, G. N., "Mycotoxins," *Ann. Rev. Pharmacology* 15:437, 1975. *This review reports on the current status of mycotoxins and the areas thought to be most relevant to human public health.*

CHAPTER 23

Antigens, Immunoglobulins, and States of Immunity

Chapter 23 presents some of the general immunological principles. The properties of antigens (foreign matter) and of the specific protein substances, immunoglobulins, produced by the body in response to antigens are discussed. This chapter also deals with the roles of the thymus gland and of the types of cells that produce antibodies and with theories of antibody production. Finally, the different states of resistance are explained.

After reading this chapter, you should be able to:

1. **Explain the general properties of antigens and antibodies.**
2. **Distinguish among the major classes of immunoglobulins.**
3. **Describe the general structural features of immunoglobulin molecules.**
4. **Explain the primary and secondary responses to antigenic stimuli.**
5. **Define the functions of the thymus gland, B-cells, and T-cells in the immune response.**
6. **List the sources and locations of normal immunoglobulins in the body.**
7. **Name and give the main features of current hypotheses for antibody formation.**
8. **Distinguish between humoral and cell-mediated immunity.**
9. **List the different states of immunity and explain their major distinguishing properties.**

As a general rule, individuals who successfully recover from an infectious disease acquire some degree of resistance toward the inciting cause. The resistance acquired may be toward a specific microorganism or toward certain microbial products that are recognized by the body's immune system as foreign. Molecules that are viewed as foreign by this system are called **antigens.** The immune system has several means of defending against such foreign substances. One of these is the formation of **antibodies** or **immunoglobulins,** which function in the specific recognition of antigens.

The nature of antigens and antibodies, selected theories concerning antibody formation, and acquired states of immunity are the major topics considered in this chapter.

Antigens and Immunogens

Macromolecules that can react with antibodies but do not necessarily stimulate the production of antibodies are generally referred to as *antigens*. Substances that provoke antibody formation and can combine with them are increasingly being referred to as **immunogens.** The stimulation of antibody production has been termed **immunogenicity.** In the interest of maintaining some degree of uniformity of expression with other chapters of this text, the terms antigen and antigenicity generally will be used for both types of responses; however, *immunogen* will be used to emphasize antibody-stimulating activity. Because many microorganisms and various types of cells are effective immunogens, they can be detected and identified by laboratory tests involving the antibodies produced in response to them. Immunogenic substances also play a most important role in the prevention of disease. They are used in the preparation of vaccines and related materials, which in turn are used to produce active states of resistance to disease agents.

Properties of Immunogens

Numerous substances can stimulate antibody production. Included in this group of both natural and synthetic macromolecules are: (1) most free proteins; (2) combinations of proteins and other substances, including nucleoproteins (nucleic acid plus protein), lipoproteins (lipid and protein), and glycoproteins (carbohydrate and protein); and (3) certain polysaccharides. The majority of lipids are not considered immunogenic. Various bacterial components, including flagella, capsules, cell walls and pili, and of course, the entire microorganism are immunogenic.

Besides these naturally occurring immunogens, synthetic ones are also possible. Such preparations result from chemical modifications of nonantigenic substances. Reactions of this sort can occur both *in vitro* and *in vivo*. Several drugs and small reactive molecules which, by themselves, do not stimulate an immune response can be chemically bonded *(coupled)* to a larger molecule, called the *carrier*, and thus become immunogenic.

Immunogens provoke their particular effects because antibody-forming *(immunopoietic)* tissues of an animal recognize them as foreign matter. The greater the incompatibility between the immunogen and the recipient's tissues, the greater the *immune response*. This is generally true, except when the toxicity of the foreign substance overwhelms the animal's recognition mechanism.

Factors That Determine Immunogenicity and Immune Responses

Immunogens generally have molecular weights greater than 5,000 and a large molecular surface with room for many ***antigenic determinant sites*** (Figure 23–1). These determinants are specific groups of atoms on the surface of the antigen that both stimulate the formation of antibodies and react with them. An antibody molecule recognizes and responds to an antigen by binding closely to the antigenic determinant. The number of determinant antigenic sites on the surface of a molecule is known as its ***valence.*** In general, an immunogen's valence is proportional to its molecular weight.

Other factors that affect the immune response include the species of animal receiving the antigen, the animal's degree of ***immunological maturity*** (the degree to which its immune mechanisms are functioning), the route of inoculation, and the use of an ***adjuvant.*** An adjuvant is a preparation that consists of material, such as mineral oil, mixed with an immunogen to prolong and intensify the antibody-provoking stimulus.

Classes of Antigens

HAPTENS

In 1921, Karl Landsteiner suggested the term ***hapten*** for substances that do not cause the production of antibodies in animals, but that combine with certain antibodies after they are formed. These properties were found to be characteristic of certain lipids and polysaccharides of animal and bacterial cells. Haptens are nothing more than single antigenic determinants. Antibody formation requires two or more antigenic determinants. Occasionally these low-molecular-weight molecules may bind to a macromolecule to form a complex that is immunogenic.

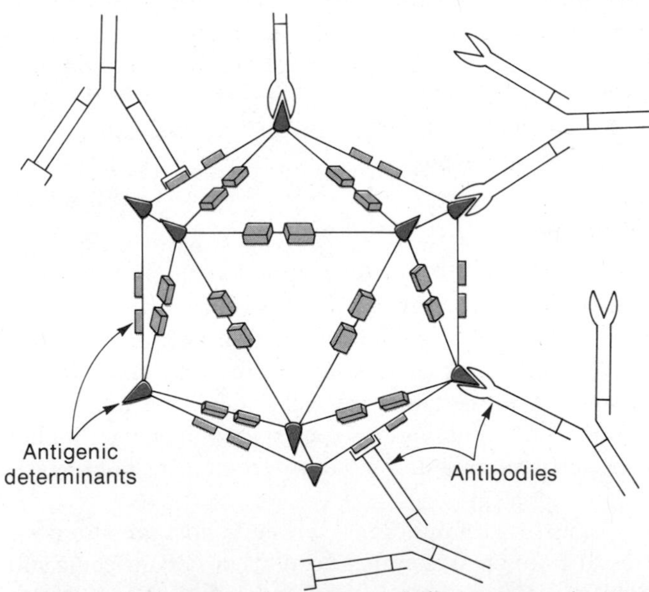

FIG. 23–1 A virus particle with two different types of antigenic determinants. Most antigens have several determinants which are bound by different antibody molecules. Such reactions are specific; that is, specific antibodies combine with specific antigens. *Hood, L. E., I. L. Weissman, and W. B. Wood:* Immunology. *Menlo Park, Calif.: Benjamin Cummings Publishing Company, 1978.*

TABLE 23-1 Some Autoimmune Disease States with the Incriminated Immunogenic Substances

Autoimmune Disease	*Immunogenic Substance*
Acquired hemolytic anemia	Red blood cells
Allergic encephalomyelitis	Myelin from the central nervous system
Aspermatogenesis	Spermatozoa
Idiopathic thrombocytopenic purpura[a]	Blood platelets
Rheumatoid arthritis	Immunoglobulins[b] (IgG)
Systemic lupus erythematosus (LE)	Deoxyribonucleic acid
Thyroiditis (Hashimoto's disease)	Thyroglobulin

[a]This disease state is characterized by bleeding in various tissues, and the presence of a rash and purpura (little areas of hemorrhaging) in the skin. It is also called purpura hemorrhagica.
[b]Other causes are believed to be operative in this disease condition.

AUTOANTIGENS ("SELF" VERSUS "NOT-SELF")

Generally, an animal does not produce antibodies against its own body substances or against cells from which they can be derived. In other words, the immunopoietic tissues recognize the individual's cells as belonging to the "self," and not as foreign matter, "not-self." In exceptional situations, however, antibodies are produced against body components. These substances are referred to as *autoantibodies,* and the antigens, as **autoantigens.** The resulting state represents the process known as *autoimmunization,* or *autoallergy.*

Under normal conditions, autoantigens are limited to the confines of particular cells and tissues and do not gain access to immunopoietic tissues. However, under certain conditions, disease states associated with the production of antibodies toward various normal cellular components are possible. Representative autoimmune diseases and the immunogenic substances believed to be responsible for each are shown in Table 23-1.

ISOANTIGENS

The erythrocytes of individuals within the same species are known to contain different antigens. In addition, antibodies capable of specifically reacting with these blood cell antigens also differ among individuals. These different factors are referred to as **isoantigens** and *isoantibodies.*

The agglutination (clumping reaction) that results from mixing antigenically different red blood cells, such as blood types A, B, or AB from one person with the normal serum of an individual of a different blood type, is called *isohemagglutination* (Color Photograph 70). Blood typing procedures are based on this phenomenon.

HETEROPHILE ANTIGENS

Various cells and tissues cause production of antibodies that react with the other tissues derived from some mammals, fish, and even plants of completely unrelated species. Forssmann, in 1911, reported that the injection of emulsions containing guinea pig tissues into rabbits caused the rabbits to produce antibodies which caused the clumping or lysis of sheep erythrocytes in the presence of complement. Antigens that stimulate production of antibodies effective against material unrelated to the original antigens are called **heterophile antigens.** Antibodies to these antigens will cross-react with the cells of various animal species and microorganisms. The best-known example of the heterophile antigens is the *Forssmann antigen.* It has been found in other animals, including birds, cats, dogs, mice, and tortoises, and has been associated with certain bacterial species, (e.g., *Bacillus anthracis, Streptococcus pneumoniae, Salmonella* spp., and *Shigella dysenteriae*). In these situations, however, the antigen might have become "implanted" in some microorganisms because of the intimate contact between pathogens and their respective hosts.

Forssmann antibodies—those that will react with sheep red cells—are present in the sera of individuals with infectious mononucleosis (IM), a fact that has been used for diagnostic purposes.

Antibodies

Blood serum contains many proteins, some of which can be distinguished on the basis of their physicochemical and immunogenic features. These properties include: (1) chemical composition, (2) chromatographic features, (3) electrical charge and migration in an electrical field, (4) molecular weight, (5) relative solubilities in alcohol, electrolytes, and water, and (6) sedimentation coefficients.

Antibodies are members of the protein group known as ***globulins***. Their presence in the blood of an immune animal was demonstrated by von Behring and Kitasato in 1890. Serum of a laboratory animal that had been injected with several small doses of diphtheria toxin was shown to have protective powers. Two experimental animals were injected with lethal doses of diphtheria toxin. In one case, the toxin was mixed with antitoxin from the immune animal. Only the recipient of the anti-serum-toxin mixture survived.

Additional experiments showed the reaction to be specific: serum from animals receiving diphtheria toxin produced antibodies specific only for diphtheria toxin; serum from animals given another toxin did not produce a protective effect against diphtheria. The results clearly demonstrated the phenomenon of ***passive immunization***, the transfer of antibodies from an immunized individual to a nonimmune recipient.

Immunoelectrophoresis (IEP)

Immunoelectrophoresis is an extremely valuable tool that enables the immunologist to separate and identify antibodies and antigens in a mixture. In the first step, the mixture is placed on a gel or gel-like material. This gel is placed in an electric field which draws any charged molecules toward either the positive or negative electrode depending on its charge. The rate at which different proteins migrate separates them into bands or spots on the gel. This separation by an electric field is the basis of electrophoresis. Next, a thin trough is hollowed out in the agar, parallel to the migration lines of the individual protein components. These steps and the appearance of a typical immunoelectrophoretic system are shown in Figure 23–2. Anti-sera against one or several proteins in the original mixtures are placed in these troughs. In areas where homologous antigen from the original mixture and antibody meet by diffusion through the gel, precipitation lines develop, usually in arcs.

IEP can be particularly valuable in analyzing and identifying a large number of different antigens present in a solution. In addition, the presence of abnormal proteins in the serum of individuals with malignancies and certain blood abnormalities can be shown with this procedure.

IEP can be applied to a variety of body fluids, including amniotic fluid, cerebrospinal fluid, human plasma and serum, respiratory secretions, saliva, animal and plant tissue antigens, and microbial antigens.

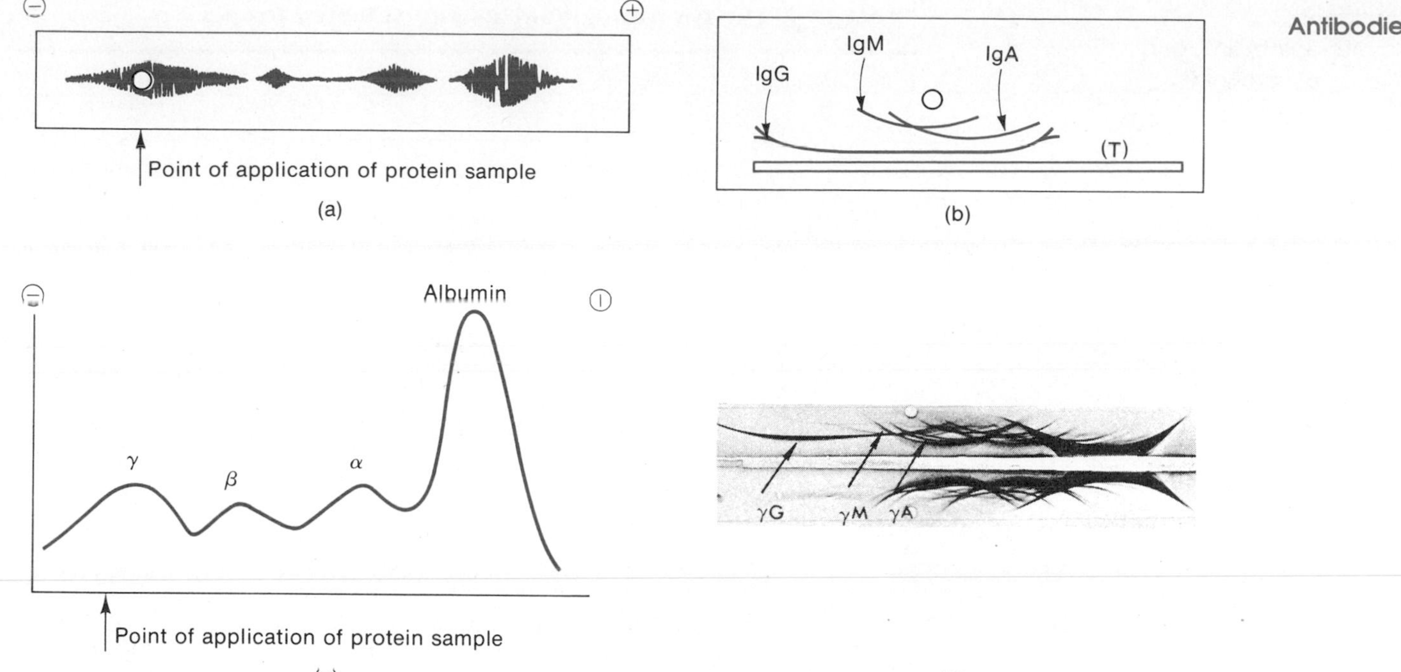

FIG. 23-2 Approaches to demonstrating the presence of various serum proteins. (a) A diagrammatic representation of ***electrophoresis*** procedure. A protein sample is placed in a prepared hole in the gel and then allowed to migrate in an electric field. (b) A graph of the locations on the gel of different proteins that migrated in the electrophoresis procedure. The four separated protein categories shown are albumin, alpha (α) globulins, beta (β) globulins, and gamma (γ) globulins. (c) Immunoelectrophoresis. Here antibodies (immunoglobulins) to serum proteins are introduced into a horizontal central trough (T). These antibodies and the separated serum proteins (which function as antigens now) diffuse toward each other to form precipitin lines as shown in (d). The diagrammatic representation in (c) shows an idealized immunoelectrophoretic pattern with only the relative positions of IgA, IgG, and IgM. (d) Immunoelectrophoretic patterns of normal serum. Although numerous serum fractions are shown, only a select few are specifically indicated. *Courtesy of Dr. M. D. Poulik, Wayne State University School of Medicine, and the Child Research Center of Michigan.*

Immunoglobulins

CLASSES

Antibodies are primarily in the slowest-moving electrophoretic fraction. Such substances were designated as gamma (γ) globulin (Figure 23–2a). Any protein exhibiting antibody activity or having antibody reaction sites in common with antibody molecules is called an ***immunoglobulin*** (Ig). The known immunoglobulins are grouped in five classes, based on differences in their antigenicity to other animals and their physicochemical properties, such as carbohydrate content, charge, and molecular size. Table 23–2 lists the classes of immunoglobins present in serum of every normal individual and some of their properties.

The most plentiful of the immunoglobulins in humans is IgG or γ (gamma) G. The IgM is next in the order of abundance. IgM immunoglobulins originally were called macroglobulins because of their large size, hence the M designation. IgD and IgE are usually present in low concentrations.

Subclasses. On the basis of antigenic reactivity and subsequent immunochemical analysis, several subclasses of immunoglobulins have been found.

TABLE 23-2 The Immunoglobulins and Selected Properties

Immunoglobulin Class	*Former Designation*	*Molecular Weight*	*Carbohydrate*	*Associated Activity*
IgA (or γA)	γ, A, or B_2A	170,000	5% to 10%	Skin-sensitizing; toxin neutralization.
IgD (or γD)	—	150,000	—	Not well defined.
IgE (or γE)	—	200,000	10.5%	Allergic reactions in humans.
IgG (or γG)	gamma globulin or γss	150,000	2.5%	Classic antibody; placental transfer, toxin neutralization, provides protection to fetus and newborn; increases phagocytosis; initiates complement reaction.
IgM (or γM)	γ_7M, or B_2M 19Sγ	900,000	5% to 10%	Frequently the first globulin with antibody activity after immunization, high bactericidal activity; increases phagocytosis; initiates complement reaction.

The four subclasses of IgG (IgG1 to IgG4) and the two subclasses each for IgA (IgA1 and IgA2) and IgM (IgM1 and IgM2) have important biological differences.

GENERAL STRUCTURE

Thousands of individual antibody molecules, differing in their primary structure, circulate in serum. Although there is great diversity in the sequence of amino acids in the molecule, all normal immunoglobulins have the same basic molecular arrangement, a unit of four polypeptide chains (Figure 23-3). Two of these are identical H (heavy) chains and two are identical L (light) chains. These components are covalently linked by disulfide bonds (S—S). These linkages also occur within the individual chains and are called ***intrachain disulfide bonds***. The formula $(L_2H_2)_n$ can be used to represent the general composition of immunoglobulins.

Two different types of light chains, designated kappa (κ) and lambda (λ), occur in immunoglobulins. A given antibody molecule contains either two κ or two λ chains (or multiples of two), but never one of each. Each class of immunoglobulin has a different type of heavy chain structure. These chains are designated by a Greek letter corresponding to the Roman capital letters used for the immunoglobulin classes. Thus, the H chain designation for IgA is α (alpha); for IgD, δ (delta); for IgE, ϵ (epsilon); for IgG, γ (gamma); and for IgM, μ (mu). Figure 23-3b shows a hypothetical comparison of the five classes of immunoglobulins.

The different subregions of the immunoglobulin are generally referred to as the "F_c domain" and the "F_{ab} domains." The F_{ab} domains, which contain the antigen-binding sites, are composed of the chemically variable portions of both

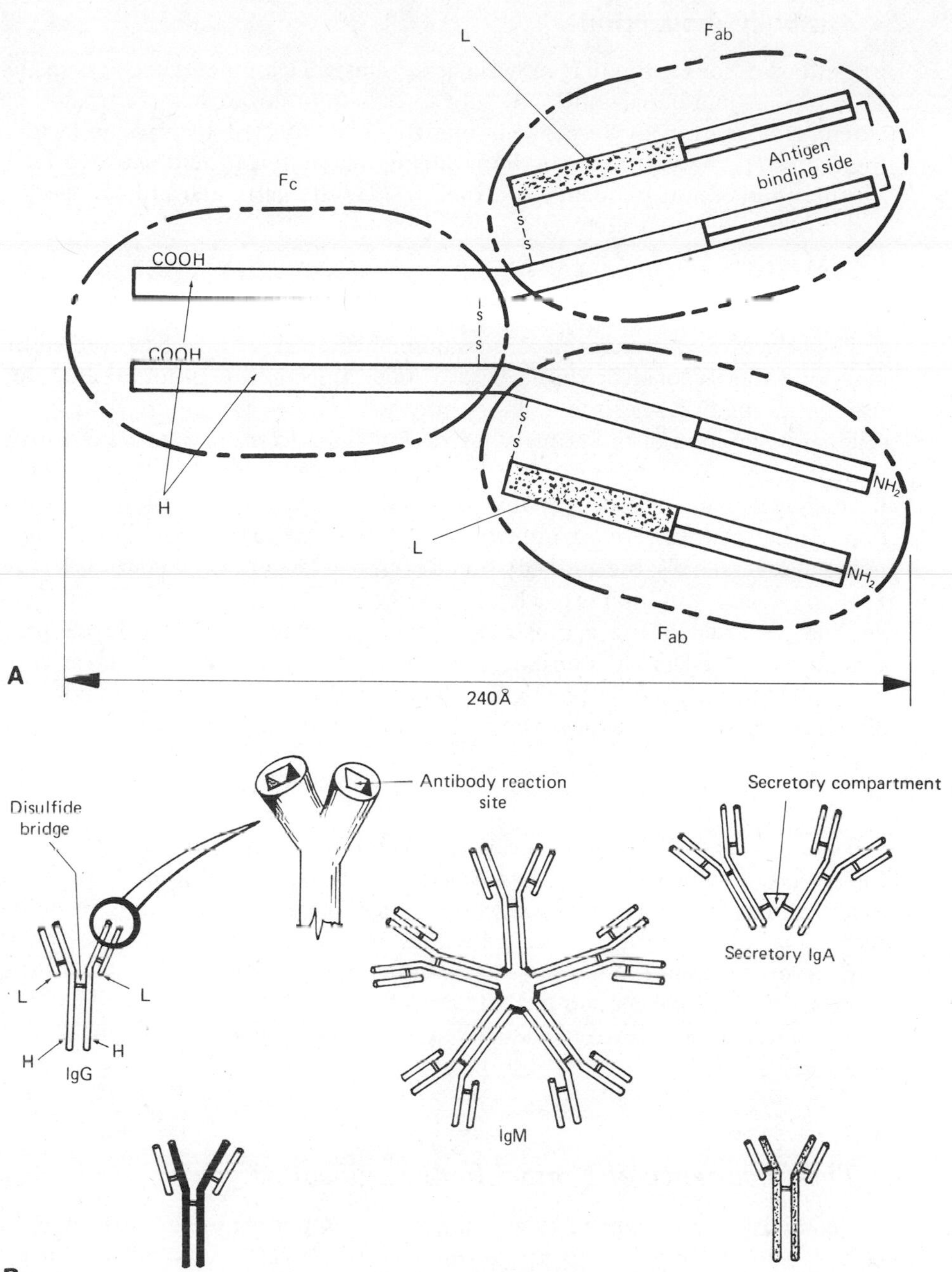

FIG. 23-3 (a) The basic immunoglobulin structure (IgG). An immunoglobulin molecule contains four polypeptide chains, two heavy (H) and two light (L) chains. These components are joined by disulfide bonds (—S—S—). The N-terminal (NH_2) portions of a light chain and the adjacent heavy chain form an antigen-binding site. These sites are contained within the F_{ab} region of the molecule. Such immunoglobulin molecules are divalent; that is, each molecule has two antigen-binding sites. The F_c portion of the molecule contains the greater constant portion of the H chains. (b) A hypothetical comparison of immunoglobulins showing their heavy- and light-chain components. The antigen-binding sites of the IgG structure also are indicated.

H and L chains. A portion of the heavy chain in F_{ab} released by enzyme treatment is called F_d. The F_c domain contains the chemically constant (c) portion of the H chain. This region participates in various biologic activities or reactions, including complement fixation and skin sensitization.

Antibody Production

Antibodies for a particular immunogenic substance are not detectable in the serum of an individual until exposure to the immunogen has occurred. The extent of the antibody response is known to be affected by various factors, including: (1) the nature of the immunizing material, (2) the dosage received, (3) the number and frequency of exposures, (4) the particular animal species, and (5) the individual involved.

The effects of immunogenic stimulation on the body can be best studied by observing the response produced with a single injection of immunogen. This reaction to the first injection of an immunogen is called *primary response*. The original description of the primary response noted a *latent* or *lag period* during which no increase in circulating antibody was detected. Improved techniques have shown that, in some instances, antibody synthesis does follow introduction of the stimulus almost immediately. After a period ranging from a few hours to several days, the antibody titer (level) reaches a peak or plateau (Figure 23–4). Peak concentration is reached when the rates of antibody production and antibody breakdown are approximately the same. Such antibody levels may remain for several months or longer and then slowly begin to decline, as antibody breakdown exceeds production. The details depend, in part, upon the animal species and immunogen material involved.

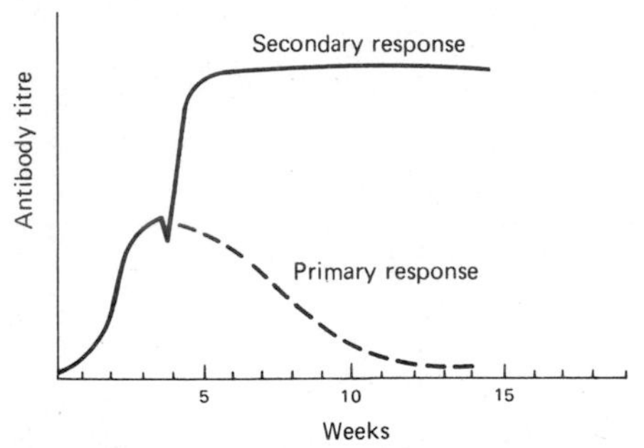

FIG. 23–4 The primary and secondary responses to an antigenic stimulus. *Gray, D. F.,* Immunology. *New York: Elsevier Publishing Company (1970).*

Some immunogens produce a sudden secondary rise in antibody titer when injected again some time after the first exposure. This effect is frequently called a *specific* **anamnestic response** from the Greek term *anamnesis,* meaning recall. The antibody titers associated with a specific anamnestic response generally are higher than those produced by the primary reaction, occur with little or no lag period, and remain for long periods.

Anamnestic reactions are produced by reimmunization with vaccines. The effectiveness of "booster shots" can be explained on this basis.

The Occurrence of Normal Immunoglobulins

Generally, after exposure to an immunogen, a temporary increase in IgM occurs, followed by a more permanent and greater IgG response. Secondary response to a second injection of the same immunogen or reimmunization usually produces IgG, although there are exceptions to this general pattern.

The immunoglobulins of the IgA class predominate in various body secretions, including colostrum (the early form of breast milk), gastrointestinal fluids, saliva, tears, and substances associated with the respiratory tract. Differences exist between IgA molecules associated with these external secretions and those found in serum. IgA immunoglobulins have been reported to increase in certain pathologic states, such as chronic liver disease.

The remaining two classes of immunoglobulins, IgD and IgE, are not well characterized. Both are present in human serum in low concentrations. The IgE globulins are associated with skin-sensitizing effects caused by certain allergens (antigens that produce allergies).

In newborn infants, the levels of IgG approach those found in adults. Most of these immunoglobulins are of maternal origin (Figure 23–5) and are transferred to the fetus across the placenta. The number of IgG molecules decreases sharply

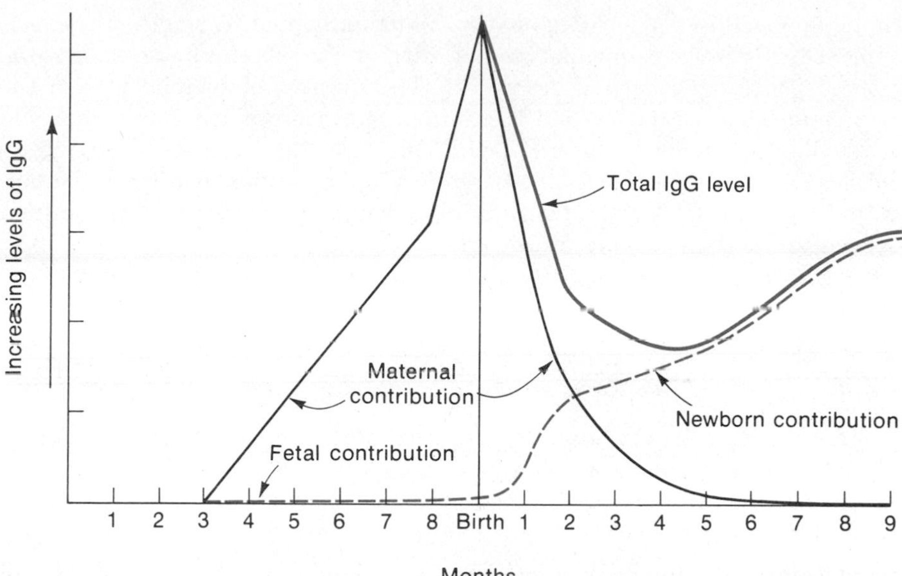

FIG. 23-5 The development of IgG levels in the human fetus and newborn. The maternal immunoglobulin contribution also is shown. The immunoglobulins in the fetus and newborn are obtained from maternal sources. After *Allensmith, M. R., et al.*, J. Pediat. *75: 1231 (1969).*

by approximately the fourth month after birth. It is about this time that the child's own IgG synthesizing machinery comes into play.

IgA and IgM immunoglobulins do not appear in the newborn's serum because they cannot pass through the human placenta. Synthesis of IgM occurs at about the same time as synthesis of IgG. IgA levels increase later, generally between the ages of 4 and 10 years.

The Development of the Immunologic System

The Thymus Gland and Its Role

The thymus is located in the chest region, between the lungs and behind the sternum or breastbone. This gland normally consists of two lobes, each of which is divided into smaller regions called ***lobules***. A lobule is made up of a ***medulla*** (center) composed of epithelial cells, lymphocytes, and Hassall's corpuscles, and a surrounding ***cortex*** consisting primarily of lymphocytes.

At birth the thymus is the most fully developed of the peripheral lymphoid tissues, with the exception of the bone marrow (the marrow is considered the central lymphoid tissue in mammals), and generally ranges in weight from 15 to 20 grams. The structure increases in size until, at puberty, its weight approaches 40 grams. Subsequently, the gland atrophies and decreases in size, until at middle-age, the thymus is a relatively insignificant tissue both physiologically and structurally.

The thymus gland is believed to be the central locale for multiplication of ***lymphocytes*** (thymocytes) during embryonic development. It is from this region that certain lymphocytes acquire a surface antigen, the theta (θ) antigen, and spread peripherally to populate the lymph nodes, the spleen, and related structures.

The importance of the thymus is indicated by the obvious defects that occur on its removal from a newborn or very young individual. When the thymus is removed from an experimental animal, such as a newborn mouse, no maturation of peripheral lymph nodes occurs. The number of lymphocytes in the peripheral blood decreases, and the antibody response is extremely poor. No antibodies are produced toward several antigenic substances. Such thymectomized animals accept foreign tissue grafts. These various defects can be corrected by grafting thymus tissue from a donor of the same inbred animal species to the thymectomized recipient.

The Immune Response in the Developing Individual

From conception to the time of birth, the human fetus develops in a highly protective environment. Beginning with approximately the third month of pregnancy, the mother begins to transfer large amounts of IgG antibodies to the fetus. The number of these maternal antibodies decreases gradually after birth (Figure 23–5). This method of passively equipping the infant with an immunologic "history" works well except in cases of Rh incompatability. Then passively transferred IgG can damage fetal blood cells, producing the condition known as the Rh baby.

It was long believed that the immune system of the newborn was immature and began to mature after birth. Currently available evidence suggests that this is not true. It appears that the maturation of the human immune system begins *in utero* sometime during the second to third month of pregnancy, and involves the differentiation of cells that will carry out both specific and nonspecific immunologic activities. These cells appear to arise from a population of stem cells or hemocytoblasts that are located with the blood-forming tissues (Figure 23–6) of the developing embryo (bone marrow, fetal liver, etc.). Depending upon the type of environment the differentiated cells enter, they will develop into either the hematopoietic or the lymphopoietic tissue. The former will result in production of blood components, such as erythrocytes, granulocytes, monocytes, and platelets. The latter can lead to still further differentiation.

Under the influence of the thymus gland, lymphopoietic cells may form a population of small lymphocytes, which participate in the tuberculin reaction, in the rejection or acceptance of certain tissue grafts, and in an individual's defense against various microorganisms. Such reactions are collectively called *cell-mediated immunity*. The cells from this type of differentiation are referred to as thymus-derived, thymus-dependent, or **T-lymphocytes.** These cells participate in antibody production.

A second type of differentiation produces a population of lymphocytes that acquire specific surface antigens known as B-antigens. These cells, called **B-type lymphocytes** and *plasma cells*, are the major ones associated with antibody synthesis, or *humoral immunity*. The B- and plasma cells are generated in, and influenced by, some site in the body other than the thymus. They are, therefore, described as thymus-independent. The identity of this location is known with certainty in birds, in which the Bursa of Fabricius serves in antibody formation.

The B- and T-cells (Figure 23–7) are the important responsive elements of an individual's immune system. Structurally B- and T-cells are identical under conventional light microscopy. However, certain differences have been revealed by electron microscopy (Figures 23–7 and 23–8). Both cell types occupy different areas within the same lymphoid tissues and both are intimately associated with another form of white blood cell, the macrophage (see Chapter 21).

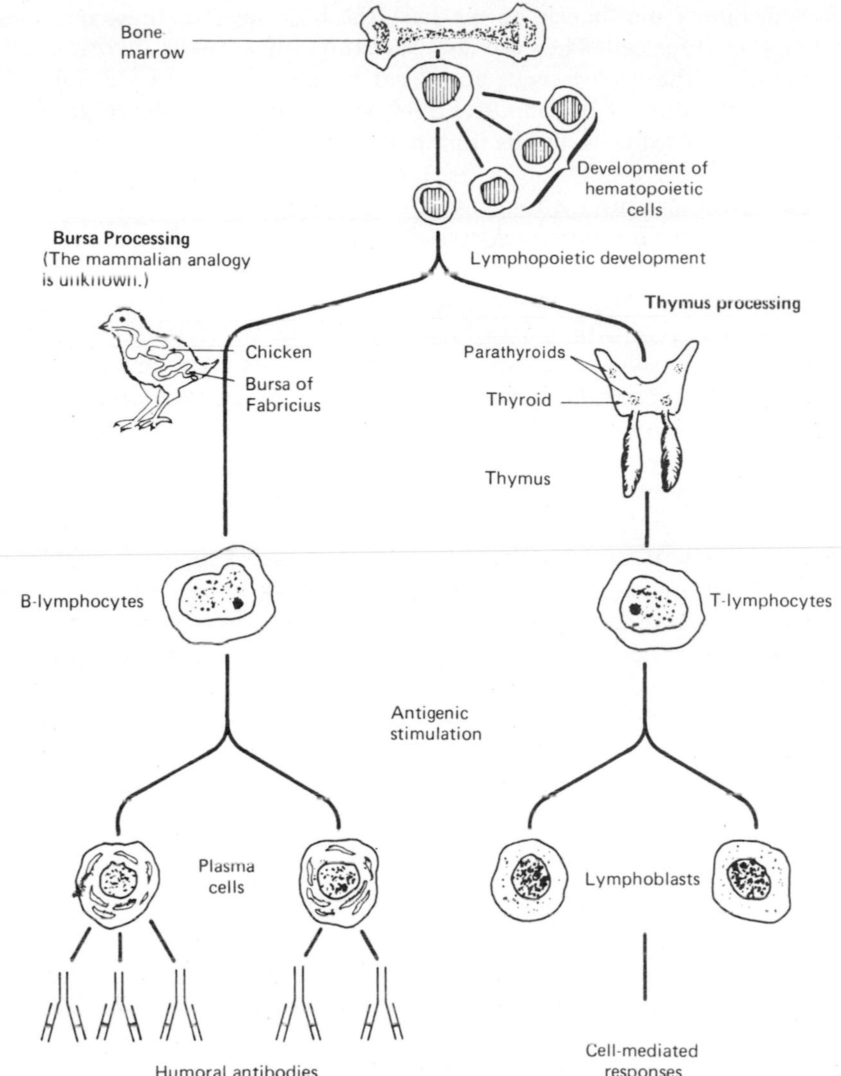

FIG. 23–6 The development of the principal cells involved in the immune response. Parent cells are differentiated into hematopoietic (blood-forming) and immunocompetent T- and B-lymphocytes. The proliferation and transformation of these cells to those of the lymphoblast and plasma-cell series occur upon antigenic stimulation.

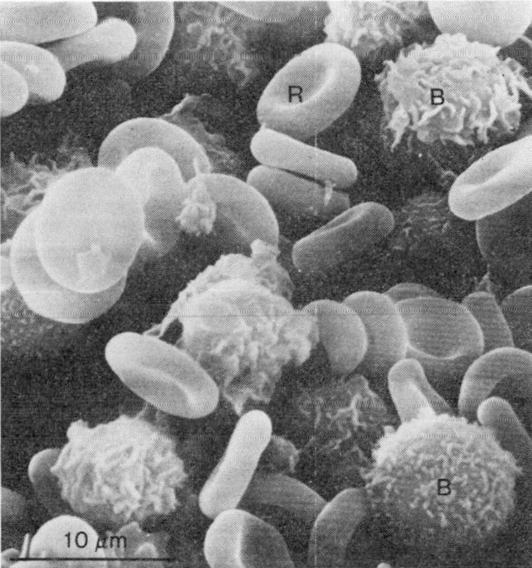

(a)

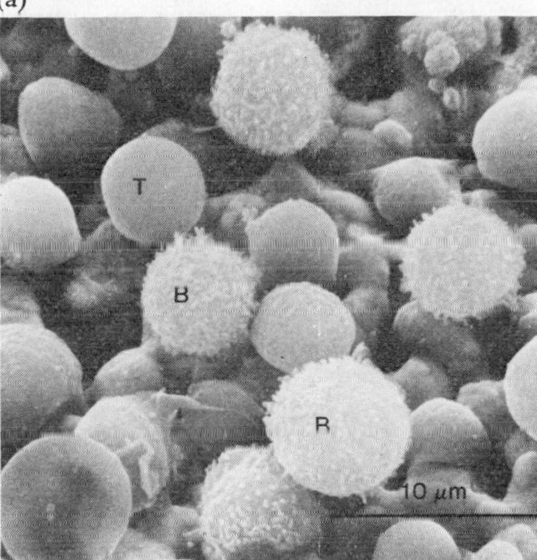

(b)

FIG. 23–7 B- and T-lymphocytes (a) A scanning electron micrograph showing the characteristics of B-type lymphocytes and red blood cells (R). (b) A scanning electron micrograph showing both B- and T-type cells. (The validity of B and T surface characteristics detected by electron microscopy has been questioned.) *Polliack, A., et al., J. Exp. Med. 138:607–622 (1973). Courtesy of Dr. Aaron Polliack, Department of Hematology, Hadassah University Hospital and Hebrew University Hadassah Medical School, Jerusalem, Israel. Work performed at Memorial Sloan-Kettering Institute for Cancer Research, New York, in Dr. de Harven's laboratory.*

B-CELLS

The B-lymphocytes tend to carry immunoglobulins on their surfaces. Although this is true even in animals not immunogenically stimulated, the response is heightened by such stimulation. Immunoglobulins are produced and secreted in large quantity by the B-cells. Some of these molecules remain attached to the cell surface. This property can be demonstrated *in vitro*. When a B-cell bearing antibody contacts erythrocyte antigens, an immune adherence occurs. Repetition of this exposure forms a rosette in which the B-cell is surrounded by adhering erythrocytes (Figure 23–8a).

T-CELLS

As indicated previously, T-type lymphocytes (Figure 22–7b) acquire a surface antigen, θ (theta), that serves to distinguish them from the B-type lymphocytes.

T-cells differ from other lymphocytes in that they do not synthesize immunoglobulins and, hence, do not have the high level of these molecules found on the B-type cell. They can also be distinguished by the *in vitro* formation of rosettes that occurs with sheep red blood cells (Figure 23–8b). This rosette develops when T-lymphocytes from nonimmune animals are incubated with sheep red blood cells. B-cells from nonimmune animals do not form such structures.

In some forms of immune response, T-cells cooperate with B-cells. While B-cells are responsible for immunoglobulin production and may be stimulated by direct contact with strong immunogens, weaker immunogens require the assistance of T-cells to create an immune response by B-cells. The T-cells, acting as helper cells together with macrophages, may concentrate immunogens and present them to B-cells, or perhaps T-cells may release substances to stimulate B-cells. T-cells can respond to a variety of antigens and participate in the control of the immune response. T-cells appear to play a crucial role in determining the amount, class, and selectivity of the immunoglobulin produced by B-cells. Both cell types develop immunological memory.

The cells are involved in cellular-mediated immunity (CMI), in which antibody, as we know it, is not secreted. Examples of such situations include the tuberculin skin response, the rejection of foreign tissue or malignant cells, and the activation of resting macrophages (phagocytic cells) into a form more capable of intracellular destruction of microbial pathogens and some tumor cells.

The roles of B- and T-cells and of macrophages in antibody production are shown in Figure 23–9. The three basic events of the immune response are shown as they occur in sequence: ***recognition,*** the binding of immunogen; ***activation,*** the stimulation of a resting cell into an active cell; ***differentiation,*** the production of the many different cell types that partake in an immune response.

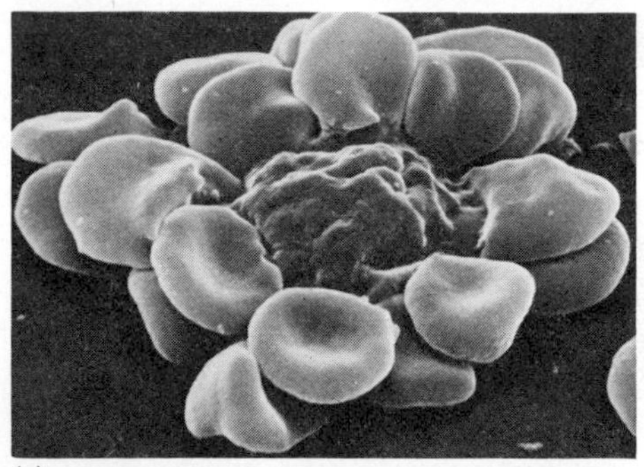
(a)

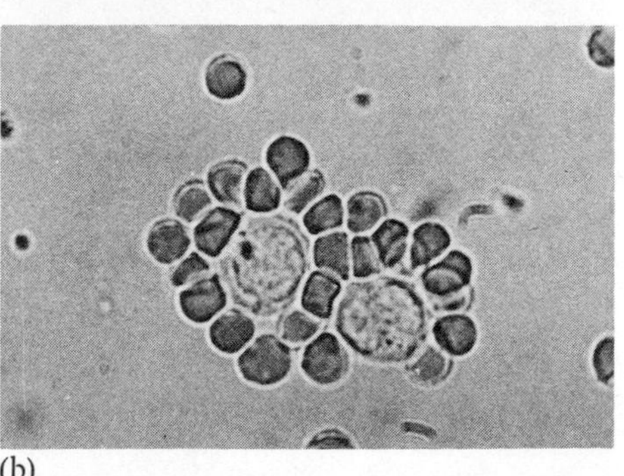
(b)

FIG. 23–8 Rosette formation. (a) A scanning electron micrograph showing a large rosette-forming cell (center) with spot-like contacts between cytoplasmic folds and erythrocytes (arrow). *Gudat, F. G., and W. Villiger:* J. Exper. Med. *137: 483–493 (1973).* (b) Spontaneous binding of sheep red blood cells demonstrating E rosette formation, as shown by light microscopy. *Aiuti, F. et al.,* Immunity *10:110 (1974).*

Mechanism of Antibody Formation

Since the 1890s much research has been aimed at finding the mechanism of antibody formation. As yet, no one hypothesis for antibody synthesis is universally accepted. These concepts fall in two general categories: ***template hypotheses*** and the ***selective hypotheses.***

TEMPLATE HYPOTHESES

There are two types of template hypotheses, the ***direct*** and the ***indirect.*** The direct template concept suggests that the immunogen acts directly as a pattern for the molding or forming of an antibody's active site. This modified portion of the antibody then would have a structural image that is the reverse of the site on the immunogen that caused its formation.

The indirect template mechanism assumes that protein synthesis (including antibody production) is under genetic control and that the specific pattern of the antibody is thereby dictated by the antibody-forming cell. The immunogen functions indirectly by causing the genetic mechanism to alter its antibody pattern or template. This genetic modification is carried by all cells descending from the first one altered by the immunogen.

While the template hypotheses account for antibody specificity, they do not satisfactorily explain certain other known immunologic phenomena, including the primary and secondary responses to immunogens and the ability of the immune system to distinguish between "self" and "not-self" components.

SELECTIVE HYPOTHESES

Selective hypotheses postulate that certain cells present in the body before the exposure to immunogens have the necessary information to synthesize a

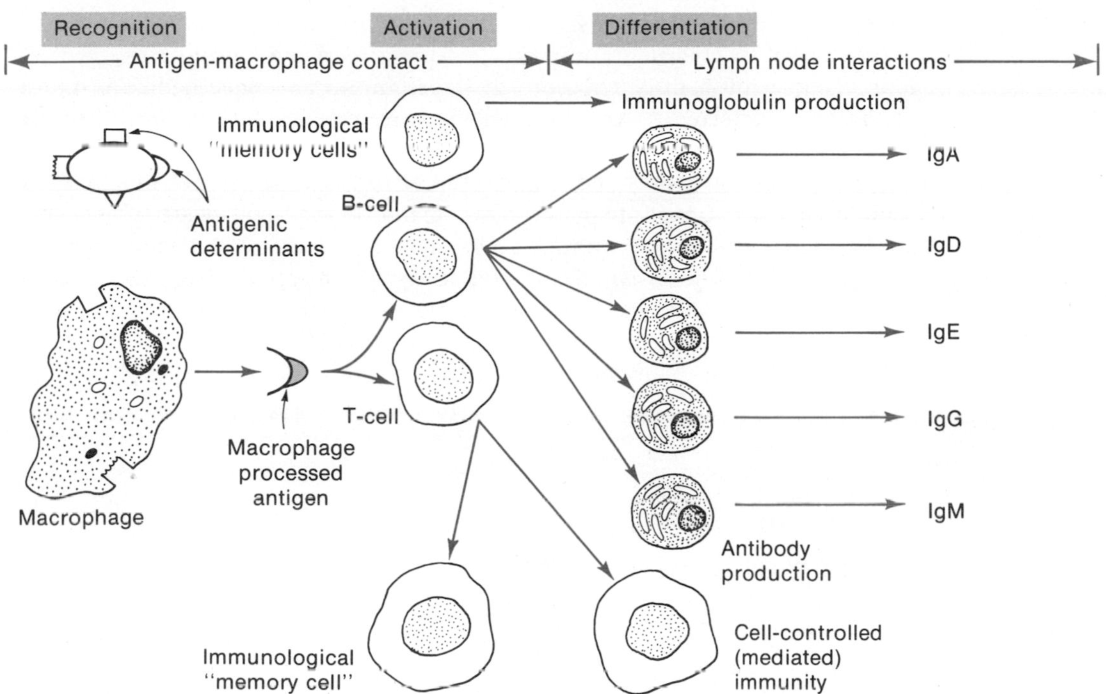

FIG. 23-9 The steps in antibody production: recognition, activation, and differentiation. When an antigen enters the body, it comes into contact with a macrophage, is processed, and is then transported through lymphatic channels to a neighboring lymph node. There, the macrophate (with processed antigen) interacts with T- and B-cells. The T-cells differentiate into memory cells and cells that control subsequent antigen recognition; the B-cells differentiate and proliferate into a clone of plasma cells. These plasma cells produce the antibody with receptor sites specific for the antigen that caused their production.

particular antibody. Such cells are capable of producing one antibody or a few antibodies. The numbers of cells necessary to meet the immunologic needs of the individual would be in the thousands, because each cell or its descendents *(clones)* could produce, at most, a few types of antibody. According to the selection hypotheses, during embryonic development, normal (self) components of the body react with and destroy those cells that could produce antibodies against them. Only those cells that survive this period constitute the antibody-producing force of the adult. Immunogens here function by combining with such cells and stimulating their antibody-producing capability. The selective hypotheses appear to better account for various observed immunologic phenomena.

Immunosuppression and Immunosuppressive Agents

The production of immunoglobulins can be suppressed in any of several ways, such as by the incorporation of chemical drugs, by the application of physical agents such as x-rays, or by the control of the antibody response by biological means. Examples of biological control of the antibody response include inhibition of the immune response to one immunogen by the introduction of a second immunogen (immunogen competition); immunoglobulin deficiency diseases in which there are pronounced losses in immunoglobulin levels as the result of deficits in B-cells or in T-cells, or a decrease in B- and T-cell functions; and a state of specific nonreactivity to a normally effective immunogenic challenge created by a prior exposure to the immunogen concerned. The latter condition is referred to as immunologic unresponsiveness, or *immunologic paralysis.*

Suppression of the immune response can be of great importance in situations such as in the survival of foreign tissue grafts (kidney and heart transplants) and in the control of autoimmune phenomena (Chapter 25). Although application of immunosuppressive agents such as x-rays or various drugs can serve a useful function, prolonged exposure to these agents can increase an individual's susceptibility to a variety of microbial pathogens. Moreover, serious infections with opportunistic microorganisms also occur among patients receiving intensive treatment with x-rays or chemical immunosuppressants.

States of Immunity

The resistance to disease displayed by individuals varies considerably because it is greatly affected by many innate or acquired factors (Figure 23–10). Generally speaking, two major categories are recognized, **innate** or **native immunities** and **acquired immunities.** Innate immunity includes species, race, and individual resistance to infection, discussed in Chapter 21. Acquired immunity may be either *natural* or *artificial,* depending on the processes involved in producing the immunity. Immunization by the injection of a bacterial vaccine is an artificially produced contact with the organism, in contrast to a natural infection.

Both of these categories are further subdivided into active and passive types. In the *active state,* an individual makes antibody in response to an immunogenic stimulus; in the *passive state,* the antibody is acquired through transfer from an immunized individual. The acquired states of immunity are described in more detail below.

NATURALLY ACQUIRED ACTIVE IMMUNITY

An individual who recovers successfully from an infection usually acquires a specific resistance to the causative agent. This immunity is produced by his antibody-synthesizing mechanism, which was stimulated into action by the infecting organism. Depending on the immunogenic nature and dosage of such pathogens and related factors, this immunity may last from a few months to several years. Although immunity is never absolute, individuals having a naturally acquired active immunity are protected against ordinary attacks by infectious agents to which they have been previously exposed. Such resistance, however, is generally not substantial enough to overcome massive infections. Some of the diseases to which an individual can develop sufficient protection as a consequence of infection include chickenpox, classic and German measles,

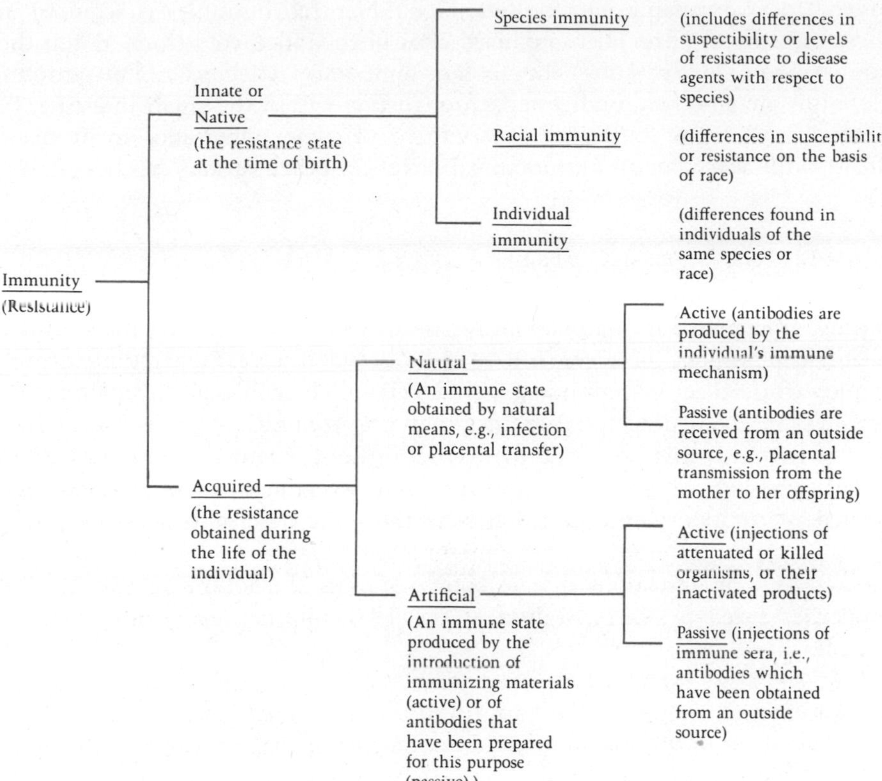

FIG. 23-10 States of immunity.

mumps, smallpox, and typhoid fever. Immunity to reinfection by certain other pathogens is either minimal or nonexistent. This group of diseases includes gonorrhea, pneumonia, and syphilis.

Subclinical or inapparent infection. Many persons experience attacks by pathogens that produce such mild symptoms that the disease goes undiagnosed. Nevertheless, the individual acquires a strong immunity through such repeated attacks. Diseases associated with this type of phenomenon include diphtheria, poliomyelitis, and scarlet fever.

NATURALLY ACQUIRED PASSIVE IMMUNITY

This form of immunity is derived through the natural transfer of antibodies from an immunized donor to a nonimmune recipient. This transfer can occur between mother and fetus as described above and via the colostrum produced by the mother immediately after birth. The duration of such immunity ranges from a few weeks to a few months. Thus, in the human species, an expectant mother having antibodies against diseases such as diphtheria, German measles, poliomyelitis, and possibly salmonellosis, imparts a share of these protective substances to her unborn child. These immunoglobulins are of the IgG class. To be sure of conferring protection on the newborn, all women should be immunized with available vaccines before pregnancy.

In humans, immunoglobulins pass easily from the maternal circulation through the placenta into the fetal circulation because of the single layer of cells separating these two systems. In lower animals, however, the placenta has several cell layers separating the two circulatory systems. Thus, antibodies are prevented from passing into the fetal blood. Natural immunity is acquired in these cases by the first milk produced after birth, called ***colostrum***. When the young ingest this secretion, they obtain temporary resistance. The immunoglobulins are absorbed, undigested, through the wall of the small intestine. In general, milk-borne antibody appears to be of some importance to humans. Breast milk also contains antimicrobial factors of other various kinds.

ARTIFICIALLY ACQUIRED ACTIVE IMMUNITY

Artificially acquired active immunity is induced by imitating nature's means: producing a mild infection. A carefully chosen immunogenic stimulus is provided without the severe effects of the actual disease. Preparations used to induce artificial active immunity include: (1) killed or inactivated microorganisms; (2) inactivated bacterial toxins, known as ***toxoids***; (3) living but attenuated (weakened) microbes; and (4) living virulent organisms administered in association with homologous antiserum. The specific types of vaccines and related preparations, immunization schedules, and descriptions of the procedures used in their preparation are presented in Chapter 26. Any vaccine to be used against an infectious disease should possess the following five general properties listed by G. S. Wilson at the 1961 International Conference on Measles:

1. Vaccination should not be harmful to the individual receiving it.
2. The effects of the vaccine should not be greater than those associated with the disease itself.
3. The vaccine must be easy to administer.
4. The benefit from vaccination should serve the community, as well as the individual.
5. The immunity conferred by the vaccine should be sufficient to eliminate the need for frequent revaccination.

In general, artificially active immune states require approximately one to two weeks to develop and are relatively long lasting.

ARTIFICIALLY ACQUIRED PASSIVE IMMUNITY

Protection against some diseases can be obtained only by provision of ample amounts of immunoglobins. Individuals exposed to botulism, diphtheria, gas gangrene, German measles (especially pregnant women), infectious hepatitis, rabies, and tetanus are treated in this way. In short, such persons must be given artificial passive immunization. Standardized doses of purified serum preparations obtained from immunized individuals are administered as soon as possible after exposure. Dosages of such protective sera are determined by the patient's body weight. The passive state of immunity that results is immediate but only temporary, because no active production of antibody toward the disease agent or its product occurs. If the immune serum used is obtained from the same animal species as the recipient, the rate of breakdown of injected immunoglobulin is approximately the same as that of normal globulins. However, if the immunoglobulins received come from another animal species, then their introduction into the individual provokes antibody production that rapidly eliminates them. Subsequent injections of the same preparation may cause severe allergic reactions, including anaphylactic shock and serum sickness.

Adoptive immunity. This immune state is primarily an experimental phenomenon. It has, at this time, no practical significance as a means of inducing antimicrobial protection. Adoptive immunity is a form of artificially acquired passive immune state produced by the transfer of cells capable of synthesizing immunoglobulins, or of directly reacting with a specific antigen, from an immunized donor to a nonimmune recipient. Such cells are referred to as being "immunologically competent."

SUMMARY

1. Individuals who successfully recover from an infectious disease generally acquire some degree of resistance toward the disease agent. This resistance results from the ability of the body's immune system to recognize disease agents or their products as foreign.
2. Molecules that the body's immune system recognizes as foreign are called *antigens.*
3. One defense response of the body to antigens is the production of antibodies or immunoglobulins.

Antigens and Immunogens

1. Antigens are molecules that react with antibodies but do not necessarily cause their production.
2. Immunogens are substances that stimulate the formation of antibodies and can combine with them. Immunogenic substances play important roles in the prevention of disease and the preparation of vaccines.

Properties of Immunogens

1. Immunogenic substances include most free proteins, combinations of proteins and other organic substances, and certain polysaccharides.
2. Cellular components of bacteria and certain synthetic substances can also stimulate an immune response.
3. Certain drugs and molecules which by themselves cannot stimulate antibody production can become immunogenic by chemically bonding to larger molecules (carriers).
4. In general, the greater the incompatibility between the foreign substance and the recipient's tissues, the greater the immune response.

Factors That Determine Immunogenicity and Immune Responses

1. Immunogens generally have molecular weights greater than 5000 and large molecular surfaces to accommodate many specific groups of atoms called antigenic determinant sites.
2. The number of antigenic determinant sites on the surface of an immunogen is known as the valence.
3. Other factors affect the immune response, including the species of animal involved, the animal's degree of immunological maturity, the route of inoculation, and the use of substances called adjuvants which prolong and intensify the antibody-provoking stimulus.

Classes of Antigens

1. Haptens are single antigenic determinants that do not stimulate antibody production but that can combine with antibodies that have already been formed.
2. Generally, antibodies are not produced in the body against its own substances or cells. The body's materials are recognized as "self," in contrast to foreign matter, or "not-self."
3. In exceptional cases, antibodies *(autoantibodies)* are produced against body components *(autoantigens)*. This type of condition is known as *autoimmunization* or *autoallergy*.
4. Isoantigens are red-blood-cell immunogens that differ among individuals of the same species. The clumping reaction (agglutination) which can be associated with these antigens serves as the basis of blood typing.
5. Heterophile antigens are substances present in the cells and tissues of some species that stimulate the production of antibodies effective against material from unrelated species.

Antibodies

Antibodies belong to a group of proteins known as globulins.

Immunoelectrophoresis (IEP)

1. Immunoelectrophoresis is used to identify antibodies or antigens in a variety of body fluids and other substances.
2. The technique combines the elements of electrophoresis and double gel diffusion.

Immunoglobulins

1. Known immunoglobulins are grouped into the five classes, IgA, IgM, IgG, IgD, and IgE, based on differences in their immunogenicity to other animals and their physicochemical properties.
2. The most plentiful of these protein substances in humans is IgG; IgM is next in the order of abundance.
3. All normal immunoglobulins share the same basic molecular arrangement, which consists of two identical H (heavy) chains and two identical L (light) chains covalently linked to one another by disulfide bonds.
4. Subregions of an immunoglobulin include the F_{ab} domains, which contain the antigen-binding sites, and the F_c domain, which contains the chemically constant portion of the H chain.

Antibody Production

1. The extent of an antibody response is affected by several factors, including (1) the nature of the immunizing material, (2) the dosage received, (3) the number and frequency of exposures, (4) the particular animal species, and (5) the individual involved.
2. The reaction to the first injection of an immunogen is called the *primary response*. Within time, the antibody level, or titer, reaches a plateau which remains for several months or longer and then slowly declines as antibody breakdown exceeds production.
3. A second injection of some immunogens will produce a secondary, or anamnestic, response which produces higher, longer lasting antibody levels than those associated with the primary reaction.

The Occurrence of Normal Immunoglobulins

1. Generally, after exposure to an immunogen a temporary increase in IgM occurs followed by a more permanent and greater IgG response. Secondary response to the same immunogen usually produces IgG.
2. IgA is the main immunoglobulin in colostrum, gastrointestinal fluids, saliva, tears, and substances associated with the respiratory tract.
3. IgD and IgE are found in low concentrations in serum. IgE is associated with skin-sensitizing effects caused by antigens that produce allergies. The functions or activities of IgD are not well characterized.
4. Most of the IgG molecules in a newborn are of maternal origin. IgA and IgM do not appear in a newborn's serum because they are too large to pass through the human placenta.
5. By approximately the fourth month after birth there is a sharp decrease in the concentration of IgG immunoglobulins, and the child's own IgG- and IgM-producing machinery begins to function.
6. IgA levels increase between the ages of 4 and 10 years.

The Development of the Immunologic System

The Thymus Gland and Its Role

1. The thymus gland, located in the chest region, is the most fully developed of the peripheral lymphoid tissue at birth, with the exception of the bone marrow.
2. After puberty, the gland begins to atrophy until at middle age it is relatively insignificant tissue both physiologically and structurally.
3. The thymus has an important role in antibody production and is believed to be the central location for the multiplication of lymphocytes (thymocytes) during embryonic development.

The Immune Response of the Developing Individual

1. The maturation of the human immune system begins *in utero*, sometime during the second to third month of pregnancy, with the differentiation of stem cells located within the embryonic blood-forming tissue.
2. Depending on environmental conditions, differentiated cells may develop into either lymphopoietic or hematopoietic tissue.
3. Lymphopoietic tissue forms either T-lymphocytes, associated with cell-mediated immunity or B-lymphocytes, associated with antibody formation.
4. T-cells are derived from the thymus; B-cells are generated in sites other than the thymus.
5. T-cells are differentiated from B-cells in two ways: first, T-cells possess the theta surface antigen and B-cells do not; second, T-cells from nonimmune animals form characteristic rosettes when incubated with sheep red blood cells, and B-cells do not.
6. T-cells, B-cells, and macrophages may act together in antibody production.
7. The three basic stages of the immune response are recognition (the cellular binding of immunogen), activation, (stimulation of a resting cell into an active one), and differentiation (production of the different types of cells required for an immune response).

Mechanism of Antibody Formation

1. Hypotheses for the mechanism of antibody formation fall into two general categories: template hypotheses and selective hypotheses.
2. The direct template hypothesis suggests that the immunogen controls the formation of an antibody's active site.
3. The indirect template hypothesis holds that antibody production is under genetic control and the specific pattern of the antibody is dictated by an antibody-forming cell. The immunogen functions indirectly by causing the genetic mechanism to change its antibody pattern. All cells descending from the first one are altered by the immunogen.
4. The template hypotheses account for antibody specificity, but do not satisfactorily explain certain immunologic phenomena.
5. Selective hypotheses postulate that certain cells present in the body before exposure to immunogens have the necessary information to synthesize a particular antibody.

Immunosuppression and Immunosuppressive Agents

1. Immunoglobulin production can be suppressed in several ways: through drugs, through physical agents, or through biological inhibition of the immune response.
2. Suppression of the immune response is important to the success of foreign tissue grafts. Immunosuppressive agents such as x rays or drugs can be used for this purpose.

States of Immunity

1. Two major states of resistance are recognized: innate, or native, immunities and acquired immunities.
2. Innate immunity includes species, race, and individual resistance.
3. Acquired immunity may be either natural or artificial depending upon the processes involved in producing the immune state.
4. Immunities can also be subdivided into active and passive immunities. In the active state, the individual produces antibodies in response to an immunogenic stimulus; in the passive state, antibodies are introduced into the individual from an outside source.

Acquired Immunity

1. A naturally acquired active immunity is generally the result of successful recovery from an infection or series of infections.
2. A naturally acquired passive immunity is obtained through the natural transfer of antibodies from an immunized donor to a nonimmune recipient. The immunoglobulins transferred from the mother to her fetus through the placenta are an example.
3. Artificially acquired active immunity is produced through immunizations. Materials used for this purpose include killed organisms, inactivated toxins, attenuated organisms, and living organisms mixed with homologous antiserum. In general, this state of immunity is rarely long lasting.
4. Artificially acquired passive immunity is produced by the injection of appropriate levels of specific immunoglobulins.

QUESTIONS FOR REVIEW

1. Define or explain the following terms:
   a. immunoglobulins
   b. adjuvant
   c. autoantigens
   d. antigen
   e. isohemagglutination

f. immunopoietic
g. immunoelectrophoresis
h. thymus gland
i. B- and T-cells
j. immunogen

2. Which components of a bacterial cell are antigenic?
3. Discuss haptens.
4. What are heterophile antigens?
5. What are the classes of immunoglobulins? How are they differentiated from one another? Draw a representative figure of an immunoglobulin and indicate the region involved in biologic activities, such as skin sensitization.
6. Describe the responses involved in antibody production. How do they differ?
7. Briefly describe one hypothesis for antibody production.
8. What are the sources of normal immunoglobulins?
9. Differentiate between native and naturally acquired immune states.
10. What host factors contribute to an individual's immunity? What accounts for differences in the immunity of individuals?
11. Distinguish between active and passive states of immunity. Which of these is longer lasting?
12. a. What types of preparations are used in producing artificially acquired active immune states?
    b. What types of preparations are used in producing artificially acquired passive immune states?
13. What are subclinical infections? What role do they play in immunity?
14. What is the thymus gland? How important is it to an individual's immune status?

SUGGESTED READINGS

Burnet, F. M. (ed.), *Readings from Scientific American Immunology*, part 1. San Francisco: W. H. Freeman and Co., 1976. *A collection of articles dealing with antibodies, their structure and function, and their role in the immune system.*

Capra, J. D., and A. B. Edmundson, "The Antibody Combining Site," *Sci. Amer.* 236:50, 1977. *An article describing how an antigen combines with an antibody molecule at a site that fits like a lock and key. The nature of this site is discussed in great detail.*

Cunningham, B. A., "The Structure and Function of Histocompatibility Antigens," *Sci. Amer.* 237:96, 1977. *An interesting article that defines histocompatibility antigens and describes how they function in tissue graft rejection and in the defense of the body againt infection and cancer.*

Davies, D. R., E. A. Padlan, and D. M. Segal, "Three-dimensional Structure of Immunoglobulins," *Ann. Rev. Biochem.* 44:639, 1975. *A general, basic article on the three-dimensional structure of antibodies and the nature of the interaction between antigens and antibodies.*

Dowling, H. F., *Fighting Infection.* Cambridge, Mass.: Harvard University Press, 1977. *This book describes many methods for fighting infection, including immunization, treatment with serum and antibiotics, and other chemotherapy methods.*

Golub, E. S., *The Cellular Basis of the Immune Response.* Sunderland, Mass.: Sinauer Associates, 1977. *This book describes the immune response and its regulation.*

Nossal, G. J. V., *Antibodies and Immunity.* New York: Basic Books, 1978. *A fairly simple book on the basic aspects of immunology.*

Old, L. J., "Cancer Immunology," *Sci. Amer.* 236:62, 1977. *Cancer cells, even though they have "foreign" labels, can escape destruction by the immune system. Results of the latest efforts to discover how cancer cells do this and how the immune system can be used for the treatment of cancer are discussed.*

CHAPTER **24**

Diagnostic Immunologic and Related Reactions

Chapter 24 applies immunological principles and techniques to the diagnosis of infectious diseases and the identification of various microorganisms and their products. We shall also show how certain immunological tests are used to determine the level of an individual's resistance to a disease agent or to follow the course of recovery from an infection.

After reading this chapter, you should be able to:

1. **Describe the importance of immunologic procedures to the diagnosis of microbial diseases.**
2. **Describe the general principles and features of commonly used diagnostic immunologic procedures.**
3. **Recognize the appearance of negative and positive reactions of immunologic reactions.**
4. **Differentiate beween hemagglutination and hemagglutination inhibition.**
5. **Describe the forms and applications of gel diffusion.**
6. **Explain fluorescent antibody techniques.**
7. **Discuss the importance and applications of investigative electron microscopy.**
8. **Define the ABO and Rh systems and their significance.**
9. **Discuss the relationship of Rh factors and disease.**

Knowing whether or not an individual has antibodies to a given antigen is valuable in establishing the identity of a disease agent, in charting a patient's recovery from infection, or in determining the effectiveness of immunization. Because of the specificity of the antigen-antibody reaction, if either the antigen or antibody is known, it is possible to identify and measure the other by employing one of a variety of *in vitro* and *in vivo* techniques.

During the past two decades, immunologic research has yielded an overwhelming body of information on humoral antibodies. The branch of immu-

TABLE 24-1 Immunologic Procedures Used in Diagnosis and/or Microbial Identification

Procedure	*Principle Involved*	*Positive Test Results*	*Applications Include:*
Agglutination	Antibody clumps cells or other particulate antigen preparations	Aggregates (clumps) of antigens	1. Diagnosis of typhus and Rocky Mountain spotted fever (Weil-Felix test) 2. Diagnosis of typhoid fever (Widal test)
Complement fixation	Antigen-antibody complex of test system binds complement, which is thereby unavailable for binding by sheep red blood cells and hemolysin of the indicator system	Cloudy red suspension	Diagnosis of various bacterial, mycotic, protozoan, viral, and helminth (worm) diseases
Ferritin-conjugated antibodies	Antibody, to which ferritin (iron-containing) particles are attached, binds various types of antigens	Presence of localized dark spheres in electron micrographs	Locating bacterial, fungal, viral, and other biological antigens by electron microscopy
Hemagglutination	Homologous antibody (hemagglutinin) aggregates of red blood cells[a]	Aggregates of red blood cells	Blood typing
Hemagglutination inhibition (viral)	Antibody inhibits the agglutination of red blood cells by coating hemagglutinating virus	Formation of a circle of unagglutinated cells	1. Determining the immune status toward German measles 2. Virus identification
Immunodiffusion	Antibody and soluble antigen diffuse toward one another through an agar gel and react where homologous antibody is in proper proportion to homologous antigen	Lines of precipitate form within the agar	Antigen and/or antibody identification
Immunofluorescent microscopy	Antibody (usually) or antigen is labeled with a fluorescent dye, which fluoresces on exposure to ultraviolet or blue light	Glowing on exposure to ultraviolet light	1. Detection of antigen or antibody 2. Identification of microbial pathogens, such as rabies, syphilis, etc.
Precipitation	Antibody and soluble antigen react where they are in proper proportion to one another	Lines of precipitate form	1. Diagnosis of microbial diseases 2. Detection of antigens
Radioimmunoassay	Antibody or antigen can be labeled with radioactive element, and the resulting complex precipitated and monitored for radioactivity	Radioactivity counts	1. Detection of antigen and/or antibody 2. Detection of hepatitis antigen
Virus neutralization	Antibody neutralizes infectivity	Absence of virus destructive effects	1. Determining neutralizing effects of antibody 2. Virus identification and diagnosis

[a]Hemagglutination reactions caused by certain viruses and bacteria generally do not involve antibody.

nology concerned with the nature and behavior of humoral antibodies is called *serology.* Because of space limitations, detailed descriptions of immunologic and serological reactions will not be given. The references listed among the suggested readings are sources for detailed descriptions of procedures and mechanisms concerned with specific antigen and antibody reactions.

This chapter surveys a number of current methods for the detection and measurement of antibodies in human serum. Many of these serological procedures, or so-called antibody detection systems, are powerful tools not only in the diagnosis of disease states, but also in the identification of microorganisms. They are based on antibodies produced *in vivo* in response to the antigenic components of microorganisms and other cells. Such microorganisms contain a wide variety of different antigens. Some of these are *type specific,* limited to a particular species, while others are *common group antigens,* antigenic to related groups of microorganisms. Certain important procedures, such as the serological tests for syphilis, have been placed in the chapter concerned with this specific disease agent. A discussion of the human blood groups and associated problems is also included in this chapter. Table 24–1 summarizes the features of several commonly used immunologic procedures.

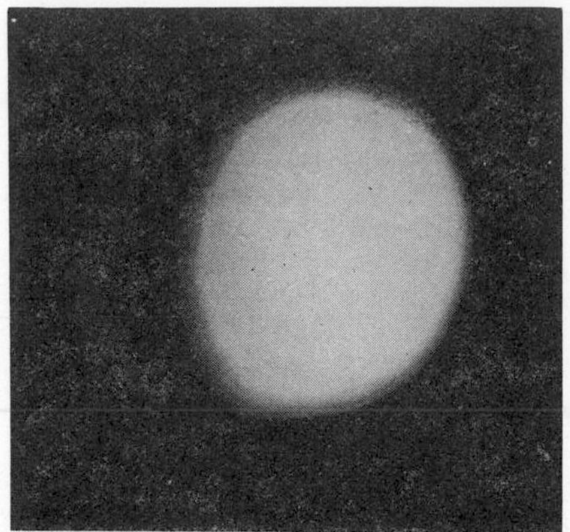
(a)

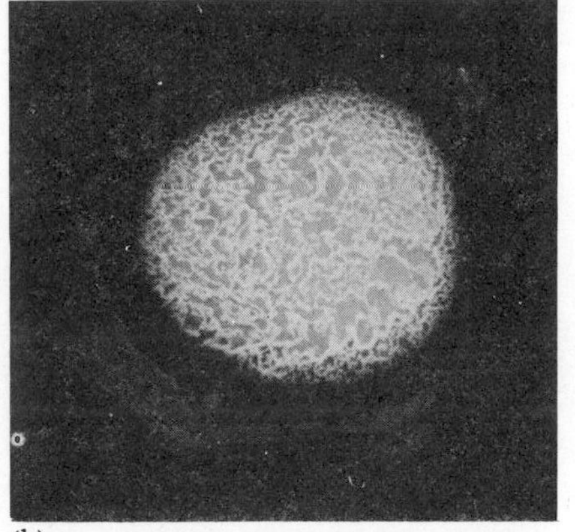
(b)

FIG. 24–1 The agglutination test for the diagnosis of brucellosis in dairy cattle. This test is based on the presence of agglutinins in the blood of infected animals. When the antigen, a suspension of *Brucella* spp. cells, is added to serum, the agglutinins clump with the antigen. In the plate, or rapid, test these mixtures are spread into thin, even layers over a glass plate. Within a few minutes, clumping can be seen with the naked eye (bottom). A negative result (absence of agglutinin) is shown at the top. *Courtesy of United States Department of Agriculture.*

Production of Antisera

To obtain potent antisera (blood serum containing antibodies) for use in diagnostic tests, an experimental animal is inoculated with suspensions of a particular antigen. Animals used for this purpose include chickens, mice, horses, rabbits, sheep, and even humans. In most laboratory situations, the course of immunization involves a series of inoculations. The immunogen may be introduced intraperitoneally, intravenously, or subcutaneously.

Determinations of the antibody level *(trial titrations)* are performed periodically by taking a blood sample from the laboratory animal. The blood is allowed to clot, and the serum is removed for testing. Once the antibody concentration reaches the desired level, the animal is bled. The immune serum obtained should contain the antibodies produced in response to the immunogenic stimulus. These antibodies are capable of binding in some manner with the antigenic determinant that caused their formation.

The Diagnostic Significance of Rising Antibody Titers

Generally speaking, the titer, or concentration of antibody in serum, fluctuates as a consequence of immunizations and of subclinical as well as full-blown current infectious states. To distinguish the antibody production associated with an actual ongoing infection from the effects of vaccination or from antibodies associated with a past infection, at least two specimens of a patient's serum are necessary. The first is obtained soon after the onset of the disease and the other approximately 12 to 14 days later. The sera from both specimens are tested to determine if a rise in concentration of the suspected antibody has occurred. If the titer has risen, as indicated by a greater antibody activity in the later specimen, identification of the causative agent is possible. If little or no antibody is detected in either specimen, it can be assumed, barring any abnormalities, that an organism other than the one being tested for is the cause of the infection. Abnormalities that could cause a lack of antibody response include: (1) the administration of immunosuppressing drugs, (2) an exposure to excessive radiation, or (3) the presence of a congenital defect such as an inability to produce immunoglobulins (agammaglobulinemia). If antibody is present in both samples with no appreciable change noted in the titers, it can be assumed that the antibody levels were present before the onset of the current infection and bear no relationship to the disease state.

The Agglutination Reaction

This classic serologic reaction was formally described by Gruber and Durham in 1896. Agglutination involves the clumping of cellular or particle-like antigens by homologous antibodies (Figure 24–1). This phenomenon is widely used for the rapid diagnosis of several infectious diseases and for the determination of blood types (Color Photograph 70). Because blood typing procedures involve reactions between erythrocytes and corresponding *hemagglutinins* (specifically *isohemagglutinins*), the phenomenon is often called **hemagglutination** (Color Photograph 70 and Figure 24–2a).

Examples of Agglutination and Related Reactions

COLD HEMAGGLUTINATION

The sera of patients with atypical primary pneumonia of mycoplasmal origin (Chapter 31) and protozoan infections, such as trypanosomiasis, contain antibodies that are capable of agglutinating erythrocytes from these patients at 2° C, but not at 37° C. Such antibodies are called *cold agglutinins*, and the phenomenon is referred to as *cold hemagglutination*. These unusual antibodies are important to diagnosis in that they appear in association with few diseases.

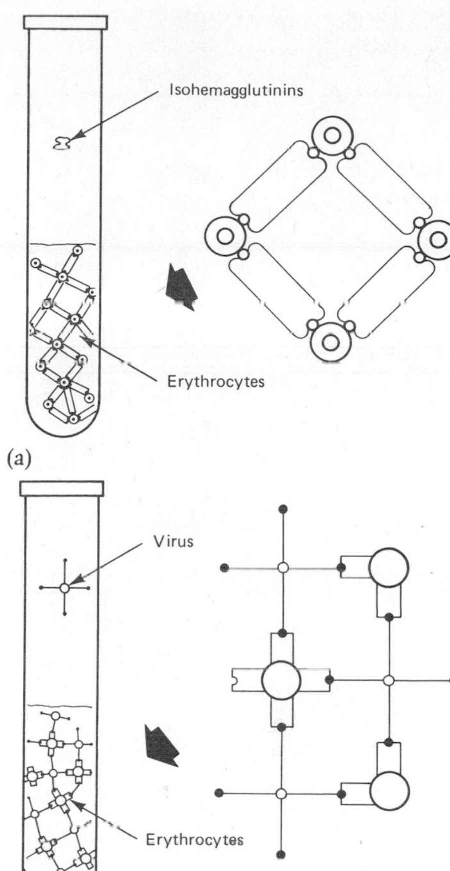

HEMAGGLUTINATION

Other forms of this biological process exist, including the agglutination of red cells by viruses and mycoplasma. Several viruses, including influenza (Figure 24–2), mumps, vaccinia, and variola (smallpox), are capable of binding to particular receptor sites of erythrocytes from suitable animal species. This activity forms a bridge between individual red cells, causing them to agglutinate.

WEIL-FELIX TEST

In 1916, E. Weil and A. Felix reported that a strain of the bacterium *Proteus*, originally isolated from the urine of a typhus fever victim, was agglutinated by the sera of patients suffering from this disease. Serum from normal persons did not produce a similar result. Later studies showed that *Proteus* spp. were not the cause of typhus fever and that antibodies against *Proteus* spp. normally occur quite commonly in humans. However, these bacteria can serve as an important tool in diagnosing various rickettsial infections.

The Weil-Felix reaction incorporates the somatic antigens (O) of *Proteus*. It is important to use nonmotile organisms because motile strains have flagellar antigens that could interfere with the test. Three strains are used in the diagnosis of various rickettsial infections: OX2, OX19, and OX-K.

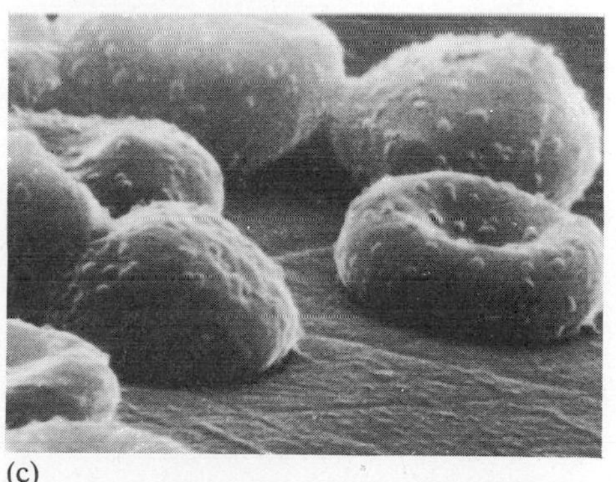

FIG. 24–2 Hemagglutination reactions. (a) A diagram of the agglutination of erythrocytes by isohemagglutinins. (b) Viral hemagglutination. (c) A scanning micrograph showing agglutination of human erythrocytes by influenza viruses. The little dot-like structures on the blood cells are the viruses. *Courtesy of Dr. L. F. Baker, Department of Microbiology, University of Southern California School of Medicine.*

WIDAL TEST

The original Widal test was a microscopic procedure used for the laboratory diagnosis of typhoid fever. This method consisted of mixing drops of the patient's blood with a loopful of a 24-hour *Salmonella typhi* culture on a glass slide or other appropriate surface. After a 30- to 60-minute incubation period, the mixture was observed microscopically for the presence of clumping, which represented a positive test. A saline control consisting of saline and *S. typhi* was always included. As performed today, the Widal test has been modified to use more than one dilution of a patient's blood.

PASSIVE AGGLUTINATION

In recent years, it has been possible to extend the agglutination reaction to a variety of soluble antigens by attaching them to the surface of insoluble particles. In passive agglutination reactions, the types of particles used include bentonite (a mineral colloid), polystyrene latex spheres, and red blood cells. Adsorption of the soluble antigens usually is achieved by simply mixing them with the insoluble particles. Diagnostic tests based upon this technique are widely used for the detection and identification of a variety of disease states such as diphtheria. Examples of procedures include latex agglutination (LA)

TABLE 24-2 Hemagglutination-Inhibition Titers of a Paired Sera Procedure

Serum Sample	*Serum Dilution Used*								*HI Titers*
	1:8	1:16	1:32	1:64	1:128	1:256	1:512	1:1024	
Acute	0	+	+	+	+	+	+	+	8
Convalescent	0	0	0	0	0	0	+	+	256

tests, which are valuable in the diagnosis of several mycotic and other infections, and the bentonite flocculation (BF) test, which is used for the diagnosis of several helminth diseases.

Hemagglutination Inhibition (HI)

In 1941, G. K. Hirst reported the phenomenon of viral hemagglutination and thereby provided a new picture and greater understanding of the relationship between viruses and host cells. His finding quickly led to the development of a new *in vitro* method, the hemagglutination-inhibition (HI) test, for the detection and titration of viral antibodies in a patient's serum and for the identification of specific viruses. Examples of viruses that clump erythrocytes and can, therefore, be tested by HI include influenza, mumps, vaccinia, smallpox, Newcastle disease, and rubella (German measles). Viral hemagglutination is inhibited by specific antibodies against the virus in a reaction called **hemagglutination inhibition.** The mechanism involved in this reaction is quite simple: The antibody molecules attach to the viral particles, thus hindering adsorption of viral particles to erythrocytes. Failure of hemagglutination to occur constitutes a positive test for antibody. Unagglutinated red blood cells slide down the sides of the container that holds the reaction materials and settle directly to its bottom, forming a compact circular red "button" or "doughnut." Agglutinated cells stick to the sides and rounded portion of the chamber's bottom, forming a ragged-edged, film-like deposit.

When HI procedure is used to monitor the antibody response during and after suspected illness, two serum specimens *(paired sera)* are taken and tested, one shortly after the onset of symptoms *(acute phase)* and the other two to three weeks later *(convalescent phase)*. Serial dilutions of the two specimens (e.g., 1:8, 1:16, 1:32, etc.) are prepared and then used to determine each specimen's titer, which is the reciprocal of the highest serum dilution that completely prevents hemagglutination. Table 24-2 shows HI titers of a paired sera procedure. The "O" indicates hemagglutination inhibition, and the "+" represents hemagglutination. The titers are 8 and 256 for the acute and convalescent samples, respectively.

Today HI is the method of choice for determining immune status against rubella (German measles). It has assumed particular importance because HI testing for the presence of rubella antibodies is recommended before any woman of child-bearing age receives rubella vaccine.

The Precipitin Reaction

Serological precipitation **(precipitin reaction)** is the reaction of a functional class of antibodies called precipitins with soluble antigens *(precipitino-*

gens). In experimental systems, a visible precipitate generally appears at the point where optimal proportions of antibody and antigen, as well as electrolytes, exist.

The main difference between precipitin reactions and agglutination reactions is the state of dispersion of the antigen used. In precipitin reactions, the molecules of precipitinogens are free in solution so that their solutions appear clear, while the molecules of agglutinogens are bound to a surface in some manner.

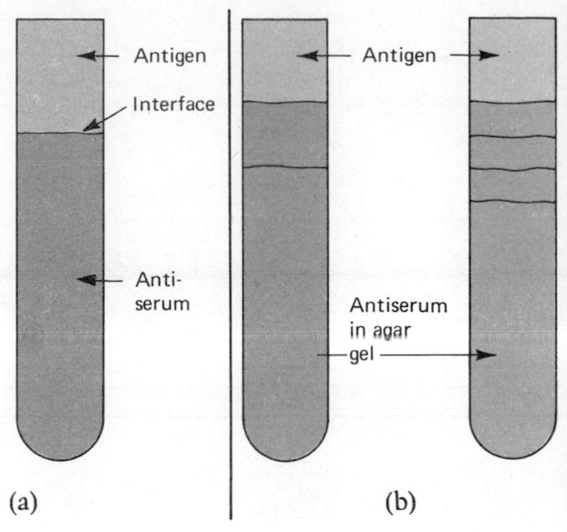

FIG. 24-3 The precipitin test and its variations. (a) The ring test. (b) The Oudin technique. The left tube contains a simple system with one type of antigen and homologous antibody. The right tube contains a complex system of multiple antigens as indicated by the multiple precipitin bands.

Ring or Interface Tests

In the course of an infection, precipitating antibody is often produced. This is usually in response to soluble microbial substances released by a disintegrative process. The presence of these antibodies can be demonstrated by the ***ring*** or ***interface*** test based on a useful form of the precipitin reactions. In this procedure, antigenic material is carefully layered over an equal quantity of antisera in a narrow tube to form a sharp liquid interface. If the antigen and antibody are homologous, a ring of precipitation develops at the interface. In this test, the reactants diffuse into one another until the optimal, immunologically equivalent proportions for precipitation are achieved. In modern practice, agar gel bases (gel matrix) are usually incorporated to stabilize the precipitates that result. Examples of such gel diffusion tests include single diffusion gel procedures, such as the *Oudin test,* double diffusion procedure, ***single radial immunodiffusion*** (RID), ***two-dimensional immunoelectrophoresis,*** and the Ouchterlony test.

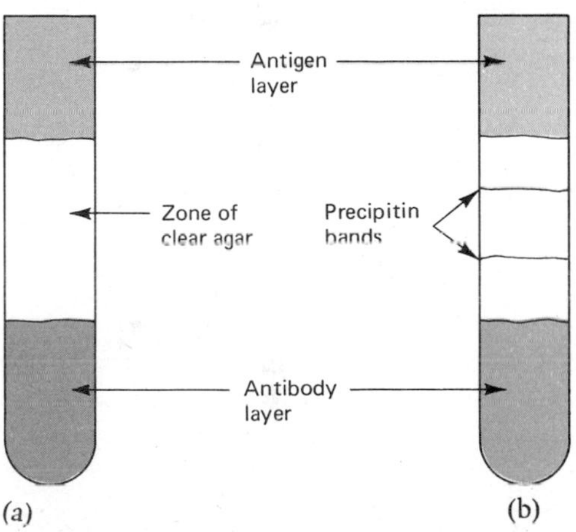

FIG. 24-4 The gel double diffusion technique. (a) The system before reactions occurs. (b) The formation of precipitin bands.

OUDIN TEST

The *Oudin* (single diffusion) test is performed by introducing antiserum into a tube of melted agar at a temperature of about 45° C. This mixture, filling a narrow tube to one-third of its height, is allowed to solidify. An antigen-containing solution is then layered on the agar preparation, and the entire system is refrigerated. Diffusion of the antigen into the agar gel takes place during this refrigeration. Depending on the number of antigenic components in the test material, one or more bands of precipitin form with homologous antibodies (Figure 24–3). One distinct band develops for each homologous soluble antigen-antibody system present. This feature of the Oudin method is a pronounced advantage.

DOUBLE DIFFUSION PROCEDURE

A variation of the single diffusion technique of Oudin is the double diffusion procedure. One new ingredient is added; a layer of clear agar is placed between the two zones containing antigen and antibody. The molecules of both antigen and antibody diffuse into the neutral zone (Figure 24–4). Precipitation bands form where there is serological equivalence, that is, where both reactants are present in equivalent proportions. This technique can be valuable in determining the number of antigen-antibody pairs present in a test specimen.

RADIAL IMMUNODIFFUSION

In recent years, radial immunodiffusion (RID) has become widely used for the measurement of a variety of proteins in serum and other body fluids. In this technique, antiserum is incorporated at a relatively low concentration in a gel on a tray. Several wells are made in the gel, and various concentrations of a test antigen and controls are placed in the wells. As antigen diffuses into the gel, it

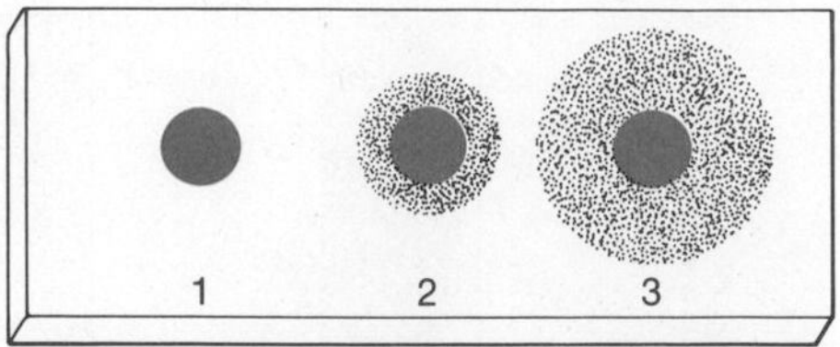

(a)

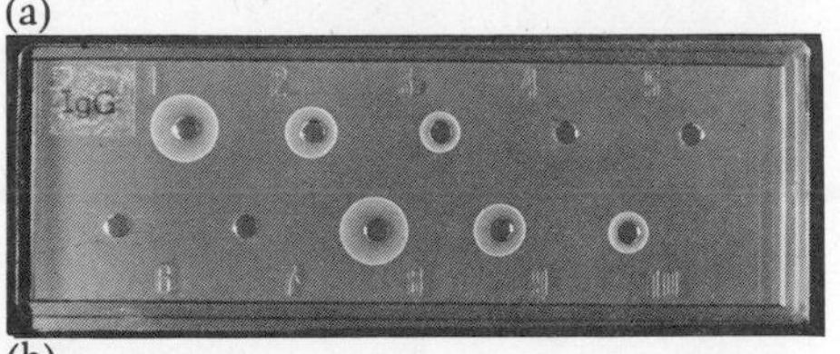

(b)

FIG. 24-5 Single radial immunodiffusion. (a) Well 1 contains no antigen, well 2 contains a low concentration of antigen as indicated by the small surrounding precipitant ring, and well 3 contains a high antigen concentration as indicated by the diameter of a large surrounding ring. (b) The results of an actual immunodiffusion assay. This technique can be very accurate and is often the best method for measuring substances such as immunoglobulin classes or subclasses and serum complement components. *Courtesy Helena Laboratories.*

forms a progressively widening circle of precipitate. The diameter of the precipitant ring is directly proportional to the antigen concentration in the well (Figure 24–5). This direct relationship between antigen concentration and ring diameter allows one to calculate the concentration of a known antigen.

TWO-DIMENSIONAL IMMUNOELECTROPHORESIS

In this technique, a serum sample is subjected to electrophoresis. The separated components are placed next to a gel that contains specific antibodies (Figure 24–6). Then the separated components are again subjected to an electric field, this one perpendicular to the original separating field. The components move into the antibody-containing gel where specific precipitant arcs are formed.

OUCHTERLONY TEST

The Ouchterlony test also incorporates gel diffusion. In this test, an agar pour plate is made without antiserum. After the agar solidifies, circular or square holes or wells are made in the surface. Solutions containing antigens are added to certain wells, while the antibody preparation is placed in another well (Figure 24–7). The plate is incubated to allow the various reactants to diffuse. Lines or bands of precipitate develop where antigenic components react with homologous antibodies from the antibody preparation. The results obtained by this technique depend upon several factors, including the relative concentrations of reactants, the incubation period, the rate of diffusion, and the molecular weight of the antigens used. The arrangement shown in Figure 24–7c has a distinct advantage over the Oudin method in that several different antigen solutions can be tested at one time.

The Ouchterlony double diffusion procedure can produce several different geometrical patterns of precipitin between the separate wells containing antigen and antibody solutions. Lines generally occur where the distance between the two reactants is at a mininum.

Much useful information can be obtained from this technique, including the detection of identical or cross-reacting components of various antigen or antibody preparations (gel diffusion analysis). Three patterns that represent possible reactions are shown in Figure 24–7. The precipitin band pattern of the ***reaction of identity*** develops when pure antigen preparations are placed in two wells adjacent to a centrally located well containing a homologous antibody solution (Figure 24–7a and d). Note that the bands fuse.

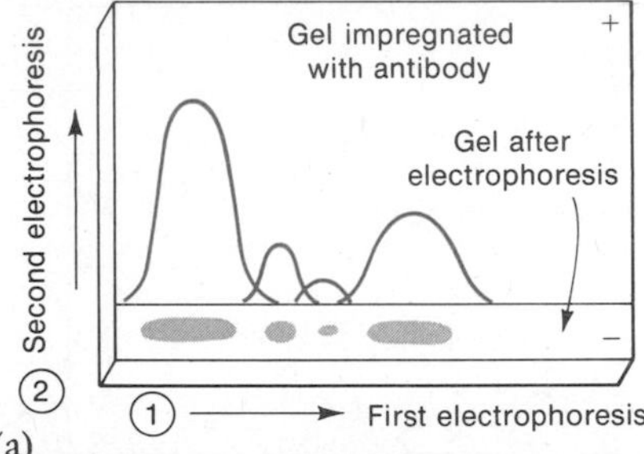

(a)

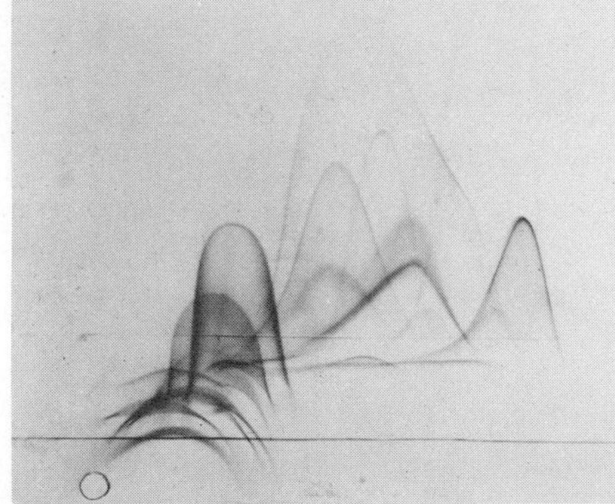

(b)

FIG. 24-6 Two dimensional electrophoresis. In this technique, components separated by normal electrophoresis are electrophoresed a second time in a gel containing specific immunoglobulins. The resulting reactions produce specific precipitant arcs. (a) The steps involved in two-dimensional electrophoresis. *Smyth, C. J., A. E. Friedmans Kien, and M. R. J. Salton*, Inf. Imm. *13:1273–1288 (1978)*. (b) The appearance of actual precipitant arcs formed in the procedure.

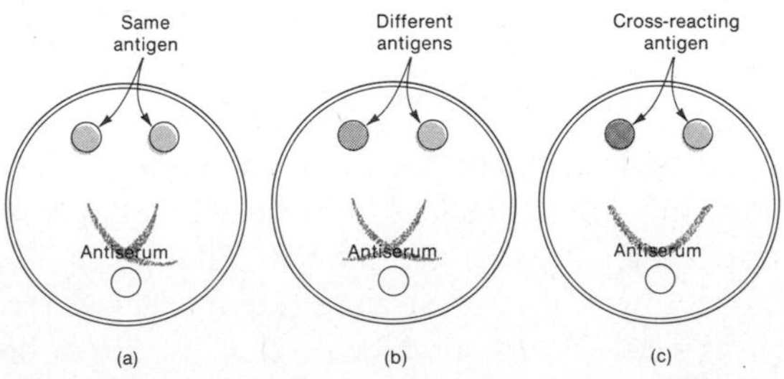

FIG. 24-7 Selected geometrical patterns that indicate double diffusion precipitin reactions. (a) Reaction of antigen identity. Both upper wells contain the same antigen, and the lower well contains homologous antiserum. (b) Reaction of antigen nonidentity. Each of the upper wells contains a different antigen and the central well holds antisera to both antigens. (c) Reaction of partial identity or cross-reaction. The upper left well contains a cross-reacting antigen, and the upper right well is filled with an antigen that is homologous for the antiserum preparation in the lower well. (d) The actual appearance of an antigen identity reaction. *Stickle, D., L. Kaufman, S. O. Blumer, and D. W. McLaughlin*, Appl. Microbiol. *23:490–499 (1972)*.

The pattern of Figure 24–7b shows the pattern formed by two unrelated antigens and an antiserum preparation that contains an antibody for each of the antigens. The arrangement of precipitin bands here is referred to as the ***reaction of nonidentity***. The antigens and antibodies diffuse toward one another from their wells, forming two distinct precipitin bands that cross.

Antiserum preparations usually react with their homologous antigen counterparts. However, some antigen preparations are so similar to the homologous antigen substance that reactions between similar ***heterologous*** antigens and an antiserum can occur. These events are referred to as ***cross-reactions***. Such reactions may be the result of several factors, including: (1) the presence of several different antigenic molecules in an antigen preparation as laboratory contaminants, (2) the presence of numerous types of antigenic molecules as natural components; and (3) the limited specificity of the antiserum preparation.

The Ouchterlony ***reaction of partial identity*** or ***cross-reaction*** is shown in Figure 24–7c. In this situation, one of the antigens and the antiserum used form a homologous system; however, the second antigen present is a cross-reacting one. The precipitin bands that develop fuse, but one of them continues toward the cross-reacting antigen preparation. This ***spur***, as it is sometimes called, is formed by those antibody molecules that have not combined with the cross-reacting antigen and have gone beyond the precipitation band facing it.

In Vitro Hemolysis Tests

Complement Fixation

The normal serum component complement is found in a variety of animals. Historically, the contribution of complement to the destruction of invading cells was first noted by Pfeiffer in 1896. His studies compared the fates of cholera-causing organisms *(Vibrio cholerae)* upon their intraperitoneal injection into normal and immunized guinea pigs. The vibrios taken from normal animals at various intervals appeared quite normal. However, those organisms taken shortly after their initial injection into the immunized guinea pigs swelled, stained unevenly, and eventually burst. The immunized animals showed no sign of infection, and apparently the vibrios underwent ***cytolysis***, cellular disruption.

The fact that serum components participated in the phenomenon was shown ***in vitro*** by exposing a hanging drop preparation of the cholera-causing vibrios to: (1) normal serum; (2) untreated immune serum; and (3) immune serum that had been heated to 56° C for 30 minutes, conditions known to inactivate complement. Only the untreated immune serum caused the lytic effect. Pfeiffer's experiments demonstrated the presence in immune serum of a thermolabile substance that contributes to the destruction of bacteria.

The reaction was one of ***immune cytolysis***. Normal sera had no effect. This type of reaction apparently is not limited to bacteria. In 1895 Bordet reported a somewhat similar phenomenon with antisera prepared against red blood cells. This observation led to the development of the complement-fixation test (Color Photograph 71).

THE COMPLEMENT-FIXATION (COMP-FIX) PROCEDURE

Recognition of the fact that various antigen-antibody combinations have the ability to fix, or combine with, complement provides a means for detecting either antibodies or antigenic substances in unknown specimens. Two systems are incorporated in this technique, the test and indicator systems. In a typical laboratory diagnostic situation, the *test system* consists of the patient's serum, an antigen preparation that may be commercially made or laboratory-produced, and complement, commonly obtained from guinea pig serum and commercially available. The components of the *indicator system* are sheep red blood cells and serum containing homologous antibodies against them. This antibody preparation is referred to as ***hemolysin***.

All sera used in complement-fixation tests are heated before use to 56° C for 30 minutes to inactivate any complement present. Reagents must be freshly and carefully prepared and must be combined in proper proportion to achieve a suitable balance between components. For example, enough hemolysin must be added to the indicator system to render the sheep erythrocytes susceptible to lysis by complement. The concentrations needed are determined before the complement-fixation is performed.

A positive test. If a particular heated serum specimen is suspected of having specific antibodies, it is diluted and the dilutions incorporated, together with antigen and complement, in the test system. Then, the components of the indicator system are added to the reaction mixture. If the serum sample contains antibody, the antibody will combine with antigen and fix the complement in the system so that no free complement remains (Figure 24–8). If the complement has been fixed, then no lysis of the sensitized sheep erythrocytes occurs when the indicator system is added. Thus a positive complement-fixation test is represented by a cloudy red suspension (Color Photograph 71). This result indicates the presence of antibody toward the antigen used in the test system.

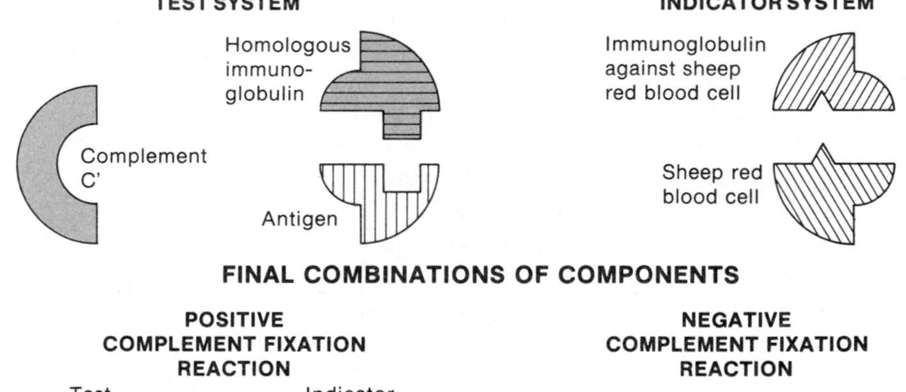

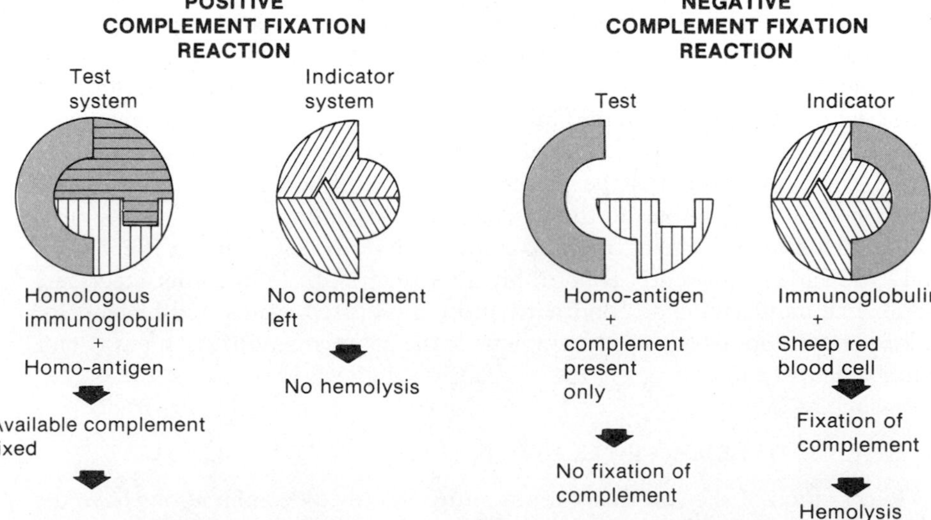

FIG. 24–8 A representation of the complement-fixation reaction. The upper portion shows the reagents used. The remaining sections indicate the combinations that occur in positive and negative tests.

A negative test. If a serum sample lacks antibody against the particular antigen used in the test system, complement fixation does not occur. Thus, complement present in solution is free to react with the components of the indicator system. The antigen-antibody complex formed by the sheep erythrocytes and hemolysin fix complement, and lysis of the red blood cells occurs, producing a clear red solution (Color Photograph 71 and Figure 24–9). A negative test result (hemolysis) indicates the absence of antibodies toward the antigen used in the test system.

Fluorescein isocyanate + Protein → Labeled protein

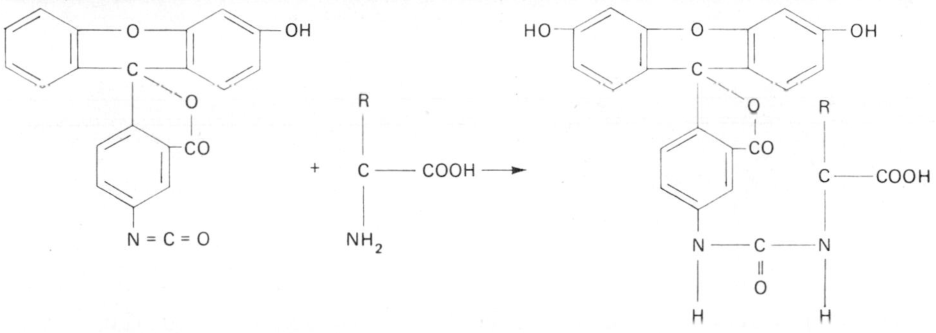

FIG. 24–9 The labeling of a serum protein with a fluorescein derivative by an isocyanurate amine linkage. *Based on Goldman, M.,* Flourescent Antibody Methods. *New York: Academic Press, 1968.*

Controls. Certain controls must be incorporated in the complement-fixation test because of the labile nature of both the complement and the erythrocytes. Antigen and patient's serum controls are used to detect any possible anticomplementary activity that might produce misleading test results. The functioning of the indicator system of sheep erythrocytes and hemolysin also are separately determined.

MECHANISM OF COMPLEMENT FIXATION

The reaction of complement with sensitized erythrocytes has been studied extensively. The basic reaction occurs in several stages, the components of complement combining with sensitized cells in a precise manner. Once antibody (principally IgM and IgG) has bound to an erythrocyte's surface, the stage is set for the subsequent events. The entire sequence of reactions produces actual holes in the cell's membrane with dimensions of about 10 nm. Through these circular lesions, small intracellular molecules escape and extracellular water enters rapidly, thus causing the cell to expand and to rupture.

APPLICATION OF COMPLEMENT FIXATION

Complement-fixation procedures have been used in the laboratory diagnosis of a wide variety of microbial infections and certain helminthic diseases (Table 24–3). The most widely recognized application has been in the Wasserman test and its modifications for the diagnosis of syphilis. The antibody-like material associated with this disease is the same as that involved with other flocculation tests, such as Venereal Disease Research Laboratory (VDRL) and Kahn.

Antistreptolysin Test

The thermolabile hemolysin of streptococci, known as streptolysin O, is antigenic in humans and most laboratory animals. In various human streptococcal diseases, antistreptolysin O titers increase during the times of infection

TABLE 24-3 Representative Diseases for which Diagnostic Complement-Fixation Tests Can Be Used

Bacterial	*Mycotic*	*Type of Disease* *Protozoan*	*Viral*	*Helminthic*[a]
Gonorrhea	Aspergillosis Blastomycosis	Amebic dysentery	ARD[b]	Echinococcosis
Syphilis	Coccidioidomycosis	Chagas' disease Leishmaniasis	Enteroviruses Influenza	Paragonimiasis Schistosomiasis
Rickettsial infections	Histoplasmosis	Malaria	Measles	Trichinosis
Tuberculosis	Sporotrichosis		Mumps	
Whooping cough				

[a]In several instances these tests are in an experimental stage.
[b]Acute respiratory diseases caused by adenoviruses.

and convalescence. In many diagnostic laboratories, the antistreptolysin test is routinely used to measure the levels of antibodies against this bacterial product.

In Vitro Immunologic Procedures Incorporating Differential Staining

Fluorescent Antibody Techniques

Fluorescent antibody methodology is a combination of the techniques of immunology and cytology. In a broad sense, the procedure involves bringing a fluorescent dye (marker) into contact with serum proteins so that they bond together chemically (Figure 24–9). This process is referred to as *labeling* or *conjugation*. The resulting preparations generally remain active biologically. These fluorescent serum-protein conjugates, containing specific antibodies, can be used to detect homologous antigens in smears or tissue sections. The most commonly used of these methods are called *direct* and *indirect* methods (Figures 24–10, 24–11 and 24–13 and Color Photographs 15 and 55).

THE DIRECT FLUORESCENT ANTIBODY METHOD

This procedure is generally considered to be the simplest one because it requires a single staining reagent and because the manipulations involved are not complex. An antigen-containing specimen is fixed to a slide with acetone, ethanol, methanol, or heat. A few drops of a standardized labeled antibody preparation are applied to the specimen. This test system (the specimen and the labeled antibody) is incubated. Following incubation, the specimen is washed free of excess antibody with saline and distilled water. The resulting preparation is usually dried, mounted in glycerol, and examined under a fluorescence microscope. If the homologous antigen is present in the specimen, the labeled antibody will unite with it and thus pinpoint its location (Figure 24–10).

Controls. To verify the immunologic specificity of the fluorescence observed with the unknown antigen-containing specimen, certain appropriate controls must be applied. These may include:

1. Exposure of the antigen-containing specimen to labeled serum that does not

contain antibody against the antigen in question. Fluorescence should not be observed.

2. Exposure of the antigen-containing specimen to homologous unlabeled antibody preparation. Here, too, fluorescence should be absent.

Purpose. Staining antigens by the direct method serves as a means of identifying unknown microbial agents and can be used to determine the distribution of antigens in tissue.

THE INDIRECT FLUORESCENT ANTIBODY METHOD

The indirect (antiglobulin) method involves formation of an "immunologic sandwich," in that nonfluorescent antibody (globulin) bound to primary antigen is, in turn, bound by fluorescent antiglobulin. The antigen itself is not directly rendered fluorescent, but rather, the nonfluorescent antibody bound to the antigen. This indirect method utilizes both the antigen-binding capability of antibodies and their protein nature, which enables them to serve as antigens. The results of this method—the microscopic appearance of the stained antigen—are generally indistinguishable from those obtained with the direct fluorescent antibody techniques. Figure 24–11 is a schematic representation of this method.

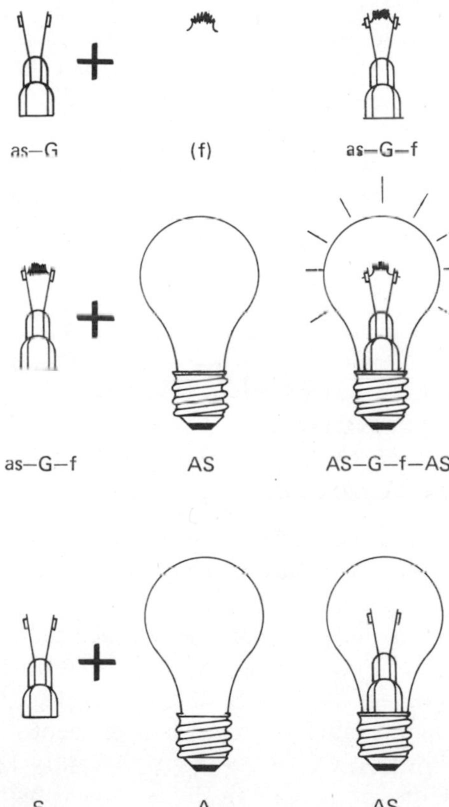

FIG. 24–11 The indirect fluorescent antibody technique. A hypothetical application of this technique is: 1. Antibodies (as) that have been prepared against sheep globulin (G) in an experimental animal such as the rabbit are labeled with a fluorescein (f) marker producing as— G— f. 2. This preparation is then applied to an antigen-containing (A) specimen that has been treated with sheep globulin (S) to form an antigen-antibody (AS) complex. The labeled antisheep globulin reacts with the antibody in this complex, causing the entire "immunologic sandwich" to fluoresce. 3. Note that the combination of sheep globulin and antigen-containing specimen does not fluoresce, and therefore, there is no indication of a reaction.

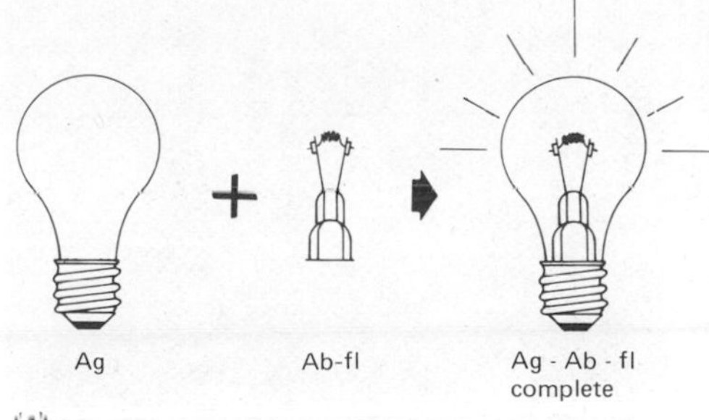

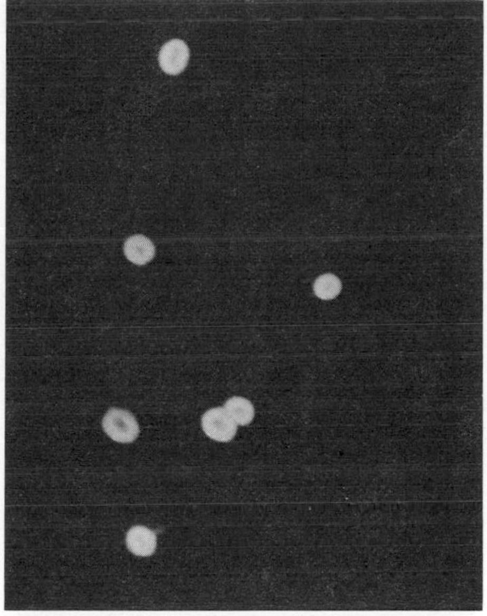

FIG. 24–10 (a) The direct fluorescent antibody technique schematically represented. Antigen and fluorescent tagged antibody are combined to form the antigens-antibody complex which will glow when exposed to ultraviolet light. (b) The appearance of noncapsulated *Haemophilus influenzae* by immunofluorescence. *Courtesy of Catlin, B. W.,* Amer. J. Dis. Child. *120:203–210 (1970).*

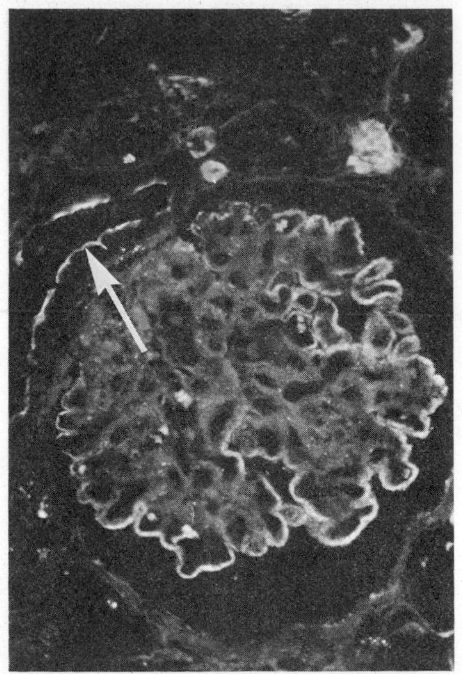

FIG. 24-12 Immunofluorescent microscopy has become an important laboratory method in diagnostic pathology, especially in diseases of the kidney and circulatory system. This micrograph shows the results obtained by the indirect method in an immunologic disorder of the kidney. The presence of immunoglobulins, IgG, is indicated by the glowing fringes and tufts in the kidney glomerulus. *Huang, S. N., H. Minassian, and J. D. More:* Lab. Inves. *35:383 (1976).*

Procedure. Standardized reagents are used. After the specimen is fixed in a manner similar to that described for the direct test, unlabeled specific antiserum (G) is applied to it. These reactants are incubated together for 15 to 60 minutes. The preparation is washed in saline, then in distilled water, and subsequently dried. Following this step, labeled antiglobulin (AG) is layered over the specimen and the preparation is incubated again for 15 to 60 minutes. Rinsing and washing steps are carried out as in the direct test. The resulting antigen-globulin-antiglobulin complex is dried, mounted, and examined with a fluorescent microscope (Figure 24–12).

Controls. This technique has much greater sensitivity than the direct method. Because of this, adequate controls are even more important to establish the specificity of the staining reaction. The possibility of nonspecific fluorescence in the test system must be ruled out. Suggested controls generally include incubating homologous antigen with combinations of the following reagents: (1) saline and labeled antiglobulin (AG); (2) normal serum and labeled antiglobulin (AG); (3) specific antiserum (G) and labeled normal serum. An additional control incubating heterologous antigen with a specific antiserum (G) and labeled antiglobulin (AG) also could be incorporated. If the fluorescence in the indirect test is specific, then fluorescence should not be observed with any of these controls.

Applications. The indirect fluorescent antibody technique has been used to demonstrate antibodies against various tissues (Figure 24–13) and microbial pathogens, including *Treponema pallidum* and Herpes simplex virus (the causative agent of fever blisters).

Variations of this basic technique exist. Test for the presence of antibody in serum, "fluorescent antibody serology," has been used in the diagnosis of syphilis and the detection of malaria antibodies.

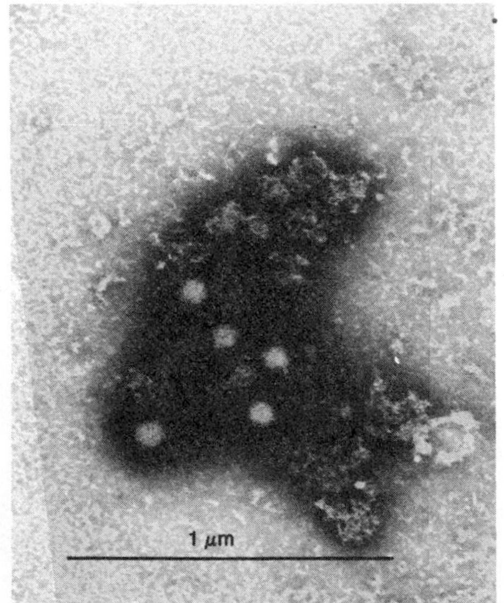

FIG. 24-13 Aggregates formed by incubation of adenoviruses with specific antibodies against them and observed by IEM, a technique that permits visualization of reactions between viruses and antibodies. *Vassall, J. H., II, and C. G. Ray,* Appl. Microbiol. *28:632 (1974).*

Diagnostic and Investigative Electron Microscopy

Immune Electron Microscopy

In recent years, the diagnostic potential and versatility of electron microscopy has been greatly extended by development of new techniques. One such technique, immune electron microscopy (IEM), was first used by Anderson and Stanley to observe the tobacco mosaic virus in the presence of a specific antibody. Immune electron microscopy has since been used to detect the presence of small amounts of antibodies (Figure 24–13), to show antigenic similarities and differences among viruses, and to identify viral particles extracted directly from human tissues and feces. Recently Feinstone, Kapikian, and Purceli found a virus-like particle in the feces of patients with hepatitis A (infectious hepatitis) using IEM. The discovery of the virus-like antigen by immune electron microscopy provides the first technique for the diagnosis and study of hepatitis A infections.

Ferritin-conjugated Antibodies

Ferritin is a protein that has a molecular weight of 700,000 and contains about 23 percent iron, largely in the form of ferric hydroxide and phosphate.

The iron is concentrated within the ferritin molecule in four particles or *micelles*. These units form a central core measuring 5.5 to 6.0 nm in diameter. Because of its composition and molecular arrangement, the ferritin molecule is electron dense and has a characteristic appearance in electron micrographs (Figure 24–15).

Ferritin can be coupled chemically to certain antibody molecules. Such preparations are used to locate bacterial (Figure 24–16), fungal, and viral antigens in tissue and to study antigen-antibody interactions.

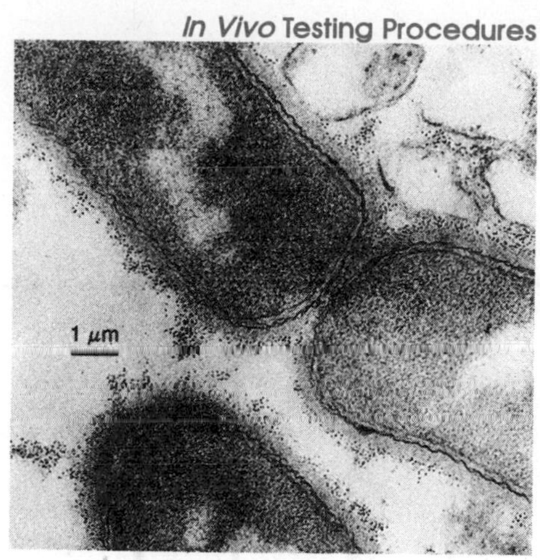

FIG. 24–15 Detecting the presence of bacterial capsules with the aid of ferritin-antibody couples and electron microscopy. Note the concentration of ferritin (dark dots) surrounding the capsules of *Salmonella typhimurium*. *Shands, J. W.,* N.Y. Acad. Sci. *133:292–298 (1966). © The New York Academy of Sciences, 1966. Reprinted by permission.*

In Vivo Testing Procedures

Virus Neutralization

Serologic reactions of various kinds are used for identifying and classifying viruses, detecting antibodies against certain viral agents in the normal population, and studying the responses of individuals to prophylactic immunization. Among the procedures so used are animal protection, complement-fixation, hemagglutination inhibition, and neutralization tests. Because the *in vitro* methods are less expensive and quicker to perform, they are more commonly used than *in vivo* tests. Nevertheless, in many situations only the more complex *in vivo* techniques are applicable.

PROCEDURES

Viral neutralization tests may use either tissue culture systems or laboratory animals, such as chick embryos, mice, or rats. The details of the procedure vary with the viral agent, the host, and related factors; however, there are two general procedures. In one of these procedures, dilutions of a virus suspension are mixed with constant volumes of undiluted serum, incubated for 1 to 2 hours, and then a specific quantity of each mixture is injected into separate groups of animals. For example, dilution mixtures ranging from 1/100 (10^{-2}) to 1/1,000,000 (10^{-6}) are each injected into four animals. The animals are observed for a specified length of time to determine any effects caused by the virus that were not inhibited by the antibodies present in the serum. Naturally, controls are also used; these include viral dilutions with serum lacking specific antibodies and without serum. In the other procedure, the viral concentration is held constant, and the serum is diluted. When tissue culture systems are used, cells are examined for any evidence of a specific inhibition or neutralization of cytopathic effects.

For general diagnostic purposes, two blood specimens should be obtained from the patient suspected of having a viral infection. One such sample should be taken during the acute phase of the disease and the second, during the convalescent period. The presence of an infection is generally indicated by a fourfold increase in antibody titer in the second blood specimen.

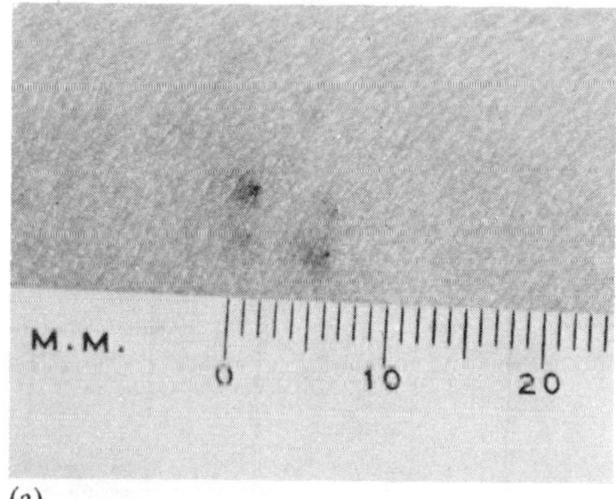

(a)

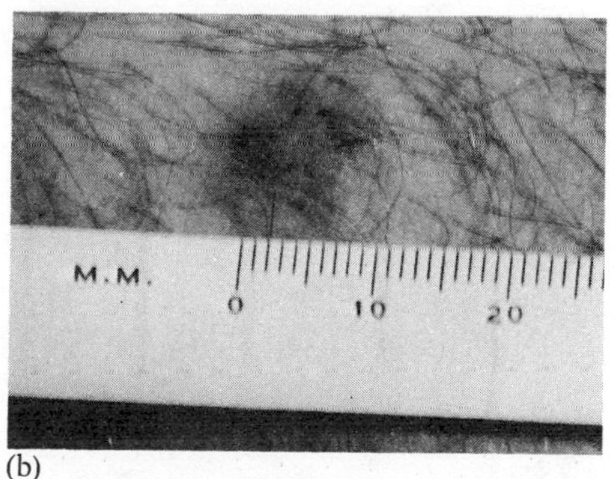

(b)

FIG. 24–16 The results of a Tuberculin Tine test. The presence or absence of induration (hardened area) can be determined by visual observation or by stroking the region around the site of injection. (a) The response to the skin testing material 48 hours and (b) 96 hours after injection. *Courtesy of Lederle Laboratories, Pearl River, N.Y.*

Diagnostic Skin Tests

The introduction of test antigens just under the skin can be used diagnostically, and to follow the progress of recovery from a disease (Table 24–4). Four such diagnostic skin tests are the Frei test for the venereal disease lymphogranuloma venereum, and the tuberculin, Mantoux, and patch tests for tuberculosis.

TABLE 24-4 **Representative Examples of Skin Diagnostic Tests**

Disease State	*Type of Infective Disease Agent Involved (If Applicable)*	*Nature of Preparation Used*[a]	*Type of Reaction*
Brucellosis	Bacterium	Brucellergin (extract of *Brucella* spp.)	Delayed
Leprosy	Bacterium	Lepromin (extract of lepromatous tissue)	Delayed
Lymphogranuloma venereum	Bacterium	Chorioallantoic membrane (extract from infected chick embryo)	Delayed
Psittacosis	Bacterium	Heat-killed organisms	Delayed
Tuberculosis	Bacterium	Purified Protein Derivative (PPD), or Old Tuberculin (OT)	Delayed
Blastomycosis	Fungus	Concentrated culture filtrate	Delayed
Coccidioidomycosis	Fungus	Coccidioidin (concentrated culture filtrate)	Delayed
Histoplasmosis	Fungus	Histoplasmin (concentrated culture filtrate)	Delayed
Leishmaniasis	Protozoan	Extract of cultured organisms	Delayed
Echinococcosis (sheep tapeworm)	Helminth	Hydatid fluid extract	Delayed
Trichinosis (pork roundworm)	Helminth	Extract of the causative agent	Immediate
Schistosomiasis	Helminth	Extract of the causative agent	Immediate
Contact dermatitis	Simple chemical compounds	Small quantities of suspected chemicals	Immediate or delayed

NOTE: The information obtained from such tests also can be used in epidemiologic surveys.
[a]Refer to the individual chapters in which these disease states are discussed for further details.

Positive responses of individuals to test antigens may be either *immediate* or *delayed*. An *immediate reaction,* which develops shortly after exposure to the test antigen, appears as an elevated, flat, pale, swollen area surrounded by a region of redness. It may be accompanied by intense itching around this **wheal and flare reaction.** The *delayed reaction* appears several hours after the introduction of the antigen (Color Photograph 73). The area around the site of inoculation becomes reddened, firm, and swollen within 24 to 48 hours (Figure 24–16). Further aspects of these immunological reactions are discussed in Chapter 25.

Skin tests can also be used to determine an individual's susceptibility to a microbial toxin. Small quantities of toxin are injected into the skin and the reaction observed. Positive responses, those showing susceptibility, are indicated by reddened areas appearing within 24 hours. The Schick test for diphtheria and the Dick test for scarlet fever are examples of this type of procedure.

Immunohematology

The ABO System

In 1900, Karl Landsteiner observed that mixing erythrocytes and sera from different human donors and incubating the mixture at body temperature resulted in the agglutination of the red cells. This phenomenon is known as *isohemagglutination* because it involves reactions between agglutinogens and agglutinins from the same *(iso-)* species. It enabled Landsteiner to demonstrate the existence of the A and B blood types. In addition, he found certain blood

TABLE 24-5 Selected Characteristics of the Major Human Blood Groups

International Designation	Agglutinogen Associated with Cells	Presence or Absence of Agglutinins within Normal Sera: anti-A or α (alpha)	anti-B or β (beta)
A	A	−	+
B	B	+	−
AB	AB	−	−
O	O	+	+

samples in which no visible reactions occurred between the reactants (corresponding agglutinogens and agglutinins). Blood cells exhibiting this negative result are designated O. The fourth and last of the major blood types, AB, was discovered by von Decastello and Sturli in 1902. AB blood is characterized by visible clumping or positive results with the reactants. The major blood types are referred to as the ABO system.

In addition to having specific blood group antigens, certain humans possess antibodies that react with the erythrocytes from individuals of other blood types, causing them either to agglutinate or to lyse. These immunoglobulins are ***isohemagglutinins*** and ***isohemolysins***, respectively. The lysis occurs as a consequence of antibody molecules (isohemolysins) sensitizing the blood cells, making them vulnerable to the hemolytic activity of complement. Usually, the antibodies in the blood serum or plasma of an individual are not directed against the blood factors present in his own blood. However, most individuals have antibodies against blood factors absent from their blood cells. For instance, a person of blood type O has antibodies against type A (anti-A) and type B (anti-B). Antibody concentrations can be increased as a result of transfusions, or, in women, by bearing children of a different blood type. Table 24–5 lists the recognized blood groups with their respective agglutinogens and agglutinins.

THE UNIVERSAL DONOR AND RECIPIENT

A transfusion reaction can occur if the concentration of agglutinins in the recipient's plasma is high enough to cause agglutination or hemolysis of erythrocytes from the donor. It is obviously advisable to transfuse a patient with blood of his particular type. However, there may be circumstances in which this is impossible, because blood of the recipient's type is unavailable. Type O blood is used in such situations, because antibodies against type O blood are very seldom encountered. While the plasma portion of O blood contains agglutinins against both the A and B antigens (Table 24–5), these antibodies would be neutralized or diluted in the recipient's circulation.

Individuals with O type blood are commonly referred to as "universal donors." Unfortunately, this designation is misleading. Transfusions of O type blood cannot be safely performed in all cases. Serious transfusion reactions can occur as a consequence of the presence in these donors of antigen-antibody systems other than the ABO system. These may be minor blood group and Rh factors. In general, transfusion reactions are prevented by performing the direct and indirect cross-matching procedures to determine the blood compatibilities of prospective donors and recipients. See the discussion of blood testing techniques later in the chapter.

Persons with an AB blood type do not have agglutinins against the A or B factors. Consequently, such individuals could receive blood from donors be-

TABLE 24-6 Reaction Patterns in Blood Type Determinations

Blood Type	*Isoagglutinins* anti-A	anti-B
A	+	−
B	−	+
AB	+	+
O	−	−

longing to any of the four major blood groups. They are, therefore, often called "universal recipients."

LABORATORY DETERMINATION OF BLOOD GROUPS (BLOOD TYPING)

Two diagnostic procedures, the tube and slide tests, are commonly used to determine blood types. The determination can be made either by testing red cells with standardized anti-A and anti-B sera, or by testing the patient's serum with standard, sensitive, known A and B red cells. For reliable results, both test systems should be employed; however, most often only the first combination is employed.

The tube technique usually incorporates erythrocytes from the person with standard test sera of anti-A and anti-B reagents. Specific proportions of each antiserum and the erythrocyte suspension are mixed, incubated at 37° C for 30 to 60 minutes, and checked for agglutination. Table 24–6 shows the pattern of reactions observed in blood type determinations.

The slide test uses the same reagents. It is performed by placing one or two drops of each test antiserum on opposite portions of a glass slide, then adding a drop of the patient's cells to each of them. The combinations are mixed separately with the aid of applicator sticks and observed for agglutination. Color Photograph 70 shows the actual reactions characteristic of the major blood types. Reactions should develop within 5 to 10 minutes.

Suitable controls include: (1) the pretesting of sera for activity, (2) dilution of cells and sera in physiological saline if a reaction has not occurred after a sufficient length of time, and (3) the incorporation of tests with known cells and antisera. The incubation temperature should also be checked, as variations in temperature can affect results.

THE ABO SUBGROUPS

Antigenic variations of the ABO system have been reported since 1935. The blood group A has been divided into the major subdivisions A_1 and A_2. The AB group is subdivided into A_1B and A_2B.

Subgroups of the B group include B_v, B_3, B_k, B_w, and B_x. The frequencies of these subgroups vary; A_1 and A_2 are more commonly encountered than others.

INHERITANCE OF THE ABO BLOOD GROUPS

The ABO blood factors constitute one example of genetic characteristics determined by a multiple allelic series. An ***allele*** is a gene belonging to a group of alternate genes that occur on a specific region of a chromosome. Inheritance of A and B characteristics follows normal Mendelian principles. An individual's blood type is determined by receiving, from each parent, one of the four allelic genes: A_1, A_2, B, or O. The specific blood group agglutinogens become permanently established, a finding readily demonstrated in fetuses and newborns. Blood group–associated isohemagglutinins, however, are not normally detectable at birth, but become so within 3 to 6 months.

The genetic composition and the observed blood type of offspring can be determined by the *Punnett square technique,* commonly called the checkerboard system. The possible types of genes of one parent appear across the top of the checkerboard square, and the genetic contributions of the other parent along the side. It is important to remember that each parent generally contributes one gene for each characteristic.

TABLE 24-7 Genotypes and Phenotypes Resulting from Selected Parental Matings (Checkerboard System)

Parental		Offspring's Possible	
Genotypes	Corresponding Phenotypes	Genotypes	Phenotypes
AA × AO	A × A	AA, AO	A
AO × AO	A × A	AA, AO, OO	A or O
BB × BO	B × B	BB, BO	B
BO × BO	B × B	BB, BO, OO	B or O
AA × BB	A × B	AB	AB
AO × BO	A × B	AO, BO, AB, OO	A, B, AB, or O
AB × AO	AB × A	AA, AO, BO	A or B
AB × BO	AB × B	AO, AB, BB, BO	A, AB, or B
AB × OO	AB × O	AO, BO	A or B

Parent 1 (genotype AB)

Parent 2 (genotype AO)

	A	B
A	AA	AB
O	AO	BO

Table 24–7 shows the possible genotypes (assortments of genes) and phenotypes (demonstrable expressions of the individual's genotype) from each possible parental mating. It can be seen from the table that the A and B alleles are dominant over the O gene. Generally speaking, the O blood type manifests itself only in persons lacking both A and B genes, that is, a homozygous O state must be present. In AB individuals, neither allele is dominant. a state of *co-dominance* exists.

The blood group substances (BGS) A and B are not limited to red cells but are found in various body fluids and tissue cells including kidney, liver, lung, and muscle. They have been detected in amniotic fluid, gastric juices, ovarian cyst fluid, perspiration, saliva, semen, tears, and urine of approximately 80 percent of the population. The other 20 percent of the population does not secrete these substances into fluids and tissue.

The Rh System

Once the ABO system was understood, it was believed that transfusion problems could not develop if the donor and recipient belonged to the same blood group. Unfortunately, between the years of 1921 and 1939, some hemolytic transfusion reactions were reported even when blood typing tests showed donor and recipient compatibility. No explanation for these reactions was offered. Moreover, prior to 1940, several reports appeared of newborns exhibiting a clinical state called erythroblastosis fetalis, with swelling and marked anemia.

In 1937, Landsteiner and Wiener, immunizing guinea pigs and rabbits with rhesus monkey blood, discovered antisera that agglutinated red cells not only from the monkey but also from approximately 85 percent of their human blood samples. A hitherto unknown human blood agglutinogen had been found. The

TABLE 24-8 A Comparison of the Designations for the Rh Blood Factors (Wiener) and Rh Agglutinogens (Fisher-Race)

Wiener System	*Fisher-Race System*
Rh_0	D
rh′	C
rh″	E
hr′	c
hr″	e
hr	d

Designations for the more recently discovered Rh factors are symbolized by various combinations of subscript or superscript letters and numerals, e.g., D_u, C_w.

new factor was designated "Rh," indicating the source of the antigen, the rhesus monkey. Further research showed it to occur in all blood groups.

The antibody response of sensitized Rh-negative individuals to the administration of Rh-positive antigens clearly demonstrated the importance of the Rh factor. In 1939, Levine and Stetson observed a transfusion reaction in a woman shortly after the delivery of her stillborn fetus. Apparently in need of a transfusion, the woman received blood from her husband. The transfusion produced a pronounced hemolytic reaction. The mother's serum was found to contain an agglutinin against the Rh factor. Levine and Stetson theorized that the presence of this agglutinin was the direct result of *in utero* immunization of the mother by antigen that the fetus inherited from the father. Later studies by Levine and his colleagues proved this to be the cause and showed that the resulting maternal antibody could pass through the placenta and cause the erythroblastosis fetalis, hemolytic disease of the newborn or "the Rh baby."

OTHER RH AND HR FACTORS

Since the original report of the Rh factor in human blood, more than twenty-five other blood factors that evidently belong to the Rh-Hr blood group system have been discovered. These blood factors have proved to be of great clinical significance, second only to the ABO system.

The Rh-Hr system is a complex one, and controversies have arisen over the nomenclature for the Rh agglutinogens. Two principal methods are currently used: the Wiener scheme (the original Rh-Hr nomenclature designations) and the Fisher-Race system (combination of the letters C, D, and E). Table 24–8 shows the comparison between these two systems of notation. The more recently discovered Rh factors are symbolized by various combinations of subscript or superscript letters and numerals, for example, D_u, C_w.

Rh typing. The Rh factors of red cells are detected by agglutination tests using the appropriate antisera, anti-Rh_0, -rh′, and -rh″. The classic and clinically most important of the factors is Rh_0 (D).

HEMOLYTIC DISEASE OF THE NEWBORN (THE RH BABY)

Hemolytic disease of the newborn, erythroblastosis fetalis, is the blood incompatibility normally encountered when differences in Rh factors exist between the mother and her child. Usually this condition develops in babies born to mothers who are negative for the Rh_0 factor and fathers who are positive for the same factor. (This specific Rh terminology is explained below.) The red cells of the child may inherit the paternal blood factor, which is foreign to the mother. If this antigen is carried across the placental barrier, it serves to immunize the mother to the Rh factor. The resulting maternal isoantibodies pass from the mother's circulation into the fetal system and attack the baby's red cells. The most common signs of the disease are anemia and yellowing or jaundice of the newborn.

Once a mother has been actively immunized against the Rh_0 factor and has given birth to one child with erythroblastosis fetalis, the disease's effects will be more severe with future Rh_0^+ offspring. If the father is heterozygous ($Rh_0^+Rh_0^-$), they may produce children lacking the Rh_0 factor. Almost all Rh_0 negative women without previous exposure to the Rh_0 factors via transfusions have given birth to one or more normal Rh_0-positive children before enough maternal antibodies were produced to cause trouble; and if the father is heterozygous ($Rh_0^+Rh_0^-$), each fetus has a 50 percent chance of being Rh negative and, therefore, not subject to the disease.

The Rh_0 (D) antigen is generally the main factor in the hemolytic disease of the newborn. However, all of the other blood antigens are capable of causing the condition.

PREVENTION OF RH ISOIMMUNIZATION

Fetal erythrocytes are commonly observed in the maternal circulation near term, and their numbers generally increase after childbirth. Much clinical evidence indicates that the processes of labor and delivery cause fetal red cells to enter the maternal circulation. Other investigators hold that there is a continual leakage of the fetal cells into the mother's system throughout pregnancy. Probably both contribute to the isoimmunization of certain Rh-negative women. The major threat of isoimmunization occurs at the end of the third trimester of pregnancy and immediately after childbirth.

A new procedure for preventing maternal Rh problems has recently been developed. The approach is to use passive immunization to suppress the antigenic stimulus provided by fetal cells during the postpartum period. An immunoglobulin G preparation that contains high titers of anti-D (anti-Rh_0) antibody is administered. Rh-negative unsensitized mothers receive this material within 72 hours after a delivery, abortion, or miscarriage involving an Rh problem. The antibody disappears after approximately 6 months, after producing a short-lived passive immunity and preventing a long-lasting active one that might endanger a later child.

Blood Testing Techniques

Compatibility Testing or Cross Matching

The primary purpose of compatability testing is to prevent a transfusion reaction as a consequence of blood incompatibility. Specifically, the cross-matching technique is designed to detect any incompatibility between the recipient's serum and the donor's cells (this is known as the ***major cross match***), or between the recipient's cells and the donor's serum (this is referred to as the ***minor cross match***). The cross-matching procedure is done after the respective blood specimens have been typed as to the ABO and Rh factors and any other factor that appears to be indicated.

Agglutination or lysis of the red cells from either the donor or recipient in their tests is considered to be indicative of an incompatible situation. However, it should be stressed that occasionally an incompatible cross match may be due to an error in blood typing of the specimens used, or to the presence of atypical antibodies in the blood of either the donor or recipient. When these causes are suspected, it is customary to investigate the possibility of error.

Coombs Tests

Two tests for the detection of incomplete antibodies, the direct and indirect Coombs tests, have great clinical importance in cases of hemolytic anemia and hemolytic disease of the newborn. Incomplete antibodies do not function in ordinary hemagglutination tests.

DIRECT COOMBS TEST

The direct Coombs test is used to determine whether or not the patient's erythrocytes have been sensitized (coated) by antibodies *in vivo*. In this test, saline-washed blood cells suspected of being sensitized are mixed with antihuman globulin serum (Coombs reagent) and observed for agglutination. A control of the patient's cells and saline is also observed. Clumping in the erythrocyte-Coombs reagent system is a positive test. This test demonstrates the presence of incomplete antibodies, but it does not identify them specifically.

INDIRECT COOMBS TEST

The indirect Coombs test is a modification of the direct procedure and is used for detecting either complete or incomplete antibodies in the serum of sensitized individuals. The procedure consists of the following three stages: (1) sensitization of erythrocytes (Rh positive) with Rh antiserum (patient's serum); (2) washing the sensitized cells to remove excess antibody; and (3) mixing the resulting preparation with the Coombs reagent. Agglutination of the Rh-antibody-coated red cells by the Coombs reagent constitutes a positive test.

The difference between these two tests is that, in the direct procedure, red cells are examined for the presence of antibody on cells (sensitization *in vivo*), while in the indirect test, Rh positive cells sensitized *in vitro* by the antibodies present in the patient's serum are used to detect the Rh antibodies.

SUMMARY

1. A variety of *in vitro* and *in vivo* techniques are available to detect and to determine the levels of antibody toward antigens.
2. Such information is important in identifying a disease agent following recovery from an infection or in determining the effectiveness of immunizations.
3. Examples of *in vitro* immunologic procedures used in diagnosis of microbial identification include agglutination, complement fixation, ferritin-conjugated antibody, immunodiffusion, precipitin tests, radioimmunoassay, and virus neutralization.

Production of Antisera

1. Antigen-containing materials to produce potent antibody-containing serum (antiserum) for diagnostic tests may be introduced intraperitoneally, intravenously, or subcutaneously.
2. Determination of antibody levels is made from blood samples removed periodically from experimental animals.
3. Once the antibody concentration reaches the desired level, sufficient blood is removed to obtain the immune (antibody-containing) serum for diagnostic purposes.

The Diagnostic Significance of Rising Antibody Titers

1. Two serum specimens of an individual are necessary to distinguish antibody production resulting from an actual ongoing infection, from the effects of immunization, or from antibodies associated with past infection. The first sample is taken soon after the appearance of disease symptoms and the other, about two weeks later.

2. If in testing such specimens for a particular disease agent, a greater degree of antibody activity occurs with the later specimen, identification of the causative agent is possible.
3. If little or no antibody activity is detected in either specimen, it can be generally assumed that an organism other than the one being tested for is the cause of the infection.
4. If antibody activity is present in both samples but no appreciable change is noted in antibody concentration, it can be assumed that such levels were present before the start of the current infection and have no relationship to the disease state.

The Agglutination Reaction

1. Agglutination involves the clumping of cellular or particulate (particle-like) antigen-containing materials by homologous antibodies.
2. Agglutination tests have been widely used for the rapid diagnosis of several infectious diseases, such as rickettsial infections and typhoid fever.
3. Examples of agglutination and related reactions include cold hemagglutination, the Weil-Felix test, Widal test, latex agglutination tests, and viral hemagglutination.

Hemagglutination Inhibition (HI)

1. The hemagglutination-inhibition (HI) test is used for the detection and titration of viral antibodies in a patient's serum and for viral identification.
2. Identification of specific hemagglutinating viruses is based on the fact that viral hemagglutination can be inhibited by specific antibodies against such viruses.
3. Adequate controls must be included in the procedure to ensure accuracy.

The Precipitin Reaction

1. Precipitin reactions involve interactions of antibodies called precipitins with soluble antigens known as precipitinogens.
2. A visible "floc" or precipitate occurs at the point where optimal proportions of antibody and antigens and related factors exist.
3. While the general form of this reaction is still functional today, it has undergone certain changes.
4. Modern-day procedures incorporate agar gel bases to stabilize the precipitates that form. Examples of these procedures include the Oudin test, double diffusion procedure, single radial immunodiffusion (RID), two-dimensional immunelectrophoresis, and the Ouchterlony test.
5. Modern-day precipitin procedures are highly accurate and are used for the quantitation of a variety of specific proteins in serum and other fluids.

In Vitro *Hemolysis Tests*

Complement Fixation

1. Various antigen-antibody combinations have the ability to fix, or combine with, complement. This type of reaction can be used to detect either antibodies or antigen-containing substances in unknown specimens.
2. The complement-fixation technique incorporates both a test and an indicator system.
3. The test system consists of a patient's serum, a commercially or laboratory prepared antigen, and complement. All serum preparations must be heated at 56° C for 30 minutes to inactivate any complement in these sources of antibodies.
4. The indicator system consists of sheep red blood cells and antibody against sheep red blood cell known as hemolysin.
5. In a positive complement fixation test, antibody combines with antigen of the test system. Complement is fixed by this combination. Thus, complement is not available to react with the indicator system. The end result is a cloudy red suspension.
6. In a negative test, complement is fixed by the indicator system resulting in a clear red solution. When complement is fixed by the sheep red blood cell–hemolysin combination, lysis of the blood cells occurs, thereby causing a release of hemoglobin.
7. Specific controls must be used in the test to ensure accuracy.
8. Complement-fixation procedures have been used in the laboratory diagnosis of a wide variety of microbial infections and helminthic diseases.

Antistreptolysin Test

1. Determination of antibody levels against the thermolabile hemolysin of streptococci, streptolysin O, is known as the antistreptolysin test.
2. Levels of antibodies against this bacterial product increase during times of infection and convalescence.

In Vitro *Immunological Procedures Incorporating Differential Staining*

Fluorescent Antibody Techniques

1. Fluorescent antibody methodology involves chemically bonding a fluorescent dye (marker) with serum proteins.
2. Such preparations contain specific antibodies that can be used for the detection of homologous antigens in smears or tissue preparations.
3. The most commonly used fluorescent antibody procedures are the direct and the indirect methods.
4. The direct fluorescent antibody method can be used to identify unknown microbial agents and to determine the distribution of antigens in tissue.
5. The indirect fluorescent antibody method can be used to detect antibodies against various microbial pathogens and those produced in certain immunologic disorders.

Diagnostic and Investigative Electron Microscopy

1. Immune electron microscopy can be used to detect small amounts of antibody, show antigenic similarities and differences among viruses, and identify viral particles in various types of specimens.
2. Ferritin-conjugated antibody preparations are useful in finding various microbial antigens in tissues and in studying antigen-antibody interactions.

In Vivo *Testing Procedures*

Virus Neutralization

1. Virus neutralization tests can use either tissue culture systems or laboratory animals, such as chick embryos, mice, or rats.
2. Tests such as these are used for identifying viruses, detecting antibodies against viruses, and studying responses to immunizations against viruses.
3. Details of the procedure vary with the viral agent, host used, and related factors.

Diagnostic Skin Tests

1. The intradermal introduction of test antigens can be used diagnostically, as well as to follow the course of recovery from a disease. Examples of such skin tests include the Frei test for lymphogranuloma venereum and the tuberculin test for tuberculosis.
2. Positive responses can occur shortly after exposure to the test antigen (immediate) or several hours later (delayed).
3. Skin tests also have value in determining an individual's susceptibility to microbial toxins. Examples of such tests include the Schick test for diphtheria and the Dick test for scarlet fever.

Immunohematology

The ABO System

1. The clumping of human red blood cells by homologous human immunoglobulins is known as *isohemagglutination*. Observing this phenomenon led to the discovery of the major blood types, A, B, AB, and O, frequently referred to as the ABO system.
2. Most individuals have antibodies against the major blood antigens that are absent from their blood cells. Thus a person of blood type O has antibodies against types A and B, a person of blood type A has antibodies against type B, and a person of blood type B has antibodies against type A. Individuals with blood type AB do not have antibodies against any of the other major blood types and are termed "universal recipients."
3. Tube and slide tests are commonly used to determine blood types.
4. These types of determinations can be made either by using an individual's red cells with standardized anti-A and anti-B sera, or by testing the individual's serum with standard known A and B type red cells.
5. Clumping or agglutination resulting with cell serum combinations identifies the particular blood antigen present. Reactions establishing a particular blood type's identity are as follows:

Blood Type	*Antiserum Used*	
	Anti-A	*Anti-B*
A	agglutination	no agglutination
B	no agglutination	agglutination
AB	agglutination	agglutination
O	no agglutination	no agglutination

6. Antigenic subgroups have been found with both A and B blood types.
7. Inheritance of ABO blood factors follows normal Mendelian principles.
8. An individual's blood type is determined by receiving from each parent one of the four alternate (allelic) genes, A_1, A_2, B, or O.
9. Major blood group antibodies become detectable within 3 to 6 months after birth.
10. Blood group substances are not limited to red cells but have been found in other cells and body fluids.

The Rh System

1. The Rh system consists of blood factors that are also important.
2. *In utero* immunization of a mother by a Rh antigen inherited by a fetus from the father may bring about the condition known as the Rh baby.
3. Since the discovery of the Rh factor in human blood, other related blood factors have been discovered.
4. Determination of Rh factors in blood is made by agglutination tests using appropriate antisera.
5. An Rh baby results from the sensitization of the mother to the Rh factor of the fetus.
6. Prevention of isoimmunization of a mother toward Rh factors can be done by the administration of anti-Rh_0 (D) antibody-containing preparations within 72 hours after delivery. This is a form of passive immunization.

Blood Testing Techniques

Compatibility Testing or Cross Matching

1. The primary purpose of compatibility testing is to prevent transfusion reactions.
2. Cross matching includes the mixing of the recipient's serum and the donor's cells (major cross match), and the mixing of the recipient's cells with the donor's serum (minor cross match).
3. Agglutination (clumping) or lysis (destruction) occurring in either the major or minor cross matches indicates an incompatibility.

Coombs Tests

1. The Coombs tests are used for the detection of incomplete antibodies. Two forms of the procedure are used, the direct and the indirect.
2. The direct Coombs test is used to determine whether or not blood cells have been coated by antibodies *in vivo*.
3. The indirect test is used to detect either complete or incomplete antibodies in the serum of a sensitized individual.

QUESTIONS FOR REVIEW

1. Differentiate between the following combinations:
   a. antigen and antibody
   b. serum and plasma
   c. toxin and antitoxin
   d. antitoxin and antibody
   e. agglutination and precipitation
   f. serology and immunology
2. What significance do serological tests have in the diagnosis of infectious diseases?
3. Construct a table listing:
   a. representative serological tests
   b. the types of reagents used
   c. the appearance of both positive and negative reactions
4. What is viral neutralization?
5. a. What is complement? Where can this substance be found normally?
   b. Describe the complement-fixation test. Include the components of the test and indication system, and the appearance of typical positive and negative tests.

6. Differentiate between the indirect and direct fluorescent antibody techniques.
7. Explain how electron microscopy can be used for diagnostic purposes.
8. a. Of what value are skin tests?
   b. List at least three that are of importance.
9. What are the major blood types, and how do they differ?
10. Distinguish between a universal recipient and a universal donor.
11. Differentiate between isoagglutinins and isohemolysins.
12. Describe the procedure used to detect ABO subgroups.
13. Give the possible genotypes and phenotypes of offspring from the following parental genotypes:
    a. AO × AB
    b. OO × AA
    c. AO × BO
    d. AO × BB
14. Discuss the major features of the Rh system and the possible complications of Rh incompatibility.
15. Identify the double diffusion precipitin reactions shown in Figure 24–17. The center well contains antigen. Each of the surrounding wells contains a different antiserum. With which of the wells is there antigen identity?

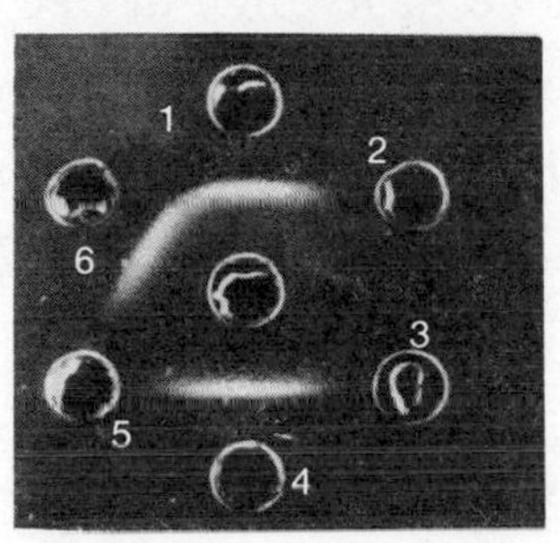

SUGGESTED READINGS

Gardener, P. S., and J. McQuillin, *Rapid Viral Diagnosis.* Great Britain: Butterworth and Co., 1974. *Viral diagnosis by immunofluorescence techniques is described. Several examples of actual procedures are given.*

Garvey, J. S., N. E. Cremer, and D. H. Sussdorf, *Methods in Immunology,* 3rd ed. Reading, Mass.: Addison-Wesley, 1977. *A methodology text containing clear presentations of principles and techniques in 'cookbook' fashion.*

Hijmans, W., and M. Schaeffer (eds.), "Fifth International Conference on Immunofluorescence and Related Staining Techniques." *Ann. N. Y. Acad. Sci.* 254, 1975. *Proceedings of a conference covering the procedures and applications of visual techniques for detecting tagged or marked antibodies.*

Kurstak, E., and R. Morisset (eds.), *Viral Immunodiagnosis.* New York: Academic Press, 1974. *Immunoenzymatic techniques, immunofluorescence, labeled antiviral antibodies in electron microscopy, and progress in viral infection diagnosis are discussed.*

Landsteiner, K., *The Specificity of Serological Reactions.* Cambridge, Mass.: Harvard University Press, 1945. *The basis of immunological specificity is described by the investigator most responsible for its definition.*

Lennette, E. H., E. H. Spaulding, and J. P. Truant (eds.), *Manual of Clinical Microbiol.,* 2nd ed. Washington, D.C.: American Society for Microbiology, 1974. *A standard reference manual that lists and describes several important immunoserological tests, including tests for syphilis, antinuclear antibody, antistreptolysin O titer, and streptococcal serology.*

CHAPTER 25

Immunologic Disorders

The immune system is impressive in its high degree of specialization and its ability to protect the body from infection. In some situations, however, the immune system can fail. Chapter 25 describes a number of such failures, involving immune-system deficiencies, exaggerated and damaging responses to immunogens, responses to drugs and various chemicals, and the transplantation of tissues.

After reading this chapter, you should be able to

1. **Define immunologic deficiency and hypersensitivity.**
2. **List and describe the general categories of hypersensitivity.**
3. **Describe the relationship of hypersensitivity to disease.**
4. **Identify the immunoglobulins associated with allergic reactions.**
5. **Outline the immunologic mechanisms and complications of anaphylaxis, atopy, cytotoxicity, allergy of infection, and graft rejection.**
6. **Describe the general approaches used in the management of allergic states.**
7. **Define histocompatibility antigens and explain their significance.**
8. **Discuss the basis for and the outcomes of autoallergic states.**

The various components of the immune system are not only important in themselves but actually indispensable. To protect and preserve the body, the immune system must be able to recognize and destroy molecules that are *foreign,* or *non-self,* while conserving those body components that are *native,* or *self.* But what happens when this system fails and actually becomes the basis of disease or contributes to the lowering of the body's protective capabilities?

Immunodeficiencies

The immunodeficiency diseases, which include a wide range of disorders, are distinguished by the inability of the immune systems to perform normally. The exact effects and symptoms of such conditions vary according to the parts of the immune system affected and the extent of the disorder. Two general categories of these disorders are recognized—**primary** and **secondary immunodeficiencies.**

Primary Immunodeficiencies

Primary immunodeficiencies (Figure 25–1) usually arise from an inherited failure of one or more immune-system components to develop. The earliest and most devastating immune defect is *bone-marrow stem-cell deficiency.* In this condition, fatal infections develop within days after birth, since neither B-type nor T-type lymphocyte components are functional. In *DiGeorge's syndrome,* the thymus gland does not develop. Here T-lymphocytes are lacking, and the infant is highly susceptible to the effects of various microorganisms such as digestive-system microbes, fungi, and atypical tubercle bacilli.

Agammaglobulinemia, the failure to produce immunoglobulins, is another congenital abnormality. This inborn error in metabolism is transmitted as a sex-linked (X-chromosome-linked) recessive trait, and therefore is primarily found in males. In the past, infants with this disease died of infection. Today, most cases are recognized during the first or second year of life. In cases of severe bacterial infections, the patients are saved with the aid of antibiotic therapy and injections of purified immunoglobulin preparations.

Electrophoretic examination of the sera from agammaglobulinemic persons shows that IgG is almost completely absent and IgA and IgM are lacking. Apparently, they are replaced by other, nonfunctional proteins in the sera.

The basic defect in persons with this condition may be either an inability to form the necessary globulins or the activation of an abnormal mechanism that destroys the globulins shortly after they are formed.

Secondary Immunodeficiencies

Secondary, or acquired, deficiencies (Color Photograph 78) occur much more frequently than the primary immunodeficiencies. The causes of the secondary deficiencies include malnutrition, malignancies (cancers), extensive exposure to radiation, burns, and various drugs that interfere with the lymphatic system. B-type lymphocyte malignancies are known to produce immunoglobulin abnormalities. For example, in certain disease states, a single cell undergoes conversion to a cancerous state. The effect is a rapid and unregulated multiplication resulting in a large family of monoclonal cells (cells with one type of offspring). This formation in turn produces a single type of uniform immunoglobulin. This condition is called a *monoclonal gammopathy* (abnormality). These proteins are found in individuals suffering from *multiple myeloma* and other can-

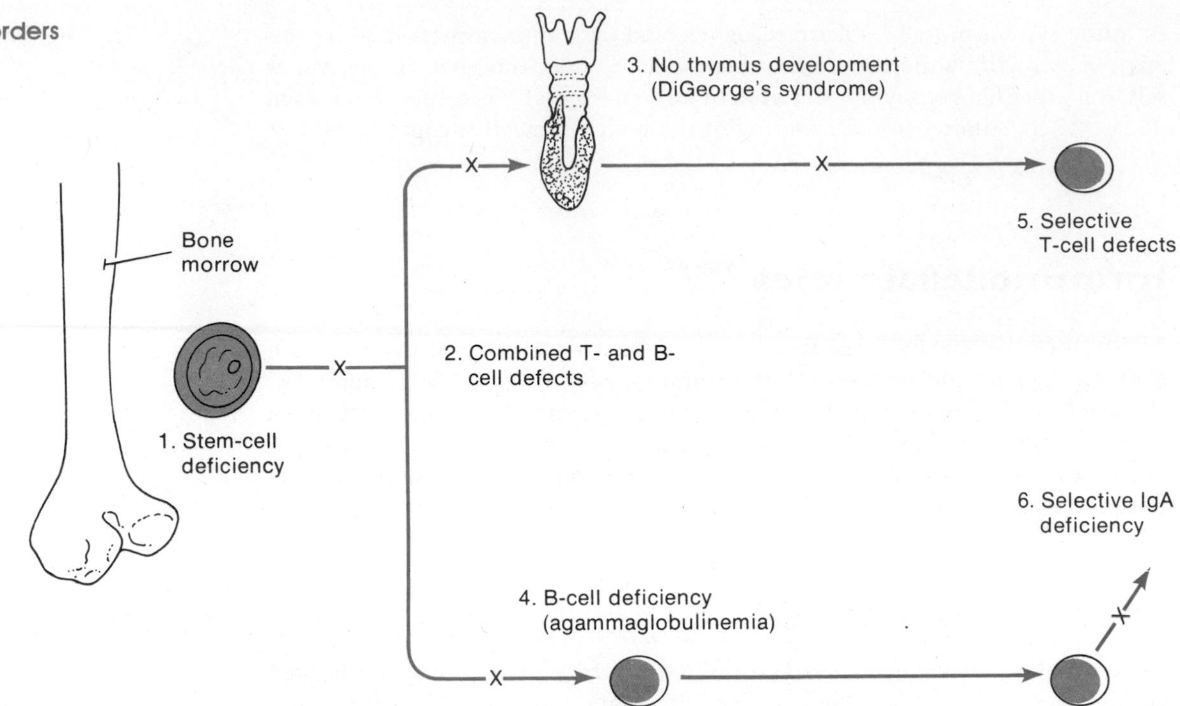

FIG. 25-1 A diagrammatic representation of primary immuno-deficiency diseases. The disorders that occur at various stages in the development of immune system are indicated by Xs. *Purtilo, D. J.* A Survey of Human Disease. *Menlo Park, Calif.: Addison-Wesley Publishing Corporation. (1978).*

cers involving the lymphatics. Immunoglobulin abnormalities may cause increases in the concentration of several or all immunoglobulins or abnormally large increases in the concentration of a single immunoglobulin type.

Hypersensitivity (Allergy)

In 1906, von Pirquet introduced the term ***hypersensitivity*** to describe the increase in reactivity that can occur when persons vaccinated with vaccinia virus are reexposed to the virus. Later, he extended the limits of hypersensitivity to include any altered activity, or ***allergy,*** caused by contact with animate or inanimate substances. This state is generally described as an acquired exaggerated response toward a specific substance that does not produce similar reactions in the majority of previously unexposed members of the same species. The inciting, or inducing, agents are referred to as **allergens.**

Initial exposure to an allergen immunologically primes, or sensitizes, the individual. Subsequent contact with the same allergen can not only lead to a secondary boosting of the immune response, but can also cause tissue-damaging reactions. Several factors influence the expressions of hypersensitive responses, including the portal of entry, the cellular and tissue responses to the allergen, and the genetic make-up of the individual.

Categories of Hypersensitivity

Historically, hypersensitivity reactions were divided into two classes on the basis of the time required for an obvious physiological response to develop upon

TABLE 25-1 Comparison of Different Types of Hypersensitivity[a]

Characteristic	Immediate (Immunoglobulin dependent) I (Classic Immediate)	II (Cytotoxic)	III (Immune-Complex-Mediated)	Delayed IV (Cell-Mediated)
Maximum reaction time for clinical manifestation (response)	30 min	Variable	3–8 hr.	24–48 hr.
Reaction mediators (regulators)	IgE, IgG, complement (C′), and pharmacological substances including histamine, SRS-A, ECF-A, kinins, and prostaglandins[b]	IgG, IgM, and complement	IgE, IgG, IgM, complement, eosinophiles, neutrophiles, and lysosomal enzymes	T-lymphocytes, macrophages, and soluble mediators such as MIF and TF[c]
Appearance of response to intradermal antigens	Wheal-and-flare		Erythema and edema	Erythema and induration
Inhibition by anti-histaminic drugs	Yes, in certain situations	No	No	No
Inhibition by cortisone	No, with normal dosages	No	No	Yes
Passive transfer with serum from sensitive donor	Generally yes	Yes	Yes	No
Examples of allergic states	Anaphylaxis, asthma, serum sickness, and drug, food, and insect allergies	Transfusion reaction, hemolytic disease of the newborn, and drug-induced allergies	Arthus reaction, serum sickness, and certain auto-immune diseases	Infection allergies, auto-immune disease, graft rejection, contact dermatitis to drugs, and tumor immunity

[a]Source: Gell, P. G. H., R. A. Coombs, and P. Lachman, (eds.) *Clinical Aspects of Immunology*. 3rd ed., Oxford: Blackwell Scientific Publications, 1974, Section IV.
[b]SRS-A is a slow-reacting substance of anaphylaxis; ECF-A is an eosinophilic chemotactic factor of anaphylaxis.
[c]MIF is a migration inhibitory factor; TF is a transfer factor.

reexposure of a sensitized individual to the allergen. Reactions that developed within a few seconds to 24 hours following allergen exposure and that involved circulating antibodies were usually classified as ***immediate***. Those that developed after 24 hours but within 48 hours and that involved the direct participation of sensitized lymphocytes were known as ***delayed*** hypersensitivity reactions. Although these designations are still used today, they are now understood to have different meanings. In 1968, R. A. Coombs and P. G. H. Gell defined four types of hypersensitivity (Table 25-1): Type I (classic immediate), Type II (cytotoxic), Type III (immune-complex mediated), and Type IV (cell-mediated, or delayed). Types I through III are immunoglobulin-dependent hypersensitivities. Type IV reactions are mediated by antigen-sensitized T-lymphocytes rather than by antibody molecules. In addition, specific interactions of sensitized T-cells with antigens are involved in the rejection of transplanted tissues and organs and in protection against cancer.

The immunoglobulin-dependent (immediate) hypersensitivities can be subdivided into two categories according to the agent primarily responsible for the immune response: the classic, heat-stable immunoglobulins, IgA, IgD, IgG, and IgM; or the heat-sensitive antibodies, IgE. Heat-stable antibodies resist destruction by heat at 56 to 60°C for periods of 30 minutes to 4 hours. It should be noted that both immunoglobulin categories may be present simultaneously.

From the characteristics listed in Table 25-1, it is obvious that hypersensitivity reactions involve several different types of physiological response by immunized cells or tissues. Nevertheless, establishing a hypersensitivity state always requires one or more exposures to the inciting allergenic substance followed by a so-called latent period in which no symptoms are shown. The hypersensitive state is then triggered by another exposure to the allergen.

The particular type of hypersensitivity acquired is determined by several factors. These include (1) the chemical nature of the allergen; (2) the route involved in the sensitization—for example, inhalation, ingestion, or injection—and (3) the physiological state of the individual. The form of the response depends on the type of contact with the precipitating allergenic dose and on the acquired hypersensitive state.

The four types of hypersensitivities are distinguished by other differences as well. These distinctions are listed in Table 25–1 and will be discussed later.

Type I—Classic Immediate Hypersensitivity

Examples of Type I allergic responses include certain forms of asthma, anaphylactic shock, hay fever ***(allergic rhinitis)***, and hives ***(urticaria)***. One of the distinguishing features of this hypersensitive state is the rapid liberation of physiologically active chemicals, such as histamine and serotonin, from affected cells. Substances of this kind are normally released from cells as a consequence of antigen and antibody interaction. Initially, immunoglobulins produced by plasma cells attach by means of their F_c portions (Figure 25–2) to basophils and mast cells. Mast cells contain heparin and histamine in cytoplasmic granules and are found in connective tissue. The F_{ab} regions of the attached immunoglobulins protrude from the cellular surfaces. When combined with the antigen, they alter the permeability of the mast cells. This reaction leads to the degranulation of mast cells and the release of histamine and serotonin.

In humans, almost all Type I reactions are associated with IgE. The liberated substances produce secondary involvement and responses in other cells. Among these effects are the destruction of blood cells, an increase in muscle activity, an increase in capillary permeability, and excessive mucus production.

The sensitivity response of Type I hypersensitivity can be transferred to a normal, nonsensitive person simply by the injection of serum or transfusion of blood from a sensitive individual.

Representative Type I Allergic States

ANAPHYLAXIS

Before approximately 1837, certain protein solutions, such as egg albumin, were used for the initial inoculation of laboratory animals and were considered to be largely harmless. In 1839, however, Magendie reported that repeated injections of such material often produced severe symptoms and even caused the sudden death of dogs. Instead of becoming immune to such foreign substances, the experimental animals became unusually sensitive to them. Moreover, death was caused by reinjection with dosages too small to affect normal laboratory animals. In essence, the effect was the opposite of protection ***(prophylaxis)***. In 1902, Richet named this phenomenon ***anaphylaxis***. The reaction has come to be known as ***anaphylactic shock***.

Two general types of anaphylactic responses are recognized—***systemic***, or ***generalized, anaphylaxis*** and ***cutaneous anaphylaxis***. Both states are temporary.

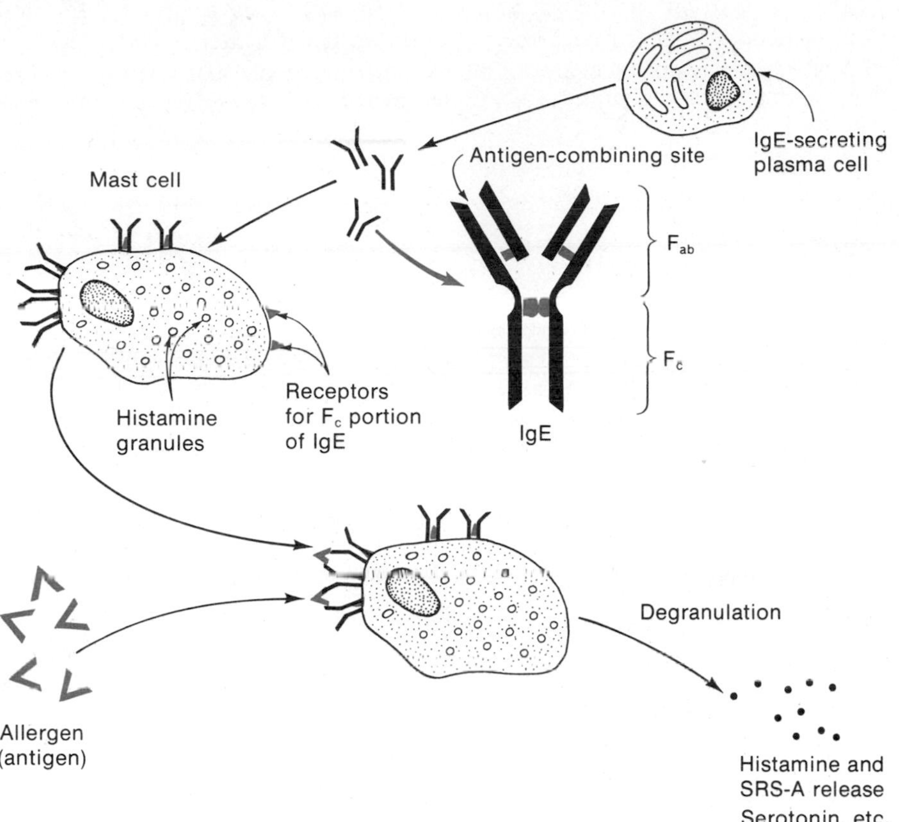

FIG. 25–2 An immune system response to an allergen. Allergens come into contact with specific IgE antibody molecules on the surface of a basophil or a mast cell. A subsequent membrane response causes the release of chemical mediators from granules in the basophil or mast cell.

If the individual does not die almost at once, recovery usually occurs within an hour.

The anaphylactic reaction results from the interaction between the specific allergen and the cell-fixed (or attached) anaphylactic antibodies. The cells specifically involved in this reaction include tissue mast cells and basophil leucocytes. Anaphylactic antibodies seem to have a special attraction for these cells. The interaction between the allergen and anaphylactic antibodies fixed to these cells triggers a process inside the cells, apparently involving several steps and ultimately leading to the release of chemical mediators (Figure 25–2). The released mediators in turn act on certain target organs or tissues, such as smooth muscles in blood vessels and portions of the respiratory passages.

Generalized anaphylaxis. The generalized form of anaphylactic response is produced by the intravenous injection of specific soluble allergens, such as horse serum or egg albumen, to which an animal has been previously sensitized. The allergens, or sensitizers, that originally cause the hypersensitive state are called *inducers.* The anaphylactic response is brought about by substances similar to the inducers called *elicitors.* Generalized anaphylaxis produces suffocation, respiratory-passage constriction, shock (failure of the peripheral circulation), engorgement of blood vessels, and other respiratory changes. The features of anaphylactic shock vary depending on the species involved.

Cutaneous anaphylaxis in humans. Cutaneous anaphylaxis results from the intradermal injection of an elicitor into a sensitized individual. The reaction begins with an intense itching at the injection site. This is shortly followed by the development of a pale, irregular wheal (a flat, elevated, swollen area) surrounded by a region of redness. The response, which usually subsides within approximately 30 minutes, is referred to as the *wheal-and-flare reaction*.

Production of active anaphylaxis. Three definite steps are required to bring about anaphylactic responses: (1) injection of the inducer substance; (2) the passage of time, referred to as the *incubation*, or *latent, period,* which leads to the sensitized state in the individual; and (3) exposure to the elicitor, generally by injection or inhalation. The elicitor is frequently called the *shocking*, or *injection, dose.* The inducer and elicitor are closely related substances.

The mechanism governing an anaphylactic response generally involves a bridging process in which an allergen links antibody molecules. For this reason, the reaction requires (1) the presence of two or more antigenic determinants on the allergen, and (2) the presence of more than one antibody molecule per cell. (Actually hundreds or thousands of such molecules usually exist in a cell.) The intensity of the response depends on both the number of antibody-antigen complexes formed and the rate at which they are formed. The more rapidly such complexes develop, the stronger is the response. The release and rapid degradation of certain active substances play a vital role in anaphylaxis and related responses.

Several active participants, or mediators, have been identified in anaphylaxis. These include cell-associated substances, histamine and serotonin (5-hydroxytryptamine), and basic peptides called *kinins.* The temporary nature of anaphylactic reactions is accounted for by the rapid degradation and excretion of these substances, which prevent them from accumulating.

The symptoms of laboratory-induced anaphylaxis differ in different laboratory animals. Such variations are explained partly by differences in the amounts of active substances in the subjects' tissues, and partly by differences in the responses of specific tissues such as smooth muscle and blood vessels.

Anaphylaxis in humans. Systemic, or generalized, anaphylactic shock can occur as a result of serum therapy or the administration of penicillin. Symptoms may include abdominal cramps, diarrhea, diffuse erythema, hives, intense itching, nausea, respiratory difficulties, and vomiting. Death may occur rapidly. The prompt intravenous or intracardial administration of epinephrine (adrenalin) will usually counter an attack of anaphylaxis.

Certain preventive measures against a fatal anaphylactic attack are available. One can skin test individuals with minute amounts of substances known as potential elicitors—for example, serum, penicillin, and the like—before administering full doses of such substances. Also, one can keep a container of epinephrine close at hand to be administered as needed.

ATOPY

About 10 percent of the population in the United States is believed to have a natural hypersensitivity, in the absence of a deliberate exposure, to a large number of environmental allergenic substances. These materials include airborne pollens of grasses, ragweeds, and trees; animal danders; foods; certain fungi; and house-dust components. Upon inhalation or ingestion of a specific allergen, a hypersensitive individual can develop various kinds of clinical syndromes, the most frequent of which are asthma, eczema, certain gastrointestinal disorders, hay fever, hives, and general cold symptoms. Coca applied the term *atopy* to these allergic disease states, from the Greek word meaning "out of place."

Apparently, the hypersensitivity develops in susceptible persons because of repeated accidental absorption of the allergenic substances. Absorption can involve the mucus membranes of the gastrointestinal or respiratory tracts or the skin. The various atopic allergic disease states are precipitated by later exposure to these allergens. The distribution of the tendency to develop diseases of this type has been shown to be familial, and the tendency is believed to be inheritable. Persons exhibiting atopic reactions are referred to as ***atopics***. Such individuals have the genetic capacity to produce blood-plasma concentrations of IgE ten times greater than those of nonatopics.

Skin testing for atopic states. Upon injection of an appropriate allergen, atopic individuals exhibit itching at the inoculation site followed by a wheal-and-flare response. The effect may persist for approximately 20 minutes. This type of response can be used to determine the substances to which the atopic is sensitive. To test an individual's susceptibility to a specific allergen, one introduces a sterile dilution into the skin either by intradermal injection or scarification (the making of a small number of superficial scratches). A sensitivity to the test substance is indicated by a wheal-and-flare response in the area of the inoculation. Intense reactions to such tests are usually considered to be associated with allergens responsible for the immediate difficulties of the subject.

Passive transfer of atopy (Prausnitz-Küstner, or P-K, reaction). The presence of antibodies in the serum of atopics was discovered in 1921 by Prausnitz and Küstner. This discovery was directly related to Küstner's pronounced sensitivity to fish. A small quantity of Küstner's serum was injected into Prausnitz's skin. After 24 hours, an extract of fish was introduced into both this site and an untreated region of Prausnitz's skin. The latter served as a control. Within 20 minutes of the fish-extract injection, a typical wheal-and-flare response developed at the site of the serum injection. The control region showed no reaction.

The P-K procedure can be used for patients who are extremely sensitive to specific allergens and cannot undergo direct testing. In this test, several hours should lapse between the injection of serum from a sensitive individual and that of the suspected allergen. The two substances should not be mixed, as no reaction will develop when a mixture is injected.

Establishing the atopic state. Not only are the IgE responses of allergic individuals to different allergens sizable, but they may also increase upon reexposure to the allergen. Nonatopics, on the other hand, do not produce significant IgE responses against common allergens. Why?

Several factors are believed to be involved in the establishment of an atopic state. Recent studies have demonstrated the existence of circulating suppressive molecules that have the exquisitely specific capacity to interfere with the activities of IgE. Although these suppressive substances are found predominantly in individuals who are not typically atopic, this does not mean that atopic individuals are unable to produce such materials. The exact nature of the suppressive molecules, and the source of production, the conditions necessary for production, and the mechanism of their action have not been precisely determined.

Immunotherapy of atopic diseases. Several approaches to the treatment of allergy exist. At present, treatment falls into two categories: (1) pharmacologic intervention—the use of medications to block release of or reduce the effects of the chemicals associated with allergic states (Figure 25-2)—and (2) immunotherapy—procedures to render an atopic individual immunologically unreactive to a particular allergen. One current immunotherapeutic approach, known as **desensitization,** or *hyposensitization,* involves the controlled administration of specific allergen preparations. Promising approaches to the future immunotherapy of allergic diseases include the stimulation of suppressor mechanisms such as those discussed earlier.

Type II—Cytotoxic Hypersensitivity

Examples of Type II responses in humans include (1) blood-transfusion reactions, in which blood-group antigens in red blood cell membranes are the inciting factors; (2) erythroblastosis fetalis (the Rh baby), in which Rh antigens on fetal or newborn red blood cells are the targets of antibodies formed by the mother; and (3) drug-caused blood loss (anemias), in which a drug forms an antigenic complex with the surfaces of blood cells and brings about the production of antibodies that are destructive for the cell-drug complex. Blood leukocytes and platelets are especially prone to these reactions. Allergens create situations that cause disruption of cells *(cytolysis)* or death of cells without disruption *(cytotoxicity)*. The antibodies primarily involved in Type II hypersensitivity responses are IgG and IgM, which can fix complement.

Type III—Immune-complex-mediated Hypersensitivity

Examples of Type III responses include the Arthus reaction, serum sickness, and certain autoimmune reactions. In this form of hypersensitivity, soluble antigen and immunoglobulins combine in the body, and the combinations can give rise to an acute inflammatory reaction. If complement (C′) is fixed by this combination, biological molecules called anaphylatoxins are produced. These molecules ultimately cause the release of histamine and the production of other active substances, which in turn set in motion a chain reaction of events that damages tissues and intensifies the inflammatory response.

The effects of immune complexes in the body depend on the absolute concentrations of antigen and antibody, which determine the reaction's intensity, and on the relative proportions of these reactants, which determine the distribution of the complex within the body. In cases of antibody excess, the immune complexes are rapidly precipitated and tend to settle around the site of antigen introduction. In cases of antigen excess, soluble complexes are produced that can result in systemic reactions. Such complexes can be widely distributed throughout the body and deposited in such sites as the kidneys, joints, and skin. Many cases of severe kidney destruction (glomerulonephritis) are due to immune complexes.

THE ARTHUS REACTION (ANTIBODY EXCESS)

In 1903, soon after the discovery of anaphylaxis, M. Arthus, a French physiologist, described the following antibody-dependent allergic reaction. When rabbits were given weekly injections of horse serum, no reaction was apparent. However, after several weeks, inoculation with the same type of material produced a localized inflammatory response. The same response was later recognized in humans and other animals.

Arthus reactions are not restricted to the skin. The phenomenon can involve most tissues in individuals having sufficiently high antibody levels. Regions exhibiting an Arthus response show the following tissue changes: (1) a marked reduction in blood flow, (2) the formation within small blood vessels of clots rich in platelets and leukocytes, (3) an escape of blood cells into neighboring connective tissue, (4) swelling, and (5) the massive infiltration of the area by polymorphonuclear leukocytes. In short, the changes that take place are those of classic inflammation. Tissue destruction occurs in the later stages of the reaction. Certain of the components of complement are believed to play a role in the Arthus reaction.

Serum sickness (antigen excess). The original description of this anaphylactic condition was made by von Pirquet and Schick in 1905. Approximately 8 to 12 days after receiving an injection of large volumes of foreign protein such as antitoxin, individuals developed the distressing condition known as serum sickness.

Symptoms of serum sickness include fever, generalized swelling of lymph nodes, itching, hives, and swelling of the ankles, eyelids, and face. The severity of these symptoms is determined by the severity of the attack. The symptoms can subside in two days, but in some cases they persist for as long as two weeks.

The various effects of serum sickness are associated with complexes involving antibodies and the injected foreign protein that causes their formation. Together these substances form toxic complexes that not only injure blood vessels, but also bring about the various symptoms noted above. As the level of antibody increases, the level of foreign protein decreases. This sequence of events ultimately leads to the disappearance of the effects of serum sickness.

THE SHWARTZMAN REACTION

In 1927, G. Shwartzman observed that local bleeding and severe tissue destruction developed from intradermal injections of bacterial culture filtrates. The reaction could be made to occur quickly if the intradermal injection was followed in 30 minutes by a second, so-called "provocative" intravenous injection. Some time later, Shwartzman proved that it was possible to induce reactions involving internal organs when both the initial and provocative injections were given intravenously.

The Shwartzman reaction is caused by the endotoxins of Gram-negative bacteria in the initial injection. The provocative injection can be either endotoxin or a variety of "immunologically unrelated" substances, including agar and starch. This reaction was shown not to be induced by an immune mechanism.

Type IV—Cell-mediated, or Delayed, Hypersensitivity

During the 80 years or so after the initial discovery of anaphylaxis, a variety of other allergic reactions were observed that appeared to be fundamentally different from those associated with Types I through III. Type IV responses do not involve the release of histamine or chemically related substances, and the sensitivity associated with this state cannot be transferred by the injection of serum from a sensitive individual to a nonsensitive one. Passive transfer of Type IV responses to nonsensitive recipients can be accomplished by means of living lymphoid cells from sensitized donors and a nonantibody-active "transfer factor." Type IV responses are not inhibited by antihistamines, but are inhibited by steroid compounds such as cortisone and hydrocortisone. *In vitro* migration of cells from sensitized animals is inhibited by the presence of antigen-specific migration inhibition factor (MIF).

Type IV responses depend upon the interaction of T-type lymphocytes with antigen. Several cell-mediated immune reactions are beneficial. They act, for example, to overcome certain types of infections such as those caused by fungi, some protozoa, viruses, and various species of bacterial genera. They also prevent foreign tissue cells from becoming established in the body (tissue-graft rejections) and stop the uncontrolled reproduction of cancer cells. When cell-

TABLE 25-2 Representative Lymphokines and Associated Functions

Lymphokine	Designation (If Appropriate)	Functions or Activities
Chemotactic factor	CF	Causes chemotaxis (chemical attraction) of macrophages
Cloning-inhibition factor	CLIF	Blocks *in vitro* multiplication of certain cell types
Dialyzable transfer factors	TF	Converts normal lymphocytes *in vivo* and *in vitro* to antigen-sensitized lymphocytes
Inhibitor RNA synthesis	IDS	Reversibly inhibits mitosis of lymphocytes
Lymphotoxin	LT	Causes cytotoxicity
Macrophage-activation factor	MAF	Partly responsible for increased lysosomal activity of macrophage
Macrophage-aggregation factor	MAF	Restricts macrophage movement and induces formation of giant cells
Macrophage-inhibition factor	MIF	Inhibits migration of macrophages
Proliferation-inhibition factor	PIF	Blocks *in vitro* multiplication of certain cell types

mediated responses cause tissue damage, the condition generally is considered to be an allergic one. Such immunologic injury, also known as **delayed hypersensitivity,** involves T-type cells bearing specific receptors on their surfaces that are stimulated by contact with antigens to release factors called **lymphokines** (Table 25–2). Whenever the receptors react with specific antigenic determinants, the T-cells become sensitized. This exposure to antigens and the sensitization are necessary for the occurrence of delayed hypersensitivity reactions.

When a sensitized T-lymphocyte interacts with the specific antigenic determinant, a cell-mediated response is initiated. The T-cell undergoes certain changes and divides, producing specifically sensitized cells and a corresponding increase in the number of reactive T-cells. This activity takes place in blastogenetic (cell-production) centers such as lymph nodes. From these areas, sensitized T-cells can enter the circulation, seed other lymphatic tissues, or accumulate at sites where the antigen is introduced.

Lymphocytes and lymphokines are not the only factors involved in delayed hypersensitivity. Under the influence of lymphokines, activated macrophages show increased phagocytic biosynthetic, and microbe-destroying properties. These macrophages are far more effective than normal macrophages in eliminating microorganisms.

Representative Type IV Allergic States

ALLERGY OF INFECTION

An allergy of infection brings about an accelerated and exaggerated tissue reaction to certain infectious agents. The most thoroughly studied example of this type of hypersensitive reaction is associated with tuberculosis. Hypersensitivity of this type was first demonstrated in 1891 by Koch. He showed that guinea pigs infected with *Mycobacterium tuberculosis* 2 or more weeks earlier, and uninfected (normal) guinea pigs reacted differently to subcutaneous injections of living, virulent tubercle bacilli. Within 2 days, the tuberculous animals developed massive inflammatory reactions at the inoculation site that gradually increased in intensity and produced areas of cellular death. The tissues of the infected animals reacted violently to the tubercle bacilli, and tended to localize the infection by walling off the area of involvement. This sequence of events is known as the *Koch phenomenon*. Uninfected guinea pigs injected with similar material normally developed progressive tuberculosis.

Koch showed that the specific inflammatory reaction and associated tissue changes could be caused by dead as well as living tubercle bacilli. Furthermore, a bacteria-free protein-fraction extract prepared from these organisms, known as *tuberculin*, produced the same response.

In actual cases of tuberculosis infection, the allergic state becomes established early, generally before the obvious signs of the infection are apparent. In 1907, Koch proposed the use of tuberculin to detect tuberculous individuals. The tuberculin skin test and variations of it are widely used today for this purpose and for the standardization of skin-testing material. However, the significance of a positive delayed-type skin test (Color Photograph 73) to an infectious disease varies with the infection. ***Reactions of this sort do not necessarily indicate current infection.***

CONTACT DERMATITIS

The form of hypersensitivity known as **contact dermatitis** includes certain types of drug allergy. It is one of the most commonly encountered human allergic diseases. The sensitization and the production of symptoms result simply from contact with various causative compounds, which combine with proteins in the skin. Included in the group of *incitants* are (1) simple chemicals, such as formaldehyde and picric acid; (2) metals, such as mercury and nickel; (3) various drugs and dyes; (4) certain cosmetics; (5) insecticides; and (6) the active components associated with poison ivy, poison oak, poison sumac, and other plants.

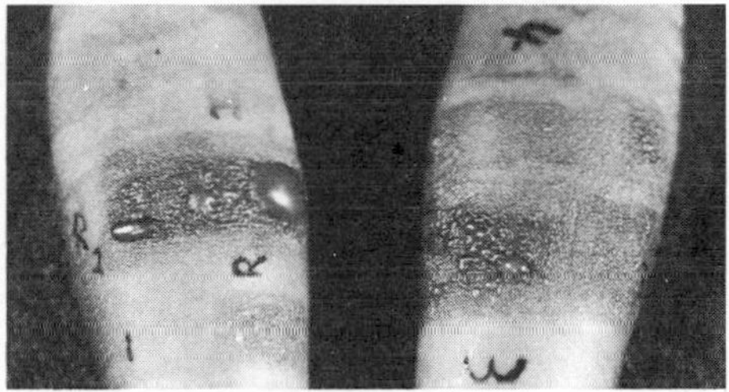

FIG. 25-3 A positive patch test for contact dermatitis. *Courtesy of Armed Forces Institute of Pathology, Washington, D.C., Neg. No. AFIP 57-15160-2.*

Two types of responses are generally recognized: *contact skin sensitivity* and *allergic contact dermatitis*. In contact skin sensitivity, exposure to the incitant causes local irritation. While these substances by themselves are not allergenic, they can become so by combining with proteins in the skin. In allergic contact dermatitis, both humans and various laboratory animals can be sensitized by skin contact with the incitant or by intradermal injection of the incitant. Approximately 5 to 20 days are needed for the development of the hypersensitivity reaction. To determine whether an individual has been sensitized, filter paper patches treated with the same sensitizing material are taped to the skin for about 24 hours. The test is generally read twice, once a few hours after the removal of the patch and again 24 hours later. A positive reaction is characterized by an erythematous region containing various-sized blisters (Figure 25-3). In the diagnosis of certain cases of contact dermatitis, examinations may have to be continued for two or more weeks.

Treating contact dermatitis requires the identification of the causative agent. Attempts to desensitize individuals have met with limited success. When the chemical involved has an oily nature, the chances for success are better. Total avoidance of the incitant is of course advisable, but it is not always practical.

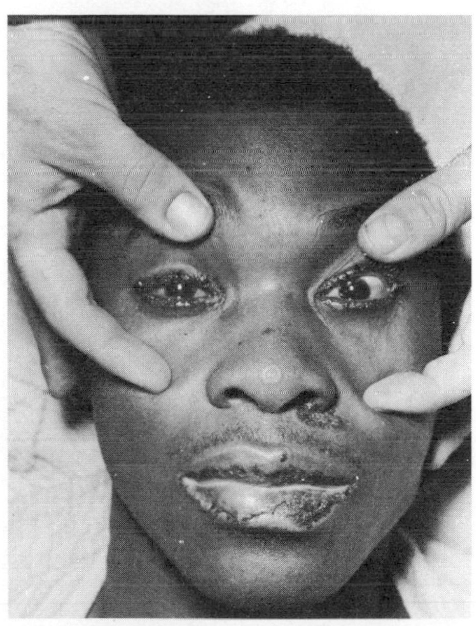

FIG. 25-4 Penicillin sensitivity. This man shows a hemorrhagic reaction involving his eyelids and nasal and oral mucosa. *Courtesy of Armed Forces Institute of Pathology, Washington, D.C., Neg. No. AFIP 54-1548-3.*

Penicillin allergy. Penicillin is considered to be among the least toxic drugs in current clinical use. Apparently, however, the antibiotic combines with certain protein derivatives in some manner to form stable inducers. These newly formed complexes can stimulate antibody production and bring about either type of hypersensitive state, immediate or delayed (Figure 25-4). Approximately 10 percent of the people who receive repeated doses of penicillin fall victim to this condition. The injection of 1 mg of the antibiotic can result in a fatal anaphylactic shock reaction in a sensitized individual.

Persons who are repeatedly exposed to penicillin in some form can develop Type IV hypersensitivity to the antibiotic. Health-care personnel and individuals involved in the preparation and packaging of penicillin fall into this category. The sensitivity develops as a drug contact dermatitis.

TISSUE TRANSPLANTATION REACTIONS

Experiments in the transplantation of animal kidneys began a chain of events that has led to an entirely new medical era. It is now possible to surgically replace or transfer a variety of tissues and organs, moving them from one site to another on the same individual or from one body to another. The transplanting of skin from one region to another in an individual is now a fairly common and usually successful operation. This procedure is used for burn victims and others who have experienced extensive skin destruction.

Other types of transplants—for example, heart, liver, or lung transplants—have proved more difficult. The transplantation of tissues involves a complex collection of cells, each of which has a large variety of antigens controlled by DNA. Except in identical twins, each individual's chromosomal DNA is unique. This uniqueness of "self" (see Chapter 23) is accompanied by a highly sensitive mechanism for sensing and recognizing foreign substances. The recognition mechanism triggers the complex response that forms an individual's immunity. Tissue transplantation activates both humoral mechanisms (circulating antibodies) and cell-mediated mechanisms of immunity.

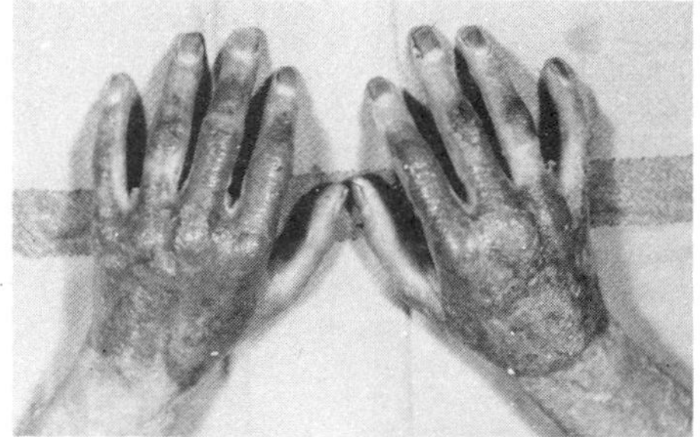
(a)

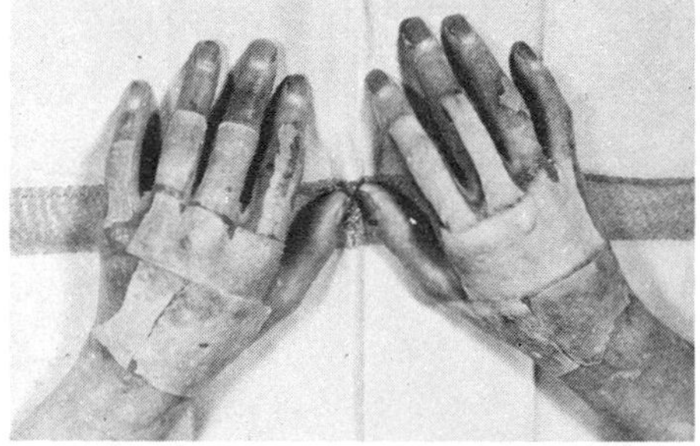
(b)

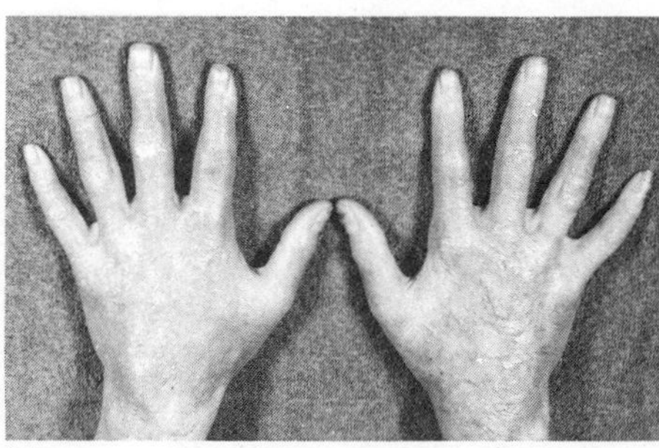
(c)

FIG. 25–5 The successful transplantation of skin in a case of severe burn. (a) Deep dermal burns affecting both hands. (b) The application of autograft. (c) The result after three transplants. *Shuck, J. M., B. A. Priutt, and J. A. Moncrief,* Arch. Surg., *98:472 (1969) © AMA.*

Transplant categories. Transplants of tissues are classified in terms of genetic relationships (identity). For example, where the tissue of one individual is involved, the transplant is called an ***autograft*** (Figure 25–5). If a graft (the tissue to be transplanted) is taken from one animal and given to another of the same species (genetically dissimilar members of the same species), the tissue is referred to as an ***allograft*** (Figure 25–6). When both individuals are genetically identical—identical twins or mice from the same highly inbred line—the tissue is an ***isograft***. Finally, a transplant involving two different species—for example, the transplantation of kidneys from a chimpanzee into a human—is referred to as a ***xenograft***.

Genetic control. The goal of transplantation is the long-term survival of the grafted tissue. The success of the procedure depends on several factors, including the degree of antigenic similarity between donor and recipient, and the nature of the transplanted tissue itself.

One approach to preventing immune rejection of transplants is careful matching of donor tissues and cells with those of the recipient. Finding the best match involves the ***histocompatibility*** of antigens. These antigens differ from individual to individual and are recognized as foreign molecules in graft rejections.

Histocompatibility antigens differ in their ability to bring about an immunological response in a graft recipient. In mice, the set of antigens known as the *H*-2 system provides by far the strongest barrier to transplantation. The system is under the control of a specific gene complex on the mouse's No. 17 chromosome (Figure 25–7a). Other parts of the *H*-2 gene complex play an important role in the functioning of the immune system and include the *I* region and the *S* region.

A series of genes within the *I* region known as immune-response ***(Ir)*** genes controls the manufacture of antibodies. Although the products of the ***Ir*** genes have not been identified, certain proteins designated ***Ia*** (*I*-region-associated) antigens have been found on the surface of lymphocytes involved in immunological reactions.

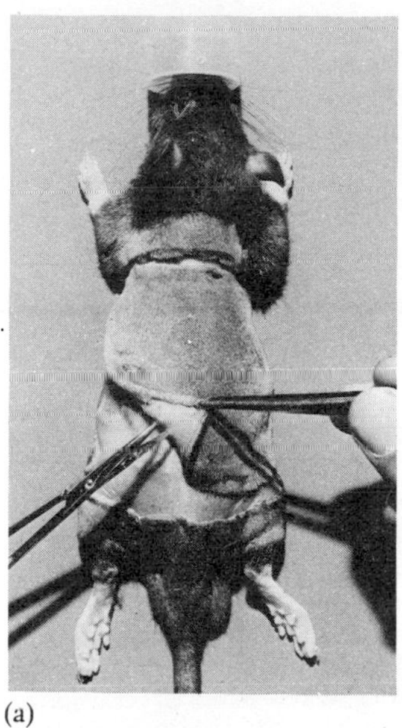
(a)

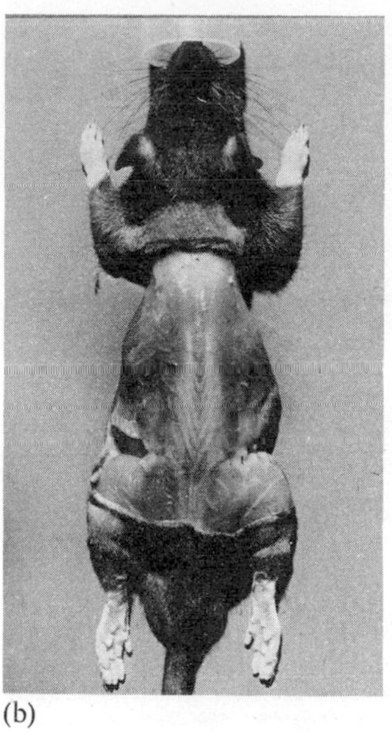
(b)

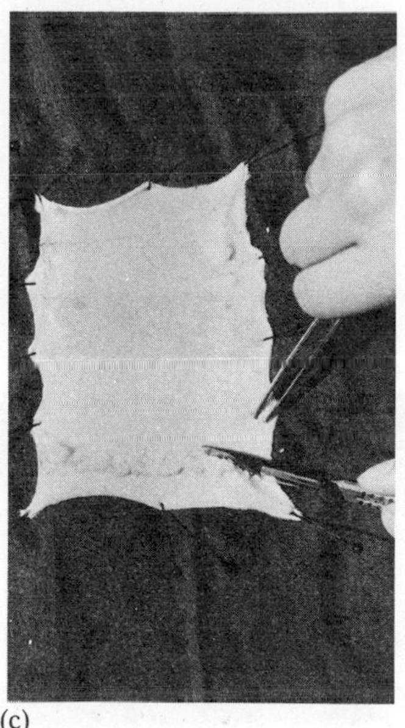
(c)

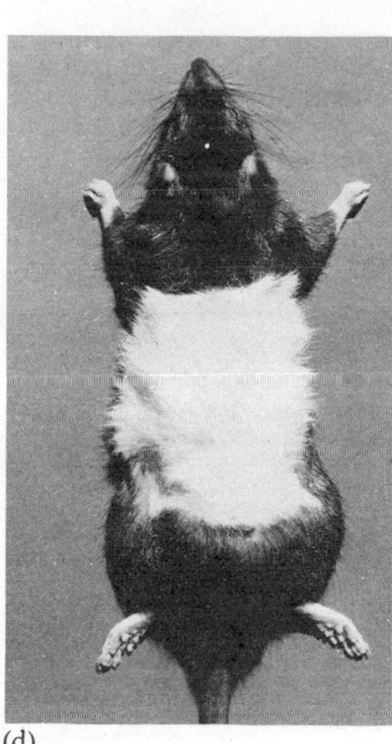
(d)

FIG. 25–6 Allograft transplantation. (a) Preparation of the recipient animal. (b) The site to receive the graft. (c) The skin graft from an animal of the same species. (d) The allograft in place 10 weeks after transplantation. *A. A. van Es,* Lab. Anim. Sci., *22: 404–406 (1972).*

The *S* region has been shown to control the manufacture of a component of serum complement. This complement acts to destroy antigenic cells such as bacteria and grafted cells once they have reacted with specific antibodies.

The strong *H*-2 antigens in the mouse have their counterpart in the human leukocyte-antigen *(HLA)* system (Figure 25–7b). This major human system is under the control of a cluster of genes on human chromosome No. 6, which controls the antigenic determinants forming the strongest antigenic barrier to transplantation between genetically nonidentical individuals. Other genes in the same chromosomal region play an important role in an individual's immune responsiveness to a wide variety of antigens.

Determining the suitability of tissue for grafting (histocompatibility testing) is accomplished by the ***lymphocyte toxicity test*** or the ***mixed-leukocyte*** (lymphocyte) ***reaction*** (MLR). The lymphocyte toxicity test is a widely applied method designed to measure the histocompatibility antigenic composition of donor and recipient. The test is performed on lymphocytes of both donor and recipient with a battery of antisera. The mixed-lymphocyte reaction test determines only the compatibility of donor and recipient and reflects incompatibilities of the major transplantation antigen.

Although *Ir* genes have not yet conclusively been shown to exist in humans, recent evidence suggests that in humans the genes of major histocompatibility have a marked effect on the susceptibility to a wide variety of diseases. Such diseases include certain forms of arthritis, multiple sclerosis, Hodgkin's disease (cancer of the lymph nodes), and the juvenile form of insulin-dependent diabetes.

Graft rejection. When tissue is transplanted from one individual to another, two distinct rejection processes can take place. The first, and traditionally the most studied, is the host rejection of grafted tissue, the ***host-versus-graft reaction.*** The second process is the reverse of this reaction, the ***graft-versus-host response.*** This reaction occurs when immunocompetent tissues are transferred to an immunologically handicapped host.

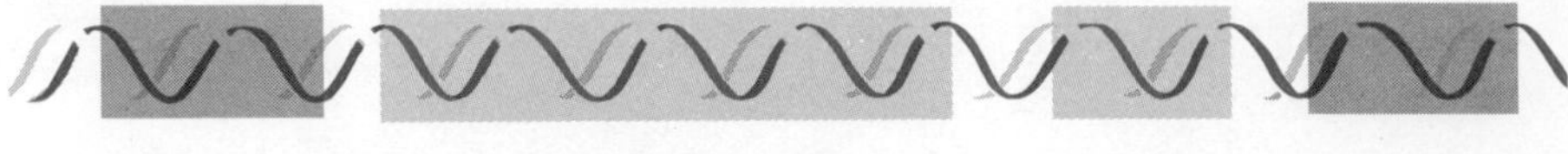

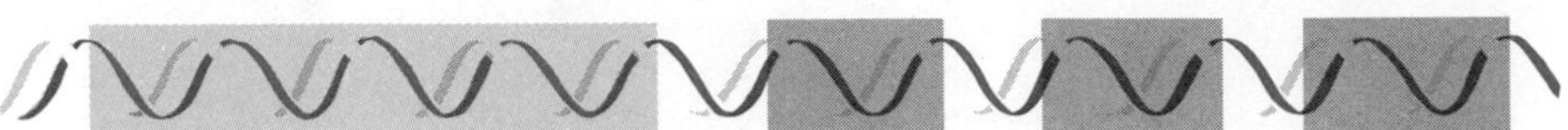

FIG. 25-7 A diagram of the chromosomes associated with histocompatibility antigens. (a) The specific genes of the mouse chromosome No. 17, with its H-2 gene complex. (b) The HLA gene complex on human chromosome No. 6. Within this region lie the four currently defined HLA genes, HLA-A, HLA-B, HLA-C, and HLA-D.

Several means are available for limiting or totally inhibiting graft rejection in certain situations. These include the injection of immunosuppressive drugs, such as corticosteroids or antilymphocytics, and whole-body irradiation. In several instances, a combination of these measures has been employed. It is important to note that, although this type of procedure can promote survival of allografts, it also lowers the individual's ability to produce immunoglobulins against pathogenic disease agents. Thus, antibiotics must be administered to prevent infection of the graft recipient.

Autoallergy (Autoimmune) Diseases

Normally in the body of an immunocompetent individual, appropriate mechanisms exist to prevent the lymphoid system from responding to "self" components as antigens. Such unresponsiveness, referred to as ***immunological tolerance,*** is essential for human survival. Unfortunately, as with all machinery, tolerance mechanisms occasionally falter and break down, thus creating autoallergic (autoimmune) disease states. In these disorders, self-antigens, or autoantigens, stimulate the production of circulating immunoglobulins (humoral response) or of specially sensitized lymphocytes (cell-mediated response), either of which will react with the autoantigen.

CAUSES OF AUTOALLERGY

Several factors may trigger an autoallergic response. These include the presence of (1) antigens that normally do not circulate in the blood; (2) the presence of an altered antigen (alterations can develop through exposure to chemicals, physical agents, or microorganisms); (3) the introduction of a foreign antigen similar to an autoantigen; (4) and the occurrence of a mutation in immunocompetent cells that results in a responsiveness to normal autoantigens. These agents may precipitate an autoallergy following such events as tissue injury, administration of drugs, or certain microbial infections. Several human viruses are enveloped with membranes that are partly derived from nuclear, intracytoplasmic, or plasma membranes of the host, but that also may include virus-specific antigens. Several of these viruses have been associated with autoallergic reactions.

Even though direct evidence is lacking, many authorities believe that autoallergic diseases largely represent Type IV, or cell-mediated, responses. Although immunoglobulins are frequently present, little or no correlation appears to exist between their presence and the autoallergic state.

Autoallergic or autoimmune diseases comprise a broad range of disorders and a confusing array of overlapping symptoms, pathological lesions, and immunological properties. Some diseases, such as Hashimoto's thyroiditis, are organ-specific. Others, such as the autoimmune hemolytic anemias, are localized but not organ-specific. Still others are nonorgan-specific. Systemic lupus erythematosis (SLE) is an example of an autoallergic disorder in which neither lesions nor autoantibodies are limited to any one organ or tissue. Autoimmunity may play an important role in rheumatoid arthritis (a common inflammatory condition of joints) and in the aging process.

Apart from the large number of currently recognized autoallergic disease states and the rather confusing signs and symptoms of these disorders, certain shared characteristics have become apparent. First, the incidence of autoallergic diseases and associated immunoglobulins tends to increase with age. Second, such diseases occur most commonly among persons with generalized immunological deficiencies. Third, autoallergy occurs most often in females. In addition, it has been observed that any given autoimmune disease may produce destructive effects that resemble those associated with the other types of hypersensitivities.

Therapy for autoallergic diseases varies widely and is influenced by several factors. These include the particular disease, the severity of the effects, and the associated hazards of prolonged therapy with corticosteroids and other immunosuppressive agents and procedures.

SUMMARY

A properly functioning immune system protects the body through its capacity to recognize and destroy *foreign*, or *non-self*, molecules.

Immunodeficiencies

1. Immunodeficiency diseases result from the inability of the immune system to perform normally.
2. Two general categories of these disorders are recognized: primary and secondary immunodeficiencies.
3. Primary, or congenital, deficiencies result from an inherited lack of development of the immune system, and include the absence of T-type lymphocytes and the inability to produce immunoglobulins.
4. Secondary, or acquired, deficiencies, occur much more frequently than primary conditions, and result from an interference with lymphatic-system activities. Factors causing such conditions include malnutrition, cancers, burns, radiation, and various drugs.

Hypersensitivity (Allergy)

1. Hypersensitivity, or allergy, is an exaggerated response by individuals exposed to a substance that does not cause similar responses in previously unexposed persons. The inciting agents are referred to as allergens.
2. Initial exposure to an allergen sensitizes the individual to future contact with the same allergen. Various harmful reactions can result from such exposures.

Categories of Hypersensitivity

1. Historically, hypersensitivity reactions were divided into two categories based on the time required for responses to occur upon reexposure to the sensitizing allergen.
2. Categories today are based on several other factors. These include the presence or absence of substances regulating the reactions, circulating immunoglobulins, the actions of B- and/or T-type lymphocytes, and the possibility of passive transfer of the hypersensitivity response.

3. Four different categories of hypersensitivity are known: Type I (classic immediate), Type II (cytotoxic), Type III (immune-complex-mediated), and Type IV (cell-mediated, or delayed).
4. The particular type of hypersensitivity acquired is determined by several factors, including the chemical makeup of the allergen, the route involved in sensitization, and the responsive and physiological condition of the individual.

Type I—Classic Immediate Hypersensitivity

1. A distinguishing feature of Type I hypersensitivity is the rapid release of physiologically active chemicals, such as histamine, from cells affected by a reaction involving allergens and specific immunoglobulins (IgE).
2. Examples of Type I allergic states include certain forms of asthma, anaphylactic shock, hay fever, and hives.
3. Atopy is an allergic response to a large variety of environmental allergic substances such as pollens of various types, foods, fungi, and house dust.
4. Several approaches to the treatment of allergy are possible, including the use of chemicals to reduce the effects of allergies, and the use of specific allergen preparations to make allergic persons immunologically unreactive to such allergens.

Type II—Cytotoxic Hypersensitivity

1. Type II conditions result in cellular destruction and involve the immunoglobulins IgG and IgM, which can fix or react with complement.
2. Examples of Type II allergies include blood-transfusion reactions, the Rh baby, and certain drug-caused blood-cell losses.

Type III—Immune-complex-mediated Hypersensitivity

1. Type III allergic states result from reactions involving specific allergens, immunoglobulins, and complement.
2. Examples of Type III responses include the Arthus reaction, serum sickness, and certain autoimmune states.

Type IV—Cell-mediated Hypersensitivity

1. Type IV allergic responses do not involve immunoglobulins or the release of chemicals such as those associated with Type I reactions. Type IV responses are dependent upon the interaction of T-type lymphocytes with antigens.
2. Situations associated with immunologic injury are known as *delayed hypersensitivity* and involve factors released by certain T-type cells known as *lymphokines.*

Representative Type IV Allergic States

1. Examples of Type IV hypersensitivity include tissue destruction in certain infectious-disease states such as tuberculosis tuberculin skin reaction, contact dermatitis, and tissue transplantation reaction.
2. The success of tissue transplants involves a group of genes that control the formation of histocompatibility antigens. In the human, these genes as well as others possibly responsible for immunological reactions are located on chromosome No. 6.

Autoallergy (Autoimmune) Diseases

1. The inability of the immune system to recognize normal parts of the body as "self" can result in disorders known as autoallergies.
2. Such conditions may develop from several factors, including exposure to chemicals, irradiation, or microorganisms, as well as aging and individual genetic defects.

QUESTIONS FOR REVIEW

1. Distinguish between primary and secondary immunodeficiencies.
2. List at least two differences among types of hypersensitivity. List and briefly describe two examples of the different states of sensitivity.
3. From what standpoint can Type IV hypersensitivity be of diagnostic importance? To which diseases is the reaction applicable?
4. What is autoimmune disease?
5. What is anaphylaxis? What accounts for the temporary nature of anaphylactic reactions? What are the symptoms of anaphylactic shock in humans?
6. a. What is atopy?
   b. Describe the wheal-and-flare response.
   c. Discuss the Prausnitz-Küstner reaction. Does it have any medical importance?
7. What are lymphokines?
8. Does the Shwartzman reaction involve an immune mechanism of the host? Explain.
9. Describe the Koch phenomenon.
10. What is contact dermatitis? What types of substances act as incitants in this condition? How can an incitant be identified?
11. Define or explain and give examples of the following:
    a. xenograft
    b. rejection
    c. allograft
    d. *H*-2 system
    e. histocompatibility
    f. *HLA* system
12. List the causes of autoallergy.
13. Differentiate between a humoral response and a cell-mediated one.
14. What is desensitization?

SUGGESTED READINGS

Billingham, R., and W. Silvers. *The Immunobiology of Transplantation.* Englewood Cliffs, N.J.: Prentice-Hall, Inc., 1971. *A short, clear presentation of the biological basis of tissue and organ transplantation.*

Crowle, A. J., "Delayed Hypersensitivity." *Sci. Amer.,* April 1960. ***A descriptive article on the type of allergy that has been identified as the cause of the pains in rheumatoid arthritis, the rash in poison ivy, and the nerve degeneration in multiple sclerosis.***

Hood, L. E., I. L. Weissman, and W. B. Wood. *Immunology.* Menlo Park, Calif.: The Benjamin/Cummings Publishing Company, Inc., 1978. *A detailed text on immunology that emphasizes the organization, regulation, and evolution of the immune system, major histocompatibility complexes, and basic aspects of cancer and associated therapy that relate to immunology.*

Norman, P. S., "The Clinical Significance of IgE." *Hospital Practice* 8:41 (1975). *A current view of the cells and chemicals responsible for allergy.*

Patterson, R. (ed.). *Allergic Diseases, Diagnosis and Management.* Philadelphia: J. P. Lippincott Co., 1972. *Describes various aspects of hypersensitivity, including classification, immunologic and cellular aspects, diagnosis, allergens, and various types of allergies.*

Snell, G. D., J. Dauset, and S. Nathanson. *Histocompatibility.* New York: Academic Press, 1976. *A detailed coverage of mammalian histocompatability.*

CHAPTER 26

Immunization and the Control of Infectious Diseases

How can the body acquire protection against infectious disease? Chapter 26 discusses various immunizing materials available for affording such protection and describes methods of vaccine preparation and administration. Some possible complications associated with vaccination are also covered, along with recommended immunization programs.

After reading this chapter, you should be able to:

1. **Describe general methods of vaccine preparation.**
2. **Distinguish between a toxoid and toxin.**
3. **Compare the advantages and disadvantages of live versus inactivated microbial vaccines.**
4. **Outline the safety precautions and measures observed in vaccine preparation.**
5. **Explain the role of immunization in the control of diseases.**
6. **Describe the general methods used for administering immunizing materials.**
7. **List and discuss the types of complications associated with vaccination.**
8. **List the preparations currently in use for both active and passive immunizations.**

Immunization with live or inactivated microorganisms and their products is one of the most fruitful approaches to preventing microbial infection. Vaccines have been successful in reducing or eliminating the disease states of diphtheria,

German measles, poliomyelitis, smallpox, and yellow fever, but they are usually effective only if administered before the infection has begun. Short-term protection or alteration of the outcome of certain infections can be achieved through passive immunization—the administration of preformed immunoglobulins. Although passive immunization is temporary, it is especially useful in the treatment of virus-exposed individuals suffering from leukemia, other forms of cancer, or immunodeficiencies.

Immunization Preparations

The biological preparations used for immunization or diagnosis can be divided into three basic categories: (1) prophylactic agents for active immunization, which include bacterial and viral vaccines, toxins, and toxoids; (2) prophylactic preparations for passive immunization, mainly globulins (gamma globulins); and (3) diagnostic reagents designed to demonstrate hyperimmune states or to detect susceptibility to disease agents. The latter include purified protein derivative (PPD) and diluted diphtheria toxin. The applications of these diagnostic reagents are discussed mainly in the chapters dealing with bacterial and mycotic infections (Chapters 30 and 31).

The Preparation of Representative Vaccines

Vaccines are preparations of either disease-causing microorganisms or certain of their component parts or products, such as toxins, rendered unable to produce disease but still antigenic. These products are used to produce an artificially acquired active immunity.

BACTERIAL VACCINES

Bacterial vaccines are generally suspensions of killed bacteria in an isotonic (physiologic) salt solution. (One exception is BCG [Bacillus of Calmette and Guérin] vaccine, which is an attenuated, or weakened, preparation for immunization against tuberculosis.) Administering such vaccines is the most common means for inducing active immunity. In the preparation of these materials, the organisms are cultured, harvested after a suitable incubation period, and then killed with heat or chemical agents.

The use of heat to kill organisms has the disadvantage of reducing the immunizing potency of preparations even where the lethal temperature and the time of exposure are kept as low as possible to insure sterilization. Chemical killing agents used for vaccine production include acetone, formalin, Merthiolate, phenol, and tricresol. The concentrations of these chemicals are adjusted to insure the antigenic effectiveness of the bacterial preparations.

Rickettsial vaccines are formalin-killed preparations of the specific pathogen (Table 26–1). For the vaccines currently in use, the rickettsia is propagated in embryonated chicken eggs, specifically in the yolk sac. As Cox, in 1938, was the first person to cultivate rickettsia in this manner, vaccines so prepared are called *Cox vaccines.*

Two general types of bacterial preparations are utilized—***stock*** and ***autogenous vaccines.*** Stock vaccine is prepared from laboratory stock cultures; autogenous vaccine is specially made from organisms freshly isolated from a patient. Autogenous vaccines are of significant value in certain staphyloccal

TABLE 26-1 Preparations Currently Used for Active Immunizations (Vaccines)

Bacterial Diseases	*Etiologic Agent*	*Means of Vaccine Preparation*
Cholera	*Vibrio cholerae*	Heat-killed suspension of *V. (comma) cholerae*.
Diphtheria	*Corynebacterium diphtheriae*	Alum-precipitated toxoid preparation of *C. diphtheriae* toxin. This antigenic material is combined with tetanus toxoid and killed *H. pertussis* in the DPT vaccine.
Epidemic typhus	*Rickettsia prowazekii*	Formalin-killed suspension of *R. prowazekii* cultivated in chick-embryo yolk sacs.
Gonorrhea[a]	*Neisseria gonorrhoeae*	
Meningitis	*Neisseria meningitidis*	Purified cell-wall polysaccharides.
Plague	*Yersinia pestis*	Formalin-killed and alum-coated suspension of *Y. pestis*.
Pneumococcal pneumonia	*Streptococcus*[a] *pneumoniae*	
Rocky Mountain spotted fever	*Rickettsia rickettsii*	Formalin-killed suspension of *R. rickettsii* cultivated in chick-embryo yolk sacs or obtained from infected ticks.
Shigellosis	*Shigella dysenteriae*	Two attenuated oral vaccines. One consists of a streptomycin-dependent mutant and the other contains a hybrid derived from a mating between an avirulent *Shigella* mutant and an *Escherichia coli*, K12 Hfr isolate (Chapter 15).
Tetanus	*Clostridium tetani*	Alum-precipitated toxoid preparation of *C. tetani* toxin. See diphtheria section above.
Tuberculosis	*Mycobacterium tuberculosis*	Bacillus of Calmette and Guérin (BCG). Prepared from a strain of *Myco. tuberculosis var. bovis* attenuated by continuous subculture on glycerol-broth-bile-potato media.
Tularemia[a]	*Francisella tularensis*	
Typhoid and paratyphoid fevers	*Salmonella typhi, S. paratyphi, S. schottmuelleri*	Heat-killed, phenol-preserved or acetone-dried preparations. Vaccines commonly contain *S. typhi* alone or in combination with *S. paratyphi* and *S. schottmuelleri* (TAB).
Whooping cough	*Bordetella pertussis*	Alum-precipitated or aluminum hydroxide- or aluminum phosphate-adsorbed, killed preparations of Phase I *H. pertussis*. See diphtheria section above.

Viral Diseases	*Means of Vaccine Preparation*
Acute Respiratory Disease (ARD)	Attenuated adenovirus (ADV)-21, strain V-270, cultivated first in human embryonic kidney (HEK) cells and then in human diploid fibroblasts. This preparation is being used primarily on military bases.
German measles (rubella)	Three attenuated vaccines are in use. These are (1) $HPV_{77}D_5$, obtained from tissue cultures of duck-embryo cells; (2) $HPV_{77}DK_{12}$, prepared from dog-kidney cells; and (3) Cendehill, obtained from rabbit-kidney cells.
Influenza	Formalin-killed preparation of prevalent viral strains. The viruses are usually grown in embryonated chick eggs.
Measles (rubeola)	Two attenuated vaccines are in use. One preparation employs the Edmonston strain in combination with measles-immune gamma globulin. The other vaccine utilizes the Schwartz strain of measles virus. A new chicken-embryo preparation is being evaluated.
Mumps	Formalin-killed preparation of virus obtained from chick-embryo cultivation. An attenuated vaccine is currently in use. It is prepared by cultivation of the virus in embryonated chicken eggs and then in chick-embryo-cell cultures.
Poliomyelitis	Two vaccines are in use. The Salk vaccine is a formalin- or ultraviolet-irradiation-inactivated preparation of the virus. The Sabin, or oral, vaccine is an attenuated preparation. Both vaccines contain types 1, 2, and 3 polio viruses.

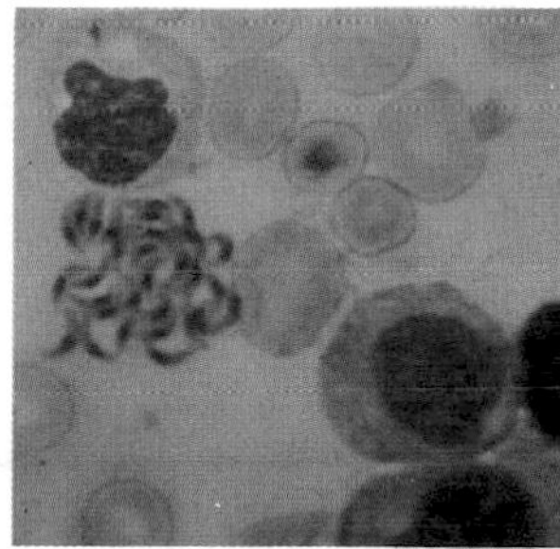

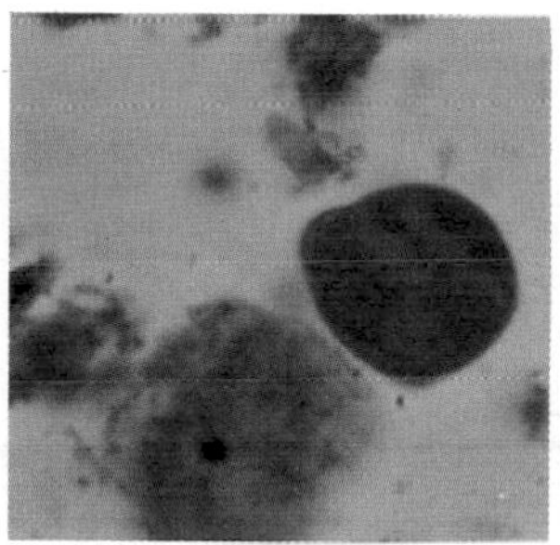

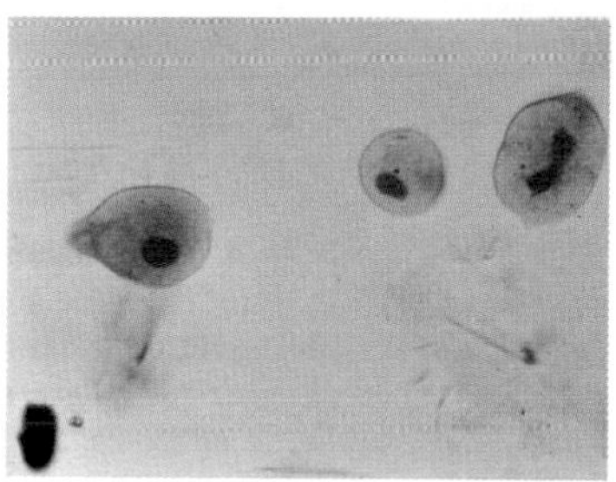

Fig. 43. *(Above left) Toxoplasma gondii* in a stained bone-marrow smear. A white blood cell and red blood cells are also shown. This protozoan can develop intracellularly as well as extracellularly; note the crescent shape of this microorganism. *From Abell, C., and P. Holland,* Amer. J. Dis. Child. *118:782–787 (1969).* **Fig. 44.** *(Above)* The trophozoite of *Entamoeba histolyica*, the cause of amoebic dysentery. This organism moves by means of pseudopods. **Fig. 45.** *(Left)* The trophozoite of the ciliate *Balantidium coli.* This organism has both trophozoite and cyst stages. It can cause gastrointestinal infections.

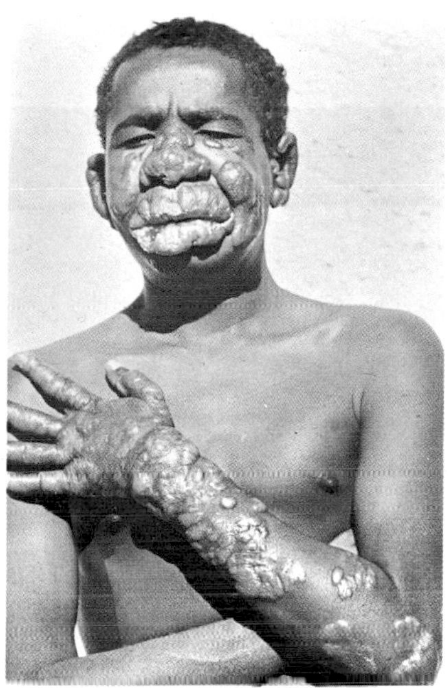

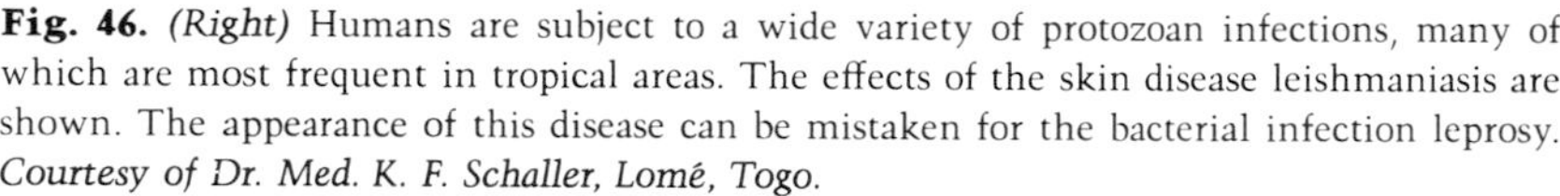

Fig. 46. *(Right)* Humans are subject to a wide variety of protozoan infections, many of which are most frequent in tropical areas. The effects of the skin disease leishmaniasis are shown. The appearance of this disease can be mistaken for the bacterial infection leprosy. *Courtesy of Dr. Med. K. F. Schaller, Lomé, Togo.*

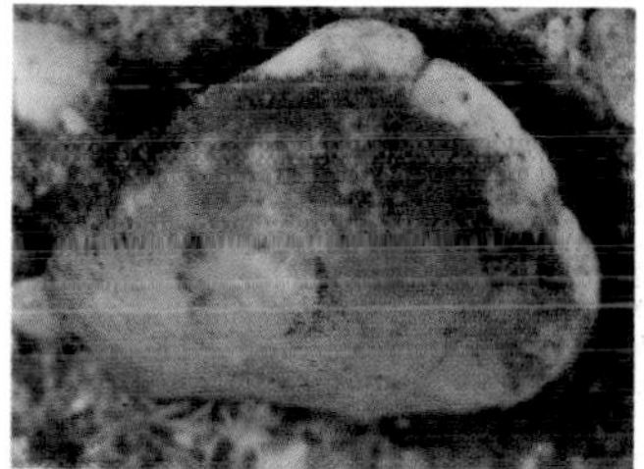

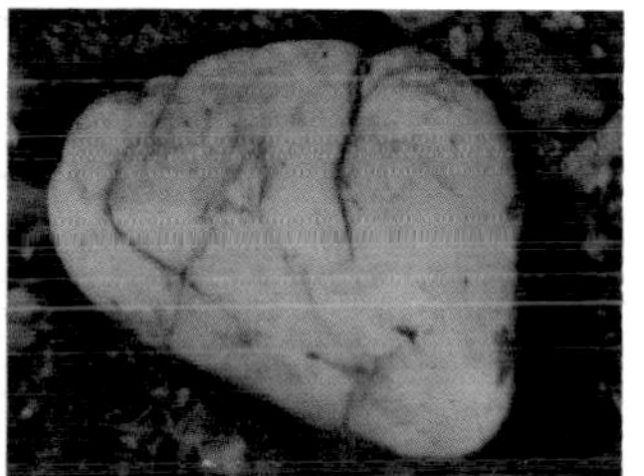

Fig. 47. Algae can be found in many varied environments. *(Above left)* In hot deserts, certain green algae colonize the microscopic air-space system a few millimeters below the surface of certain porous rocks. *(Above right)* For the quartz shown here, the main source of water is dew, which is absorbed and retained by the porous rock. With the cooling of the desert at night, the dew condenses and provides a source of moisture for the algae. With the appearance of the sun, the algae carry out photosynthesis, providing various minerals and other necessary factors are present.

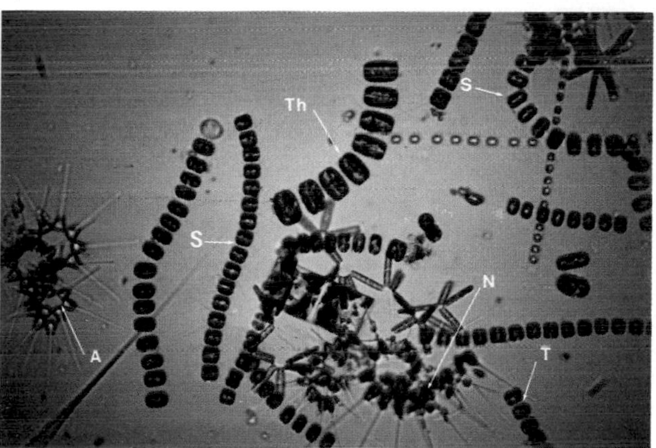

Fig. 48. This marine phytoplankton community of various diatom genera, including *Asterionella* (A), *Navicula* (N), *Rhizosolenia* (R), Skeletonema (S), *Thalassionema* (T), and Thalassiosira (Th), flourishes during the winter months. *Courtesy of Dr. Paul Hargraves, University of Rhode Island.*

HELMINTH INFECTIONS; INDUSTRIAL, FOOD, AND WASTE-TREATMENT MICROBIOLOGY

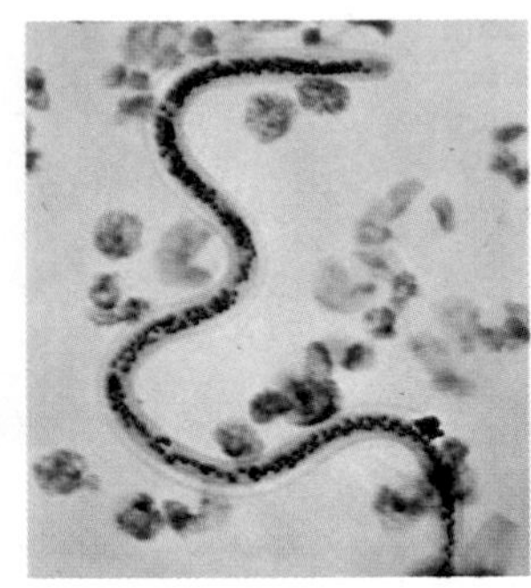

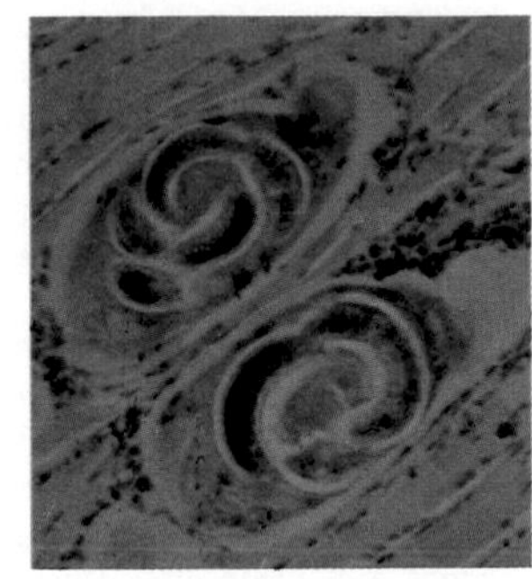

Fig. 92. *(Above left)* A blood smear showing the presence of the microfiliarian parasite *Wuchereria bancrofti.* This helminth is the causative agent of filiariasis. *Culex* spp. are frequently the mosquito vectors for the disease agent. **Fig. 93.** *(Above right)* Muscle tissue containing the larvae of the pork roundworm *Trichinella spiralis.* These roundworms may live ten to twenty years in this state. If tissue containing the larvae is consumed raw or if it is not cooked properly, the larvae are released into the digestive system, where they mature and cause the disease known as trichinosis.

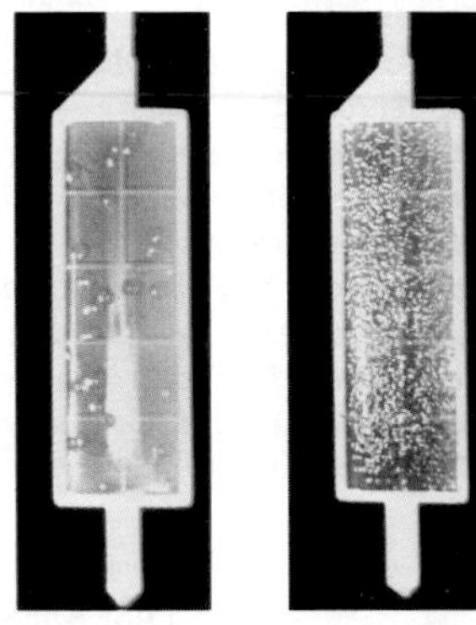

Fig. 94. *(Left)* The selective and differential medium MacConkey Agar can be used on urine dip-slides to provide a rapid test for infection. Colonies of lactose fermenters appear red on the medium. Low-colony *(left)* and high-colony *(right)* results are shown. *From Pazin, G. J., A. Wolinsky, and W. S. Lee,* Amer. Fam. Phys. *11:85–96 (1975).*

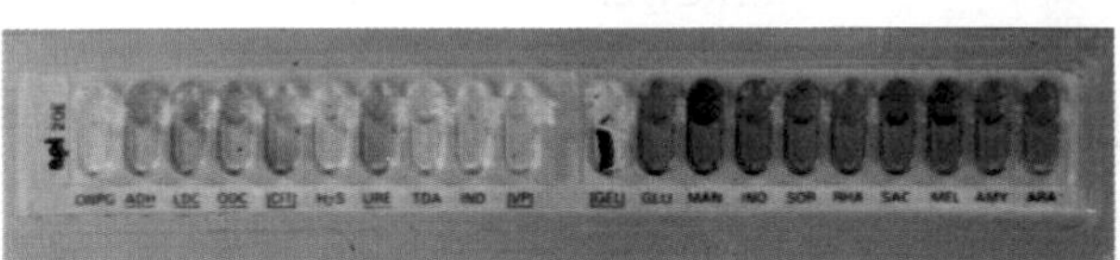

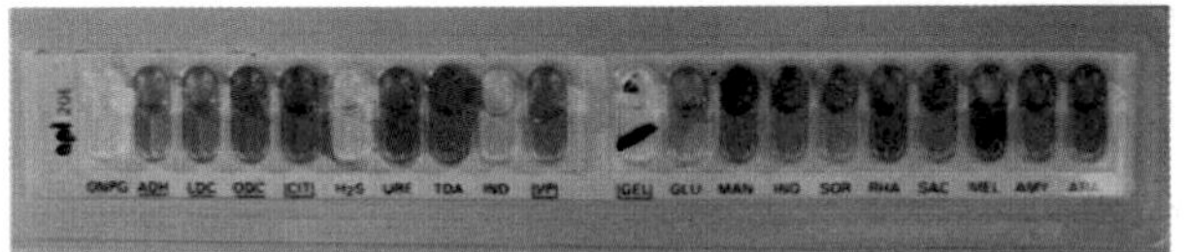

Fig. 95. *(Left)* A 20 Enteric ready-to-use system manufactured by Analytab Products, Inc. (API). The combination of substrates in this system allows the user to perform twenty-two standard biochemical tests. The tests in the top row show the appearance of uninoculated systems. The tests in the bottom row demonstrate examples of the color changes indicating positive reactions.

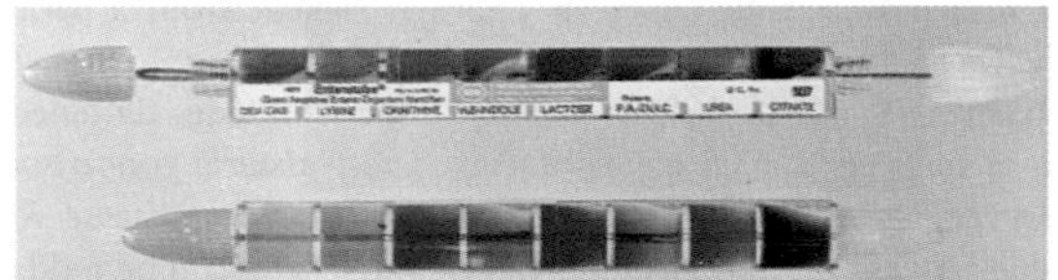

Fig. 96. *(Left)* Roche Diagnostics' Entero-Tube (ENCISE) Identification System. This photograph shows another multiple-test system; this system allows the user to perform eleven standard biochemical tests. The top system shows the appearance of an uninoculated set of tests. The bottom system demonstrates examples of the color changes associated with positive reactions.

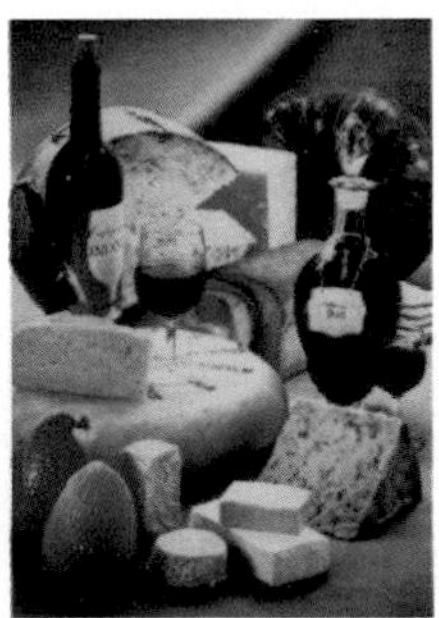

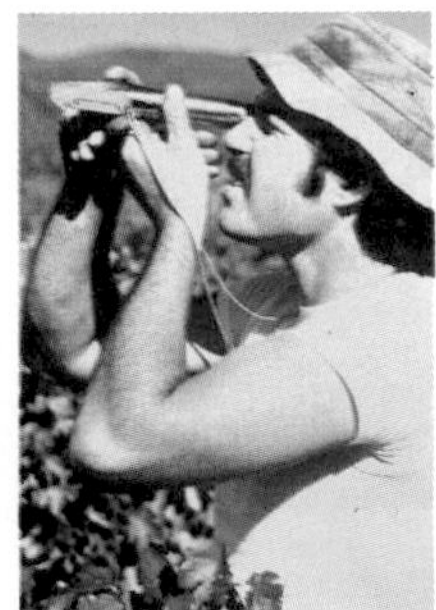

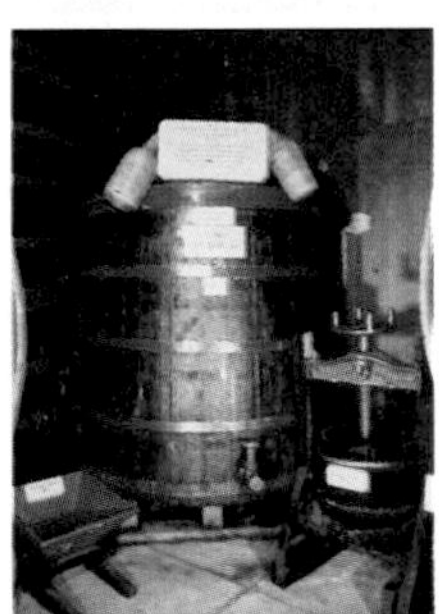

Fig. 97. *(Above left)* Each of the foods and beverages shown is a product of microbial fermentation. *Courtesy of the Wine Institute, San Francisco.* **Fig. 98.** *(Above center)* Before grapes are harvested, they are field-tested for sugar content. Each variety of grape is harvested when the sugar content reaches 20.5–24.0 percent. *Courtesy Sebastiani Vineyards.* **Fig. 99.** *(Above right)* Some devices used to make wine, including a fifty-gallon redwood fermentation tank, a grape crusher, and a press used in early California winemaking. *Courtesy of Sebastiani Vineyards.*

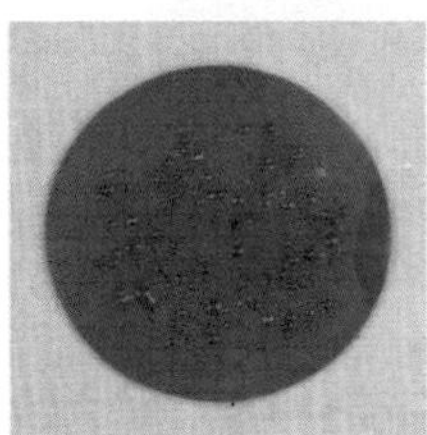

Fig. 100. Coliforms on the surface of a milipore filter. *Courtesy of Milipore Filter Corporation.*

TABLE 26–1 Preparations Currently Used for Active Immunizations (Vaccines) (Continued)

Viral Diseases	*Means of Vaccine Preparation*
Rabies (hydrophobia)	Two vaccines are available. The duck-embryo vaccine (DEV) is a beta-propiolactone-inactivated preparation of fixed virus obtained from duck-embryo cultivation. A nervous-tissue vaccine (NTV) consists of fixed virus obtained from injected rabbit-brain tissue and inactivated by either phenol at 37° C (Semple Vaccine) or ultraviolet irradiation. (See Chapter 37 for a more thorough discussion.) A new vaccine prepared from virus grown in human diploid cells and inactivated by tri (n)-butyl phosphate is under study.
Smallpox[b] (variola)	Attenuated cowpox obtained from calves.
Yellow fever	Attenuated strain of the virus (17D) cultivated in chick embryos.

[a]Vaccines that are under development or soon to be released.
[b]Hospital personnel should receive vaccines every three years, but smallpox vaccination is being discontinued for the general population. See a later section of this chapter for the explanation.

infections. Before killed vaccines are released for human use, they are thoroughly tested for safety and potency.

Microbial components. At present, several preparations consisting of different parts of microorganisms are being tested for their immunizing properties. Examples of these include the pili of *Neisseria gonorrhoeae* and the ribosomes of *Escherichia coli* and *Vibrio cholerae*. At the time of this writing, no commercial preparation involving these materials has been made available for human immunizations.

Toxoids. The toxins of several bacteria can be converted into nontoxic but still immunogenic preparations called **toxoids.** Heat or formalin are used in the production of toxoids.

In most commercial preparations, 0.2 to 0.4 percent formalin is added to a bacterial toxin such as diptheria or tetanus. The resulting mixture is incubated until detoxification is complete. Inert protein is then removed. The resulting preparation is called *natural fluid* or *plain toxoid.*

Another type of toxoid is prepared through the incorporation of certain aluminum compounds, such as alum, aluminum hydroxide, or aluminum phosphate. When alum is added to the toxin, the immunogenic component of the toxin precipitates. This material is washed and suspended in sterile physiologic saline. A diphtheria toxoid prepared in this way would be called *diphtheria toxoid, alum precipitated.* When aluminum hydroxide or phosphate is added to a toxin, the immunogenic components adsorb onto the particles of these compounds. The resulting toxoid preparation is *aluminum hydroxide,* or *aluminum-phosphate-adsorbed toxoid.*

Both types of toxoids, alum-precipitated and aluminum-hydroxide-adsorbed, produce a prolonged and relatively continuous antigenic stimulus. The aluminum compounds function as adjuvants that slowly release the immunizing substances.

Currently available toxoids are shown in Table 26–1.

VIRAL VACCINES

Several viral vaccines are composed of viruses whose virulence has been greatly reduced or eliminated. Such organisms are referred to as being **attenuated,** or weakened.

The virulence of viruses and other microorganisms can be reduced by several

See Chapter 12.

methods. These methods include (1) cultivation at temperatures above normal for the organism, (2) desiccation, (3) the use of unnatural hosts—for example, tissue culture or mice—for propagation of the microorganisms, and (4) continued and prolonged serial passages through laboratory animals. The first two techniques listed were discovered and used effectively by Louis Pasteur to combat anthrax and rabies.

An example of the procedures involved in the preparation of an attenuated viral vaccine is the preparation of the measles vaccine currently in use.

Inactivated vaccines. Some viral vaccines consist of killed (inactivated) viruses. These include Salk polio vaccine, IPV (inactivated poliomyelitis vaccine), and influenza vaccine (Table 26–1). Formalin is usually the chemical killing agent.

The Safety of Live versus Inactivated Preparations

The acceptability of a vaccine depends upon the general need for the preparation and the degree of protection it can provide. As severe and life-threatening bacterial diseases such as diphtheria and pneumococcal pneumonia progressively disappear, public expectation for a greater freedom from viral diseases can be expected. Almost all the effective viral vaccines now used consist of living, attenuated viruses. Live vaccines produce a high level of immunity, usually in a single dose. However, though such immunizing preparations have obvious advantages when compared to inactivated ones, live vaccines are subject to certain problems. These disadvantages include the following possibilities: (1) that infectious viruses will remain due to insufficient weakening; (2) that the viruses will spread from the vaccinated individual to susceptible contacts; (3) that contaminating viruses are present; (4) that a genetic change will take place resulting in a highly virulent viral strain; and (5) that the vaccine will be inactivated by heat in facilities that lack adequate refrigeration. Inactivated vaccines, on the other hand, are free from most of these potential hazards. However, producing a level of immunity using inactivated vaccines comparable to that produced by live preparations requires larger amounts of antigen and several injections.

Vaccine Safety

The risk of accidents with vaccines has been considerably reduced by the development of elaborate series of tests of vaccine safety and effectiveness. For example, virus vaccines containing specific immunologically active virus components, both infectious (live) and inactivated, are checked for immunologic and pathogenic properties at all stages of preparation. The fate of viruses in the vaccinated organism is also studied. If the viruses are eventually shed, the possibility that they might act as pathogens for susceptible contacts is checked.

Vaccines Currently in Use

The principal objective of immunization is to produce a solid degree of protection against infectious disease. Vaccine-conferred immunity should provide as much or more resistance as would follow an actual infection. Preparations used

TABLE 26–2 A Recommended Schedule for Active Immunization and Tuberculin Testing

Recommended Age	*Immunizing Agent*
2–3 months	Diphtheria toxoid, Pertussis vacine, Tetanus toxoid } DPT (combined preparation) Oral polio vaccine (TOPV)
3–4 months	DPT OPV (Type III or Trivalent Preparation)
6 months	DPT TOPV (optional)
15 months	Measles, mumps, and rubella vaccine. These vaccines can be used in combined form or as individual preparations.[a] Tuberculin testing also is included at this point.[b]
16–18 months	DPT booster TOPV
4–7 years	DPT booster TOPV
14–16 years	Td (adult) booster[c]
Thereafter every 10 years at 10-year intervals (except in case of injury)	Smallpox vaccine[d] Td (adult) booster[c]

[a]Children between the ages of 12 months and puberty may be vaccinated either with combined vaccines or with single-vaccine preparations.
[b]Initial testing is recommended at 1 year of age. The frequency of testing thereafter depends on the risk of exposure and the prevalence of tuberculosis in the community.
[c]Adult form of tetanus and diphtheria toxoids. The diphtheria toxoid dosage is reduced because of possible undesirable reactions in individuals with several previous inoculations.
[d]Routine immunization is not recommended by the American Academy of Pediatrics (AAP) or the U.S. Public Health Service (USPHS).

for immunization should be safe, free from unpleasant side effects, and relatively simple to administer. Table 26–2 provides a schedule for active immunization based in part on the recommendations in the Red Book of the American Academy of Pediatrics.

Combined Vaccines

The appearance of new vaccines makes the use of combined forms of immunizing preparations desirable. Combined forms are simpler to administer, less expensive to produce, and require fewer visits by the subject to health-care facilities than single-immunogen preparations. Examples of combined preparations include DPT (diphtheria-pertussis-tetanus); MMR (measles-mumps-rubella viruses vaccine); TOPV trivalent oral poliomyelitis vaccine, which contains all three immunologically distinct strains of attenuated polio viruses; and TAB (typhoid and paratyphoid A and B). Several studies have demonstrated excellent antibody responses to combined vaccine preparations. The combined vaccines provide simple, safe, and effective means of immunizing against important infectious diseases.

BCG and Tuberculosis Prevention

The proper use of ***Bacillus of Calmette and Guèrin*** (BCG) in the prevention of tuberculosis has long been a controversial and emotionally charged issue in the United States. Although available in this country, the attenuated bacterial preparation has been used infrequently for disease prevention. In contrast, BCG vaccination has been a major part of the World Health Organization's effort to control tuberculosis in countries with high rates of transmission. This group has been notably successful in reducing the incidence of new cases of tuberculosis. Control of tuberculosis in the United States is already quite successful, as evidenced by a low transmission rate. For this reason, there appears to be no reason for instituting mass BCG vaccination in the United States. However, under some circumstances, a BCG-vaccination program might be of great value, especially when the usual surveillance and treatment programs have failed or cannot be readily applied. Such situations might involve (1) infants who are unavoidably exposed to family contacts with active cases of pulmonary tuberculosis; (2) such groups as ghetto dwellers, migrants, alcoholics, and others, which have no regular health-care services and for which the usual methods of disease detection and treatment are inadequate; (3) populations with a known high frequency of tuberculosis; (4) health-care personnel working where an endemic incidence of tuberculosis is relatively high; and (5) individuals with negative tuberculin-skin-test results who are at high risk of repeated exposures to infected persons.

Passive Immunization

Passive immunization is effective, acts immediately, and is temporary in its effect. The preparations used for passive immunization are of two basic types: **antitoxins** and *antimicrobial sera*. Many of these preparations are produced in lower animals. They should only be used in clinical situations in which human sources of antitoxins and sera are not available, since these preparations present the possibility of hypersensitivity reactions.

Antitoxins

Antitoxins are antibodies capable of neutralizing the toxin that stimulated their production. These protein substances may be referred to as constituting an *immune serum*. An antitoxin is specific in its action against its toxic counterpart, but it does not exert any effect on the microorganism that produced the toxin. Most commercial preparations used for the passive immunization of humans are produced in horses, although antisera from cows are available for use with individuals sensitive to horse products.

PREPARATION

The preparation of antitoxins, such as those of diphtheria and tetanus, involves administration of toxin solutions to a horse or other appropriate animal until sufficient antitoxin titers are produced. The animal is then bled and its serum or plasma processed to concentrate the antitoxin and eliminate a large proportion of native horse-serum protein.

Removing as many of the horse-protein components as possible reduces the likelihood of sensitizing individuals receiving antitoxin or of precipitating anaphylaxis or serum sickness in already sensitized persons. (Sensitization of an individual develops in response to the native horse-serum protein, not to the antitoxins in the serum preparation.)

STANDARDIZATION

Before antitoxin preparations are released, they are sterilized, usually by filtration, treated with a chemical preservative to maintain the sterility of the preparation, and standardized. Three procedures are used for standardizing most antitoxins: animal- *(in vivo)* protection procedures, tube-flocculation tests, and skin-challenge tests.

The first step in the ***animal-protection test*** is the injection into test animals of different quantities of a particular toxin mixed with 1 unit of the corresponding standard antitoxin prepared by a central controlling agency, such as the National Institutes of Health, in Bethesda, Maryland. This procedure determines the dose of toxin lethal to a laboratory animal of a certain weight after a specified length of time in the presence of 1 standard unit of antitoxin. This quantity is called L_+. For example, in the standardization of diphtheria and tetanus toxins, the L_+ dose is the quantity of toxin needed to kill a 250-gm guinea pig on the fourth day following the injection of the toxin-antitoxin combination. Once the L_+ dose of the toxin has been obtained for the unit of standard antitoxin, the toxin is used to standardize the newly processed antitoxin. Standardization is achieved when the quantity of the new preparation producing the same results as 1 unit of the standard antitoxin is found.

In the ***flocculation test,*** certain proportions of the respective toxin and antitoxin preparations are mixed in test tubes. A flocculent precipitate generally forms in the tube that contains the proportions of toxin and antitoxin needed for neutralization.

The ***skin-challenge test*** (or simply ***skin test***) resembles the animal-protection procedure except that the standard is not death of the animal but the production of skin reactions by toxin-antitoxin combinations.

Commercial antitoxin preparations have been used principally in cases of diphtheria and tetanus. The designations for tetanus antitoxin preparations include ATS (antitetanic serum) and TAT (tetanus antitoxin). However, antitoxins have also been used to treat other diseases, including botulism and gas gangrene.

A physician should be present when antitoxin is administered, and the patient's blood pressure and pulse should be checked during and after the treatment to detect any hypersensitive reaction.

IMMUNE SERUM GLOBULIN (GAMMA GLOBULIN)

Immune serum globulin (ISG), also referred to as gamma globulin, is derived from human blood, plasma, or serum, and contains most of the antibodies found in whole blood. The concentrations of specific antibodies vary among different preparations. Immune serum globulin contains primarily IgG (γG) immunoglobulins. Conspicuously absent are IgM-associated antibodies, important to the body's defense against bacterial pathogens, and secretory IgA (γA) immunoglobulins, important to the protective mechanism on mucous membranes. Nevertheless, ISG preparations have advantages. These include (1) the absence of serum hepatitis virus, (2) the presence of a large amount of antibodies in a small volume, and (3) stability during long-term storage. The value of human serum globulin has been shown unequivocally in cases of measles and certain congenital immune-deficiency disease states. ISG can be useful in cases of posttransfusion hepatitis, German measles during the first trimester of pregnancy, and exposure to chickenpox of patients receiving immunosuppressive drugs. The variable success rates observed with immune serum globulin in these situations are probably due to differences in the amounts of specific antibody molecules among the preparations used.

SPECIFIC IMMUNE SERUM GLOBULIN (SIG)

Specific immune serum globulins (SIG) have a higher concentration of specific antibody to the agent in question than immune serum globulin preparations. The specific immune globulins, which are used more frequently, include those for measles, mumps, whooping cough, tetanus, shingles, and the Rh_0 blood factor. These globulin preparations are made from sera obtained from individuals recently recovered from an active infection or from individuals who are hyperimmunized to a given material. Serum globulins are injected into persons infected with the disease or recently exposed to it.

The Role of Allied Health Science Personnel

All allied health-science personnel, especially nurses, need a basic understanding of immunologic principles. Immunization against preventable diseases is one of the most important means of preventing or controlling communicable-disease epidemics. Nurses not only maintain and sterilize the instruments used in immunizing procedures, but also frequently administer vaccines and related preparations. In addition, they often have the responsibility of maintaining the immunization records of patients and informing parents as to the importance for their children of certain immunizations and of completing immunization schedules (Table 26–2).

To perform these duties efficiently and intelligently, health-science personnel must be aware of the nature of the material to be administered, the correct method for administration, the anticipated results, and the contraindications and possible side effects (Table 26–3) of the material to be used.

Administering Vaccines

PREPARING FOR ADMINISTRATION

Aseptic precautions must be taken during any type of inoculation procedure. These procedures include the proper cleaning and sterilizing of all non-disposable equipment and the washing and drying of the inoculator's hands. The containers for the immunizing preparations should also be disinfected. The cap or any other part of the container to be used should be wiped with 70 percent alcohol or other appropriate agent.

ROUTES OF ADMINISTRATION

Injection. In order for antibody production to occur, the antigenic material must be introduced beneath the epithelial tissues. Among the possible injection routes for humans are the intradermal (intracutaneous), intramuscular, and subcutaneous injection routes. For the primary immunization of humans, the intramuscular route of injection is most commonly used. The intradermal procedure is often used in the revaccination of previously inoculated individuals. Other routes of injection, such as intraperitoneal, intrathecal, and intravenous, have been used in certain situations requiring the administration of antisera and related materials, but such applications are rare. In the case of experimental animals used for the production of antibodies, the intraperitoneal and intravenous routes are generally employed. Both of these methods give excellent antisera.

Oral administration. With the development of the Sabin live poliomyelitis vaccine, oral administrtion has come into widespread use in the mass immuniza-

TABLE 26-3 Representative Reactions, Their Possible Causes, and Prevention

Reaction	*Possible Cause*	*Prevention*
Anaphylaxis	1. Immunologic interaction between antigen and skin-sensitizing antibody causing the release of reaction-mediating substances, including histamine and serotonin (See Chapter 25)	1. Skin testing with diluted materials 2. Conspicuously labeling a patient's record for his allergic nature
Encephalomyelitis (inflammation of central nervous system)	1. Immunologic basis of antigen-antibody reaction 2. Possible predisposition to reaction because of neurologic disorders, mental retardation, and so on	1. Avoiding revaccination to prevent recurrence of this reaction
Fetal injury	1. Effects of live vaccines	1. Avoiding administering live vaccines during pregnancy
High fever	1. Possible intolerance of vaccine 2. Reduction of tolerance to heat stress	1. Not exceeding recommended dosages 2. Avoiding administration of multiple toxic vaccines on the same day 3. Using fever-reducing medication, such as salicylates, after vaccinations
Induction of disease	1. Existence of a subclinical infection with the disease agent against which vaccination is being given 2. Susceptibility of individuals with immunologic deficiency states, such as hypogammaglobulinemias or of patients under steroid or immunosuppressive therapy	1. Avoiding inoculations of patients appearing to be symptomatic for the disease against which vaccination is to be given 2. Avoiding administering live vaccines to such persons
Serum-sickness-like reactions	1. Immunologic basis of antigen-antibody reaction	1. Using epinephrine and antihistamines in treatment
Severe local injury (abscess formation)	1. Bacterial contamination 2. Inadequate depth of vaccine administration	1. Proper cleansing of inoculation site 2. Proper injection technique
Sepsis	1. Secondary abscess formation 2. Contaminated needles, syringes, or vaccines	1. Proper cleansing of inoculation site 2. Using disposable needle and syringes 3. Preventing vaccine contamination during storage and subsequent use
Toxic reactions	1. Sensitivity of individual to vaccine	1. Reducing immunizing dosages

tion of whole community populations. In this technique the vaccine is usually given to the recipient in a small disposable cup, filled from a premeasured plastic packet or a calibrated dropper.

Intranasal administration. It has been suggested that to be effective immunization procedures should stimulate the immune responses induced by natural infection. In the case of viral upper respiratory disease, natural infection leads to the appearance of specific antibodies both in the serum and in the secretions at the local site of infection. This finding has given rise to the use of the nose spray as a mode of vaccine delivery. In certain parts of the world, preparations for diseases such as German measles and influenza are currently being administered intranasally.

TABLE 26-4 Frequently Reported Reactions to Certain Vaccines

Vaccine	*Selected General Features of Side Reactions and Potential Dangers*	*Prevention or Treatment*
BCG (Bacillus of Calmette and Guérin)	1. Regional lymph node enlargement followed by pus formation and perforation with prolonged drainage in individuals under 1 month of age receiving dosages greater than 0.025 cc 2. Possible activation of quiescent tuberculosis	1. Avoiding administering vaccine to persons with positive tuberculin skin reactions
DPT and Td[a] (Diphtheria, Tetanus Toxoids, and Pertussis Vaccine)	1. Toxic reactions 2. Encephalitis, when it occurs, is more commonly associated with the Pertussis component	1. Not exceeding recommended dosages, or reducing (tenfold) diphtheria toxoid in Td preparation 2. Most adverse effects averted through immunization of healthy children, and administering the final DPT dose at 3 to 4 years of age 3. Skin testing beginning with the tetanus toxoid
Measles (attenuated)	1. Fever, malaise, and regional lymph node enlargement	1. Immunizing healthy children only 2. Administering adequate fluids and salicylates between the fifth and eighth day to children known to have histories of high-fever reactions
Rabies (duck-embryo preparations)	1. Local redness, induration, and heat 2. Systemic reactions uncommon	1. Skin testing for individuals with hen-egg sensitivity; some degree of cross-reactivity may exist between the two egg sources
Rubella	1. Fever, rash, and mild local reactions 2. Pain, swelling, and stiffness in joints 3. Numbness and tingling sensation	1. Avoiding administering vaccine during pregnancy or where a possibility exists of pregnancy within 3 months of vaccination or where evidence exists of a fever, respiratory disease, or cancerous state

[a]Td adult dosages.

Complications Associated with Vaccinations

Undesirable, though apparently inevitable, side reactions to immunization procedures have been reported ever since Jenner introduced vaccination in 1796. Before any vaccine is administered, patients should be questioned as to the history of previous reactions associated with vaccinations. Obtaining such information is especially important where immunizations involve vaccines produced in eggs. A full and careful documentation of the circumstances surrounding any adverse reaction is important. Data obtained should include the type of vaccine, its lot number and other pertinent features, the quantity of material administered, the route and site of injection, and as full a description as possible of any reaction from the time of onset to its termination. Details of the patient's health, age, and family history may also be significant. When an unfavorable reaction occurs after a specific immunization vaccine has been administered, the fact must be noted on the patient's record. Finally, the dangers involved with an additional exposure should be fully explained to the individual.

TABLE 26–5 Recommended Immunization for American Travelers

Preparation	*Areas Involved*	*Qualifying Remarks*
Cholera	Countries requiring vaccination for entry	Not recommended during pregnancy
Diphtheria and tetanus (Td)	Recommended universally	
Immune serum globulin	Africa, Asia, Central and South America	Used to prevent infectious hepatitis
Plague vaccine	Cambodia, Laos, Viet Nam	Should be used where sylvatic plague exists
Poliomyelitis	Other than usual tourist routes, remote sections of tropical areas, where the disease is common	
Rabies (duck-embryo vaccine) *(preexposure)*	Africa, Asia, South America	Recommended only for personnel resident in these areas; not for short-term visitors
Typhoid fever	In endemic areas or regions where outbreaks are occurring	Not recommended during pregnancy
Typhus fever vaccine	Endemic areas for the disease include Asia, Africa, Central and South America, Europe	Should be used only for persons remaining in endemic regions for long periods of time
Yellow fever	Countries that require vaccination for entry, include parts of Africa and South America	Not recommended during pregnancy or for individuals with documented hypersensitivity to eggs

Representative reactions, their possible causes, and the complications that have been encountered with selected vaccines are summarized in Tables 26–3 and 26–4. Preventive measures and, in some cases, treatments are also listed.

The vaccines for cholera, typhoid fever, typhus, and yellow fever are not regularly used in the United States, except by military personnel or persons intending to go into endemic regions where certain vaccines are required. Unfavorable reactions from these preparations include fever (cholera, typhoid, and yellow fever), anaphylaxis (rare with the typhus vaccine), and inflammation of the nervous system (yellow fever). The latter reaction occurs most frequently in children under 1 year old.

Immunization for International Travel

Several infectious diseases are considered "quarantinable" under WHO International Sanitary Regulations. These regulations require that individuals traveling to, through, or from certain specified regions must be immunized against specific diseases. Verification of vaccination is required by some countries at the time of entry, and in certain situations may be needed for reentry. For example, individuals traveling through regions considered to be "yellow-fever country" are required to present verification of vaccination against that viral disease. Certain immunizations are recommended for American travelers. These are listed in Table 26–5. Immunizations against poliomyelitis and typhoid fever are generally not needed if the usual tourist facilities are used.

Eradication Through Immunization

Smallpox was the first of the great human scourges to yield to preventive measures. Vaccination with cowpox or vaccina virus (Figure 26–1), introduced by Edward Jenner in 1798, has eradicated the disease. This achievement is attributable to the WHO Smallpox Eradiction Campaign. Even though the virus of smallpox apparently no longer exists anywhere on earth, governments will continue to maintain a surveillance system and, in some cases, the requirement that individuals traveling to certain regions of the world be vaccinated.

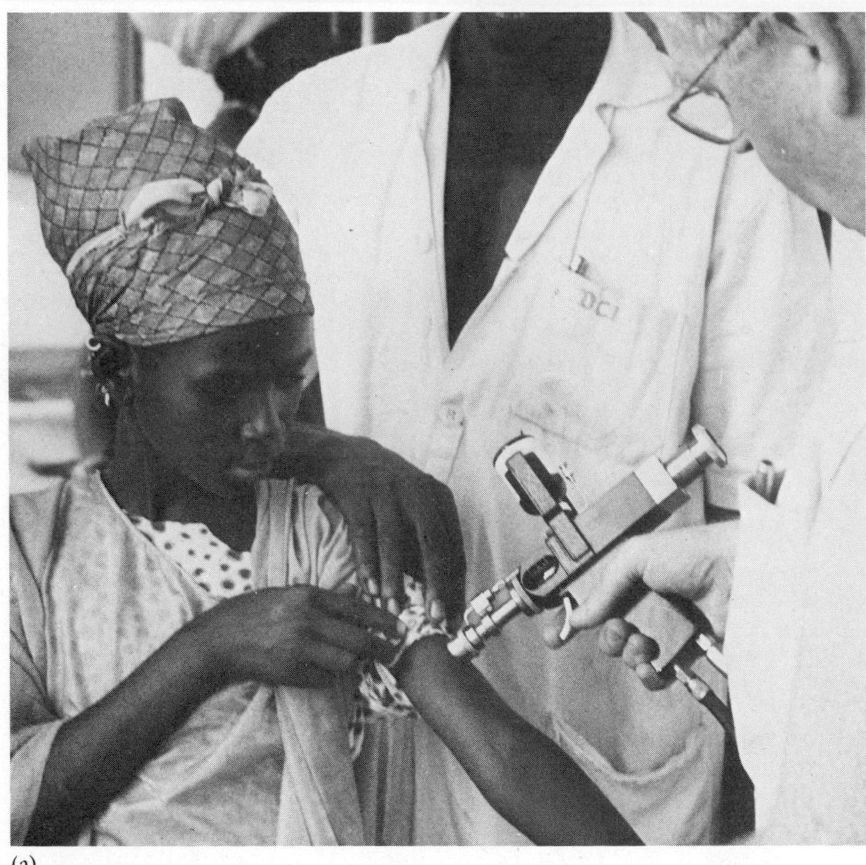

(a)

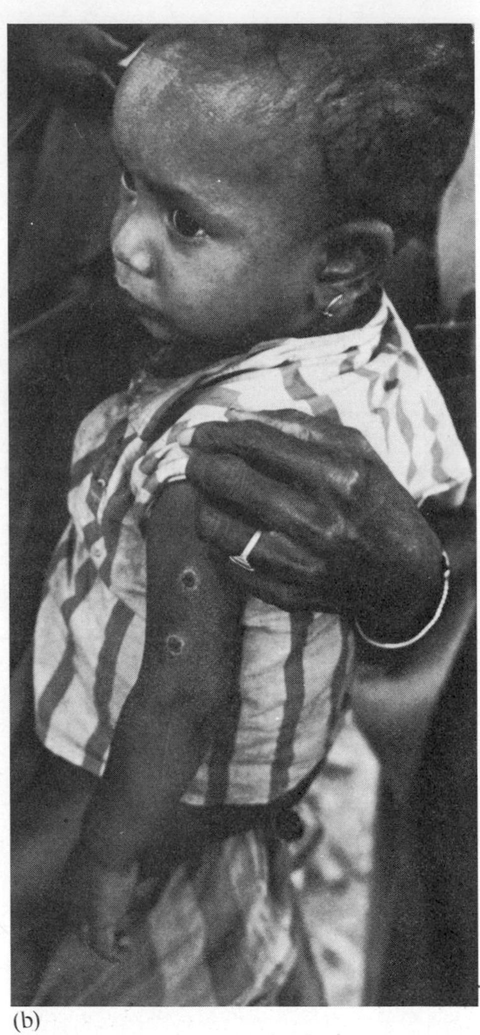

(b)

FIG. 26-1 Smallpox vaccination. (a) Vaccination against smallpox with a jet injector. (b) A positive reaction to smallpox vaccination showing scab formation. This child was revaccinated. Both photos courtesy World Health Organization, Geneva.

SUMMARY

1. One current approach to the prevention of microbial infections involves the use of live or inactivated microbes or their products.
2. Such preparations are usually effective if they are used before a specific infection has begun.

Immunization Preparations

Biological preparations for immunization or diagnosis can be divided into three categories: (1) preventive agents for active immunization, (2) protective preparations for passive immunization, and (3) diagnostic reagents.

The Preparation of Representative Vaccines

1. Most preparations of bacterial vaccines consist of killed organisms in isotonic salt solution.
2. Organisms used for vaccines are killed with the aid of heat or chemical agents such as formalin.
3. Newer vaccines consisting of bacterial parts, including pili and ribosomes, are being tested.
4. Toxins converted by heat or chemical agents into nontoxic antigenic preparations are called *toxoids*.
5. Immunizing materials against virus disease contain either attenuated (weakened) or killed viruses.

The Safety of Live versus Inactivated Preparations

1. The live vaccines now in use generally produce a high level of immunity and are usually given in single doses, but they are also more subject to problems than inactivated vaccines.
2. Problems encountered with live virus vaccines include (1) insufficient weakening of the pathogen, (2) spread of viruses to susceptible contacts, (3) contamination, (4) genetic changes, and (5) inactivation due to inadequate storage conditions.
3. Larger amounts of antigen and multiple injections are needed with killed vaccines to produce levels of immunity comparable to those of live preparations.
4. The risk of accidents has been reduced by the establishment of better safety controls.

Vaccines Currently in Use

1. Immunizations should produce a solid degree of protection against infectious diseases.
2. Preparations should be safe, free from unpleasant side effects, and relatively simple to use.
3. Several vaccines consist of combined forms of immunizing preparations. Combined forms are simpler to use, less expensive to produce, and require fewer visits to the health-care facility than single vaccine preparations.

BCG and Tuberculosis Prevention

1. The proper role of the Bacillus of Calmette and Guérin (BCG) in tuberculosis prevention has been controversial.
2. The preparation is considered appropriate in several situations, including those in which the usual surveillance procedures (skin testing, etc.) and treatment programs have failed or cannot be readily applied.

Passive Immunization

1. Passive immunization is effective, acts immediately, and is temporary in its effect.
2. Preparations used for passive immunization are of two basic types: antitoxins and antimicrobial sera (immune serum globulin).
3. Antitoxins are antibodies capable of neutralizing the toxin that stimulated their production.
4. Immune serum globulin is one product obtained from human blood, plasma, or serum. It contains most of the types of immunoglobulins (antibodies) found in whole blood.
5. Specific immune serum globulin (SIG) contains a higher specific antibody concentration to the disease agent than that found in immune serum globulin preparations.

The Role of Allied Health Science Personnel

1. Immunization is one of the most important means available for preventing and controlling infectious diseases.
2. Individuals responsible for administering immunizing materials must be aware of the nature of the vaccine, the correct method of administration, anticipated results, and contraindications and possible side effects.

Administration of Vaccines

1. Aseptic precautions must be taken during any type of inoculation procedure.
2. Several injection routes can be used for immunizations; these include intradermal, intramuscular, and subcutaneous routes. Oral and intranasal administration are two other techniques for administering vaccines.

Complications Associated with Vaccinations

1. Side reactions to vaccinations occur in certain individuals.
2. When an unfavorable reaction occurs, it should be fully described on the medical records of the individual.

Immunization for International Travel

The immunization requirements for international travel vary according to the specific regions to be visited.

Eradiction Through Immunization

Smallpox was the first human infectious disease to be completely eradicated by a vaccination program.

QUESTIONS FOR REVIEW

1. Define or explain the following terms:
   a. attenuated viruses
   b. active immunity
   c. artificially acquired immunity
   d. toxoid
   e. gamma globulin
2. What general types of immunizing agents are currently available?
3. What is the difference between a toxin and a toxoid?
4. What is the nature of the immunizing material used with each of the following infectious diseases?
   a. typhoid fever
   b. whooping cough
   c. measles
   d. yellow fever
   e. tuberculosis
   f. influenza
   g. smallpox
   h. tetanus
   i. mumps
   j. polio
   k. rabies
   l. diphtheria
5. Describe at least three routes of administration for vaccines.
6. Does the administration of immune serum globulin have any value in combating the effects of disease agents? If so, with which diseases does this beneficial effect occur?
7. What complications may develop as a consequence of vaccinations? Describe several common examples.

SUGGESTED READINGS

Henderson, D. A., "The Eradication of Smallpox," *Sci. Amer.* 235:25 (1976). *A description of the World Health Organiza-*

tion's efforts to eradicate smallpox.

Langer, W. L., "Immunization against Smallpox before Jenner," *Sci. Amer.* 234:64 (1976). *Before Jenner introduced the inoculation with cowpox, smallpox was prevented by the inoculation with material from smallpox victims. This article tells how this procedure was performed before Jenner's time in the eighteenth century.*

Philips, C. F., "Cytomegalovirus Vaccine: A Realistic Appraisal," *Hosp. Pract.* 14:75–80 (1979). *A discussion of the possible benefits, limitations, and dangers of a vaccine program for cytomegalovirus infection, stressing the logical approach and the steps involved in vaccine development.*

White, R. G., "The Adjuvant Effect of Microbial Products on the Immune Response," *Ann. Rev. Microbiol.* 30:579–600 (1976). *An examination and evaluation of some of the mechanisms associated with the ability of microbial products to stimulate antibody production. Stresses common principles of adjuvant activity.*

Wishnow, R. M., and J. L. Steinfeld, "The Conquest of the Major Infectious Diseases in the United States: A Bicentennial Retrospect," *Ann. Rev. Microbiol.* 30:427–450 (1976). *This article tells of past successes in controlling diseases such as smallpox, tuberculosis, cholera, typhoid fever, malaria, yellow fever, poliomyelitis, and diphtheria in the United States.*

PART FIVE

Microorganisms and Infectious Diseases

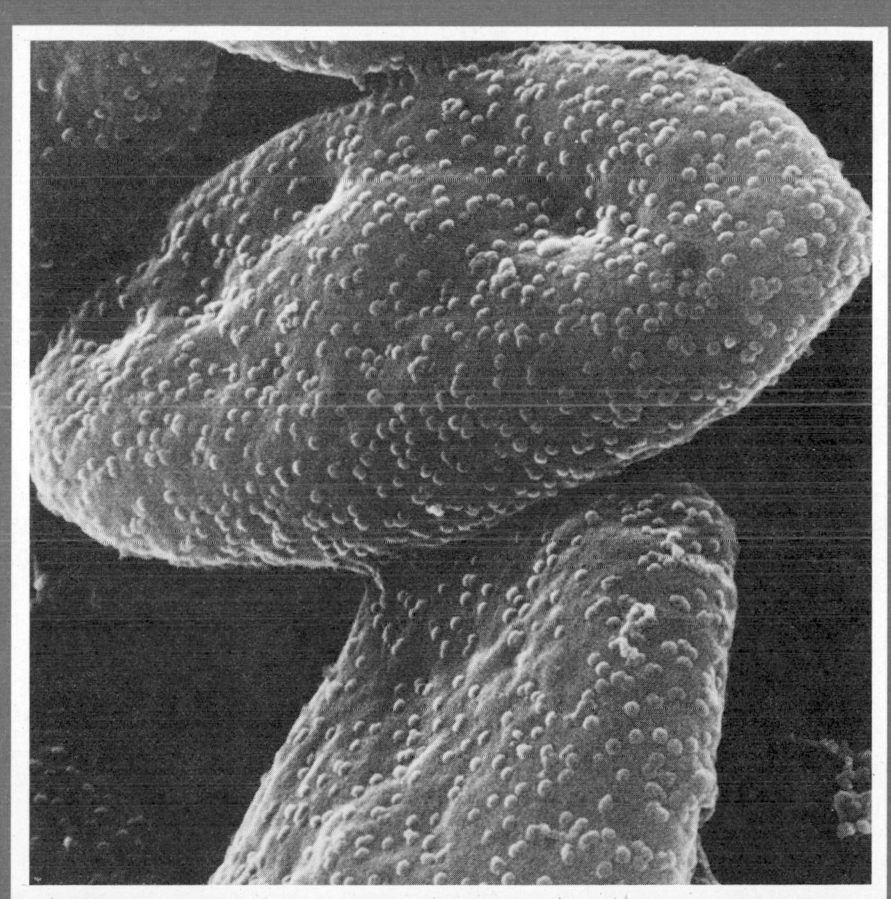

CHAPTER **27**

Principles of Disease Transmission

How is an infectious disease spread? What are the principles underlying the patterns of occurrence? How can the spread of pathogenic microorganisms be controlled in health-care facilities such as hospitals and in the population at large? Chapter 27 covers these and other topics related to the transmission of disease.

After reading this chapter, you should be able to

1. **List six sources of infectious body fluids.**
2. **Distinguish between an incubatory and a convalescent carrier.**
3. **Define zoonosis, and give six examples.**
4. **List and explain five principal modes of transfer for infectious disease agents and describe appropriate control measures for each.**
5. **Describe the role played by arthropods in the transmission of infectious diseases.**
6. **Name a disease spread by each of the following arthropods: cockroaches, fleas, lice, mites, mosquitoes, and ticks.**
7. **Describe the contributions of Theobald Smith and Ronald Ross to the understanding of disease transmission.**
8. **Describe how plants become infected.**
9. **Define the following terms:**
   a. **epidemic**
   b. **pandemic**
   c. **morbidity**
   d. **fomite**
   e. **nosocomial**
   f. **asepsis**
   g. **mortality rate**
   h. **biological means of disease transmission**

Humans, lower animals, and plants can be successfully parasitized by a variety of microorganisms and by such forms of animal life as worms, mites, and ticks. The transmission of such agents from host to host is essential both to their survival and their biological success as pathogens. Pathogens are transmitted from the source of infection to susceptible hosts by many means and mechanisms. In this chapter, we describe some means of transfer and a variety of measures by which disease transmission can be controlled.

Epidemiology is the study of the distribution and causes of disease prevalent in humans. Epidemiologists approach problems of disease inductively. That is, they collect and analyze data from many individuals to reach conclusions about the epidemiology of a particular disease. It should be noted that this area of investigation is not necessarily limited to the ***communicable/infectious*** type of disease only. The so-called noninfectious diseases—for example, cancer, cardiovascular conditions, congenital defects, diabetes mellitus, emphysema, vitamin deficiencies (such as pellagra, rickets, and scurvy)—have been and continue to be studied epidemiologically.

Communicable diseases are known to be infectious—that is, to interfere with normal function. However, some infectious diseases are not necessarily communicable, that is, transmittable. Examples include leprosy and certain forms of tuberculosis. Therefore, to prevent any misconceptions as to the nature of such diseases within the scope of epidemiology, the combined term *communicable/infectious* is used.

For centuries, the patterns of occurrence among various communicable/infectious diseases have differed noticeably. The following are the usual terms used to describe the prevalence of diseases:

1. **Endemic.** This term describes a disease that is constantly present but involves relatively few persons. Examples of such diseases, drawn from various localities, include coccidioidomycosis, leprosy, and tuberculosis.
2. **Epidemic.** An epidemic is an unusual occurrence of a disease involving large segments of a population for a limited period of time. Examples are influenza and poliomyelitis epidemics.
3. **Pandemic.** A pandemic is a series of epidemics affecting several countries, or even the major portions of the world. The influenza pandemic of 1918–1919 exhibited such a worldwide distribution.
4. **Sporadic.** Sporadic diseases are uncommon, occur irregularly, and affect only a relatively few persons. Infections such as diphtheria and whooping cough (pertussis) occur sporadically. These and other communicable/infectious diseases may ordinarily be sporadic or endemic, but, depending upon factors such as the immunity of the population and sanitation, they can sometimes assume epidemic proportions.

Morbidity and Mortality Rates

When an outbreak of a communicable disease occurs, or even when a single case appears, epidemiologists gather many types of data. Some of the principal findings are frequently expressed in terms of morbidity and mortality rates. **Morbidity** is generally defined as the number of individuals having the disease per unit of the population within a given time period. Usually, 100,000 is taken as the unit of population for such calculations. The *mortality rate* is the number of deaths attributable to a particular disease per unit of the population (usually 1000) within a given time period. Reports may be compiled weekly, monthly, yearly, or for even longer periods, depending on the purpose of the study.

Occasionally, outbreaks of disease occur that are more or less limited to particular segments of a population. Consequently, morbidity and mortality rates may be calculated for that population segment alone. An *infant mortality rate* is an example. Figure 27–1 summarizes some of the factors involved in reducing the morbidity and mortality of infectious diseases.

Reporting Communicable/ Infectious Diseases

State administrative codes require that actual or even suspected cases of certain communicable/infectious diseases be reported to local health authorities. The number and kinds of such reportable diseases vary among the states. The specific reportable infections in California are listed in Table 27–1; this state's list is a fairly comprehensive one. Individuals charged with the responsibility of notifying local health authorities include physicians, coroners, directors of hospitals, clinics, and laboratories, and any persons knowing of a disease's existence.

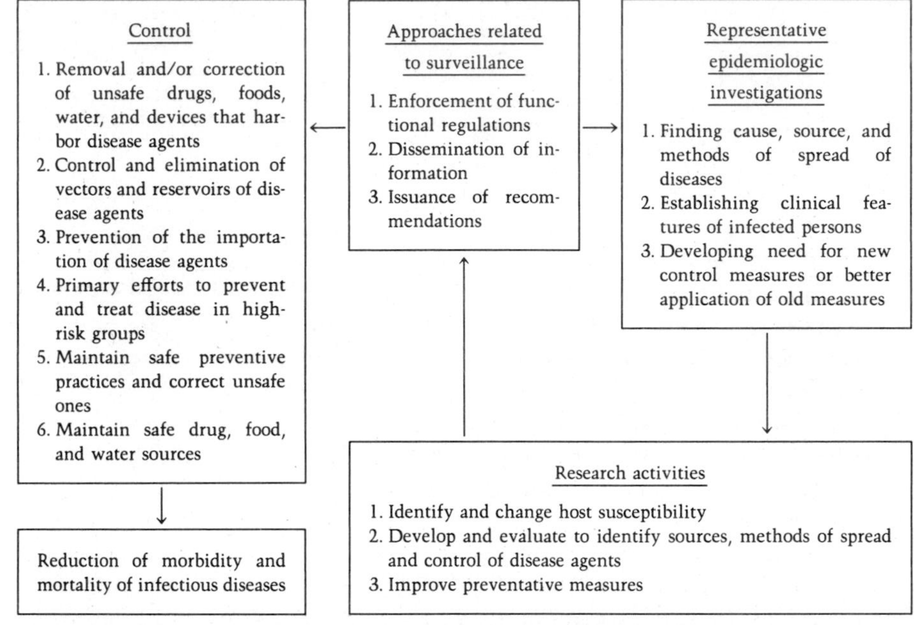

FIG. 27–1 Factors involved in the reduction of morbidity and mortality of infectious diseases. The figure exhibits the interrelationships among control measures, epidemiologic investigations, and research. After *Bennett, J. V.*, Annals Internal. Med. *89:761–763 (1978)*.

Sources and Reservoirs of Infection

The sources of infectious-disease agents are many and varied (Figure 27–2). Generally speaking, however, the most disabling and most common infections among humans are caused by microorganisms capable of living and reproducing in human tissues. Where these organisms are present, human tissues and

TABLE 27-1 Communicable/Infectious Diseases Reportable in California

Disease	*Nature of Causative Agent*	*Disease*	*Nature of Causative Agent*
Acute infectious conjunctivitis of the newborn (includes gonorrheal ophthalmia)	Bacterial (B)	Scarlet fever	B
Anthrax	B	Shigella infections	B
Asiatic cholera	B	Streptococcal infections (including streptococcal sore throat)	B
Botulism	B	Syphilis	B
Brucellosis	B	Tetanus	B
Chancroid	B	Trachoma	B
Diarrhea of the newborn	B	Tuberculosis	B
Diphtheria	B	Tularemia	B
Dysentery (bacillary)	B	Typhoid fever (both actual cases and carriers)	B
Food poisoning (excluding botulism)	B	Typhus fever	B
Gonorrhea	B	Coccidioidomycosis	Fungal
Granuloma inguinale	B	Trichinosis	Helminth
Leprosy	B	Malaria	Protozoan
Leptospirosis	B	Dengue fever	Viral (V)
Meningitis (meningococcal or meningococcemia)	B	Encephalitis (acute form)	V
Paratyphoid fever A, B, and C	B	Infectious hepatitis	V
Pertussis (whooping cough)	B	Measles (rubeola)	V
Plague	B	Mumps	V
Psittacosis	B	Poliomyelitis	V
Q fever	B	Rabies (both human and lower animal)	V
Relapsing fever	B	Serum hepatitis	V
Rheumatic fever (acute)	B	Viral exanthema in pregnant women	V
Rocky Mountain spotted fever	B	Yellow fever	V
Salmonella infections (exclusive of typhoid fever)	B		

Source: Adapted from "Morbidity and Mortality Reportable Diseases," 14th Report (week ending April 11, 1970), County of Los Angeles Health Department.

secretions serve as a reservoir of infection. The sources of infectious body fluids are referred to as *portals of exit*. They include (1) the gastrointestinal tract, (2) the genitourinary system, (3) the oral region, (4) the respiratory tract, (5) the blood and blood derivatives, and (6) lesions of the skin and other areas.

The individual who harbors infectious agents of disease is called a **carrier.** A carrier who apparently suffers no ill effects is called a *healthy carrier.* The individual who is in an incubating state, undergoing the beginning disease but without exhibiting symptoms, is referred to as an *incubatory carrier.* Such persons may be infectious during the last stages of their incubation periods. Another category of carrier is the *convalescent:* in certain situations, patients recovering from an infection may serve as sources of pathogens.

Several other reservoirs of infectious agents are recognized. These include lower animals, arthropods, soil, and inanimate contaminated objects. Some of these sources may also serve as a means of disease transmission.

Zoonoses

Various warm-blooded animals are recognized as reservoirs of infectious-disease agents for humans. Such sources include bats, birds, cattle, cats, dogs, horses, mice, monkeys, rabbits, rats, skunks, and various wild mammals. Rats, for example, are implicated in the transmission of plague, rat-bite fever, and certain tapeworms (Figure 27–3). Diseases that primarily affect lower animals but can also be transmitted to human beings by natural means are referred to as **zoonoses** (Table 27–2). Several animals also serve as sources of parasites that affect human beings.

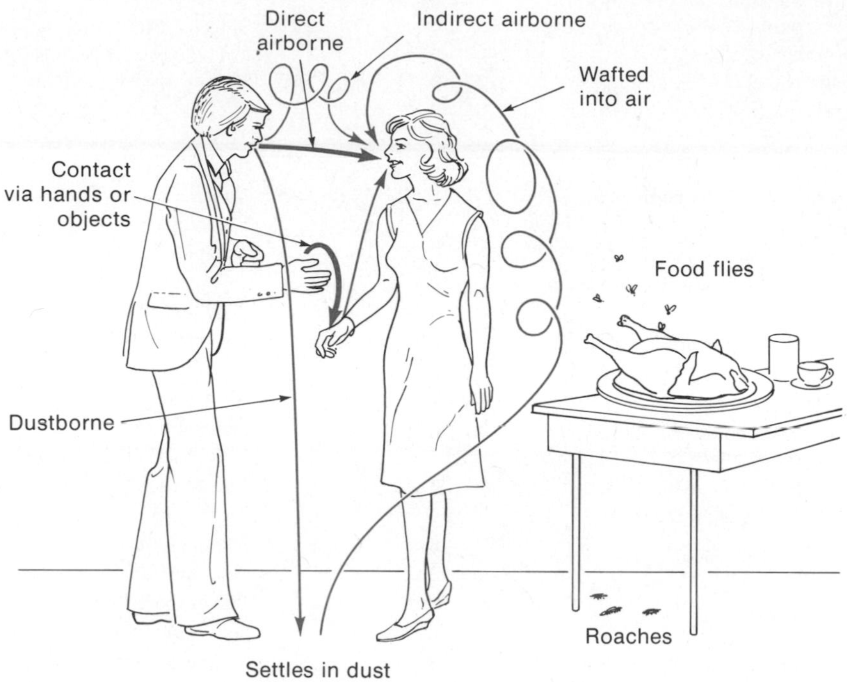

FIG. 27–2 Some common sources of infection and portals of exit. Note that certain of these can also function as means of disease transmission.

Certain infectious agents can be transmitted by the bite of warm-blooded animals. Perhaps the best known of these is rabies. The chief vectors of this viral infection include cats, coyotes, dogs, foxes, jackals, skunks, and a variety of bats. Since the turn of the century, vampire bats have been incriminated as vectors of rabies among cattle in various regions of the world, including Central and South America. When in a rabid state, these bats can bite one another as well as cattle and humans. The reports of bat- and skunk-associated rabies in humans has been steadily increasing. Figure 27–4 shows some types of bats found in the United States.

Most species of bats are colonial in nature, congregating together in buildings, caves, mines, or trees. In general, bats are considered beneficial to humans, because they consume large quantities of insects and rodents. However, rabies has been reported to occur in more than 20 species of bats, including fruit-eating, insectivorous, and vampire varieties. Rabies may also be latent in these animals. Bats with latent rabies may serve as carriers, excreting the viral agents in their saliva and feces for several months.

Bat colonies can be removed by means of repellents, batproofing procedures, or simple physical destruction. Substances used as repellents have included napthalene and paradichlorobenzene. Toxic chemicals such as chlordane have been employed for the destruction of bat colonies. However, batproofing, if feasible, is apparently the only truly satisfactory method for the removal of bats. To batproof a building, one must determine the bats' actual roosting site and seal off the various means of access. A knowledge of the migratory habits of the colony is useful in this regard. It is necessary to guard against the possibility of trapping bats before they have had an opportunity to leave and of overlooking a possible entry to the site.

TABLE 27-2 Representative Zoonoses Produced by Microorganisms

Disease	*Associated Animals*	*Major Mode of Transmission*
Bacterial and Related Infections		
Anthrax	Domestic livestock	Direct contact with infected and contaminated soil
Brucellosis (undulant fever)	Domestic livestock	Direct contact with infected tissues; ingestion of milk from diseased animals
Bubonic plague	Rodents	Fleas
Leptospirosis	Dogs, rodents, wild animals	Direct contact with infected tissues and urine
Relapsing fever	Various rodents	Lice and ticks
Rocky Mountain spotted fever	Dogs, rodents	Ticks
Salmonellosis	Dogs, poultry, rats	Ingestion of infected meat; contamination of water
Tularemia	Wild rabbits	Direct contact with infected tissues; deer flies, ticks
Fungus Infections		
Several forms of ringworm	Various domestic animals, e.g., cats, dogs	Direct contact
Protozoan Infections		
African sleeping sickness (trypanosomiasis)	Humans, wild game animals	Tsetse flies
Chagas' disease	Humans, wild animals	Kissing bugs
Kala-azar leishmaniasis	Cats, dogs, rodents	Sandflies
Toxoplasmosis	Birds, wild rodents, domestic animals, e.g., cats	Generally unknown; possibly contamination of food and water
Viral Infections		
Eastern equine encephalitis (EEE)	Birds; horses and related animals	Mosquitoes
Influenza	Humans, swine, horses	Direct contact with droplets
Jungle yellow fever	Various species of monkeys	Mosquitoes
Rabies	Bats, cats, dogs, humans, skunks, wolves, etc.	Bites, contamination of wounds with infectious saliva

Principal Modes of Transfer for Infectious-disease Agents

Infectious-disease agents may be transmitted to susceptible individuals in a variety of ways. These include (1) direct contact with obviously infected persons or carriers; (2) indirect contact with inanimate objects, food, or water contaminated by infected individuals; (3) inhalation of airborne dust or droplet nuclei containing infectious agents; (4) inoculation; and (5) arthropods, which may serve either as mechanical or biological vectors. *Mechanical transmission* refers to the situation in which an insect physically transports a pathogen from contaminated material such as food or water to other objects. Cockroaches and flies are good examples. In ***biological transmission***, a portion of the pathogen's life cycle is carried out in the vector. Transmission of the malarial pathogen by the anopheline mosquito is an example of biological transmission.

The mechanical means of disease transmission includes the 5 Fs: food, fingers, flies, feces, and fomites. The biological means of transmission include the injection of blood and blood products, warm-blooded animal bites, arthropod bites, and the introduction of arthropod feces into bites or wounds. It is important to note that many diseases can be spread in a variety of ways.

Direct Contact

Individuals who come into direct contact with infectious lesions such as open sores, boils (Color Photograph 78), and draining abscesses (Color Photograph 79) obviously run the risk of acquiring the disease agent. Contagious diseases—from the Latin word ***contagio***, meaning touch or contact—include anthrax, syphilis, and gonorrhea. Many of the disease states spread by direct contact gain access to the body through the nose and throat.

Pathogens can be transmitted through hand shaking or kissing. Examples of diseases spread in this manner include poliomyelitis, chickenpox, the common cold, bacillary dysentery, and streptococcal infections. Certainly washing hands after blowing the nose, defecating, urinating, or working with infected persons helps to limit the spread of disease agents.

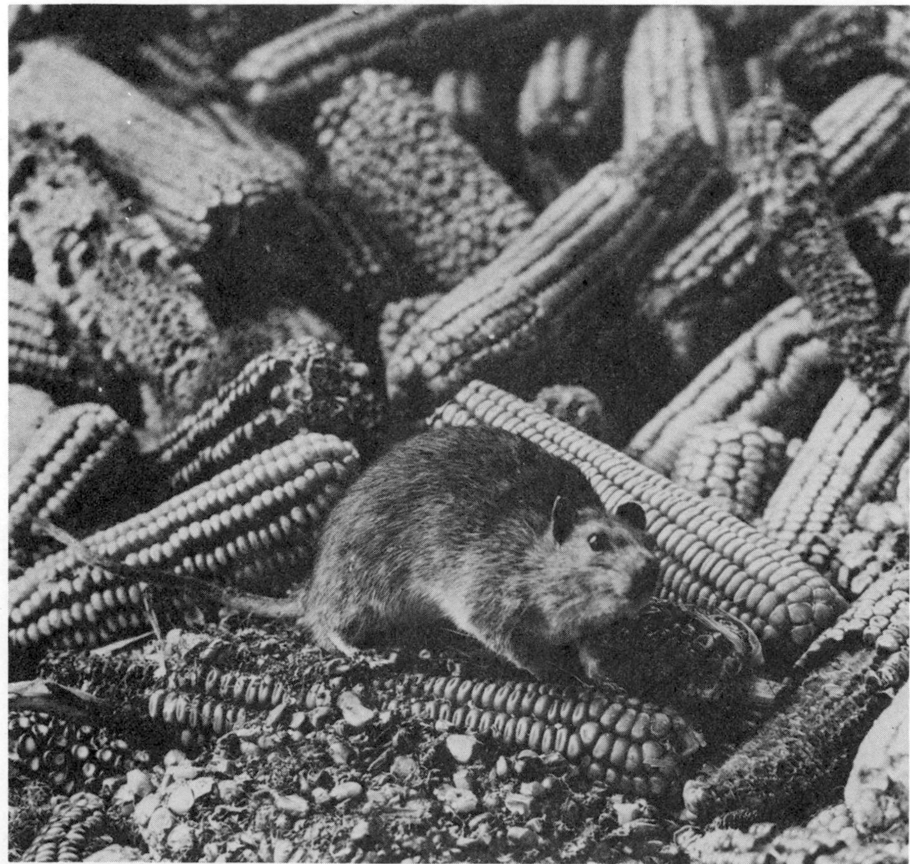

FIG. 27–3 Rats, which are not only involved with the transmission of several diseases such as plague, rat-bite fever, and certain tapeworms, but are also responsible for the destruction of stored and other foodstuffs. *Courtesy U.S.D.A.*

Indirect Contact

Various microorganisms can be transmitted by food, water, and, quite often, contaminated inanimate objects. Moist foods that are not highly acid can serve as excellent culture media for pathogenic microorganisms, including the causative agents of amebic dysentery, bacillary dysentery (shigellosis), cholera, and typhoid fever. These diseases can also be spread through contaminated water supplies.

Raw or inadequately cooked meat from infected animals is a well-known source of disease agents. In addition to microorganisms, such products can contain helminths capable of causing trichinosis (Color Photograph 93) and tapeworm infections. Proper sanitary measures and adequate meat inspection substantially reduce the possibility of these diseases being transmitted. Many states have stringent requirements of sanitation for the farms and ranches that supply meat for human consumption. Such measures are also important for bacterial disease control. Included in this category are infections such as undulant fever (brucellosis) and bovine tuberculosis, both of which can be transmitted by milk from infected cows.

The handling of food for human consumption by undiscovered carriers is always a serious hazard. The carriers may cough or sneeze onto food or handle utensils or food without washing their hands after using the toilet or blowing the nose. Also, food handlers or dishwashers might have draining abscesses or boils, which serve as other sources of disease agents. Eating utensils and drinking glasses can also be important factors in the transmission of diseases. The thorough washing and proper disinfecting of such items is essential to good sanitation. Various types of commercial dishwashing equipment are available that clean and disinfect utensils mechanically.

Regular inspection of restaurant personnel and equipment, including dishwashing machines, is necessary for the effective prevention of infections spread by food. Standardized methods exist for bacteriological examination of dishes and related items. Specimens can be taken directly by means of a sterile cotton swab or, if possible, the utensil can be introduced directly into sterile media. The American Public Health Association publishes appropriate methods, media, and other details for this purpose.

Maintenance of adequate sanitation in restaurants can be difficult, costly, and time-consuming. It is therefore not surprising that fast-food restaurants are increasing their use of disposable paper and plastic dishes and eating utensils. This practice greatly reduces operation costs and, more importantly, markedly increases sanitation levels. Pathogens are seldom found in bacterial counts of these plastic and paper products.

Air- and Dustborne Infections

Particles bearing microorganisms are released into the general environment in two major ways. Some are produced during normal activities involving the respiratory tract—for example, talking, coughing, and sneezing. Significantly larger numbers of organisms are liberated by sneezing than by the other two activities. Microorganism-bearing particles from the skin, clothing, and even dressings covering wounds are also generated by normal body movements.

The second major means by which particles are introduced into the general environment is the redistribution of accumulated particles in room dust. Dustborne infections include the fungal diseases of coccidioidomycosis and histoplasmosis. Once droplets are released into the air, they fall to the ground at a rate determined by their size. On the ground, these droplets stick to or become mixed with the variety of animal, plant, and mineral debris, commonly known as "house dust." Evaporation, or drying, takes place next. The rate of evaporation depends on the size and composition of the droplets and the rela-

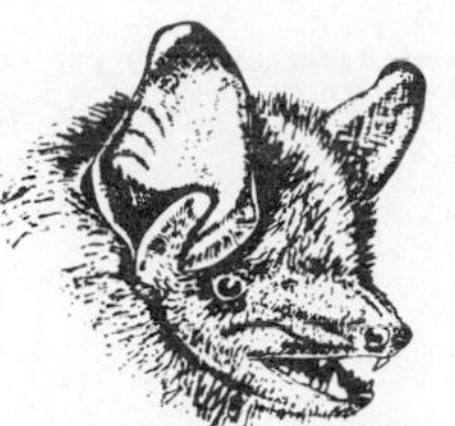

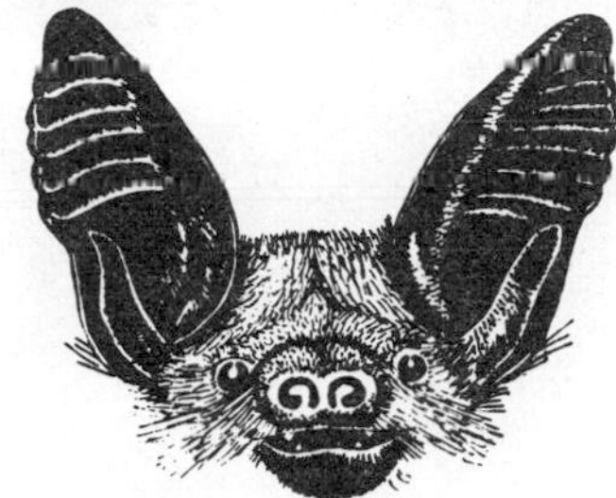

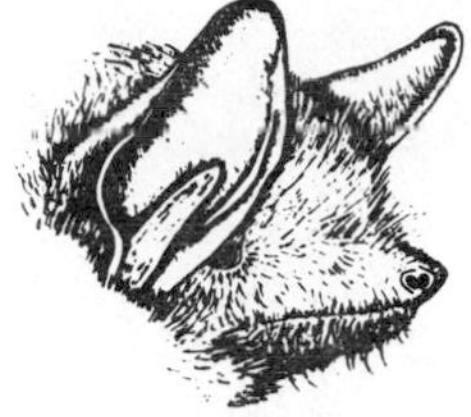

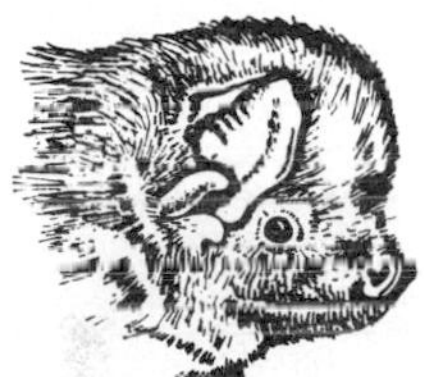

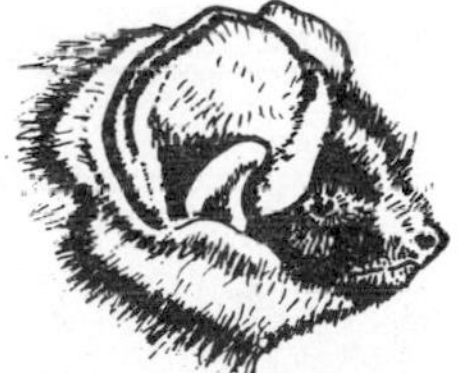

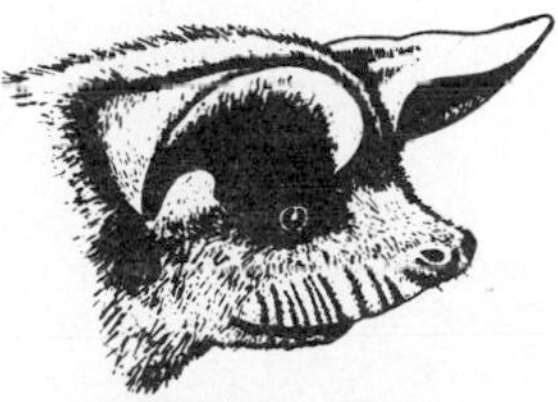

FIG. 27-4 Some common bats. *Courtesy of K. E. Murray, Bureau of Vector Control, California State Department of Public Health. Drawn by Joe E. Brooks, Bureau of Vector Control.*

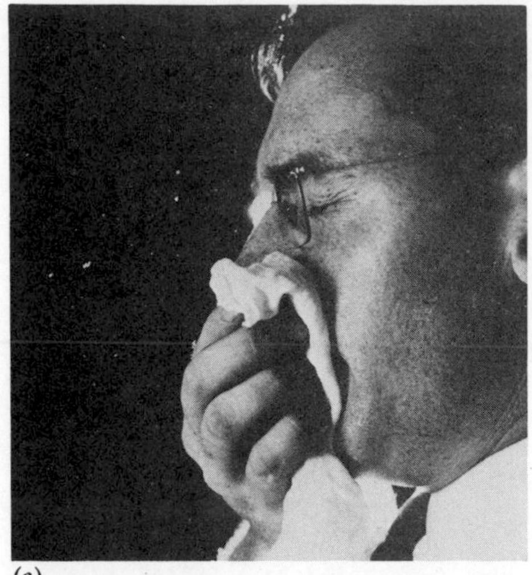
(a)

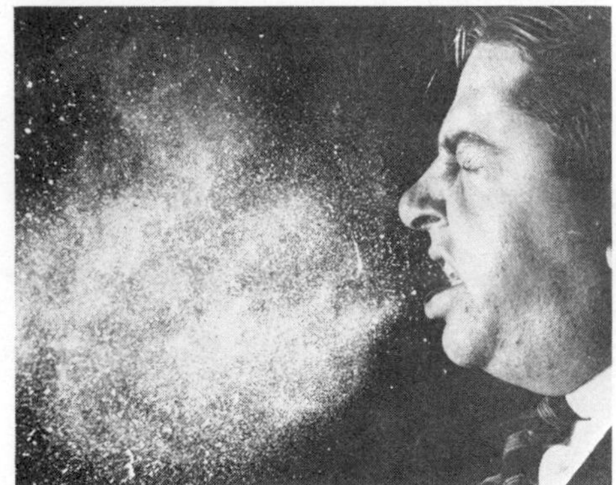
(b)

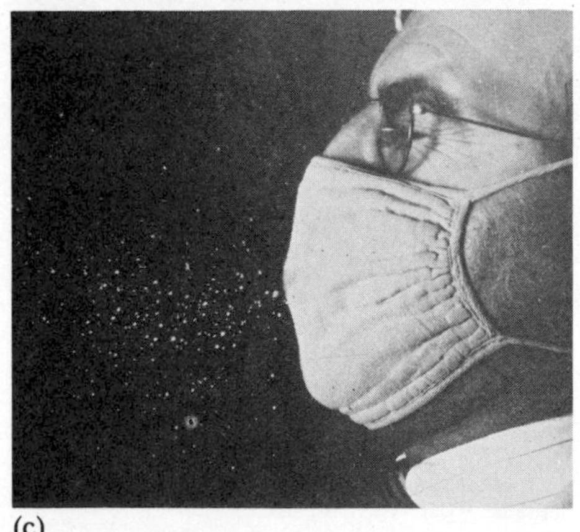
(c)

FIG. 27–5 Sneezing. (a) Even this stifled sneeze produces many droplets. It is clear from the photo that the hands and arms can easily become contaminated with nasal secretions. (b) A full-blown, unstifled sneeze. Note the heavy cloud of material introduced into the air. (c) Despite the presence of a surgical mask, droplets from an unstifled sneeze are still propelled into the air. *Courtesy of M. W. Jennison, Department of Bacteriology and Botany, Syracuse University, and the American Society of Microbiology, LS-5, LS-15.*

tive humidity of the atmosphere. The higher the humidity, the slower is the rate of evaporation.

Depending on the types of microorganisms and the composition of droplets present, bacteria and related organisms may survive for long periods of time. This is especially true with droplets containing saliva, sputum, or other discharges. What remains of a droplet after evaporation is called the *droplet nucleus.* Droplet nuclei do not settle quickly after being disturbed, but remain suspended in the air for long periods of time, thus potentially giving rise to *droplet nucleus airborne infections.* This means of transmission contrasts with dust-particle-borne microorganisms, which settle quickly. Droplet nuclei are reported to settle at a rate of 0.04 feet per minute, while dust particles settle at a rate of 1 to 5 feet per minute.

Obviously, coughs or sneezes, stiffled or not, produce a microbial spray (Figure 27–5). In an effort to prevent hospital-acquired **(nosocomial)** infections, hospital personnel frequently wear masks to reduce the possibility of producing droplet nuclei. Unfortunately, preventing such sprays is impossible. Procedures and practices used to minimize disease transmission by such means include the application of bactericidal compounds to floors and the use of special floor coverings to help trap dust.

Fomites

Inanimate objects or substances capable of absorbing and transferring infectious microorganisms are called **fomites.** A wide variety of materials can spread human diseases. These include clothing, eating utensils, instruments, bed linens, toys, and even fossils (Figure 27–6). Reports indicate that Indian relics and fossils from endemic areas pose a definite public health hazard. Dust and dirt that have accumulated on such objects may contain spores of infectious agents. Individuals could inhale this material while cleaning the relics.

Plant pathogens are transmitted by such fomites as gardening tools, gloves, and soil.

Accidental Inoculation

Infections can develop from the direct introduction of pathogens during surgery. Occasionally, individuals working with clinical specimens may introduce a pathogen into their bodies through a preexisting cut or an accidental wound with a contaminated hypodermic needle or inoculating loop. Any work with infectious materials should be done with great care. In the laboratories associated with microbiology, carelessness can lead to many possible hazards. Among the situations too often encountered are improperly sterilized inoculating needles, culture tubes or flasks left unplugged in incubators, partially opened culture flasks, inadequately disinfected microbial-culture spills, and eating and drinking in laboratories.

Arthropods and Disease

Throughout the centuries, "bugs" have thwarted human efforts to establish stable and safe environments. As new cities or agricultural communities developed, devastating diseases associated with arthropods made their appearance. During the sixth century B.C., malaria and plague flourished in newly established cities. One of the few recourses left to human beings was to escape from these centers of disease, to return only long after the epidemic dangers had passed.

Although various arthropods were known to live on the outer surfaces of mammals, until the nineteenth century little was known of the relationship between insects and disease agents. Toward the end of the nineteenth century, scientists launched an intensive, systematic study of infectious diseases. One product of this work was the demonstration in 1893 by T. Smith and F. L. Kilbourne that ticks transmit the protozoa *Babesia bigemina*, which causes Texas cattle, or red-water, fever. This disease had been recognized in the United States since 1796, but its true etiology or cause was masked until the investigations by Smith and Kilbourne.

The discovery of this arthropod-microbial association provided a model that investigators could use to show the significance of other arthropods to disease epidemiology. Sir Ronald Ross (Figure 27-7) applied the model in this way, demonstrating the importance of *Anopheles* spp. mosquitoes to malaria.

In recent years, knowledge of arthropod-borne diseases has increased immeasurably. Along with several areas of related research, this knowledge forms the specialization referred to as medical entomology. This field of study is concerned with the recognition and description of arthropods, the distribution of arthropod-associated diseases, the effects of disease agents on the arthropod vector, the effects of the disease agent on the host, and the control of arthropods.

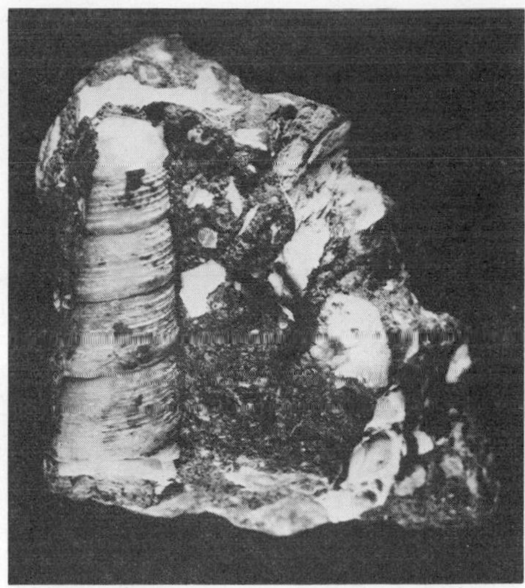

FIG. 27-6 A fossilized sea shell, taken from a dry creek bed in Simi Valley, California. This shell was incriminated as a source of the fungus *Coccidioides immitis*, the causative agent of cocccidioidomycosis. A case of this disease apparently developed from the inhalation of fungal spores during the cleaning of the shell. *Rothman, P. E., et al.*, Amer. J. Dis. Child. *118:792 (1969)*. Sir Ronald Ross (1857–1932). *Courtesy of the National Library of Medicine, Bethesda, Maryland.*

THE ARTHROPODA

Arthropoda is the largest of the animal phyla. As of 1964, about 740,000 species of this phylum were known. Many of these species are of medical and economic importance. Partially their significance lies in their ability to produce serious injuries, or even sensitization, as in the case of centipedes, wasps, and spiders. But Arthropoda is also important because several arthropods serve either as intermediate hosts for parasites or as vectors for pathogenic microorganisms. It is the latter aspect that concerns us in this section.

Although arthropods vary greatly, they all share several major characteristics: (1) a rigid or semirigid exoskeleton composed of chitin; (2) a complete digestive tract; (3) an open circulatory system (with or without a dorsally situated heart) that forms a body cavity (hemocoel); and (4) excretory, nervous, and respiratory systems. Members of the class Insecta have segmented bodies and jointed legs.

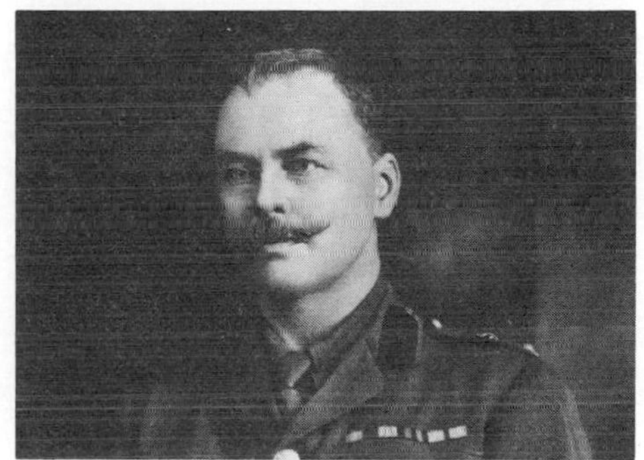

FIG. 27-7 Sir Ronald Ross (1857–1932). *Courtesy of the National Library of Medicine, Bethesda, Maryland.*

A classic example of an arthropod that transmits disease agents mechanically is the common house fly, *Musca domestica*. The etiologic agents of such diseases as infectious hepatitis, polio, and salmonellosis may be picked up by flies during contact with fecal matter containing viable infectious microorganisms. These pathogens may contaminate various body parts of the fly and may be deposited on food when the fly rests or feeds on it. Factors affecting the survival of pathogens, the availability of arthropods, and the rapidity of transfer are all important in the mechanical transmission of pathogens by arthropods.

Most arthropod-borne diseases are transmitted biologically. Many animal and plant pathogens require an arthropod for purposes of development, multiplication, or both. Susceptible hosts become infected through the bites of such pathogen-carrying arthropod vectors.

ARACHNOIDEA OR ARACHNIDA

Ticks and mites. Ticks and mites are important medically because they can (1) serve as reservoirs of infection, (2) transmit infectious disease agents (Table 27-3), and (3) directly cause disease, such as tick paralysis. Two main groups of ticks are recognized, the hard- and soft-shelled ticks (Figure 27-8).

The life cycle of both ticks and mites begins with an egg. Six-legged larvae hatch from the eggs and develop into eight-legged nymphs. These forms later become adults. Certain infectious disease agents are known to pass into the eggs of infected ticks (through *transovarian passage*, or *transmission*) and into the larvae of mites. In this way, the disease agents are transmitted to succeeding

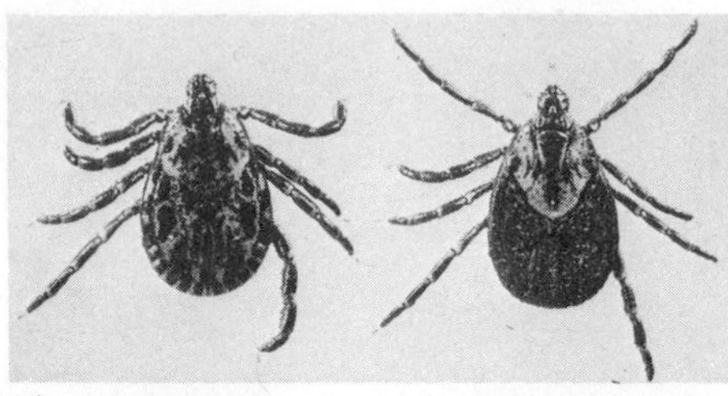
(a)

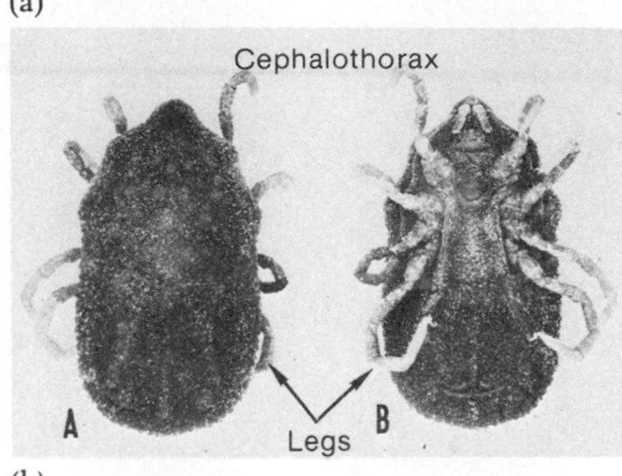

(b)

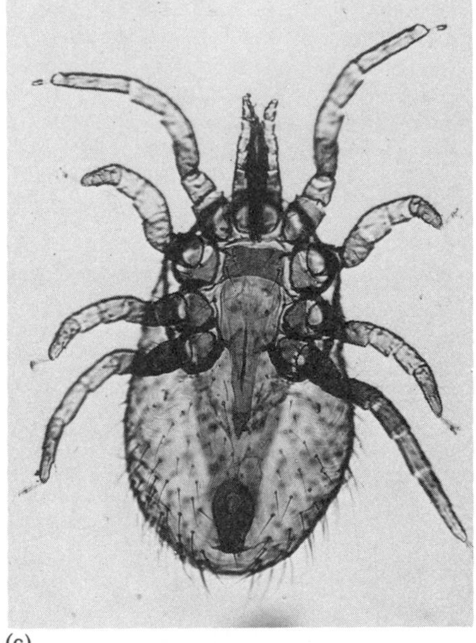
(c)

FIG. 27-8 Ticks and a mite. (a) A dorsal (top) view of a male and a female hard-shelled dog tick *(Dermacentor variabilis)*. (b) Dorsal and ventral views of a female soft-shelled tick *(Ornithodoras concanensis)*. (c) A female mite *(Liponyssus bacoti)*. *Courtesy of the Rocky Mountain Laboratory, U.S. Public Health Service, Hamilton, Montana.*

TABLE 27-3 Representative Tick-Borne Diseases of Humans

Vector	*Disease*	*Etiologic Agent*	*Geographic Distribution (Endemic Areas)*
Americanum spp. *Dermacentor* spp. *Amblyomma* spp.	Q fever	*Coxiella burnetii*	Worldwide
Ixodes spp.	Queensland tick typhus	*Rickettsia australis*	Australia
Hyalomma spp. *Dermacentor* spp.	Tick-borne hemorrhagic fever	*Flavivirus*	Asia Minor, Southeastern Europe, U.S.S.R.
Ornithodoros spp.	Tick-borne relapsing fever	*Borrelia recurrentis* and *Borrelia* spp.	Central and Northern America, Central Asia, Rocky Mountains and Pacific Coast in the United States
Amblyomma spp. *Haemaphysalis* spp. *Hyalomma* spp. *Rhipicephalus* spp.	Tick-borne typhus	*Rickettsia conori*	Africa, Mediterranean areas
Amblyomma spp. *Dermacentor virabilis* *Dermacentor* spp.	Rocky Mountain spotted fever	*Rickettsia rickettsii*	Portions of Canada and South America, Mexico, the United States
Amblyomma spp. *Americanum* spp. *Dermacentor* spp. *Haemaphysalis* sp. *Rhipicephalus* sp.	Tularemia	*Francisella tularensis*	Western United States

Source: Adapted from Cheng, T. C.: *The Biology of Animal Parasites.* Philadelphia: W. B. Saunders Company, 1964.

generations. Thus, these particular arthropods represent important reservoirs of infectious-disease agents.

Distinguishing between mites and the two classes of ticks can be confusing. The following characteristics differentiate them: (1) ticks are larger than mites; (2) ticks have little or no body hairs while long hairs are present on the membranous body of mites (when ticks do have hairs, the hairs are short); (3) the bodies of ticks are leathery in appearance; and (4) ticks have an exposed, teeth-bearing ***hypostome*** (a rodlike organ at the base of the beak) used for attachment purposes.

Several species of mites infest humans and can thereby transmit certain diseases, including rickettsialpox and scrub typhus. Furthermore, sarcoptic acariasis, a noninfectious disease, is caused by the skin-burrowing mite *Sarcoptes scabies.* The term ***acariasis*** is used to denote a mite infestation (Figure 27–9).

THE INSECTA

Lice. Lice are parasitic on the surfaces of birds and several mammalian species—cats, cattle, dogs, goats, horses, and man. Generally, the mouth parts of lice are adapted either for sucking the blood and tissue fluids of mammals or for chewing epitheloid structures associated with the skin of their hosts.

Two genera of lice (Figure 27–10) are associated with humans, *Pediculus* and *Phthirus.* Members of the latter genus are known as the pubic, or crab, lice. The two recognized forms of *Pediculus* are *P. humanus var. corporis* (body louse) and *P. humanus var. capitis* (head louse). The two varieties are distinguished on the

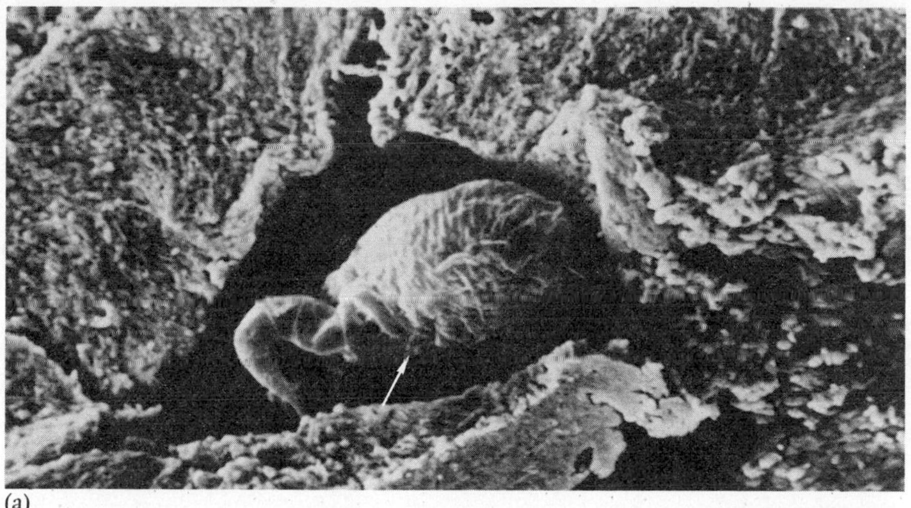

(a)

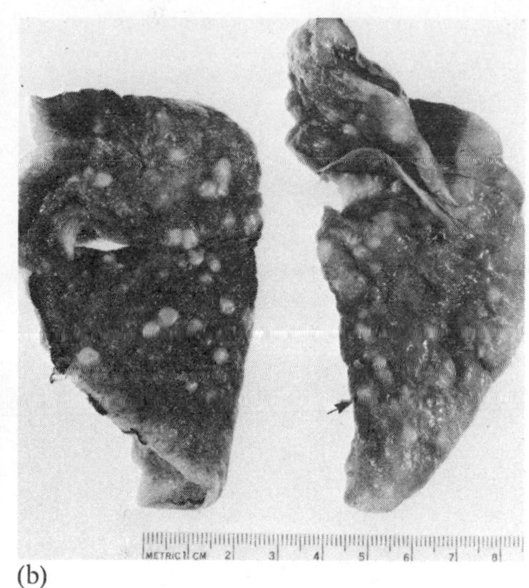

(b)

FIG. 27–9 A mite. These arthropods are frequently considered to be disease agent vectors, but traditionally they are neglected as disease agents in their own right. (a) This scanning micrograph shows a mite (arrow) in lung tissue. *Kim, J. C. S.,* J. Med. Primato *5:3–12 (1976).* (b) The lung damage in this Rhesus monkey was caused by mite infestation. *Kim, J. E. C., et al.,* Inf. Immun. *5:137–142 (1972).*

basis of size (head lice are slightly smaller), and the fact that body lice seldom infest the head region of the host. Head lice apparently roam over the entire body.

Several infectious diseases are transmitted by these lice. Diseases such as cholera, impetigo, and trachoma are spread by mechanical means. The rickettsial diseases of epidemic typhus and trench fever, and the bacterial infection of relapsing fever are biologically transmitted.

The life cycle of lice is composed of the egg (nit), nymph, and adult stages. Male and female organs are in separate insects. Blood meals can be taken by both the nymph and adult forms. Human lice can be found clinging to hair or clothing. A primary measure for controlling human lice is effective personal cleanliness. This precaution is especially important in crowded areas and during disasters such as earthquakes and floods. Control of these insects can also be accomplished through the judicious use of appropriate chemical agents.

THE HEMIPTERA

Most of the hemiptera are plant-eaters. However, several species apparently have abandoned plant feeding, and now eat insects. Probably no other group of arthropods exerts as pronounced an effect on human welfare as these insects. Several species, such as aphids (Figure 27–11) and plant lice, cause extensive plant destruction. Others are vectors for viral plant disease agents and for protozoan pathogens of man and animals. Certain reduviid insects, commonly referred to as "assassin bugs," attack higher forms of animals, including man. Chagas' disease (American trypanosomiasis) is transmitted by species of the genera *Panstrongylus, Rhodnius,* and *Triatoma.*

These bloodsucking insects vary in size. They are usually black or brown and occasionally have bright red or yellow markings (see Color Photograph 91). Life cycles of the reduviid bug comprise an egg, nymph, and adult stage. Male and female organs are in separate insects.

FIG. 27–10 The body louse *(Pediculus humanus var. corporis).*

Fleas. Fleas (Figure 27–12) are bloodsucking ectoparasites ("outer-surface" parasites) with long, compressed, wingless bodies ranging in size from 1.5 to 4.0 mm (males are generally smaller than females).

During their life cycle, fleas pass through the egg, larva, pupa (cocoon), and adult stages. The pattern of development is an example of complete metamor-

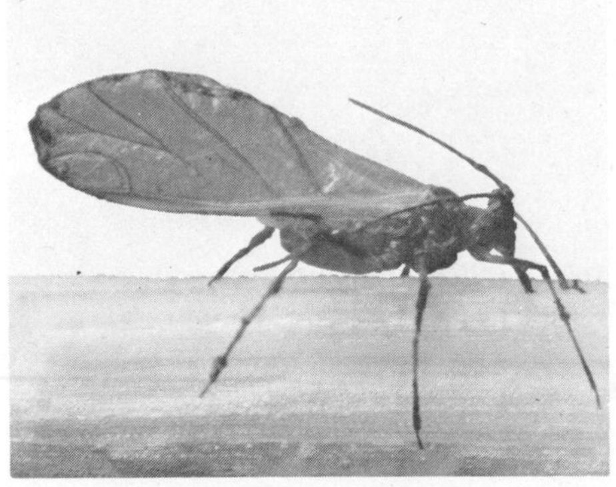

FIG. 27-11 An aphid feeding on a juicy plant. This insect is a transmitter of a variety of plant pathogens. *Courtesy of W. F. Rochow, Cornell University, Ithaca, N.Y.*

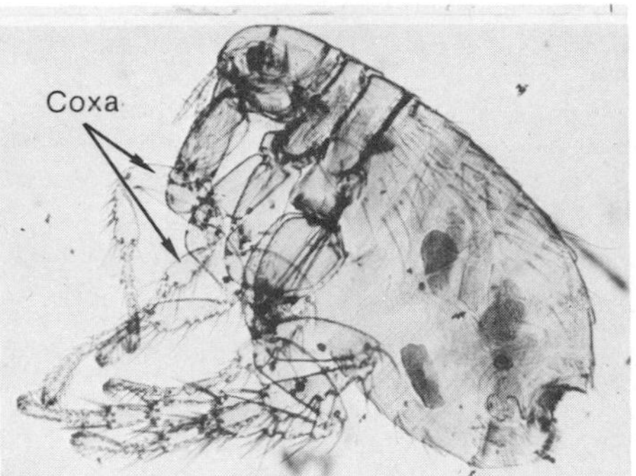

FIG. 27-12 The human flea *(Pulex irritans). Courtesy of the Bureau of Vector Control, California State Department of Public Health.*

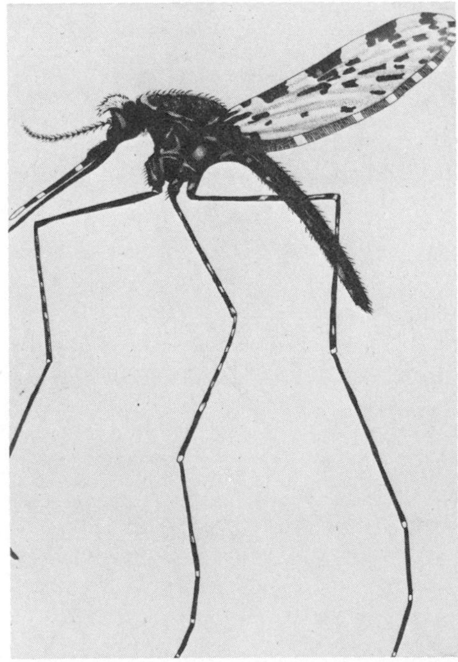

FIG. 27-13 One vector of malaria, *Anopheles gambiae. Courtesy of World Health Organization, Geneva.*

phosis; inside silky cocoons the larvae are transformed into highly complex adult female and male fleas. When the pupal development is complete, adult fleas emerge. The larvae feed mainly on any nutritive debris, including blood-containing feces of adult fleas. Adults feed on their particular hosts.

Fleas are of medical interest primarily because they are involved in the transmission of plague and endemic typhus. *Xenopsylla cheopis* (rat flea) is considered the most important vector for both of these diseases. *Nosopsyllus fasciatus* as well as any other species of flea associated with rats may also act as common vectors of endemic typhus.

Fleas serve as mechanical vectors for a number of helminths, such as the dog tapeworm *(Dipylidium caninum)* and the rat tapeworm *(Hymenolepis diminuta)*. Flea infestations also cause skin irritations. The chigger, or burrowing flea (*Tunga* spp.), burrows into the skin of mammals, including humans, and produces intense itching that can lead to ulceration.

Mosquitoes. Several species of mosquito are known to transmit helminthic, protozoan, and viral diseases of humans and lower animals (Table 27–4). These insects are probably best known as the vectors for *Plasmodium* spp., which cause malaria. Approximately 2000 mosquito species have been described, many in almost every country.

TABLE 27-4 Representative Human Viral Diseases Transmitted by Mosquitoes

Major Arthropod Vector	*Disease*	*Geographical Distribution*
Aëdes aegypti	Dengue fever (breakbone fever)	Caribbean area, Southeast Asia, Southwest Pacific
Aëdes sollicitans *Culex salinarius* *Mansonia perturbans*	Eastern equine encephalitis (EEE)	In the United States along the Atlantic coast to the Gulf coast, and occasionally in Kansas and Wisconsin; Mexico; South America
Culex tritaeniorhynchus	Japanese B encephalitis	Far East
Culex annulirostris *C. tarsalis*	Murray Valley encephalitis	North Australia, New Guinea
Culex quinquefasciatus *C. tarsalis*	St. Louis encephalitis	Western and Mid-western United States
Mansonia titillans	Venezuelan equine encephalitis (VEE)	South America, including Colombia, Ecuador, and Venezuela; Panama and Trinidad
Culex spp.	West Nile encephalitis	Egypt, India, Israel, Sudan
Aëdes spp. *Anopheles* spp. *Culex tarsalis* *Culiseta* spp.	Western equine encephalitis (WEE)	Western United States
Aëdes aegypti *Haemagogus mesodentatus* *Haemagogus* spp.	Yellow fever	South America; epidemic in Central and North America

Source: Adapted from Cheng, T. C., *The Biology of Animal Parasites.* Philadelphia: W. B. Saunders Company, 1964.

These "delicate flies of evil reputation" have long legs and slender bodies (Figure 27–13). Other distinguishing features of mosquitoes include (1) the elongated mouth parts (proboscis) of adult females, in most cases adapted for blood-sucking; (2) the bushier (plumose) antennae in the males (Figure 27–14); and (3) the characteristic wing veins and scales.

The life cycle of mosquitoes comprises the egg, larva, pupa, and adult stages. Moisture is a major factor in development of the larval form, or *instar.* Most mosquitoes live in fresh water, but species of certain genera—*Aëdes, Culex,* and *Mansonia,* for example—breed in brackish or salt water. These three genera, plus the ***Anopheles*** and ***Haemagogus***, are also the genera mainly involved with transmission of disease agents among humans and lower animals. Generally speaking, the most effective measures for controlling mosquitoes include elimination of breeding sites and the destruction of larval and adult mosquitoes.

COCKROACHES

The German cockroach is believed to be an important vector in the mechanical transmission of several infectious diseases. These include amebic dysentery, infectious hepatitis, salmonellosis, and shigellosis. Cockroaches are widely distributed and survive under a great variety of conditions.

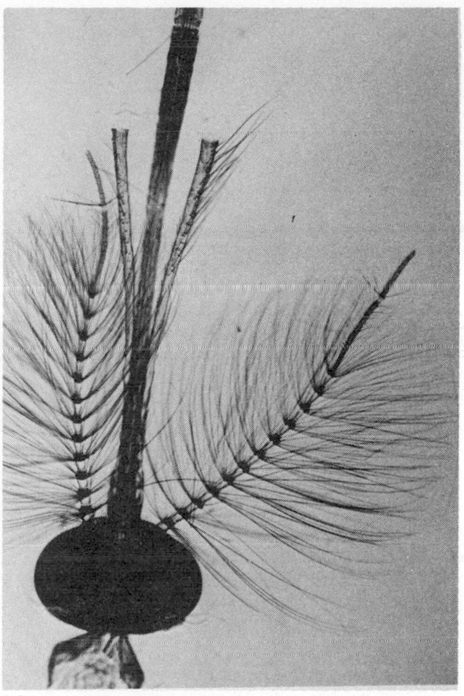

(a)

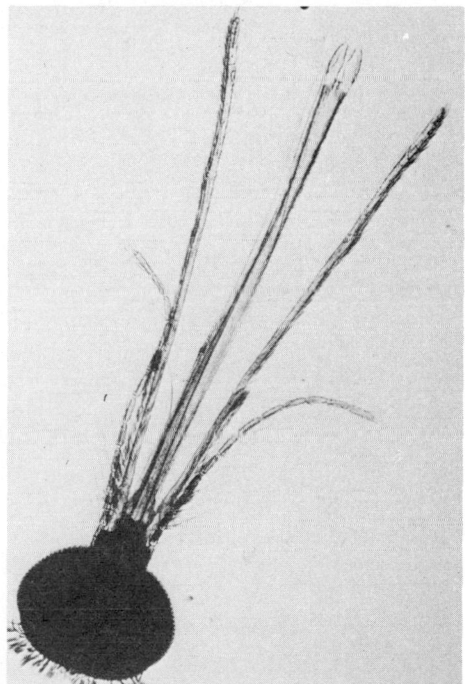

(b)

FIG. 27–14 A comparison of anopheline mosquito antennae. Note the jointed nature of these structures. (a) Male antennae. (b) Female antennae.

The Hospital Environment

Hospital Infections

The hospital environment is a potential reservoir of infection, for it houses both patients with a variety of pathogenic microorganisms and a large number of susceptible individuals. Today, ***nosocomial***, or hospital-acquired, infections pose serious and far-reaching problems. For example, since 1950 marked increases have been noted in bacteremia and deaths caused by staphylococci and Gram-negative organisms such as *E. coli*, ***Enterobacter*** spp., ***Pseudomonas*** spp., and ***Proteus*** spp.

Many factors contribute to the problem of nosocomial infections (Figure 27–15). They include: (1) overcrowding and staff shortages in hospitals; (2) the closing of most communicable-disease hospitals; (3) the indiscriminate, frequent, and prolonged use of broad-spectrum antibiotics; (4) the tendency toward longer, more complicated surgical procedures; (5) a false sense of security that has fostered neglect of aseptic techniques; and (6) the use of immunosuppressing agents such as steroids, anticancer drugs, and irradiation. Such practices have provided fertile fields for previously harmless bacteria, which have emerged as the cause of more than 60 percent of all hospital-acquired infections. It is estimated that approximately 5 percent of all patients admitted to hospitals for reasons other than infectious states develop nosocomial infections.

Reported sources of contamination in outbreaks of nosocomial infections have included intravenous infusion products, respiratory therapy equipment, stethoscopes, medicinals and lotions, catheters, and shaving brushes used in the preoperative shaving of patients. A recent study has implicated rolls of adhesive tape, which are exposed to a variety of patients, as potential sources of nosocomial infections. This finding is not surprising, since adhesive tape is used in a variety of ways, used and unused portions of tape are exposed to patient secretions, and contaminated rolls of tape may in turn contaminate the hands of personnel.

Hospital personnel are considered to be important sources of infectious agents, as various parts of their bodies and clothes may serve to transport pathogens. In fact, nosocomial diseases may involve a major proportion of the individuals, equipment, and materials with which patients come into contact.

Certain areas of hospitals are considered to involve an especially high risk regarding the transmission of diseases. Among these areas is the central supply unit, where most equipment used in patient care is cleansed and stored until needed again. Nurseries are another such area, because of the limited resistance of newborn infants to infection. Also, operating rooms and obstetrical delivery rooms are considered to be high-risk areas in disease transmission, since broken skin is a common portal of entry for pathogenic organisms.

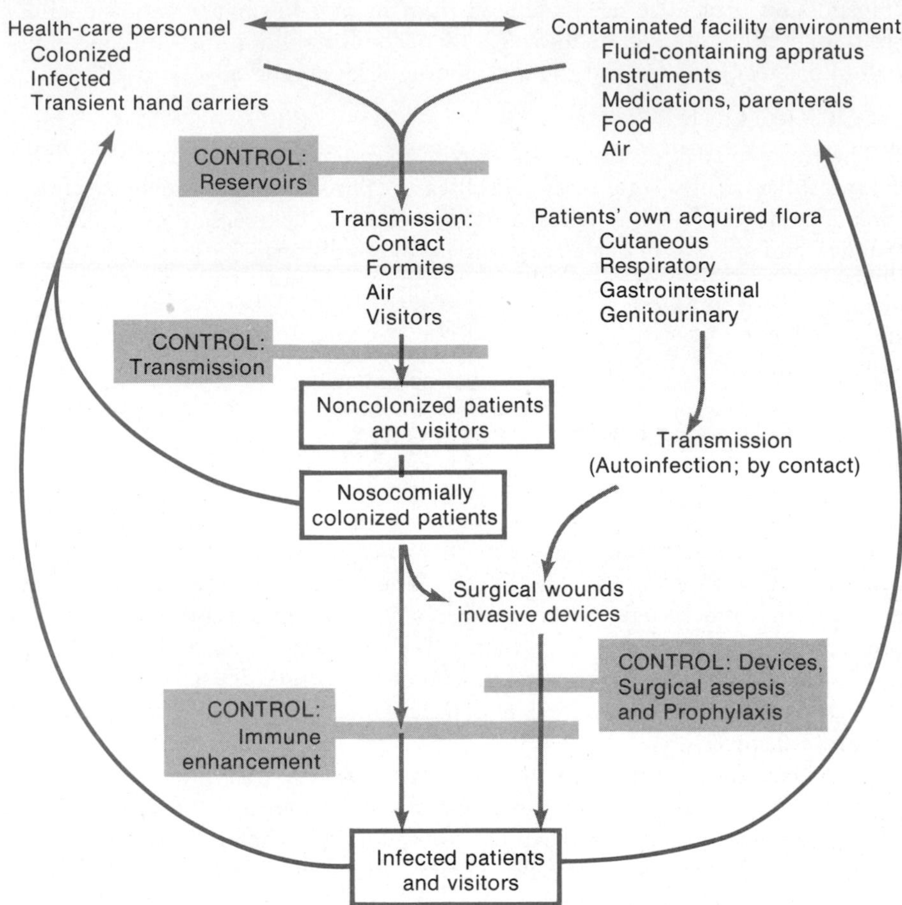

FIG. 27-15 The epidemiology of nosocomial infection including sources of infections agents and some control measures.

MEDICAL DEVICES AND INFECTION

The use of various medical devices for diagnosis or treatment increases the risk of infection. These foreign objects, which are placed in contact with a patient's tissues, either temporarily or semipermanently, represent one of the most important factors in the transmission of nosocomial infections. Interestingly enough, device-related infections appear to be the most preventable of the hospital-acquired infections.

Medical devices can bring about infections by (1) damaging or invading skin or membrane barriers to infection; (2) supporting the growth of microorganisms and thus serving as reservoirs of disease agents; (3) interferring with host defense mechanisms; and, (4) when contaminated, directly infecting individuals. Table 27–5 lists several types of medical devices associated with infections. Most often, device-related infections are caused by Gram-negative organisms.

Principles of Control

Health-care personnel (and perhaps the nurses more than any other category) are responsible for patients 24 hours a day. To safeguard the well-being of patients and prevent the transmission of infectious diseases, health-care personnel use the basic measures of ***medical asepsis*** and ***surgical asepsis***.

MEDICAL ASEPSIS

The term medical asepsis refers to those techniques used to reduce the direct or indirect transmission of pathogenic microorganisms—both by reducing their number and hindering their transfer from one person or place to another. A variety of techniques are used. These include washing, dusting, disinfection, and isolation.

SURGICAL ASEPSIS

Surgical asepsis involves those practices that make and keep objects and areas sterile, that is, free from *all* microorganisms. Aseptic techniques are necessary in all surgical procedures or other procedures involving the body's deeper tissues. During injections, for example, a break is made into the body tissues, rendering them more susceptible to infection. Surgical asepsis is also used throughout operating and delivery rooms and in nurseries to protect susceptible newborns. It is applied to the care of surgical wounds for several days following an operation, or until the injured tissues are healed sufficiently.

All materials used during these procedures are sterilized. Certain articles, such as linen or gauze, are obtained from the stock supply of sterile packages. The surgeon and all other personnel involved in the procedure limit the introduction of microorganisms into the operative area by wearing sterile gowns, caps, masks, and rubber gloves, and by washing their hands and associated areas adequately.

Surgical asepsis exacts very high standards of sterility to materials used in the hospital. Any object—including the outside wrappings of even known sterile supplies—not known to be sterile is assumed to be unsterile. In addition, sterile objects and packages must be kept dry, since moisture can carry bacteria to the sterile area.

In protecting patients from infection, nurses must understand and be able to apply the principles of sterile technique, since a breach in technique may become a threat to the patient's life. Even mild infections delay recovery and are expensive.

TABLE 27–5 Nosocomial Infections Related to Common and Specialized Medical Devices

Infection	*Related Medical Devices*
Circulatory system, including inflammation of veins	Arterial pressure monitors; intravenous catheters; and needles
Deep-wound infections	Artificial hip
Inflammation of heart tissue	Prosthetic heart valve
Eye infection	Prosthetic lens
Eyelid inflammation	Humidifier
Gastrointestional inflammation	Suction machine
Hepatitis	Kidney-machine equipment
Pneumonia	Respiratory equipment
Urinary tract infections	Examination equipment (cystoscope); urinary catheter

Measures of Control

HAND WASHING

Personnel should wash their hands before and after each patient contact, especially with patients considered to be potential sources of infectious agents. All areas of the hands should be well lathered and scrubbed, with special attention given to the nails and nail beds. All rinsing should be performed under running water. The washing and rinsing steps should be repeated and followed by adequate drying. A sterile cream or lotion may be applied to prevent chapping. Soaps used for purposes of hand washing should contain a bacteriostatic agent, most commonly hexachlorophene. Although the value of hexachlorophene has been questioned, this material is still widely used to control straphylococcal infections.

ISOLATION

The purpose of isolating a patient is to contain an infectious agent within a prescribed area, thus preventing the spread of infection. A patient is placed in isolation for one of two reasons—either to prevent the spread of a communicable disease to other persons, or to protect an unusually susceptible patient from exposure to disease agents. The decision to isolate a patient may be based on a particular syndrome or microorganism or the dictates of a specific hospital service, such as pediatrics or geriatrics.

Isolation by microorganism. The more significant communicable diseases that should be considered for isolation are caused by such microorganisms as *Staphylococcus aureus, Pseudomonas aeruginosa,* Group A beta hemolytic streptococci, *Mycobacterium tuberculosis, Treponema pallidum, Neisseria meningitidis,* and *Salmonella* and *Shigella* spp. Less common but still important organisms include *Bacillus anthracis, Vibrio cholerae, Corynebacterium diphtheriae, Yersinia pestis, Pseudomonas pseduomallei, Actinobacillus mallei, Leptospira* spp., and the agents of psittacosis (parrot fever) and rabies.

Isolation procedures for patients with communicable diseases are not rigid routines but depend in part on the microorganism involved and its virulence. The procedures are determined by the mode or route by which the organism is transmitted from one person to another, by the location of the microorganism within the host, and by its portal of exit, (e.g., feces, wound drainage, or respiration secretions). The type of precautions taken also depend upon the usual portal of entry of the organism into the body (e.g., the skin, gastrointestinal tract, or respiratory tract).

The nurse must explain to the patient, as well as immediate family members and visitors, the reasons for the isolation and the procedures to be followed.

Reverse isolation. To shield highly susceptible patients from pathogens in the hospital environment, reverse isolation is employed. Such patients include premature infants, organ-transplant patients, severely burned patients, leukemia patients, and individuals receiving radiation therapy. The person in reverse isolation is placed in a single room that has been thoroughly cleaned and disinfected prior to his or her admission. Everyone entering the room wears a gown to prevent pathogens from being carried into the room on clothes. No one with a known infection is allowed to enter the room.

If a more strict reverse isolation procedure is needed, the patient may be placed in an isolator, or plastic tent, which provides a germ-free environment. The isolator has a sterile air supply, and only sterile equipment is passed into it through special portholes. Attached to the sides of the plastic tent are rubber gloves with long sleeves. These features permit nursing and other personnel to render adequate care while still protecting the patient from exposure to pathogens.

Institutional Policies for Control

Health-care facilities vary greatly in the specific policies they maintain for the isolation and control (which includes prevention) of communicable diseases (Figure 27–16). Each institution should put its policies in writing, and complete details of care should be available to all staff members. Some of the generally accepted policies are listed below:

1. Correct hand washing is one of the most important measures in preventing the spread of infection.
2. Isolation gowns should be worn by persons giving direct nursing care to the patient or by persons whose uniforms are likely to come into contact with contaminated material.
3. There is no consistent policy on the use of masks, but it must be remembered that a wet or ill-fitting mask provides little or no protection.
4. Disposable equipment and supplies should be used whenever possible. Nondisposable equipment should be disinfected and/or sterilized where feasible. All used equipment should be disinfected as soon as possible and with a minimum of handling. Such items should be removed from the patient's room for sterilization or, if disposable, for incineration.
5. All contaminated material, including equipment, trash, linen, and specimens, should be removed from the patient's room by a double-bagging technique. In this method, contaminated material is placed in a paper or plastic bag, which is then passed into another clean bag held by someone outside the patient's room. The outside bag is then properly labeled "isolation" and identified as to contents (Figure 27–16).
6. Terminal disinfection is performed when a patient has recovered, been transferred, or died. This procedure includes sterilizing or disinfecting all possibly contaminated material and equipment, such as mattresses, pillows, furniture, floors, and walls.

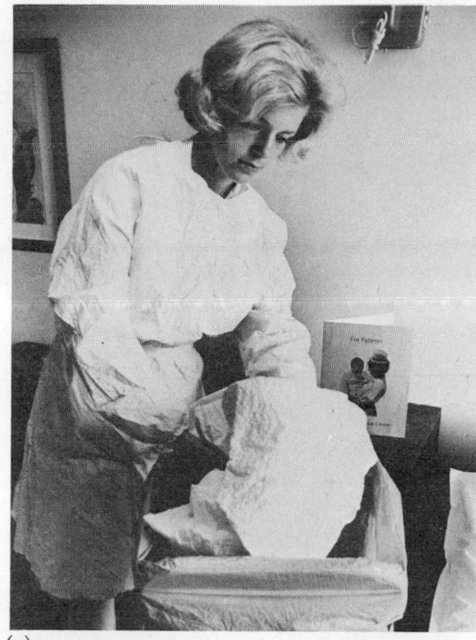

(a)

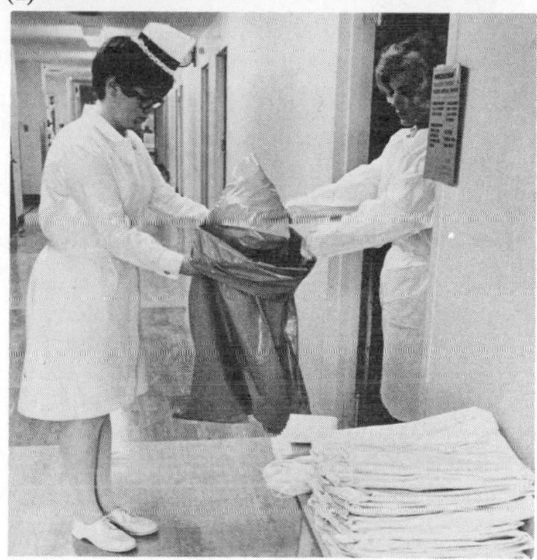

(b)

FIG. 27–16 The double-bag technique. (a) A nurse discards disposable paper bed linen and a patient gown in a plastic hamper. The nurse also wears a disposable paper gown, which she deposits in the hamper before leaving the room. (b) The bag is secured at the top and placed in an uncontaminated bag at the unit door for transmittal to the incinerator. *Courtesy of Andrew McGowan, St. Luke's Hospital Center, New York.*

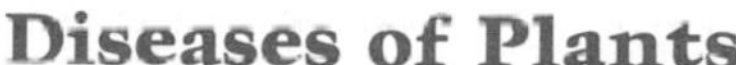

Diseases of Plants

The causative agents of plant infections and crop spoilage are for the most part of the same general types as those responsible for animal infections—bacteria, fungi, viruses, and parasitic nematodes (Color Photographs 3B and 6B). Fortunately, however, none of the organisms affecting plants has thus far been shown to be capable of producing infections in humans or other animals. Plant-disease agents are transmitted in a wide variety of ways—for example, by arthropods, through contaminated soil and tools, during grafting procedures, mechanical inoculation (the rubbing of abrasives on the surfaces of leaves), and by seeds and even certain species of fungi and nematodes. Many factors, such as host resistance, temperature, moisture, and virulence of the disease agent, are important to the development of plant diseases. In many ways, the disease process in plants closely resembles that in animals.

SUMMARY

1. Humans, lower animals, and plants can be successfully parasitized by a variety of microorganisms, worms, mites, and ticks.
2. Essential to the survival of such disease agents as pathogens is their transmission from sources of infection to susceptible hosts.
3. Epidemiology is the study of the distribution and causes of disease, both infectious and noninfectious.
4. Several terms are used to describe the prevalence of diseases: (1) *endemic* which refers to a disease that is constantly present but that involves a relatively small number of victims; (2) *epidemic*, an unusual occurrence of a disease involving large segments of the population for a limited time period; (3) *pandemic*, a series of epidemics affecting

several areas of the world; and (4) *sporadic*, which describes diseases that appear at unusual or irregular periods.

Morbidity and Mortality Rates

1. Morbidity is the number of individuals per 100,000 having a disease within a given time period.
2. The mortality rate refers to the number of deaths due to a particular disease per 1000 individuals within a given time period.

Reporting Communicable/Infectious Diseases

State administrative codes require that actual and suspected cases of certain diseases be reported to local health authorities. Variations exist among states as to specific diseases that should be reported.

Sources and Reservoirs of Infection

1. Sources of infectious agents are many and varied.
2. The most disabling and common human infections are caused by microbes capable of using human tissues for their own needs and thus making these tissues into sources of infectious material.
3. Individuals harboring disease agents without any ill effects are called healthy carriers.
4. Persons in an incubating state but still without symptoms are called incubatory carriers.
5. Individuals recovering from an infection and secreting disease agents in body fluids are referred to as convalescent carriers.

Zoonoses

Diseases that primarily affect lower animals but that can also be transmitted to humans by natural means are called zoonoses.

Principal Modes of Transfer for Infectious-disease Agents

1. Infectious disease agents can be transmitted to susceptible individuals by (1) direct contact, (2) indirect contact with contaminated food or inanimate objects or substances known as fomites, (3) inhalation of airborne dust or other particles, (4) inoculation, and (5) arthropods.
2. Arthropods, which include fleas, ticks, and mosquitoes, transmit disease agents either mechanically or biologically.
3. Mechanical transmission is the simple physical transporting of a pathogen from one location to the next. In biological transmission, a portion of the pathogen's life cycle is carried out in the transporting body. These two forms of transmission are not limited to arthropods.
4. Disease agents can be mechanically transmitted by (1) fingers, (2) flies, (3) contaminated foods and water, (4) feces (waste materials), and (5) fomites.

Direct Contact

Individuals can acquire disease agents through direct contact with open sores and other lesions, through shaking hands, and even through kissing.

Indirect Contact

Various microorganisms can be transferred by contaminated food, water, and fomites.

Air- and Dustborne Infections

Individuals can release particle-bearing microorganisms into the environment by normal activities involving the respiratory system such as talking, sneezing, and coughing. Another source of release is the redistribution of existing particles in room dust.

Fomites

1. Fomites are inanimate objects or substances capable of absorbing and transferring pathogens.
2. Examples of potential fomites include eating utensils, toys, instruments, and soiled bed clothes.

Accidental Inoculation

Infections can develop through the direct inoculation of pathogens into the body by means of contaminated needles and inoculating instruments.

Arthropods and Disease

1. Many arthropods can produce severe injuries to several body organs, cause allergies, and transmit disease agents.
2. Arthropods involved with the transmission of disease agents include ticks, mites, lice, fleas, mosquitoes, and cockroaches.

The Hospital Environment

1. The hospital environment is a potential reservoir of infection.
2. Hospital-acquired, or nosocomial, infections are the result of several factors, including (1) patient overcrowding, (2) staff shortages, (3) indiscriminate and improper usage of antibiotics, (4) longer and more complicated surgical procedures, and (5) the use of such immunosuppressive agents as anticancer drugs and irradiation.
3. The use of medical equipment and devices, either for diagnosis or treatment, increases the risk of infection.

Principles of Control

Hospital-acquired infections can be controlled through the use of techniques that reduce the direct or indirect transmission of pathogens (medical asepsis), and practices that make and keep objects and areas involved in surgical procedures sterile (surgical asepsis).

Diseases of Plants

1. The causative agents of plant infections and crop spoilage are similar to agents of diseases in animals.
2. Plant pathogens can be transmitted by a variety of means, including arthropods, contaminated soil and tools, seeds, grafting procedures, and even fungi and roundworms.

QUESTIONS FOR REVIEW

1. Define or explain the following terms:
   a. epidemic
   b. sporadic infection
   c. pandemic
   d. communicable disease
   e. endemic
   f. epidemiology
2. Differentiate between morbidity and mortality rates.
3. What is a carrier? What types of diseases are associated with such individuals?
4. What are the five Fs, and why are they important?
5. What are fomites?
6. What types of fomites might one encounter in the following situations?
   a. a physician's office
   b. a dormitory
   c. a dentist's office
   d. a restaurant
   e. a hospital room
   f. a clinical laboratory

7. List at least six infectious diseases that can be transmitted by fomites.
8. Periodically, newspapers report the occurrence of both natural and manmade disasters. Discuss the types of conditions favorable for the spread of diseases and the particular infectious diseases that might prevail in the following situations:
   a. an earthquake
   b. a war
   c. a flood
   d. a famine
   e. a fire
   f. a blizzard
9. Differentiate between biological and mechanical means of disease transmission.
10. What contributions did the following individuals make toward the understanding of disease transmission and processes?
    a. Sir Ronald Ross
    b. Theobald Smith
11. What dangers do bats pose for the well-being of human beings and the various domestic animals in their environment?
12. What arthropod vectors are associated with the following diseases?
    a. malaria
    b. Rocky Mountain spotted fever
    c. Western equine encephalitis
    d. plague
    e. typhus fever
    f. dog tapeworm
13. What methods are commonly available for the control of arthropods?
14. Discuss medical asepsis.
15. What practices are involved in surgical asepsis? How does it differ from medical asepsis?
16. What is reverse isolation?
17. Associate specific infectious diseases with the following potential means of disease transmission (mark your answers down on paper and keep for future reference).
    a. flies
    b. ticks
    c. water (contaminated)
    d. mosquitoes
    e. hypodermic syringe
    f. cockroaches
    g. mouthpiece (used)
    h. nasal secretions
    i. milk
    j. kissing
    k. fleas
    l. sexual relations
    m. dogs
    n. soil
    o. mites
    p. lice

SUGGESTED READINGS

Burnet, M., and D. O. White, *Natural History of Infectious Disease.* London: Cambridge University Press, 1972. *Interesting accounts of the history of various infectious agents—bacteria, protozoa, and viruses—and the spread and control of infections.*

Cundy, K. R., and W. Ball, (eds.), *Infection Control in Health Care Facilities: Microbiological Surveillance.* Baltimore: University Park Press, 1977. *Describes the control of disease agents in various hospital settings.*

Gibson, G. L., *Infection in Hospital.* New York: Churchill Livingstone, 1975. *Describes several sources of hospital infection involving both personnel and the hospital environment. Describes the types of infection that may be encountered from each source and covers possible control methods.*

Harris, K. F., and K. Maramorosch (eds.), *Aphids as Virus Vectors.* New York: Academic Press, 1977. *A text (one of a series) organized according to the arthropods associated with the transmission of pathogens to plants. Provides an understanding of vector-borne plant diseases.*

Kaplan, M. M., and R. G. Webster, "The Epidemiology of Influenza," *Sci. Amer.* 237:88 (1977). *Describes how genetic recombination between human and animal strains of influenza virus may be responsible for the appearance of new subtypes of virus and thus new epidemics.*

CHAPTER **28**

The Identification of Disease Agents

The first step in disease control is the identification of pathogenic microorganisms. Chapter 28 discusses general approaches to the isolation and identification of various disease-causing microbes.

After reading this chapter, you should be able to:

1. **Outline general approaches used to identify pathogenic bacteria, fungi, protozoa, and viruses.**
2. **List seven types of specimens used for the diagnosis of bacterial infections.**
3. **List five types of specimens used for the diagnosis of mycotic infections.**
4. **Discuss the precautions necessary for the transport of microbe-containing specimens for diagnosis.**
5. **Compare the general approaches and techniques used in the isolation and identification of aerobic and anaerobic bacteria.**
6. **Describe the advantages and disadvantages of multiple-test and rapid-method systems in the identification of microorganisms.**
7. **Discuss quality control and its importance in a diagnostic laboratory.**

Approaches to Identifying Pathogens

The isolation and identification of an unknown pathogen is extremely important, not only to adequate treatment, but also to disease control. Laboratory diagnosis involves the collection and transport of appropriate specimens; prompt microscopic examination of such specimens (whenever practical); the selection and use of culture media in the isolation, identification, and determination of the antibiotic sensitivity of a pathogen; and the use of both specific and nonspecific diagnostic serological tests. In recent years, there has been a trend toward developing simple prepared systems for the rapid identification of microorganisms, and toward the automation of various aspects of procedures to decrease the time required for diagnostic tests.

Upon recognizing the clinical symptoms of a particular infectious disease, a physician will request that certain specimens be taken and sent to the laboratory for processing and examination. With the proper handling, the organisms in the specimen can be identified. Careful attention to details and good communication between members of the allied health team are necessary for the most rapid and accurate identification of disease agents. Once the pathogen has been identified, laboratory findings are transmitted as quickly as possible to the attending physician.

Protozoa and Helminths

The procedures required for identification of a disease agent vary significantly with the type of organism involved. For example, the examination of feces for helminth (worm) ova and other forms of parasites usually involves preparation of a wet mount of fresh or preserved material. A permanent, stained preparation may be made to assist in identification. The identification of protozoa such as the malarial parasites involves the examination of Wright or Giemasa stained blood smears. With extensive searching, a single smear of this type may be sufficient to locate various stages in the parasite's life cycle (Color Photograph 85). Thus, repeated blood samples and examinations are rendered unnecessary.

Fungi

Fungi are inoculated on a selective medium and incubated at room (25° C) and body (37° C) temperatures. Once growth appears, these organisms can usually be differentiated through microscopic examination. Structures such as hyphae and spores plus the arrangements of spores and other structures identify the pathogen. Yeasts may require one or several additional steps. For example, ***Cryptococcus neoformans*** from clinical specimens has a broad capsule, and the presence of the enzyme urease distinguishes it from other yeast cells. This genus is the only one among the pathogenic yeasts that has the enzyme. Yeasts of ***Canadida*** species (spp.) are generally differentiated from similar organisms by the formation of pseudomycelia. Here, in a culture of corn meal Tween 80, cells remain together, forming a chain of yeasts. Thus, species in this genus are identified by the presence of pseudomycelia. Sugar fermentation and oxidation tests confirm the identification.

Bacteria

The isolation and identification of pathogenic bacteria may require relatively few or many different tests and media. For this reason, and also because many laboratories only occasionally encounter parasites and fungi, the differential identification of bacteria is stressed in this chapter. Some common problems involved in the collection and handling of specimens as well as the isolation and identification of possibly significant microorganisms are discussed in the following sections. The purpose of this chapter is to provide the reader with an overall view of the problems associated with diagnostic microbiology. Addi-

TABLE 28-1 Representative Types of Specimens Used for the Laboratory Diagnosis of Certain Bacterial Infections

Infection	*Autopsy Material*	*Biopsy Material*	*Blood*	*Spinal Fluid*	*Sputum*	*Stool*	*Vesicular Fluid or Skin Scraping*	*Throat Swab*	*Throat Washing*	*Urethral Discharge*	*Urine*
Actinomycosis (lumpy jaw)		+			+						
Boils		+					+				
Diphtheria								+	+		
Enteritis (salmonellosis)			+			+					+
Gas gangrene	+	+									
Gonorrhea										+	
Meningitis	+		+	+							
Shigellosis						+					
Syphilis		+	+	+							
Tuberculosis	+	+		+	+			+			+
Urinary-tract infection		+								+	+

tional details on individual organisms described here are provided in later chapters.

Collecting and Handling Specimens

Initially, the physician must decide which type of specimen or specimens will enable him or her to confirm the clinical diagnosis. Next, these specimens are taken from the patient as ordered and sent to the laboratory. Transport involves appropriate precautions to keep the specimen in good condition.

It is a good practice for physicians to indicate the particular reasons for the specimen on the order slip. Information of this sort can aid laboratory personnel in selecting the media and/or conditions that will make recovery of a suspected pathogen more likely. The proper media and conditions are particularly important where certain fastidious, unusual, or slow-growing organisms are involved.

In a hospital situation, most specimens are collected by physicians or nurses, but blood samples are generally obtained by medical technologists. Many different types of specimens are used in laboratory diagnosis. Representative specimens, together with the bacterial and mycotic diseases with which they may be associated, are listed in Tables 28–1 and 28–2. Additional information concerning specimens for other pathogenic types is provided in later chapters.

Certain types of specimens are taken with swabs. If these dry out after collection or during transit to the laboratory, they may prove to be unsatisfactory. The introduction of dacron swabs has greatly improved this situation, since many organisms survive well on dry dacron. One method for transporting a throat-swab specimen from the patient to a laboratory is shown in Figure 28–1. It is still advisable to transport a swab specimen in a tube containing a holding medium: any of several liquid or semisolid media that prevent desiccation of the pathogenic organisms without allowing overgrowth of normal flora or contaminants.

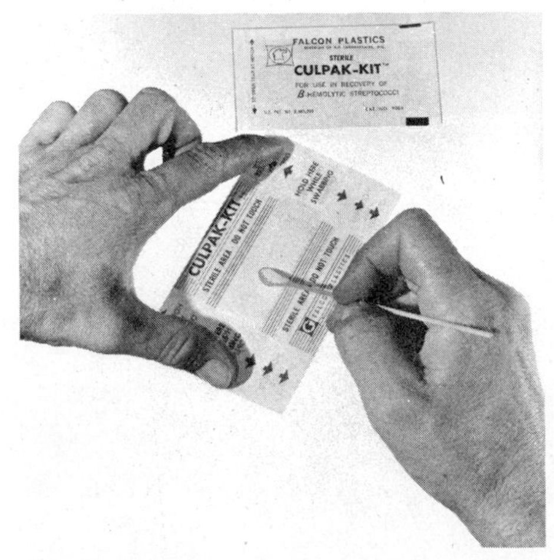

FIG. 28–1 A special plastic pack that aids in the recovery of pathogenic *Streptococci* from a throat swab when the specimen must be transported some distance to a laboratory. The organisms survive well for a day or more. *Courtesy of Falcon Plastics, Division of BioQuest, Los Angeles.*

TABLE 28-2 Representative Types of Specimens Used for the Laboratory Diagnosis of Certain Mycotic (Fungal) and Related Infections

	Autopsy Material	*Biopsy Material*	*Blood*	*Hair*	*Mucous Membranes or Skin Scrapings*	*Nail Material*	*Sputum*	*Vaginal Smear*
Athlete's foot *(Tinea pedis)*					+	+		
Coccidioidomycosis	+	+	+				+	
Histoplasmosis	+	+	+				+	
Moniliasis *(oral thrush)*					+		+	
Nocardiosis	+	+					+	
North American blastomycosis	+	+					+	
Ringworm of most skin and hair surfaces				+	+			
Vaginal thrush								+

Most specimens remain adequate for culturing for several hours if they are refrigerated prior to planting. However, bacteria such as *Neisseria meningitidis* are sensitive to the cold, so a cerebrospinal-fluid specimen suspected of containing this organism must be cultured immediately. Wound specimens should also be processed immediately, since any anaerobes present die rapidly upon exposure to oxygen. Refrigeration is generally adequate for urine, stools (feces), and sputum. Sputum collection is best done in the collection kit shown in Figure 28-2.

Urine is the only specimen for which a bacterial count is performed as a clinical test. Urine must be collected in a sterile container (Figure 28-3).

Samples of several types of clinical specimens (throat swabs, feces, blood serum) can be rapidly frozen and kept in this state for later viral examinations. Frozen samples may also be shipped in dry ice to a reference laboratory for further study. Serum for such viral or other serological testing must be separated from the whole blood and sent in a sterile tube. Whole blood if frozen proves unsatisfactory for serological tests. Clotted blood for examination should be refrigerated or transported in ice. Because some parasitic forms degenerate rapidly, stool specimens must be placed in preservative solutions to insure that the organism will be recognizable.

This brief discussion has barely touched on the problems of proper collection and handling procedures. Because many microorganisms have unique requirements, laboratory personnel must be familiar with the specific organisms in order to find them in clinical specimens.

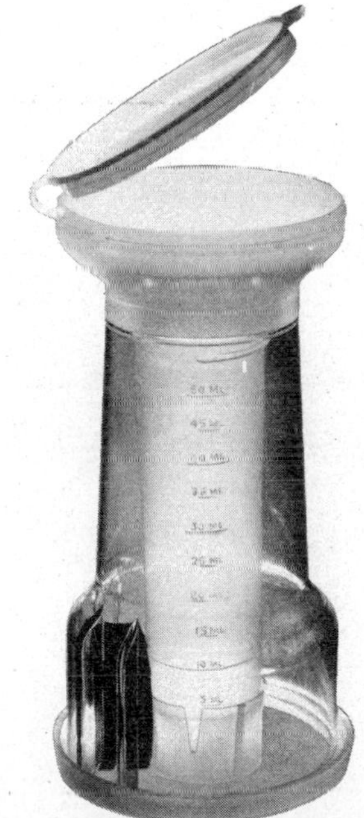

FIG. 28-2 A sputum collection kit. A tight-fitting lid covers a funnel into which sputum is coughed. The funnel directs the specimen into a graduated, threaded plastic centrifuge tube. The screw cap is shown near the bottom of the tube. To process the sputum for culture, the clinician merely removes the bottom cap and detaches the centrifuge tube from the screw cap. *Courtesy of Falcon Plastics, Division of BioQuest, Los Angeles.*

Transporting Microbe-containing Specimens

The rapid isolation and subsequent identification of microbial pathogens are important in determining the appropriate chemotherapy for the disease. Most microbial pathogens are fragile and short-lived. Because they deteriorate in transit or under unfavorable conditions, clinical specimens should be shipped to a laboratory by the most rapid means available.

Since specimens containing pathogens pose a clear danger to human life, such specimens must be packaged properly whether they are to be transported by commercial aircraft or by other means. Adherence to all requirements specified by current federal guidelines is essential to the safeguarding of all persons.

Laboratory Procedures

A small clinical laboratory that processes only a few specimens per day generally can be academic in its approach to identifying microorganisms. Each specimen can be examined soon after its arrival, and, depending on the type of organism observed in wet mount or stained smear, an appropriate isolation medium can be selected and inoculated. In examining the growth that appears, an experienced microbiologist may note several important clues to the identity of the suspected disease agent. Included in this group of properties would be odor, colonial appearance, and staining reactions.

As the volume of specimens in a laboratory increases, the amount of time that can be spent on each decreases. In this case, the laboratory must adopt some general procedures. Often, specimen smears cannot be stained and observed soon enough to allow the selection of appropriate isolation media. In such situations, media must be chosen that will isolate the significant pathogens usually associated with a particular type of specimen.

Media

A wide variety of media are available to assist the microbiologist. However, these should not be used as a substitute for careful observation. The fact that a certain organism grows and produces a characteristic colony on a medium is only presumptive evidence as to its identity. Biochemical testing and in some cases serotyping may be necessary for adequate identification.

MULTIPLE-TEST AND RAPID-METHOD SYSTEMS

The identification of bacterial species is based on schemes or keys that take into consideration a variety of characteristics, such as differential-staining reactions and colonial properties. Biochemical tests determine the ability of a particular organism to utilize or attack certain substances and to produce chemical products that can be analyzed. Traditionally, the use of a variety of well-chosen biochemical tests has offered the best means of specific or near-specific identification of unknown bacterial cultures. Reference works and identification schemes describe the results of key reactions obtained with known bacterial species.

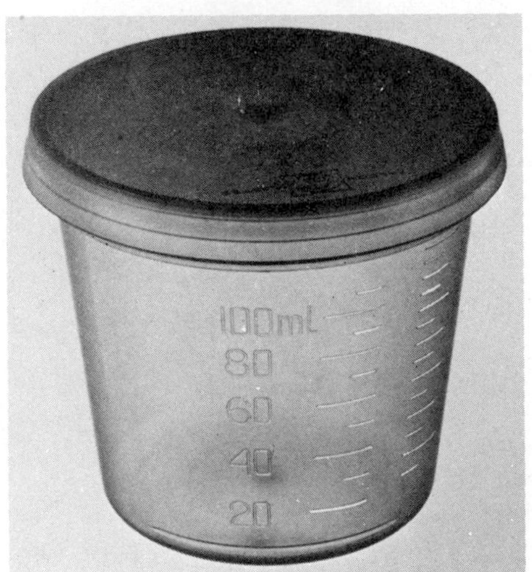

FIG. 28-3 A sterile container with a tight-fitting lid used for urine specimens. This type of container is satisfactory for sputum specimens as well. *Courtesy of Falcon Plastics, Division of BioQuest, Los Angeles.*

In many cases, the biochemical tests used to identify unknown cultures are performed in separate Petri plates and/or test tubes (Color Photographs 63 through 65). These procedures are not only costly but also time consuming. Efforts to minimize both the expense and the routine drudgery of microbiological methods have led to development of at least three types of improved biochemical testing procedures and materials. Descriptions of the innovations follow:

1. Combinations of several test substrates in one or two tubes. These are inoculated and incubated in the conventional manner. Triple Sugar Iron Agar (Color Photograph 65) is used for the differentiation of Gram-negative enteric organisms by their ability to ferment dextrose (glucose), lactose, or sucrose and to reduce sulfites to sulfides. It is dispensed in the form of an agar slant.
2. Miniaturized, multicompartmental devices that perform separate biochemical tests. These arc inoculated by unconventional methods but incubated according to standard practices (Color Photographs 94 and 95). Figure 28-4 shows several commercially available miniaturized multiple-test systems and devices. Complete instructions and identification keys are provided by the manufacturers. Several systems, including API 20 Enteric (Analytab Products, Inc.), consist of a plastic strip that holds 20 miniatur-

ized compartments, or capsules, each containing a dehydrated substrate for a different test (Color Photograph 94). The dehydrated substrates are inoculated with a bacterial suspension and subsequently incubated according to a procedure described by the manufacturer.

3. Paper strips impregnated with biochemical substrates. These are inoculated by unconventional methods and produce reactions in significantly less time than do conventional tests (Figure 28–4). One example is represented by Pathotec strips, shown in the figure. This system consists of paper strips impregnated with a test substrate. The test area is exposed to a heavy bacterial suspension during incubation. A color reaction appears within a short period of time.

The various systems and techniques such as those described are intended to make more convenient the traditional biochemical tests for identifying unknown bacterial cultures. Each has certain advantages and disadvantages, and these should be weighed before a decision is made to adopt a particular system.

The Blood Culture

Bacteremia, the presence of bacteria in blood, may be of clinical importance. Various microorganisms gain access to the circulatory system, thus spreading from a diseased area by direct extension. Once the bloodstream is invaded by pathogens, potentially any or eventually all organ systems can become involved. The speed with which a positive blood culture is recognized and the attending physician notified is of critical importance to proper patient treatment. When a patient exhibits an elevation of temperature that is unexplainable on a clinical basis, blood cultures are usually taken. Although techniques vary, in one common practice three blood specimens are taken at approximately 2-hour intervals, and these are used to inoculate appropriate culture media. Careful preparation of the skin before obtaining the blood specimens is mandatory. Although many antiseptic preparations are available, the use of tincture of iodine is still probably the best choice for adequate skin disinfection. After the tincture of iodine is applied, it is first allowed to dry and then wiped off with isopropyl alcohol. Proper technique at this point minimizes the possibility of contamination of the blood specimen by skin bacteria.

MEDIA

A variety of media are available for blood culture; these include Trypticase Soy and Tryptic Soy broths, Thiol, and Liquoid. The growth-inhibiting effects of natural sera, various antimicrobial compounds, and antibiotics can be reduced or even eliminated through dilution of the blood specimen, which is accomplished when the blood is added to the broth medium in a ratio of 1 to 10. Some microbiologists believe that adding **anticoagulants** to the media enhances the isolation of organisms. Certain compounds may also be added to neutralize antibiotics that a patient may have received prior to collection of the blood specimen.

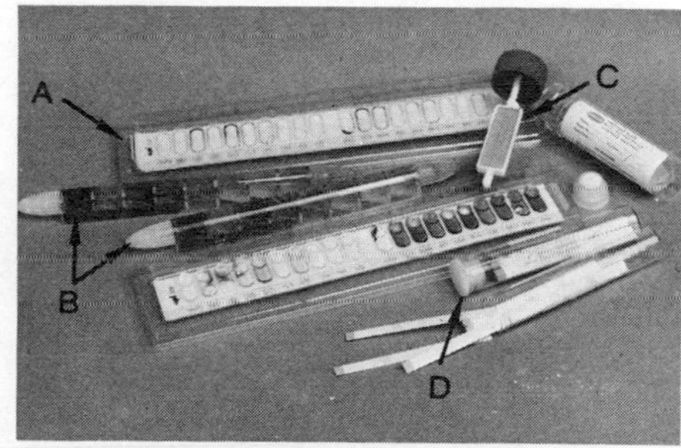

FIG. 28–4 Representative examples of multiple- and rapid-test systems used in the identification of unknown bacterial cultures. (a) API Enteric 20. *Analytab Products Inc.* (b) Enterotube. *Roche Diagnostics.* (c) Urine dipslide. *Oxoid, Ltd.* (d) Pathotec strips. *Photo by C. Righter.*

EXAMINATION

In the case of bacterial infections, blood cultures must be examined daily for the presence of growth or any indication of a microorganism's presence. If growth is detected, subcultures should be made with fresh media. These subcultures are incubated under aerobic and anaerobic conditions and microscopic examinations of the positive cultures are made. At this point, the attending physician is notified so that he or she can evaluate the patient's treatment in light of this new information. Any and all additional information, including tentative identification of the isolated organism and antibiotic sensitivity, should also be passed on to the physician as quickly as possible. The examination procedure outlined above is critical to the analysis of blood cultures.

Alternate methods for analyzing blood cultures have been proposed. Some involve the use of membrane filtration. In a more exotic procedure, liquid culture media are used that incorporate radioactive carbon (^{14}C). Bacterial metabolic activity releases radioactive carbon as $^{14}CO_2$. A special sensing device can detect the gas in this form. Figure 28–5 illustrates the principle of a radiometric BACTEC instrument, which is available commercially, and Figure 28–6 shows the BACTEC system. This device is a fully automated model that analyzes multiple cultures in a controlled environment.

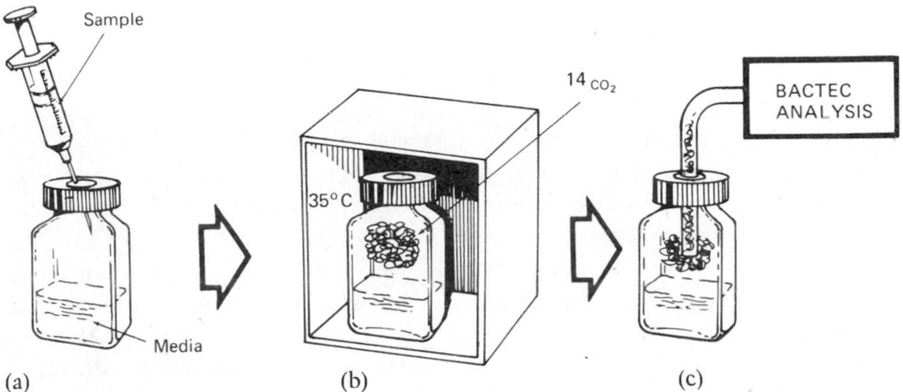

FIG. 28–5 The BACTEC principle. (a) A specimen is inoculated into a culture medium containing ^{14}C substrate. (b) Bacterial metabolism produces ^{14}CO by exploiting the organisms' own use of the ^{14}C-containing substrate. (c) The BACTEC instrument (Figure 28–6) is used to measure the released $^{14}CO_2$.

General Identification Procedures

FIG. 28–6 The BACTEC 225 automated system. *Courtesy of Johnston Laboratories, Cockeysville, Maryland.*

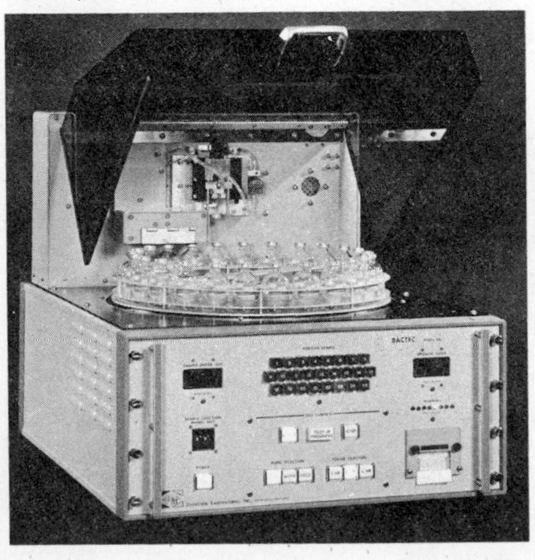

Familiarity with the pathogens most likely to cause particular clinical symptoms and with the organisms most likely to be present in a certain specimen is important to good clinical microbiology. Other chapters of this book cover the various microorganisms encountered in the disease states and associated specimens. This chapter describes the acceptable techniques associated with various specimens.

Each specimen must be handled aseptically. After the specimen is used for the inoculation of appropriate media, one or more smears should be made of it for microscopic examination. Smears or wet mounts are usually omitted with fecal specimens, except when examination for worms' ova or parasites is requested. However, some clinical microbiologists recommend the routine examination of a Gram stain of feces or rectal swabs. The purpose of this practice is to acquaint the medical technologist with the typical assortment of Gram-negative and Gram-positive organisms so that he or she will recognize an atypical assortment that might be diagnostic. For example, this would be important in cases of staphylococcal enterocolitis or *Clostridium perfringens* food poisoning.

A Gram stain of sputum is routinely prepared. A second smear for acid-fast staining may disclose an undiagnosed case of tuberculosis.

Guidelines for the Identification of Selected Microorganisms

Gram-positive Aerobic Bacteria

Certain characteristics, including colonial and cellular morphology, hemolytic reactions, and various biochemical tests, are useful in making a limited clinical identification of Gram-positive aerobic bacteria such as *Staphylococcus aureus, S. epidermidis, Streptococcus* spp., *Streptococcus pneumoniae, Corynebacterium diphtheriae,* diphtheroids, and *Bacillus* spp.

PATHOGENIC COCCI

Staphylococci. Staphylococcus aureus is often distinguished from *S. epidermidis* on the basis of coagulase production alone. Other characteristics, such as pigmentation and mannitol fermentation (Color Photograph 74), help to confirm the identification.

The following procedure illustrates how these properties are used. Specimens suspected of harboring *S. aureus* may be planted on Mannitol Salt Agar and on blood agar. Both species of staphylococci grow on these media. *S. aureus,* however, produces acid from mannitol; this process causes the medium to turn yellow around the bacterial colonies (Color Photograph 74). On blood agar plates (BAP), these organisms may cause a breakdown of hemoglobin, recognized by the appearance of clear zones around the colonies (Color Photograph 58B) indicating beta hemolysis. Organisms exhibiting these effects are tested further for the production of coagulase characteristic of pathogenic staphylococci (Color Photograph 75). Mannitol fermentation agrees well with coagulase production; pigment production is somewhat less reliable. Rare cultures of *S. aureus* fail to produce coagulase on initial isolation from a clinical specimen, but when these are subcultured, typical results appear.

While *S. epidermidis* is not considered to be a significant pathogen, it has been implicated in a number of disease states, including abscesses and bacterial endocarditis. Thus, *S. epidermidis* should be treated with respect.

Streptococci. During the primary isolation of pathogenic bacteria on BAP, the luxuriant growth of staphylococci often distinguishes them from streptococci, which form pinpoint colonies. However, in some cases all colonies will be small and the Gram-stain reactions difficult to interpret. These circumstances may be due to the selection of a specimen for a smear from mixed colonies, or to inadequate time being allowed for careful observation.

In this type of situation, the test for the enzyme catalase is useful, since streptococci do not produce catalase. This enzyme rapidly degrades hydrogen peroxide (H_2O_2) into oxygen and water. When staphylococci are removed from a culture and emulsified in 3 percent H_2O_2, the resulting activity is sufficiently vigorous to cause bubbling. A drop of H_2O_2 on a colony will also cause vigorous oxygen-gas release.

The hemolytic reaction (Color Photograph 58B) is very useful for identification of streptococci in clinical specimens. Most human pathogens are group A beta hemolytic organisms, which are sensitive to a low concentration of the antibiotic bacitracin. Thus, the reaction to this antibiotic is used to differentiate group A members from other beta streptococci that are resistant to this level of the antibiotic. In practice, the beta streptococci are restreaked on BAP, and a disk containing 0.04 units of bacitracin is placed on the streaked area. Formation of a zone of inhibition is interpreted as positive identification of the group A beta hemolytic streptococcus (Color Photograph 58B).

Other streptococci of clinical significance include group B and D beta, and several gamma and alpha hemolytic strains. The enterococci or group D beta hemolytic strains should be differentiated from other non-group A organisms, since the susceptibility of the former to chemotherapeutic agents differs greatly from that of the others. They are generally resistant to sulfa drugs and tetracyclines, and sensitive to the penicillins and streptomycin. The other groups are generally sensitive to sulfonamides and tetracyclines as well.

Pneumococci. The Gram-positive ***Streptococcus pneumoniae*** forms colonies that closely resemble those of the α-hemolytic viridans streptococci. Microscopically, *S.* ***pneumoniae*** appear as ovoid diplococci.

In one procedure for *S.* ***pneumoniae*** isolation and identification, a disk containing optochin (ethylhydrocupreine hydrochloride) is applied to a portion of a streaked area on a primary isolation plate, that is, BAP or blood azide. Optochin is a chemotherapeutic drug that was used for treatment of pneumococcal infection before sulfonamides were known. *S.* ***pneumoniae*** colonies are similar to those of alpha streptococci, but they will not grow in the immediate area about the optochin disk.

If the results are not definitive, a bile solubility test can be performed, since pneumococci are noted for their susceptibility to lysis by bile. A drop of a 10 percent desoxycholate solution or a small crystal of the compound is placed next to the colonies in question. Within 5 or 10 minutes, pneumococci lyse and their colonies disappear. Streptococci are unaffected in this procedure.

Gram-positive bacilli (rods). From a clinical standpoint, the most significant aerobic, non-spore-forming bacterium in this category is ***Corynebacterium diphtheriae***. This organism generally resides in the upper respiratory tract of healthy carriers or infected persons. Rarely, if ever, is it found elsewhere. Blood or chocolate agar supplemented with tellurite or Loeffler serum medium is used in isolating this organism. Tellurite salts inhibit most contaminants from growing and make possible differentiation among the three generally accepted varieties of *C.* ***diphtheriae***.

Several distinguishing morphological features of this pathogen are helpful in diagnosis. These include the arrangements of several cells forming letters such as L, X, and V and the demonstration of metachromatic granules by Loeffler methylene blue staining. When diphtheria is suspected on the basis of clinical signs, the laboratory must notify the attending physician immediately of any confirmatory findings. Furthermore, the local public health department must also be notified. Generally, the health-department authorities also require that a subculture of the suspected culture be sent to them so they can determine if the isolate produces diphtheria toxin.

Three other species of ***Corynebacterium*** that may be found in clinical specimens are *C.* ***pseudodiphtheriticum***, *C.* ***acnes***, and *C.* ***xerosis***. These organisms are commonly called ***diphtheroids***. They are also found in water and surface contamination studies of hospitals, restaurants, and clinics, and may be implicated occasionally in disease states. This group is usually identified through the observation of Gram-positive club-shaped rods growing on routine isolation media. Findings of diphtheroids are also reported to health-department authorities.

Other common contaminants in surface specimens, and occasionally in clinical specimens, are the spore-forming rods of ***Bacillus*** spp. These organisms are distinguished from diphtheroids by their colonial and cellular morphology. Moreover, after 24 to 48 hours of incubation, the cultures usually contain spores (Color Photograph 12). Unless there is reason to suspect the presence of *B. anthracis* in a clinical specimen, the isolated organisms are considered to be soil or dust contaminants and are reported as *Bacillus* spp.

Gram-negative Aerobic Enteric Bacteria

Gram-negative aerobic enteric bacteria are extremely common in clinical specimens and probably make up the major portion of the laboratory workload. Unfortunately, these organisms look very much alike and Gram stains of organisms from primary isolation media such as blood agar do not serve to distinguish them. Biochemical testing procedures are used to differentiate and identify specific bacteria.

The procedure for identifying Gram-negative aerobic enteric bacteria depends largely upon circumstances. If the source of the organism is stool, then the primary concern is with the major enteric pathogens *Salmonella* and *Shigella* spp. for children and adults, and with enteropathogenic *Escherichia coli* for children under three.

Whenever enteric Gram-negative bacteria are encountered in specimens other than stool, they may be significant and should be identified. They are especially serious in specimens of urine, blood, sputum or bronchial aspirates, spinal fluid, and wounds. Sometimes they are in small numbers relative to organisms such as *S. aureus*, streptococci, and pneumococci, and may not seem important. Nevertheless, they should be identified and reported to the physician. She or he can then determine the best treatment to combat the possibility that opportunistic bacteria will continue the infection after a chemotherapeutic agent has brought the primary pathogen under control.

NONFERMENTATIVE AEROBIC GRAM-NEGATIVE BACTERIA

Often when a Gram-negative rod is found and inoculated onto routine media, the colonies formed do not ferment the respective sugars in selective and differential media, such as Eosin Methylene Blue, MacConkey, or Hektoen-Enteric Agars (Color Photographs 62 and 63). When this is so, the organisms are suspected of being *Salmonella, Shigella, Proteus,* or *Providencia* spp.

Enteric Gram negative bacteria ferment the glucose in the Triple Sugar Iron Agar slant medium (Color Photograph 65). The lack of any acid production indicates that organisms from some other group are involved. *Pseudomonas aeruginosa* and *Alkaligenes faecalis* are two common nonfermenters. Of these, *P. aeruginosa* is the more important as a pathogen. The properties of several of these organisms are given in later chapters.

GRAM-NEGATIVE AEROBIC DIPLOCOCCI

This grouping is comprised mainly of the genus *Neisseria*. In the clinical laboratory, various nonpathogenic species are found in sputum, throat swabs, and cervical and vaginal swabs. These same specimens may be submitted in cases of suspected meningococcal meningitis, or of gonorrhea, which are caused by the two pathogenic *Neisseria* species. It is therefore important to differentiate these organisms from nonpathogens. The pathogenic species *N. gonorrhoeae* and *N. meningitidis* usually require blood or chocolate agar and 3 to 10 percent CO_2 for isolation. In contrast, nonpathogenic *Neisseria* species generally grow on ordinary nutrient agar in the absence of CO_2.

When gonorrhea is suspected, the specimen should be planted onto Thayer-Martin chocolate agar containing a mixture of antibiotics formulated to prevent the growth of practically all organisms but *N. gonorrhoeae* or *N. meningitidis*. Any other organisms that may grow on this medium can be differentiated on the basis of cellular morphology and the oxidase test (Color Photograph 86B). The neisseriae are oxidase-positive, as are *Pseudomonas* spp. and certain others, but the growth of oxidase-positive, Gram-negative diplococci on Thayer-Martin medium is presumptive evidence for one of the pathogenic neisseria.

Although the specimen or source of the organism is certainly indicative for species identification, most laboratories still prefer, and correctly so, to perform sugar fermentation tests. As a memory aid, note that *N. (g)onorrhoeae* ferments (g)lucose only, while *N.(m)enin(g)itidis* ferments (m)altose and (g)lucose.

FASTIDIOUS AEROBIC GRAM-NEGATIVE BACILLI (RODS)

The fairly broad grouping of bacteria called fastidious aerobic gram-negative bacilli includes species of *Hemophilus, Bordetella, Brucella, Pasteurella,* and *Francisella.* Except for *H. influenzae,* these organisms are not routinely encountered in the clinical laboratory. The reader should refer to the individual descriptions and references in other chapters.

Anaerobic Bacteria

Anaerobic bacteria are generally cultured from wound and blood specimens. They may be cultured from other types of specimens (e.g., urine) and biopsies if their presence is suspected from clinical findings.

Representative cultivation procedures for anaerobic bacteria have been discussed earlier. Generally, specimens are inoculated into thioglycollate broth and on a BAP. The latter medium can be incubated in a special anaerobic incubator, Brewer jar, or Gas Pak system.

CLOSTRIDIA

Clostridium spp. are characterized as Gram-positive, anaerobic, spore-forming rods, and are differentiated from one another on the basis of hemolytic patterns and sugar fermentations. Formation of spores by clostridia usually requires a slightly alkaline, high-protein medium, for example, Trypticase Agar-Base.

PEPTOSTREPTOCOCCI

Peptostreptococcus spp. (anaerobic streptococci) may appear in specimens from wounds, sinus and ear infections, and abscesses. Their identification is usually based upon the observation of Gram-positive chained cocci growing anaerobically but not aerobically.

BACTEROIDES

The group of anaerobic, Gram-negative bacteria known as *bacteroides* includes organisms that are non-spore-forming, rodlike, and have rounded or pointed ends. Some are filamentous or have spherical bodies. Most of these organisms are very difficult to isolate because of their extreme sensitivity to free oxygen. Genera included in this group are *Bacteroides, Sphaerophorus, Fusobacterium,* and *Streptobacillus.* Species of *Bacteroides* and *Sphaerophorus* are probably encounted most often as pathogens. They are generally differentiated by colonial and cellular morphology and selected biochemical tests.

Acid-fast Bacteria

The two bacterial genera that are routinely acid-fast (Color Photograph 11A) are *Mycobacterium* and *Nocardia.* (On rare occasions isolates of the genus *Corynebacterium* may be acid-fast and thus may create some confusion.)

MYCOBACTERIA

Mycobacteria can be isolated from various types of specimens. These include bronchial and gastric lavage (washings), spinal fluid, sputum, tracheal aspiration, and lung tissues. With the exception of tissues and spinal fluid, most specimens are digested and decontaminated routinely. One of the procedures used to isolate mycobacteria involves breaking up the mucus in the specimen, not only to separate mycobacteria from this material, but also to kill contaminating organisms. The latter aspect is accomplished by raising the pH of the preparation. Mycobacteria survive these treatments and thus can be isolated.

After a specimen has been suitably prepared, it is generally used to inoculate two different media. The media currently recommended are an egg-base medium and a clear agar medium. To speed development of the cultures, they are incubated under increased CO_2 tension of 5 to 10 percent.

Characteristically, *M. tuberculosis* has a nonpigmented, tan-to-buff, heaped colony that appears in about 2 to 3 weeks. Whenever any growth appears on the media, acid-fast stains should be performed to determine if a mycobacterium or some contaminant is present.

NOCARDIA

Specimens suspected of containing nocardiae are usually planted onto BAP and Sabouraud's dextrose agar slants and incubated at room temperature and at 35° C. Since these organisms may survive the decontamination and digestion procedures, they may be found on routine mycobacteria media. They are differentiated from mycobacteria and other bacteria by their colonial morphology and the presence of branching acid-fast mycelia, and through biochemical tests.

Unfortunately, the usual acid-fast staining procedures may not show these organisms to be acid fast. The nocardia are only slightly more resistant to decolorization than non-acid-fast organisms, and therefore greater care must be exercised.

Various species of *Nocardia* appear on BAP in several days as small colonies resembling *M. tuberculosis*. Within 5 to 10 days, the colonies become waxy, folded, and yellow to orange. Identification of species is based upon colonial morphology and selected biochemical tests.

Quality-control Considerations

The interpretation of any test result depends upon the degree of confidence the investigator has in the quality of materials used and in the personnel who performed the testing. To insure high quality, all media reagents and staining solutions should be frequently checked under suitable control conditions. For example, you cannot rely upon the interpretation of a Gram stain unless you have performed the procedure with the same reagents on known Gram-positive and Gram-negative organisms. Prepared smears of a *Bacillus* species and a *Neisseria* species are good controls, since these organisms are particularly sensitive to deviations in technique. Federal regulations prescribe quality-control tests that all laboratories engaged in interstate commerce must perform (Table 28–3).

Periodically, laboratory personnel should be required to identify microbial unknowns to test their technical ability. The College of American Pathologists and the American Society for Clinical Pathologists have developed a survey program for this purpose, but individualized programs could be developed through the cooperative efforts of local and regional laboratories of universities and public health departments.

Periodic internal controls are also important. For example, routine specimens might be submitted to the clinical laboratory by the chief microbiologist in cooperation with hospital staff physicians. The specimen submitted would not

TABLE 28-3 Quality Control Required for Laboratories Engaged in Interstate Commerce

Item	*Particular Requirements*
Laboratory Manual	1. Keep current 2. Note dates on which procedures go into effect 3. List complete references 4. List criteria for quality control
Records	1. Show any and all changes in procedure 2. Give evidence of monitoring of materials and methods 3. Indicate remedial action when necessary
Stains	1. Incorporate procedures for control
Media	1. Incorporate procedures for testing prior to or concurrent with use
Serology	1. Test positive controls 2. Test negative controls 3. Test selected weak or variable controls

differ in appearance from many others, but it would be specially designed to familiarize the technologists with unusual organisms or pathogens not often encountered—for example, *Pasteurella multocida, Brucella* spp., or *Bordetella pertussis.*

One important aspect of quality control is the preventive maintenance of equipment and the routine monitoring of equipment performance. Centrifuges must be checked periodically to see that operating speeds are accurate. Also, the minimum and maximum temperatures of all incubators, refrigerators, freezers, water baths, and thermal blocks should be monitored frequently. Significant deviations from the norm usually indicate a pending failure of the control mechanism. Such a failure could result in the cooking of cultures or spoilage of expensive frozen serological reagents.

SUMMARY

Approaches to Identifying Pathogens

1. The isolation and/or identification of an unknown disease agent is extremely important to adequate treatment and disease control.
2. The numbers and types of procedures used in identifying disease agents vary significantly with the type of organism involved.

Collecting and Handling Specimens

1. The many different types of specimens used in laboratory diagnosis include blood, feces, sputum, stool, urine, and throat swabs.
2. Specimens must be obtained with care and kept in good condition during delivery to the laboratory. Holding media (nutrient preparations) and special containers are used for the transport of some materials such as throat swabs.
3. Specimens should be sent to laboratories by the most rapid means available and according to federal guidelines. Proper handling of such materials is essential to protecting all persons.

Laboratory Procedures

The general procedures adopted by a diagnostic laboratory depend in part upon the volume of specimens it must handle.

Media

1. Differential media are used to distinguish among organisms, but complete identifications generally involve further testing and other methods.
2. A variety of traditional or standardized biochemical tests have been combined in order to reduce time and materials used in microbial identification.
3. Examples of these systems include: the combination of several tests in one or two tubes; miniaturized, multicompartment devices; and biochemical substrates impregnated in paper strips.

The Blood Culture

1. The detection of bacteria or other microbial types in blood

may be of major importance.

2. Various media and devices are available for the rapid processing of specimens.

General Identification Procedures

1. All specimens must be handled aseptically.
2. Routine identification begins with staining procedures such as the Gram-stain and acid-fast procedures.

Guidelines for the Identification of Selected Microorganisms

1. Cellular and colonial appearance, hemolytic reactions, and various biochemical tests are important to the identification of Gram-positive aerobic bacteria such as *Staphylococcus aureus* and species of *Streptococcus.*
2. Biochemical tests are of major importance in differentiating and identifying Gram-negative aerobic enteric bacteria, as well as most other aerobic Gram-negative bacteria.
3. Anaerobic bacteria include both Gram-negatives and Gram-positives. Since these organisms are sensitive to the presence of free oxygen, care must be taken to grow them under anaerobic conditions.
4. Acid-fast bacteria are also identified on the basis of staining reactions, colonial appearance, and biochemical tests.

Quality-control Considerations

Quality-control measures consist of the monitoring of equipment, materials, and personnel involved in the performance of diagnostic tests.

QUESTIONS FOR REVIEW

1. What importance do you attach to
   a. correct procedure in obtaining specimens?
   b. prompt delivery of specimens to the laboratory?
   c. proper inoculation of specimens?
   d. routine examination of smears and wet mounts?
   e. accurate identification of pathogenic organisms?
   f. prompt communication of information concerning a specimen?
2. Why is the careful transport of specimens containing microorganisms important?
3. Of what value are multiple-test and rapid-media systems?
4. Are there any disadvantages to using multiple-test media?
5. With the aid of media, staining procedures, and other related materials, indicate how you would distinguish between the following pairs of organisms:
   a. *Staphylococcus aureus* and streptococci
   b. *Bacillus* species and clostridia
   c. Pneumococci from other streptococci
   d. Pneumococci from *Neisseria* species
   e. Mycobacteria from *Bacillus* species
6. How important is quality control to a laboratory? Describe three aspects of quality control in a microbiological laboratory.

SUGGESTED READINGS

Bodily, H. L., E. L. Updyke, and J. O. Mason, *Diagnostic Procedures for Bacterial, Mycotic, and Parasitic Infections.* 5th ed. New York: American Public Health Association, Inc., 1970. *A good reference describing recommended methods for microbiological examination of clinical specimens from many different types of infections.*

Kurstak, E., and R. Morisset (eds.), *Viral Immunodiagnosis.* New York: Academic Press, Inc., 1974. *A contributed volume dealing with immunological techniques and their application in the identification of viruses.*

Lennette, E. H., E. H. Spaulding, and J. P. Truant (eds.), *Manual of Clinical Microbiology.* 2nd ed. Washington, D.C.: American Society for Microbiology, 1974. *An excellent reference for several fields. Covers procedures for the collection, handling, and processing of a wide variety of specimens.*

Mutruka, B. M., and M. J. Bonner, *Methods of Detection and Identification of Bacteria,* Cleveland, Ohio: Chemical Rubber Co. Press, 1976. *A collection of biochemical tests performed on certain groups of bacteria. Covers new methods of detecting and identifying bacteria and automated and computer methods of identifying bacteria.*

Phillips, I., and M. Sussman (eds.), *Infection with Non-sporing Anaerobic Bacteria.* New York: Churchill Livingston, 1974. *Contains a number of excellent chapters on the isolation and identification of nonsporing anaerobes, culture media, and biochemical tests. Stresses the importance of finding and identifying these types of organisms.*

CHAPTER **29**

Microbial Diseases of the Skin, Nails, and Hair

Chapter 29 describes several microbial diseases associated with the skin, nails, and hair. The effects of bacteria, fungi, protozoa, and viruses and the methods by which these microbes are spread, identified, and controlled are discussed.

After reading this chapter, you should be able to:

1. **Outline the general structure and organization of the skin and indicate the areas attacked by pathogenic microorganisms.**
2. **Distinguish among the general effects caused by pathogenic bacteria, fungi, protozoa, and viruses associated with the skin.**
3. **Discuss at least two each of bacterial, mycotic, protozoan, and viral diseases of the skin, including the causative agent, means of transmission, and control measures.**
4. **List the general differences of approaches used for the identification of microorganisms pathogenic for the skin, nails, and hair.**
5. **Discuss the roles of opportunistic fungi in causing disease.**
6. **Distinguish between superficial mycoses and deep-seated mycoses.**
7. **Explain the relationship of varicella-zoster virus to chickenpox and shingles.**
8. **Describe the general types of complications that can be associated with microbial diseases of the skin, nails, and hair.**

Human beings are both the primary source and the target of various pathogenic, or potentially pathogenic, microorganisms. From birth to death we live in an environment that is rarely free of such organisms. Moreover, many body regions such as the gastrointestinal tract, nose, skin, and throat serve as additional sources of pathogens. Diseases of the skin are caused by a variety of bacteria, fungi, protozoa, viruses, and worms. Many organisms capable of causing localized infections of the skin also may cause injury of internal tissues and organs (systemic infection).

The Organization of the Skin

The skin, together with hair, nails, and various glands, makes up the covering of the human body. As Figure 29–1 shows, the structural arrangement of the skin consists of two main parts, the ***epidermis*** (outer layer) and, underneath this layer, the ***dermis.*** A ***subcutaneous tissue*** layer composed of loose connective tissue is located below the dermis and serves to attach the skin to underlying structures. The thickness of the skin and of the individual layers varies in different parts of the body.

The dermis region contains dense, irregularly arranged connective tissue and various types of cells, including fibroblasts, histiocytes (phagocytes), mast cells, blood and lymphatic vessels, and nerves. Hair follicles, sweat glands, superficial sebaceous glands, and a variable amount of muscle are also found in this layer.

The subcutaneous layer contains a large number of components, including fat tissue, blood vessels, special nerve endings, nerve trunks, hair follicles, sebaceous glands, and sweat glands.

In addition to its functions of excretion, reception of external stimuli, secretion, and temperature regulation, intact skin serves as a natural protective barrier to the majority of infectious disease agents, as discussed in Chapter 21. However, hair follicles and the openings of secreting glands constitute potential portals of entry for pathogens (Figure 29–2). Certain physiologic factors are important in providing barriers to skin-invading microorganisms. These include the acidity of the skin, the presence of an indigenous flora, and a temperature that may prevent the growth of certain disease agents. Another extremely important factor, which applies not only to skin invasion but to injuries of other body regions, is the inflammatory reaction. The outcome of an infection is largely determined by this local response.

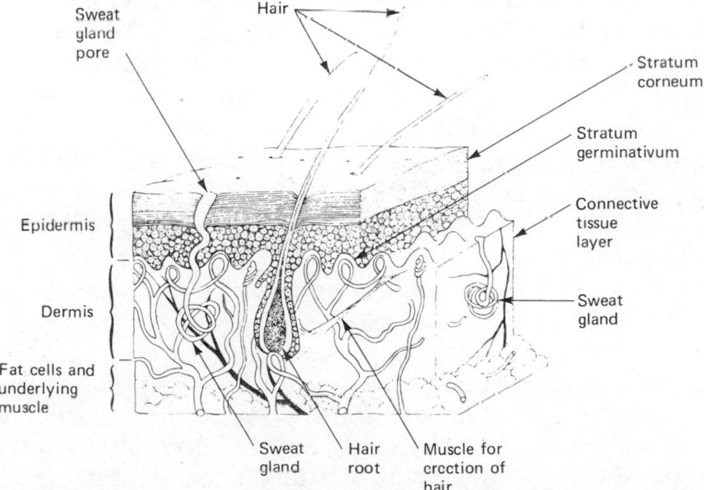

FIG. 29–1 A vertical section of human skin, showing its structural arrangement. Sites of certain infections also are indicated.

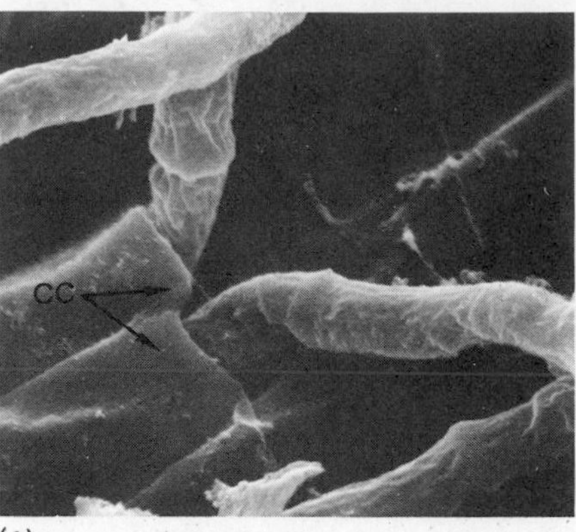

(a)

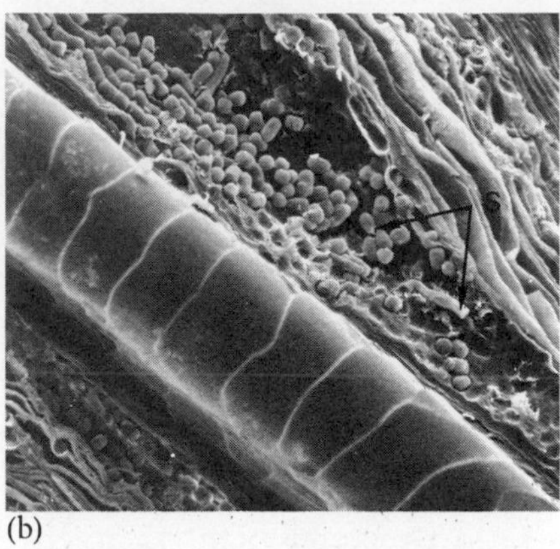

(b)

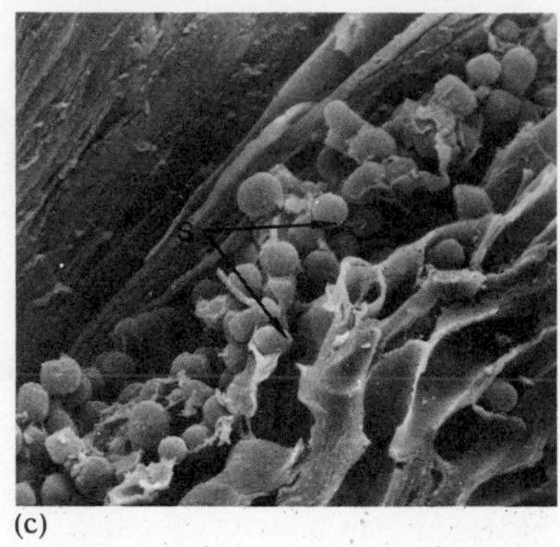

(c)

FIG. 29–2 Scanning micrographs showing the intricate invasion pattern of skin- and hair-destroying fungi (dermatophytes). (a) Hyphae can be seen here wedging under the free edges of overlapping cuticle cells, which encase the hair shaft. (b) Spore formation from hyphae in progress next to a hair follicle. (c) Invasive hyphae carve tunnels in hair that resemble wormholes in wood. Note the presence of spores in the space between the hair shaft and follicle. *Hutton, R. D., S. Kerbs, and K. Yee.*, Inf. Imm. *21:247–253 (1978).*

Skin Lesions

The breaks in the skin that occur during the course of normal living provide opportunities for infectious agents to enter the body. The nature and extent of injuries affect host-parasite relationships to varying degrees. So-called minor infections can develop into serious problems if they (1) spread and involve neighboring tissues; (2) cause bleeding; (3) produce local anemia due to stoppage of circulation; or (4) result in edema (swelling). Table 29–2 provides brief descriptions of infectious diseases of the skin.

This chapter will discuss some of the microbial skin infections in more detail.

Bacterial Diseases

The signs, symptoms, and pathological features associated with skin infections vary from localized effects, such as those listed in Table 29–1, to extensive involvement and penetration of deeper tissues (Color Photograph 79) and even death. The identification of microbial pathogens of the skin frequently depends on the isolation and cultivation of the pathogen and the results of various biochemical tests of the types mentioned in Chapter 28. Skin tests or other immunological procedures may also be useful in the diagnosis. Table 29–2 describes selected bacterial skin infections, including their diagnosis and treatment.

Anthrax

Anthrax is primarily an infection of domestic animals such as cattle, goats, and sheep. It has also been reported in other warm-blooded animals, including camels, cats, chickens, elephants, horses, rodents, and wild deer. Although the human form of the disease (Figure 29–3) was first reported in the mid-eighteenth century, it was not recognized as related to the disease of animals.

TABLE 29-1 Brief Descriptions of Selected Skin Lesions

Type of Lesion	*Description*
Blebs, blisters	Thin-walled, rounded or irregularly shaped blisters containing serum or a combination of serum and pus
Carbuncle	A deep sore or ulcer lesion of the skin and subcutaneous tissue; usually a hardened border and draining of pus are evident
Crusts (crustae or scabs)	Dried accumulations of blood, pus, or serum combined with cellular and bacterial debris; detachment of thin crusts may leave dry or moist red bases; these generally heal, resulting in a smooth skin surface; scar formations are usually associated with thick crusts covering ulcers
Furuncle	Localized inflamed regions that develop soft centers and eventually discharge pus
Macules (maculae, spots)	Usually round, circumscribed alterations in the color of the skin; the lesion is neither elevated nor depressed; the outline of a spot or macule may either be quite distinct or may blend into the surrounding region
Maculopapules	Slightly raised macules
Papules (papulae or pimples)	Circumscribed, solid, elevated lesions without visible fluid contents; the color, consistency, and size of papules vary
Pustules (pustulae)	Small elevated skin lesions containing pus; they may develop from papules; these lesions also vary in color, size and contents (pus, blood or both); pustules may consist of a single cavity or several compartments with fluid
Scars	Newly formed connective tissue that replaces tissue lost through injury or disease; these secondary lesions tend to be pink at first, then they assume a glistening appearance; scars are normal components of the healing process
Ulcers	Rounded or irregularly shaped depressions or excavations; these lesions vary in size
Vesicles (small blisters)	Elevations that may occur irregularly or in groups or rows; they may contain blood, pus, or serum; the color of the lesion depends upon its contents; vesicles may arise from a macule or papule and develop into pustules

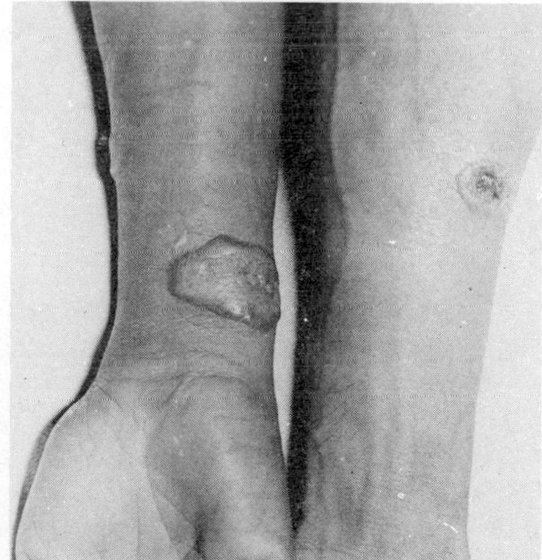

FIG. 29-3 Malignant (destructive) pustule of anthrax. *Courtesy of the Armed Forces Institute of Pathology, Washington, D.C., Neg. No. D-45409-10.*

TABLE 29-2 Features of Selected Bacterial Diseases Associated With The Skin

Disease	*Causative Agent*	*Gram Reaction*	*Morphology*	*Incubation Period*	*General Features of the Disease*	*Laboratory Diagnosis Includes*	*Possible Treatment*
Anthrax	*Bacillus anthracis*	+	Rod	Less than 1 week	A reddened, elevated, swollen pimple develops at site of infection; it may lead to bloodstream invasion (septicemia) and tissue death; oral lesions are reddened and swollen; pulmonary infection causes severe lung damage and death	1. Demonstration of organisms in tissue biopsy 2. Isolation, and finding of "curled hair lock" or medusa head colonies 3. Preciptin reaction to show presence of anthrax antigens in tissue	Chloramphenicol, erythromycin, penicillin, tetracyclines
Boils, carbuncles	*Staphylococcus aureus*	+	Coccus	4–10 days	Localized swollen areas of tissue destruction in deeper skin layers; may lead to bloodstream invasion; fever and general malaise	1. Smear 2. Isolation on blood, and mannitol-salt agars[a] 3. Coagulase positive reaction (Color Photograph 75)	Appropriate antibiotics; for penicillin-resistant organisms, semi-synthetic penicillins not affected by penicillinase
Erysipelas	Beta-hemolytic group A streptococci	+	Coccus	Unknown, probably 2 days	Fever, headache, stinging or itching at site of infection developing into widespread thickened, reddened areas	1. Smear 2. Isolation on blood agar with typical beta-hemolysis (Color Photograph 58B) 3. Bacitracin sensitivity test 4. Serological tests	Penicillin, or erythromycin, symptomatic
Furuncles	*S. aureus*	+	Coccus	Several days	Localized swollen areas which develop soft centers and eventually discharge pus	Same as listed earlier for this organism	Same as listed earlier for this organism
Gas gangrene[b]	*Clostridium perfringens* and other clostridia	+	Rod	1–3 days	Usually affects muscle tissue; fever, fast heartbeat, severe pain; infected wounds smell foul, have a discharge and accumulate gas within tissues	1. Demonstration of Gram-positive sporeformers in specimens 2. Anaerobic culture 3. Biochemical tests	Surgical removal of devitalized tissue, polyvalent antitoxin, appropriate antitoxin
Green-nail syndrome and toe web infection	*Pseudomonas aeruginosa*	–	Rod	1 week or longer	Greenish discoloration of nail plate (Color Photograph 80) Formation of thick, white scaling areas between toes	1. Demonstration of organism in specimens 2. Isolation, culture, and demonstration of pigment production	Sulfonamides, carbenicillin, gentamicin
Impetigo contagiosa	*S. aureus*	+	Coccus	4–10 days	Crust, scabs; localized pain and fever accompany the disease	Same as listed earlier for this organism	Same as listed earlier for this organism
	Beta-hemolytic group A streptococci	+	Coccus	Same	Less severe form than for *S. aureus*	Same as listed earlier for this organism	Same as listed earlier for this organism

Disease	Causative Agent	Gram Reaction	Morphology	Incubation Period	General Features of the Disease	Laboratory Diagnosis Includes	Possible Treatment
Leprosy (Hansen's disease)	*Mycobacterium leprae*	Not done; acid-fast	Rod	1–5 years or longer	Four different types of the disease are recognized: *lepromatous*—round, nonelevated patches showing skin color changes (macules); *tuberculoid*—well-defined, reddened or nonpigmented areas, loss of sensation, and nerve destruction; *intermediate*—macules, and nerve involvement, lepromin skin test may be positive; *borderline*—infectious form of the disease showing the features of both lepromatous and tuberculoid leprosy	1. Demonstration of acid-fast bacilli in smears from skin scrapings or biopsy preparations 2. Demonstration of nerve damage 3. Lepromin skin test	Sulfones, including 4, 4′—diaminodiphenyl-sulfone (DDS)
Pseudomonas pyoderma	*Pseudomonas aeruginosa*	—	Rod	1 to several days	Eroded and macerated skin surface, producing a bluish green pus and grape odor.	1. Demonstration of Gram-negative rods in specimens 2. Isolation and culture 3. Pigment demonstration 4. Biochemical tests	Same as listed earlier for this organism
Scarlet fever	Beta-hemolytic group A streptococci	+	Coccus	4–10 days	Fever, headache, sore throat, vomiting, raised reddened rash, "strawberry tongue"; peeling of body surface and tongue may occur	1. Serological tests 2. Disease symptoms are usually enough	Same as listed earlier for this organism
Tetanus (lockjaw)	*Clostridium tetani*	+	Rod	2–4 days or longer	Sudden and violent involuntary contractions of voluntary muscles, convulsions, locking of jaw muscles; fever and pain may be present	1. Demonstration of Gram-positive, spore-forming rods in specimens 2. Demonstration of toxin production	Tetanus antitoxin, appropriate antibiotics, surgical debridement
Wound botulism	*Clostridium botulinum*	+	Rod	Unknown, possibly 12–36 hours	Fever, double vision, difficulty in talking and swallowing, neck weakness	Generally the same as listed for tetanus	Specific botulism antitoxin, surgical removal of dead tissue, drainage and irrigation of the wound site, appropriate antibiotics

[a]Pathogenic *Staphylococcus aureus* produces acid from mannitol and a positive coagulase test (Color Photographs 74 and 75).
[b]*Staphylococcus aureus* and *Streptococcus pyogenes* functioning together can produce a form of this disease referred to as synergistic gas gangrene.

Robert Koch, applying the procedure now described in Koch's postulates, showed clearly that anthrax is caused by *Bacillus anthracis*.

Transmission. Anthrax is found world-wide, but is most prevalent in Africa, Asia, and central and southern Europe. Most human cases of the disease are acquired by handling infected animals and their products, such as meat, hides hair, wool, bristles, bones, and manure. Oral forms of anthrax have developed from use of unsterilized toothbrushes made from bristles contaminated by *B. anthracis* spores. Infection results from direct contact (Color Photograph 79), inhalation, or even possibly the ingestion of the etiologic agent. Insect bites have also been implicated as a means of transmission.

Control. In 1881, Pasteur demonstrated the effectiveness of a vaccine against anthrax. The preparation contained organisms attenuated by cultivation at higher than optimal temperatures, 42° to 43°C. Today, similar vaccines are routinely used. Unfortunately, these preparations do not produce long-lasting immunity—protection ranges from 9 to 12 months—so vaccination affords only partial control.

Other anthrax control methods include the disposal of infected carcasses, either by cremation or deep burial, and the disinfection of infected animal products by boiling or the use of formaldehyde.

Gas Gangrene

Several species of the genus *Clostridium* are known to cause gas gangrene. Among them are *C. novyi*, *C. perfringens*, and *C. septicum*. Most are not highly invasive, but they secrete highly injurious toxins during their growth in damaged tissues. Such toxic substances may be of a hemolytic, tissue-destroying, or lethal nature. The growth of clostridia in tissues often results in the accumulation of gas, mainly hydrogen, and of toxic breakdown products of tissues. The latter can bring about extensive connective and muscle tissue destruction, as well as serious systemic involvement.

Transmission. Infection occurs by the contamination of open wounds (incisions or lacerations) by clostridial spores. The process continues when the spores of the causative agent germinate in tissues that provide anaerobic conditions. Germinated cells undergo multiplication, grow, and secrete toxins. Infections have been associated with wounds resulting from attempted abortions, automobile accidents, frostbite, and military combat.

Leprosy (Hansen's Disease)

Leprosy is a chronic infectious disease of humans caused by the acid-fast rod *Mycobacterium leprae* (Figure 29–4). This microorganism was first observed in the skin lesions of leprosy patients in 1873 by Armauer Hansen. Although *M. leprae* was one of the first microorganisms reported to cause a human disease, so far it has not been convincingly cultured *in vitro*. Moreover, its introduction into experimental animals has only recently resulted in the development of a typical disease state. Thus after more than one hundred years, Koch's postulates are close to being fulfilled.

Several of the early descriptions of leprosylike diseases have made it very difficult to determine when the infection first appeared. Contrary to common opinion, the skin eruptions described in the Old Testament (Leviticus) were not what we now call leprosy. The word "lepra" was applied by early physicians to all scaly skin eruptions. The purpose of this practice was simply to avoid confusing such disease states with any of the better-recognized infections. Despite the vagueness of early descriptions, leprosy is thought to have been present in various parts of Africa and the Far East before the Christian era. Leprosy subsequently spread through the European continent as a consequence of military actions and an increase in migration.

It appears likely that leprosy was introduced into the American continent from Europe and Africa. Today, the disease occurs mainly in tropical areas.

Predisposing factors. Leprosy is usually acquired during childhood, although exposure and resultant infections are known to occur in adults. In general, the longer and more intimate the contact is with infectious persons, the more likely the infection will be transmitted.

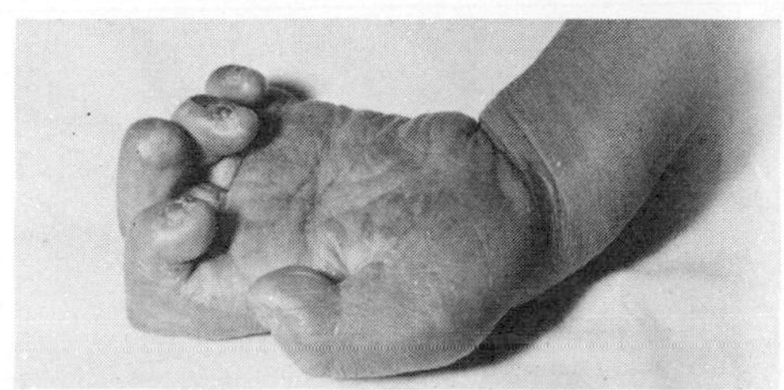

(a)

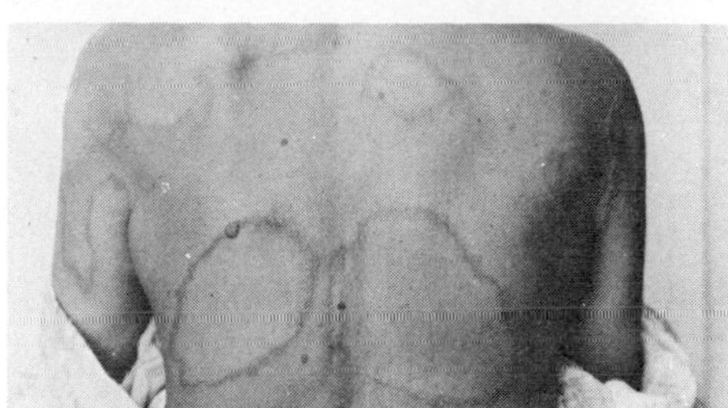

(b)

FIG. 29–5 (a) The deformed "claw" hand associated with lepromatous leprosy. *Courtesy of the Armed Forces Institute of Pathology, Washington, D.C., Neg. No. AFIP 56-14075-2.* (b) In tuberculoid leprosy, the skin within the nodules (arrows) is completely without sensation. *Courtesy of the Pathology Research Laboratory, Leonard Wood Memorial, Armed Forces Institute of Pathology, Washington, D.C.*

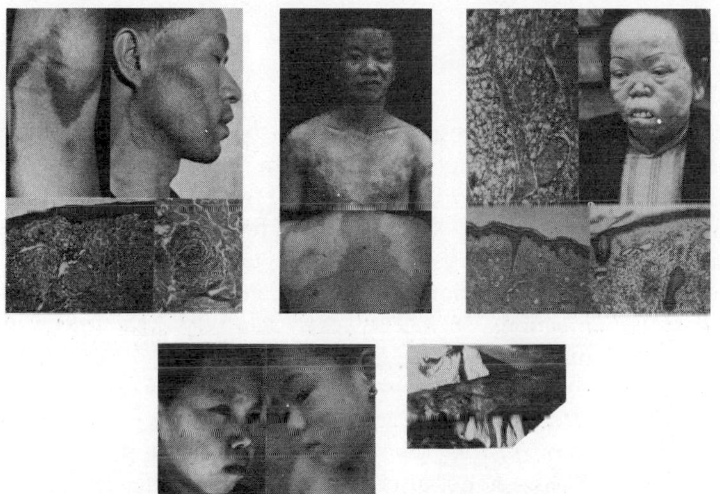

FIG. 29–4 The classification of leprosy. The composite photo shows the various forms of leprosy after contact with *Mycobacterium leprae.* An indication of the degree of immunity and the number of bacilli in these different types of leprosy is shown. *Skinsnes,* O. K., Ann. N.Y. Acad. Sci. *154:19 (1968). The New York Academy of Sciences, 1968; reprinted by permission.*

Sources of infection and the mode of transmission. Sources of human infection are human cases. There is no relationship between human and rat leprosy. Rat leprosy is caused by another microorganism, *M. lepraemurium.*

Leprosy is usually transmitted by prolonged direct contact with infected (lepromatous) patients (Figure 29–5) or by inhalation of organisms from sputum, nasal, or other types of discharges. Indirect contact via contaminated objects or various insects has also been implicated. The portal of entry is open to question; the skin and the mucous membranes of the nose and throat have been suspected.

Prevention. Naturally the reporting of leprosy cases and the hospitalization of the patients is desirable. Hospitalization is especially important for all individuals with the lepromatous (progressive or infectious) form of the disease (Figure 29–4). One important aspect of hospitalization that is frequently overlooked is that it offers an opportunity to inform and educate patients, especially with respect to their treatment.

Contaminated articles should be adequately disinfected in all cases of suspected or known leprosy.

Pseudomonas Infections

Pseudomonas aeruginosa has been largely ignored as a causative agent of several specific skin diseases. This Gram-negative rod has been reported to produce a variety of skin infections associated with epidermal destruction (Color Photograph 78), such as with burns. *Pseudomonas* septicemia may develop from these cases or from changes in the normal human flora or immune mechanisms of the individual, brought on by the use of antibiotics or drugs capable of suppressing antibody production. In healthy persons the pathogenic effects of this organism are limited. Examples of these dermatologic infections include "green nail" syndrome (Color Photograph 80) and toe web infection.

Staphylococcal Infections

Staphylococcus aureus is a Gram-positive, spherical bacterium that usually appears in grapelike clusters (Color Photograph 10A). In humans, staphylococci produce a variety of infections that involve any and all tissues of the body. The disease states are characterized by pus formation. They include carbuncles (Color Photograph 2), deep tissue abscesses, empyema, endocarditis, furuncles, boils, impetigo contagiosa (Color Photograph 2), meningitis, osteomyelitis, pneumonia, and wound infections. In recent years, staphylococcal infections have gained additional significance because of the appearance of drug-resistant mutants of *S. aureus.*

Transmission and predisposing factors. The exact mode of transmission involved in staphylococcal diseases is not always clear. Droplet nuclei, airborne organisms, carriers, and direct contact with individuals having open infected wounds have all been implicated as sources of disease agents. Hospital environments and hospital personnel in particular serve as sources of staphylococci in epidemic situations. Intimate contact with attendants, nurses, and physicians harboring these organisms in their nasopharyngeal regions poses serious problems in control. Carriers who happen to be food handlers constitute another difficult control situation.

In general, infections caused by *S. aureus* occur in persons whose local and general defense mechanisms are significantly lowered. Individuals with chronic debilitating diseases, such as cancer, diabetes mellitus, and cirrhosis of the liver, are prone to staphylococcal infections. Furthermore, infections can result from exposure to skin irritants or as a complication of burns or of wounds produced either accidentally or from surgical operations.

Frequent recurrent skin-limited infections often occur during the years of puberty. Examples of such diseases include inflammations of hair follicles (folliculitis) and acne vulgaris. The latter state is a chronic condition that appears as inflammations of the sebaceous glands located on the back, chest, and face.

Prevention. Great care must be exercised in treating staphylococcal infections. The proper handling and disposal of contaminated objects must be observed in hospital, as well as home, environments. Individuals with infections of this type should be made aware of the potential danger they can pose to others if adequate hygienic habits are not observed.

FURUNCLES AND CARBUNCLES

Poor hygiene and nutrition, as well as the irritation produced by the rubbing of clothing, can contribute to the formation of both boils, or furuncles, and carbuncles (Figure 29–6).

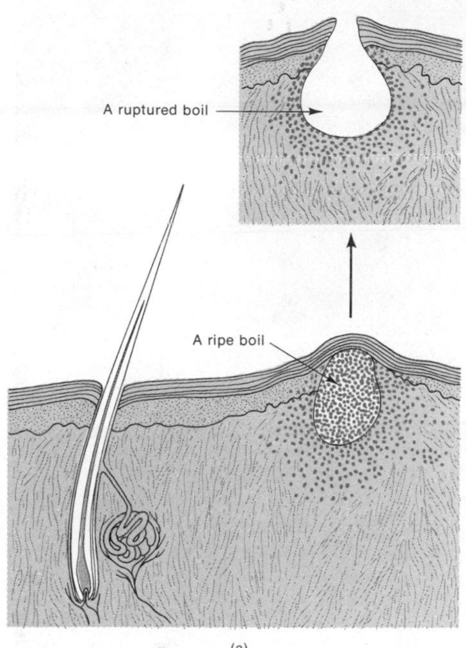

FIG. 29–6 Staphylococcal infections of the skin. (a) A boil, its general formation and eventual rupture with the release of bacteria. After *Brock, T. D., and K. M. Brock, Basic Microbiology. Englewood Cliffs, N.J.: Prentice-Hall (1978).* (b) Chronic Furunculosis. This patient also has inflammations of hair follicles and the accumulation of tumorous growths called *keloids.* All of these conditions are due to staphylococcal infections. *Courtesy of the Armed Forces Institute of Pathology, Washington, D.C., Neg. No. AFIP 53-12335.*

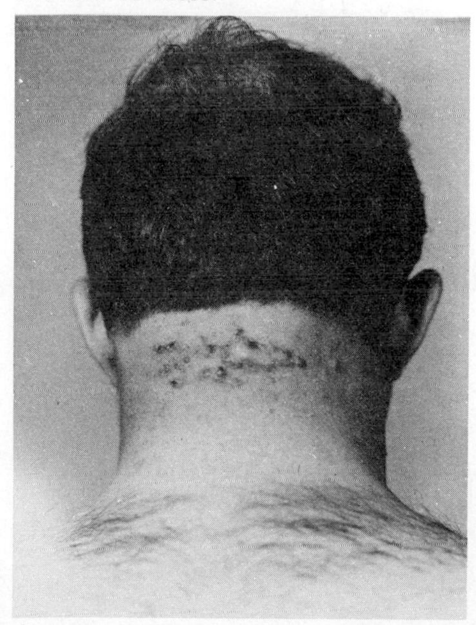

(b)

IMPETIGO CONTAGIOSA

This communicable infection of the superficial skin layers is commonly encountered in areas where hygienic conditions are poor. Occasionally the disease is epidemic, but in most situations it is sporadic with children under ten the most common victims (Color Photograph 2). Orphanages and nurseries offer favorable environments for the spread of impetigo.

Transmission. Impetigo contagiosa is spread by direct contact with infected persons or indirectly by contact with fomites such as bed sheets, handkerchiefs, pencils, or towels. The crusts from lesions also serve as a source of *S. aureus.* Staphylococci are usually introduced into the body through some form of abrasion or other lesion. The premature removal of scabs or crusts of viral skin infections, for example, chickenpox or smallpox, may provide additional portals of entry.

Streptococcal Infections

The streptococci include several organisms that, under the right conditions, are capable of infecting virtually all areas of the body. Primary infections can involve the respiratory, circulatory, or central nervous systems, as well as the skin and genital and urinary tracts. Streptococci are known for their frequent secondary invasion of body tissues. Various strains of these organisms can cause the same disease state, and, conversely, a single given streptococcal species can produce several kinds of infections.

The virulence of streptococci (as in the case of many other 'parasitic' microorganisms) seems to depend upon their cellular products, surface components, and related substances. These factors are important in the organism's ability to establish itself in the host.

In 1895, Mamorek first observed that streptococci were capable of causing the *in vivo* as well as *in vitro* destruction (lysis) of red blood cells. In 1903, Schottmuller suggested that this hemolytic activity be utilized for classification purposes. This suggestion wasn't fully explored until J. H. Brown undertook an intensive study in 1919. Based on his findings and those of others, streptococci were categorized into one of three groups on the basis of their hemolytic activity on blood agar plates. These categories were (1) ***alpha* (α) *hemolytic***, generating a greenish zone surrounding the bacterial colony (Color Photograph 58 a); (2) ***beta* (β) *hemolytic***, generating a clear zone surrounding the colony (Color Photograph 58 b); and (3) ***gamma* (γ) *hemolytic***, causing no obvious change on the medium (Color Photograph 58 c).

In the early 1930s, R. Lancefield further subdivided the hemolytic streptococci into groups based on immunological differences. These groups were designated by the capital letters A through O. The group A beta hemolytic streptococci contain the greatest number of human pathogens.

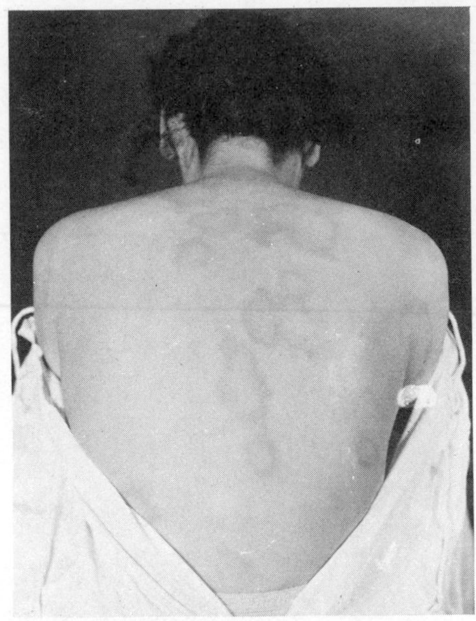

FIG. 29-7 Erysipelas caused by group A streptococci. *Courtesy of the Armed Forces Institute of Pathology, Washington, D.C., Neg. No. AF 18 58-6180.*

Transmission. Humans are the "ultimate" sources of pathogenic streptococci. Factors involved in the transmission of these organisms to susceptible persons include climate, crowding, improper sanitation, and the creation of aerosols.

ERYSIPELAS

This disease occurs world-wide, but with greater frequency in the temperate zone. Erysipelas (Figure 29–7) is an acute infection arising as a complication of surgery or of accidental wounds. Usually victims of the disease show a history of minor injuries. Group A streptococci are the ones most often found causing this disease.

SCARLET FEVER

Various strains of group A beta hemolytic streptococci are known to cause scarlet fever. Many of these organisms also produce other infections, including septic sore throat, erysipelas, tonsillitis, puerperal fever, and wound abscesses. Typically, scarlet fever is an acute inflammation of the upper respiratory tract that may be accompanied by a generalized rash. In recent years this infection appears to be milder in its effects. The term *scarlatina* is often used to designate the milder forms of scarlet fever. The various effects of the infection are directly related to a toxin produced by streptococci infected by a temperate bacterial virus. The toxin usually spreads from the infected site to other parts of the body.

Transmission. Scarlet fever infection is spread by means of (1) droplet nuclei, (2) aerosols, (3) contaminated food and water, and (4) direct contact with carriers, individuals in the acute stage of the disease. Fomites have been implicated, but it is believed such contaminated objects are not commonly involved.

Predisposing and related factors. This infection is world-wide. However, the development of a rash occurs more frequently in the temperate zones. Scarlet fever occurs most commonly during the fall, winter, and early spring months.

Studies indicate that this disease appears more frequently in Caucasians. Scarlet fever infection may occur in persons of any age. In general, however, it is most common in children under ten years of age.

One aid in the diagnosis of scarlet fever is the Schultz-Charlton, or "blanching," test. This procedure involves the injection of either 0.1 ml of the scarlet fever antitoxin or 0.2 to 0.5 ml of convalescent serum into an area with pronounced rash. A clearing or blanching will occur around the site of injection within 4 to 8 hours if the rash is associated with scarlet fever infection.

IMPETIGO CONTAGIOSA

Although impetigo contagiosa is usually caused by staphylococci (Color Photograph 2), the streptococci have also been associated with the condition. The streptococci are considered to act more as secondary invaders. Group A organisms appear to be the ones most often involved.

Streptococcal impetigo is a universal disease that usually occurs in areas where sanitation and personal hygiene are poor. The disease mainly affects young children, although when the above-mentioned conditions exist during natural disasters and war, adults can also develop the infection.

The infectious agents can be transmitted by means of fomites (napkins, bed clothes, pencils) or by direct inoculation with infectious discharges from persons having the disease.

CONSEQUENCES OF GROUP A STREPTOCOCCAL INFECTIONS

Several consequences, or *sequelae,* can develop from streptococcal infections, especially throat involvement. Acute hemorrhagic glomerulonephritis and rheumatic fever are the most common complications. These conditions are discussed in later chapters.

Other Clostridrial Infections

TETANUS

Tetanus was described by Hippocrates some 24 centuries ago. Its effects, sudden contractions of voluntary muscles and convulsions, are caused by a neurotoxin known as tetanospasmin, which is among the most poisonous substances known, second only to botulinus type A toxin. Tetanospasmin is produced by the widely distributed anaerobic bacterium *Clostridium tetani*—an organism present in dust, soil, and the feces of both domesticated and wild animals.

Transmission. Tetanus is associated with wounds of all types. Any break in the skin, whether a superficial scratch or a puncture, is subject to contamination by the spores of *C. tetani* (Color Photograph 12B). Once these spores gain access to the injured area, if there is enough dead or dying tissue to provide reduced oxygen concentration, they may germinate into the growing cells that produce the tetanus-causing toxin.

Clostridium tetani is considered, for the most part, a relatively noninvasive organism. Foreign objects, including glass and slivers of metal or wood, can introduce spores into the deeper tissues. A newborn infant may develop *tetanus neonatorum* from infection of its severed umbilical cord. Tetanus can affect people of all ages and can develop from abortions, circumcisions, ear-piercing, injections of drugs, and negligent surgical procedures.

Immunization is the only effective means of controlling tetanus. An initial course of three injections of tetanus toxoid is generally used, followed by a single booster injection after one year. Immunization schedules and the use of toxoid and antitoxin preparations are discussed in Chapter 26.

WOUND BOTULISM

Although wound botulism is a relatively rare disease, the marked increase in reported cases should serve as a signal of its potential danger. The causative agent of wound botulism as well as of the more familiar food poisoning is *Clostridium botulinum.* The spores of this bacterium are commonly found in the soil. Most infections are caused by contamination of wounds with soil. Although *C. botulinum* is noninvasive, it produces a potent exotoxin.

Mycotic Infections

Human skin, nails, and hair are particularly vulnerable to attack by certain pathogenic fungi. Of the 50,000 to 200,000 known species of fungi, about 50 are recognized as human pathogens. Most pathogens are of the class Deuteromycetes (Fungi Imperfecti). Several of these agents are capable of affecting the skin and related tissues that also contain the protein keratin (Color Photographs 40, 42 and 81). These fungi are also called *dermatophytes,* and most are found world-wide.

It is customary and useful to group the fungal diseases, or *mycoses,* according to the tissues and organs affected and the disease pattern or patterns. Our consideration of these diseases follows the terminology observed in the *Ciba Foundation Symposium, Systemic Mycoses* (1968).

Classification of Mycotic Infections

SUPERFICIAL MYCOSES

Fungi that attack mainly the epidermis, hair, nails, and mucosal surfaces are called *superficial fungi.* The diseases caused by such agents include the various forms of ringworm, or tinea (from the Latin meaning "growing moth" and *Candida* infections of mucosal surfaces, such as thrust and vulvovaginitis. These infections are frequently referred to as the *superficial mycoses* or *surface mycoses.*

Superficial mycoses are further classified on the basis of the location of the effects produced by the causative fungus (Table 29–3). For example, ringworm of the scalp is *tinea capitis;* that of the feet *tinea pedis,* more commonly known as "athlete's foot."

DEEP-SEATED, OR SYSTEMIC, MYCOSES

Infections in which the causative agents invade the subepithelial tissues (dermis and deeper regions) are known as *deep-seated, deep, or systemic mycoses* (Color Photograph 82).

OPPORTUNISTIC FUNGI

Some fungi are *opportunistic* pathogens. They are not normally pathogenic to healthy persons, but under certain conditions, they can produce severe infections. Included among these opportunistic agents are species of *Aspergillus, Candida, Cryptococcus, Geotrichum, Mucor,* and *Rhizopus.* Factors that have been found to predispose individuals to opportunistic infections include chronic anemia, leukemia, metabolic disorders (such as *diabetes mellitus*), and intensive treatment with broad-spectrum antibiotics and drugs that suppress antibody formation.

Diagnostic and Related Features of the Dermatophytes

Unlike some systemic fungi, dermatophytes are not dimorphic; they do not have yeast and hyphal stages. Most dermatophytes look alike in skin lesions. Culturally, however, their properties are quite different (Color Photographs 35B and 41). One of the most widely used media for the cultivation of fungi is Sabouraud's dextrose agar. This acidic medium (pH approximately 5.6), is especially suited for most fungi because they are able to survive in this environment while certain bacteria are prevented from growing. Media can be made

TABLE 29-3 Representative Superficial Mycoses

Disease	Causative Agent	Source of Infection	Geographical Distribution	Possible Treatment
Tinea barbae (ringworm of the beard)	*Microsporum canis* (rare); *Trichophyton mentagrophytes; T. rubrum, T. sabouraudi, T. verrucosum, T. violaceum*	Infected animals and children	World-wide	Griseofulvin; application of warm saline compresses; antibiotics to prevent secondary bacterial infections
(ringworm of the scalp)	*audouini, canis, gypseum, T. mentagrophytes, T. sabouraudi, T. schoenleinii, T. sulfureum, T. tonsurans, T. violaceum*	Infected animals, people, and fomites	World-wide	Griseofulvin; antibiotics to prevent secondary bacterial
Tinea corporis (ringworm of the body)	*M. audouini, M. canis, M. gypseum, T. concentricum, T. mentagrophytes, T. sabouraudi, T. schoenleinii, T. sulfureum, T. tonsurans, T. violaceum*	Infected animals and articles of clothing	World-wide	Griseofulvin; for small lesions, fungicides such as Tinactin, Verdefam, or Whitfield's ointment
Tinea cruris (ringworm of the groin)	*Candida albicans, Epidermophyton floccosum, mentagrophytes, rubrum*	Infected articles of clothing or athletic supports	World-wide	Whitfield's ointment; 1
Tinea manuum and Tinea pedis (ringworm of the hands and feet)	*C. albicans, E. floccosum, M. canis, T. mentagrophytes, T. rubrum, T. schoenleinii*	Direct contact with fungi in moist environments including showers, swimming and wading pools	World-wide	Aqueous potassium permanganate soaks; Griseofulvin; antifungal ointments and powders
Tinea nigra (ringworm of the palms)	*ladosporium werneckii*		orld-wide	
Tinea unguium (ringworm of the nails)	*C. albicans, E. floccosum, T. mentagrophytes, T. rubrum, T. schoenleinii, T. violaceum*	Infected individuals or regions of the body	World-wide	Griseofulvin
Tinea versicolor (branny scaling of the skin involving)	*alassezia furfur*		World-wide	percent sodium hyposulfite, or 1 percent
Black piedra	*Piedraia hortai*	Infected hair (beard, mustache, scalp)	Tropical countries	Shaving infected area, or adequate cleaning of hair followed by application of a mild fungicide
White piedra	*Trichosporon beigelii*	Infected hair (beard, mustache, scalp)	Temperate and tropical regions	

more selective by adding antibiotics that discourage the growth of bacteria and saprophytic fungi. Other common laboratory media are also used for fungal cultivation.

The identification of several fungi is based on the presence and characteristics of hyphae and spores in culture.

Detection of fungi in specimens involves techniques for their isolation and cultivation and also may include a direct microscopic examination of tissues. One of the procedures usually employed involves digesting specimens such as infected hairs in 10 percent potassium or sodium hydroxide with the aid of heat. This is performed on a slide, which is then inspected under the microscope for the fungus.

Staining procedures including the Gram stain and the periodic acid-Schiff (PAS) stain are also used. Reactions obtained with Wood's light (a form of ultraviolet light) are also of diagnostic value with certain infections.

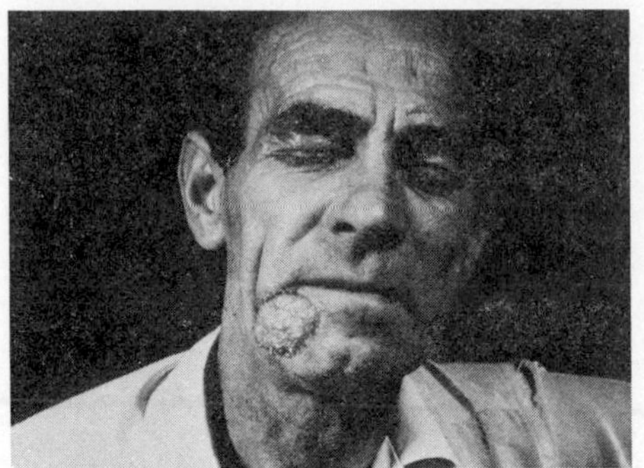

FIG. 29–8 Tinea barbae. Note the localized, boggy appearance of this infection. *Courtesy of the Armed Forces Institute of Pathology, Washington, D.C., Neg. No. 56-4858.*

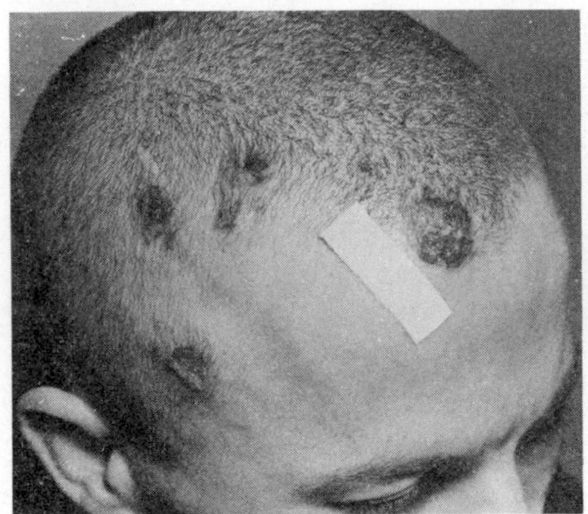

FIG. 29–9 Favus, a severe form of tinea capitis, or ringworm of the head. *Courtesy of the Armed Forces Institute of Pathology, Washington, D.C., Neg. No. 8-535-1.*

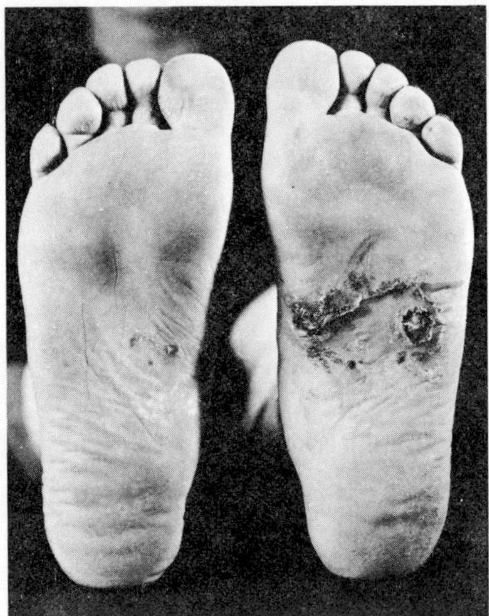

FIG. 29–10 Tinea pedis, or ringworm of the foot. *Courtesy of the Armed Forces Institute of Pathology, Washington, D.C., Neg. No. 53-14665-1.*

Representative Dermatophycoses

TINEA BARBAE

The fungal infection known as tinea barbae is a chronic condition involving the bearded regions of the face and neck (Figure 29–8). Only men are affected.

Fungi that attack hair or hair follicles can produce *ectothrix* or *endothrix* infections. With the ectothrix condition, growth of the fungal agent (in the form of arthrospores) occurs in and on the hair shaft (Color Photograph 42). In an endothrix infection, the organism grows only within the hair shaft.

TINEA CAPITIS

An infectious mycotic condition, tinea capitis involves the scalp (Figure 29–9) and the follicle and shaft of the hair. Tinea capitis may be acquired by direct contact with infected animals, humans, or fomites. The disease is commonly found among individuals living in overcrowded areas and having poor hygiene. Children are most often affected.

Prevention. Preventive measures are important with tinea capitis. Parents should be made aware of its contagious nature. Shampooing after haircuts may help prevent the disease.

TINEA CORPORIS

The nonhairy skin of an individual's body is affected in the chronic mycotic disease known as tinea corporis (Color Photograph 81). The infection is found in both sexes, with a greater frequency in moist, warm regions of the body. The disease agent in children is often *M. canis*; in adults several *Trichophyton* species produce the infection (Color Photograph 41).

TINEA CRURIS

Tinea cruris is a chronic, superficial infection usually confined to the inner surfaces of the groin. Perianal and armpit involvement can also occur.

TINEA MANUUM AND TINEA PEDIS

Tinea manuum and tinea pedis infections are long lasting and usually develop when fungi acquired through contact with contaminated showers, swimming and wading pools, and wet, tropical terrain is spread from the toe webs (Figure 29–10). The toenails and fingernails may become involved as a secondary effect (onychomycosis).

As fungal products are absorbed by the infected person, various nonfungal eruptions may occur on the extremities and trunk. These indicate the so-called "id" or trichophytid reaction, an allergic reaction to the products of the causative fungus, *Trichophyton* spp. Reddened areas appear on the skin far from infected regions. No fungi are present in these eruptions.

Prevention. As with all tinea infections, preventive measures are important in the control of tinea pedis. These include keeping potential areas of infection clean and dry.

TINEA VERSICOLOR

Malassezia furfur is the causative agent of the chronic fungus infection tinea versicolor. The condition is usually asymptomatic, although it may cause mild itching and loss of skin pigment (Figure 29–11). The disease is most commonly associated with young adults.

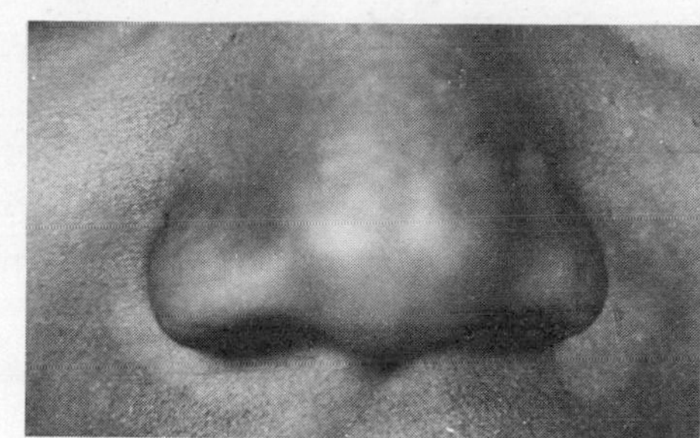

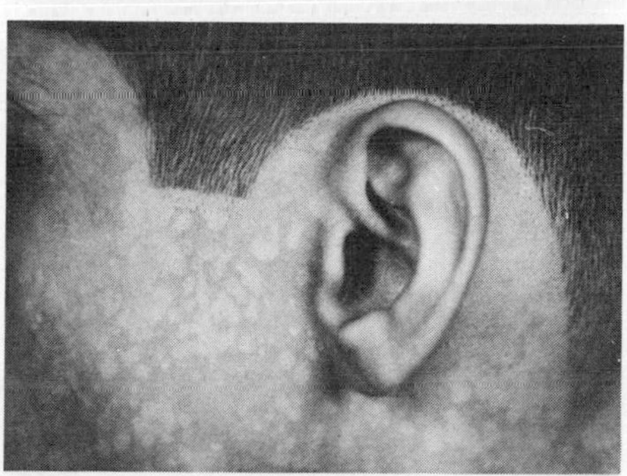

FIG. 29–11 Tinea versicolor. The appearance of the fungus infection involving the face. Areas with a loss of pigment are quite obvious. *Kamalam, A., and A. S. Thambiah,* Sabouraudia *14:129–148 (1976).*

PIEDRA

Piedra is characterized by fungal growths securely attached to the hair's surface, forming firm black, brown, or white nodules. Two forms of the infection are recognized, black and white piedra. All ages and both sexes appear to be vulnerable to the infection.

Other Diseases Caused by Fungi

Several superficial fungi are capable of attacking tissues other than the skin.

CANDIDIASIS

Candidiasis dates back to the beginnings of microbiology. Its effects range from simple, localized infections to uncontrollable, fatal septicemias. *Candida albicans* is considered the usual causative agent of bronchopulmonary candidiasis, skin and nail candidiasis (Figure 29–12), oral thrush, vaginitis, and paronychia, that is, inflammation of the nail bed.

Thrush is a candidal infection of the mouths of infants. It may be contracted from an infected birth canal or from contaminated equipment in the nursery.

It should be noted that the mere presence of the fungus is not enough to cause disease, since *C. albicans* has often been isolated from the skin, oral cavity, and intestinal tract of healthy individuals. However, it can cause infection when host resistance is lowered, as when there is some form of nutritional deficiency, or as a complication of bacterial or viral diseases. Candidiasis is commonly seen at both extremes of life, in the very young and the very old, as well as in debilitated persons. Predisposing factors include diabetes mellitus, pregnancy, obesity, and vitamin deficiencies. The infection has shown an increase in recent years as a complication of therapy with antibiotics, corticosteroids, and cytotoxic drugs (used in cancer therapy). *Candida* species have been, in many instances, grouped with the opportunistic fungi.

Prevention. Preventive measures are directed toward keeping susceptible skin areas as dry as possible. Rubber gloves and the avoidance of excessive exposure to detergents and related substances may help in controlling the disease.

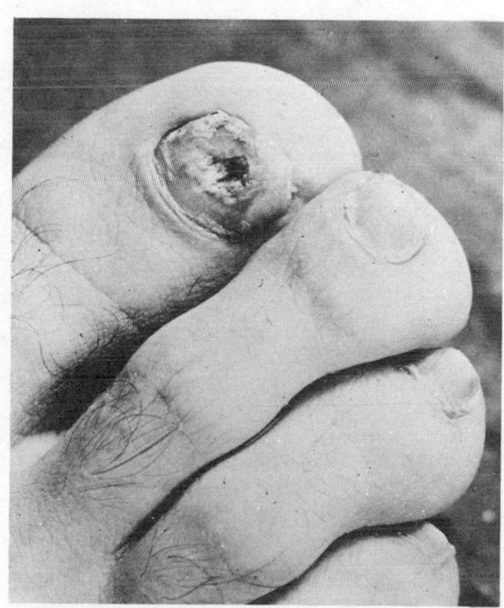

FIG. 29–12 *Candida*-caused onychomycosis. Note the brittle appearance of the infected toenail. *Courtesy of the Armed Forces Institute of Pathology, Washington, D.C., Neg. No. 58-13966-4.*

Viral Infections

Several viral infections are either limited to the skin or involve it in the course of disease development (Table 29–4). Some of the better-known viral diseases, including chickenpox, cold sore, measles, smallpox, and warts, will be discussed.

The clinical features associated with viral skin diseases vary widely. Yet certain diseases may possess identical features, creating a problem in diagnosis.

Knowing the terminology of skin diseases presented in Table 29–1 is helpful, not only in diagnosis, but also in following the development of a disease process. Table 29–4 lists general symptoms and approaches to laboratory diagnosis for several common viral diseases.

Although promising results have been obtained in treating some viral skin infections (Table 29–4), treatment is often limited to preventing secondary bacterial infections and relieving the victim's discomfort (symptomatic treatment).

TABLE 29–4 Representative Viral Diseases of Humans That Affect the Skin

Disease	*Causative Agent*	*Incubation Period*	*General Features of the Disease*	*Laboratory Diagnosis*	*Possible Treatment*
Chickenpox (varicella)	Varicella zoster virus	2–3 weeks	General red rash leading to vesicles; different forms of rash appear in successive crops and are distributed mainly over the trunk and face; slight fever and itching are commonly experienced	1. Detection of giant cells in specimens[a] 2. Serological tests, such as fluorescent antibody 3. Tissue culture	5-iodo-2′ deoxyuridine (IUDR); symptomatic treatment
Fever blister (cold sore, herpetic gingiostomatitis, herpes simplex virus infection)	Herpes simplex virus *(Herpesvirus hominis)*	Unknown, possibly 4–7 days	Localized skin and/or mucous membrane lesions that appear as blisterlike eruptions on the lips, face, ears, etc.	1. Demonstration of typical inclusion bodies in specimens[a] 2. Viral isolations 3. Serological tests	5-iodo-2′ deoxyuridine (IUDR) (promising medication); other DNA synthesis inhibitors and certain dyes, such as neutral red and proflavine
German measles (rubella)	Rubella virus	14–21 days	Slight fever, general discomfort, swollen lymph nodes, and macular rash (Color Photograph 00)	1. Tissue culture[a] 2. Viral isolation 3. Serological tests, such as hemagglutination inhibition	Immune globulin preparations
Measles (morbilli)[b]	Measles virus	14–21 days	Rash appears about 14 days after exposure; fever, cough, muscle pains, general discomfort, photophobia, redness of eyelids, characteristic lesions in mouth, Koplik's spots (red ulcers with bluish white center on the mucous membrane of inside cheek surfaces)	1. Viral isolation in tissue culture[a] 2. Serological tests	Antibiotics to prevent secondary bacterial infections; symptomatic treatment
Shingles (herpes zoster)	Varicella-zoster virus	2–3 weeks	Blisters along nerve trunk, pain (sometimes extreme), slight fever, and general discomfort	Same as for chickenpox[a]	5-iodo-2′ deoxyuridine (IUDR); zoster immunoglobulin
Smallpox	*Orthopoxvirus*	6–22 days	Fever, headache, back pain, aching limbs and general prostration, small red rash in and around groin area; rash proceeds from macular to pustule to scab formation	1. Virus isolation by tissue culture, and chick embryos[a] 2. Serological tests, such as complement fixation 3. Electron microscopy	Hyperimmune serum; antibiotics to prevent secondary bacterial infections; self-healing
Warts (papilloma)	*Polyomavirus*	Unknown	Growths on the back of hands, palms, soles, and other body regions; generally no pain or fever	1. Electron microscopy[a] 2. Tissue culture	Surgical or chemical removal of warts; certain vaccines being developed

[a]The typical features of the disease are usually sufficient for diagnosis.
[b]Rubeola is also used as a synonym for this disease. Unfortunately, the term has been used as a synonym for German measles (rubella).

The Herpesvirus Group

The viruses of the herpes group have several distinguishing properties, including (1) the possession of double-stranded DNA, (2) the presence of a nucleocapsid with cubical symmetry, (3) inactivation by chloroform and ether, (4) viral mutiplication in the nucleus of infected cells, (5) the production of clinical effects such as blister eruptions of the skin (Figure 29–13) and mucous membranes, with occasional nerve involvement, and (6) the formation of intranuclear inclusions known as Lipschütz or type A inclusions (Figure 29–14).

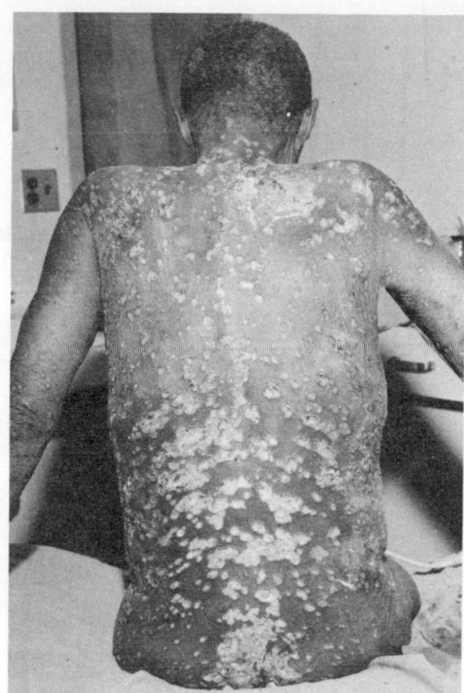

FIG. 29–13 Patient with generalized herpes simplex infection. The individual's immune state was altered by a cancerous condition. Identification of the viral agent was made by tissue culture studies of vesicle fluid. *Hospital, Brooklyn. Photo by F. G. Hertling.*

HERPESVIRUS TYPE I (HERPES SIMPLEX VIRUS)

The most common form of herpes simplex virus infection is an inflammation of the gums ***(herpetic gingiostomatitis)***. This condition occurs on the individual's first encounter with the viral agent (primary infection), chiefly in children between the ages of one and five. Similar primary involvement in adults may be quite severe. After recovery, the virus assumes a latent form. However, infections involving the skin and mucous membranes producing blisterlike lesions (Table 29–4) can recur quite readily as a consequence of precipitating causes, such as emotional disturbances, infections, lymphoma, menses, and sunburn. Although persons with recurrent herpes have circulating antibodies, they do not prevent the disease effects (Figure 29–15).

Transmission of the virus can occur by direct contact, including kissing, hand touching, and sexual relations, and by fomites.

VARICELLA (CHICKENPOX)-HERPES ZOSTER (SHINGLES) VIRUS

A variety of immunologic tests—agglutination, complement-fixation, and viral neutralization—have shown the viruses that cause chickenpox (varicella) and shingles (herpes zoster) to be immunologically identical. Furthermore, the morphological examination of the virions, inclusion bodies and cytopathic effects associated with these agents found them to be physically indistinguishable. The identity of these agents has been further established by the production of typical cases of chickenpox in children following inoculation of shingles blister fluid. On the basis of these and related studies, the majority of investigators believe that varicella and herpes zoster represent different forms of infection with the same agent, the V-Z virus.

VARICELLA (CHICKENPOX)

Chickenpox is one of the most common diseases in residential schools. It is primarily a childhood infection, but approximately 20 percent of cases are adults. Varicella is the primary disease state produced in an individual without immunity. Infections are transmitted via droplets of respiratory secretions and contact, either direct or indirect, with infectious skin surfaces. As noted above, an individual with shingles (herpes zoster infection) is also a source of infectious material for an outbreak of chickenpox.

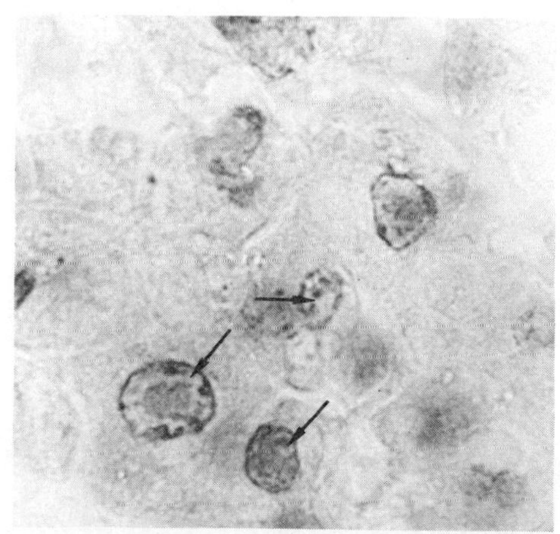

FIG. 29–14 A liver specimen from a 10-day-old child, showing typical inclusions of herpes simplex virus (arrows). During the early stages of viral development, the inclusions stain blue when they contain viruses. The red state results after the viruses have been released. Thus the Lipschütz inclusion body is an empty shell, a 'token' of viral infection. *Courtesy of the Armed Forces Institute of Pathology, Washington, D.C., Neg. No. 56-2952.*

Immunity. Recovery from an attack of chickenpox usually provides a relatively long-lasting active immune state. Recurrent infections are extremely rare.

Control. Control measures for this disease include isolation of infected persons and the administration of immunoglobulin to exposed individuals. Both of these means, however, are of limited effectiveness. No effective vaccine exists at present.

HERPES ZOSTER (SHINGLES)

Herpes zoster is uncommon in children; most cases occur in adults (Figure 29–16). At least 70 percent of adults have had previous exposure to the

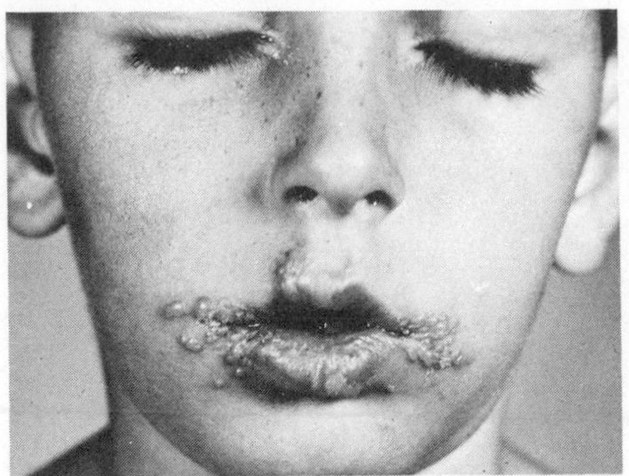

FIG. 29–15 Common features of herpes simplex virus infection. Involvement of the lips. *Courtesy of the Armed Forces Institute of Pathology, Washington, D.C., Neg. No. 55–11961–1.*

varicella-zoster virus, as indicated by the presence of circulating antibodies. Shingles represents a reinvasion, or recurrence, of varicella-zoster virus in persons partially immune to varicella.

The natural means of transmission for shingles is not known. The virus may gain entrance to the body by way of the throat. From here it enters the bloodstream and then localizes in ganglionic nerve cells. In this location the virus remains inactive for varying periods. Activation may be caused by several factors, including cancer, trauma, and certain drugs, such as those containing antimony or arsenic.

Warts (Papilloma Virus Infection)

HUMAN (PAPILLOMA) WARTS

Verruca vulgaris, otherwise known as the common wart or condyloma (Figure 29–17), is caused by human papilloma virus, which is a DNA virus.

Warts appear to be transferred by scratching. In addition, indirect spreading of viruses has been reported to occur by contact with contaminated bathroom and swimming pool floors, communal washroom facilities, and gymnastic equipment. Barbers, chiropodists, and masseurs also have been implicated in spreading the disease. Genital warts, or condylomata acuminata, are transmitted by venereal contact.

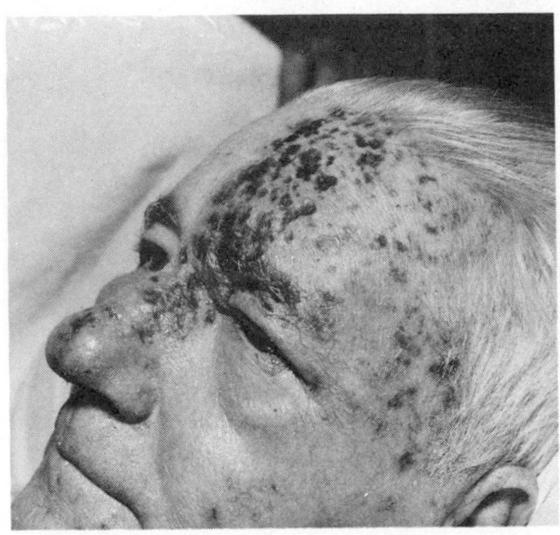

FIG. 29–16 Shingles in an adult patient, showing involvement of the ophthalmic nerve. *Courtesy of the Armed Forces Institute of Pathology, Washington, D.C. Neg. No. 58–15409–4.*

The Paramyxoviruses

The paramyxoviruses have several properties, including (1) the possession of one large molecule of single-stranded RNA, (2) an envelope with a lipid composition similar to that of the host's cell membrane, (3) replication in the cytoplasm, and (4) for most strains, hemagglutinating activity. The paramyxoviruses include the agents of classic measles (morbilli), mumps, Newcastle disease, and several human and lower animal respiratory infections.

MEASLES (MORBILLI)

Measles is a highly contagious disease usually contracted by exposure to respiratory secretions. As a rule, the virus causes disease in areas where large numbers of unimmunized young children reside. Outbreaks primarily affect children, as older persons have usually acquired some immunity from previous exposures to the virus. When susceptible adults are infected, symptoms are generally more severe than in children.

Complications may follow a measles virus infection, the most common being bacterial secondary infections such as pneumonia and middle ear infection. In general, it is advisable to administer antibiotics to protect infected children under three years of age and other persons with debilitating diseases such as bronchitis and tuberculosis against bacterial pathogens.

The virus can also produce serious complications such as infection of the central nervous system, sometimes leading to mental retardation. Fortunately, such cases are infrequent.

Pooled human immune globulin preparations can help modify the course of the disease. Timing and dosages are crucial.

Recovery from measles usually provides a long-lasting state of naturally acquired active immunity. Second bouts with the virus are uncommon.

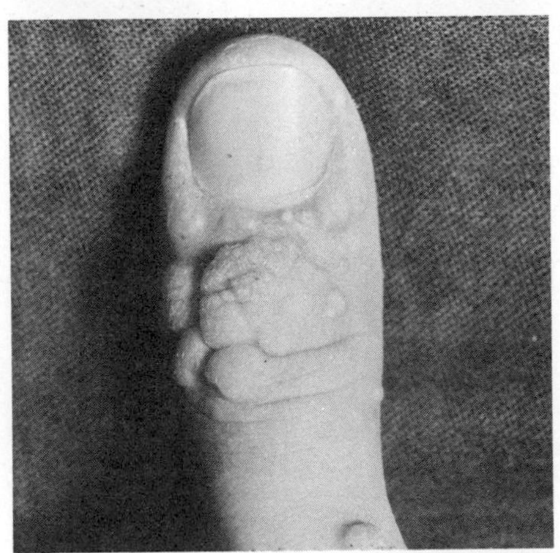

FIG. 29–17 The common wart, *verruca vulgaris.* This infection is commonly found on the backs of hands, usually in the area of the nail folds. *Courtesy of the Armed Forces Institute of Pathology, Washington, D.C., Neg. No. AMH 10737-2.*

Prevention. Several types of vaccines and programs have been developed for the express purpose of eradicating measles. One major approach involves immunization of all children at one year of age, administration of a vaccine to any unimmunized children upon their entry into school, and administration of measles immune globulin to all "exposed susceptible persons." To further this program, many schools now refuse entry to children not immunized against measles (unless the failure to immunize is for religious or medical reasons).

A Togavirus Representative

Rubella virus is a typical togavirus in all respects, except that it is not transmitted by arthropods. It contains a single-stranded RNA molecule.

GERMAN MEASLES (RUBELLA)

Rubella occurs in either epidemic or sporadic form world-wide. German measles is typically a mild disease with few and rare complications. However, among pregnant women the disease takes on an entirely different perspective because of the defects the viral agent can induce in fetuses during the early stages of pregnancy. The effects of the disease on the fetuses, referred to collectively as the rubella syndrome, include cataract formation, congenital heart disease, permanent deafness, mental retardation, spontaneous abortion, and stillbirth. The consequences of rubella are not only varied, but unpredictable. It appears that virtually any organ of a developing fetus may fall victim to the effects of the virus.

The mechanism or mechanisms contributing to these embryopathic effects are unknown. Studies of autopsied rubella infant victims show underdeveloped organs, and tissue culture shows pronounced chromosome breakage in lymphocytes from one-year-olds demonstrating the rubella syndrome. Based on these findings, several investigators have suggested that the virus may inhibit cell multiplication in the fetus.

Transmission of rubella usually occurs by direct contact with persons harboring inapparent infections. The nasal secretions of infected individuals are highly contagious. In addition, normal-appearing infants born to women who have had clinical rubella during the first three months of pregnancy excrete virus at birth. Such newborns come into close contact with various health care personnel, expectant mothers, and other children.

Control. Recovery from German measles generally imparts a long-lasting active immunity to the viral agent, and vaccines are also available. If teenaged girls have not yet had German measles, vaccination is recommended, since it is highly desirable for young girls to be exposed to the viral agent before reaching childbearing age.

Pooled preparations of immune globulin are administered to pregnant women as soon as possible after exposure if these women are in their first trimester. The effectiveness of this procedure is questionable, especially in relation to the prevention of congenital defects. Some physicians recommend a therapeutic abortion to their patients in the event of a rubella infection during the first trimester of pregnancy.

The Poxviruses

Agents of more than two dozen diseases in humans and lower animals belong to the poxvirus group. In the past the two poxviruses of greatest significance for humans were the agents of smallpox and vaccinia, the virus used in smallpox vaccination. The first of these is believed extinct, but immunization with vaccinia is still sometimes advisable.

Most members of the poxvirus group (1) multiply and produce inflammatory lesions (pocks) after inoculation onto the chorioallantoic membranes of chick embryos (Color Photograph 53), (2) have double-stranded DNA, (3) replicate in the cytoplasmic regions of cells, (4) agglutinate fowl or mouse red blood cells, and (5) are resistant while in dried form to a wide variety of adverse environmental conditions.

SUMMARY

1. Diseases of the skin are caused by a variety of microorganisms and worms.
2. Organisms producing localized skin infections also may cause injury of internal organs.

The Organization of the Skin

1. The skin, nails, and hair make up the covering of the human body.
2. The skin consists of the outer, *epidermis,* layer and the lower, *dermis,* layer.
3. The functions of the skin include excretion, receiving external stimuli, secretion, temperature regulation, and serving as a natural barrier to most microbial disease agents.
4. Barriers to skin-invading microorganisms include skin acidity, indigenous microbial flora, temperature, and the inflammatory reaction.
5. Breaks in the skin during normal living can provide opportunities for microorganisms to gain entrance into the body.
6. The type and extent of injuries to the skin and the microorganisms involved influence the seriousness of the infections.

Bacterial Diseases

1. The signs, symptoms, and destruction of skin infections may vary from localized effects to rather extensive involvement and penetration into deeper tissues.
2. Identification of microbial pathogens of the skin frequently is dependent on the isolation, cultivation, and results of various biochemical tests.
3. Bacterial diseases associated with the skin include anthrax, erysipelas, gas gangrene, impetigo, green-nail syndrome, leprosy, scarlet fever, tetanus, and wound botulism.

Mycotic Infections

1. Human skin, nails, and hair are particularly susceptible to attack by certain pathogenic fungi known as *dermatophytes.*
2. Fungus infections or *mycoses,* are grouped according to the tissues or organs affected.

Classification of Mycotic Infections

1. Fungi that mainly attack the skin, hair, nails, and mucosal surfaces are called *superficial* or *surface fungi.*
2. *Deep-seated* or *systemic* mycoses are associated with the deeper tissues.
3. Some fungi that normally are not pathogenic but take advantage of lower host resistance are called *opportunists.*

Diagnostic and Related Features of the Dermatophytes

1. The identification of several fungi is based on their growth characteristics and the presence and microscopic properties of their hyphae and spores.
2. The use of Wood's light (a form of ultraviolet light) is of diagnostic value with certain infections.

Representative Dermatophycoses

1. Fungal infections of the skin, hair, and nails are examples of ringworm (tinea).
2. Examples of such conditions include ringworm of the body (tinea corporis), feet (tinea pedis), head (tinea capitis), and groin area (tinea cruris).
3. Prevention of ringworm includes keeping potential or susceptible areas clean and dry.

Other Diseases Caused by Fungi

The yeast infection, thrush, is caused by *Candida albicans.* This condition occurs in individuals with lowered resistance or suffering from complications of treatment or other microbial diseases.

Viral Infections of the Skin

1. Several viral infections are either limited to the skin proper or involve it in a disease process.
2. Examples of viral diseases of the skin include chickenpox, cold sore, measles, smallpox, and warts.

QUESTIONS FOR REVIEW

1. a. What types of microorganisms make up the flora of the normal skin (see Chapter 21)?
   b. Are any of these organisms capable of invading normal skin? Explain.
   c. Does the microbial flora of the skin serve any useful function? Explain.
2. Select five bacterial species that are associated with diseases of the skin. Construct a table and compare these agents with respect to the following properties:
   a. morphology
   b. Gram reaction
   c. method of diagnosis

d. determination of pathogenicity (if applicable)
e. preventive and control measures

3. Does there appear to be any form of immunity toward bacterial agents capable of causing skin infections? If so, toward which ones? Are vaccines available against these organisms?
4. a. What types of microorganisms are associated with wounds? Are any of these agents aerobic?
   b. With what types of wounds, for example, abrasions, lacerations, etc., is tetanus associated?
5. Compare the properties of an endotoxin with that of an exotoxin (see Chapter 22).
6. a. What is gas gangrene? How does it differ from an ordinary case of gangrene?
   b. How is gas gangrene treated?
7. a. What is leprosy?
   b. How is it transmitted?
   c. Where does this disease occur?
8. How does wound botulism differ from botulism associated with food?
9. Differentiate between superficial and deep-seated mycoses.
10. What is a dermatophyte? Give six examples.
11. How can one distinguish between endothrix and ectothrix infections?
12. How can the following diseases be contracted?
    a. tinea capitis
    b. tinea cruris
    c. tinea pedis
    d. tinea corporis
    e. tinea versicolor
    f. tinea unguium
    g. white piedra
13. What methods are generally used in the diagnosis of dermatophytosis?
14. Discuss the diseases of *Candida albicans* as to their various forms and possible means for their prevention.
15. a. If you were traveling in a tropical or subtropical area of the world, what mycotic infections might you find?
    b. How could these diseases be prevented?
16. Differentiate between the following terms:
    a. macule and pustule
    b. vesicle and scar
    c. maculopapule and crust
17. Describe the various disease states caused by herpes simplex virus *(Herpesvirus hominis)*. Are there any precipitating causes?
18. a. Compare the modes of transmission of the viral skin diseases discussed in this chapter.
    b. What control measures could be employed to limit infection?
19. What is the relationship between varicella and shingles?
20. What types of complications are associated with viral skin disease?
21. Differentiate between German measles and morbilli.
22. With which of the viral skin diseases discussed in this chapter is a laboratory diagnosis essential?
23. Can all viral pathogens cause congenital defects? Explain.
24. Which of the infections discussed in this chapter have you experienced?
25. Against which viral diseases of the skin are vaccines currently available?
26. Define or explain the following terms:
    a. vaccinia
    b. Lipschütz body
    c. rubella syndrome
    d. verruca vulgaris
    e. poxvirus

SUGGESTED READINGS

Benenson, A. L. (ed.), *Control of Communicable Diseases in Man.* 12th ed. Washington, D.C.: American Public Health Association, 1975. *An excellent, useful reference to human microbial diseases. Emphasis is given to diagnostic aspects and public health control measures.*

Cooper, L. Z., and S. Krugman, "The Rubella Problem," *Disease-a-Month*, Feb. 1, Yearbook Medical Publishers Inc., Chicago (1969). *A detailed review of the various effects of rubella virus.*

Eckmann, L., *Principles of Tetanus.* Bern and Stuttgart: Hans Huber Publishers, 1967. *A well-written presentation of tetanus and its mechanism of action.*

Henderson, D. A., "The Eradication of Smallpox," *Sci. Amer.* 235:25–33 (1976). *A detailed description of the measures used to eliminate one of the historically important and serious diseases of humans. The article includes discussions of basic immunological and epidemiological topics.*

Marples, M. J., "Life on the Human Skin," *Sci. Amer.* 220:108–115 (1969). *A well-illustrated article describing the skin as a habitat for microorganisms.*

Moss, E. S., and A. L. McQuown, *Atlas of Medical Mycology.* Baltimore: Williams & Wilkins Co., 1970. *A functional reference dealing with a variety of human fungus infections.*

CHAPTER **30**

Oral Microbiology

Chapter 30 discusses specific microbial diseases affecting teeth, gums, and other supporting tissues. Attention is also given to the microbial flora of the oral region and the complications that can develop from disease states associated with the mouth.

After reading this chapter, you should be able to:

1. **Describe the general organization and components of the human mouth, and indicate the areas susceptible to attack by pathogenic microorganisms.**
2. **Discuss the relationship of the microorganisms in the mouth to the health of the individual.**
3. **List the general properties of four different microorganisms that make up the oral flora.**
4. **Describe the causative agent, means of transmission, and control measures for at least two each of bacterial, mycotic, and viral diseases affecting the oral regions.**
5. **Distinguish among the following disease states of the oral region as to general appearance or symptoms and treatment:**
    a. **gingivitis**
    b. **periodontal disease**
    c. **necrotizing ulcerative gingivitis**
    d. **periodontitis**
6. **Define or explain plaque formation and calculus.**
7. **Describe the cause, development, and control of dental caries.**

The mouth is continually exposed to organisms from the external environment, beginning with passage through the birth canal. In time, an ecological balance is reached that serves to establish a resident microbial flora that remains fairly stable throughout life. Oral infections result from disturbances in the relationship of this resident flora to the tissues of the mouth.

Structure of the Mouth

The oral cavity, or mouth, is situated at the beginning of the gastro-intestinal tract. This space is enclosed on the sides by the lips and cheeks, above by the hard and soft palates, and below by the floor of the mouth and the tongue. The lips are covered on the outside by skin and on the inside by mucous membrane. Small glands are present beneath the mucosa, and there are many muscle bundles within the lips.

The palate is divided into a hard palate at the front of the mouth and a soft palate at the back. The bones of the hard palate are covered by a thick layer of firm but soft tissue. The soft palate connects with the passageway from the mouth to the throat. It is continuous with the tissues encircling the opening to the pharynx.

The floor of the mouth lies in a horseshoe around the tongue, and is continuous with the *gingiva* (the gum) and with the tongue. Near the front end are the openings of the submandibular and sublingual *salivary glands*.

The human develops two sets of teeth, the deciduous and the permanent. There are 20 teeth in the first set, also called the milk teeth; the permanent set usually contains 32 teeth. Teeth are categorized into four groups: *incisors, canines, premolars* or *bicuspids*, and *molars*. Incisors are used for cutting food, canines for tearing food, and premolars and molars for grinding. Each tooth has three parts (Figure 30–1): the *crown*, the portion above the gum; the *root*, the structure embedded in the jaw; and the *neck*, which is the narrower region between the crown and the root.

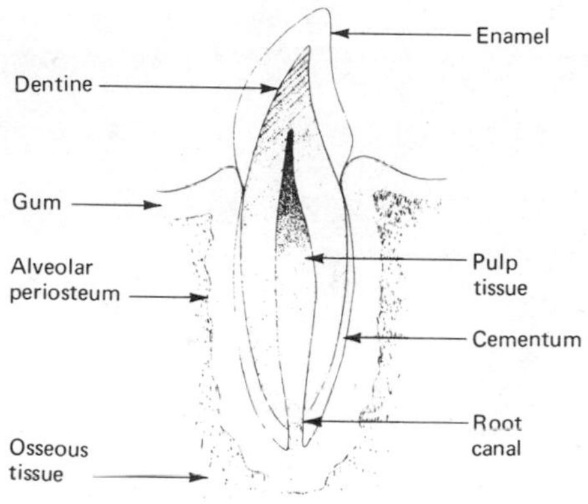

Enamel
Dentine
Gum
Alveolar periosteum
Pulp tissue
Cementum
Root canal
Osseous tissue

FIG. 30–1 The structure of a human tooth.

A tooth's crown is coated with *enamel*, the hardest substance found in the body; the rest of the tooth is covered by a layer of modified bone called the *cementum*. Under the enamel coating is an ivorylike tissue called *dentine*, which comprises the bulk of the tooth. The dentine is quite hard and striated. Within this layer is a cavity, the *pulp chamber*, containing blood vessels, connective tissue, and nerve endings. The contents of this chamber are frequently referred to as the *dental pulp*.

Teeth tend to become covered with a gummy accumulation of salivary mucin and bacteria, called *dental plaque* (Figure 1–13c), which can be seen by the naked eye. It has been suggested that the early growth of aerobes and the buildup of plaque may be necessary to provide a suitable environment for the growth of anaerobes that predominate in older plaque.

The Oral Flora

Because the mouth is warm and moist and has a regular supply of fresh food, it makes an ideal growth environment for microorganisms. The study of *oral ecology* is both interesting and complex. Microscopic examination of plaque from a tooth's surface usually reveals a wide variety of bacteria (Figure 30–2). Many studies have been conducted to find which organisms, and in what concentration, predominate in the oral cavity.

The oral cavity of the fetus is essentially germ-free until it passes through the birth canal. At this time, lactobacilli, micrococci, alpha and gamma anaerobic streptococci, coliforms, corynebacteria, yeasts, viruses, and protozoa are obtained from the vaginal and urogenital tract. Staphylococci and pneumococci may be added from the air. Feeding and contact with people and new environments add many more organisms.

The assortment of organisms in the oral flora is relatively stable, though subject to change with aging. Although other microorganisms may be introduced, perhaps with food, they are usually transient and seldom take up permanent residence.

The organisms present at any one time exist in balance with one another, and any change in this balance may result in disease. Attempts to study the oral microbiota in the laboratory have proved most difficult, since duplication of the oral environment is almost impossible. Mixed culture studies have yielded some information, but so far no one has developed a system capable of duplicating the environment required by oral microorganisms.

The organisms of the human mouth fall into three groups with regard to their tolerance of, or requirement for, oxygen: the strict anaerobes, strict aerobes, and the "facultatives." This last group includes everything between the two extremes—all those microorganisms that can tolerate some concentration of oxygen, from very high to very low.

Although bacteria are the most obvious inhabitants of the oral cavity (see Table 30–1), other microorganisms are often seen. These include several species of fungi, viruses, and protozoa.

Of the fungi, probably those most commonly found are of the genus *Candida*. It has been estimated that in approximately 40 percent of the "normal" population, these organisms can be cultivated from saliva. In a healthy mouth, they make up only a small percentage of the total oral flora. However, in children, the aged, and the debilitated, they are of major importance. Oral *Candida* infections often follow heavy dosages of antibiotics. This is undoubtedly because of the change in bacterial population and the resulting imbalance in oral ecology.

Viruses, both human and bacterial, have been recovered from the oral cavity. The causative organisms of cancer sores, herpes simplex, and measles can be found in oral lesions during obvious disease. Little is known about the place of viruses in the normal ecology of the human mouth, but no doubt many types are present.

Nonspecific Infections of the Oral Region

Infections of the face, oral cavity, and neck may be extremely serious, depending upon their location and the microorganisms involved. Specific infections caused by bacteria, fungi, or viruses occur here as well as in other body sites. More commonly, there are mixed bacterial infections in deep cavities in teeth or as a result of tissue injury.

Focal Infections

A localized area of infection anywhere on the body is called a *focus of infection*. When organisms or their toxic products spread from this focus to distant tissues, either to form another site of infection or to produce a hypersensitive reaction, the process is known as a **focal infection.**

The concept of focal infection has had a long and stormy history. Shortly after the concept was introduced, medical and dental practitioners enthusiastically condemned infected teeth and oral tissues as the cause of many unexplained conditions in the body, using it to justify the extraction of teeth and related procedures. Countless thousands of teeth were sacrificed to the cause. Then the pendulum swung too far to the other side, and the oral regions were almost ignored as a source of focal infection. At present, certain conditions are known to be related to oral foci of infection. The importance of good oral

TABLE 30-1 Microorganisms in the Oral Flora[a]

Microorganism	Gram Reaction	Morphology	Characteristics and/or Associated Activities
Actinomyces	+	Rod to coccoid	Most are facultative anaerobes; organisms can be found between teeth and in gum grooves; certain species are pathogenic
Bacterioides	−	Rods	Strict anaerobes; some species are pathogenic and are associated with gum disease (necrotizing ulcerative gingivitis)
Borrelia	−	Spirals	Strict anaerobes; some species may cause diseases involving supportive tissues in the mouth
Branhamella catarrhalis	−	Cocci	Aerobic; parasites of the human mucous membranes
Candida[b]	+	Large oval cells	Represent only a small percentage of the organisms in the total oral flora; known to cause oral infections in individuals with diabetes or cancer or persons receiving large doses of antibiotics
Corynebacterium	+	Rods	Aerobes and facultative anaerobes; picket fence arrangement of cells is a common feature; some pathogenic species *(C. diphtheriae)* produce exotoxins
Diphtheroids	+	Rods	Aerobes to microaerophilic; club-shaped cells arranged in patterns resembling Chinese characters; normal inhabitant of the mouth
Fusobacterium	−	Rods	Strict anaerobes; normally found in mouth and other human cavities
Lactobacilli	+	Rods	Facultative organisms that produce large amounts of acid from carbohydrates; pathogenicity unusual
Leptotrichia	−	Rods	Highly anaerobic; found in recesses and crevices between teeth; appear as very thick, long, nonbranching rods with rounded ends (Figure 30–2c)
Mycoplasma	−	Variable shapes	Mostly facultative anaerobes; highly variable in shape (pleomorphic); certain species are parasitic as well as pathogenic
Neisseria	−	Cocci	Aerobes or facultative anaerobes
Nocardia	+	Coccoid to rods	Strict aerobes with branching; certain species are pathogenic
Streptococci	+	Cocci	These organisms make up the largest bacterial group in the oral cavity; streptococci are associated with plaque formation and the production of acids from carbohydrates; alpha-hemolytic streptococci (viridans group) pose danger in cases of tooth extraction and heart valve damage; beta streptococci are noted for diseases such as strep throat and scarlet fever
Treponema	−	Spirochete	Strict anaerobes; some species normally found in mouth
Veillonella	−	Cocci	Parasitic anaerobes

[a]Various protozoa and viruses also are found in the mouth.
[b]Yeast.

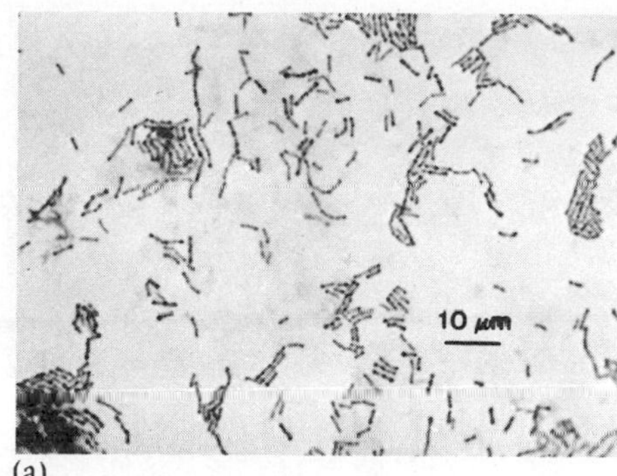

(a)

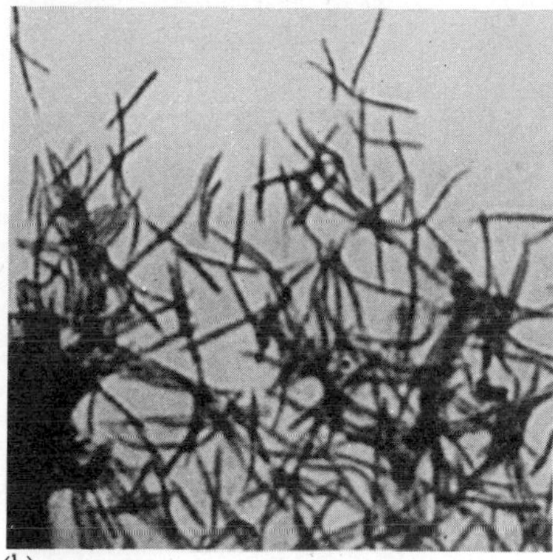
(b)

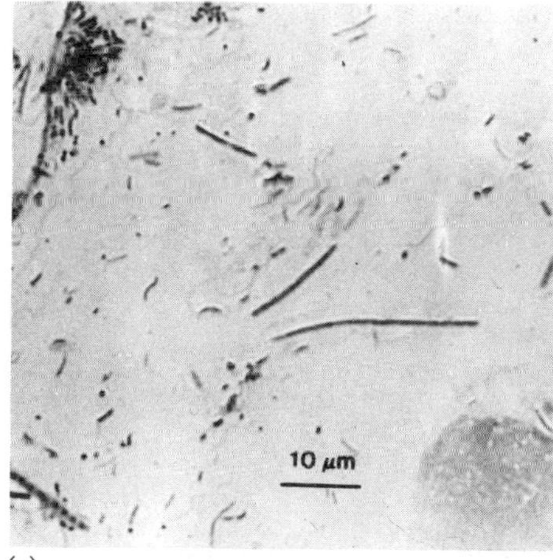

(c)

FIG. 30–2 Representatives of the oral flora. (a) A pure culture of lactobacilli. Note the polar staining in these organisms. (b) Fusobacteria, another rod, with tapered, pointed ends. *Courtesy of Dr. Richard Parker.* (c) Mixed oral flora. The long, granular organisms are *Leptotrichia.* A few rods, diplococci, and threadlike forms are also seen.

hygiene, along with elimination of infection, is considered an important part of restoring and maintaining good health.

Selected examples of nonspecific oral foci of infection in the periodontium or supporting structures of the teeth are discussed in Table 30–2. Resultant changes in the tissues of infected teeth include abscesses and apical granulomas (a form of tumorous growth). Examples of disease states specifically related to oral foci are discussed later.

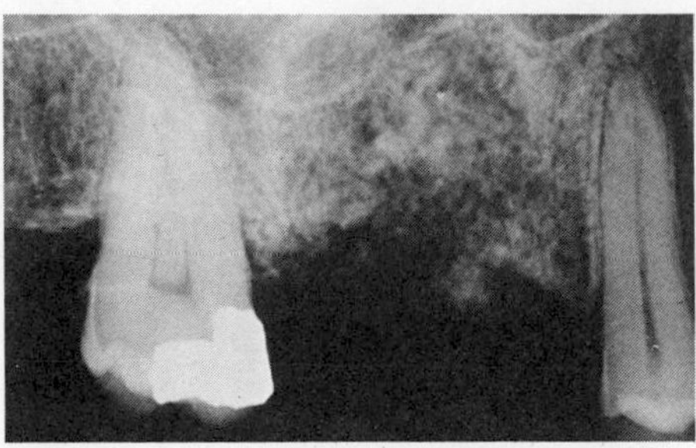

FIG. 30-3 Chronic osteomyelitis involving the maxilla. This x-ray shows the moth-eaten appearance of the bone. *Courtesy of Dr. N. H. Rickles, Pathology Department, University of Oregon Dental School.*

DRY SOCKET

With dry socket, the blood clot that formed following the removal of a tooth has been dislodged and lost from the extraction site, thus exposing the bone and allowing some degree of infection to develop. Any of the factors listed in Table 30–2 have been implicated as causes of dry socket. The bony walls of the socket often show signs of tissue death and become infiltrated with bacteria of many types. A foul odor also develops.

OSTEOMYELITIS

Inflammation of the bone *(osteo)* marrow *(myelo)* may occur from the introduction of many different types of bacteria either as pure or mixed cultures (Figure 30–3). The resulting infection leads to inflammation, cellular degeneration, and necrosis of the tissues involved, often including the bone (osteitis) and the ***periosteum*** or surrounding membrane (periostitis).

Several different factors may cause osteomyelitis (Table 30–2).

The disease may be of short duration (acute) or long lasting (chronic), depending upon many factors, such as the type and number of organisms involved, their virulence, and the age and resistance of the host. Since the teeth in the area may be loose, pain and difficulty in eating can occur. Thus the patient's nutritional status can also be affected.

PERICORONITIS

Pericoronitis may begin in a flap of tissue overlying an erupting tooth or around an impacted or partially erupted third molar. Pericoronitis, or inflammation *(-itis)* around *(peri-)* the crown *(coronal)* of the tooth, may spread into the surrounding tissues, resulting in a cellulitis, or diffuse inflammation of the soft tissues. The bacteria involved here produce large amounts of the enzymes hyaluronidase and fibrinolysins, which are capable of breaking down tissue cohesiveness, thus allowing the spread of the infection. As infection spreads, that side of the face begins to swell and the firm tissues may become discolored.

TABLE 30–2 Features of Nonspecific Oral Foci of Infection

Infection and/or Condition	*Causes (C) and/or Contributing Factors (CF)*	*Brief Description*	*Signs and Symptoms*
Dental caries	*CF:* Climate, composition and amount of saliva, hormonal balance, nutritional state, oral hygiene, fluoride level in drinking water, diet, genetic makeup *C:* Interactions between the host tissues and specific caries-producing microorganisms, e.g., *Streptococcus* species	Loss of calcium salts (decalcification) of inorganic substances of teeth, followed by disintegration of organic portions	General pain, chronic irritation, headache, and complications resulting in infections of surrounding areas
Dry socket	*C:* Contamination of the extraction area, excessive injury, rinsing with hot fluids, dislodging of blood clot by vigorous rinsing, lowered host resistance, implanting bacteria or foreign material	Dislodging of a blood clot and exposure of bone from a tooth extraction site	Foul odor, swollen and inflamed gums, pain, and a mass of dead tissue (slough) along the margin nearest the socket

TABLE 30-2 Features of Nonspecific Oral Foci of Infection (Continued)

Infection and/or Condition	*Causes (C) and/or Contributing Factors (CF)*	*Brief Description*	*Signs and Symptoms*
Gingivitis	*C:* Improper or inadequate oral hygiene, food impacting between poorly closing teeth or around teeth badly broken from decay	Inflammation of gums	Swollen, reddened, and bleeding gums; pus formation may occur
Necrotizing ulcerative gingivitis	*CF:* Fatigue, anxiety, and other forms of stress, debilitating illnesses, such as cancer or diabetes, severe vitamin deficiency diseases, local irritation of gums, calculus, and overhanging gums *C:* Implicated bacteria include *Borrelia vincentii* and *Fusobacterium fusiforme*	This disease is also known as trench mouth or Vincent's disease; destruction of gums and associated tissues	General pain in gums, slight fever, malaise, ulceration of gums, bleeding, loss of dead tissue, foul odor, and metallic taste; bone involvement may occur in untreated cases
Osteomyelitis	*C:* Infected pulp, residual infections, severe periodontal disease with extension into the bone, many forms of destructive injury, and specific infections such as actinomycosis, syphilis, and tuberculosis	Inflammation and eventual destruction of bone and surrounding tissues	Severe pain, elevated temperature, swollen lymph nodes associated with the area, loose teeth, and difficulty in eating
Pericoronitis	*C:* Contaminated instruments, infections following extractions, and specific bacteria including *Streptococcus* species	Inflammation around the crown of the tooth; the condition may spread to other surrounding tissues	Face swollen on the side involved, discoloration of tissue, draining of pus from involved area
Periodontitis	*C:* Untreated gingivitis *CF:* Various factors acting together are important considerations, including plaque formation, calculus, allergic responses to bacterial antigens, poor oral hygiene, injury by dental floss, genetic factors, hormonal balance, and poor closure of jaw (malocclusion)	This condition is also known as pyorrhea. It is an inflammation of the periodontium, the directly supporting tissue of the tooth	Inflamed gums, bleeding, loss of bone around the teeth, loose teeth; many cases exhibit few symptoms

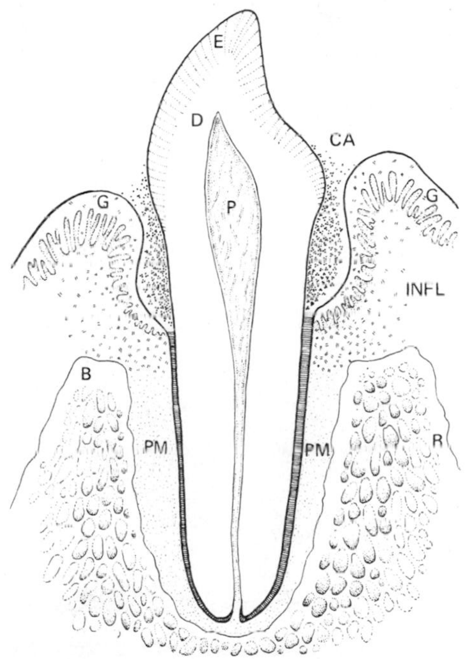

FIG. 30-4 In periodontal disease, the gingival tissue, (G), shows inflammation, swelling, and loss of stippling, and plaque (CA) and calculus extend down the root, creating a marked inflammation reaction with resultant loss of bone (B). Pus may be expressed from the pocket. Also shown are tooth enamel (E), dentine (D), pulp (P), periodontal membrane (PM), and cementum (C). *Courtesy of Dr. N. H. Rickles, Pathology Department, University of Oregon Dental School.*

PERIODONTAL DISEASE

The diseases of the tissues surrounding and supporting the teeth, gingivitis and periodontitis in their many forms, can be grouped under the general heading of periodontal disease (Figure 30-4).

Periodontal disease, a world-wide affliction of humans, appears clinically as an inflammation of the soft tissues around the teeth. The disease may affect all of the tissues around the teeth, or it may involve only isolated areas. In the

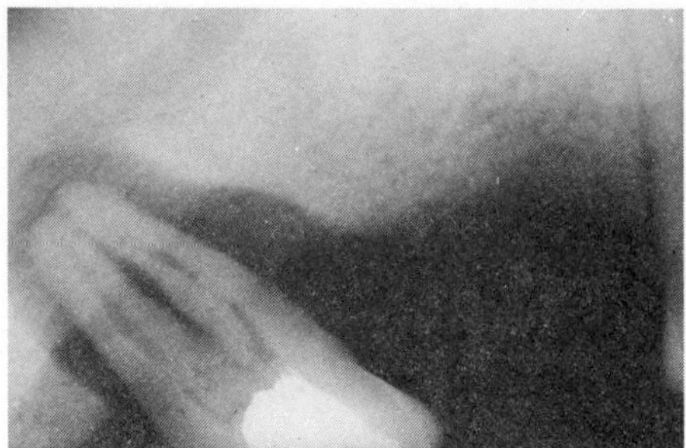

FIG. 30-5 Periodontal disease has caused almost total destruction of the bone surrounding this lower molar. Clinically the patient has a periodontal abscess with swelling and acute inflammation. *Courtesy of Dr. N. H. Rickles, Pathology Department, University of Oregon Dental School.*

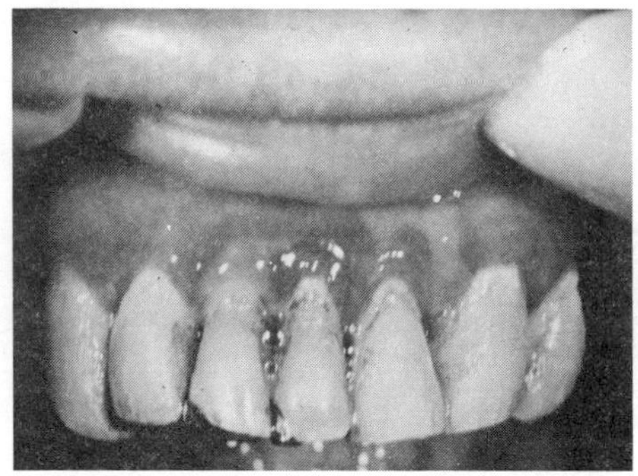

FIG. 30-6 Gingivitis. Note the severe involvement of the gingiva around the teeth, where there is also heavy building of plaque and calculus. *Courtesy of Dr. N. H. Rickles, Pathology Department, University of Oregon Dental School.*

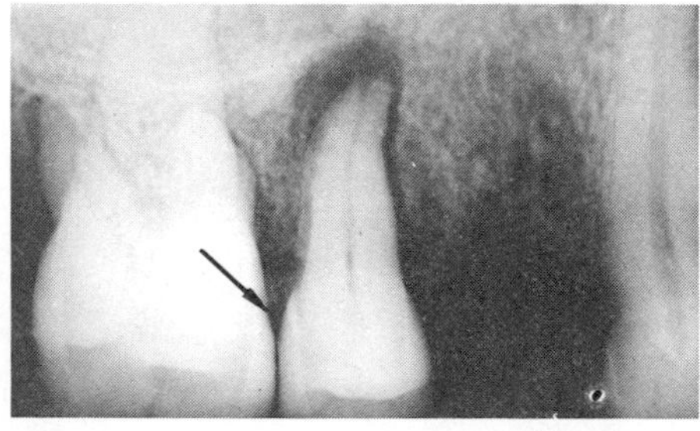

FIG. 30-7 The very dark area at the apex and along the root surface of the tooth represents total destruction of the normal tissue. The area is an abscess that drains to the surface along the side of the tooth (arrows). Calculus is evident between the bicuspid and molar. Note that the teeth are free from evidence of decay. *Courtesy of Dr. N. H. Rickles, Pathology Department, University of Oregon Dental School.*

advanced stages, destruction of cementum and periodontal membrane accompanied by loss of alveolar bone occurs (Figure 30–5). The net result is the formation of a pocket between the root and the overlying soft tissue, usually with marked inflammation and pus formation. Unfortunately, there are few clinical symptoms, and the disease progresses relentlessly until the teeth are lost. In people over 35 years of age, this disease—not tooth decay—is the major cause of tooth loss.

It is quite possible that no single factor is responsible for the infection, but rather many factors acting in concert (Table 30–2). One current hypothesis is that periodontal disease is caused not by a particular bacterial species, but rather by certain enzymatic and related activities of organisms in intimate contact with tissues surrounding the teeth.

In recent years the roles of dental plaque and calculus (Figure 30–6) in the process have been studied. Dental plaque formation is of great importance, especially since it may well be the initiator of dental decay as well as periodontal disease. Plaque is a mixture of bacteria embedded in an accumulation of saliva and bacterial products sticking to the tooth surface. Calculus is an almost constant companion of periodontal disease and is considered by many to be the major causative factor in its development (Figure 30–7).

Calculus is a hard, calcified substance that sticks firmly to the teeth or to appliances worn in the mouth. The external environment together with systemic factors of the host apparently determine whether the plaque will calcify or become associated with dental decay. Calcification of plaque begins in small areas that enlarge and combine to form large areas of calculus. The rough, ragged calculus further increases the irritation to the periodontium, the supporting tissue surrounding the teeth.

The possibility that certain types of periodontal lesions in humans are virus-induced has been suggested. Yet another possible etiological mechanism involved is allergic inflammation produced by bacterial antigens in gingival tissues.

GINGIVITIS

Gingivitis is an inflammation of the gingiva (that portion of the oral mucous membrane that surrounds a tooth). It is the most common disease affecting the soft tissues of the oral cavity. If unchecked, the inflammatory process eventually leads to severe periodontal disease.

NECROTIZING ULCERATIVE GINGIVITIS (N.U.G.)

Necrotizing ulcerative gingivitis (N.U.G.) is also called Vincent's infection or trench mouth, a name earned during World War I when it was common among soldiers (Figure 30–8). The outbreaks of N.U.G. among soldiers and in other crowded groups under emotional or physical stress convinced many clinicians that it was an infectious and communicable disease. However, recent studies have shown that N.U.G. is not communicable, and it is no longer required that physicians and dentists report cases of the disease.

The infection is found among adolescents and young adults. Fatigue and anxiety evidently play a most important role in predisposing the mouth to this tissue-destroying (necrotizing) condition.

The infection may involve the gums as Vincent's infection, the oral mucosa as Vincent's stomatitis, or extend to the throat as Vincent's angina.

PERIODONTITIS

Untreated gingivitis leads to periodontitis, inflammation of the periodontium. Another name for this condition is ***pyorrhea***.

DENTAL CARIES

Tooth decay is a world-wide problem, although not all areas and peoples are affected equally. Dental caries is a disease of the calcified tissues of the teeth characterized by a decalcification, or loss of calcium salts, of the inorganic substance. This is either followed by or accompanied by disintegration of the organic portion of the tooth. The etiology is complex, and considerable controversy exists over the exact mechanism of caries development. Dental decay in teeth is the result of an interaction between the host tissues and extremely specific cariogenic (caries-producing) microorganisms that utilize nutrients provided by the host's diet.

All bacteria known to cause decay on the smooth surfaces of the teeth are plaque-formers, secreting the complex polysaccharides of plaque, which are derived chiefly from sucrose (table sugar). Three polysaccharide-producing streptococci are found in large numbers in humans: ***Streptococcus mutans, Streptococcus sanguis,*** and ***Streptococcus salivarius.*** The extracellular polysaccharides that these organisms produce from sucrose enable them to adhere to one another and thus form colonies on the tooth's surface. Although the streptococci are not the only bacteria known to synthesize polysaccharides, they are the only ones that form plaque. Various experiments have shown that these streptococci and certain others, of human or rat origin, can produce tooth decay in germ-free rats. The process is shown in Figure 30–9.

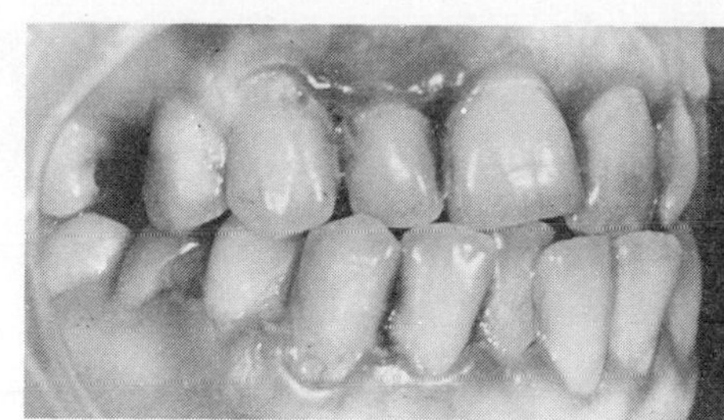
(a)

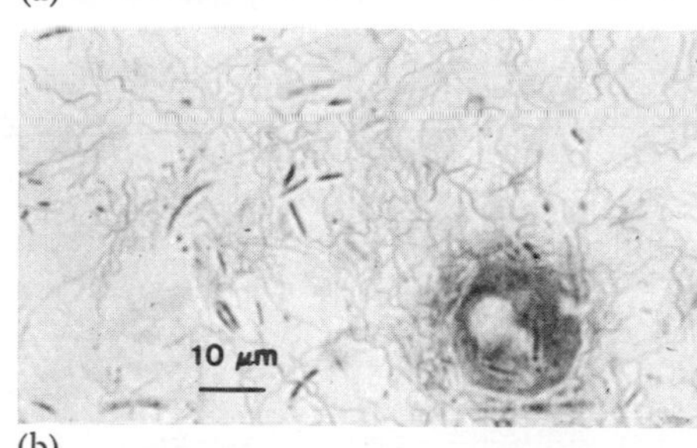

(b)

FIG. 30–8 Trench mouth, or N. U. G. (a) The appearance of Vincent's infection with "punched-out" necrotic projections, accompanied by swollen and inflammed gingiva. *Courtesy of Dr. Francis Howell, Pathology Department, University of Oregon Dental School.* (b) This smear was taken from a patient suffering from Vincent's infection. Note the large numbers of *Borrelia* and a variety of other cells. The large dark cell is a phagocytic inflammatory cell. *Courtesy of Dr. N. H. Rickles, Pathology Department, University of Oregon Dental School.*

Dental decay (Figure 30–10) and the defects produced by caries can be treated and the tooth restored to proper form and function in most cases. In recent years greater effort has been expended on measures to prevent this costly and often painful disease of humans. At present, plaque is most effectively eliminated by mechanical means such as brushing and flossing. An anti-plaque chemotherapeutic agent contained in an easy-to-use, palatable vehicle would greatly simplify effective oral hygiene. Such a drug could drastically reduce periodontal disease while also reducing dental caries.

At this time, however, there is no chemotherapeutic agent that can be safely administered for long-term control of bacterial plaque. Antibiotic compounds can be considered only for short-term plaque control because of their systemic side effects and limited spectrum of activity. All other compounds are limited in their usefulness by unpleasant or toxic side effects, by limited lack of effectiveness, or by inadequate experimental evidence.

Many substances have been tested as to their ability to eliminate or reduce the numbers of bacteria, change the flora to harmless non-acid-formers, inhibit enzyme activity, and alter the tooth surface. One of the most popular, but still controversial, compounds is sodium fluoride. When used in proper amounts, this material has been shown to have significant effects on caries incidence without causing ill effects in the user.

Diseases Related to Oral Foci of Infection

LUDWIG'S ANGINA

Certain serious complications can develop from infected teeth. One of these states, Ludwig's angina, involves beta-hemolytic streptococci (Figure 30–11). Microorganisms from such sites of infection pour into the surrounding tissues of the oral cavity. Ludwig's angina is a particularly dangerous infection of the throat and neck, since the swelling that develops may eventually block the air passages.

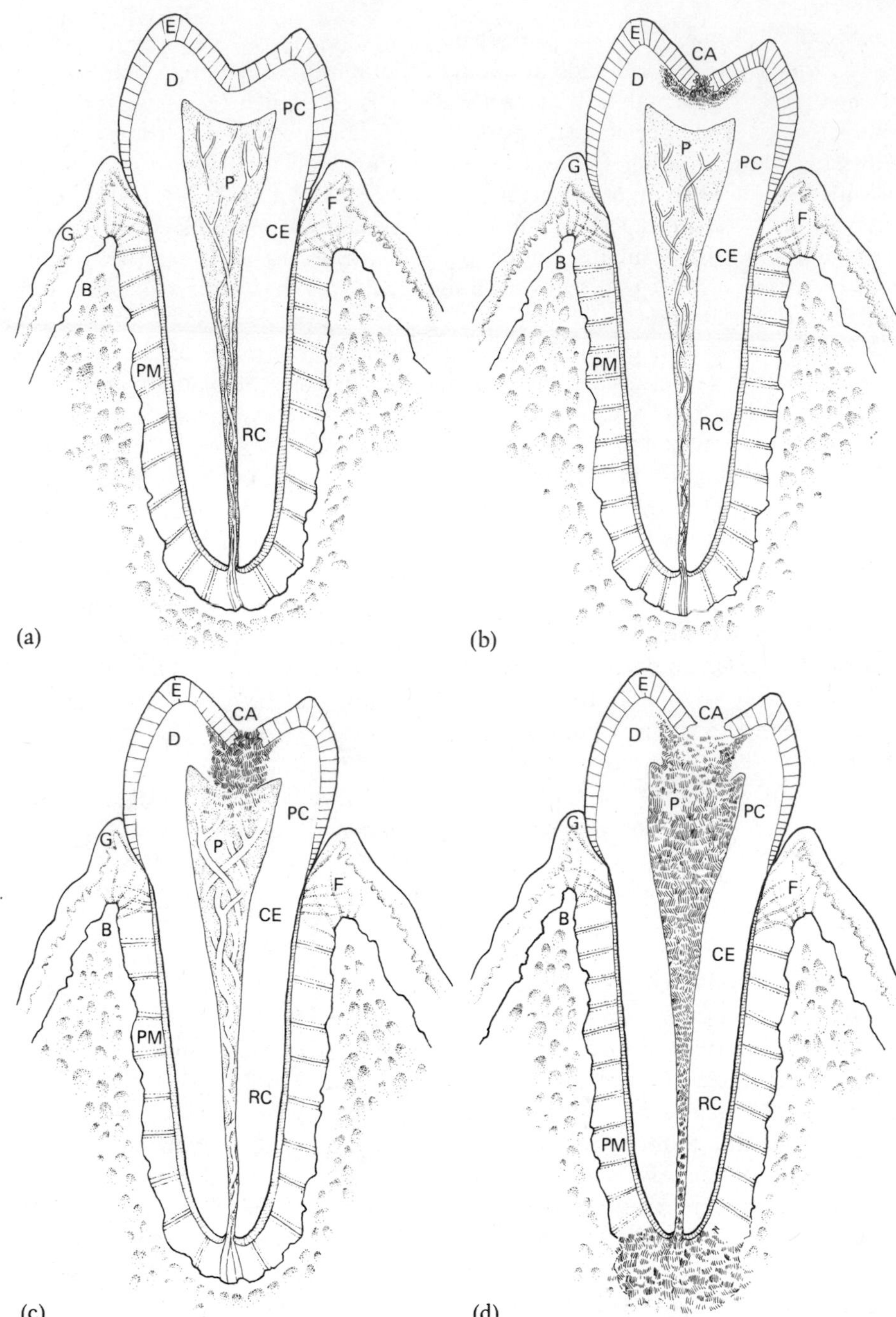

FIG. 30–9 Diagrammatic representation of a section through a premolar tooth, showing the progress of decay on the chewing surface. (a) A normal tooth and its surrounding tissues. (b) A carious lesion. (c) The decay has passed through the dentine into the pulp, which has become inflammed, with many engorged vessels. (d) The decay has spread to involve the tissues around the end of the root. At this stage there is some destruction of bone. Symbols: enamel barrier (E), dentine (D), gingiva (G), cementum (C), pulp tissue (P), pulp chamber and canal (PC), root canal (RC), alveolar bone (B), periodontal membrane (PM), fibers (F), cemento-enamel junction (CE), carious lesion (CA). *Courtesy of Dr. William B. Wescott, Pathology Department, University of Oregon Dental School.*

Bacterial Infections

Various bacterial pathogens involve the oral cavity at some time during their development cycles (Table 30–3). A representative number of such agents are

TABLE 30-3 Bacterial Infections Involving the Oral Cavity

Disease Entity	*Causative Agent*	*Gram Reaction*	*Symptoms and Clinical Appearance*	*Treatment*
Actinomycosis	*Actinomyces israelii, A. bovis*	+	Facial swelling, usually involving the jaw, with hardened and draining sinuses	Penicillin Sulfonamides Incision and drainage
Leprosy	*Mycobacterium leprae*	[a]	Tumorlike masses of tissue involving the oral lining, tongue, lips, or palate	Diaminodiphenylsulfone Sulphetrone Sulfoxone sodium Glucosulfone sodium Diphenylthiourea
Syphilis	*Treponema pallidum*	[a]	Primary oral chancres, secondary mucous patches, tertiary gummas; chronic, spreading, inflammatory, destructive lesions	Benzathine penicillin G Procaine penicillin G with 2% aluminum monostearate Tetracycline Erythromycin in penicillin-sensitive patients
Tuberculosis	*Mycobacterium tuberculosis*	[a]	Ulcerated punched-out lesions on mucosa or tongue; primary oral tuberculosis lesions are rare; fatigue, malaise, night sweats, productive cough when respiratory system involved	Streptomycin Isoniazid Tetracycline Para-aminosalicylic acid
Yaws	*Treponema pertenue*	[a]	Oral lesions "daughter yaws" secondary to skin lesions; affecting mucous membranes	Penicillin

[a]Grain stain reactions are not significant.

discussed in other chapters of this division.

Mycotic Infections

Fungus pathogens, as well as bacterial and viral agents of disease, involve the oral cavity either in a superficial manner or as a consequence of systemic disease. One common mycotic infection is discussed to illustrate this point; others are briefly characterized in Table 30–4.

CANDIDIASIS (MONILIASIS)

In 1965, Cohen reported that vitamin deficiencies, iron deficiency anemia, pregnancy, and diabetes may predispose an individual to the development of monilial stomatitis (candidiasis). Woods suggested in 1951 that the growth of *Candida* spp. appears to be restricted by the coexisting bacterial flora, but when this flora is suppressed by antibiotics, the *Candida* grow without restraint. As a result, patients may develop monilial infections of the oral cavity (Figure 30–12) or a more severe, generalized monilial infection of the blood involving the heart valves, respiratory system, gut, and brain. The oral lesions involve the tongue, palate, cheeks, and lips, and may further extend to the tonsils, pharynx, and larynx. *Candida* spp. may enter tissues at the time of tooth extractions. The diagnosis of candidiasis may include a direct examination of freshly obtained clinical specimens (Figure 30–13) and specimen cultivation.

TABLE 30-4 Mycotic (Fungus) Infections Involving the Oral Cavity

Disease Entity	*Causative Agent*	*Symptoms and Clinical Appearance*	*Treatment*
Candidiasis (moniliasis, thrush)	*Candida albicans*	Superficial lesions of skin or mucous membranes in skin folds or creases, often involves inside surfaces of lips; oral lesions are soft, grayish white, and strip off, leaving raw, bleeding surfaces; may accompany denture sore mouth	Nystatin Amphotericin B Gentian or crystal violet Potassium iodide
Coccidioidomycosis	*Coccidioides immitis*	Approximately 60% show no symptoms; 40% have symptoms of influenza; pulmonary lesions, skin, and oral mucosal granulomatous lesions	Symptomatic treatment Bed rest Amphotericin B
Cryptococcosis (torulosis)	*Cryptococcus neoformans*	Fever, cough, and pleural pain following inhalation of dusts containing the organism; oral lesions usually seen in systemically debilitated as ulcerations or sores	Amphotericin B Sulfadiazine Sulfapyridine
Geotrichosis	*Geotrichum candidum* (other *Geotrichum* species)	White patches on oral mucosa; may develop pulmonary and intestinal lesions	Nystatin Amphotericin B
Histoplasmosis	*Histoplasma capsulatum*	Lesions of the skin and involvement of reticuloendothelial system; nodules may occur in the mouth or throat and involve the respiratory tract	Amphotericin B
Mucormycosis	*Absidia* *Rhizopus* *Mucor*	Purulent nasal discharge; inflammatory, gangrenous mucosa; progressive systemic involvement with fatal outcome if untreated; rarely involves the oral region	Amphotericin B Correction of diabetes mellitus or underlying disease
North American blastomycosis	*Blastomyces dermatitidis*	Hard or wavy swellings often with sores, drainage	Amphotericin B
South American blastomycosis	*Blastomyces brasiliensis (Paracoccidioides brasiliensis)*	Fever, rales, and cough; chronic granulomatous lesions on the skin or mucous membranes and in various organs; oral lesions common	Amphotericin B
Sporotrichosis	*Sporotrichum schenckii*	Primary nodule often with ulceration; infection spreads along lymph channels and involves lymph nodes; may have oral nodules with ulceration	Potassium iodide Sulfonamides Amphotericin B

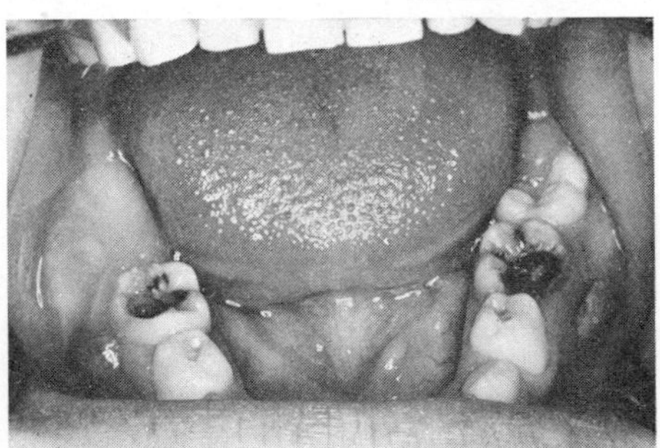

FIG. 30-10 A child with extensive caries of the primary second molars. The dark areas of the teeth represent advanced caries, which have infected the pulp. Note the pus-containing swelling on the gingiva of these teeth. *Courtesy of Dr. N. H. Rickles, Pathology Department, University of Oregon Dental School.*

TABLE 30-5 Viral Infections Involving the Oral Cavity

Disease Entity	*Causative Agent*	*Symptoms and Clinical Appearance*	*Treatment*
Chickenpox (varicella)	Varicella-herpes zoster virus	Vesicles with a surrounding erythematous zone appear on the mucosa and soon ulcerate	Symptomatic
Hand, foot, and mouth disease	Coxsackie virus Group A, Types 16, 6, and 10	Vesicles and ulcerations involving buccal mucosa, tongue, gingiva, and lips; ulcers are painful and interfere with eating; lesions also present on hands and feet	Symptomatic
Herpangina (aphthous pharyngitis)	Coxsackie virus Group A, Types 2, 4, 5, 6, 8, and 10	Sudden onset of high fever, headache, and sore throat, accompanied by papules, vesicles, and later ulcers on the pillars of the fauces, the uvula, and soft palate	Symptomatic
Herpes simplex (fever blister)	Herpes simplex *(Herpesvirus hominis)*	Primary lesions usually in oropharyngeal mucosa as multiple, very small vesicles, which rupture and ulcerate; a bright red zone is present around the periphery; fever, malaise, anorexia, and lymphadenopathy are present; recurrent lesions of mucosa on lips common	Supportive *Lactobacillus acidophilus* preparations, certain drugs that inhibit DNA synthesis (currently under study)
Herpes zoster (shingles)	Varicella-herpes zoster virus	Vesicles form along the distribution of a sensory nerve and soon ulcerate	Symptomatic
Hoof and mouth disease	Foot and mouth disease virus	Vesicles and ulcerations involving lips, tongue, palate, and mucosa; heal within two weeks	Symptomatic
Measles (rubeola)	Paramyxovirus	Koplik's spots appear on buccal mucosa as bluish white spots with a reddish surrounding zone, followed in a few days by a diffuse rash, fever, and catarrhal inflammation	Symptomatic
Molluscum contagiosum	Molluscovirus	Usually on skin of face; may rarely involve the intraoral tissues with slightly elevated lesions showing a superficial purulent discharge	Curretage Electrodessication
Mumps	Mumps virus	Painful swollen salivary glands, usually the parotid	Symptomatic Convalescent serum
Smallpox (variola)	Orthopoxvirus	Ulcerations of the oral mucosa; the tongue may be involved; severe symptoms with fever, headache, nausea	Hyperimmune vaccinia Gamma globulin Thiosemicarbazone

Viral Infections

A representative group of viral infections of the oral cavity are listed in Table 30-5 and discussed here.

HERPANGINA (APHTHOUS PHARYNGITIS)

Herpangina is specific and highly contagious, transmitted by direct contact. Sporadic outbreaks of the infection have been reported in many parts of the United States, usually during the summer months. It begins during the warm weather and disappears with the first plant-killing frost. Children up to 15 years of age are commonly affected.

HERPES SIMPLEX

The herpes simplex lesion has been called by many names, including canker sore, fever blister, cold sore, aphthous ulcer, and herpes labialis. This common viral disease affects the oral tissues (Figure 30–14), often remains localized, and produces considerable pain and discomfort for the patient.

Many factors may stimulate the virus *(Herpesvirus hominis)* to produce clinical lesions. Among these are excessive exposure to sun, fever, allergy, mechanical trauma, gastrointestinal upsets, and certain psychological factors.

MUMPS (EPIDEMIC PAROTITIS)

This world-wide acute, communicable disease is caused by a paramyxovirus. Humans are the only natural hosts for the causative agent. The virus apparently is spread as a droplet infection or by direct contact with saliva and respiratory secretions.

Mumps most frequently affect children between 8 and 15 years of age, with an overall incidence of at least 60 percent of the population. Adults who develop mumps often suffer severe complications, including infections of the testes (orchitis) in young men, and of the brain and its coverings (meningoencephalitis). The oral tissues involved are the salivary glands, most commonly the parotid glands. These are the largest of the salivary glands, found slightly below the ear. The immunity resulting from having the disease is of long duration and may develop following subclinical infections. Subsequent attacks have rarely been reported. Swelling of one salivary gland produces the same immunity as multiple gland involvement.

Temporary passive immunity toward the virus may be obtained by giving injections of gamma globulin from serum known to contain mumps antibody in high concentrations. Active immunization by vaccination is also possible.

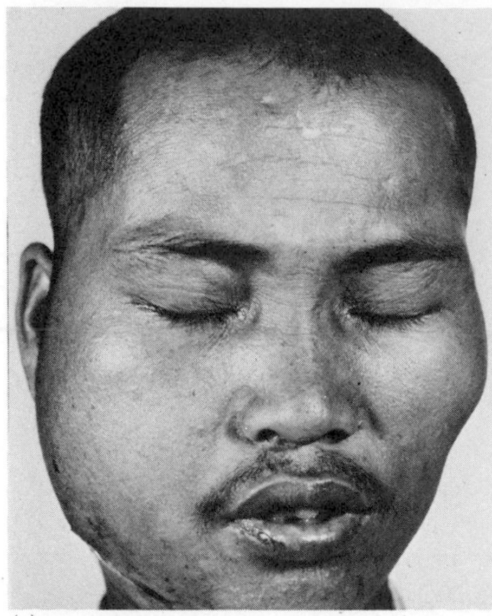

(a)

(b)

FIG. 30–11 Ludwig's angina. (a) This photograph shows the typical swelling that can occur. The infection probably developed from an infected tooth on the left side of the individual's face. (b) The result of treatment, which included an incision to produce drainage. *Courtesy of the Armed Forces Institute of Pathology, Washington, D.C., Neg. Nos. AFIP 44713–1 and 44713–2.*

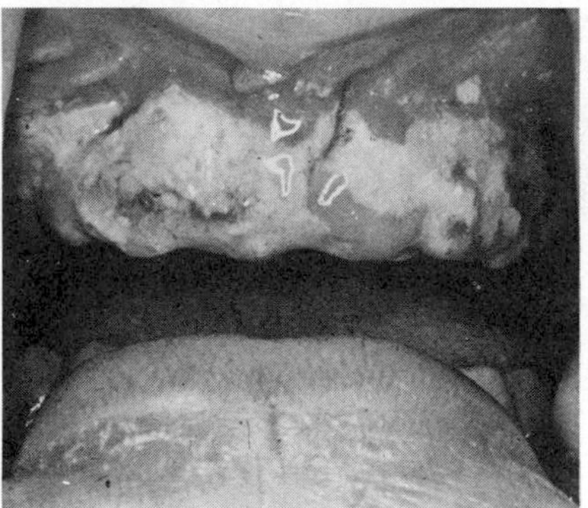

FIG. 30–12 Candidiasis. Forward view of the gingiva, showing the extent of the grayish white membranous growth. *Courtesy of Dr. N. H. Rickles, Pathology Department, University of Oregon Dental School.*

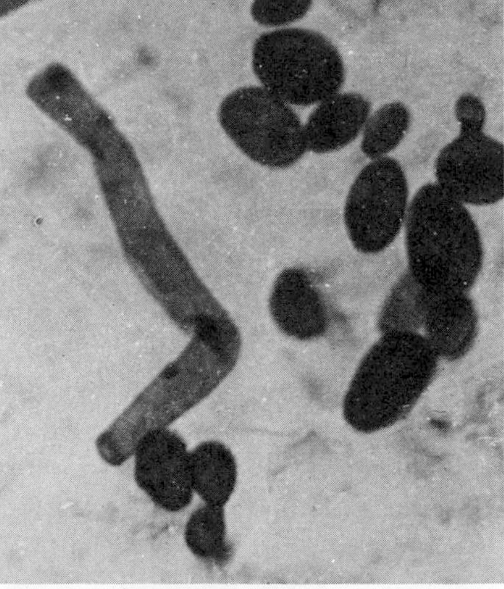

FIG. 30–13 *Candida albicans* in a direct smear from sputum. *Kozinn, P. J., and C. L. Taschdjian,* JAMA, *198/2:170–172 (1966).*

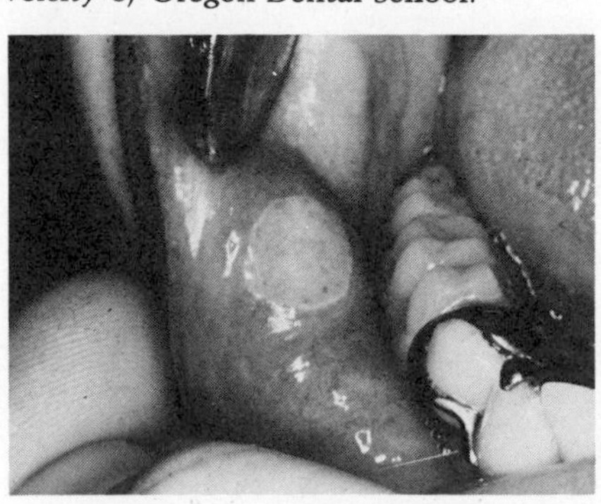

FIG. 30–14 Herpex simplex virus involving the inner surface of the lip. This is an older lesion with secondary infection and a thin layer of necrotic tissue over the surface. *Courtesy of Dr. N. H. Rickles, Pathology Department, University of Oregon Dental School.*

SUMMARY

Oral infections result from disturbances in the relationship of the individual's resident flora to the tissues of the mouth.

Structure of the Mouth

1. The human mouth has four groups of teeth, cutting *incisors*, tearing *canines*, and grinding *bicuspids* and *molars*.
2. Each tooth has three parts: the *crown*, the major exposed portion; the *root*, the portion below the gum and embedded in the jaw; and the *neck*, the constricted region between the crown and root.
3. A tooth's crown is coated with enamel; the rest is covered by modified bone layer called the *cementum*. Dentine underlies the enamel.
4. The gummy accumulation of salivary mucin and various types of bacteria is called *dental plaque*.

The Oral Flora

1. The microorganisms normally found in the human mouth can be divided into three groups on the basis of their oxygen requirements: strict anaerobes, strict aerobes, and facultative organisms.
2. The oral flora is relatively stable as to the types of organisms present. In addition to bacteria it includes several species of fungi, viruses, and protozoa.

Nonspecific Infections of the Oral Region

Infections of the face, oral cavity, and neck may be extremely serious, depending upon their location and the microorganisms involved.

Focal Infections

1. A localized area of infection anywhere on the body is called a *focus of infection*.
2. Oral foci of infection include those conditions that exist in the supporting structures of the teeth and the changes resulting from infected teeth. Examples include tooth decay (caries), infected gums (gingivitis), inflammation and destruction of the bone (osteomyelitis), and inflammation of tissue directly supporting the teeth (periodontitis, or pyorrhea).

Diseases Related to Oral Foci of Infection

Several serious complications can develop as a consequence of infected teeth or other portions of the mouth and various dental procedures. One such complication is Ludwig's angina.

Bacterial Infections

Various bacterial pathogens involve the mouth and related structures at some time during their development cycles. Examples of disease states of this kind include anthrax, syphilis, and tuberculosis.

Mycotic Infections

Pathogenic fungi also can involve the mouth. Examples of associated diseases include the yeast infection candidiasis.

Viral Infections

Viral infections of the mouth include chickenpox, fever blister (herpes simplex), herpangina, and mumps.

QUESTIONS FOR REVIEW

1. List at least five structures of the oral cavity and a particular infection or disease state associated with each of them.
2. What types of bacteria make up the largest microbial group of the oral cavity? Which one can cause diseases?
3. What is N.U.G.?
4. Discuss the following clinical states as to general features, causes, and treatment, if any:
   a. dry socket
   b. Vincent's infection
   c. osteomyelitis
   d. periodontitis
   e. pericoronitis
   f. dental caries
   g. periodontal disease
   h. sub-acute bacterial endocarditis
5. What is the role of calculus in periodontal disease?
6. What mechanisms have been offered to explain how periodontal disease develops?
7. What is pyorrhea?
8. What is a focal infection? How important is it to the general health of the body?

SUGGESTED READINGS

Dunlap, C. and B. Barker, Oral Lesions, Needham, Massachusetts, Hoyt Laboratories. *A highly illustrated reference to the diagnosis and treatment of a wide variety of oral lesions.*

Fenner, F., and D. O. White, *Medical Virology*. 2nd ed. New York: Academic Press, 1976. *An understandable book on viral diseases, including those of the skin, such as measles, and the herpesvirus infections, chickenpox, and shingles.*

Holt, S. C. and E. R. Leadbetter, "Comparative Ultrastructure of Selected Oral Streptococci: Thin Sectioning and Freeze-etching Studies," *Can. J. Microbiol.*, 22:475–485, 1976. *An electron microscopic study of the internal organization of streptococci associated with cariogenic activities.*

Long, S. S. and R. M. Swenson, "Determinants of the Developing Oral Flora in Normal Newborns," *Appl. Environ. Microbiol.*, 32:494–497, 1976. *A study of the factors that are important determinants in establishing the ecological place of bacteria in the oral microflora.*

Phillips, I., and M. Sussman (eds.), *Infection with Nonsporing Anaerobic Bacteria*. New York: Churchill Livingstone, 1974. *Contains several chapters on anaerobic infections of skin, soft tissue, and muscle. The publication is descriptive and easily understood, with several good references and tables.*

Roizman, B., and T. Buchman, "The Molecular Epidemiology of Herpes Simplex Viruses," *Hosp. Pract.* 14:95–104 (1970). *Descriptions of a straightforward enzymatic method to herpesvirus identification. This article emphasizes the need for exact identification of causative agents, especially in legal and epidemiologic situations.*

Wannamaker, L. W., and J. M. Matsen, eds. *Streptococci and Streptococcal Diseases*. New York: Academic Press, 1972. *Descriptions of several streptococcal infections of skin, the oral cavity, and kidney.*

CHAPTER **31**

Microbial Infections of the Respiratory Tract

What are common respiratory tract infections? How can they be prevented or controlled? Chapter 31 describes several major respiratory microbial diseases, including diphtheria, influenza, tuberculosis, whooping cough, and the pneumonias.

After reading this chapter, you should be able to:

1. **Describe the general organization of the human respiratory tract and indicate the areas susceptible to attack by pathogenic microorganisms.**
2. **Discuss measures used to control and treat respiratory infections.**
3. **Discuss at least three each of bacterial, fungus, and viral diseases of the respiratory system with respect to the causative agent, means of transmission, and general symptoms.**
4. **List general approaches to the diagnosis of bacterial, fungus, and viral infections of the respiratory system.**
5. **Describe the effects of the protozoan disease agent *Pneumocystis carinii*.**
6. **Describe the types of complications associated with microbial diseases of the respiratory tract.**
7. **List and explain at least two approaches to the prevention of viral infections of the respiratory system.**
8. **Discuss the value of antibiotics in the treatment of virus-caused respiratory infections.**
9. **List factors that can predispose respiratory infections.**

The human respiratory tract starts at the nose, passes through the various parts of the respiratory tree, and ends in the air sacs, or alveoli. This entire system is adapted to making air containing oxygen available to the circulatory system, and by it, to the whole body. Unfortunately, the respiratory tract is a frequent portal of entry for various microorganisms. Diffferent organisms gain access to different levels in the system, thus accounting in part for the differences in the types of infections occurring in the upper and lower portions of the respiratory tract. The respiratory system also provides a means of transmitting microbes to other individuals during speaking, coughing, and sneezing, when droplets of microbe-containing secretions are released.

The human respiratory tract provides an extensive area, approximately 60 square meters, of contact between the environment and the body. It includes the nose, pharynx (throat), larynx (voice box), trachea (windpipe), bronchi, and lungs (Figures 31–1 and 31–2). In addition to its protective roles against foreign particles and microorganisms, the respiratory system is designed for the efficient exchange of gases between the blood and the atmosphere.

Structures of the Respiratory System

The Pharynx

The pharynx, or throat, is a tubelike structure that, in addition to other functions, serves as a passageway for both food and air. It is associated with certain lymphoid tissues consisting of the pharyngeal ***tonsils*** (adenoids) and the lingual tonsils. A total of seven openings lead to or from the throat. There is one with the mouth, two with the nose, one with the larynx, one with the esophagus, and two with the Eustachian tubes. The ***Eustachian*** (auditory) ***tubes***, which connect the middle ear with the throat region, equalize the air pressure in the middle ear with atmospheric pressure. These tubes also serve as channels for middle ear drainage.

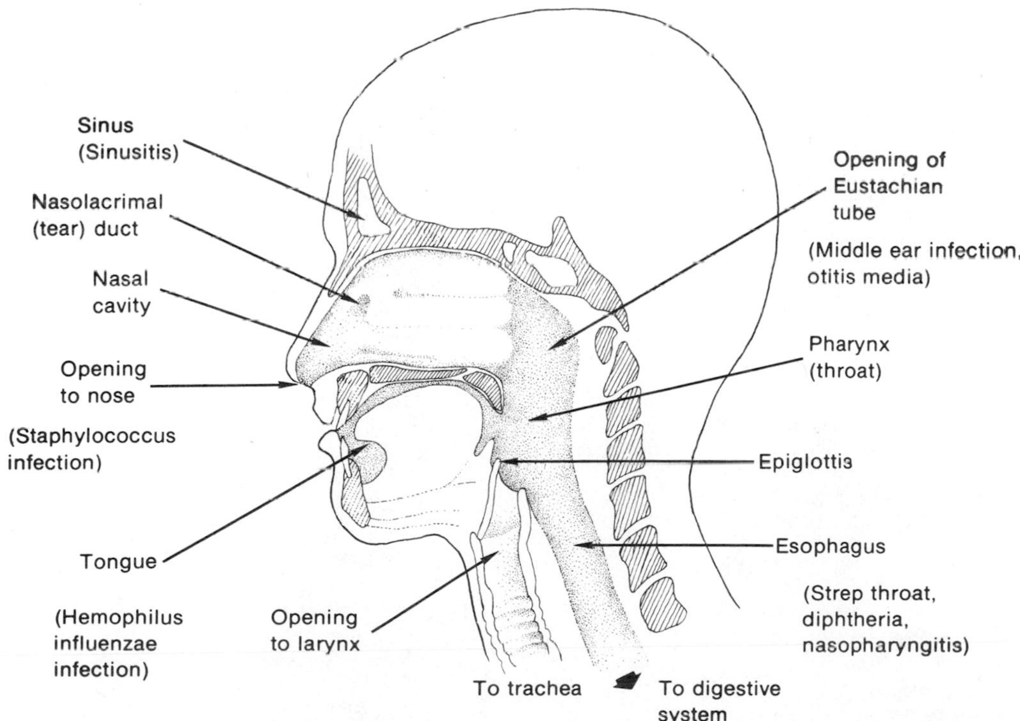

FIG. 31–1 The human respiratory system showing sites with which microbial infections are associated. The upper respiratory system is shown here.

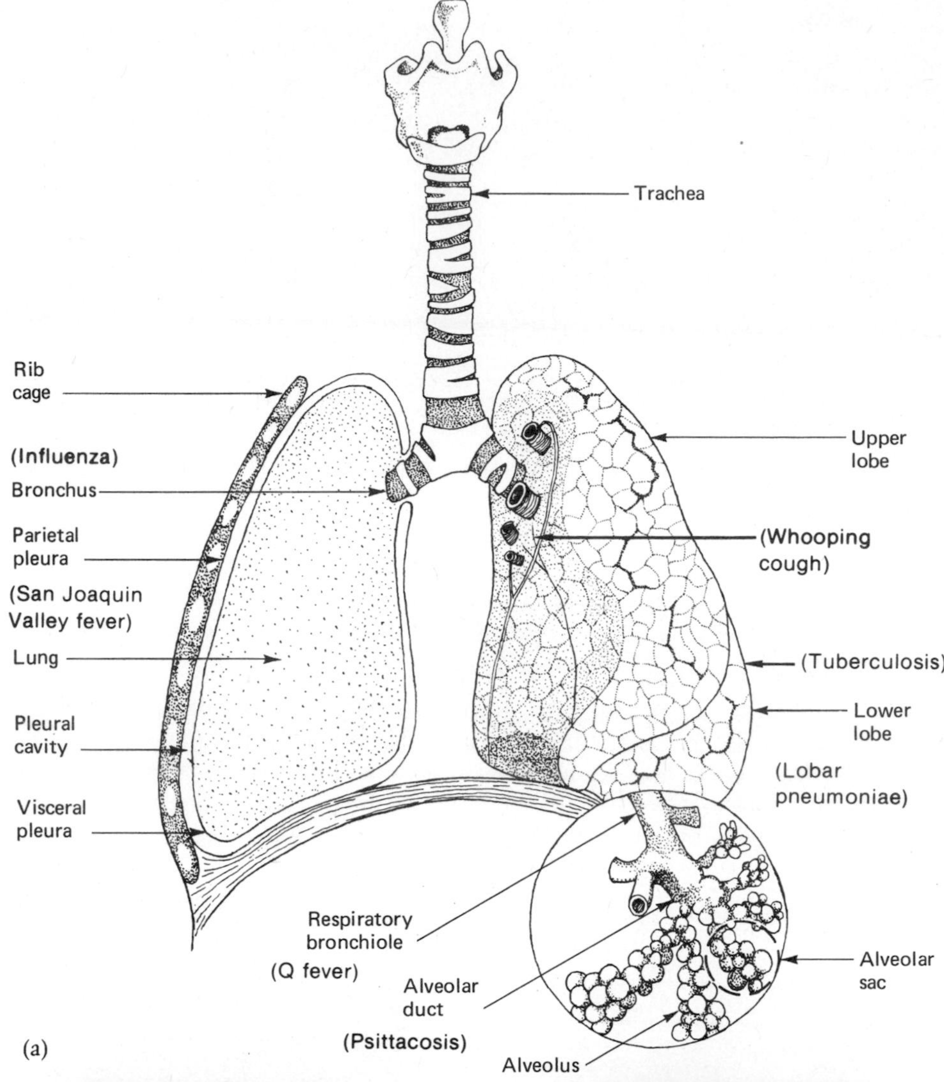

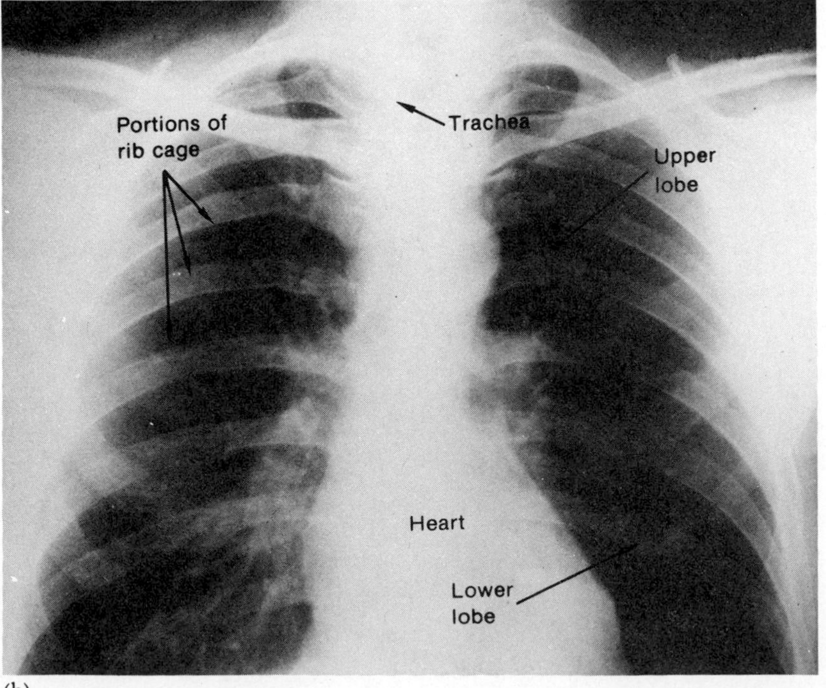

FIG. 31-2 Portions of the respiratory tree. The relationship of the pleura, the membranes covering the lungs, is also shown. (a) The lower portion of the system. The alveoli (air sacs), which participate in gaseous exchanges, are emphasized. Specific sites associated with microbial infections are indicated. A depression on the middle surface of each lung is the region through which the primary bronchus, blood vessels, lymphatics, and nerves penetrate the structure. (b) An x-ray showing the appearance of normal lungs. *Kay, K.* Trans. N.Y. Acad. Sci. *36:511 (1974).*

The Trachea

The trachea, commonly called the windpipe, is a thin tube averaging about 2.5 cm in diameter. It passes from the voice box, or larynx, into the thoracic, or chest, cavity, where it divides into the two primary ***bronchi***. The trachea is lined by ciliated ephithelial cells.

The Lungs and the Primary Bronchi

The cone-shaped organs of respiration, the lungs, are soft and spongy. Each lung is divided into ***lobes***. The right lung is composed of three lobes, the left lung two. Most of the chest is taken up by the lungs.

The bronchial tree (Figure 31–2) is formed from both bronchi dividing and subdividing into smaller bronchi, leading into several sizes of tubelike structures called ***bronchioles***. The smallest of these, approximately 0.5 mm, are known as ***terminal*** bronchioles. These divide and give rise to ***respiratory*** bronchioles, which in turn branch into several alveolar ducts. Alveolar sacs develop from the ducts. The walls of these sacs form the ***alveoli*** in which gaseous exchange (external respiration) occurs. Because of the narrower passages, air moves much more slowly in this lower portion of the system than in the upper portion. Two membranes form a closed sac that envelops the lungs. The inner membrane, the ***visceral pleura***, covers the outer lung surface. The outer membrane layer, the ***parietal pleura***, lines the inner surface of the chest wall. The potential cavity between these two membranes is called the ***pleural cavity***. A serumlike fluid found in this region enables the two pleurae to glide over one another during respiratory movements.

Normal Flora of the Respiratory Tract

The normal flora of the human nose includes species of *Bacterioides, Branhamella, Corynebacterium, Haemophilus, Micrococcus, Staphylococcus,* and *Streptococcus*. Some of these microorganisms can pose serious problems and cause disease. At birth the throat, windpipe, and bronchi are sterile. However, within 24 hours after birth, these sites become colonized by streptococci and other bacteria. In the adult, the respiratory tract below the level of the epiglottis (Figure 31–1) is normally sterile.

Introduction to Microbial Infections of the Respiratory Tract

Several microorganisms can cause respiratory tract infections. Many of the resulting diseases are quite common and are among the most damaging of any that affect humans.

Various microbial pathogens—bacteria, fungi, and viruses—find suitable avenue for entry and site for multiplication in the respiratory tract. Even though they use the respiratory tract as a portal of entry and at times a portal of exit, the resulting infectious process may easily extend to other regions of the body.

The various secretions associated with the respiratory system can be infectious. Relatively few microorganisms are introduced into the environment during normal breathing, even by an infected individual. However, an infected person or carrier not covering the nose or mouth while sneezing or coughing can easily contaminate the environment with disease agents. The communicability of infectious diseases is influenced by several factors, including (1) the survival of respiratory pathogens on fomites or in the air, (2) the number of microorganisms inhaled, (3) the duration of contact, and (4) the anatomical site involved in the localization of the infectious agents.

Control Measures

In the past fifty years, many advances have improved the control and prevention of infectious diseases involving the lungs. The future appears to hold additional promise, especially for the effective control of respiratory diseases such as pneumococcal pneumonia.

Many of the measures used to control respiratory tract infections are similar, if not identical, to those described in Chapter 27 for other types of diseases. The procedures are largely determined by the characteristics of the pathogen or particular disease it causes. Control of respiratory tract infections may include (1) isolation of infected persons, (2) concurrent disinfection or sterilization of contaminated equipment, such as mouthpieces, thermometers, rubber tubing, and any and all contaminated articles such as eating utensils and dishes, (3) the use of and proper disposal of gowns following contact with infectious individuals, (4) the disinfection of rooms or associated facilities used by infected persons, and (5) the washing and disinfecting of hands before and after contact with patients or with any and all articles handled by patients, such as blankets, dishes, laundry, or pillows.

Representative Microbial Diseases

Several infections of the respiratory tract are of great concern because of the ease with which they are transmitted and contracted and the difficulty in eradicating their disease agents. A number of these microbial pathogens and the diseases they cause are described in Tables 31–1 through 31–8. Treatment, which includes the use of antibiotics in certain cases, is also indicated in several of these tables.

FIG. 31–3 Lung abscess formation caused by *Staphylococcus aureus*. X-ray shows cloudy lung area (arrow) with abscess before treatment. Compare this view with Figure 31-2b. *Courtesy of Dr. Marcel Bilodeau, Hospital Laval, Quebec, Canada.*

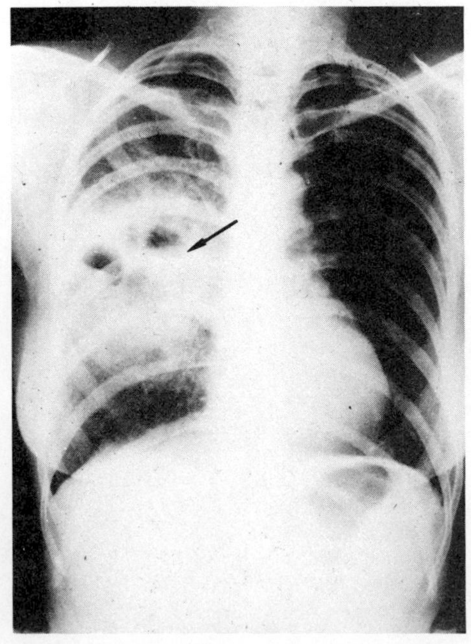

Diagnosis

Respiratory tract infections can often be diagnosed on the basis of x rays (Figure 31–3), the patient's history, and examination. Confirmation is made by laboratory work, including microscopic examination of sputum, blood, and other specimens; isolation of pathogens from specimens; serological tests; and animal inoculations. Most of the tables in this chapter present the general diagnostic approaches used in respiratory tract infections.

Upper Respiratory Infections

The upper respiratory region, which includes the middle ear, the small air cells behind the ears called the mastoids, the sinuses, and the nasal corner of the

TABLE 31-1 Features of Selected Bacterial Upper Respiratory Tract Infections

Disease	Causative Agent	Gram Reaction	Morphology	Incubation Period	General Features of the Disease	Laboratory Diagnosis	Possible Treatment
Diphtheria	*Corynebacterium diptheriae* (Klebs-Löffler bacillus)	+	Rods appearing in aggregates resembling X's, Y's, and Chinese letters	1–10 days	Symptoms appear suddenly and include fever, sore throat, general discomfort, formation of diphtheritic pseudomembrane on tonsils, throat, or in the nasal cavity; complications such as heart and kidney failure can develop	1. Gram stain of throat specimen 2. Demonstration of metachromatic granules (Figure 7–2d) 3. Isolation and culture 4. Demonstration of toxin production production	1. Diphtheria antitoxin therapy combined with antibiotic therapy 2. Antibiotics include erythromycin, penicillin, and tetracyclines
Middle ear infection (otitis media)	*Hemophilus influenzae* *Staphylococcus aureus* *Streptococcus pneumoniae*	− + +	Rod Coccus Coccus	1–2 days	Pain first limited to ear, then spreads to other head regions; other symptoms include varying degrees of deafness, dizziness, noises, feelings of revolving in space or of surroundings rotating, pus formation, and difficulty in swallowing	1. Gram stain of specimen 2. Isolation and culture 3. Serological tests	Ampicillin, cephalothin, erythromycin, penicillin, vancomycin
Sinus infection (sinusitis)	*Bacterioides* species *Hemophilus influenzae* *Streptococcus pneumoniae*	− − +	Rod Rod Coccus	1–2 days	Accumulation of mucus in the sinuses; pain, headache, general discomfort, difficulty in breathing	1. Gram stain of specimen 2. Isolation and culture from specimens 3. Biochemical tests	Chloramphenicol, penicillin, vancomycin
Streptococcal (strep throat)	*Streptococcus pyogenes*	+	Coccus	1–3 days	Chills, fever, headache, nausea or vomiting, rapid pulse, reddened and swollen throat and uvula, and presence of a gray or yellow white material covering the throat; complications include middle ear infections, kidney infections, and blood poisoning	1. Gram stain of specimen 2. Isolation and culture from specimens 3. Serological tests for streptococci	Antibiotics, penicillin, and tetracyclines

eyes (Figure 31–1), are exposed to a variety of pathogens when air is inhaled. These organisms can establish infections in these sites (Tables 31–1 through 31–3) and spread to other regions of the respiratory tract.

Bacterial Diseases

DIPHTHERIA

Diptheria, an acutely infectious communicable disease, has been known since ancient times, but its specific nature was not recognized until the nineteenth century. The bacterial cause of diphtheria was identified from stained smears by Edwin Klebs in 1883 and successfully cultivated and shown to produce the disease soon after by Friedrich August Löffler.

Löffler, who first demonstrated that *Corynebacterium diphtheriae* causes the disease, concluded from his studies that when the bacteria are injected into guinea pigs, they produce a powerful toxin. The disease state developed as a consequence of the poisonous material being transported via the bloodstream to other parts of the animal's body. By separating organisms from their liquid environment, Pierre Paul Émile Roux and Alexandre Émile John Yersin in 1888 showed the presence of the *C. diphtheriae* toxin in the liquid phase of the medium.

In 1951, V. J. Freeman offered further insight into the course of diphtheria when he discovered that only those *C. diphtheriae* strains infected with a specific bacteriophage could produce the toxin that causes diphtheria.

Toxin-producing *C. diphtheriae* produces a severe inflammation of the throat. A tough membranelike structure, pseudomembrane, forms on the tonsils and spreads to lower portions of the respiratory tract or upward into the nasal passages. This membrane may cause suffocation. The absorption of the toxin into the bloodstream can cause complications such as paralysis and cardiac arrest (Table 31–1).

The discovery of the diphtheria toxin had great immunological significance. By 1890, Emil von Behring and his associates were immunizing laboratory animals with a heat-attenuated toxin preparation and obtaining antitoxin with which to treat human victims of the disease. Unfortunately, their heat-attenuated form of diphtheria toxin proved too toxic for human immunization purposes. Not until 1923 was an effective and safe modified toxin for immunization prepared by treating the toxin with formalin. The resulting toxoid retains its antigenicity but is incapable of disease production.

Transmission. Most instances of diphtheria result from direct contact with droplets. *C. diphtheriae* is a hardy organism, able to withstand cold, heat, and drying.

Diphtheria occurs world-wide, mainly among individuals over six months but not past middle age. Among the major sources of *C. diphtheriae,* carriers, individuals showing no outward signs of the disease, are believed to account for approximately one fourth of the known cases. However, exposure to a recognizably infected person is far more likely to result in a case of diphtheria than exposure to a carrier. Infected persons may be a source of disease agents for as long as one to two weeks.

Predisposing factors associated with the disease include chilling, poor nutrition, overcrowded conditions, and operations involving the nose and throat. In the last case, diphtheria may result from the exposure of a noninfected individual to the pathogen, or from a carrier of *C. diphtheriae*.

Immunity and Prevention. A relatively long-lasting acquired immunity results from one attack of diphtheria. Infants born to mothers immunized against *C. diphtheriae* infection usually have temporary protection. Because such immunity only lasts for a few weeks after birth, widespread immunization of infants is practiced. In the United States, the DPT vaccine (diphtheria, pertussis, and tetanus) is used to induce immunity. Later booster injections and exposure to infected persons contribute to maintaining adequate antitoxin levels in the individual. It is important to note that the antibody response of individuals varies widely. Therefore, it may be necessary to administer several booster shots during childhood and later in life to bring a person's degree of immunity up to a functional level.

Schick test. The Schick test, a skin test that determines susceptibility to diphtheria, is used in testing large groups of people. It is reliable in most, but not all, situations. The procedure involves injection of 0.1 ml of a standardized preparation of diphtheria toxin just under the skin of the inside of the arm. Appearance of a reddened, swollen, tender area around the site of injection indicates susceptibility.

Hypersensitivity to the toxin preparation has been reported. This reaction may result from sensitivity to other components of the skin test material. To distinguish such responses from a true indication of susceptibility, toxoid is injected into the opposite arm. Hypersensitive individuals will react to both types of preparations.

Among the measures adopted by health agencies to protect susceptible individuals are large-scale immunization programs. The quarantine of carriers and the daily use of appropriate antibiotics help prevent transmission of the disease until their systems are free of *C. diphtheriae.* Carriers should be quarantined until bacterial cultures are negative.

DISEASES OF THE EAR

Various microorganisms can cause infections of the ear. This section will be primarily concerned with those involving bacterial pathogens. Table 31–2 lists some of the diseases associated with such microorganisms.

It is well known that individuals with nasopharyngeal (nose and throat) diseases are often predisposed to ear infections. This is especially true in cases of adenoid growths, Eustachian tube obstructions, and various forms of middle ear and sinus infections. Treatment must be directed not only toward the ear disease but also against the predisposing condition.

Pus-Producing Middle Ear Infection (Suppurative Otitis Media). Pus-forming ear infection is a common childhood disease, although it is quite frequently overlooked. The infection usually results from inflammatory conditions involving the upper air passages (Table 31–2). Contaminated swimming water entering the middle ear from the nose or nasopharynx, injuries to the tympanic membrane, skull fractures associated with the temporal bone, and certain complications of epidemic cerebrospinal meningitis all may produce this condition. Apparently children are predisposed to acute suppurative otitis media if they have adenoids in the nasopharynx and if they possess a hereditary tendency toward nasal congestion (catarrhal) and pus formation of the upper air passages.

Staphylococcus aureus, Hemophilus influenzae, and beta-hemolytic streptococci are the most common etiologic agents of this disease (Table 31–2). *Streptococcus pneumoniae* also is known for its ability to produce this form of otitis media.

TABLE 31-2 Representative Microbial Diseases of the Ear

Disease	Causative Agent	Gram Reaction	Morphology (if applicable)	Possible Treatment
Boils	*Staphylococcus aureus*	+	Coccus	Cephalothin, lincomycin, methicillin, nafcillin, vancomycin
Inflammation of the eardrum	Mixed infections involving hemolytic streptococci and viruses	+	Cocci	Ampicillin, cephalothin, erythromycin, penicillin, symptomatic
Inflammation of the outer ear	*Escherichia coli, Proteus* spp., *Pseudomonas* spp.	−	Rods	Chloramphenicol, gentamicin, kanamycin, penicillin, polymycin, tetracyclines
	Hemolytic streptococci, S. aureus	+	Cocci	Ampicillin, cephalothin, erythromycin, penicillin, vancomycin
Otitis media (middle ear infection)	Mixed infections *Streptococcus pneumoniae*, beta-hemolytic streptococci, *S. aureus*	+	Cocci	Ampicillin, cephalothin, erythromycin, penicillin, vancomycin
	Hemophilus influenzae	−	Coccobacillus	Chloramphenicol, kanamycin, penicillin, streptomycin, tetracyclines
Mycotic infection of the external ear and ear canal	*Aspergillus niger*	Not useful	Mold	
	Candida albicans	+	Yeast	Amphotericin B
Throat abscess	Beta-hemolytic streptococci, *S. aureus*	+	Cocci	Ampicillin, cephalothin, erythromycin, penicillin, vancomycin

STREPTOCOCCAL SORE THROAT

Streptococcal sore throat is an acute, severe inflammation of both the tonsils (tonsillitis) and the throat (pharyngitis). Strep throat can be caused by several strains of Lancefield's group A, beta-hemolytic streptococci (Table 31–1).

Transmission. Strep throat usually occurs in epidemic form and is associated with contaminated milk products and water. The nasopharynxes of individuals suffering from the disease during the acute or convalescent stage serve as the source of infectious agents. There are also carriers.

Milk products may be contaminated by human handling or as a consequence of infection in the cows. In epidemics involving milk consumption, the source of contamination can usually be traced to a single dairy. Furthermore, strep throat is more common in regions where pasteurization of milk is not practiced. Epidemics may last from 2 to 6 weeks. The incidence of this disease is greater during the winter and spring months.

Prevention. Control measures for strep throat include pasteurization of milk, isolation of infected persons, and proper disinfection or disposal of objects contaminated by the discharges of infected persons. Such persons should not be allowed to come into contact with products for consumption during either the acute or convalescence stage of the disease.

Virus Diseases

This section deals with common viral agents for which the respiratory tract is both the principal site for replication and the site of their cytopathic effects (Table 31–3). It is important to make this distinction because several viruses can grow in the respiratory tract or use the tract for entry into the body without producing their effects there. These viruses are not discussed here.

In 1968, A. J. Rhodes and C. E. Van Rooyen reviewed the major viral respiratory infections. They wrote that the number of viruses causing respiratory illness in humans and other animals is steadily increasing. Identification of the virus associated with a given disease is complicated by the fact that one viral agent may produce more than one set of symptoms. The antigenic characteristics of several respiratory viruses such as influenza change periodically, and there are no sharp distinctions in the symptoms of the various respiratory diseases; symptoms of many diseases overlap. Rhodes and Van Rooyen also concluded that susceptibility to respiratory illness is influenced by developmental, immunologic, and physiologic features of the host.

USE OF ANTIBIOTICS

In the treatment of various viral respiratory diseases, antibiotics are given primarily to prevent secondary bacterial infections. This is done even though there is no clear evidence that these drugs reduce or eliminate the effects of the causative agents. Additional aspects of treatment are directed toward relieving the discomfort of the disease victim.

THE COMMON COLD

According to many authorities, acute afebrile diseases (those without fever) of the upper respiratory tract are the most frequent of human afflictions. As a group they cause the loss of millions of hours of work each year. In most cases these infections are not serious, only extremely uncomfortable. Many studies have led to the view that several different viruses can cause the common cold. Several of these etiologic agents have been designated as the *rhinoviruses* (from the Greek *rhino* meaning "nose"). It is important to note that these viruses are not the sole cause of the common cold.

The rhinovirus-caused common cold appears to have a wide geographic distribution, as judged from the presence of antibodies in persons throughout the world. The transmission of rhinovirus infections seems to require a close and continued contact among individuals.

Control. Attempts to develop vaccines against cold viruses have so far not been successful. Another approach to the problem of control has concentrated on the active inhibitor of viral activities, *interferon*. Here again, effective application has not been attained. The intake of large quantities of vitamin C has been suggested as an effective means of providing resistance toward respiratory illness under normal conditions. Further studies are currently underway to evaluate this control measure.

Attempts to control the spread of common cold agents by use of disinfectant aerosols, irradiation with ultraviolet light, or the quarantine of infected persons are usually of little value.

TABLE 31-3 **Viral Agents and Commonly Associated Upper Respiratory Tract Infections**

Respiratory Tract Infection	*Virus by Generic Designation*[a]	*General Features of the Disease*	*Laboratory Diagnosis*
Common cold	*Coronavirus* *Rhinovirus*	Cough, watery nasal discharge, head cold (coryza), headache, nasal obstruction, sneezing, sore throat	Isolation and identification of causative agent using tissue culture (not routinely done)
Croup (acute laryngotracheo-bronchitis)	*Adenovirus* *Orthomyxovirus* *Paramyxoviruses* Respiratory syncytial virus	Symptoms range from mild to severe and can be grouped into the following types: *Type 1*—cough, hoarseness, harsh breathing high-pitched sounds *Type 2*—fever, toxic effects, vomiting *Type 3*—convulsions, bluish coloration (cyanosis), dehydration, and restlessness	1. Isolation and identification of causative agent using tissue culture 2. Serological tests
Minor respiratory illnesses	Adenoviruses Echoviruses Paramyxoviruses Reoviruses	Fever, sore throat, swollen lymph nodes in neck, persistent cough	1. Isolation and identification of causative agent using tissue culture 2. Serological tests

[a]Based on the results of isolations from cases of respiratory infections.

CROUP

Croup, or acute laryngotracheobronchitis, is an acute infectious disease of children under three years of age. Males are affected more often than females. Croup may be mild or severe in its effects (Table 31–3).

Lower Respiratory Infections

The lungs inhale many pathogenic microorganisms that normally are eliminated efficiently by the defenses of the host. However, several diseases of the lower respiratory tract are life-threatening if not treated quickly and adequately (Tables 31–4, 31–6, and 31–7).

Bacterial Pneumonias

Several bacterial species can cause pneumonia (Tables 31–1 and 31–4). One of the most recently discovered forms of the condition is Legionnaire's disease. This pneumonia earned its name and notoriety by striking many individuals, some fatally, who attended an American Legion convention in Philadelphia in 1976. Since that first report of Legionnaire's disease, other outbreaks have been noted. The general features of this disease together with those of other types of pneumonia (Figure 31–4) are given in Table 31–4. Because of space limitations, only pneumococcal pneumonia will be presented in greater detail.

FIG. 31–4 The appearance of the human lung in staphylococcal pneumonia. *Courtesy of the Armed Forces Institute of Pathology, Washington, D.C., Neg. No. AFIP 55-6150.*

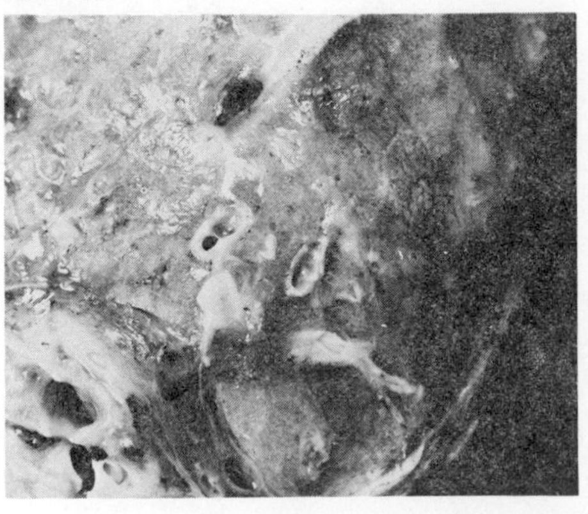

PNEUMOCOCCAL PNEUMONIA

Streptococcus pneumoniae has caused by far the majority of pneumonia cases in which a whole lobe or more than one lobe is involved, referred to as *lobar pneumonia*.

Over 75 different serological types of *S. pneumoniae* have been reported. Differentiation among the various types is based on the existence of immunologically distinct polysaccharides, which form the capsules of these organisms (Color Photograph 13). The designation of each type is by number, such as type 3, type 7, and so on.

S. pneumoniae is also capable of causing diseases other than pneumonia. These include infection of the middle ear (otitis media), pneumococcal meningitis, and inflammation of the sinuses (sinusitis). Antibiotic-resistant strains are being found, making treatment difficult. The development in 1977 of a polyvalent vaccine effective against the most common types of *S. pneumoniae* should greatly reduce the incidence of these diseases.

Other microorganisms that have been known to produce lobar pneumonia, though far less frequently, are *Klebsiella pneumoniae, Mycobacterium tuberculosis, Yersinia pestis,* which causes pneumonic plague, *Francisella tularensis,* which causes tularemia or rabbit fever, and *Serratia marcescens.*

Transmission and Predisposing Factors. Pneumonia produced by *S. pneumoniae* occurs during the winter months in temperate zones, usually among those between 15 and 45 years of age. Although this disease is not considered highly communicable, its incidence has been noted to be greater where close personal contact exists, as in households, barracks, dormitories, hospital wards, prisons, and similar group living quarters. Mortality rates have been substantially reduced, especially in the young, by early and adequate administration of antibiotics.

Pneumococci are usually spread by droplet nuclei from nasal or pharyngeal secretions. Individuals exposed to such infectious material may contract the disease or become carriers. It is interesting to note that 40 to 70 percent of normal adults have *S. pneumoniae* as normal inhabitants of their throats.

Several factors have been reported to predispose individuals to pneumococcal and other bacterial pneumonias. Among these so-called secondary causes are viral infections of the upper respiratory tract and local or generalized pulmonary edema (fluid in the lungs). Pulmonary edema can be brought about by irritating anesthetics, cardiac failure, and influenza. More general predisposing causes that have been implicated include increasing age, debilitating disease states (such as diabetes or malignancies), fatigue, and chilling. With many, if not all, of the factors mentioned the underlying feature is impairment of the lung's defense mechanism, its phagocytic activity by tissue macrophages.

Complications. Unfortunately, complications arise with at least 15 to 20 percent of the pathogen's victims. Commonly encountered complications include recurrence of the disease, inflammation of the pleura, otitis media, and sinusitis.

Immunity and Prevention. Individuals who have recovered from pneumococcal pneumonia often carry the causative agents in their upper respiratory tracts for long periods, despite the fact that they also have antibodies circulating in their bloodstreams. These antibodies remain for several months. If an individual suffers a second attack of pneumonia, it is probably due to a serological type of *S. pneumoniae* other than the one that caused the first infection.

Preventive measures against pneumococcal diseases include immunization and the adequate treatment and isolation of infected persons. Indiscriminate use of antibiotics should be avoided because it can induce drug reactions and can enhance the survival of drug-resistant organisms.

MYCOPLASMA INFECTIONS

Mycoplasma have been known for years to cause diseases of lower animals, but only recently have investigations demonstrated that one species is pathogenic for humans. This is *Mycoplasma pneumoniae,* the etiologic agent of primary atypical pneumonia (Table 31–4).

PSITTACOSIS

Psittacosis, or parrot fever, is the term generally given to respiratory infections contracted from psittacine birds (canaries, cockatoos, lovebirds, parakeets, parrots, and thrushes). It is caused by strains of *Chlamydia psittaci.* In general, psittacosis is considered to be *zoonotic,* spread by lower animals through natural means to humans. However, some cases of human disease have resulted from direct contact with infected persons (Table 31–4).

Transmission. In psittacine birds, the infection is usually spread by direct contact, droplets, and droppings. Latent disease states are common with these animals, and under conditions of stress—chilling, dampness, or overcrowding—the inactive infection is known to develop into overt psittacosis. The symptoms of infected birds include diarrhea, emaciation, and a mucopurulent discharge from the mouth. Many cases of human disease develop in pet owners, animal handlers, and pet store attendants. Great care must be exercised in handling specimens suspected of containing the psittacosis agents.

Control. Control measures against psittacosis usually include the imposition of a six-month quarantine on shipments of psittacine birds, the use of spot laboratory examination on shipments of these animals, and the incorporation of antibiotics into the feed for psittacines. Chlortetracycline has proved extremely efficient in reducing the incidence of the disease in birds.

Q ("QUERY") FEVER

Q fever, a zoonotic rickettsial infection, was first described in 1933 by Derrick in Australia. The etiologic agent for the disease is *Coxiella burnettii* (Table 31–4). Arthropods do not play a major role in transmission of the disease to humans. However, ticks are considered important to the cycle of infection in wild rodents. Human infections, as well as those of other animals, occur through the inhalation of infectious discharges (droplet transmission) from diseased cattle, goats, and sheep. Milk and eggs have also been implicated in disease cycles.

TUBERCULOSIS AND OTHER MYCOBACTERIAL DISEASES

Tuberculosis (TB) has been a plague of humanity for centuries, especially among populations suffering from malnutrition and poor sanitary conditions. The clinical manifestations as well as the communicable nature of this infectious disease have been known since at least 1000 B.C. Both Aristotle and Hippocrates described tuberculosis. The name of the infection probably arose from the postmortem observation that nodular lesions, or tubercles, were in the lungs of victims of the disease.

In 1882 Robert Koch, fulfilling the dictates of his famous postulates, clearly proved *Mycobacterium tuberculosis* (Color Photograph 11A) to be the cause of this infection. Since Koch's discovery, a number of other species of the genus *Mycobacterium* have been reported to cause similar disease states in humans and other animals. Tuberculosis is still the preferred term for the mycobacterial diseases caused by *M. tuberculosis, M. bovis,* and rarely *M. avium* infections. In their 1969 publication entitled *Diagnostic Standards and Classification of*

Tuberculosis, the National Tuberculosis and Respiratory Disease Association recommends that other mycobacteria-caused diseases be reported in a manner that specifies the etiological agent (for example, lung infection caused by *M. kansasii*).

Transmission and Predisposing Factors. Today, infection with *M. tuberculosis* occurs primarily through inhalation of droplet nuclei. Sputum, "coughing sprays," and droplets released by the sneezing of infected persons serve as common sources of the disease agent. So does contaminated dust.

Other ways by which mycobacteria may gain entrance into the susceptible individual include ingestion and direct inoculation. Tubercle organisms may be swallowed by children when they place contaminated objects in their mouths or consume food containing these bacteria. The danger of acquiring tuberculosis from infected dairy products has been largely eliminated in many countries by the pasteurization of milk products and by the tuberculin testing of dairy cattle. (On rare occasions, butchers may become infected through handling diseased meats, or pathologists may become infected in examining infected tissues.) Congenital tuberculosis appears to be rare, as the placenta is usually an effective barrier to *M. tuberculosis*.

Predisposing factors of tuberculosis include advanced age, chronic alcoholism, poor diet, certain metabolic diseases, some occupations, race, and prolonged stress. Tuberculosis itself is not inherited. The question of whether air pollution and cigarette smoking predispose one to tuberculosis has not been settled.

Active pulmonary tuberculosis among infants and children has been substantially reduced in the United States. In general, however, the disease is severe in infants. Susceptibility to tuberculosis increases with age after adolescence. For some unknown reason, the typical victims of the disease in the United States are white males 40 years of age or older. However, the ratio of death to active cases of tuberculosis is substantially higher in the nonwhite members of the population. This is true for both sexes of American Indian, Eskimo, and black members of the population.

Tuberculosis is a disease associated with poverty. Overcrowding, poorly ventilated rooms, and malnutrition favor the establishment of *M. tuberculosis* infection. Quite possibly, factors such as these may account for the greater mortality among nonwhites.

Among the metabolic diseases, diabetes mellitus appears to be the most frequently encountered one that predisposes to pulmonary tuberculosis.

Other significant predisposing factors include prolonged periods of fatigue or overexertion and chronic alcoholism, which is closely related to poor nutrition. Whether or not other respiratory diseases influence susceptibility to tuberculosis has not been firmly established. Frequent colds have been implicated, however.

The properties of several mycobacteria strains have been recorded for many years. From these records, it appears that the characteristics have remained relatively constant. Subsequently, several strains have been utilized as standards in studies and as material for human prophylactic immunization. The bovine tubercle bacillus *Bacille Calmette and Guêrin*, or BCG, is used for immunization.

The Pathogenesis and Pathology of Tuberculosis. The pathogenesis and pathology of tuberculosis are relatively complex subjects. The discussion here will emphasize the characteristic responses of the body to tubercle bacilli. Additional information can be obtained from the reference sources given at the end of the chapter.

The response of the individual to tubercle bacilli is dependent primarily upon the body's resistance and the organism's virulence. The size of the initial

TABLE 31-4 **Features of Selected Bacterial Lower Respiratory Tract Infections**

Disease	*Causative Agent*	*Gram Reaction*	*Morphology*	*Incubation Period*
Atypical primary pneumonia	*Mycoplasma pneumoniae* (Eaton's agent)	[a]	Pleomorphic	7–21 days
Legionnaire's disease	*Legionella pneumophila*	−	Rod	2–10 days
Pneumonia	*Klebsiella pneumoniae* (Friedlander's bacillus)	−	Rod	1–2 days
	Staphylococcus aureus	+	Coccus	1–2 days
	Streptococcus pneumoniae	+	Coccus	1–3 days
	Streptococcus pyogenes (Group A, beta-hemolytic)	+	Coccus	1–2 days
Psittacosis	*Chlamydia psittaci*	−	Rod	6–15 days
Q fever	*Coxiella burnetii*	−	Rod	14–28 days
Tuberculosis	*Mycobacterium tuberculosis*	[d]	Rod	28–42 days for primary infection
Whooping cough (pertussis)	*Bordetella pertussis* (Bordet-Gengou bacillus)	−	Rod	7–10 days

[a]Gram reactions are of little value with this pathogen.
[b]This is a more severe form of pneumonia than that caused by *S. pneumoniae*.

General Features of the Disease	*Laboratory Diagnosis*	*Possible Treatment*
Cough, chills, headache, sore throat, general discomfort, thick sputum with pus	1. Isolation of organisms from specimens 2. Serological tests, e.g., cold agglutinins	Antibiotics, tetracyclines
Chills, rapidly rising fever, abdominal pains, slight headache, muscle aches, nonproductive cough; complications leading to respiration failure can occur	1. Isolation of organism from specimens 2. Gram stain 3. Serological tests	Antibiotics including erythromycin, gentamicin, rifampin and streptomycin
Fever, chest pains, thick reddish brown sputum	1. Gram stain 2. Isolation and culture organisms from specimens 3. Biochemical tests	Chloramphenicol, streptomycin, tetracyclines
High fever, blue coloration (cyanosis), frequent cough, pus-containing discharge from nose, eyes, and rapid breathing;[b] a complication of certain viral infections such as measles	1. Gram stain 2. Isolation and culture organisms on blood agar 3. Mannitol salt agar and coagulase test (Color Photographs 74 and 75)	Penicillin, tetracycline
Sudden onset of symptoms, including severe chills and shaking, high fever, chest pain, thick rust-colored sputum, dry cough, and vomiting	1. Gram stain of sputum 2. Isolation organism from specimens 3. Biochemical tests, e.g., bile solubility, optoochin tests 4. Serological test, e.g., Quellung test[c]	Penicillin, broad-spectrum antibiotics
Chills, cough, difficulty in breathing, fever, general discomfort; complications include infections of the central nervous system and kidneys	1. Gram stain 2. Isolation and culture from specimens 3. Serological tests for streptococci	Penicillin, tetracycline
Sudden onset of symptoms, including cough, difficulty in breathing, fever, pain, and headache	1. Demonstration of organism in specimens 2. Isolation by animal inoculations, e.g., chick embryos and mice 3. Serological tests	Chloramphenicol, oxytetracycline
Sudden onset of symptoms, including dry cough, fever, headache, and general stiffness	1. Isolation of organism in tissue culture or chick embryos 2. Serological tests, e.g., complement fixation	Antibiotics
Wide variety of symptoms, including fever, general discomfort, weight loss, productive blood, formation of tubercle (nodule in lung tissue); skin test eventually becomes positive	1. Demonstration of acid-fast bacilli in specimens (Color Photograph 11A) 2. Isolation and culture 3. Animal inoculations 4. Biochemical tests 5. Skin testing and x ray	Isoniazid (INH), P (para) aminosalicylate (PAS), Streptomycin, rifampin, and the combination of two or more drugs for drug-resistant tubercle bacilli
Disease occurs in three stages: *Catarrhal*—persistent dry cough, slight fever, poor appetite, excessive mucous secretions, tearing, and vomiting *Paroxysmal*—coughing attacks referred to as "whooping,"[e] a production of thick, stringy mucous masses *Convalescent*—coughing attacks decrease in severity.	1. Isolation and identification of organism with cough plates using Bordet-Gengous agar 2. Serological test, e.g., agglutination	1. Antibiotics, including chloramphenicol, oxytetracycline, and penicillin 2. Symptomatic

[c]The Quellung (German, "swelling") test is diagnostic for infections caused by various encapsulated bacteria, including *Streptococcus pneumoniae*, *Hemophilus influenzae*, and *Klebsiella* spp. The procedure involves treating encapsulated cells with specific antisera that combine with the capsular polysaccharide, causing the capsule to swell.
[d]The Gram-stain reaction is not used diagnostically. The acid-fast staining procedure is used instead.
[e]The characteristic "whoop" is caused by rapidly inhaling air, which passes quickly over the vocal cords.

inoculum and the location of the infection are also important factors. In humans, a wide range of responses can occur. The tissue changes that develop are mainly those associated with inflammation and repair.

An inflammatory process is produced by the presence of *M. tuberculosis*. This tuberculosis inflammation is unusual in that it incorporates wandering tissue phagocytes known as *macrophages*, or histiocytes, and phagocytic pneumocytes. Most other inflammatory processes utilize polymorphonuclear leukocytes (PMNLs).

The initial and characteristic lesion of tuberculosis, called the *tubercle*, appears as a nodule in the lung tissue. Infection sites may be found in any portion of the lung (Figure 30–2). However, the pleura appear to be frequently involved. In most cases, single localized lesions (single foci) form, although multiple foci are known to occur.

Pulmonary lesions develop in the most aerated regions of the lungs. The presence of a high oxygen concentration, which *M. tuberculosis* requires, may account for the development of lesions in the top parts of the upper lobes of human lungs. In cattle, the dorsal region of the lower lung lobes is involved.

Healing. The healing of tuberculous lesions may occur in several ways. These include calcification, fibrosis, and resolution. Usually, all three types of healing are combined.

Calcification is the deposit of calcium within the semisolid centers of older tuberculous lesions. Calcification usually occurs after two years.

Fibrosis, or *scarring*, accompanies the healing of most tuberculous lesions. Collagen is deposited during the process.

Resolution probably accompanies the healing of all tuberculous lesions. This process includes the disappearance of infiltrating macrophages and even of the tubercles described earlier.

When healing does not take place, the tuberculosis is considered to be progressive. Established lesions can extend into surrounding tissue simply by enlargement or can spread to other areas by means of the circulatory system.

Skin Tests. Robert Koch's discovery of the tuberculin reaction in 1890 provided one of the most valuable diagnostic procedures for the control of tuberculosis. In addition to its obvious importance from the standpoint of differential diagnosis, the test is an extremely important epidemiological tool.

The basis of the tuberculin reaction is the development during the course of an infection of a specific delayed hypersensitivity to certain products of *M. tuberculosis* and related mycobacteria. These products are contained in culture extracts and are referred to as *tuberculins*. The sensitivity that occurs in individuals may develop one month or more after infection, usually remaining for several years or for an entire lifetime.

The tuberculin test reveals previous infection but does not prove the presence of an active disease state. Confirmation of an active case of tuberculosis is done with x-ray examination, and isolation of *M. tuberculosis*.

Preparations Used for Testing. Two types of tuberculin, Old Tuberculin (OT) and Purified Protein Derivative (PPD), are widely used for skin testing. The first material was originally described by Robert Koch and incorporates the heat-sterilization of an *M. tuberculosis* culture. The active component in Old Tuberculin is a protein noted for its heat stability and retention of specificity for several years.

The second preparation, PPD, is a slightly more refined testing substance than OT. It is preferred because its strength lends itself to standardization of dosages; skin tests performed with the same dose are comparable. PPD contains an active protein obtained from filtrates of autoclaved tubercle bacilli cultures.

Techniques for Administration. Three procedures are currently used in the tuberculin test: (1) intradermal injection (Mantoux test), (2) jet injection, and (3) multiple puncture. The first of these methods, intradermal injection, serves as the standard procedure for comparison purposes with all other tests. Moreover, more accurate control of dosage is possible with the Mantoux test. The other two methods are utilized for epidemiological (survey and screening) purposes.

Interpretations of Skin-Testing Reactions. The following interpretations and recording of skin test results are in keeping with the current recommendations of the National Tuberculosis and Respiratory Disease Association.

The intradermal introduction of tuberculin into sensitized persons usually causes the formation of a hard area (Color Photograph 73) that may or may not be associated with a surrounding reddened area (erythema). The intensity and size of the reaction varies according to the individual's sensitivity and the quantity of skin-testing material introduced. Those persons exhibiting tuberculin sensitivity are called *reactors*. The degree of sensitivity can be determined from the size and accompanying features of the skin reaction, for example, erythema and tissue destruction. Reports from many parts of the world indicate a relationship between the size of the skin reaction and the risk of developing active tuberculosis: the larger the reaction, the greater the possibility of active disease. Skin reactivity to the introduction of skin-testing material may be suppressed by several factors or conditions. These include advanced age, terminal or severe, acute diseases (such as cancer), and the administration of large quantities of cortisone. Infectious diseases such as measles and smallpox, vaccination against these diseases, or a rapidly progressive case of tuberculosis may also cause suppression of skin reaction.

The tuberculin test is practical not only because it can serve as a diagnostic tool but also because it can screen large groups of people for tuberculosis and detect infections and their sources. After initial infection with tubercle bacilli, the sensitivity to tuberculin develops in approximately 2 to 10 weeks. Once this sensitivity is acquired, it usually persists. The various factors that can affect its expression have been discussed earlier.

Prevention. Preventive measures used for tuberculosis include casefinding and mass survey programs conducted among populations of apparently "healthy" individuals. Tuberculin testing and x-ray examinations are used for these purposes. Location of active cases can thereby be adequately determined.

The prophylactic use of chemotherapeutic agents (chemoprophylaxis) has been quite successful in reducing the incidence of active tuberculosis. This approach has been used with high risk groups, such as recent contacts, infants, and tuberculin converters (individuals whose skin tests turn positive). BCG vaccination has also been used to protect uninfected persons in contact with known tuberculous patients when normal measures of chemoprophylaxis can not be performed. Because BCG vaccinations influence the diagnostic value of tuberculin testing, its use is being questioned.

The prevalence of tuberculosis in many Western countries has been greatly reduced. Unfortunately, however, despite the availability of treatment and early detection measures for tuberculosis, the infection is far from being eradicated, especially in the tropics and in the Far East. This is the result of several factors, including the nature of the disease itself (healthy-appearing persons may actually be infected and thereby serve as reservoirs for *M. tuberculosis*), limitations of detection and diagnosis, a general disinterest among a community, an unwillingness of infected individuals to be isolated and adequately treated, and the development of drug-resistant infections. The antibiotic rifampin used in combination with other antituberculous agents has been successful in the treatment of drug-resistant infections.

WHOOPING COUGH (PERTUSSIS)

First described in 1578 by Baillou, pertussis is today found world-wide but appears to be more prevalent in colder regions. Children under five years of age, especially newborns, are the primary victims, with females being affected more frequently than males. However, aged and debilitated individuals are also quite susceptible.

Transmission. Whooping cough is characterized by spasmodic coughing attacks and the whooping that accompanies rapid air intake during the coughs. With this prominent feature of the disease, transmission is no doubt mainly by droplet infection. However, fomites should not be ruled out. Isolation of the causative agent is obtained by holding a Petri dish containing glycerin-potato-blood agar in front of an ill child's mouth during a coughing attack.

The etiologic agent, ***Bordetella pertussis*** (formerly known as ***Hemophilus pertussis***) was isolated by Jules Bordet and Octave Gengou in 1906. It is a small, nonmotile, Gram-negative rod. Capsules are formed by virulent organisms.

Complications that may occur with whooping cough include collapsed lung, bronchopneumonia, interstitial emphysema, convulsions, and bleeding in various regions of the body (brain, conjunctivae, eyes, or skin).

Prevention. Active immunization is the most widely used practice for the control of pertussis. As noted earlier, this is accomplished by the use of the combined DPT (diphtheria, pertussis, and tetanus) vaccine.

Susceptible contacts are isolated and administered human hyperimmune serum. Exposed individuals who have been vaccinated one year or more previously should be given a booster.

Fungus Diseases

Several fungus species are associated with respiratory diseases in humans (Table 31–5). Humans acquire these infections by inhaling spores from such reservoirs as dust, bird droppings, and soil. Certain fungi, *Coccidioides immitis*, for example, are not widely distributed in nature, but appear to be found only in particular geographic regions (Color Photograph 83). Other agents are more widely distributed (Table 31–6). Some of these pathogens are discussed in this chapter; others are presented elsewhere in the text. Diseases and treatments are presented in Tables 31–5 and 31–6.

FIG. 31–5 The typical nodular skin lesion of coccidiodomycosis. *Courtesy of Dr. N. H. Rickles, Pathology Department, University of Oregon Dental School.*

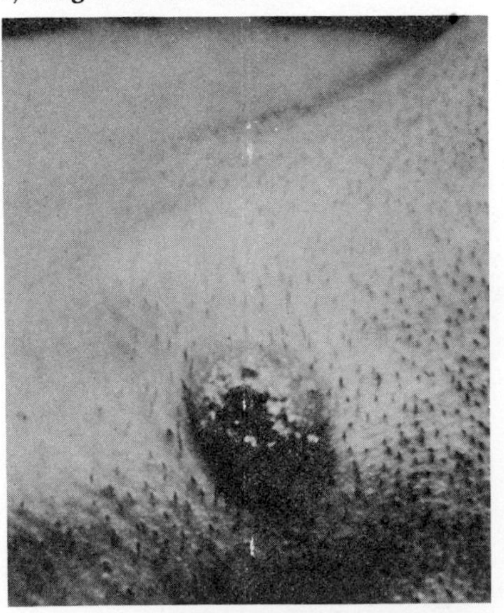

DIAGNOSIS

The laboratory identification of fungi-causing respiratory infections includes demonstration of the causative agent in various types of specimens and subsequent culture of the fungus. Skin tests and serological procedures as described in Chapter 24 are of value in some cases. Table 31–6 indicates approaches to diagnosis for several pathogenic fungi.

COCCIDIOIDOMYCOSIS

The fungus disease coccidioidomycosis (Figure 31–5) is also known as desert fever, San Joaquin fever, and valley fever. Three distinct forms are known with this infection: the ***acute***, the ***chronic pulmonary***, and the ***disseminated*** forms (Color Photographs 82 and 83B). The incidence of infection is related to climatologic conditions in the endemic areas (Table 31–6), the peak of infection

TABLE 31–5 Fungi Associated with Human Respiratory Diseases

Respiratory Disease	*Fungus Species*	*Possible Treatment*
Aspergillosis, asthma, bronchiectasis, rhinitis	*Aspergillus fumigatus*	Amphotericin B
Bronchopulmonary candidiasis	*Candida albicans*	Amphotericin B
Chronic pneumonitis	*Cryptococcus neoformans*	Amphotericin B
Coccidioidomycosis	*Coccidioides immitis*	For disseminated form, Amphotericin B
Geotrichosis	*Geotrichum candidum*	Potassium iodide (orally), sodium iodide (intravenously)
Histoplasmosis	*Histoplasma capsulatum*	1. Amphotericin B 2. Surgical removal of oral lesions
North American blastomycosis (Gilchrist's disease)	*Blastomyces dermatitidis*	1. Amphotericin B 2. Hydroxystilbamidine 3. Surgical procedures together with chemotherapy
Sporotrichosis of the lungs (rare)	*Sporotrichum schenckii*	Amphotericin B

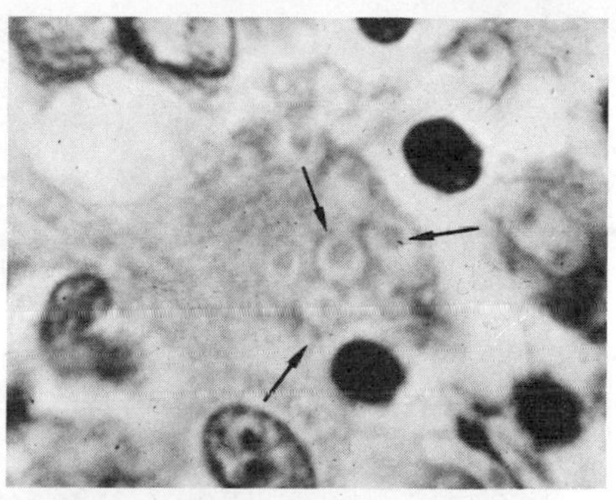

(a)

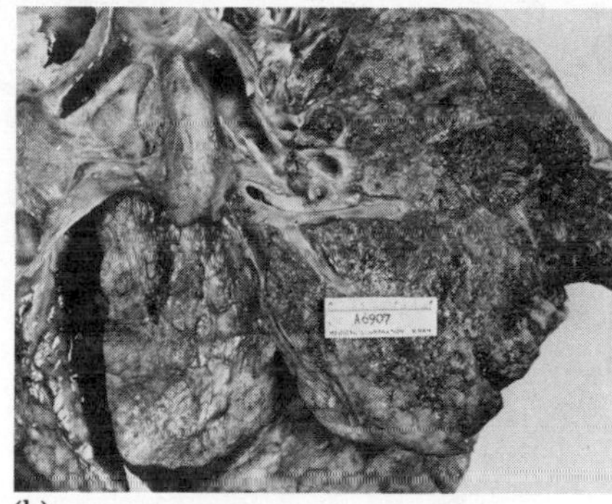

(b)

FIG. 31–6 (a) *Histoplasma capsulatum* in the parasitic stage within tissue. Note the clear areas (arrows) that result from shrinkage of the cytoplasm away from the rigid walls. (b) The gross effect of *H. capsulatum* on the lung. *Courtesy of the Armed Forces Institute of Pathology, Washington, D.C., Neg. No. 58-1455-854965.*

occurring in the dry, dusty summer months, especially after a rather rainy winter season.

Transmission. Coccidioidomycosis is usually contracted from the inhalation of soil or dust containing the characteristic arthrospores of the causative agent, ***Coccidioides immitis*** (Color Photograph 83A). Domestic animals and rodents can develop the disease and may be partially responsible for its persistence in some areas.

Immunity. Recovery from primary coccidioidomycosis confers a solid, permanent immunity to further infection.

HISTOPLASMOSIS

The fungus disease histoplasmosis is caused by ***Histoplasma capsulatum***. (Figure 31–6) Histoplasmosis occurs throughout the world, with a relatively high incidence in certain countries (Table 31–6). Histoplasmosis is no longer thought of as a rare and fatal disease, but rather as one that is widespread and generally mild. The organism appears localized within macrophages and reticuloendothelial cells (Figure 31–7a). The disease may affect one or several organs. It may be difficult to diagnose, since it presents a broad spectrum of effects, ranging from an asymptomatic or mild infection, to an acute, severe disease to a chronic pulmonary disease of long duration.

Transmission. Histoplasmosis is disseminated to human beings by spores (Figure 31–7) from the fungus, which grows readily in acidic soil in areas with proper temperature and moisture. Spores are also found in bird droppings.

NORTH AMERICAN BLASTOMYCOSIS (GILCHRIST'S DISEASE)

The chronic systemic fungal disease known as North American blastomycosis occurs only on the North American continent and is usually secondary to pulmonary involvement. Sporadic cases have been reported in all states. Males aged 20 to 40 are most often affected.

The causative agent, ***Blastomyces dermatitidis,*** appears as yeast cells in infected tissues or in cultures at 37°C and as a mold in cultures at room temperature. At least three clinical states of the disease are known, namely, pulmonary and disseminated blastomycosis and a skin infection.

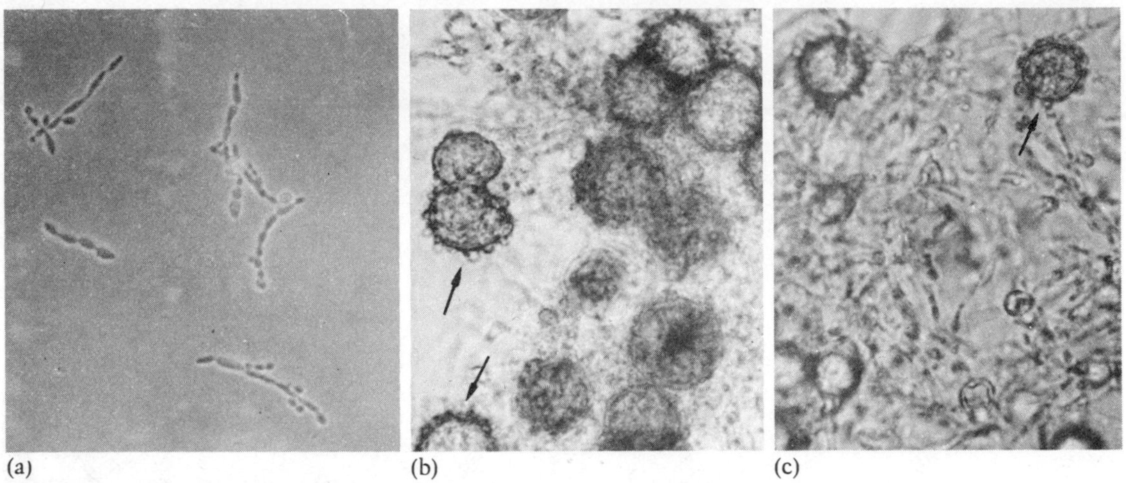

FIG. 31-7 (a) Yeast phase of *H. capsulatum* strain A811 under dark phase. (b and c). Mycelial phase of *H. capsulatum* showing individual tuberculate macroconidia (arrows). *Pine, L.,* App. Microbiol. *19:413–420 (1970).*

Influenza Virus Infection

Epidemics of influenza (Table 31–7) have plagued humans and other animals for centuries. Widespread epidemics, or pandemics, occurred in 1847–1848, 1889–1891, and 1918–1919. The last of these caused approximately 20 million deaths. Young adults between 20 and 40 were affected to a very large extent. Although a significant accumulation of data incriminated a virus as the causative agent of the pandemic of 1918–1919, ***Hemophilus influenzae,*** the so-called influenza bacillus, was still regarded as the cause of the disease. Subsequent research firmly established the viral nature of the disease. Moreover, it became clear that *H. influenzae*—as well as numerous other bacterial species, including *Streptococcus pneumoniae* and *Staphylococcus aureus*—were secondary invaders in patients with influenza and quite often were responsible for the fatal forms of pneumonia that developed.

The original strains of human influenza viruses, isolated in 1933 and prevalent for about 10 years, are referred to as Type A or A classic. As additional strains were discovered on the basis of antigenicity studies, other designations were created (Table 31–7).

Complications. Unfortunately, influenza epidemics have been accompanied by a rise in mortality. The greatest proportional rise in deaths from complications has been caused by bronchitis and pneumonia. Complications have also been reported in organs other than the lungs, such as the components of the circulatory and central nervous systems. The development of chest complications during an influenza epidemic is determined by several factors, including the viral strain involved, the age and general health of the host, and the severity of the original attack of the disease.

Immunity. Persons recovering from an infection usually acquire resistance to the particular antigenic strain responsible for the respiratory illness. Unfortu-

TABLE 31-6 Features of Selected Fungus-Caused Lower Respiratory Tract Infections

Disease	*Geographical Distribution (General)*	*Incubation Period*	*General Features of the Disease*	*Laboratory Diagnosis*[a]
Coccidioidomycosis (San Joaquin Valley fever)	Southwestern United States (southern California), Central and South Americas	10–21 days	General flulike symptoms including chills, cough, fever, malaise, chest pain, and a pus-containing sputum in the case of pneumonia[b]	1. Demonstration of nonbudding spherules in clinical specimens 2. Culture and demonstration of arthrospores (Color Photographs 00 83A and 83B) 3. Serological testing, e.g., complement fixation, immunodiffusion (see Chapter 24) 4. Skin test
Histoplasmosis	Widespread in the United States, endemic in Missouri, Tennessee, Kentucky, Kansas, Iowa, Indiana and Southern Illinois, Panama, Argentina, Brazil, Phillipines, and Java	5–18 days	Either no detectable illness or mild effects; small calcified growths appear in several body organs upon recovery	1. Demonstration of typical yeast forms in specimens (Figure 31-7a) 2. Isolation and cultivation 3. Serological test, e.g., complement fixation, immunodiffusion, latex agglutination 4. Skin test
North American blastomycosis (Gilchrist's disease)	North America, more prevalent in south central and mid-Atlantic United States and Ohio-Mississippi River Valley	Several weeks	Symptoms are usually quite mild and self-healing and include cough, fever, and general discomfort; complications and spread to other body regions can occur	1. Microscopic demonstration of multinucleated, nonencapsulated yeast cells in specimens 2. Isolation and cultivation

[a]Tentative diagnosis is possible based on disease (clinical) symptoms.
[b]The spread of the disease throughout the body (disseminated form), usually starts from the respiratory system.

TABLE 31-7 Features of Human Influenza—A Viral Disease of the Lower Respiratory Tract

Influenza Virus Type or Subtype	*General Features of the Disease*	*Laboratory Diagnosis*
A (classic) A_1 (A prime) A_2 (Asian)[a] B C	Uncomplicated influenza symptoms include backache, chills, fever, headache, general discomfort, nasal congestion, cough, dry and sore throat, loss of appetite, nausea, and vomiting; complications include pneumonia	1. Isolation of causative agent using chick embryo 2. Detection of viral antigens by immunofluorescence 3. Serological test, e.g., hemagglutination inhibition, complement fixation (see Chapter 24)

[a]Often incorrectly called 'Asiatic.'

nately, new strains with new antigens develop and consequently cause successive attacks of influenza.

Prevention. Immunization of certain key individuals, such as police officers, nurses, physicians, and other health care personnel, is recommended before an epidemic strikes. Pregnant women, the elderly, and persons with debilitating diseases, such as chronic heart or respiratory diseases, should also be immunized. Mortality rates in persons 45 years of age and over have been higher than in other age groups. As influenza can spread rapidly among residents of homes for the aged or nursing homes, the prophylactic use of vaccines is important there.

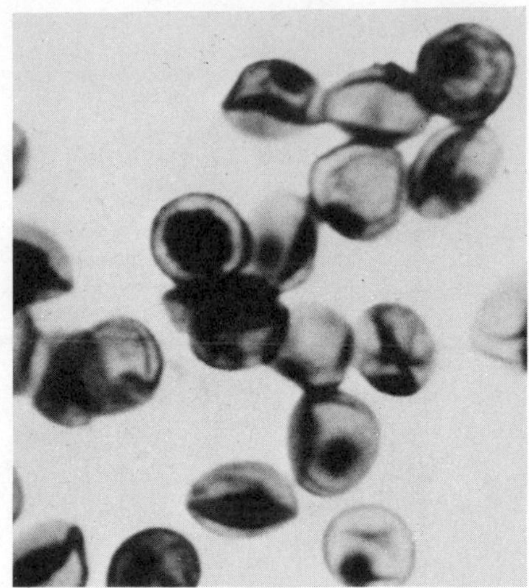

FIG. 31–8 Clusters of *Pneumocystis carinii* cysts. There are three developmental stages of *P. carinii:* cyst, trophozoite, and sporozoite forms. Cysts are round, measure about 4 to 10μm in diameter, and contain 1 to 8 sporozoites (Color Photograph 84). The trophozoites vary in shape and range in size from 2 to 5 μm in diameter. A small amount of nuclear material in these forms, usually V-shaped, is located eccentrically. The three stages of *P. carinii* can be demonstrated through the use of Giemsa, Wright, or polychrome methylene blue stains. It should be noted, however, that knowledge of the morphology of *P. carinii* in the various stages of its life cycle is essential for the recognition of the organism with these stains. *Courtesy of Kim, H. K., and W. T. Hughes,* Amer. J. Clin. Path. *60:462–466 (1973).*

Pneumocystis carinii

The tissue parasite *Pneumocystis carinii* (Figure 31–8) has received considerable attention in recent years as the cause of a respiratory infection involving the pulmonary alveolar spaces and surrounding supporting structures. *P. carinii* infections have occurred almost exclusively in children with congenital immunologic disorders, in patients with certain generalized circulatory disorders, in debilitated infants, in newborn and premature infants, and in patients receiving immunosuppressive therapy. The causative agent, originally discovered in the guinea pig several years ago, has since been found in other animals, including cats, dogs, mice, monkeys, and sheep. There are several similarities between human and animal *P. carinii* pneumonitis with respect to the morphology and pathogenicity of the protozoan (Table 31–8) and histology of the diseased tissue. The organism infects the intraalveolar space of the lung as an opportunist and rarely penetrates tissue. To date, all attempts at *in vitro* isolation have failed. This inability to cultivate *P. carinii* has prevented more extensive studies of the organism in relation to its habitat, life cycle, pathogenesis, and epidemiology. Various reports, however, clearly indicate that *P. carinii* has a world-wide distribution.

TABLE 31–8 Features of *Pneumocystis carinii* Infection

Disease	Incubation Period	General Features of the Disease	Laboratory Diagnosis
Pneumonia	Unknown, possibly 7 days	Course of the disease ranges from 4 to 6 weeks; symptoms include cough, bluish coloration of the skin, fever, rapid breathing, and lung consolidation	1. x-ray 2. Demonstration of *P. carinii* cysts in specimens (Color Photograph 84) special stains

There are three developmental stages of *P. carinii:* cyst, trophozoite, and sporozoite forms. Cysts are round, measure about 4 to 10 μm in diameter, and contain 1 to 8 sporozoites (Color Photograph 84). The trophozoites vary in shape and range in size from 2 to 5 μm in diameter. A small amount of nuclear material in these forms, usually V-shaped, is usually located off-center in the organism. The three stages of *P. carinii* can be demonstrated through the use of Giemsa, Wright, or polychrome methylene blue stains. However, one must be able to recognize *P. carinii* in each stage of its life cycle in order to use these stains.

Transmission. Although the mode of transmission for *P. carinii* is not definitely established, the inhalation of the parasite into the respiratory tract appears to be the most probable means.

SUMMARY

1. The human respiratory tract starts at the nose, passes through various parts of the respiratory tree, and ends in the air sacs, or alveoli.
2. The system is not only susceptible to microbes that can cause infections at different levels, but it can aid in the transmission of pathogens.

Structures of the Respiratory System

The Pharynx (Throat)

1. The pharnyx, or throat, is a passageway for food and air.
2. It is associated with the tonsils (lymphoid tissue) and is connected with the middle ear by means of the Eustachian tubes.

The Trachea (Windpipe)

The trachea, or windpipe, is a thin tube that passes from the voice box, or larynx (or voice box), into the chest cavity. Here it divides into two primary bronchi.

The Lungs and the Primary Bronchi

1. Each lung is divided into lobes, with the right lung consisting of three and the left lung two.
2. The bronchial tree is formed from two large bronchi, each of which divide and subdivide into smaller *bronchi.*
3. The smaller bronchi in turn lead into tubelike structures of varying sizes, the *bronchioles.*
4. Bronchioles branch into alveolar ducts. Gaseous exchanges occur in the air sacs, or *alveoli,* which develop from these ducts.
5. Two membranes, the inner (visceral) and the outer (parietal) pleura, form a sac that encloses the lungs. The potential cavity between these membranes is called the *pleural cavity.*

Normal Flora of the Respiratory Tract

1. The normal flora of the human nose includes a variety of bacterial species, some of which have the potential to cause disease.
2. In the adult human, the respiratory tract below the level of the epiglottis is normally sterile.

Introduction to Microbial Infections of the Respiratory Tract

1. Various microbial pathogens—bacteria, fungi, and viruses—can enter and multiply in the respiratory tract. Moreover, the various secretions associated with the respiratory system can be a source of disease agents.
2. The communicability of infectious diseases of the respiratory system is influenced by several factors such as survival of the pathogen on fomites or in the air, the number of microbes inhaled, the duration of contact, and the anatomical site involved in the infection.
3. Control measures for respiratory tract infections are similar, if not identical, to those of other types of diseases.

Representative Microbial Diseases

1. Respiratory tract infections are of great importance because of the ease with which they are transmitted and contracted and the difficulty in eliminating disease agents.
2. Diagnosis is frequently based on the disease picture, which includes x rays, patient's history, and examination, and on the laboratory isolation and identification of the disease agent.

Upper Respiratory Infections

1. The upper respiratory region, which includes the middle ear, mastoids, sinuses, and the nasal corners of the eyes, are exposed to a variety of pathogens.
2. Infections in these sites can spread to other regions of the respiratory tract.
3. Examples of bacterial infections of this region include the toxin-associated diphtheria, suppurative otitis media (pus-producing middle ear infection), and streptococcal sore throat.
4. Viral diseases of the upper respiratory tract include the common cold, croup, and minor infections.

Lower Respiratory Infections

1. Several diseases of the lower respiratory tract are life-threatening if not treated quickly and adequately. These diseases are usually acquired through the inhalation of the disease agent.
2. Bacterial infections of this portion of the respiratory system include the pneumonias caused by such organisms as *Streptococcus pneumoniae,* mycoplasma infections, psittacosis (parrot fever), Q fever, tuberculosis, other mycobacterial diseases, and whooping cough.
3. Fungus infections of the lower respiratory tract include coccidioidomycosis, histoplasmosis, and North American blastomycosis.
4. Influenza epidemics have caused severe infections in humans and other animals for centuries. These virus infections can be complicated by secondary bacterial invaders.
5. The protozoan *Pneumocystis carinii* causes infections of the air sacs and supporting structures. The disease agent infects individuals having some form of impairment of their immunologic systems.

QUESTIONS FOR REVIEW

1. Compare the different bacterial respiratory infections. Construct a table for this purpose and include the following categories:
   a. specific causative agent
   b. distinguishing clinical features
   c. Gram reaction
   d. region of the tract involved
   e. means of transmission
   f. availability of diagnostic skin test
2. a. What general measures are used in the prevention and control of respiratory diseases?
   b. Why are certain diseases of this type difficult to eradicate? Explain.
3. What significance does the acid-fast staining procedure have in the diagnosis of respiratory disease? Which, if any, respiratory system pathogens are noted for their acid-fast reaction?
4. List examples of complications that can develop from a bacterial respiratory infection. How can such problems be prevented?
5. What are the reservoirs and sources of infectious agents of the following diseases?
   a. tuberculosis
   b. psittacosis
   c. diphtheria
   d. whooping cough
   e. influenza
   f. atypical primary pneumonia
   g. lobar pneumonia
   h. the common cold
6. What distinguishing property or properties does *Mycoplas-*

ma pneumoniae have in comparison with other bacterial pathogens?

7. a. What fungus pathogens cause respiratory disease? Where can these diseases be found?
   b. What factors contribute to a person's susceptibility to fungal diseases?
8. List five viral respiratory tract infections, together with their respective causative agents.
9. Discuss the measures used in the diagnosis, treatment, and prevention of viral respiratory system diseases.
10. Can complications develop from influenza? Explain.
11. If you were planning a world trip, including Arabia, southern California, Egypt, Greece, Japan, and India, to which respiratory diseases would you be exposed?

SUGGESTED READINGS

Ciba Foundation Symposium, *Pathogenic Mycoplasmas.* New York: Associated Scientific Publishers, 1972. *Contains topics from a symposium on the mycoplasmas. Specific areas considered include the structure, pathogenicity, isolation, characterization, and treatment of this bacterial group.*

Cohen, A. B., and W. M. Gold, "Defense Mechanisms of the Lungs," *Ann. Rev. Physiology* 37:325 (1975). *Antimicrobial and immune defenses of the lungs and air passages are reviewed in this article.*

Eichenwald, H. F., "Respiratory Infections in Children," *Hosp. Pract.* April, 81–90 (1976). *A review of infectious diseases associated with the respiratory tracts of children.*

Pappenheimer, A. M., Jr., "Diphtheria Toxin," *Ann. Rev. Biochem.* 46:69 (1977). *A detailed article dealing with the toxin of* Corynebacterium diphtheriae. *Its production, structure, and mode of action are discussed.*

Stuart-Harris, C. H., and C. Andrewes, *Influenze and Other Virus Infections of the Respiratory Tract.* Baltimore: Williams & Wilkins Company, 1965. *A short but fairly complete description of several viral respiratory infections.*

Microbial Diseases of the Gastrointestinal Tract

CHAPTER 32

Food and water are important vehicles for the transmission of microbial disease agents that affect the gastrointestinal tract. Several infections and poisonings involving this human system are discussed in this chapter. Attention is also given to the identification, prevention, and control of disease states such as amebic dysentery, Asiatic cholera, typhoid fever, various forms of food poisoning, and virus infections.

After reading this chapter, you should be able to:

1. **Describe the general organization of the human gastrointestinal system and indicate the areas attacked by pathogens and their products.**
2. **Distinguish between bacterial food poisoning and food infection.**
3. **Discuss the general features of the microbial ecology of this system.**
4. **Discuss at least three each of bacterial, protozoan, and viral diseases of the gastrointestinal system with respect to the causative agent, means of transmission, and general symptoms.**
5. **List and explain specific measures used to prevent or control bacterial food poisoning.**
6. **Distinguish among the various microorganisms associated with causing hepatitis.**

7. **Explain the significance of bacterial spores and protozoan cysts to disease states of the gastrointestinal system.**
8. **Discuss the general approaches to the treatment of diseases associated with the gastrointestinal system.**

Microbial diseases of the gastrointestinal tract usually result from the ingestion of food or water containing pathogenic microorganisms or their toxins. Despite the availability of functional control measures, diseases such as amebic dysentery, cholera, and salmonellosis still occur frequently in some parts of the world. The incidence of these and related diseases is greatly affected by various factors, including poverty, crowding, malnutrition, and natural reservoirs for pathogens.

The gastrointestinal (GI) tract (Figure 32–1), also called the digestive tract, is a canal consisting of the mouth, oropharynx, esophagus, stomach, small and large intestines, and the rectum, and anus. It runs through the body from the mouth to the anus and is approximately 9.5 meters long. The wall of the digestive tract contains absorptive surfaces, glands, and muscles. Variations in diameter and structures occur along the length of the tract. Certain glands and structures, including the liver and pancreas, which are outside the digestive tract, contribute secretions important to the digestive process. The function of the digestive system is to supply food and water to the body's internal environment. Once inside the body, basic substances such as amino acids, simple sugars, and fatty acids are carried to the cells via the circulatory system.

Because various portions of the digestive system are vulnerable to direct attack by microbial pathogens or may be secondarily involved in a disease process, a brief survey of this system's parts will be presented as a frame of reference.

Parts of the Gastrointestinal Tract

The Stomach

This portion of the digestive system has a shape somewhat resembling a thick-walled J. The stomach is on the left side of the body just under the lower ribs. The inner layer mucous membrane of the stomach, the *mucosa,* contains millions of glands that secrete mucus and the various components of the gastric juice. Hydrochloric acid secreted by the stomach keeps the pH of the stomach contents low and kills many microorganisms that are ingested.

Food entering the stomach from the esophagus passes through a *sphincter,* a one-way constricting device, which remains closed until it receives the proper

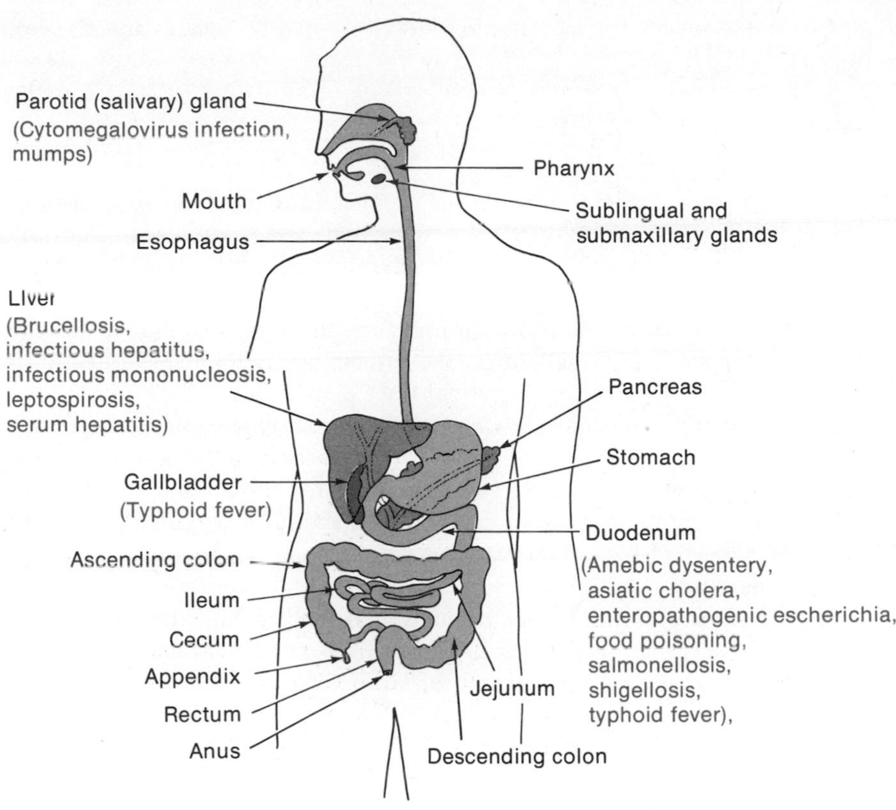

FIG. 32-1 The human gastrointestinal tract showing specific locations at which pathogenic microorganisms and their infections can be found.

stimulus to open. The sphincter prevents food from passing back into the esophagus.

The Small Intestine

The small intestine is a coiled tube about 7 meters, or 25 feet, long and 2.5 cm in diameter in an adult. The small intestine is divided into three portions or loops, the ***duodenum*** (0.3 meters or 1 foot long), the ***jejunum*** (1.5 meters or 5 feet long), and the ***ileum*** (approximately 5.5 meters or 19 feet long).

Food leaving the stomach passes first into the duodenum. There the entering acidified material is mixed with secretions produced by the liver and pancreas, as well as those secreted by the small intestine itself. Much of the entering material is composed of mucus, which aids the passage of the digesting food material through the intestine.

Most enzymatic digestion and absorption take place in the small intestine. (Only alcohol and certain poisons, such as strychnine, are absorbed through the stomach wall.) The highly absorptive nature of the small intestine is closely linked to its enormous surface area, which is composed of millions of small, fingerlike structures called ***villi*** (Figure 32-4a). Each of these units contains capillaries and a *lacteal*, a small lymph vessel. The capillaries absorb amino acids and simple sugars; the lacteals are concerned with fatty acids and glycerol absorption.

The Large Intestine (Colon)

For convenience, the large intestine is divided into the following regions: ***ascending colon***, ***transverse colon***, ***descending colon***, and ***rectum***. Food from the small intestine passes into the thicker-walled, larger-diameter ascending colon. The small intestine opens into the large intestine from the side, not the top, thus leaving a "blind sac" at the beginning of the large intestine called the ***caecum***. The ***appendix***, a small fingerlike projection, is located at the tip of the caecum.

The large intestine is primarily involved with the processing, storage, and elimination of food material remaining after digestion and absorption have occurred. Such material consists of an indigestible residue and large quantities of water. One of the functions of the large intestine is to absorb much of this water.

The rectum functions in storing the waste products of digestion, or ***feces***, and the anus serves in eliminating such material. In addition to the indigestible food elements, fecal matter contains large quantities of bacteria (some of which may be pathogenic), heavy metals, and certain body secretions such as bile.

The Liver

One of the largest organs or glands found in the body, the liver is vitally important to the well-being of the individual. The liver is located in the upper portion of the abdominal cavity just beneath the diaphragm.

Bile, or ***gall***, is produced by all parts of the liver and stored in the gall bladder. Bile emulsifies fats so they can pass through the intestines, prevents food from decaying there, and stimulates the intestinal muscles. It enters the small intestine by way of the ***bile duct***. If this duct becomes clogged or blocked, the condition known as ***jaundice*** (a yellowing of body tissues) develops. This condition has a variety of causes, including gallstones and various worm and microbial diseases, such as viral hepatitis.

Diseases of the liver cause destruction of its cells (hepatocytes), preventing them from carrying out important activities. Fortunately, the liver's immense capacity for regeneration makes it resistant to permanent damage. However, in cases of severe injury, the organ heals with the formation of nonfunctioning scar tissue, a condition known as ***cirrhosis***.

LIVER FUNCTION TESTS

Since the general observable signs and symptoms of liver, or hepatic, disease states are nonspecific, laboratory tests of liver function are required for a specific diagnosis. Such tests are used to detect causes, specifically diagnose, follow recovery, and evaluate various forms of treatment in liver disease.

Gastrointestinal Microbial Ecology

The structure of the gastrointestinal tract determines the localization of the microbial flora and, to some extent, the composition of the flora as well.

TABLE 32–1 Microorganisms Isolated from Various Regions of the Human Gastrointestinal System[a]

Microbial Type	Gastrointestinal Region Stomach	 Small Intestine	 Large Intestine
Actinobacillus	+	+	−
Bacillus species	−	−	+
Bacteroides	+	+	+
Bifidobacteria	+	+	−
Candida[b]	+	−	−
Clostridia	+	+	−
Coliforms	+	+	+
Lactobacilli	+	+	+
Peptostreptococcus	+	−	−
Staphylococcus	+	+	−
Streptococcus	+	+	+
Torulopsis[b]	+	−	−
Veillonella	+	+	−

[a]The microorganisms isolated and the numbers found vary to some extent, depending upon the diet, environmental factors, methods used for isolation, and geographical location of the subjects.
[b]Yeast.

Microbial habitats may exist in any area from the esophagus to the anus. Each habitat provides a different kind of environmental or nutritional challenge.

The gastrointestinal tract is sterile in the normal fetus up to the time of birth. During normal birth, the baby picks up microorganisms from portions of the mother's reproductive tract and from any other environmental source to which it is exposed. Many of these microbes are not able to establish themselves in the neonatal tract and disappear soon after birth. Other microbial types are pioneers, producing the offspring that eventually form the established communities in the adult.

Soon after birth, in most suckling infants, the microorganisms commonly found are primarily lactic acid bacteria. In breast-fed babies, species of *Bifidobacterium* (Figure 32–2) predominate. With further development, a variety of complex interactions involving the individual, environment, diet, and even microorganisms themselves regulate the events that establish the microbial flora of the gastrointestinal tract. Table 32–1 lists microorganisms isolated from various portions of this system. Interestingly enough, *Escherichia coli* is a minority, rather than the chief inhabitant of most gastrointestinal ecosystems. A wide variety of microorganisms, such as strict anaerobes, normally outnumber *E. coli*.

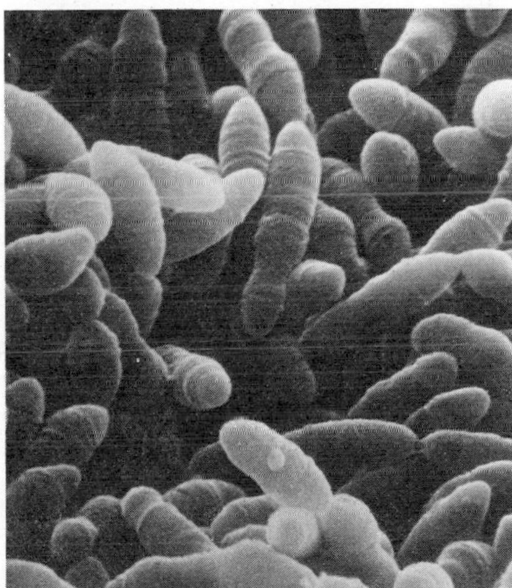

FIG. 32–2 The bifidobacteria. These anaerobic organisms are important members of the natural microflora of the human gastrointestinal system. *Bauer, H., and H. Sigarlakie,* Can. J. Microbiol. *21:1305–1316 (1975).*

Bacterial Diseases

The World Health Organization Expert Committee on Enteric Infections has adopted the designation *acute diarrheal disease* for disease conditions in which there is a disturbance of intestinal functions, and which once started may produce dehydration and the passage of liquid stools. The specific bacterial pathogens that can cause such conditions are shown in Table 32–2 along with other agents of gastrointestinal disease. Among the organisms associated with acute diarrheal disease are the agents of cholera, gastroenteritis, bacillary dysentery, and traveler's diarrhea.

It is now apparent that intestinal microflora may induce diarrhea in three ways: they may change dietary foodstuffs or host secretions into substances that affect gut fluid movement; they may penetrate the intestinal lining and damage the bowel wall; or they may produce exotoxins (Color Photograph 72) that cause an emptying of large amounts of water and electrolytes into the intestines without damaging the mucosa. It now appears that this last process may be implicated in many serious and not-so-serious diarrheal disorders. The features of representative disease states will be described in this chapter.

A representative approach and selected biochemical reactions involved in the isolation and identification of gastrointestinal bacterial pathogens are presented in Figure 32-3 and Table 32-3. The approaches to laboratory diagnosis, treatment, and the general features (signs and symptoms) of microbial diseases can be found in other tables in this chapter.

Asiatic Cholera

In the nineteenth century, pandemics of Asiatic cholera spread from the Far East to Africa, other parts of Asia, Europe, and North America. During the

TABLE 32-2 General Features of Bacterial Diseases of the Gastrointestinal Tract

Disease	*Causative Agent*	*Gram Reaction*	*Morphology*	*Incubation Period*	*General Features of the Disease*	*Laboratory Diagnosis*	*Possible Treatment*
Asiatic cholera	*Vibrio cholerae*	–	Vibrio	Usually 2–5 days	The disease ranges from mild to severe and symptoms include large amounts of mucus in stools (rice-water stools), sudden loss of water and electrolytes, and dehydration; collapse, shock, and death can occur without treatment	1. Gram stain and culture of specimens (Color Photograph 10B) 2. Biochemical tests (Table 32-3) 3. Serological tests 4. Phage typing	1. Maintain proper fluid and electrolyte balance 2. Antibiotics, including tetracyclines
Brucellosis (Malta Fever, undulant fever)	*Brucella abortus, B. melitensis, B. suis*	–	Coccobacilli	1–3 weeks	Variable symptoms may include general discomfort, weakness, muscle aches and pains, elevated temperature late in the day, falling during the night, enlarged lymph nodes, spleen and liver involvement; disease may become chronic; residual tissue damage can occur	1. Gram stain and isolation of organism from specimens 2. Animal incubations for isolations 3. Serological tests, e.g., agglutination, fluorescent antibody 4. Skin testing with *Brucella* antigens 5. Phage typing (Color Photograph 77)	Tetracyclines
Salmonellosis (gastro-enteritis)	*Salmonella typhimurium* and other *Salmonella* spp.	–	Rod	8–10 hours, possibly up to 48 hours	Symptoms appear suddenly and include abdominal pain, diarrhea, dizziness, fever, headache, nausea, vomiting, and poor appetite	1. Isolation of organism on appropriate media (Color Photographs 63A and 63B) 2. Biochemical tests (Table 32-3) 3. Serological test, e.g., specific agglutination reactions	1. Restoration of fluid and electrolyte balance 2. Antibiotics, including chloramphenicol
Shigellosis (bacillary dysentery)	*Shigella boydii, S. dysenteriae, S. flexneri, S. sonnei,* and other *Shigella* spp.	–	Rod	1–14 days	Symptoms appear suddenly and include abdominal pain, diarrhea, high fever, general discomfort, stools containing mucus, blood, and pus ('red currant jelly' appearance), rectal burning, and dehydration; complications include massive bleeding and perforation of the large intestine	1. Isolation, Gram stain, and culture from specimens 2. Biochemical tests (Table 32-3)	1. Antibiotics, including ampicillin, chloramphenicol, and tetracyclines 2. Maintain fluid and electrolyte balance
Traveler's diarrhea	Enterotoxin-producing *E. coli* strains	–	Rod	Usually 2–5 days	Symptoms appear suddenly and include abdominal pain, diarrhea, dehydration, nausea, chills, vomiting, jaundice, possible convulsions, and weight loss; complications do not usually develop	1. Isolation, Gram stain, and culture from specimens (Color Photograph 62B) 2. Biochemical tests (Figure 32-3 and Table 32-3) 3. Serological tests, e.g., agglutination, fluorescent antibody	Symptomatic
Typhoid fever	*Salmonella typhi*	–	Rod	1–2 weeks or longer	Symptoms appear gradually and include abdominal distention, constipation, rising fever, headache, loss of appetite, nausea, vomiting, diarrhea, and appearance of a rash (rose spots) on abdomen; complications include inflammation of gall bladder, perforation of small intestine, intestinal bleeding, and pneumonia	1. Gram stain 2. Isolation and culture from specimens 3. Biochemical tests (Figure 32-3 and Table 32-3) 4. Bacteriophage typing (Color Photograph 77)	Antibiotics, including chloramphenicol
Weil's disease (spirochetal jaundice, leptospirosis)	*Leptospira interrogans*	Usually not done	Spiral	2–20 days	Symptoms appear suddenly and include lack of appetite, chest pains, head cold, difficulty in swallowing, swollen lymph nodes, fever, vomiting, and jaundice; complications are severe involvement of the skin, central nervous system, kidneys, and liver	1. Isolation of organism from specimens 2. Serological tests, e.g., specific agglutination, complement fixation (see Chapter 24)	1. Antibiotics, including penicillin and tetracyclines 2. Symptomatic 3. Restore fluid and electrolyte balance

TABLE 32-3 Selected Properties of Gram-negative Bacterial Species Associated with Gastrointestinal Disease States

	Tests[a]												
									Fermentations				
Organism	*Indole*	*MR*	*VP*	*Citrate*	*Urease*	*PD*	*OD*	*Glu*	*Lac*	*Man*	*Su*	*H_2S*	*Mot.*
Alcaligene faecalis	–	–	–	–	–	–	–	NC	NC	NC	NC	–	+
Escherichia coli	+	+	–	–	–	–	±	AG	AG	AG	AG	–	+
Enterobacter (Aerobacter) aerogenes	–	–	+	+	–	–	–	AG	AG	AG	AG	–	±
Proteus mirabilis	–	–	±	±	±	+	+	AG	NC	NC	AG	+	+
P. morgani	+	+	–	–	+	+	+	AG	NC	NC	NC	–	+
P. vulgaris	+	+	±	±	+	+	–	AG	NC	NC	AG	+	+
Pseudomonas aeruginosa	–	–	–	+	–	–	–	NC	NC	NC	NC	NC	+
Salmonella typhi	–	+	–	–	–	–	–	A	NC	A	NC	+	+
S. paratyphi A	–	+	–	–	–	–	+	AG	NC	AG	NC	–	+
S. schottmulleri (paratyphi B)	–	+	–	+	–	–	+	AG	NC	AG	NC	+	+
Shigella dysenteriae	±	+	–	–	–	–	–	A	–	–	–	–	–
Vibrio cholerae	+	–	–	–	–	–	–	A	NC	A	A	+ (Slow)	+
V. parahaemolyticus	+	+	–	+	–	–	+	A	NC	A	NC	–	+
Yersinia enterocolitica	±	+	–	–	+	–	+	A	NC	A	NC	–	+

[a]Explanation of symbols: MR=methyl red; VP=Voges Proskauer; PD=phenylalanine deaminase; OD=ornithine decarboxylase; Glu=glucose; Lac=lactose; Man=mannose; Su=sucrose; H_2S=hydrogen sulfide; Mot=motility; –=negative; +=positive; ±=variable, dependent upon the strain of the organism; A=acid; AG=acid and gas; NC=no change or negative.

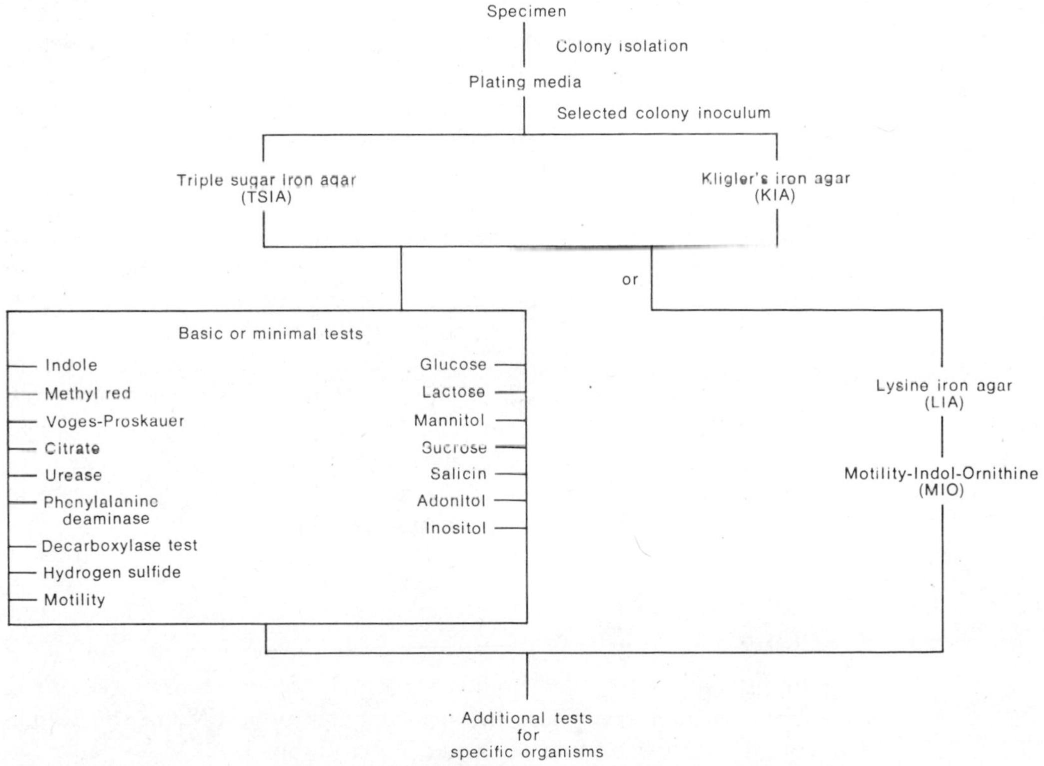

FIG. 32-3 A representative preliminary biochemical approach to the identification of common gastrointestinal bacterial pathogens. Many of the reactions, either individual or combined in multiple test systems, are shown in Color Photographs 63, 64, 65, 95, and 96. It should be noted that identification schemes vary among facilities and institutions. The decarboxylation tests listed are practical procedures for detection of decarboxylases (enzymes) that remove carboxyl groups (COOH) from the amino acids arginine, lysine, and ornithine. *Differentiation of Enterobacteriaceae by Biochemical Reactions, p. 12, Center for Disease Control, Atlanta, Georgia 30333, 1974.*

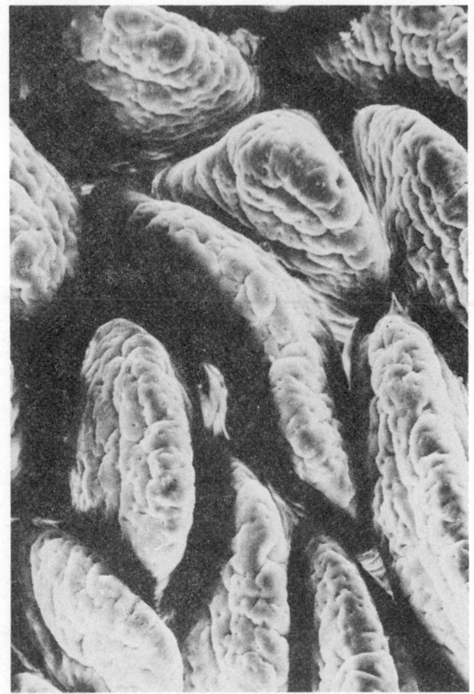

(a)

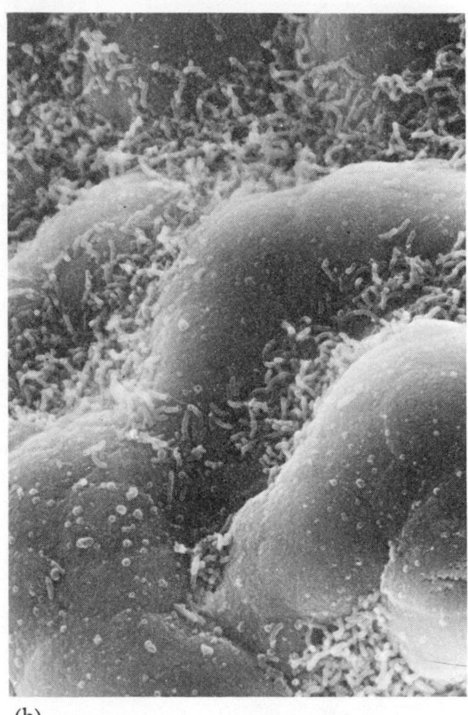

(b)

FIG. 32-4 Cholera is caused by a toxin produced by *Vibrio cholerae* in the human small intestine. The ability of the bacteria to adhere to the intestinal lining and establish themselves in this area (bound organisms) is thought to be an important aspect in producing the disease. (a) A portion of the intestine free of disease agents. (b) Large patches of *V. cholerae* on the adult villus. *Nelson, L. T., J. D. Clements, and R. A. Finkelstein,* Inf. Imm. *14:527-547 (1976).*

present century, the disease appears to have been more or less limited to India and surrounding areas, although epidemics have occurred in other parts of the world, including Egypt, Indonesia, Korea, and the Philippines.

Transmission. The causative agents of cholera are the Gram-negative, slightly curved rods *Vibrio cholerae* (Figure 32–4). Individuals acquire cholera (Table 32–2) through the ingestion of the causative organisms in sewage-contaminated food or water or by coming directly into contact with an infected person's feces. Houseflies may also spread the vibrios. Epidemics are usually associated with such sources of infection. There appear to be no long-term carriers.

Contamination of water supplies is usually caused by recent introduction of cholera organisms rather than the persistence of the agents in such an environment. Fish obtained from contaminated waters and eaten without sufficient cooking are also a source of disease agents.

Cholera epidemics have been described as either ***protracted*** or ***explosive***. Explosive epidemics occur when the pathogenic agents are transmitted by means of contaminated food or water. The protracted forms of cholera occur when disease-causing organisms are spread by direct contact or by fecal-contaminated objects (fomites).

Cholera is more frequent during the warmer months of the year. Very few cases of this disease are found in the winter. In the endemic areas of the Far East, cholera appears to be related to a warm climate, high absolute humidity, and large population. When the monsoons bring heavy rainfall to these regions, the incidence of cholera drops substantially because the heavy rains wash away contaminated matter.

It is fairly well accepted now that the diarrhea of cholera is due to the action of an exo-enterotoxin, choleragen, on an intact intestinal wall. It is believed that the ability of *V. cholerae* to adhere to the intestinal lining and to establish themselves in this area may be an important aspect in producing cholera (Figure 32–4b).

Prevention. A cholera vaccine consisting of heat-killed organisms can provide protection. Unfortunately, this immunity is not long-lasting. Around 4 to 6 months of protection is believed possible. The vaccine is given in two 1-ml doses, 7 days apart.

Probably the most effective measure to protect against cholera infection is to establish and maintain purified water supplies. In the areas where the disease prevails, this would greatly help in reducing the incidence of infection. In addition, of course, the elimination of flies, suitable treatment of patients during convalescence, and education of the general population as to the means of transmission are effective preventive measures.

Brucellosis

Brucellosis, commonly called undulant or Malta fever, occurs in countries bordering the Mediterranean Sea, the islands of Cyprus and Malta, the Scandinavian countries, Mexico, and the United States (Table 32–2).

Transmission. Humans acquire brucellosis through contact with the tissues or excretions of infected animals or by the ingestion of contaminated meat or unpasteurized dairy products. Sixty percent of human infections in the United States in 1975 involved meat-processing workers. Accidental inoculations of brucellae also have been reported. In general, the disease is not readily transmitted from human to human.

Causative Agents. The causative agents belong to the genus *Brucella,* which was named after Sir David Bruce, who first isolated the causative agent of Malta fever. The genus contains the closely related species *B. abortus, B. canis, B. neotomae, B. ovis, B. suis,* and *B. melitensis. B. canis* causes Bang's disease, or bovine brucellosis; *B. suis* causes swine (porcine) brucellosis; and *B. melitensis* causes goat (caprine) brucellosis, or Malta fever.

The brucellae are small, pleomorphic, Gram-negative coccobacilli. These organisms are nonmotile and non-spore-forming. All species are obligate parasites capable of maintaining an intracellular existence.

Prevention. Prevention of brucellosis centers on the elimination of reservoirs of the disease. This involves immunization of natural reservoirs, such as cattle, goats, and hogs, and the segregation and even the destruction of infected animals. Vaccination of humans against this disease has been limited.

The routine pasteurization of dairy products is another effective means of prevention. This procedure has markedly reduced the number of human cases of brucellosis in the United States.

Leptospirosis

Leptospirosis is produced by distinct and slender spirochetes of the genus *Leptospira* (Table 32–2). Human leptospiral disease is a severe illness accompanied by a high fever, jaundice, some bleeding, and involvement of the kidney. The spirochetes may become established in the urinary system and thus serve as a major source of contamination of water.

Causative Agents. Strains of *Leptospira* can be found in various bodies of water, such as lakes, ponds, and rivers, on decaying matter, and sometimes even in tap water. Leptospires measure approximately 4 to 20 μm in length and 0.1 μm in width. These organisms are quite thin (*leptos* is from the Greek, meaning "thin"), elongated structures consisting of many small coils tightly set together (Figure 8–9). Quite often leptospires are shaped like the letters C, S, and J. Finely tapered or "hooked" ends are characteristic of these organisms.

Leptospires may be stained with a Giemsa stain preparation or with silver stains.

Transmission. Leptospirosis is considered a zoonosis. Several species of wild rodents and domestic animals, including cattle, cats, and dogs, serve as reservoirs of infection. The natural hosts may experience a mild infection, but they seldom die of the disease. A particular *Leptospira* strain is usually quite well adapted to its host and is capable of inhabiting portions of the animal's kidney without inflicting damage. Thus the periodic release of large numbers of leptospires in the animal's urine is not unusual. Humans acquire the disease agent by coming into contact, either directly or indirectly, with this infected urine. *Leptospira* infections may result from bathing in, or falling into, stagnant bodies of water contaminated by the infectious urine of rodents. The spirochetes may gain access to the body tissues by penetrating the mucous membranes of the eyes and nasopharynx or by entering through skin abrasions or cuts. Cases involving ingestion of contaminated food and water have also been reported.

Several factors seem to affect the incidence of human infections, among them age, sex, occupation, and seasonal variations. In general, adults are more likely to acquire leptospirosis because of a greater possibility of exposure. For example, newborn infants are not exposed to contaminated bodies of water that might be used for swimming, boating, or fishing. The age most commonly involved is between 20 and 30 years. The higher percentage of cases among males is due to greater occupational exposure. Occupations that have previously been typically male—such as plumbing, meat packing, and farming—afford a greater chance of exposure to infected animals and contaminated bodies of water. No difference in susceptibility between males and females has been reported.

In tropical areas, leptospirosis occurs throughout the year. In general, leptospira require moisture and warmth for survival. These conditions also increase the use of outdoor facilities for both pleasure and work, thereby creating greater exposure.

Prevention. Because the natural reservoirs of leptospirosis are varied and numerous, eradicating them would be quite difficult. An effective vaccine for this disease is not available for humans, and preventive measures are directed toward reducing human contact with contaminated water or urine from infected animals. Preventive measures include wearing protective clothing, such as gloves and rubber boots, while working with objects or water supplies that may be contaminated; avoiding bodies of water that might be contaminated by infected animals; and not using or ingesting water and food that may be contaminated. Because dogs may be exposed to infected animals or their urine, they are commonly immunized against the disease.

Salmonellosis: Food Infection

This disease, which bears no relationship to salmon, is primarily limited to the gastrointestinal tract. Outbreaks of salmonellosis are usually explosive in nature, and are associated with banquets, weddings, or other group meals. The suddenness of the disease tends to distinguish it from other infectious diseases involving the gastrointestinal system, such as amebic or bacillary dysentery (Tables 32–2 and 32–6).

Causative Agents. Several species of *Salmonella* are known to produce salmonellosis. Included in this group are *S. choleraesuis, S. enteritidis*, and *S. typhimurium*. These organisms are Gram-negative, motile, non-spore-forming rods. At the present time the members of the genus *Salmonella* are divided into serological groups based on their antigenic properties. All these organisms have the same somatic or O antigens, which are components of their cell walls. They are of several hundred serological types based on differences in their flagellar or H antigens. Another antigen found with certain salmonellae is the Vi or virulence antigen, another somatic antigen.

Transmission. Humans acquire salmonellosis through consumption of contaminated food or water. A variety of foods have been implicated as sources in outbreaks; these include cream-containing bakery goods, ground meats, poultry, sausages, and eggs. Rodents such as mice and rats are often infected by salmonellae. Such animals, after recovery, may become carriers and by means of their excreta contaminate foods. This possibility should be guarded against in establishments where food is stored or prepared. Contamination by human carriers also occurs.

Prevention and Control. Measures that can be taken against salmonellosis include (1) the proper cooking of foods obtained from animal sources, such as ground meat and sausages; (2) poultry refrigeration and covering of prepared foods; (3) protection of food from contamination by mice, rats, or flies and related insects; (4) the periodic inspection of food handlers; and (5) proper sanitation.

Salmonella food poisoning is a reportable disease. Reporting cases to public health authorities is important, in order that suitable measures may be taken to prevent an epidemic.

Shigellosis (Bacillary Dysentery)

The principal causes of this acute infectious disease are the pathogenic shigellae. Shigellosis is distinct from amebic and viral dysentery. The various species of ***Shigella*** are widely distributed but are found primarily in human intestines and occasionally in the intestinal tracts of monkeys and other mammals. The most common causes of bacillary dysentary are ***Shigella dysenteriae*** (discovered by Japanese bacteriologist Kiyoshi Shiga in 1896) and *S. flexneri*. In general, the shigellae are far less invasive than the salmonellae.

Classifying shigellae on the basis of fermentation reactions has proved difficult in certain cases (Table 32–3). The use of newer methods has simplified classification (Color Photographs 95–96). Separation into species and serological types on the basis of antigenic composition has been successful.

Transmission. Since the fourth century B.C. when it was first described, shigellosis has been reported during several major military campaigns. This disease seems to occur with greater frequency than other forms of dysentery.

The human is the sole reservoir of infection; no lower animal reservoir is known. Although all age groups are susceptible to infection, children and males between the ages of 20 and 30 are most commonly infected. Predisposing factors include lowered states of resistance, malnutrition, overcrowding, and poor sanitation.

Bacillary dysentery is usually contracted through the ingestion of contaminated food or water. The causative agents can be transmitted by feces, fingers, flies, or food.

Individuals recovering from bacillary dysentery may become carriers of shigellae. This is an important consideration in the control and prevention of shigellosis, as these persons serve as reservoirs between outbreaks.

Complications known to occur with shigellosis include the perforation of the large intestine and massive bleeding.

The particular factors responsible for the pathogenicity in shigellosis have been fully determined only for infections produced by ***Shigella dysenteriae***. In addition to producing an endotoxin characteristic of all shigellae, *S. **dysenteriae*** is known to form an exotoxin. This soluble, heat-labile protein, called the Shiga neurotoxin, is one of the most powerful poisons known. When injected into experimental animals, the toxin causes bleeding, fever, diarrhea, paralysis, and death.

Prevention. The control of shigellosis involves far more than the appropriate use of antibiotics. Since human beings serve as the only source of infectious agents, preventive measures must be directed toward infected persons, carriers, and items that may have been contaminated. The elimination of flies, the proper sanitary disposal of excreta, and the protection of food and water are also important.

Unfortunately, vaccines have not been developed that could increase individual resistance. Thus, in situations of widespread shigellosis, the use of mass chemoprophylaxis may be necessary.

Typhoid Fever

The various species of *Salmonella* are associated with at least three distinguishable human disease states: enteric fever, blood poisoning *(septicemias)*, and the acute forms of infectious food poisoning discussed earlier.

Individuals suffering from septicemia exhibit a high fever and the presence of bacteria in the blood. *Salmonella choleraesuis* is a common causative agent. All of these conditions are collectively called *salmonellosis*. Typhoid fever is the classic example of enteric fever. It is caused by the Gram-negative, motile, non-spore-forming rod *Salmonella typhi*.

Transmission. Humans acquire typhoid fever by ingesting contaminated food or water. Flies and fomites have also been implicated. In countries where sanitation is adequate, typhoid fever appears either sporadically or in an endemic form. Often the source of infectious agents is traced to carriers. In regions with poor sanitation, impure water, improper waste disposal, and lack of pasteurization, typhoid epidemics are more likely to occur. All ages may be attacked.

Salmonella typhi can gain access to various tissues and organs via the bloodstream. Thus the bone marrow, gall bladder, and spleen can serve as future sources of reinfection. This gives rise to the relapses observed with typhoid fever when organisms gain access to the bloodstream from other foci of infection.

Two Bacterial Disease States of Increasing Frequency

Several enteric or so-called coliform bacilli are normal, nonpathogenic inhabitants of the gastrointestinal tract. However, other related strains or species are associated with pathological states involving the human urogenital and intestinal system. This group of Gram-negatives includes *Citrobacter freudii*, enteropathogenic *Escherichia coli*, enterotoxin-producing *E. coli*, *Providencia* spp., *Serratia* spp., *Vibrio parahaemolyticus*, and *Yersinia enterocolitica*. Two of the most important will be discussed here.

INFANT EPIDEMIC DIARRHEA (ENTEROPATHOGENIC *ESCHERICHIA COLI*, EPEC)

Epidemic diarrhea in newborn and young infants has often been reported. Most of these outbreaks have been associated with specific enteropathogenic strains of *Escherichia coli* (EPEC). However, studies from India, Vietnam in 1971, and Japan in 1967 showed that EPEC can cause disease not only in children, but in adults as well. There are at least two mechanisms of disease production: formation of a choleralike enterotoxin and invasion of intestinal epithelial lining.

Transmission. Incidents of infant epidemic diarrhea pose a definite threat in hospital nurseries. Unfortunately, outbreaks of this kind may be accompanied by a high mortality rate. Controlling the spread of enteropathogenic strains is a difficult problem because they develop resistance to commonly used antibiotics.

Epidemic diarrhea usually affects newborns and infants under two years of age. Premature babies are attacked most severely. Although the disease can occur in older children and adults, the effects are not serious.

Sources of enteropathogenic *E. coli* include convalescent infant carriers, cats, dogs, certain foods, and fomites.

TRAVELER'S DIARRHEA

In recent years evidence has shown that enterotoxin-producing *Escherichia coli* can cause an acute dehydrating diarrhea known as traveler's diarrhea. Traveler's diarrhea, as the name suggests, is acquired by individuals traveling from one part of the world to another and being exposed to different strains of *E. coli,* some of which have virulence factors such as enterotoxin production. Recovery from the condition is usually without complications.

Food Poisoning (Intoxications)

The clinical state of food poisoning discussed here refers to the symptoms resulting from the consumption of food or drink contaminated by pathogenic bacteria or their toxic products. "Naturally" poisonous foods and conditions arising from the ingestion of foods sprayed with pesticides will not be considered here.

In the past, certain gastrointestinal upsets were generally labeled *ptomaine poisoning.* The designation was used synonymously with food poisoning. This practice has declined as careful studies have shown the presence of pathogenic microorganisms or their products in foods consumed by stricken persons.

The agents of common bacterial food poisoning are well established. Among the conditions they produce are botulism, perfringens poisoning, salmonellosis, and staphylococcal poisoning. Salmonellosis is an example of an active infection (infectious food poisoning); the other three states are examples of poisonings or bacterial intoxications. In poisoning, it is the toxins alone that produce the symptoms (Table 32–4).

Microorganisms have been implicated in causing other gastrointestinal upsets; these microorganisms include *Bacillus cereus,* certain *Escherichia coli* strains, and members of the Arizona group. Moreover, viruses have been incriminated in certain cases of food-borne illnesses.

BOTULISM

The name *botulism* is derived from the Latin *botulus,* meaning "sausage." Uncooked sausages were associated with disease for years. *Clostridium botulinum,* the causative agent of this disease, produces a powerful neurotoxin when it grows under appropriate anaerobic conditions. Botulism is not considered an infectious disease. *C. botulinum* is not an invasive microorganism. However, persons who eat foods containing *C. botulinum* toxin develop an intoxication. Botulism has been associated with a variety of food products, including improperly preserved or prepared home-canned fruits and vegetables, smoked fish, and uncooked fish and meats. Outbreaks of the disease have also occurred with commercial products. The neurotoxin causing botulism can usually be completely inactivated through heating at 100°C for 10 minutes. This fact accounts for the relatively low incidence of the disease. It should be noted, however, that this procedure may not always be effective, as toxin inactivation also depends on the toxin's concentration.

It is important to note that foods contaminated by the toxin do not necessarily appear or smell any different from uncontaminated products. Furthermore, neither the gastric secretions of the stomach nor the protein-digesting enzymes of the duodenum inactivate the toxin. This poison is absorbed both from the stomach and the small intestine.

Six exotoxin types are known. Types A, B, E, and F are associated with human diseases; types C and D are reported to affect fowl and cattle, respectively. Most human cases and the highest mortality are caused by types A and E.

Botulinum toxin acts by becoming attached to the endings of efferent nerves. There it blocks the release of acetylcholine by nerve fibers when a nerve impulse passes through the peripheral nervous system. Antitoxin cannot neutralize the neurotoxin once it is attached. Thus treatment should begin as soon as possible if botulism is suspected. A new and distinct form of this intoxication has been uncovered, infant botulism. The critical and frightening difference between the infant and adult forms of botulism is that children appear to become ill without having ingested toxin-containing foods. What is ingested are spores. Once in the intestine, *C. botulinum* spores germinate into vegetative cells, and toxin production begins. The exact number of cases of infant botulism that occur is not known. Awareness of this condition as a cause of infant deaths is quite limited.

STAPHYLOCOCCAL FOOD POISONING

As we have seen, staphylococci are normally found in various regions of the human body, including the nose, skin, and throat. These bacteria cause one of the most common types of food poisoning. The active agent of staphylococcal food poisoning is one of several enterotoxins produced by certain *Staphylococcus aureus* strains. At least five different enterotoxins have been reported. They are designated as enterotoxins A, B, C, D, and E.

Transmission. Staphylococcal food poisoning occurs world-wide and is not a communicable disease. Age, race, and sex do not play a role in the occurrence of the condition. Humans show symptoms of the disease after consuming food in which these organisms have grown and produced a sufficient quantity of the toxin. Types of food that serve as growth media for staphylococci include bakery goods, especially those with custard or cream filling; cured, processed, or leftover meats; fish; and dairy products. Staphylococci grow in such foods when they are left unrefrigerated. In order for enterotoxin to be produced in sufficient concentration, food must remain at or above room temperature for several hours. Because the toxin is not inactivated by heat, cooking foods that have previously been left unrefrigerated provides no protection against staphylococcal food poisoning.

The sources of disease agents include individuals with staphylococcal infections, human carriers, infected animals, and milk or milk products contaminated by carriers.

Complications or deaths associated with this disease are rare.

TABLE 32-4 A Comparison of Common Bacterial Food Poisonings (Intoxication)

Condition	Causative Agent	Gram Reaction	Morphology	Incubation Period	General Features of Intoxication	Laboratory Diagnosis	Possible Treatment
Botulism	*Clostridium botulinum*	+	Rod	12–96 hours	Difficulty in speaking, double vision, inability to swallow, nausea, vomiting, and paralysis of urinary bladder and all voluntary muscles; death caused by stoppage of heart action and/or breathing may occur	1. Gram and spore stains 2. Anaerobic culture of suspected foods 3. Toxicity testing with mice	1. Antitoxin 2. Antibiotics to prevent secondary infection
Perfringens poisoning	*Clostridium perfringens*	+	Rod	Within 18 hours	Abdominal cramps, chills, bluish coloration of the skin, diarrhea, headache, nausea, and vomiting	1. Gram stain and spore stains 2. Anaerobic culture of suspected foods	1. Measures to replace salt and water loss 2. Symptomatic
Staphylococcal intoxication	*Staphylococcus aureus*	+	Coccus	1–6 hours	Severity of symptoms depends on amount of enterotoxin ingested and include abdominal cramps, chills, bluish coloration of the skin, diarrhea, headache, nausea, and vomiting	1. Gram stain 2. Isolation of *S. aureus* on mannitol salt agar (Color Photograph 74) 3. Demonstration of coagulase positive 4. Enterotoxin detection in foods	1. Measures to replace salt and water loss 2. Symptomatic

Prevention. Preventive measures against food poisoning include the proper covering and refrigeration of all foods and the exclusion of persons with obvious skin infections or disorders from food handling during preparation or serving.

The true problems with staphylococcal food poisoning are not associated with food processing, but instead are related to the mishandling of food in food service establishments and in the home.

PERFRINGENS POISONING

Clostridium perfringens is more widely spread than any other pathogenic bacterium. Its principal habitats are the soil and the intestinal contents of humans and animals. This organism has been recognized since the late 1800s, when reports linked it with food poisoning; however, it was not until 1945 that *C. **perfringens*** food-borne illness was reported. The illness received considerable attention in Great Britain in 1953 and has been recognized as a very important food poisoning organism in the United States since that time.

Strains of this bacterial species are divided into six types, A through F. The basis for this classification is the immunologically specific toxin produced by each strain. ***Clostridium perfringens,*** type A, is known to cause a form of intoxication analogous to that associated with staphylococcal enterotoxin. A more severe form of disease, enteritis necroticans, is produced by *C. **perfringens,*** type F.

Transmission. Outbreaks of perfringens poisoning have been associated with several types of food, including cooked meats and poultry dishes.

Prevention. Preventive measures are similar to those described for staphylococcal poisoning.

Viral Infections

Various viral pathogens may infect portions of the gastrointestinal system (Table 32–5). Sometimes symptoms of a disease process may not be evident. When an infection does occur, the effects do not necessarily produce gastrointestinal disturbances, but may cause reactions involving other body structures, such as those of the nervous and respiratory systems.

Certain viruses invade the gastrointestinal system and utilize its parts for purposes of replication only. Viral involvement may accompany other types of infections, but direct evidence showing the relationship of viruses to outbreaks of gastrointestinal upsets, such as summer diarrhea, is usually lacking. Discussion here is limited to the main groups of pathogens known to invade the GI system.

Picornavirus Infections

Coxsackie-, echo-, and polio viruses are recognized as capable of infecting the gastrointestinal system. Originally, these specific agents were named enteroviruses because of their obvious association with this system. It soon became apparent, however, that several viruses in the group could infect the respiratory tract and central nervous system as well. Another group of pathogens primarily

TABLE 32-5 General Features of Viral Diseases of the Gastrointestinal Tract

Disease	*Incubation Period*	*General Features of the Disease*	*Laboratory Diagnosis*	*Possible Treatment*
Cytomegalovirus inclusion disease	Unknown	Symptoms of infected newborns include hepatitis, jaundice, increased size of liver and spleen, decreased number of blood platelets, and loss of sight; postnatally infected individuals may show no symptoms or may develop pneumonia; death can occur[a]	1. Demonstration of intranuclear inclusions (Figure 32-5) in specimens 2. Isolation of organism in tissue culture 3. Serological test, e.g., immunofluorescence, complement fixation	No specific treatment; however, immune globulins and steroids have been used
Hepatitis A virus disease (infectious hepatitis)	15–40 days	Symptoms show a wide range and include abdominal discomfort, muscular pains, jaundice, dark urine, light-colored stools, fever, chills, and sore throat	1. Liver function tests 2. Serological tests to eliminate other disease states	No specific therapy; supportive treatment including avoidance of physical stress, administration of vitamins and substances necessary to maintain caloric, fluid, and electrolyte balances; immune globulins have been used
Hepatitis B virus disease (serum hepatitis)	60–160 days	Symptoms are similar to those of hepatitis A disease; however, hepatitis B symptoms tend to be more severe	1. Liver function tests 2. Serological tests, e.g., complement fixation, hemagglution inhibition, radio immunoassays (RIA)[b] 3. Demonstration of viral antigen (HB_sAg)	Same as for infectious hepatitis
Infectious mononucleosis	19–49 days	Symptoms include mild jaundice, slight fever, enlarged and tender lymph nodes, sore throat, headache, and general weakness; complications can occur and include convulsions, anemia, and inflammation of heart tissue	1. Demonstration of atypical T-lymphocytes 2. Liver function tests 3. Serological tests, e.g., specific agglutination tests, heterophile antibody	Bed rest; use of anti-inflammatory agents in cases of hemolytic anemia; hospitalization of severe cases

[a]Several other infectious diseases may produce identical symptoms. These include the TORCH group (toxoplasmosis, rubella, herpesvirus) and syphilis.
[b]Radioimmunoassays are versatile, sensitive procedures that use antigens with radioactive labels for the measurement of antibody levels (titers) and/or the detection of antigens.

affecting the respiratory system was consequently designated the rhinoviruses. All of these various viruses were classified in a more adequate group, the ***picornaviruses. Pico*** means "small" and ***rna*** comes from the type of nucleic acid found in this group. Coxsackieviruses were named after Coxsackie, New York, where the first isolations took place in 1948. The name ***echo*** was derived from certain of the properties of these viruses: E = enteric location; C = capable of causing cytopathic changes in tissues cells; H = human source; and O = orphan. At one time there were more viral agents than diseases, hence the term ***orphan***.

Several pathogenic viruses of lower animals are also in the picornavirus group. These include the agents of encephalo-myocarditis of mice, Teschen disease of pigs, and foot-and-mouth disease (FMD).

In general, picornaviruses enter the human body via the oral route. A few, however, enter by means of the respiratory tract. The disease states produced by this group differ in the tissues involved, the types of lesions resulting from infection, and the severity of the attack. Similar disease states (for example, aseptic meningitis) may be caused by different picornaviruses. Most of the infections produced by picornaviruses are discussed in greater detail elsewhere in the text.

Cytomegalovirus Inclusion Disease

The cytomegaloviruses (CMV), also known as the salivary gland viruses, are a group of highly species-specific infecting agents. Humans, monkeys, and other animals can fall victim to them. Both *in vitro* and *in vivo*, these viral pathogens produce a cellular response characterized by ***cytomegaly*** (increases in cellular size) and by the presence of intranuclear inclusion bodies (Figure 32–5).

Transmission. Young infants appear to acquire CMV congenitally. Some instances of postnatal infection have also been reported. When CMV infection occurs with older individuals, it has been associated with leukemia or other cancerous diseases. Some cases have been reported in which generalized cytomegalic inclusion disease (CMID) produced complications in drug-caused suppression of the immune response with organ transplantations. There is a strong suggestion that the use of hormones and related drugs may bring about an activation of a latent CMV infection.

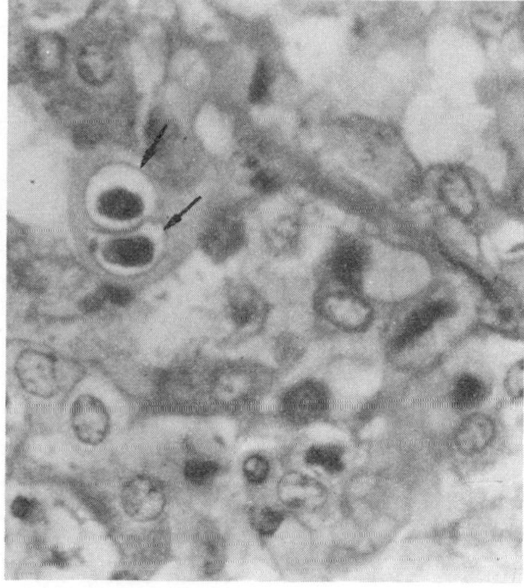

FIG. 32–5 Cytomegalovirus infection, showing the presence of intranuclear inclusions (arrows) in giant cells. *Cangir, A., and M. P. Sullivan,* JAMA *195:1042 (1966). Courtesy of the University of Texas M.D. Anderson Hospital & Tumor Inst., Houston, Texas.*

Viral Hepatitis

Viral hepatitis is an infectious enteric and systemic disease that characteristically involves the liver. Jaundice, a yellowing of tissues, is the most prominent symptom. The features of viral hepatitis are many (Table 32–5), ranging from viremia (viruses in the bloodstream) that does not seriously affect the liver, to a destructive disease state ending in death within a few days.

It is customary to designate viral hepatitis in relation to a special causative agent, such as hepatitis A virus, formerly infectious hepatitis (IH), and hepatitis B virus, formerly serum hepatitis (SH). The type A and type B microorganisms are separate viruses. Although they have several features in common, they differ in several respects. The most important of these include (1) the method of transmission, (2) the manner in which symptoms occur, (3) the incubation period, and (4) the chemical composition of the virus.

Humans are the only known natural hosts for viral hepatitis. Many infectious hepatitis cases have been associated with closed community environments such as camps, nurseries, housing tracts, and schools. Outbreaks have also occurred in hospitals. Infectious hepatitis virus is spread by the fecal contamination of food or water. Serum hepatitis virus, on the other hand, is usually transmitted by almost any type of injection, including those self-administered by drug addicts using contaminated needles and syringes. Moreover, doctors, nurses, technologists, or research technicians who handle blood or blood products are particularly vulnerable to this disease agent. Before the significance of the proper sterilization of syringes and needles in preventing serum hepatitis was realized, several outbreaks were reported in clinics giving routine injections. Unfortunately, even when suitable procedures are used, cases of the disease occur, especially in association with transfusions. Cases have also been traced to instruments used in oral surgery and to the practice of tattooing.

Experimental studies have shown mosquitoes to be potential transmitters of the disease agent.

PROPERTIES OF THE HEPATITIS VIRUSES

At this time, information on hepatitis A virus is limited. More is known of the type B virus.

Through electron microscopy, several viruslike particles of hepatitis B have been demonstrated. The first of these, originally referred to as the Australia

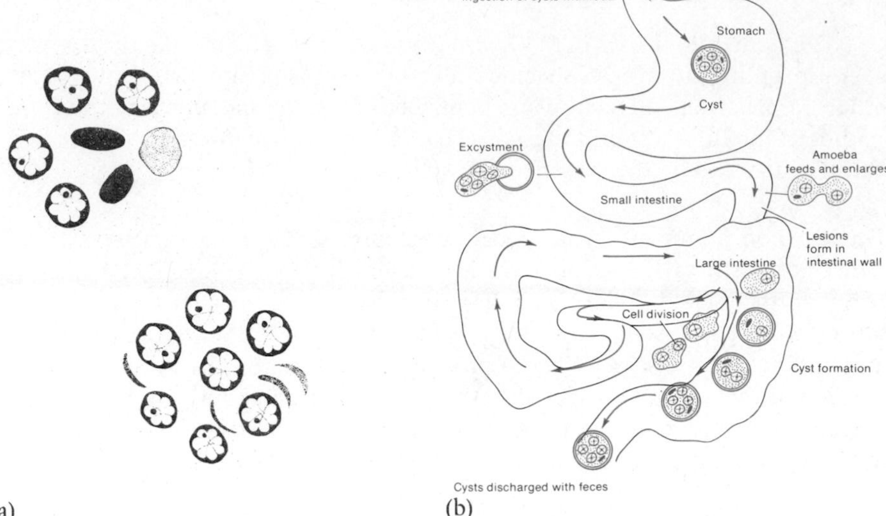

FIG. 32-6 Intestinal protozoa. (a) ***Entamoeba histolytica*** trophozoite and cyst stages. Average diameter of these protozoans is slightly over 20 μm. (b) The life cycle of ***Entamoeba histolytica***, the causative agent of amebic dysentary. The cycle shows the importance and role of protozoan cysts in disease transmission.

(Au) antigen, appears only in patients with serum hepatitis. It was found to be a spherical particle (probably actually icosahedral) with an average diameter of 20 nm. It contains no nucleic acids. A second particle, called the Dane particle, measures approximately 42 nm in diameter and is composed of an outer protein coat (which reacts with antibody specific for the viral surface antigen) and an inner DNA core of 27 nm in diameter. The outer coat of the Dane particle contains the hepatitis B surface antigen or HB_sAg. This surface antigen is a lipoprotein found in the serum of many patients with serum hepatitis. A third particle, called the Juang particle, has a diameter of 23 to 27 nm. It was discovered in the nuclei of liver cells from liver transplant patients who contracted hepatitis.

The emerging view of the relationship among these different particles is that the Juang particle is the DNA- or RNA-containing viral core. It replicates in the liver cell nucleus and there presumably causes the tissue damage associated with hepatitis B. Through some as-yet-unknown mechanism, the viral core migrates to the cell cytoplasm, where it is sheathed in the viral protein coat to become the Dane particle. This is believed to be the form in which the virus is transmitted. This mode of replication is similar to that of mouse leukemia and of herpesviruses, whose protein coats are also synthesized in the cytoplasm.

Other Types of Viral Hepatitis

Other viral agents may also produce liver injury. Epstein-Barr virus, the cause of infectious mononucleosis, and cytomegalovirus are examples of recognized viral agents that produce hepatic damage, occasionally severe enough to be clinically recognized as hepatitis. In addition, it is well to keep in mind the possibility that agents as yet undiscovered (hepatitis virus types C, D, and so on) may account for several cases of hepatitis.

Prevention and Control

Since under most circumstances it is impossible to differentiate between the two types of viral hepatitis, the preventive and control measures are applicable to both infectious and serum hepatitis.

In dealing with suspected or known cases of viral hepatitis, it is customary to observe "enteric precautions." Such measures include (1) the hygienic disposal of feces, (2) the careful cleansing and disinfection of bedpans and toilet bowls, and (3) the proper sterilization of all dishes, eating utensils, bedclothes, and linen.

Preventing the transmission of viral hepatitis requires other important precautions as well. Nondisposable syringes, needles, tubing, and other types of equipment used for obtaining blood specimens or for the administration of therapeutic agents should be adequately sterilized before reuse. Most common means for chemical sterilization are not reliable for destroying hepatitis-causing viruses. Physical methods employed for this purpose are boiling in water for at least 20 minutes, heating in a drying oven at a temperature of 180°C for one hour, or autoclaving. Whenever possible, disposable equipment should be used for routine hospital and clinic procedures. *Disposable items should be properly sterilized before being discarded.*

The possibility of transmitting viral hepatitis by means of blood or plasma transfusions is yet another problem facing physicians and hospitals. An individual with a history of jaundice should not be used as a blood donor. Unfortunately, no method used today is effective in rendering whole blood containing hepatitis virus totally free of the agent, but treating plasma with the chemical agent betapropiolactone shows great promise. Plasma exposed to this chemical viricide and ultraviolet irradiation has been given to patients without adverse reactions.

When given shortly after exposure, or early during the incubation period, the use of immune serum globulin has proved effective in the prevention of infectious hepatitis. Immune (gamma) globulin usage in cases of serum hepatitis is questionable at this time.

VACCINE PRODUCTION

One of the most important steps in producing a vaccine is the ability to grow the pathogen in question. Unfortunately, no one has been able to grow either of the hepatitis viruses. However, a vaccine that sidesteps this requirement has been prepared by using viral antigens isolated from human carriers of hepatitis. The viral component in the vaccine is the hepatitis B surface antigen (HB_sAg). It is readily found in the blood plasma of patients with hepatitis B. Research with a variety of laboratory animals, including chimpanzees, has shown that the vaccine stimulates antibody production and provides protection against challenge doses of live virus. A preparation of this type has great significance for humans. Additional testing is necessary before it can be made available for general usage.

Parasitic Protozoan Infections

Amebiasis (Amebic Dysentery)

Amebiasis, caused by ***Entamoeba histolytica*** (Table 32–6), occurs world-wide with a higher morbidity rate in warmer climates where opportunities for exposure to the protozoan are greater.

Transmission. Transmission of *E.* ***histolytica*** is most often by contaminated water supplies, flies, infected food handlers, and person-to-person contact. Communities with poor sanitary conditions provide opportunities for repeated exposure.

Life Cycle. Fully developed cysts (Figure 32–6a and Color Photograph 44) are ingested by humans. These forms undergo excystment, division, growth, and multiplication (Figure 32–6b). The resulting trophozoites in the alimentary canal may penetrate the wall of the large intestine and multiply there. The parasites are known to feed well on red blood cells. Destruction of tissues may or may not produce the classic symptoms of amebic dysentery. Involvement of the liver and other organs may also occur as a result of bloodstream invasion by the protozoan. Cyst formation results when trophozoites enter the intestine and find unfavorable conditions. It should be noted that if trophs are rapidly discharged from this region, as in the acute diarrhea stage, these parasites die quickly.

Prevention. Improvement in sanitation is the most important step toward disease prevention. Access to food by flies and cockroaches should be eliminated, and infected persons should not be allowed to handle food. Inadequate purification of water supplies must also be eliminated. Furthermore, education in personal hygienic habits and in the dangers of using as fertilizer human fecal matter that may be from infected persons should be expanded.

Balantidiasis

Balantidium coli (Color Photograph 45) is the only ciliate considered parasitic for humans. Geographically, ***Balantidium coli*** is found practically world-wide. The parasite lives in the large intestine, where it can invade the mucosa and submucosa, causing ulceration and frequently a fatal form of dysentery.

Transmission. Humans acquire *B.* ***coli*** by ingesting viable cysts from contaminated food. Once *B.* ***coli*** becomes established in a human host, its transmission from person to person is greatly enhanced in areas where sanitation is poor.

Life Cycle. After cysts are ingested, the parasites in the host's intestine excyst, and the newly emerged trophozoites feed on various forms of organic matter, including starch grains, bacteria, and the host's cells. Invasion of the surrounding tissue may occur. Encystment of *B.* ***coli*** trophs takes place with the dehydration of fecal matter containing them, either before or after feces evacuation from the large intestine. Subsequent contamination of food or water with such material may start the cycle again.

Prevention of Infection. Generally speaking, the most practical methods for the control of *B.* ***coli*** infection are improvement of sanitary facilities, effective treatment of all infected persons, and increased education on the dangers of contaminated food and water.

Giardia (Lamblia) Intestinalis

A large percentage of individuals harboring ***Giardia (lamblia) intestinalis*** (Figure 32–7) have no symptoms. However, reports of some cases have definitely indicated involvement of the gall bladder and the production of gastroenteritis. The disease can be found in most environments, apparently more

TABLE 32-6 General Features of Protozoan Infections Associated with the Gastrointestinal System

Disease	*Causative Agent*	*Incubation Period*	*General Features of the Disease*	*Laboratory Diagnosis*	*Possible Treatment*
Amebiasis (Amebic dysentery)	*Entameoba histolytica*	Usually 3–4 weeks	Abdominal cramps, flatulence, diarrhea, feces containing blood and mucus, weight loss, and general fatigue; complications such as invasion of the liver (amebic hepatitis) may develop	1. Demonstration of trophozoites and cysts in specimens (Color Photograph 44) 2. Serodiagnostic tests, e.g., immunodiffusion, fluorescent antibody (Chapter 23)	Chloroquine hydrochloride, metronidazole, maintenance of fluid and electrolyte balance
Balanitidiasis	*Balantidium coli*	Unknown	Intense abdominal pain, diarrhea, loss of weight, and vomiting; rapid destruction of tissue and death may occur	Demonstration of cysts in stool specimens (Color Photograph 44)	Antibiotics, including aureomycin and terramycin; Carbarsone
Giardiasis	*Giardia intestinalis*	Unknown	Generally no symptoms. In some cases, abdominal cramps, flatulence, nausea, and alternating constipation and diarrhea	Demonstration of cysts in specimens (See Figure 32-7)	Quinacrine hydrochloride (Atabrine), metronidazole

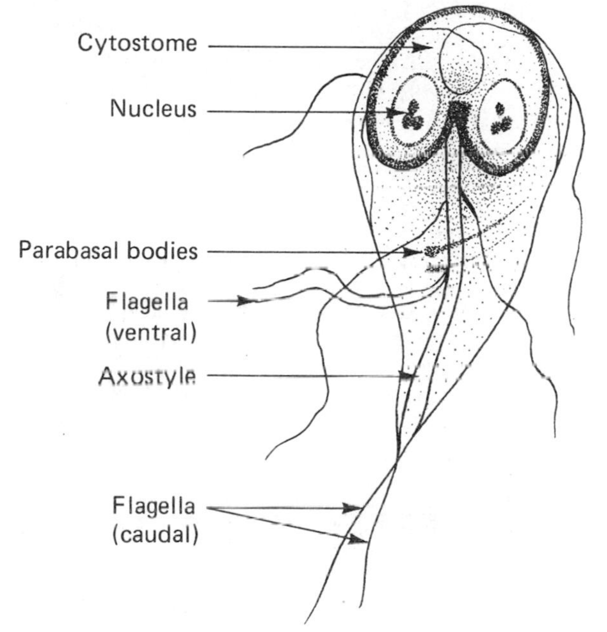

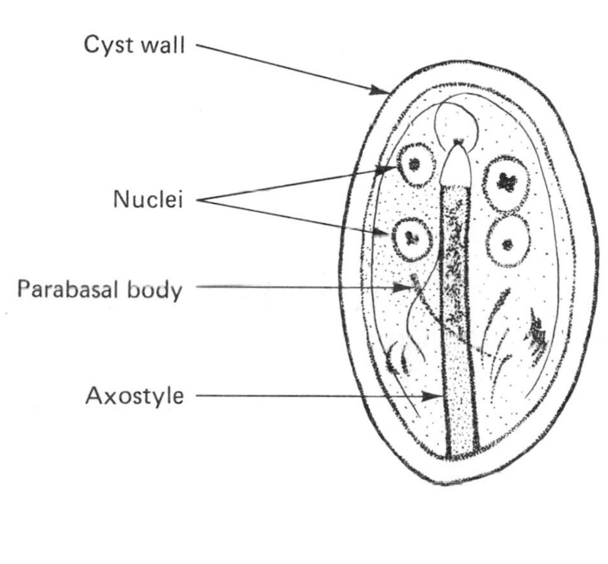

FIG. 32-7 Composite sketches of the stages of *Giardia intestinalis.* (a) A typical trophozoite. The length of this form ranges from 9 to 21 μm, while the width can vary from 5 to 15 μm. (b) An ovoid cyst. These structures vary in length from 8 to 14 μm and in width from 7 to 10 μm.

commonly in children than in adults. Outbreaks of *Giardia* infections are being found with greater frequency in ski resort areas in which sewage facilities have become overloaded.

SUMMARY

Structure and Function

1. The human gastrointestinal (GI) system includes the mouth, oropharnyx, esophagus, stomach, small and large intestines, the rectum, and several accessory organs such as the liver and pancreas.
2. The system serves as the means by which food and water are processed to meet the needs of the body.

Parts of the Gastrointestinal Tract

The Stomach

The stomach contains millions of glands that secrete mucus and gastric juice.

The Small Intestine

1. Most enzymatic digestion and absorption take place in the small intestine.
2. Small, fingerlike processes called villi contain capillaries and small lymph vessels. Capillaries absorb amino acids and carbohydrates. Lacteals absorb fatty acids.

The Large Intestine (Colon)

1. This organ is primarily involved with the processing, storage, and elimination of food remaining after digestion and absorption.
2. Water absorption is the major function of the large intestine.
3. Waste products of digestion are *feces*. This material contains indigestible food, large quantities of bacteria, and various other substances.

The Liver

1. The liver is one of the largest organs in the body.
2. Bile is produced by all parts of the liver and stored in the gall bladder.
3. Blockage of the bile duct causes *jaundice*, or a yellowing of body tissues.
4. Liver function tests are necessary for diagnosis of disease states of this organ.

Gastrointestinal Microbial Ecology

1. The structure of the GI tract determines the location and the composition of the microbial population of the system.
2. Prior to birth the tract is sterile. During birth, and thereafter, the system is exposed to a variety of microbes, some of which establish themselves (colonize) in specific locations.

Bacterial Diseases

1. Conditions in which there is a disturbance of intestinal functions accompanied by dehydration and the passage of liquid stools are referred to as *acute diarrheal disease*. Examples of diseases in which this condition exists are cholera, gastroenteritis, bacillary dysentery, infantile diarrhea, and traveler's diarrhea.
2. The practical identification of bacterial pathogens includes extensive biochemical tests for the detection of specific enzymes.
3. Several other bacteria can infect different regions of the system and cause serious illness. Examples of such disease are brucellosis, leptospirosis, and typhoid fever.

Food Poisoning (Intoxications)

1. Microbial food poisoning or intoxication refers to symptoms resulting from the consumption of food or drink contaminated by pathogens or their toxins.
2. Examples of bacterial intoxications are botulism, perfringens poisoning, and staphylococcal food poisoning.

Viral Infections

1. Various viruses, as well as certain other microorganisms, invade the GI system, use its parts for replication purposes only, and then invade other body structures.
2. The pathogens that infect the GI system include the coxsackie-, echo-, and polio viruses, cytomegalovirus, infectious hepatitis virus (type A), and the virus of infectious mononucleosis.

Parasitic Protozoan Infections

1. Several protozoans can invade and infect the various parts of the gastrointestinal system. Examples of resulting protozoan infections are amebic dysentery, balanitidiasis, and giardiasis.
2. These parasitic microbes exhibit two forms, the *cyst* (environmental resistant form) and the *trophozoite* (active feeding and invasive form).
3. Prevention of protozoan diseases and of diseases caused by other microbial types includes immunization (if available), improvements of sanitation, and adequate treatment of infected individuals.

QUESTIONS FOR REVIEW

1. Could antibiotics taken by mouth affect an individual's intestinal flora? Explain.
2. Differentiate between bacterial food poisoning and bacterial intoxication. Give examples of each.
3. a. Would the heating of foods containing an enterotoxin inactivate the toxin? Explain.
   b. What types of foods provide good growth conditions for staphylococci? For *Clostridium perfringens?*
   c. List at least two measures to prevent staphylococcal poisoning.
4. Discuss "ptomaine poisoning." Is it related to bacterial gastrointestinal diseases?
5. If you were going to tour Spain, Egypt, India, Peru, and Mexico, what diseases associated with the gastrointestinal system might you encounter? What precautionary measures would be advisable?
6. What disease outbreaks would you expect as a consequence of natural disasters such as earthquakes and floods?
7. Compare reservoirs for the following diseases:
   a. Asiatic cholera
   b. bacillary dysentery
   c. staphylococcal poisoning
   d. enteropathic *Escherichia coli*
   e. brucellosis
   f. leptospirosis

   g. amebic dysentery
   h. infectious hepatitis

8. What protective mechanisms against viral and bacterial diseases are provided by the human gastrointestinal system?
9. Propose an approach to the identification of a bacterial pathogen of the gastrointestinal tract.
10. a. Distinguish between infectious and serum hepatitis.
    b. What control measures can be used to effectively prevent both diseases?
    c. Why do these diseases pose a particular problem as well as a danger to hospital personnel and patients?
11. Are vaccines or immunization procedures used for any gastrointestinal associated diseases? If so, list them.
12. What is cytomegalic inclusion disease (CMID)? Are there any predisposing factors associated with it?
13. Discuss infectious mononucleosis with respect to the following topics:
    a. causative agent
    b. age group affected
    c. treatment and prevention
14. a. Is the liver vulnerable to infectious agents? Explain.
    b. List other parts of the GI system vulnerable to such attacks.
15. What general types of diagnostic methods are used for viral infections of the gastrointestinal tract?
16. What diseases are associated with the various members of the picornaviruses?

SUGGESTED READINGS

Balows, A., R. M. DeHaan, V. R. Dowell, Jr., and L. B. Guze (eds.), *Anaerobic Bacteria: Role in Disease*. Springfield, Ill.: Charles C. Thomas, 1974. *A collection of papers, including several on anaerobic infections of the digestive tract.*

Feinstone, S. M., and R. H. Purcell, "Non-A, Non-B Hepatitis," *Ann. Rev. Med.* 29:359 (1978). *Describes a new agent found to be one cause of human hepatitis. Its clinical characteristics, attempts to isolate a causative agent, and approaches to prevention are also discussed.*

Melnick, J. L., G. R. Dreesman, and F. B. Hollinger, "Viral Hepatitis," *Sci. Amer.* 237:44 (1977). *Discusses the recent advances in the epidemiology and immunology of viral hepatitis. Vaccine development against hepatitis B is also described.*

Reed, J. S., and J. L. Boyer, *Viral Hepatitis: Epidemiologic, Serologic, and Clinical Manifestations*. Chicago: Year Book Medical Publishers, Inc., 1979. *A detailed but clear presentation of the current state of viral hepatitis. Of particular interest are the sections concerned with hazards, principles of management, future developments, and hepatitis vaccines.*

Savage, D. C., "Microbial Ecology of the Gastrointestinal Tract," *Ann. Rev. Microbiol.* 31:107–133 (1977). *The current level of understanding of the microbial ecology of the gastrointestinal (GI) tract is discussed. Other topics in this article include the succession of organisms in infants and the factors that influence the composition of microbial populations in the GI tract.*

CHAPTER **33**

Microbial Infections of the Circulatory System

Chapter 33 describes briefly the various components of the cardiovascular system, emphasizing the structure and functions of the heart and blood vessels. Among the microbial infections that affect this system are malaria, plague, typhoid fever, and certain rickettsial diseases.

After reading this chapter, you should be able to:

1. **Describe the general organization of the human circulatory system and indicate the areas attacked by microbial pathogens.**
2. **List and discuss at least six bacterial diseases associated with the circulatory system, specifying the causative agent, means of transmission, preventive measures, and methods of control for each disease.**
3. **Discuss one viral disease and one protozoan disease that involve the circulatory system.**
4. **Distinguish among the general effects resulting from bacterial, protozoan, and viral infections of the circulatory system.**
5. **Describe the approaches to the diagnosis of rickettsial diseases, infectious mononucleosis, and malaria.**

The development of many infectious diseases follows a consistent pattern. Once pathogens enter the body and establish a local, or main, site of infection, they may spread to other regions of the body by means of the circulatory system, forming secondary sites of infection. Depending on the properties of the disease agent, the circulatory system may spread toxins released by the pathogen. Certain microbial disease agents also attack and destroy tissues of the cardiovascular system.

The circulatory system meets the needs of humans and other vertebrates for internal transport and intercommunication between the various cells of the body. Blood, the transport medium, carries nutrients and hormones, removes cellular waste products, assists in the regulation of body temperature, and aids in the control and elimination of foreign organisms. The blood flows under pressure in a one-way path through the vessels (arteries, veins, and capillaries) and heart directly to the tissues and organs where it is needed. The blood is pumped from the heart into the *aorta*, the artery leading from the heart, then into other arteries and on to the smaller capillaries. Upon serving its purpose, the blood is returned to the heart through the veins.

The heart functions as a pump, providing the force necessary to maintain adequate blood flow throughout the body. Actually it is a double pump: the right side receives blood from the body and pumps it to the lungs, where carbon dioxide in the blood is exchanged for oxygen, and the left side receives the freshly oxygenated blood from the lungs and pumps it to other body organs. Figure 33–1 shows the general direction, or path, followed by the blood through the human circulatory system.

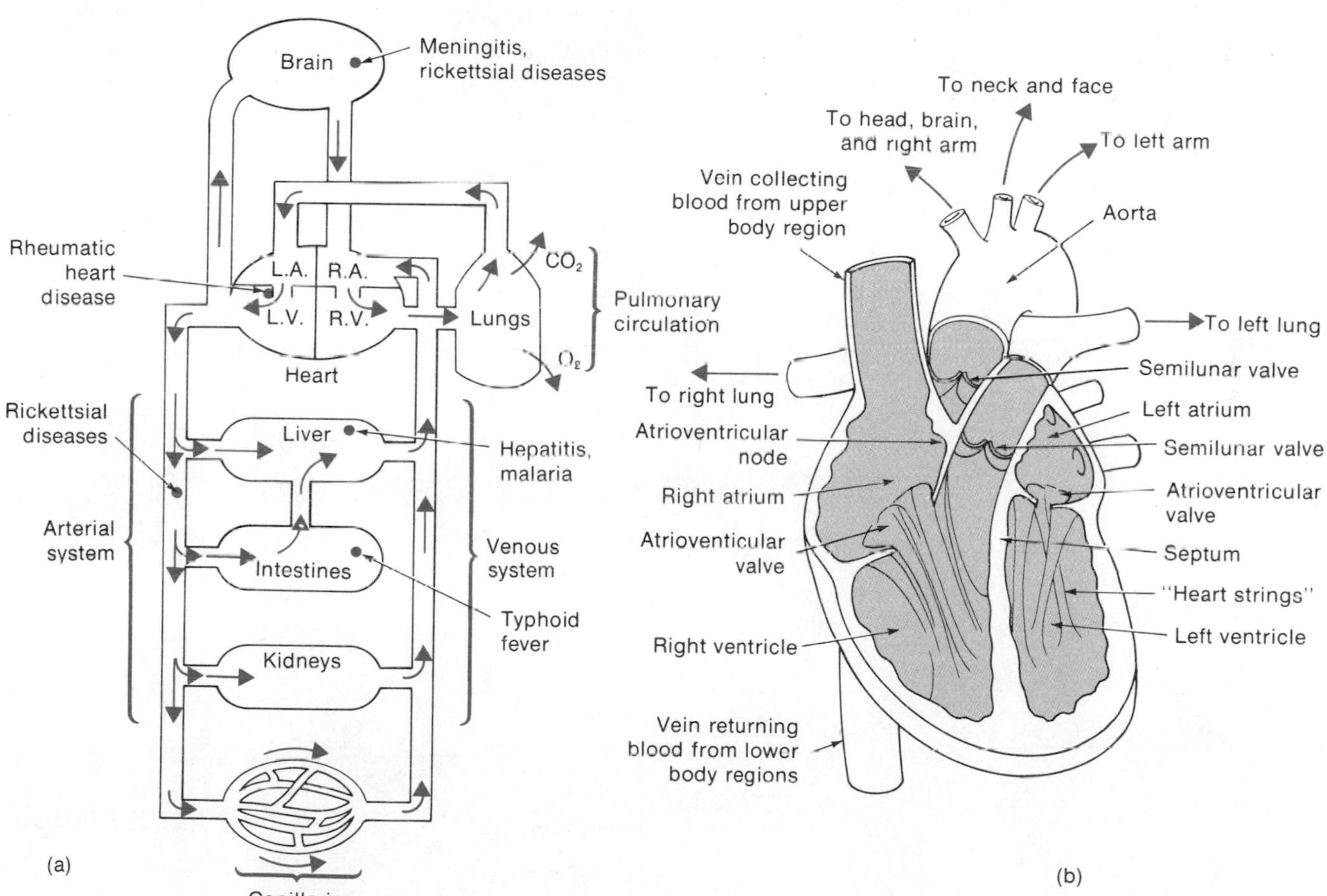

FIG. 33–1 (a) The structure and general direction of the human circulatory system. This closed system is really a double one consisting of the pulmonary system, which serves the lungs, and the systemic system, which serves the rest of the body. Specific organs with which microbial infections are associated are indicated. (b) An interior view of the heart, showing its various parts.

Components of the Circulatory System

The Heart

The heart (Figure 33–1b) is a cone-shaped, muscular organ about the size of a fist. It is situated between the lungs, directly behind the breastbone, or sternum, and is tilted so that the tip, or apex, is directed to the left. The heart is mainly striated muscle called *cardiac muscle* or *myocardium*. The individual muscle fibers making up the myocardium are branched and tightly joined to one another. The inner surface of the heart is lined with endothelial tissue called *endocardium*. The outside of the heart is covered with an epithelial tissue called *pericardium*. The pericardium also forms the *pericardial sac* within which the heart is located. Normally, this sac contains a small amount of fluid to lubricate the heart. Because the heart moves freely when it beats, it needs this sacular structure to separate it from the surrounding organs; otherwise, friction might produce lesions on the rubbing organs.

The human heart consists of four separate chambers (Figure 33–1b). The two upper chambers are the *atria* (singular, *atrium*), and the two lower chambers are the thick-walled, larger, highly muscular *ventricles*. Valves between the atria and ventricles and between the heart and attached vessels allow blood to flow in only one direction, preventing the backward flow of blood. The valves between the atria and the ventricles are the *atrioventricular valves*. The valve on the right side is called the *tricuspid valve* because it has three flaps; the valve on the left is the *bicuspid*, or *mitral*, valve because it has two flaps. *Semilunar valves* that resemble half moons prevent backward flow into the ventricles from their attached blood vessels.

Arteries, Veins, and Capillaries

Blood vessels are divided into three main categories: *arteries*, *veins*, and *capillaries*. Structural and functional characteristics distinguish these vessels. Of the three types, the arteries have the thickest, strongest walls, made up of three

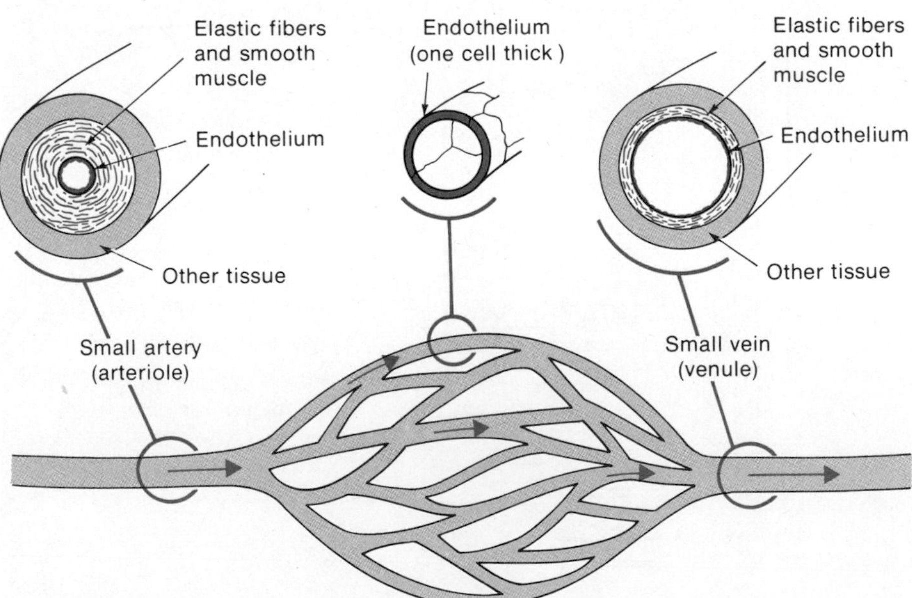

FIG. 33–2 A comparison of artery, vein, and capillary structure shows that arteries have thicker walls than other vessels, and capillaries are much smaller and have walls one cell thick. They are the most important part of a closed circulatory system because exchange of nutrient and waste molecules takes place across their walls.

layers (Figure 33–2). The inner layer, or endothelium, lines the vessels; the middle layer contains smooth muscles and elastic tissues; the outer layer, also elastic, is made of various supporting tissues.

The main function of the arteries is to conduct blood from the heart to the capillary network where the exchange of material between blood and tissue cells occurs (Figure 33–2). The veins collect blood from the capillaries and return it to the heart for a new cycle.

The heart and blood vessels form a closed system, so that blood is always contained within this series of vessels and never runs free. If the heart stops beating for only a few minutes, death can result. The amount of blood pumped with each beat is small. However, by beating about 70 to 75 times a minute, the heart pumps 10 to 12 pints of blood per minute, equal to the total amount of blood in an adult body.

Diseases of the Heart

In most developed countries of the world, heart disease is the leading cause of death. The activities of the heart can be impaired in at least three ways: (1) **endocarditis,** including infection and damage of the heart's valves and associated tissues; (2) insufficient nourishment for cardiac muscle, due to a narrowing of the arteries of the heart, sometimes associated with a blood clot (thrombus) within these vessels; and (3) over-exertion of the heart, resulting in exhaustion. Any one of these situations can cause enlargement of the heart, one of the most important signs of heart disease.

The heart can suffer from infection just as any other part of the body can. Of the various infections of the heart, rheumatic heart disease and subacute bacterial endocarditis are the most common.

Rheumatic Fever and Rheumatic Heart Disease

Many diseases, including those of the eye, skin, throat, gastrointestinal tract, bones, and joints are known also to affect the heart. Rheumatic fever is one such disease. It is a hypersensitivity state that develops in a small percentage of individuals following such streptococcal infections as sore throat. Because proteins of group A hemolytic streptococci are antigenically similar to the proteins in the heart and other tissues of susceptible persons, the antibodies formed attack not only the bacteria but also the host's heart tissues. While the resulting inflammation is usually mild, it may produce rheumatic fever and serious involvement of the heart. The consequences of one or more episodes of rheumatic fever cause the heart valves, particularly the mitral valve, to become inflamed. Abnormal growths of connective tissue (fibrosis) form on portions of the valves, scarring and deforming them. This condition is known as rheumatic heart disease. The valve damage is produced by narrowing of the valve opening *(stenosis)* or failure of the valve to close completely (valvular insufficiency). In short, the valves do not function properly. If the damaged valves cannot be repaired surgically, they may be replaced with an artificial valve (Figure 33–3). Fibrosis of the mitral valve, the valve most commonly involved, usually leads to left heart failure.

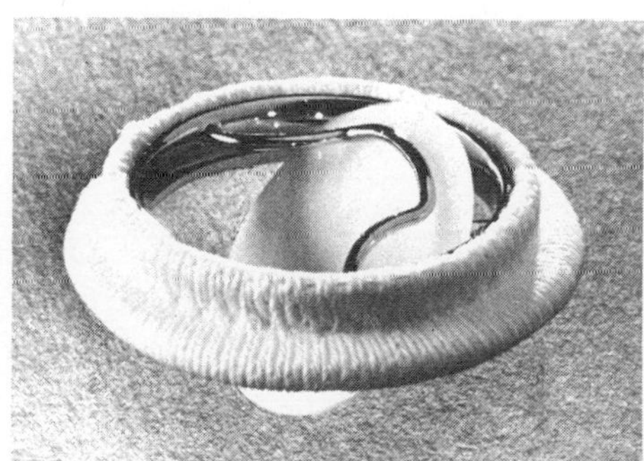

FIG. 33–3 An artificial replacement valve. The device is surgically inserted into the area of the damaged valve. Note the centrally located movable valve.

Prevention. To prevent rheumatic heart disease, sore throats and other disease states caused by group A hemolytic streptococci should be diagnosed (Table 31–1) and treated with antibiotics to minimize the development of antibodies to the streptococcal antigens.

The popular belief that rheumatic heart disease is restricted to young persons of low-income groups in cold, wet countries is incorrect. It is a disease of universal distribution, found among all climates, races, social strata, and ages.

Subacute Bacterial Vegetative Endocarditis (SBE)

Heart valves that have been scarred by rheumatic fever are readily implanted with bacteria, which can lodge in the irregular and roughened portions of these valves. These organisms produce an inflammatory condition of the heart known as endocarditis.

Less commonly, this condition may develop in valves altered by congenital malformations, infections other than rheumatic fever, and roughened irregular areas resulting from hardening of the arteries (arteriosclerosis).

Subacute endocarditis may be a very serious complication of any dental procedure that allows bacteria to enter the bloodstream of a person with heart valve damage. Bacteria often enter the blood ***(bacteremia)*** from extractions, endodontics, surgical procedures associated with gums, deep scaling (removing infected material from the tooth's surface), and currettage (removal of material by scraping). Any manipulation of infected or inflammatory vascular tissues within the gums, even by chewing, can open small capillaries or force microorganisms into the bloodstream. The greater the injury, the greater the incidence of bacteremia.

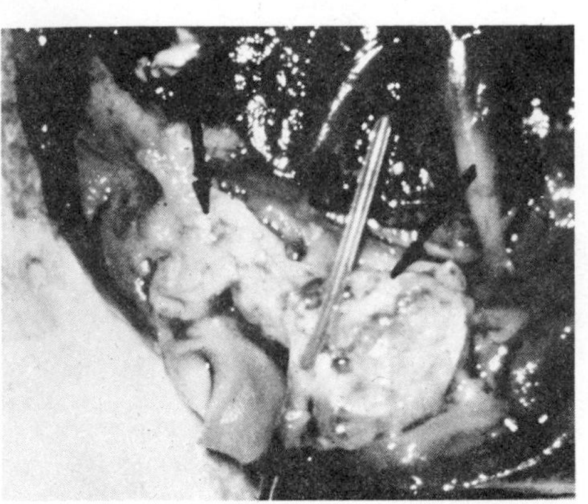

FIG. 33–4 The appearance of heart valve vegetation associated with endocarditis. *Santoro, J., and M. E. Levison,* Inf. Immun. *19:915–918 (1978).*

Individuals with subacute bacterial endocarditis experience prolonged fever, a changing heart murmur, and the growth of bulky, bacterial "vegetations" on the heart valves (Figure 33–4). These accumulations consist of tangled masses of fibrin strands, platelets, and blood cell fragments along with the bacterial masses. Infected individuals may also develop uncontrolled infections by antibiotic-resistant organisms, or organisms may be dislodged from damaged valves and travel to other organs, resulting in further destruction and even death.

Control and prevention. The successful control of bacterial endocarditis includes prevention of rheumatic heart disease and prompt diagnosis and treatment.

Other Microbial Diseases of the Circulatory System

Signs and Symptoms of Infections

The signs and symptoms of various infectious diseases involving the circulatory system are nonspecific. However, in some cases the features of the disease are highly specific and suggestive of an infection. Tables 33–1 and 33–2 list characteristics of certain microbial diseases with laboratory diagnosis and possible treatment also given in Table 33–1.

Bacterial Infections

PLAGUE

For centuries, *Yersinia pestis* has caused pandemics that have ravaged Asia and Europe. The Great Plague, which began in A.D. 542 (Figure 33–5) is believed to have been responsible for the deaths of over 100 million people in fifty years. The pandemic that reached its height of severity during the fourteenth century and became known as the Black Death has been considered the

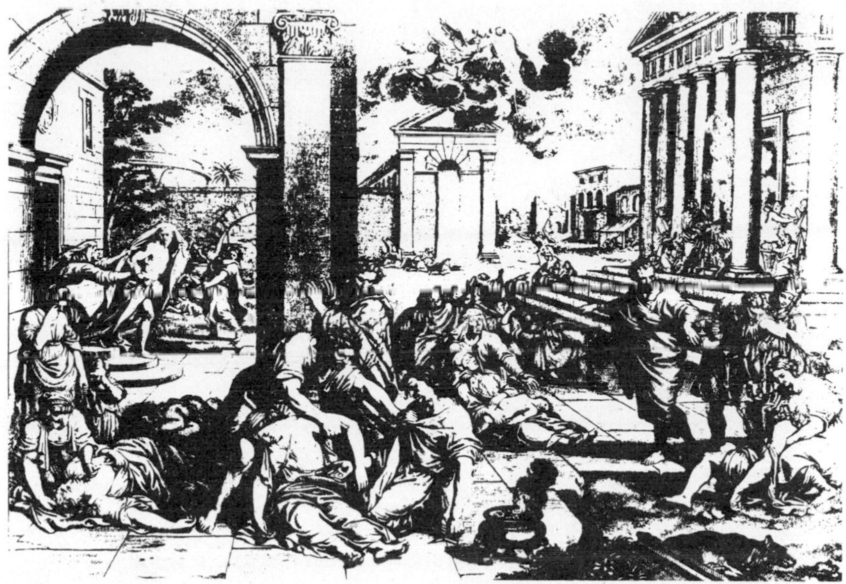

FIG. 33–5 This painting of "The Plague of Epirus" by Pierre Mignard depicts the havoc and destruction of human life caused by the bacterial disease that became known as the Black Death. Records of this first adequately described pandemic, which occurred in the sixth century A.D., indicate that plague killed more than 100 million people within a fifty-year period. *Courtesy National Library of Medicine.*

worst catastrophe to strike Europe, and perhaps the world. An estimated one third of the world's population died in it. Serious outbreaks of plague continued to appear in Europe and Asia from 1360 to 1400. The name Black Death was coined because of the severe cyanosis (blue or purple color of the skin) that developed in the terminal stages of the disease (Table 33–1). The last pandemic of the nineteenth century started in central Asia in 1871 and spread to other parts of the world. Epidemics continue to occur occasionally in many regions of Asia and Africa. There have also been reports of sporadic infections in South Africa, South America, and the southwestern United States. Plague was apparently spread to South Africa from South America in 1899.

Y. pestis (Figure 33–6a) was identified as the causative agent of plague in 1894 by Alexandre Yersin. In the same year, Shibasaburo Kitasato also reported finding the plague bacillus.

This bacterial infection is primarily a disease of rodents, both domestic and wild. However, several other mammalian species, including cats, deer, kangaroos, and monkeys can be infected. Recurrent outbreaks apparently occur among various species of wild rodents, such as pack rats, prairie dogs, rabbits, and squirrels. This form of the disease, known as *sylvatic plague*, poses a serious threat to human well-being, since such infected animals are a source of disease agents for future epidemics.

Transmission. The major direct sources for humans are house rats, *Rattus rattus* and *R. r. dairdi*, and the "ship's" rat, *R. r. alexandrinus*. *Y. pestis* is transmitted by the bite of rat fleas primarily belonging to the genera of *Nosopsyllus* and *Xenopsylla*. Infected fleas regurgitate microorganisms together with aspirated blood into the wound caused by their bites and may deposit feces. *Y. pestis* does not reproduce within the tissues of the insect vector.

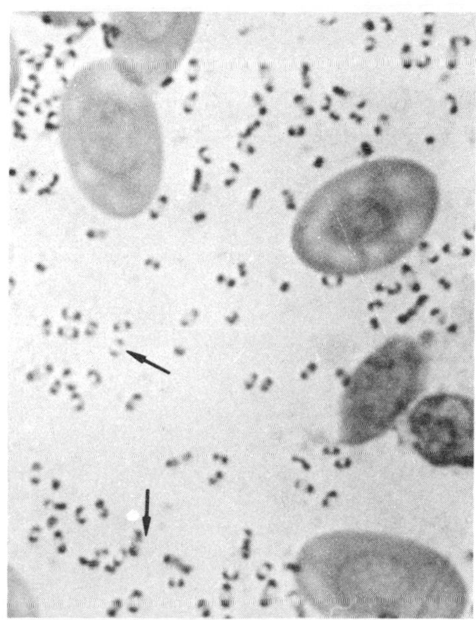

(a)

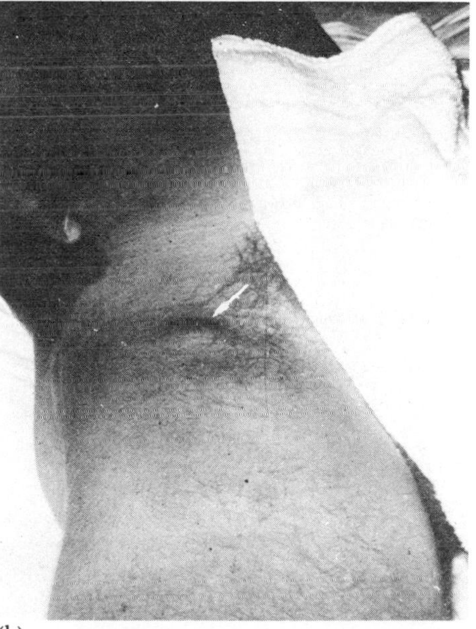

(b)

FIG. 33–6 (a) The bipolar, or "safety pin," appearance of *Yersinia* and *Pastuerella* species. *Courtesy of Drs. C. A. Manthei and K. L. Heddleston, USDA.* (b) The appearance of a plague bubo (arrow) on a victim's leg. *Courtesy of Mycology Section, Laboratory Division, Center for Disease Control, U.S. P.H.S.*

TABLE 33-1 Selected Bacterial Diseases Associated with the Circulatory System

Disease	Causative Agent	Gram Reaction	Morphology	Incubation Period	Signs and Symptoms	Laboratory Diagnosis	Possible Treatment
Plague	*Yersinia pestis*	—	Rod	2–6 days	*Bubonic plague:* formation of enlarged lymph nodes *(buboes)*, fever, chills, severe headache, and exhaustion; *Pneumonic plague:* contagious, coughing, chest pains, difficulty breathing, and bluish coloration of skin (cyanosis)	1. Isolation and culture 2. Gram stain of specimens 3. Animal inoculations 4. Fluorescent antibody technique	Chloramphenicol, streptomycin, sulfonamides, tetracyclines
Relapsing fever	*Borrelia recurrentis*	Not done	Spirochetes	3–10 days	Sudden appearance of fever, which lasts 4 days and ends suddenly, continued fever attacks (relapses) with each one milder than previous ones	1. Staining blood specimens 2. Animal inoculation	Chloramphenicol, tetracyclines
Rickettsialpox	*Rickettsia akari*	—	Rod	10–24 days	Formation of a small, red, hard blister at site of mite bite, followed by sudden appearance of backache, chills, fever (104° F), and rash	1. Tissue culture and chicken embryo isolation 2. Serodiagnostic tests such as Weil-Felix and complement fixation[a]	Chloramphenicol, tetracyclines
Rocky Mountain spotted fever	*R. rickettsi*	—	Rod	3–10 days	Backache, chills, fever, and rash, which develops on ankles, forehead, and wrists and spreads to trunk	Same as for other rickettsia in this table	Chloramphenicol, tetracyclines
Scrub typhus	*R. tsutsugamuchi*	—	Rod	10–20 days	A localized sore site of mite bite followed by backache, chills, fever (102–105° F), and rash; deafness and mental disturbances can be complications	Same as for other rickettsia in this table	Chloramphenicol, tetracyclines
Tularemia	*Francisella tularensis*	—	Rod	3–10 days	Fever, headache, general discomfort, and enlarged lymph nodes with pus formation	1. Isolation of causative agent and culture 2. Gram stain 3. Fluorescent antibody technique and other immunological tests	Kanamycin, streptomycin
Typhoid fever	*Salmonella typhi*	—	Rod	7–14 days	Abdominal swelling, constipation, loss of appetite, nausea, vomiting, fever (104° F), diarrhea with possible blood in stools, rash on abdomen (rose spots); complications include gall bladder infection	1. Isolation and culture 2. Biochemical tests 3. Serological testing, agglutination[a] 4. phage typing	Ampicillin, chloramphenicol, trimethoprimsulfamethoxazole
Typhus (endemic) fever	*R. mooseri*	—	Rod	6–15 days	Symptoms similar to other typhus fevers	Same as for other rickettsia in this table	Chloramphenicol, tetracyclines
Typhus (epidemic) fever	*R. prowazekii*	—	Rod	10–15 days	Symptoms similar to other typhus fevers; the rash begins on the trunk and spreads to the arms and legs	Same as for other rickettsia in this table	Chloramphenicol, tetracyclines

[a]Refer to Chapter 24 for descriptions of these procedures.

TABLE 33-2 Representative Human Rickettsioses

Group Category and Disease	*Causative Agent*	*Principal Vector or Means of Transmission*	*Geographical Distribution*	*Mammals Concerned in Normal Cycle*
Louse-borne Group				
Epidemic typhus	*R. prowazekii*	*Pediculus capitis*, *P. corporis*	World	Humans
Brill's disease	*R. prowazekii*	None	Europe, North America	Humans
Trench fever	*Rochalimaea quintana*	*P. corporis*	Africa, Europe, North America	Humans
——[a]	*R. canada*	*Haemaphysalis leporispalustris* (tick)	Eastern Canada	Humans
Flea-borne Group				
Endemic (murine) typhus	*R. mooseri (typhi)*	*Xenopsyllus cheopis* (rat flea)	World	Rodents
Tick-borne Group				
Boutonneuse fever	*R. conorii*	*Amblyomma variegatum*, *Rhipicephalus sanguineus*, others	Africa, Europe, India, Middle East	Dogs, wild rodents
Queensland tick	*R. australis*	*Ixodes holocyclus*	Australia	Marsupials, wild rodents
Rocky Mountain spotted fever	*R. rickettsii*	*Amblyomma* spp., *Dermocentor* spp., *Rhipicephalus sanguineus*	Western hemisphere	Dogs, wild rodents
Mite-borne Group				
Rickettsialpox	*R. akari*	*Allodermanyssus sanguineus*	Europe, North America	Wild rodents
Tsutsugamushi fever (scrub typhus)	*R. tsutsugamushi (R. orientalis)*	*Trombicula* spp.	Asia, Australia, Pacific Islands	Wild rodents
Q fever	*Coxiella burnetii (R. burnetii)*	Primarily droplet infection, although certain species of ticks have been implicated	World	Cattle, goats, sheep, wild rodents

NOTE: The specific rickettsial infections listed are arranged according to the arthropod vectors. This approach is commonly employed.
[a]The disease has not been named.

Forms of plague. Plague takes two main forms in human beings: ***bubonic plague*** and ***primary pneumonic plague***. In untreated cases the mortality rate for bubonic plague varies from 70 to 90 percent. For primary pneumonic plague, it is 100 percent. Death occurs quickly if treatment is not administered.

Bubonic plague is acquired through the bite of an infected flea. The injected microorganisms gain entrance to the regional lymph nodes, usually in the groin. These lymph nodes become enlarged and extremely tender, thus resulting in **bubo** formation (Figure 33–6b).

Prevention. Vaccines either of an attenuated or killed type have been used to produce an artificially acquired active immunity.

RELAPSING FEVER

Relapsing fever caused by the spirochetes of *Borrelia* (Figure 33–7a) are either louse- or tick-borne infections. Louse-borne disease is usually epidemic in nature, occurring in the crowded conditions that develop during times of war and natural disasters. *Pediculus humanus var. capitis* and *var. vestimenti* are the louse vectors involved. The tick-borne infections are endemic and are primarily limited to regions in which the vectors *Ornithodorus* spp. (Figure 33–7b) live. Human infections with tick-borne borreliae are few and largely confined to field workers, hunters, soldiers, and tourists. Repeated attacks of fever, referred to as relapses, give the disease its name (Table 33–1). Each of the successive episodes tends to be less severe than the previous ones, until they subside altogether.

No natural animal reservoir of *B. recurrentis* has been uncovered, although a variety of rodents have been implicated. A similar situation exists with *B. duttonii* (one of the tick-borne borreliae). A reservoir is created, however, when female ticks pass the borreliae to some of their eggs (transovarial passage).

Tick-borne fevers have been reported to be more intense, shorter in duration, and involve the central nervous system more often than the louse-borne variety. In addition, the relapse episodes are greater in number.

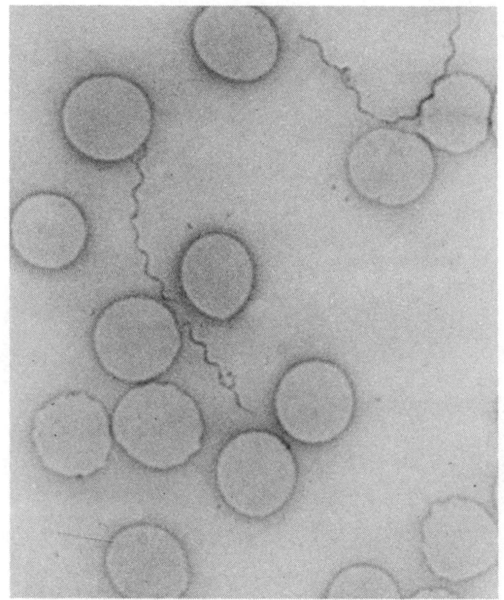
(a)

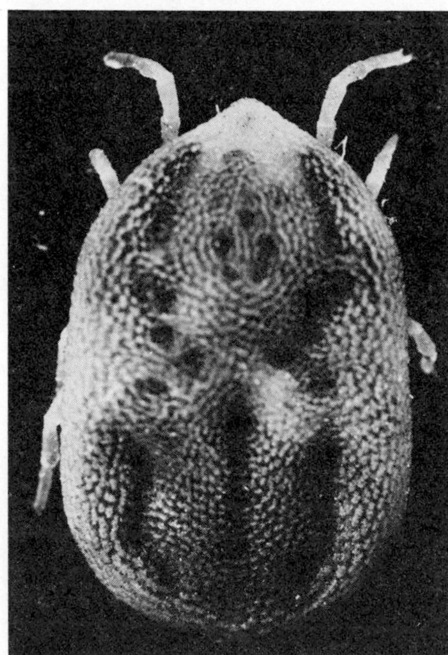
(b)

FIG. 33–7 (a) Stained blood smear preparation of *Borrelia recurrentis*. This organism ranges from 8 to 40 μm in length and from 0.2 to 0.5 μm in width. (b) *Ornithodorus* sp., a vector for tick-borne relapsing fever. *Courtesy of the Bureau of Vector Control, Berkeley, California.*

RICKETTSIAL INFECTIONS

The first discovery of rickettsia was largely a consequence of certain investigations by Howard Taylor Ricketts in 1909. While studying various aspects of the so-called Rocky Mountain spotted fever, he observed the presence of extremely small, distinct, rodlike formations in the blood of patients and certain associated ticks. This pathogen later was named *Rickettsia rickettsii*, in honor of its discoverer, who contracted and in 1910 died of typhus fever.

Subsequent work has identified more than 30 varieties of rickettsia that are pathogenic for humans or lower animals. This research has also provided techniques for the isolation and cultivation of rickettsia, as well as methods for their identification and control, including vaccines and insecticides against vectors.

Transmission. One distinctive feature of most rickettsia is that their transmission, under natural conditions, is dependent upon a variety of arthropods, such as fleas, lice, mites, and ticks (Table 33–2). An exception to this mode of spread is Q fever, which is primarily a droplet-transmitted infection. As the rickettsial agents multiply in the arthropod responsible for their transmission, the arthropods can be considered true natural vectors. Humans are the only vertebrate reservoirs for the rickettsia causing Brill's relapsing typhus (Brill's disease), epidemic typhus, and trench fever. In all other rickettsioses humans act as accidental hosts only (Table 33–2). Therefore, the rickettsial diseases, with the exceptions previously noted, are zoonoses.

General clinical features. Most rickettsial infections involve the circulatory system. Effects may extend to other tissues and organs as well (Table 33–1).

Epidemic typhus fever. The occurrence of *R. prowazekii* is traditionally linked to natural disasters, especially severe winters, famine, and war. In all of these situations, overcrowding makes maintenance of adequate personal hygiene difficult. The opportunities to bathe and wash clothes are limited. This provides an environment for body lice to flourish and for the transmission of typhus fever.

The transmission of epidemic typhus involves a human-to-louse-to-human cycle. The disease can develop in persons of any age. However, the effects of the infection are more severe in older individuals (Figure 33–8). Under normal conditions, the rickettsia are introduced into humans as a body or head louse obtains a blood meal. While the arthropod feeds, it defecates, releasing infective organisms. As the bite of the louse causes extreme itching, the natural tendency is to scratch the affected area, thereby inoculating oneself with the infectious feces. Although this is the way in which epidemic typhus is usually contracted, it is also possible to acquire an infection by inhaling dried, infected louse fecal matter, or by having it blow into the eye, across the conjunctiva.

Trench fever. The rickettsial disease trench fever, also known as His-Werner disease, Polish-Russian intermittent fever, and shank (or shin) fever, is also commonly associated with wartime conditions. Widespread during World Wars I and II, it has also been reported in Mexico and Tunisia. Transmission of the disease is similar to that of epidemic typhus.

Flea-borne (murine) tyhus fever. Flea-borne typhus fever is a rickettsiosis found mainly in tropical and subtropical regions and is caused by *R. typhi.* As this disease is common in rats, the infection can occur wherever these rodents and the tropic rat flea *Xenopsyllus cheopsis* exist. Localities such as granaries, storehouses, and waterfront areas are likely breeding sites.

The general transmission cycle of endemic typhus is from an infected rat to a flea to another rat. Humans acquire the infection accidentally; if a susceptible rat is not available, the infected rat flea uses the human as its new host. As in epidemic typhus, rickettsia are introduced by the contamination of an infected flea bite with feces containing the infectious agents.

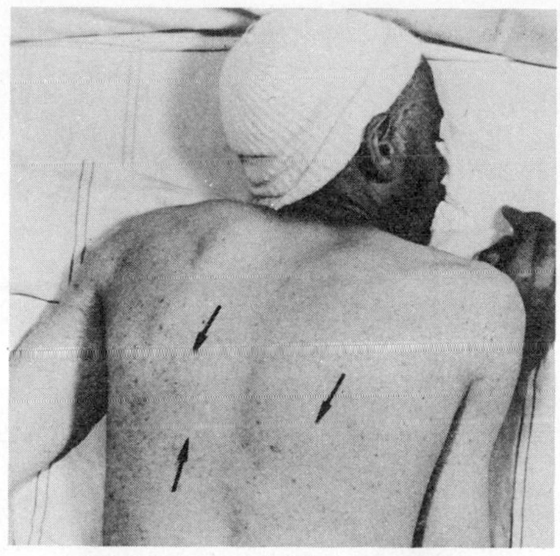

FIG. 33-8 Rash on the back of a victim of epidemic typhus. *Courtesy of the Armed Forces Institute of Pathology, Washington, D.C., Neg. No. 60-1011A.*

Rocky Mountain spotted fever. Rocky Mountain spotted fever, caused by *R. rickettsii,* was first recognized during the 1870s in Montana. Dogs, field mice, hares, rabbits, and squirrels all serve as reservoirs. Moreover, the tick vector itself serves as a reservoir, transmitting the rickettsia to future generations of ticks through transovarial passage. Representative tick vectors (Figure 33–9) and the geographic regions involved are identified in Table 33–2. Tick borne rickettsial species (such as *R. rickettsii*) that cause spotted fevers (Figure 33 10) characteristically multiply in both the cytoplasmic and nuclear regions of infected cells (Figure 33–9b). Other rickettsia pathogenic for humans reproduce only in the cytoplasm of cells.

Scrub typhus (tsutsugamushi fever.) Scrub typhus is an example of a **zoonosis** associated with rodents. The causative agent, *R. tsutsugamushi,* is also known as *R. orientalis.* Humans acquire the disease when bitten by infected mites, such as *Trombicula akamushi* and other *Trombicula* species (Figure 33–11).

Rickettsialpox. R. akari is the causative agent for rickettsialpox. The disease was first reported in 1946. Humans acquire the infectious agents through the bite of a common mouse mite, *Allodermanyssus sanguineus.* In the United States, the usual host for *A. sanguineus* is the common house mouse *Mus musculus.* Although *R. akari* is not transmitted by ticks, it is grouped with other rickettsia comprising the Rocky Mountain spotted fever category, because it has several properties in common with the group, including antigenicity and pattern of multiplication.

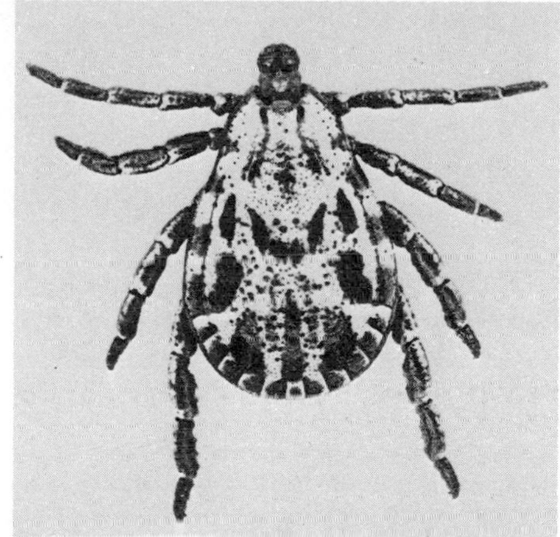

(a)

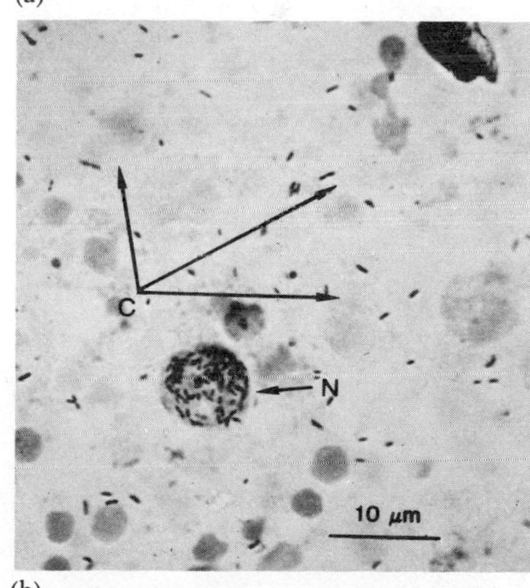

(b)

FIG. 33-9 (a) An adult male *Dermacentor andersoni,* the Rocky Mountain wood tick. (b) *R. Rickettsii.* Note the appearance of these rickettsia in both the cytoplasmic (C) and nuclear (N) regions of the cell. *Courtesy of the Rocky Mountain Laboratory, U.S. Public Health Service, Hamilton, Montana.*

TULAREMIA (DEER-FLY FEVER, RABBIT FEVER, AND OHARA'S DISEASE)

Tularemia, caused by *Francisella (Pasteurella) tularensis,* was first reported in ground squirrels from Tulare County, California (hence its name) in 1911. The first human case of the disease was reported in 1914.

Transmission. Human beings can acquire tularemia by handling the carcasses of infected animals (Figure 33–12) or by contact with water contaminated by them. They may also be infected by the bites of infected flies and ticks (Figure 33–12b), *Amblyomma* spp. and *Dermacentor* spp., or by inhalation of infectious

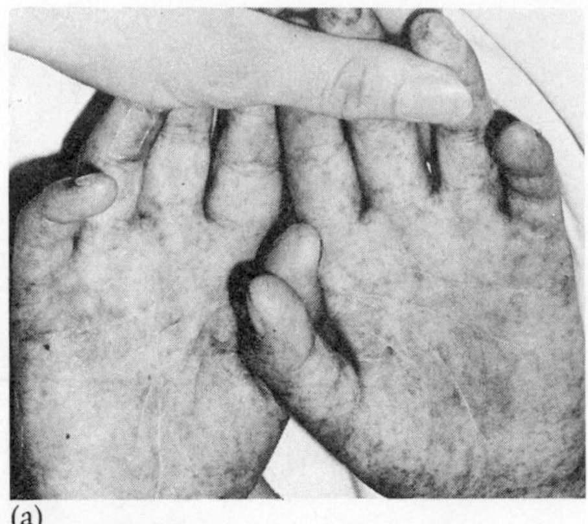

(a)

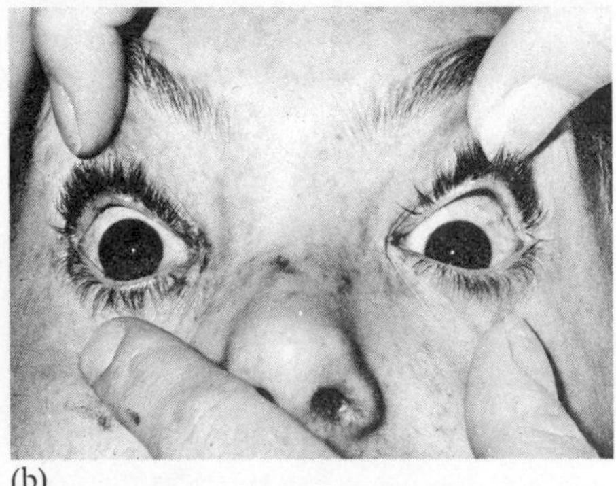

(b)

FIG. 33-10 Clinical features of Rocky Mountain spotted fever in children. A severe rash on a patient's hands. The skin on the fingertips of this child later became gangrenous. In general, the rash is most severe on the palms of the hands and soles of the feet. (b) Another feature of the disease is conjunctivitis, regularly noted in children. The photograph also shows the facial rash and hemorrhagic crusts in the nose. *From Haynes, et al.,* J. Pediatrics *76:685-693 (1970).*

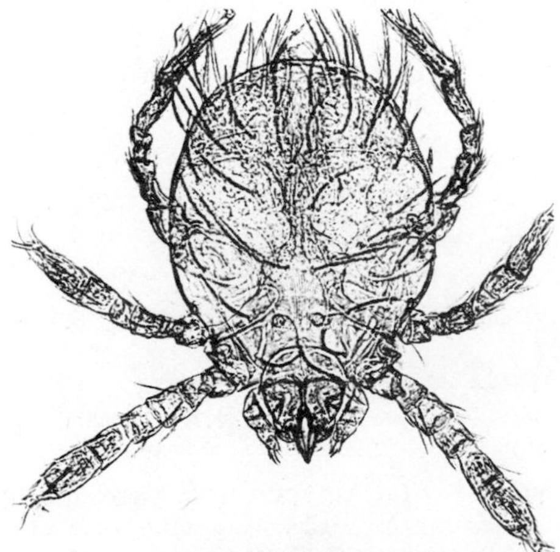

FIG. 33-11 *Trombicula akamushi*, the mite vector for tsutsugamushi fever. *Courtesy of the Rocky Mountain Laboratory, U.S. Public Health Service, Hamilton, Montana.*

aerosols. Infections also have resulted from the bites of animals that have fed on diseased rabbits.

Immunity. Recovery from tularemia usually produces a relatively permanent, naturally acquired active state of immunity. However, second episodes of infection have been reported. Relapses may occur even though high antibody titers are present in the infected individual. This situation is probably due to the fact that the organisms are normally inside the body cells, preventing access to them by antibodies.

TYPHOID FEVER

The various species of the genus *Salmonella* are associated with at least three clinically distinguishable disease states in humans: enteric fever, septicemias, and acute forms of infectious food poisoning. Septicemias of this kind usually do not involve the gastrointestinal tract but they do produce a high fever and bacteremia. *Salmonella cholerasuis* is a common causative agent. All of these conditions are collectively called *salmonellosis*. Typhoid fever is the classic example of the enteric fevers (Table 33–1).

Transmission. Ingestion of contaminated food or water causes the infection of humans. Flies and fomites have also been implicated as sources of the disease agent. In countries where adequate sanitation is maintained, typhoid fever appears either sporadically or in an endemic form. Quite often the source of infectious agents is traced to carriers, individuals who do not have symptoms of the disease but who harbor the causative agent. In regions with poor sanitation, no purification of water supplies, improper waste disposal, and lack of pasteurization, typhoid epidemics are more likely to occur. All ages may be attacked.

The causative agent, *S. typhi*, can gain access to various tissues and organs (such as the bone marrow, gall bladder, and spleen) via the bloodstream. These areas can serve as future sources of reinfection. Thus another complication of typhoid fever is the relapse that occurs when organisms gain access to the bloodstream from foci of infection.

Protozoan Infections

The destructive effects of protozoans depend on their number, size, degree of activity, location, and toxic products. Consequently, symptoms may be absent, few, or severe (Table 33–3).

KALA AZAR

The genus of flagellates that causes *kala azar* is named in honor of William Leishman, who discovered them in 1900. Morphologically, *Leishmania donovani* cannot be readily distinguished from other *Leishmania*. However, differentiation can be made on the basis of the effects of the disease state.

At present, closely related forms are described as either *dermotropic* or *viscerotropic* (Figure 33–13), according to the part of the body they invade (Table 33–3). The dermotropic species are said to belong to the *L. tropica* species-complex, and cause the classical skin form of leishmaniasis called the Oriental sore.

Transmission and life cycle. L. donovani is spread by the bite of various sandfly species of the genus *Phlebotomus.* The arthropod acquires the leishmanial form of the parasite by feeding on an infected host (human or other suitable mammal).

Prevention. Control measures include: (1) the use of insecticides to eliminate the arthropod vector, (2) treatment of infected individuals, and (3) the use of personal prophylactic devices such as insect repellents and sandfly nets. In addition, contaminated materials, such as dressings, clothing, and bedding, should be properly disinfected.

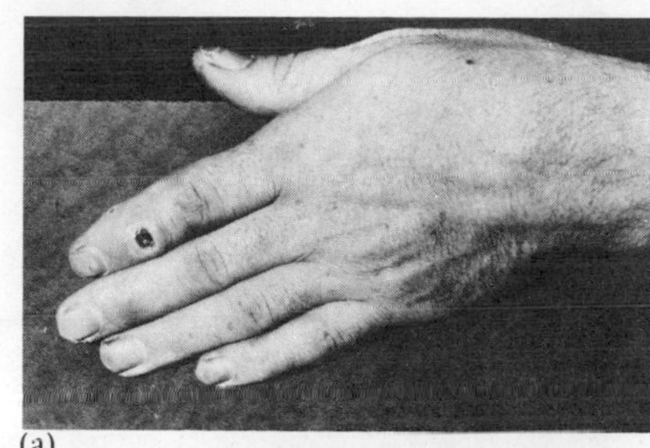

(a)

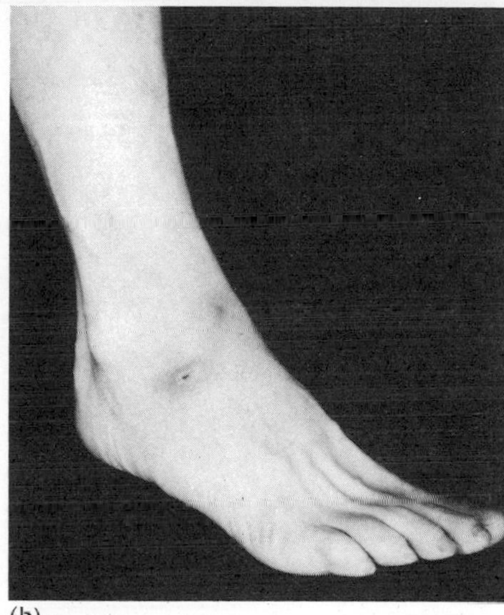

(b)

FIG. 33–12 Tularmia. (a) An infection resulting from the handling of an infected rabbit carcass. (b) Site of primary involvement, probably resulting from an infected arthropod bite. *Courtesy of the Armed Forces Institute of Pathology, Washington, D.C., Neg. Nos. 85387-2 and AN 1147-1A.*

MALARIA

Nearly a century has passed since the discovery of the first malarial parasite. Considered to be among the greatest killers of the human race, malaria has been known from antiquity. Accounts of the disease's observable effects date back to at least 1500 B.C. While in Egypt, Hippocrates utilized the earlier records of malaria and noted the existence of differentiating fever cycles and other clinical features. With this information, he was able to divide the disease into quotidian, benign tertian, and quartan fevers. These designations denoted 24-, 48-, and 72-hour fever cycles, respectively. It is now known that they (and some other tertian fevers) are caused by infections with different species of the malarial parasite of the genus *Plasmodium*. Human malaria may involve any area where *Anopheles* mosquitoes capable of supporting the parasite breed and are present in significant numbers, where reservoirs of the malarial parasite are available, and where control measures directed against mosquitoes are not adequate.

Four species of *Plasmodium* are known human pathogens: *P. falciparum, P. malariae, P. ovale,* and *P. vivax*. Their respective distributions are shown in Table 33–3.

Life Cycle. A typical life cycle of malaria (Figure 33–14) begins with the sexual phase, **sporogony,** developing within the invertebrate host (anopheline mosquito).

Infective units **(sporozoites)** enter the human bloodstream through the bite of a parasite-harboring female mosquito and readily pass from the peripheral circulation into the parenchymal cells of the liver. There the parasites grow and undergo repeated divisions, eventually releasing *merozoites,* forms capable of invading red blood cells and thereby beginning the *erythrocytic* portion of the asexual cycle. Variations in this general cycle occur, depending upon the *Plasmodium* species.

Schizogony (asexual development in red cells) begins with invasion of the red blood cells by merozoites. One such parasite assumes the shape of a signet ring in its new environment, grows, and develops into an ameoboid, single-nucleus feeding form, known as a *trophozoite.* (See Color Photographs 85A, 85B, and 85C for representation of these blood stages.) When the parasite attains its full size, mitotic division accompanied by cytoplasmic segmentation occurs. Ultimately a solid body composed of a varying number of merozoites forms. This structure is referred to as a *mature schizont.* The parasite-supporting red cell ruptures, releasing the merozoites, the toxic metabolic products of the parasite, and the remains of the host cell into the general circulation. This group of substances is responsible for the chills and fever characteristic of the malarial syndrome (Table 33–3).

Certain merozoites, instead of continuing the asexual cycle, invade red cells and develop into female and male *gametocytes.* These forms circulate in the peripheral bloodstream, becoming available for ingestion by an anopheline mosquito. Under normal conditions, a large number of parasites are present when mosquitoes take their blood meals. In the mosquito, they undergo transformation into mature sex cells and participate in the sexual cycle, or sporogony. Fertilization of a mature female cell *(macrogamete)* by a male cell *(microgamete)* forms a *zygote.* This becomes an *oökinete,* which is elongated and capable of movement. The oökinete penetrates the mosquito's stomach wall, rounds out, and develops into a stationary form known as a *oöcyst.* A series of divisions within this structure produces many slender, threadlike,

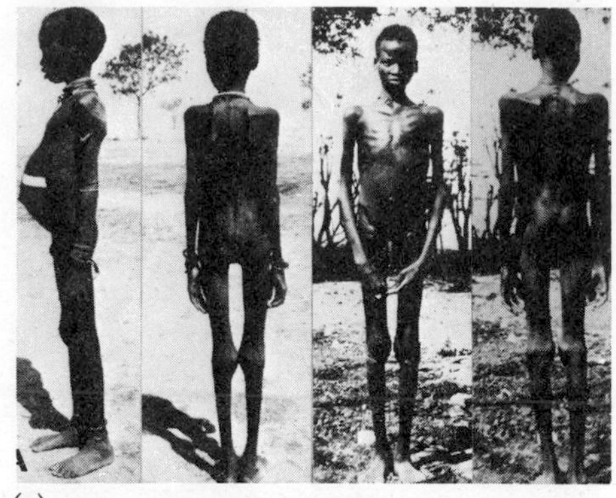

(a)

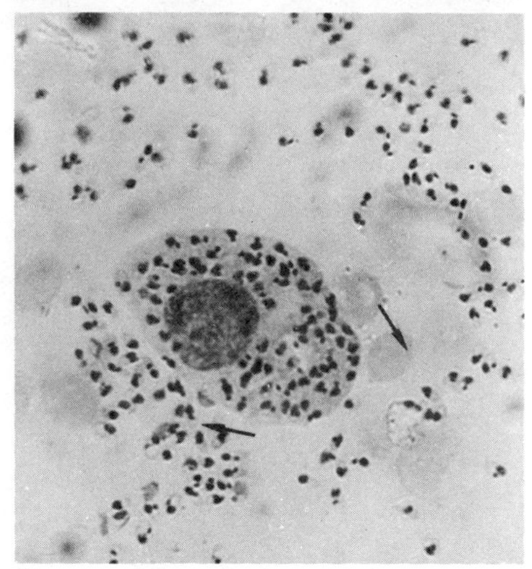

(b)

FIG. 33-13 (a) Two victims of kala azar. *From Hoogstraal, H., and D. Heyneman,* Amer. J. Trop. Med. & Hyg. *18:1091 (1969).* (b) *Leishmania donovani* in blood. *Courtesy of the Armed Forces Institute of Pathology, Washington, D.C., Neg. No. AFIP 55-17580-3.*

potentially infective sporozoites. Rupture of the oöcyst releases the sporozoites, which migrate throughout the mosquito's body. Those infective units entering the salivary glands of the arthropod can be introduced into another human when the mosquito obtains a blood meal. The malarial asexual cycle can then begin again.

Treatment. Several drugs are effective against malaria (Table 33-3). The choice of medication is determined by the particular situation, whether it is for termination of an acute primary attack, suppressive or prophylactic therapy, or treatment of relapsing malaria. Intelligent therapy also depends upon an accurate diagnosis and thorough knowledge of the effects of antimalarial drugs.

Prevention. Control of malaria involves measures directed against the vector of the disease and against the spread of disease by the definitive host, human beings. Eradication of the mosquito vector requires the destruction and elimination of breeding areas as well as larval and adult stages of the vector. Control measures in the case of humans include the use of suppressive and prophylactic medications in endemic areas, prompt and adequate treatment of overt clinical attacks, and avoidance of mosquito bites.

During late 1970 and early 1971, several cases of malaria in California were traced to heroin addicts who had had contact with one of the major sources of the malarial parasite, a Vietnam veteran. Since addicts frequently share unsterilized syringes and needles, the disease was easily transmitted. Suitable vectors are known to exist in California, but fortunately, mosquitoes were not plentiful during these outbreaks of the disease. Had these cases appeared in the summer months, statewide epidemics might have developed.

Infectious Mononucleosis

Infectious mononucleosis (IM) is an acute leukemialike infection caused by the Epstein-Barr virus (EBV). This virus was originally detected in cell cultures obtained from a cancerous state of children called Burkitt's lymphoma. Infectious mononucleosis has been found primarily in young adults, especially college students. It has often been called the "student's disease." The disease involves components of the reticuloendothelial system (RES), including the lymph nodes and spleen. An increase in lymphocytes is also associated with the illness. These cells are abnormal and can be classified on the basis of certain cytoplasmic and nuclear features. Such atypical lymphocytes are called Downey cells, and at least three classes are recognized. In general, the leukocyte levels are related to the course of the disease. Epstein-Barr virus infects B-type lymphocytes, while T-type lymphocytes together with antibodies produced in response to the virus kill the infected cells.

Transmission. Infectious mononucleosis is transmitted chiefly by kissing (direct oral means) or by drinking from a shared bottle or glass (indirect oral means) with the exchange of saliva and perhaps leukocytes. Experimental attempts to transmit the infection to animals and humans using various specimens, e.g. blood, gargle washings, and lymph nodes, have been unsuccessful.

Victims of the disease may experience symptoms such as mild jaundice, slight fever, enlarged and tender lymph nodes, sore throat, headache, and general weakness. Some individuals may have abdominal pains, bleeding gums, and a slight cough. Usually, once a person has had infectious mononucleosis an immunity is established. Definite recurrences are rare.

TABLE 33-3 Protozoan Diseases Associated with the Circulatory System

Disease	Causative Agent	Geographical Distribution	Incubation Period	General Features of the Disease	Laboratory Diagnosis	Possible Treatment
Kala azar (dum-dum fever)	*Leishmania donovani*	Central and South America	From 10 days to several months	Fever, bleeding from gums, lips, and nose; enlarged liver and spleen; pneumonia can be a complication	1. Microscopic demonstration of causative agent in blood, bone marrow, and spleen specimens 2. Serological tests, e.g. complement fixation, fluorescent antibody test[a]	Sodium antimony gluconate, ethylstibamine, amphotercin B
Malignant tertian malaria	*Plasmodium falciparum*	Tropical and subtropical areas	12–30 days (depends on species)	Headache, nausea, abdominal pain, vomiting, chills,[b] prolonged fever stage, little sweating, convulsions, and coma; enlarged liver and spleen, heart failure, and bloody urine are complications	Demonstration of parasites in blood smears (Color Photograph 85)	Amodiacquine hydrochloride (acute infection), quinine dihydrochloride
Quartan malaria	*P. malariae*	Tropical and subtropical areas, including Africa and Ceylon	12–37 days (depends on species)	A relatively mild form of the disease with some chills, fever, headache, nausea, and abdominal pain	Demonstration of parasites in blood smear	Chloroquine phosphate (acute infection), quinine dihydrochloride
Tertian (ovale) malaria	*P. ovale* (rare)	East and west Africa, South America, United States	12–30 days (depends on species)	Periods of shaking chills, fever, headache, nausea, muscular pain, and vomiting	Demonstration of parasites in blood smears	Chloroquine phosphate (acute infection), quinine dihydrochloride
Tertian (vivax or benign) malaria	*P. vivax*	Reported to be established in central and western Africa and Philippines; also occurs sporadically in China, Greece, and Iran	12–30 days (depends on species)	Periods of shaking chills (cold stage), followed by fever (104–106° F or 40–41° C) with profuse sweating, nausea, vomiting, headache, and muscular pains	Demonstration of parasites in blood smear	Chloroquine phosphate (acute infection), quinine dihydrochloride

[a]Refer to Chapter 24 for a description of these procedures.
[b]The chill stage here is usually milder than that of other malarial infections.

Diagnosis and treatment. In addition to the symptoms of this disease, certain laboratory findings are used for diagnostic purposes. These include the presence of atypical, large T-lymphocytes and a characteristic positive test for heterophile antibodies—those which agglutinate red blood cells in sheep. Liver function tests may also be performed. Infectious mononucleosis is rarely fatal. Treatment procedures usually include bed rest and the hospitalization of individuals with severe complications, such as convulsions and rupture of the spleen.

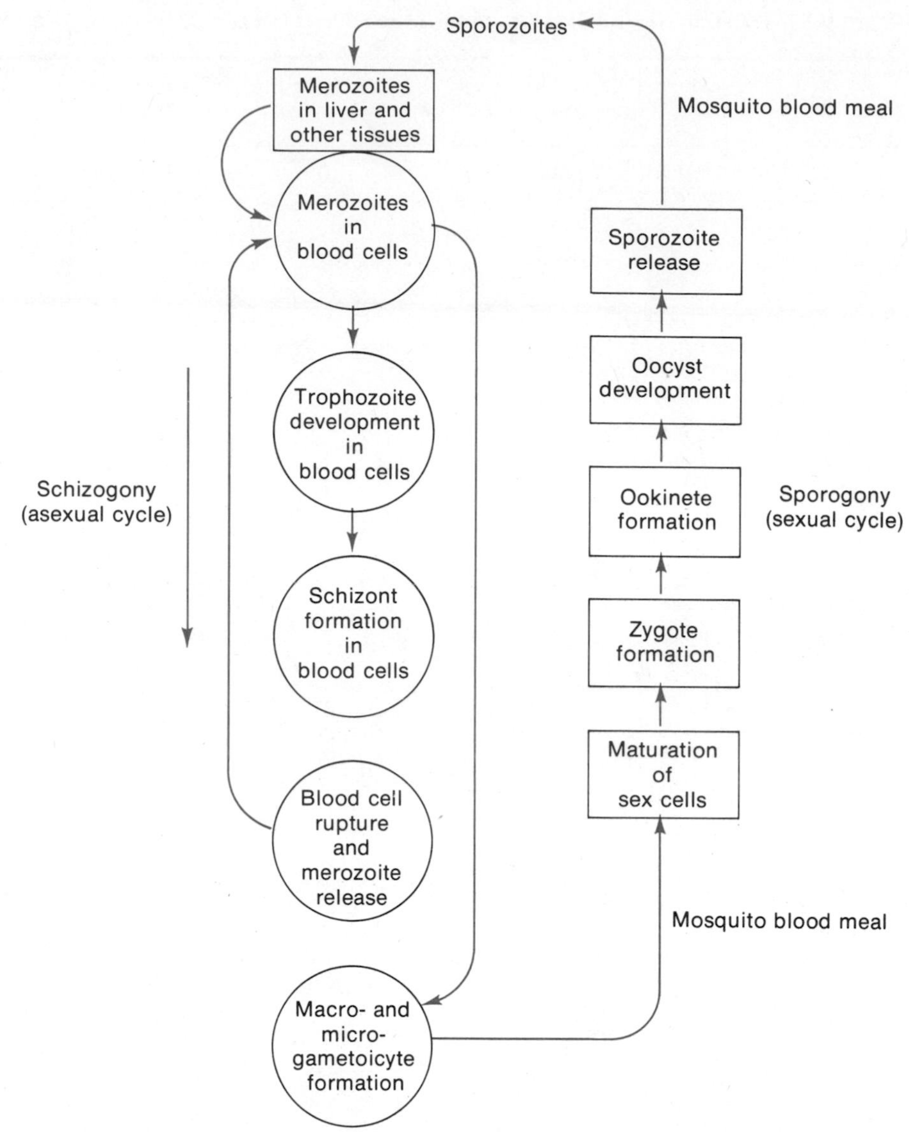

FIG. 33-14 The life cycle of the malaria parasite. Refer to Figure 10-20 and Color Photograph 85 for additional details and views of the protozoans involved.

SUMMARY

1. The circulatory system, in addition to being susceptible to microbial diseases, can serve to spread disease agents and their products to other regions of the body.
2. The circulatory system meets several needs of vertebrates including internal transport of nutrients and hormones, removal of cellular wastes, regulation of body temperature, and control and elimination of foreign organisms.
3. Blood flows through a closed system that consists of the vessels—arteries, veins, and capillaries—and the heart.

Components of the Circulatory System

1. The heart is a highly muscular organ lined with endothelial tissue called *endocardium*. The outside is covered with epithelial tissue called *pericardium*.
2. Internally the heart consists of four chambers: the two upper chambers are called the *atria*, the two lower ones, the *ventricles*.
3. Arteries, the vessels with the thickest walls, conduct blood from the heart to the capillary network, where the actual exchange between blood and tissue cells occurs. The veins collect blood from the capillaries and return it to the heart for a new cycle.

Diseases of the Heart

1. Activities of the heart can be affected by endocarditis (which includes infection of its tissues), by insufficient

nourishment for heart muscle, and by over-exertion of the heart, resulting in exhaustion.

2. The heart can be subjected to infections, just as any other part of the body can.
3. Two infections of the heart are rheumatic heart disease and subacute bacterial endocarditis (SBE).
4. Rheumatic heart disease is a hypersensitivity state that develops in a small percentage of individuals having a history of streptococcal infections.
5. Subacute endocarditis results from inflammation of the endocardium by bacteria lodged in irregular or damaged heart valves. Subacute endocarditis may be a complication of any dental procedure that allows bacteria to enter the bloodstream of a person with damaged heart valves. Accumulation of formless masses of fibrin strands, blood cell fragments and bacterial masses called *vegetations* develop in damaged valves.

Other Microbial Diseases of the Circulatory System

Bacterial Infections

1. Several bacterial infections involve the circulatory system, including plague, relapsing fever, tularemia, and rickettsial diseases such as rickettsialpox, Rocky Mountain spotted fever, scrub typhus, and endemic and epidemic typhus fevers.
2. Many bacterial infections of this system are transmitted by arthropods such as fleas, lice, mites, or ticks.
3. Preventive measures include immunizations (if available) and elimination of the arthropod vectors.

Protozoan Infections

1. As with other microbial disease agents, the destructive effects of pathogenic protozoans depend on their number, size, degree of activity, location, and toxic products.
2. Examples of protozoan diseases involving the circulatory system include kala azar (spread by sandflies) and malaria (spread by anophelene mosquitoes).
3. Preventive measures are usually directed toward the elimination of the arthropod vector.

Infectious Mononucleosis

1. Infectious mononucleosis (IM) is an acute leukemialike infection caused by the Epstein Barr virus (EBV). The virus was originally detected in cell cultures from children with the cancerous condition called Burkitt's lymphoma.
2. EBV involves the lymph nodes and the spleen and attacks B-type lymphocytes. T-type lymphocytes together with specific antibodies produced in response to the virus kill infected cells.
3. Transmission of the disease agent can occur through kissing or using a contaminated glass or other object that comes into contact with the mouth.

QUESTIONS FOR REVIEW

1. What are the functions and activities of the human circulatory system?
2. Why is the circulatory system regarded as being "closed"?
3. a. How do arteries, veins, and capillaries differ?
   b. How are these blood vessels similar?
4. How do infectious disease agents affect the various components of the circulatory system?
5. Give the general means of transmission for each of the following diseases:
   a. typhoid fever
   b. malaria
   c. plague
   d. typhus fever
   e. tularemia
   f. rheumatic heart disease
6. Distinguish betwen bubonic and pneumonic plague.
7. What is subacute bacterial endocarditis?
8. If you were assigned to speak to a group of representatives from developing countries on the transmission and control of arthropod-transmitted diseases, which diseases would you select? What major means of control would you recommend to this group?
9. What components and mechanisms of the circulatory system contribute to the elimination of disease agents? (Refer to Chapter 22 for assistance in answering this question.)
10. Of what particular importance is infectious mononucleosis to college students?

SUGGESTED READINGS

Aikawa, J. E., *Rocky Mountain Spotted Fever.* Springfield, Ill.: Charles C. Thomas, 1966. *An excellent short reference on Rocky Mountain spotted fever, including its history and discovery, clinical picture, control of the disease, and diagnostic and immunologic studies.*

Bartlett, R. C., P. D. Ellner, and J. A. Washington, II, *Blood Cultures.* Cumitech I, American Society for Microbiology, Washington, D.C., 1974. *A short publication describing general procedures for the isolation of bacterial pathogens from blood (blood cultures).*

Brown, H. W., *Basic Clinical Parasitology,* 4th ed. New York: Appleton-Century-Crofts, 1975. *A good general text, containing an extensive chapter on parasitic diseases involving the blood, such as trypanosomiasis, leishmaniasis, and malaria.*

Davis, E., *Rheumatic Fever.* Springfield, Ill.: Charles C. Thomas, 1969. *A basic discussion of rheumatic fever, including aspects of infection, the rheumatic population, family histories, and features of hemolytic streptococci.*

Gregg, C. T., *Plague! The Shocking Story of a Dread Disease in America Today.* New York: Charles Scribner's Sons, 1978. *In addition to covering the properties of* Yersinia pestis, *the causative agent of plague, this book discusses in detail such topics as the biology of rats and other rodents, historical accounts of epidemics, control methods, and several unanswered questions about plague.*

Jelijaszewicz, J. (ed.), *Staphylococci and Staphylococcal Disease.* New York: Gustav Fischer, 1976. *A collection of specialized articles dealing with an extensive number of staphylococcal infections and their associated treatment.*

Krug, S., and D. J. Gocke, *Viral Hepatitis. Major Problems in Internal Medicine.* Philadelphia: W. B. Saunders Co., 1978. *A short but highly informative text dealing with the cause, transmission, diagnosis, and consequences of viral hepatitis. New developments in electron microscopy and biochemical approaches to the characterization of hepatitis A virus are also described.*

CHAPTER **34**

Microbial Diseases of the Reproductive and Urinary System

Urinary tract infections represent a major source of human discomfort. The most common diseases of this system are bacterial. Most of these infections remain limited to the urinary tract, but some can develop into extensive disease processes involving other organs and sometimes leading to death. Venereal diseases are also common in humans. Left untreated and unchecked, these conditions pose serious threats to human well-being. Chapter 34 considers various genitourinary tract infections.

After reading this chapter, you should be able to:

1. **Describe the general organization of the human urinary system and indicate the areas attacked by microbial pathogens.**
2. **Describe the microbial flora of the human urinary tract.**
3. **Discuss predisposing factors and routes of transmission associated with urinary tract infections.**
4. **List and describe three infections of the urinary system, including their causative agents, means of transmission, and control measures.**
5. **Explain the importance of anaerobes to urinary tract infections.**
6. **Distinguish among the seven most common human venereal diseases as to causative agents, areas of the reproductive system attacked, general effects, and measures for treatment and control.**

7. **Discuss the significance of venereal infection in pregnancy.**
8. **Compare the general approaches to diagnosis of urinary tract and reproductive system infections.**
9. **Explain the complications associated with diseases of the urinary tract and reproductive system.**

The many functions of the urinary system include eliminating waste products, regulating the chemical composition and acid-base balance of the body tissues, and keeping the water content of the body constant. In general, the system is constructed and organized to prevent invasion by microorganism. However, certain circumstances, such as obstruction of the flow of urine or the use of various medical devices, can promote infection. Many of the microbial agents are opportunists that are actually members of the body's normal flora.

The organs of the reproductive system are also subject to infection by a variety of agents. Of these, the **venereal diseases,** so termed because they are usually transmitted through sexual activities, are of particular importance. This is because of the discomfort and disability (including blindness, disfigurement, and sterility) that they can cause.

Anatomy of the Urinary System

The human urinary system includes two *kidneys,* two *ureters,* the *urethra,* and the *urinary bladder* (Figure 34–1). The bean-shaped kidneys are compound tubular glands that secrete urine. This excretory product goes by way of two muscular tubes, the ureters, to the bladder, which stores the product until its elimination. Urine is discharged by way of the urethra to the outside. The female urethra functions only in urination; the male counterpart serves for the passage of both urine and semen.

A kidney consists of an outer cortex and inner medulla (Figure 34–1). The basic functional unit of the kidney is the *nephron,* which is composed of a *glomerulus* (blood filter) and a long tubule (concentrator and urine collector). The glomerulus, a tuft or collection of capillaries, is surrounded by a spherically expanded portion of the nephron, the *Bowman's capsule* (Figure 34–2). Blood is filtered through the glomeruli and concentrated by the tubules, which empty into the ureters (Figure 34–2). The renal capsule filters dissolved substances and some water out of the blood plasma; the renal tubule reabsorbs water, electrolytes, and other substances to help maintain the body's normal internal environment. The kidneys establish and help to maintain the concentration of electrolytes (for example, chloride, potassium, sodium, and bicarbonate) in the human body and excrete poisonous substances.

Several of the components of the urinary system are subject to infection.

The Flora of the Normal Urinary Tract

Experiments with various animals have shown that the normally sterile kidney is highly resistant to bacteria. Many well-known urinary tract pathogens are unable to invade the kidney and produce infection there. There are a few exceptions to this finding, including certain enterococci strains, *Escherichia coli, Proteus* spp., and staphylococci.

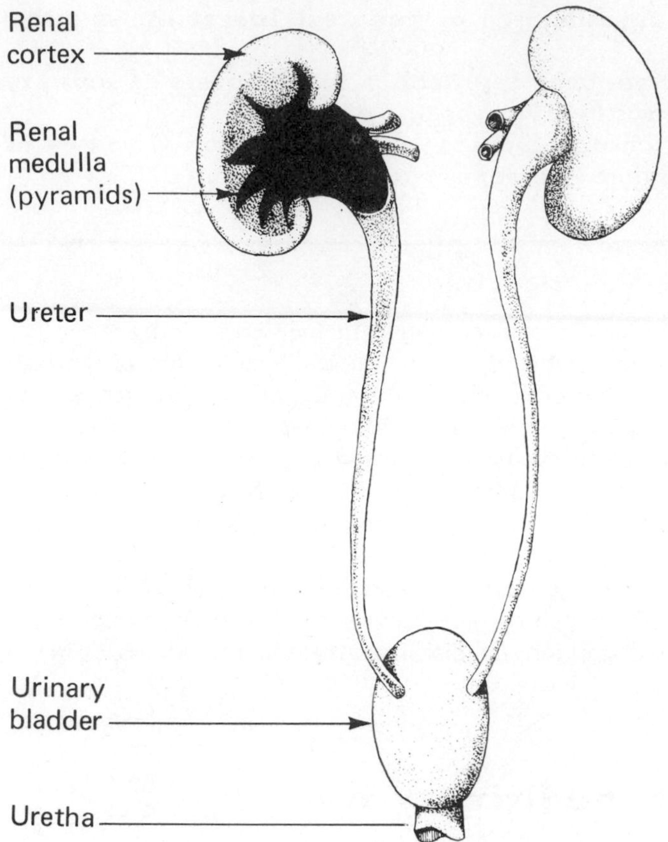

FIG. 34-1 The human urinary system. Specific pathogens and their associated sites of infection are also indicated.

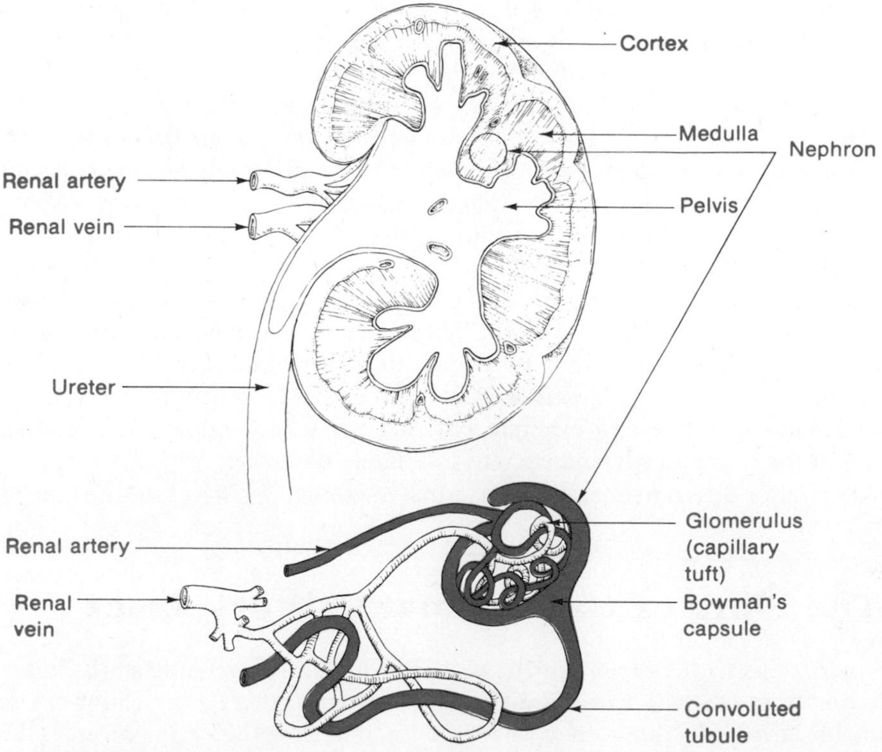

FIG. 34-2 A human kidney and a renal nephron. The pathway of urine formation is also shown in the enlarged view of the nephron.

In humans, bacteria are commonly present in the lower urethra. However, their numbers decrease in regions near the bladder. This is apparently caused by some antibacterial effect exerted by the urethral lining and the frequent flushing of the epithelial surface of the urethra by urine, which is normally sterile. Urinary tract infections are more frequent in females than in males. This may be because the male urethra is longer and, by virture of its location, less likely to be subject to fecal contamination.

Diseases of the Urinary Tract

An Introduction to Urinary Tract Infections

Common urinary infections are summarized in Table 34-1. The bacteria commonly associated with urinary tract infections are intestinal flora called **coliforms.** Coliforms have been isolated from 80 percent of the cases that have developed in the absence of urinary obstructions or that have been unaffected by antibiotic therapy or urologic manipulations such as *catheterization* (the insertion of a surgical tubular device into organs or body cavities).

TABLE 34-1 Representative Diseases of the Urinary System

Disease	Causative Agent	Gram Reaction	Morphology	Possible Treatment
Cystitis (inflammation of the urinary bladder)	*Escherichia coli, Proteus vulgaris, Pseudomonas aeruginosa*	−	Rods	Sulfonamides, chloramphenicol, kanamycin, oral penicillin G, polymyxin
Glomerulonephritis (inflammation of kidney glomeruli)	*Streptococcus pyogenes*	+	Coccus	Chloramphenicol, erythromycin, lincomycin, penicillin, vancomycin
Kidney cortex infections	*Staphylococcus aureus*	+	Coccus	Cephalothin, lincomycin, methicillin, nafcillin, vancomycin
Nonspecific urethritis (inflammation of the urethra)	*Candida albicans*	+	Oval yeast	Amphotericin B
	Mycoplasma hominis and T-strains	−	Pleomorphic	Erythromycin, tetracyclines
	Staphylococci and streptococci	+	Cocci	
	Trichomonas (vaginalis) hominis	Not useful	Protozoan	Cephalothin, lincomycin, methicillin, penicillin, vancomycin
Prostatitis (inflammation of the prostate gland)	*E. coli, P. aeruginosa*	−	Rods	Sulfonamides, gentamicin, oral penicillin G, polymyxin
	Neisseria gonorrhoeae	−	Coccus	Penicillin, erythromycin, tetracyclines
	Staphylococci and streptococci	+	Cocci	Cephalothin, lincomycin, methicillin, penicillin, vancomycin
	Mixed infections of the above organs			Appropriate antibiotics
Puerperal sepsis (child-bed fever)	Anaerobic streptococci	+	Cocci	Chloramphenicol, erythromycin, penicillin, vancomycin
	Clostridia	+	Rods	Chloramphenicol, penicillin, tetracyclines
	E. coli, Proteus spp.	−	Rods	Sulfonamides, chloramphenicol, gentamicin, kanamycin
	Neisseria gonorrhoeae	−	Coccus	Erythromycin, penicillin, tetracyclines
Pyelonephritis (inflammation of the kidney and pelvis)	*Bacteroides* spp., *Enterobacter aerogenes, E. coli, Proteus* spp., *Pseudomonas aeruginosa*	−	Rods	Chloramphenicol, gentamicin, kanamycin, polymyxin, tetracyclines
	Staphylococci and streptococci	+	Cocci	Chloramphenicol, kanamycin, methicillin, penicillin, vancomycin
Pyonephrosis (inflammation of the kidney with pus formation)	Anaerobic streptococci	+	Cocci	Chloramphenicol, penicillin, vancomycin
	Bacteroides spp.	−	Rods	Chloramphenicol, penicillin, tetracyclines

When infection follows catherization, *Pseudomonas* spp. infections are found in greater numbers. Infections caused by enterococci, *Proteus* spp. and staphylococcus are believed to result from direct contact with infected individuals or with contaminated articles, such as bedpans and catheters.

Anaerobic bacteria and several species of fungi are also known to cause urinary tract infections. The relationship of venereal diseases to this category of disease will be discussed later.

PREDISPOSING CONDITIONS

Several clinical factors have been implicated as predisposing individuals to urinary tract infections. These include diabetes mellitus, neurologic diseases (for example, poliomyelitis and spinal cord injuries), toxemia of pregnancy, and lesions that interfere with urine outflow. Kidney stones, stricture, and tumors are examples of such urinary obstructions.

ROUTES OF INFECTION

Although a controversy exists as to the pathways by which bacteria gain access to the kidney, three major routes of infection have been listed: ***hematogenous*** (via the blood), ***lymphatic***, and ***ascending urogenous*** (via the ureter). Most clinical and experimental evidence indicates that the last-mentioned route is the most common pathway in pyelonephritis (inflammation of the kidney and pelvis). The infecting organism in large part determines the form and intensity of the resulting infection.

Sometimes it is possible to establish how causative agents are acquired. For example, infections that develop in women shortly after marriage may be the consequence of mechanical injury to the urethra during sexual intercourse. The onset of a typical acute infection is commonly associated with urinary tract instrumentation.

In the bladder cavity, several factors provide a favorable environment for bacterial persistence in urine. These include (1) the availability of adequate nutrients, (2) the absence of surface phagocytosis (which commonly occurs in other tissues), (3) an optimal temperature for growth, and (4) the fact that some bacteria remain in the bladder after urination. Apparently the film composed of remaining urine and bacteria, which coats the bladder surfaces, serves as an inoculum for newly formed urine. Evidence indicates that such contaminated urine can also be a source of infectious agents for other regions of the urinary tract. Pathogens have been found capable of traveling in a direction opposite to normal urine flow.

SELECTED ASPECTS OF DIAGNOSIS

The presence of bacteria in freshly voided urine may have little or no significance unless they happen to be microorganisms such as *Mycobacterium tuberculosis* or *Salmonella* spp. Such urine, having passed through the urethra, will usually contain members of the region's normal flora, such as *Bacillus* spp., coliforms, diphtheroids, *Proteus* spp., staphylococci, streptococci, and yeasts.

Catheterized specimens may also be contaminated, since the equipment used can come into contact with the urethra and consequently collect normal urethral flora. Since members of the normal flora can cause cystitis, prostatitis, pyelonephritis, and other severe urogenital infections, their presence in a urine specimen is not very helpful in identifying pathogens.

Standard procedures. The presence of more than 100,000 bacteria per milliliter of urine is strongly indicative of acute disease. Diagnostic culturing systems are available not only to determine the concentrations of bacteria in specimens, but also to detect the presence of specific medically important microorganisms (Figure 34–3), including the following: *Candida albicans* (a yeast), *Escherichia coli*,

Neisseria gonorrhoeae, Pseudomonas aeruginosa, Staphylococcus aureus, Streptococcus faecalis, and *Trichomonas* (vaginalis) *hominis* (a protozoan).

SYMPTOMS OF URINARY TRACT INFECTIONS

The following symptoms usually signal the presence of urinary tract disease: blood in the urine, accumulation of fluid in tissues, pain, kidney enlargement, and blood loss, causing anemia. Such symptoms are usually found with infections of the kidney, urinary bladder, ureter, and urethra.

Kidney (Renal) Diseases Caused by Bacteria

Two major types of infections affect the kidney—those that cause a diffuse inflammation of the tissues, *pyelonephritis,* and those that primarily involve the organ's cortex. Detailed discussion of clinical and diagnostic features and the treatment of these disease states can be found in the texts listed in the reference section at the end of this chapter.

ACUTE PYELONEPHRITIS

Acute pyelonephritis is probably the most common disease of the kidney. It is an inflammation of one or both kidneys, involving the tubules. It is generally not considered a primary infection, but rather a complication brought on by an infectious process, such as respiratory disease or sepsis elsewhere in the body.

Escherichia coli is the major cause of this condition. Some 60 to 80 percent of acute pyelonephritis is attributed to this organism. Other bacteria that have been associated with this infection include *Enterobacter aerogenes, Proteus* spp.,

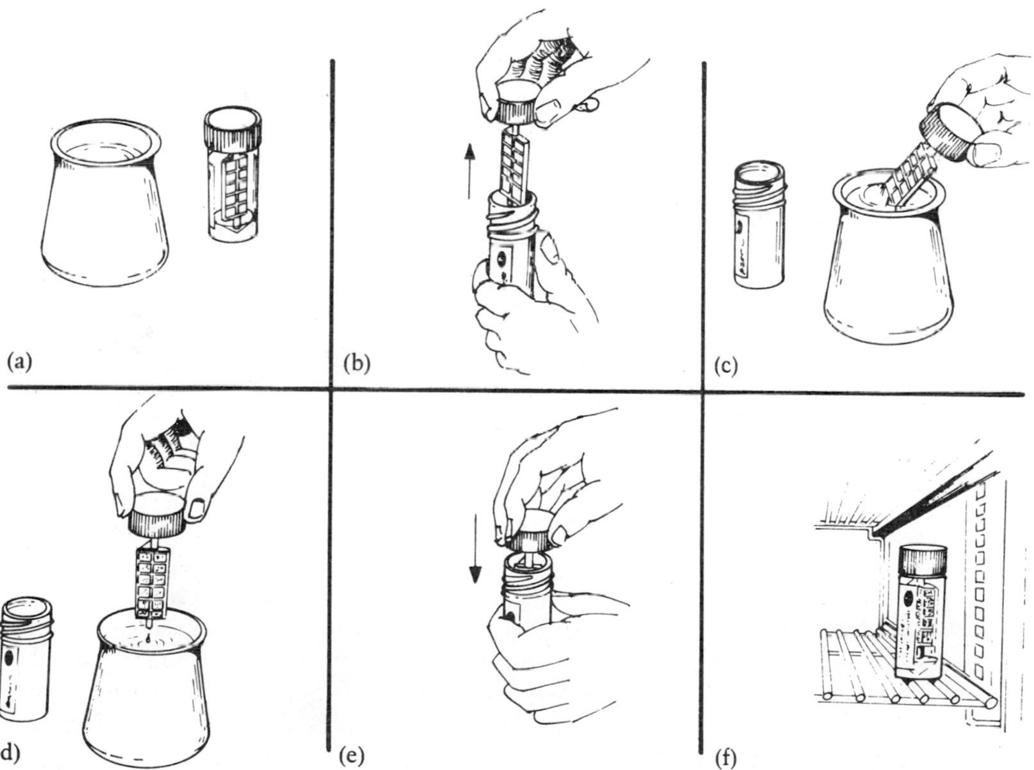

FIG. 34-3 One type of diagnostic culture system, the urine dip-slide procedure. The components of the procedure, voided urine and a dip-slide in its container. (a) The dip-slide is removed from its container (b) and inserted into the urine specimen (c). Excess urine is allowed to drip back into the container (d), and the dip-slide is placed back into its container (e) for incubation (f). *After Pazin, C. J., A. Wolinsky, and W. S. Lee:* Amer. Fam. Phys. *11:85–96 (1975).*

Pseudomonas aeruginosa, staphylococci, and *Streptococcus pyogenes*. Most causes of acute pyelonephritis are "blood-borne." However, some infections have been reported to develop after the instrumentation of the urinary tract.

This kidney infection appears to occur more often in females than in males. In the female, acute pyelonephritis is a common complication of lower urinary tract infections. However, the majority of cases are of a harmless nature. Lesions usually heal spontaneously, leaving only small scars in the kidney tissue. Nevertheless, it is important not to underrate these infections, as they may recur or become chronic, eventually producing serious kidney damage.

KIDNEY CORTEX INFECTIONS

Infections of the renal (kidney) cortical regions are quite different from pyelonephritis in several ways. The former are localized infections of the cortex that are definitely spread via the blood. Pyelonephritis, on the other hand, is a diffuse infection that is not necessarily acquired from the bloodstream.

In cortical infections, the microorganism most frequently present is *Staphylococcus aureus*. *E. coli* may be a secondary invader.

Diseases of the Urinary Bladder

The bladder exhibits considerable resistance to infection. However, it can succumb to disease.

CYSTITIS

The inflammation of the bladder that characterizes cystitis can be either acute or chronic. The acute form is one of the most common urinary tract lesions. However, it is a symptom rather than a specific disease. Thus, the underlying causative factor of acute cystitis must be uncovered if treatment is to be effective. Attacks are common among women.

Sources of bladder infection in the female include the gastrointestinal tract, the cervix (cervicitis), the uterus (endometritis), the urethra, and vaginal involvement by the protozoan *Trichomonas hominis*. In males, the condition may be associated with several body structures, including the gastrointestinal tract, the kidneys, and the urethra. A frequent source of cystitis is an infection of the prostate. Several other factors that can contribute to the development of acute cystitis are foreign bodies self-introduced, certain diseases involving the blood, and diabetes mellitus.

Microorganisms commonly associated with acute cystitis include *E. coli*, *P. vulgaris*, and *Ps. aeruginosa*.

Diseases of the Ureter

Infections of the ureter may develop independently or may be a consequence of disease states involving the bladder, intra-abdominal organs, or kidneys. Inflammatory lesions of the ureter are usually associated with disease and related states of the kidney. These include acute and chronic pyelonephritis, tuberculosis, and various changes produced by kidney stones. Involvement occurs mostly through a direct extension from the other organs. Treatment usually includes the elimination of the original source of the problem. Therefore, depending on the clinical diagnosis, procedures such as antibiotic therapy or surgery may be necessary.

NONSPECIFIC URETHRITIS

Inflammation of the urethra, nonspecific urethritis (NSU), is caused by microorganisms other than *Neisseria gonorrhoeae* and by other factors including chemical agents (ingestion of alcoholic beverages or certain chemotherapeutic agents) and trauma, such as passage of a **catheter.** Nonspecific urethritis is a very common disorder among females. Microorganisms that have been associated with the condition include the yeast *Candida albicans*, hemolytic staphylococci and streptococci, *Mycoplasma hominis*, T-strains of mycoplasma, and *Trichomonas hominis*. Mixed infections also occur.

Urinary Tract Infections Caused by Anaerobes

Several anaerobic organisms are known for their ability to cause renal infections. These anaerobes include members of the genera *Actinomyces, Bacteroides, Clostridium,* and *Streptococcus.* Diseases can come about from several causes, including ascending infection with bowel organisms, bacteremia, the introduction of organisms during instrumentation and surgical procedures, and the lymphatic spread from the intestinal region.

Kidney stones are usually found in instances of anaerobic kidney infections. Although *C. perfringens* has been isolated from such stones, it is believed that the majority of infections develop in the dead tissue associated with the stones. Anaerobes may complicate various clinical states, such as congenital defects and renal or bladder **tumors.**

Immunological Kidney Injury

ACUTE GLOMERULONEPHRITIS

Kidney injury often develops following mild or moderate streptococcal infections. The intensity of the disease varies from a slight involvement of the kidney to severe injury ending in death. Most victims recover with varying degrees of kidney damage. This complication is a case of immunologic hypersensitivity. Two types of reactions can occur: (1) antibodies can form against the individual's kidney tissue; and (2) antigen-antibody complexes can become trapped in the glomerulus and cause inflammation (glomerulonephritis).

Anatomy of the Reproductive System

The Female Reproductive System

The female reproductive system consists of two "button-shaped" organs called the *ovaries*, two *oviducts (Fallopian tubes)*, the *uterus (womb)*, and the *vagina* (Figure 34–4). The ovaries are situated near the kidneys on either side of the uterus.

Each ovary consists of a *medula* (interior) and of a *cortex* (outer region). Ova, or eggs, in various stages of development, are contained within the cortex. In addition to producing sex cells, the ovaries produce important hormones, such as estradiol and progesterone.

When an ovum is released *(ovulation)*, the egg is transported to the opening of the oviducts. The oviducts convey the egg to the uterus. In case of fertilization, the developing embryo attaches itself in the uterine wall after about a week. The vagina is both a birth canal and a copulatory canal. A thin fold of mucous membrane, called the *hymen*, may be found covering the external opening of the vagina. As Figure 34–4 shows, the uterus projects into the upper portion of the vagina. This region is referred to as the *cervix*, or *neck*, of the uterus.

The external genitalia of the female, collectively referred to as the *vulva*,

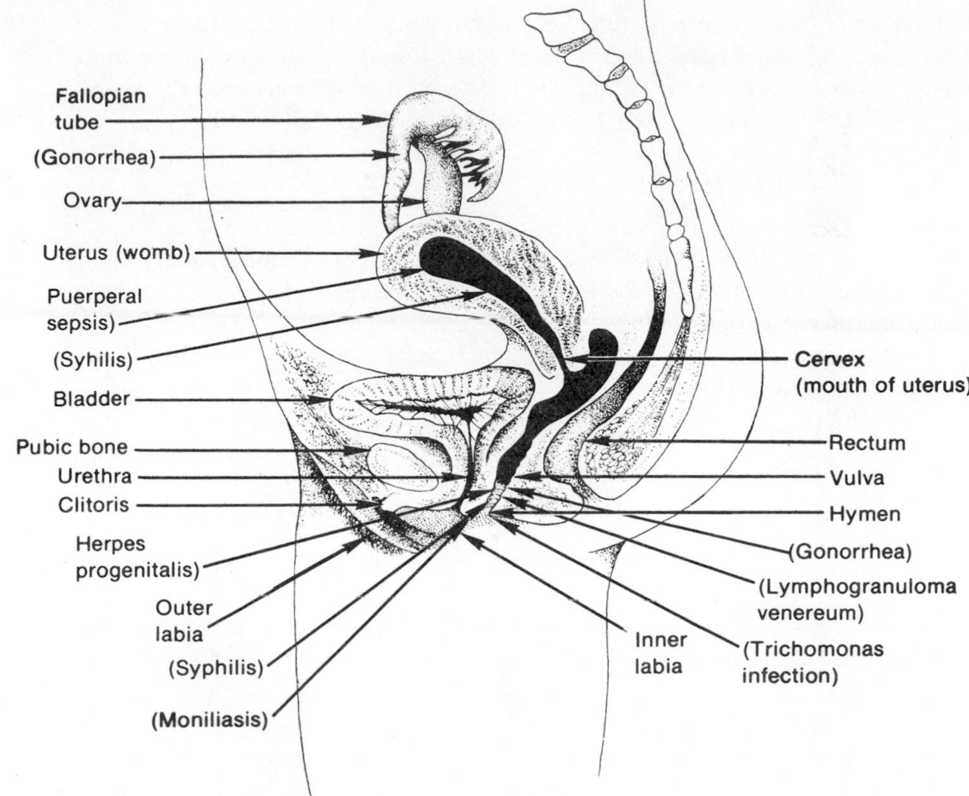

FIG. 34-4 The female reproductive organs and related structures. Sites of infection and disease agents are also indicated.

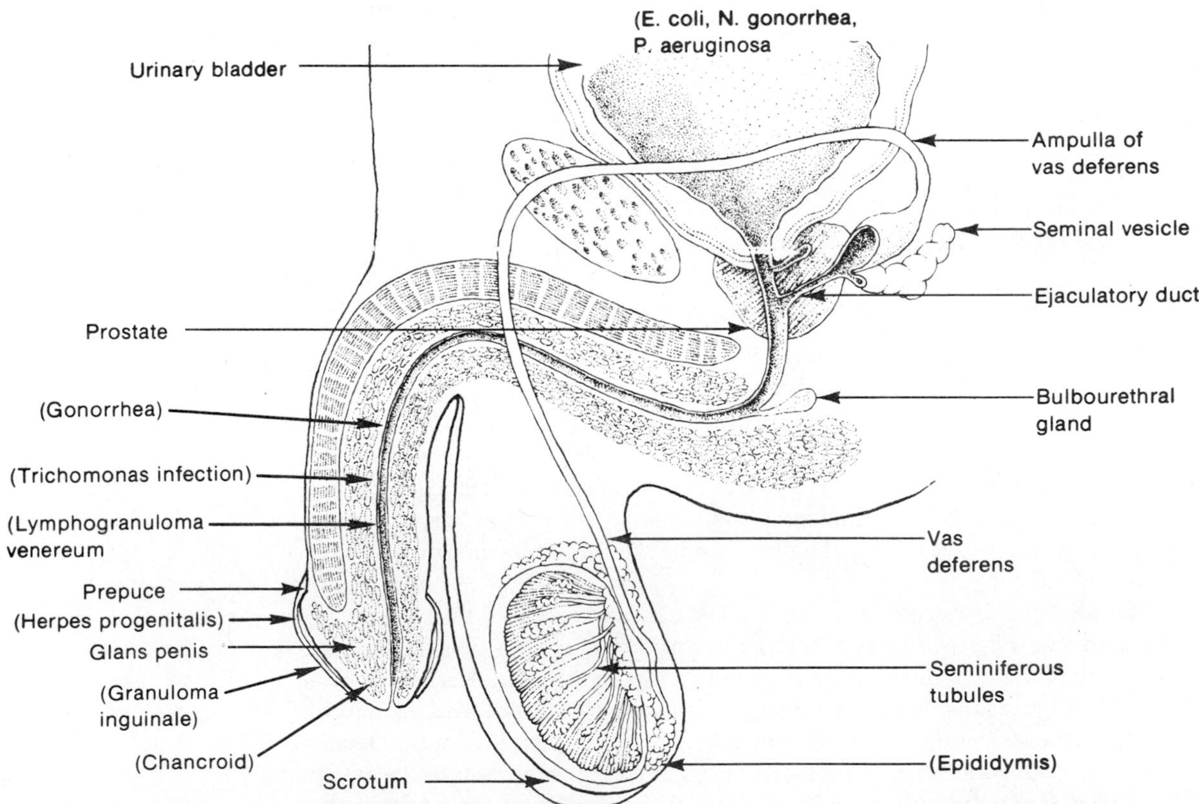

FIG. 34-5 The male reproductive system. Sites of infection and structures attacked by microorganisms are also shown.

include the *clitoris, labia majora, labia minora,* and vestibule. The clitoris, a small erectile organ homologous to the male penis, is located toward the front of the vulva. The labia majora and the labia minora are folds of skin that line the vaginal opening. The labia minora, which are situated between the labia majora, contain the *glands of Bartholin.* These glands are responsible for the secretion of an alkaline fluid that functions as a lubricant during copulation.

The Male Reproductive System

This system includes two oval glandular *testes,* a system of *ducts,* auxiliary glands, and the *penis* (Figure 31–5). The testes are located outside of the abdominal cavity suspended by the *spermatic cords* in a saclike structure. The testes are divided into lobes that contain several *seminiferous tubules.* They produce *spermatozoa* and *testosterone* (male sex hormone). Mature sex cells (sperm) go from the seminiferous tubules to the duct called the *vas deferens,* or *ductus deferens,* by way of the *epididymis.* This latter structure is a coiled duct located on the upper surface of each *testis.* The vas deferens carries the sperm to the *urethra.*

The three auxiliary glands, namely, the *seminal vesicles,* the *prostate gland,* and the *bulbourethral glands of Cowper,* are involved with the formation of *seminal fluid,* or *semen.* The secretions of the seminal vesicles empty into the vas deferens, while those of the prostate and bulbourethral glands empty into the urethra.

Diseases of the Reproductive System

The reproductive organs and associated structures are subject to a wide variety of inflammatory conditions. The remaining portion of this chapter describes the reproductive system and a number of representative nonvenereal and venereal (or genitoinfectious) diseases.

Anaerobic Infections of the Female Genital Tract

The normal bacterial flora of the vaginal region can include several anaerobic species belonging to the genera of *Bacteroides, Clostridium* and *Streptococcus.* From this location, these microorganisms, as well as others, may penetrate the uterine or pelvic cavity when suitable anaerobic conditions prevail, causing severe infections. Most of these result from complications of the confinement period following labor, the *puerperium,* or from complications of septic abortion. Clostridia gain entrance to the uterus by means of unsterile instruments or other materials used in the performance of the abortive procedure.

PUERPERAL (CHILDBIRTH) SEPSIS

Puerperal sepsis is an infection that develops from the invasion of open wounds that occur normally or as the result of surgical procedures in the genital tracts of women who have just given birth. Postpartum (after-birth) hemorrhage, premature rupture of membranes, and prolonged labor predispose mothers to puerperal sepsis. Microorganisms reported as causative agents include anaerobic streptococci, clostridia, *Escherichia coli, Neisseria gonorrhoeae,* and *Proteus* spp.

Infections are acquired through direct contact with persons harboring pathogens in their upper respiratory passages. Even the patient herself may be the source of pathogens. Droplet nuclei and fomites also may serve as sources of infectious agents.

Diseases of the Male Reproductive System

SURFACE INFECTIONS OF THE PENIS

Several nonvenereal infections are known to affect the penis. Inflammation of the glans penis *(balanitis)* and a similar condition of both the glans and the prepuce *(balanoposthitis)* are common examples. A variety of microorganisms can produce such infections. The usual treatment is circumcision and the administration of appropriate antibiotics. Diseases caused by other pathogens, such as herpesviruses, are discussed elsewhere.

DISEASES OF THE PROSTATE

The prostate, which is composed of glandular tissue and smooth muscle, surrounds a portion of the male urethra. It is one of the most important of the male sex glands. Unfortunately, it is subject to various types of diseases. Two of these diseases associated with microorganisms are acute and chronic prostatitis.

Acute prostatitis. Neisseria gonorrhoeae was once considered to be the chief cause of acute inflammations of the prostate gland. Now several other microorganisms, including *E. coli, P. aeruginosa,* staphylococci, and streptococci, have also been identified as causative agents of prostatic infections. Mixed infections have been commonly encountered.

Bacterial pathogens reach the prostate by routes similar to those listed for kidney infections. In cases of nonspecific urethra infections and gonorrhea, the prostate gland becomes involved as a consequence of an acute urethral inflammation. Blood-borne infections of the prostate may occur as complications of boils, carbuncles, osteomyelitis, and epidemics of acute respiratory tract infections. The seminal vesicles may also be affected.

Chronic prostatitis. This infection of the prostate manifests itself more commonly in middle-aged males. Chronic prostatitis is usually sequel to an acute infection of the gland. The bacteria producing this condition are similar to those associated with acute prostatitis.

The Venereal (Genitoinfectious) Diseases

Venereal diseases are those diseases that are sexually transmitted (Table 34–2). The infectious agents that cause these diseases are important both because they cause discomfort and disability and because some may result in sterility or life-threatening situations. The signs and symptoms of common venereal diseases are given in Table 34–3.

CHANCROID (SOFT CHANCRE)

The Gram-negative coccobacillus *Hemophilus ducreyi,* which is occasionally called Ducrey's bacillus, is the causative agent of chancroid. The disease is highly contagious, specific, and appears as a venereal ulcer on the genitals. Chancroid bears no relation to the primary lesion of syphilis (hard or Hunterian chancre). Generally, *H. ducreyi* is transmitted by sexual contact. However, some reports implicate dressings and surgical instruments as possible sources of infection. Poor sanitary habits are considered a predisposing factor.

TABLE 34-2 Sexually Transmissible Diseases

1. Chancroid (B)[a]
2. Condyloma acuminata (genital warts) (V)
3. Gonorrhea (B)
4. Granuloma inguinale (B)
5. Herpes progenitalis (V)
6. Lymphogranuloma venereum (B)
7. Molluscum contagiosum (V)
8. Monilial vaginitis (Y)
9. Nongonococcal urethritis (B)
10. Pediculosis pubis (L)
11. Reiter's syndrome (arthritis, and inflammations of the eyelid and urethra) (B)
12. Scabies (L)
13. Syphilis (B)
14. Trichomonas infestation (P)

[a]B = bacterial; L = lice; P = protozoan; V = virus; and Y = yeast.

Diagnosis. Chancroid is usually diagnosed on clinical grounds. This involves excluding other types of venereal infections and examining specimens microscopically. The absence of hard chancres and the failure to detect spirochetes by means of dark-field microscopic examination usually eliminate the possibility of syphilis. *H. ducreyi* may be detected in Gram-stained smears prepared from ulcer specimens. Culturing specimens in media containing blood or its derivatives is also a standard procedure. *H. ducreyi* is a Gram-negative bacillus and produces hemolysis on blood agar.

A skin test with a killed suspension of the causative agent is used in Europe to differentiate between chancroid and other venereal diseases. Usually 48 hours are needed to demonstrate a positive reaction. It is characterized by redness and hardening at the site of injection.

GONORRHEA

Gonorrhea, a highly infectious, pus-producing disease, is often referred to as a ***specific urethritis***. Gonorrhea is the most common communicable disease in the United States today. It outnumbers syphilis by about 40 to one. The disease is caused by the Gram-negative "biscuit-shaped" diplococcus, *Neisseria gonorrheae* (Color Photographs 86A and 86B), which is usually situated intracellularly. The disease primarily involves the genitourinary tract. However, various complications can develop, among them endocarditis, meningitis, and pyelonephritis. Once the disease is acquired, it may persist for many years if treatment is not administered.

The most common means by which adults contract gonorrhea is through sexual intercourse. In the male, the disease initially remains limited to the lining of the front portion of the urethra (Figure 34–6). However, with additional sexual relations, improper instrumentation during examinations, or self-medication, the infectious agents can be introduced into the deeper, or posterior, portion of the urethra. From this focus, other parts of the urogenital system can be readily invaded.

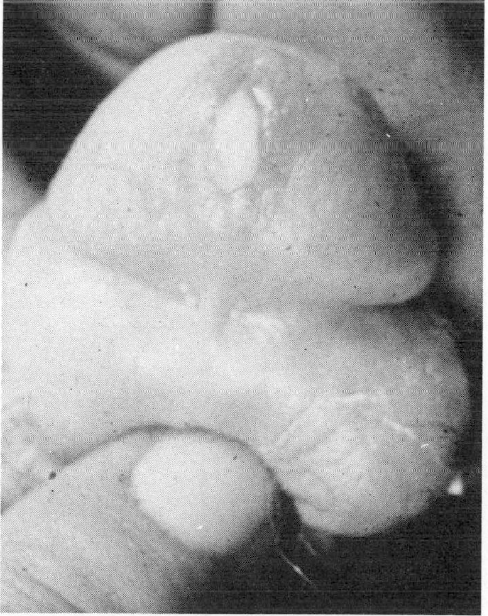

FIG. 34–6 The urethral discharge in an acute case of gonorrhea. *Courtesy of the Armed Forces Institute of Pathology, Washington, D.C., Neg. No. 218663-5-96.*

In the female, *N. gonorrhoeae* causes not only urethritis, but also inflammations of the cervix and Fallopian tubes. In adult females, the designation of ***external gonorrhea*** is used when gonococcal involvement includes glands and related parts near the vagina and the urethra. If the infection spreads from these structures to the mucous membrane that lines the uterus, the membrane lining of the Fallopian tube, the ovaries, or the peritoneum, the term *internal*

TABLE 34-3 Features of the Venereal Diseases

Disease	*Causative Agent*	*Gram Reaction*	*Morphology*	*Incubation Period*	*Type of Discharge*	*General Features of Disease*	*Laboratory Diagnosis*	*Possible Treatment*
Chancroid	*Hemophilus ducreyi*	–	Small rod (coccobacillus)	1–3 days	Pus-containing and bloody	Symptoms include small elevated lesions that form irregular soft-edged sores, soft chancres (Color Photograph 90), and some pain	Gram stain and culture of specimens	Sulfonamides, chloramphenicol, streptomycin, tetracyclines
Gonorrhea	*Neisseria gonorrhoeae*	–	Coccus	3–9 days or as late as 2 weeks	Mucous and pus-containing	Symptoms in the male include uncomfortable sensation along the course of the urethra and painful and frequent urination; the majority of females do not show definite symptoms	1. Gram stain and CO_2 culture of specimens 2. Biochemical testing 3. Fluorescent-antibody test (Color Photograph 55)[a]	Penicillin, erythromycin, tetracyclines
Granuloma inguinale	*Calymmatobacterium granulomatis*	–	Small rod (coccobacillus)	Unknown	None	The appearance of a moist pimple (papule) on or in vicinity of external genitalia	Smears of specimen and isolation of organism using chick embryos	Chloramphenicol, streptomycin, tetracyclines
Herpes progenitalis (genital herpes)	*Herpesvirus hominis* type 2	Not done[b]	Virus	At least 36 hours	None	Itching and rash occur followed by clusters of blisterlike lesions that break and form sores	Similar to those for other *herpes* viruses[a]	DNA synthesis inhibiting drugs symptomatic, generally quite limited
Lymphogranuloma venereum (LGV)	*Chlamydia trachomatis*	– or variable (not useful)	Small rod (coccobacillus)	3–21 days	Mucous discharge containing pus and blood	Swollen lymph nodes, which become filled with pus and eventually rupture and drain; these and other lesions occur in the vulvovaginal and/or rectal areas of females; leathery patches also occur	1. Serological tests, e.g., specific complement fixation 2. Skin test, Frei test	Sulfonamides
Monilial *(Candida)* vaginitis	*Candida albicans*	+ (usually not done)	Yeast cell	Unknown	Thick, yellow, cheesy consistency	Severe itching in and around involved areas[c]	1. Microscopic examination of discharge 2. Culture	

Syphilis	*Treponema pallidum*	Not useful	Spirochete	9–90 days	Generally none	*Primary:* Formation of a hard sore (Hunterian chancre at infection site) (Color Photograph 87); healing occurs without scarring *Secondary:* Occurs about two months after chancre; symptoms due to generalized spreading of the disease include swollen lymph nodes, general discomfort, fever, headache, and skin rash (Color Photograph 88); large numbers of organisms may be found in mucous patches in various mouth parts *Tertiary:* Soft, gummy, swollen areas, or tumors, the ***gummas*** (Color Photograph 89) may form in any tissue *Congenital:* Involvement of skin (Figure 34–8), teeth (Figure 34–9), and mucous membranes; anemia, enlarged liver and spleen, deafness, and blindness	1. Demonstration of organism in dark-field preparation of primary chancre 2. Serodiagnostic tests, e.g., Venereal Disease Research Laboratory (VDRL), Reiter complement fixation, fluorescent treponemal antibody absorption (FTA-ABS)[a]	Penicillin, erythromycin, tetracyclines
Trichomiasis	*Trichomonas hominis*	Not done	Flagellated protozoan	Unknown	Green-whitish, foamy, foul-smelling discharge	Profuse discharge and irritation	Microscopic examination and staining of specimens, e.g., Gram, acridine orange	Metronidazol, trichomycin, hamycin

[a]Refer to Chapter 24 for descriptions of these procedures.
[b]Virus infection: the Gram stain is not done.
[c]Monilial vaginitis is common in pregnant women and has been associated with the use of oral contraceptives.

gonorrhea is employed. Many infected women and some men show no symptoms of the disease, however.

There are clear indications that the use of birth control pills increases the possibility of infection by establishing conditions more favorable to the survival of *N. gonorrhoeae*.

Unfortunately the eyes of newborns can become infected with *N. gonorrhoeae* as the newborns pass through the birth canal passage. This disease, known as ***opthalmia neonatorum***, was once the major cause of blindness in many parts of the world. The administration of a 1-percent silver nitrate solution or antibiotics immediately after birth has greatly reduced the incidence of this infection.

Children can experience another manifestation of *N. gonorrhoeae, vulvovaginitis*. This type of gonococcal involvement is looked upon as an "institutional disease," as it has been found to be transmitted by contaminated towels or similar articles in hospitals, orphanages, and schools. It appears that the conjunctiva and vagina of children are quite vulnerable to gonococcus infections. In adults it is the internal genital organs and associated structures that have particular susceptibility. Vulvo-vaginitis is not exclusively caused by *N. gonorrhoeae*. Hemolytic staphylococci and streptococci, as well as other microorganisms, have also been isolated from cases of vulvo-vaginitis. A new problem is presented by *N. gonorrhoeae* L-forms.

Prevention. Preventive measures for gonorrhea are directed toward detecting and treating the sexual contacts who transmitted the disease to the patients and educating the public as to the means of transmission, availability of treatment, and other pertinent details. Since 1976, penicillin-resistant strains of *N. gonorrhoeae* have been isolated from patients in several regions of the world. Such organisms make control of this disease more difficult.

GRANULOMA INGUINALE (GRANULOMA VENEREUM)

Granuloma inguinale is caused by the Gram-negative *Calymmatobacterium (Donovania) granulomatis*. Originally the infection was believed limited to the tropics; however, several reports have proved it to be endemic in parts of the United States. The organism is presumed to be spread through sexual intercourse, although other means are thought possible. The disease itself is not highly contagious.

LYMPHOGRANULOMA VENEREUM (LGV)

This disease is caused by *Chlamydia trachomatis*. Under normal conditions this microorganism is transmitted by sexual intercourse. However, infections can be acquired through nonvenereal contacts, such as hands.

Lymphogranuloma venereum is also known by a variety of other names, including Duran-Nicholas-Favre disease, lymphogranuloma inguinale, fifth venereal disease, and venereal bubo. The last term refers to the enlarged regional lymph nodes that develop approximately 1 week to 2 months after the initial disease symptoms.

As healing proceeds, scars form and eventually obstruct lymph channels. Characteristic effects of this phase of LGV include elephantiasis (massive enlargement) of the external genitalia in males and rectal narrowing in females (Figure 34–7).

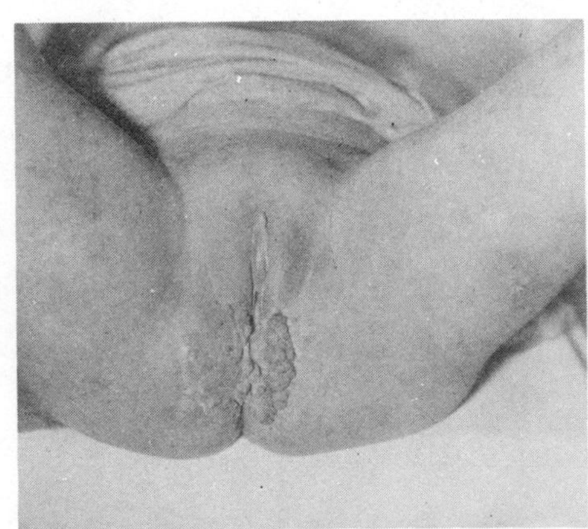

FIG. 34–7 Perianal lesions of lymphogranuloma venereum. *Courtesy of the Armed Forces Institute of Pathology, Washington, D.C., Neg. No. D4542–1.*

SYPHILIS AND THE OTHER TREPONEMATOSES

Most health experts regard the treponematoses as one of the world's worst communicable disease problems. During the late 1940s and early 1950s, a remarkable decrease in the incidence of venereal syphilis was widely noted. This event coincided with the increased availability and use of penicillin. The gen-

TABLE 34-4 A Comparison of Selected Epidemiologic Features of the Treponematoses

Microorganism	Disease	Geographical Distribution	Age Group Affected	Mode of Transmission: Biological: Venereal	Nonvenereal	In utero	Mechanical: Flies, fomites, etc.
Treponema pallidum	Venereal syphilis	World	Sexually mature individuals and some newborns	Common	Not usually	Not uncommon	Extremely rare
T. pallidum	Endemic syphilis (Bejel)	Rural regions, prevalent in Africa, Australia, Mediterranean countries	Children 2 to 10 years of age	Not usually	Common	Rare	Probably not uncommon
T. pertenue	Yaws	Rural regions, mostly tropical areas	Children 4 to 15 years of age	Not usually	Common	Questionable	Possibly not uncommon
T. carateum	Pinta	Rural regions, humid, tropical areas, only in the Americas	Individuals ranging in age from 10 to 30 years	Not reported	Common	Implicated	Implicated

eral view held that syphilis was well on the road to eradication and would be relegated to the groups of historical diseases.

Unfortunately, during the 1960s this downward trend of reported cases reversed abruptly, and syphilis is occurring in near epidemic proportions. The numbers of cases in the United States increased from 6399 in 1956 to 22,962 in 1964. These numbers are only minimum estimates, because, according to many public health authorities, numerous cases go unreported. An extremely unfortunate aspect of the current status of syphilis is the increased involvement of teenagers and young adults 13 to 24 years of age.

The first recorded occurrence of syphilis in its present form was a great pandemic that erupted in Europe in 1497. One theory suggests that it was brought to Europe from Haiti by Columbus's crew and the six Indians whom they brought with them, but the origin of syphilis in the New World is by no means established. (See the chapter-end references for a Public Health Service publication on the history of syphilis.)

Morphological and cultural properties. The causative agent of syphilis, *Treponema pallidum,* was discovered in 1905 by Fritz Schaudinn and Erich Hoffman. This treponeme belongs to the order of Spirochaetales and the family of Treponemataceae.

The microorganism is one of three principal human pathogenic agents belonging to the genus *Treponema.* The others are *T. pertenue* and *T. carateum,* the causative agents of yaws and pinta, respectively (Table 34-4). The three species are morphologically and serologically indistinguishable. *T. pallidum* is a thin, delicate, spiral bacterium ranging from 6 to 15 μm in length with a uniform cylindrical thickness of about 0.25 μm, arranged in a number of tight body coils (6 to 14 turns or spirals). Upon dark-field examination of clinical specimens from primary and secondary syphilitic lesions, the spirality of the organism and its well-known corkscrewlike rotation are easily recognized (Figure 2-11b).

Up to the present time all attempts to culture *in vitro* the treponemes pathogenic for humans have been unsuccessful. *T. pallidum* can be grown in the testes of rabbits and it has been maintained in fluid media containing carbon dioxide, pyruvate, a reducing agent such as cysteine, serum albumin, and serum ultrafiltrate.

Transmission. Syphilis is transmitted through direct contact with infectious lesions in both the primary and secondary stages of the disease. These lesions may be either genital, oral, or on skin. *T. pallidum* is capable of passing through abraded skin and intact mucous membranes. From the lesions, the spirochetes gain access to the circulatory system of the individual and are carried to every organ. Outside the body, this microorganism is extremely vulnerable to the effects of both physical and chemical agents. These destructive forces include heat, drying, storage at refrigerator temperatures (approximately 3 to 4° C), and ordinary soap and water.

Clinical features. The laboratory diagnosis and several clinical features of this venereal disease are compared with those of other treponeme infections in Table 34–3.

The clinical manifestations of syphilis may conveniently be divided into three stages: primary, secondary, and tertiary.

Primary syphilis. The primary lesion, or chancre, develops at the site of entry of *Treponema pallidum* within 2 to 6 weeks after exposure and lasts for approximately 6 weeks. During this stage, the treponemes invade lymph nodes, enter the bloodstream, and are distributed throughout the body, producing a *spirochetemia*. Extragenital chancres commonly involve the lip (Color Photograph 87) but also may involve the tongue or other mucosal sites. Such lesions are relatively painless.

The organisms are transmitted directly from an individual with syphilitic lesions of this nature. The immediate rapid spread of organisms throughout the body makes all attempts at local disinfection after contact ineffective and of no prophylactic value.

The primary chancre, which is also known as the *hard* or *Hunterian chancre,* begins as a single small, slightly elevated, round, red nodule on the tissue surface. It is usually painless. The central area breaks down, and the nodule ulcerates and discharges a fluid containing numerous treponemes.

These organisms can be demonstrated by dark-field examination and are fully capable of infecting others. The spirochetes cannot be demonstrated in tissue sections except with special stains such as silver impregnation. Diagnostic blood tests do not become positive until at least a week after the appearance of the chancre. The chancre heals spontaneously, leaving very little scarring unless there has been a superimposed secondary bacterial infection.

Secondary syphilis. One to two months following the appearance of the chancre, the generalized spread of the disease and widespread swelling of lymph nodes may become evident. Malaise accompanied by a rise in temperature, headaches, and various skin rashes are common symptoms (Color Photograph 88). Swollen grayish-white areas may develop on the mucous membranes of the lips, soft palate, tongue, or other areas. The typical mucous patch is a slightly elevated and flattened grayish-white area that can be removed, leaving a red zone of erosion and ulceration. In the throat the chancres may have a creeping outline; they have been called "snail track ulcers." Such lesions contain large numbers of *T. pallidum* and are slow to heal.

In the secondary stage of syphilis, the mouth often contains many treponemes, a ready source of infection for dentists, their assistants, or anyone else who places an unprotected finger in the mouth of one of these infected individuals. Highly contagious skin lesions also occur.

Spotty eruptions may also occur in the mouth and on the skin. The oral lesions are often on the palate, but they may involve the entire oral mucosa as nonelevated or slightly elevated reddish areas. Microscopically, the tissue shows a nonspecific chronic inflammation, often associated with capillaries having thickened walls.

The secondary stage of syphilis can be confirmed clinically by demonstrating *T. pallidum* from mucous patches or by diagnostic blood tests, which are positive in almost all cases. This stage can disappear, be latent, and then reappear several times before finally disappearing.

Tertiary syphilis. The **gummas,** which are soft, gummy tumors (Color Photograph 89), and nodules of tertiary syphilis usually take 5 to 20 years to appear, but they may occur, though rarely, within a short time after the secondary stage. Of the many changes that become apparent within tissues, two are most commonly seen: (1) ***syphilitic arteritis,*** in which the small arteries become narrowed as a result of a fibrous thickening of their walls; (2) ***gummas,*** lesions that are a type of tissue death followed by scarring and are assumed to be the result of a longstanding, progressive decrease in the blood supply to the tissue (Color Photograph 89). Gummas may form in any tissue. Some involve the tongue, palate, and facial bones. These gummas ulcerate, leaving typically rounded, "punched out" edges. When they occur in the palate they may eventually perforate, leaving an irregular opening into the nasal area, which will interfere with speech.

The third stage of the venereal disease includes conditions known as latent syphilis, neurosyphilis, late benign syphilis, and cardiovascular syphilis.

The lesion of ***late benign syphilis,*** which is the gumma, usually does not produce death or total physical incapacity. However, when lesions arise in vital organs, the complications that occur certainly are not benign. The gumma is believed to be a consequence of a hypersensitivity reaction to *T. pallidum.* It can involve any body organ. In addition, gummas may be found associated with the bones and skin of an infected individual. Serologic tests are usually highly reactive in this form of syphilis.

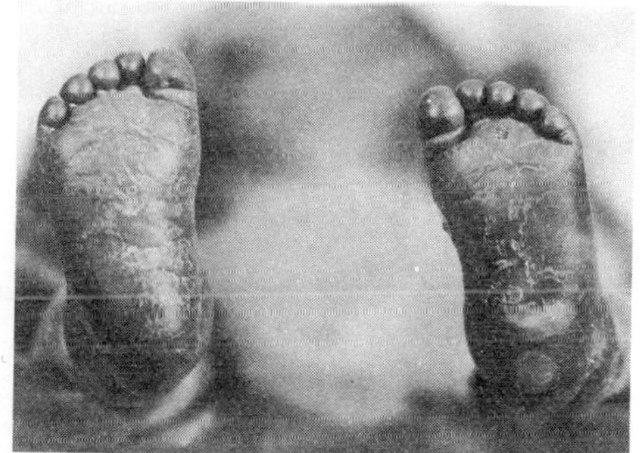

FIG. 34–8 Skin lesions of congenital syphilis appear soon after birth, frequently in the form of vesicles. These lesions can progress to superficial, crusted erosions. *Courtesy of the Armed Forces Institute of Pathology, Washington, D.C., Neg. No. 54-2488-7.*

Congenital syphilis. Congenital syphilis occurs when *T. pallidum* crosses the placenta and infects the fetus. A situation of this nature may arise after the eighteenth week of gestation, when atrophy of the Langhan's cell layer of the placenta takes place. However, adequate treatment of an infected mother before this time usually prevents involvement of the fetus. If a woman conceives while she is in the primary or secondary stages of syphilis, her pregnancy in all probability will end in a stillbirth. When pregnancy occurs during the later stages of this infection, newborns may exhibit a variety of clinical manifestations ranging from fulminating fatal congenital infections to a normal, uninfected state.

Congenital syphilis is divided into two principal stages, early and late congenital syphilis. A primary stage is not present, as *T. pallidum* is directly introduced into the fetus via the placenta.

The effects of early congenital syphilis may include skin (Figure 34–8) and mucous membrane lesions, hemolytic anemia, enlarged liver and spleen, and the involvement of teeth (Figure 34–9), bone, and the central nervous system. These symptoms appear before the child reaches 2 years of age.

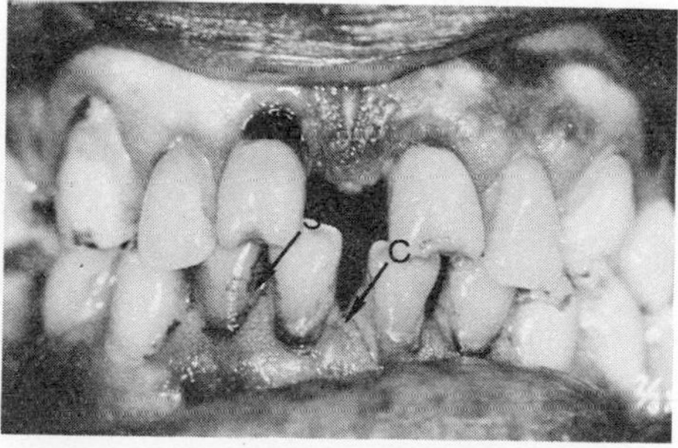

FIG. 34–9 Characteristic notched incisors (I) of congenital syphilis. Poor hygiene with considerable calculus (C) and stain (S) is also evident.

The late form of congenital syphilis is defined by the persistence of these effects beyond the age of 2. In approximately 60 percent of cases, the disease is latent, and is characterized by reactive diagnostic immunologic reactions. However, several signs of this stage of syphilis may appear. These include rare cardiovascular lesions, Clutton's joints (a painless involvement of the joints, usually the knees), inflammation of the eyes, involvement of the bones and skin, Moon's molars (poor development of the cusps of the first molars), and neurosyphilis. Clutton's joints, eighth-cranial nerve deafness, and eye inflammation usually occur together near the beginning of puberty and appear to be produced as a consequence of a hypersensitivity response rather than by the purely destructive effects of *T. pallidum*.

Endemic syphilis, pinta, and yaws. Endemic syphilis is known by several other names, including Bejel and Skerljevo. The disease, found primarily in tropical areas, is believed to be transmitted through direct contact. The causative spirochete produces lesions during the early and late periods of the disease. Involvement of the cardiovascular and central nervous systems as well as the skin usually occurs.

Pinta, a contagious disease caused by ***Treponema carateum***, seems to be limited to tropical and subtropical regions, like Central and South America. The infection is believed transmitted by direct contact. Flies have also been implicated as vectors. The lesions (which primarily involve the feet, hands, and scalp) are described as dry, scaly, and exhibiting a variety of colors. The name of the disease is derived from the Spanish verb ***pintar***, which means "to paint." These lesions at first are highly pigmented, and then, after several years, lose color. Other body tissues are not usually invaded. *T. **carateum*** is morphologically indistinguishable from *T. **pallidum***. Wassermann antibodies are commonly detected, especially in the secondary and late stages of pinta. Penicillin is effective in the treatment of the disease.

Yaws is also a contagious disease, caused by *T. **pertenue***. The infection is not transmitted by sexual contact, but by direct contact and possibly by flies. Yaws is found in tropical areas, especially those with heavy rainfall. The characteristic lesion resembles a raspberry and consequently it has been referred to as a ***framboise***. This disease is known by several other names, including ***bouba*** (Portuguese), ***buba*** (Spanish), ***framboesia*** (Dutch and German), and ***pian*** (French). **Ulceration** of the lesion eventually occurs, followed by formation of a dry crust and healing. Secondary eruptions usually manifest themselves within 2 to 4 weeks. The late stage of the disease is characterized by the involvement of the skin and bones. Congenital yaws is apparently a rare phenomenon. Serologic tests for syphilis are positive in yaws infections. Penicillin is effective in the treatment of diseased persons. Unfortunately, *T. **pertenue*** infections occur in areas where medical services are extremely limited.

GENITAL HERPES (HERPESVIRUS TYPE 2 INFECTION)

Ten years ago, a sexually transmitted viral infection called genital herpes was a rare condition, certainly considered minor compared to the better-known and more virulent venereal bacterial diseases gonorrhea and syphilis. Currently, the incidence of this viral infection is increasing dramatically and is causing genuine alarm among public health experts. ***Herpesvirus*** type 2 has been recognized as the causative agent of primary and recurrent infections involving the genital tract.

TRICHOMONAS HOMINIS, A GENITAL PROTOZOAN

Many flagellates capable of inhabiting humans have been found in human fecal matter, in the mouth, and in the genital tract. For the most part their pathogenicity is doubtful, and many authorities consider them harmless commensals. However, one species, ***Trichomonas hominis***, is pathogenic. ***Trichimonas hominis*** is found only in the genitourinary system and has been acknowledged as the causative agent of genitourinary trichomoniasis. Several recent investigations have proved this disease to be a true venereal infection.

The disease seems to be as frequent in adult males as in females. In women, the acute stage involves a noticeable discharge; the symptoms in males are generally latent and therefore not obvious. Prostate involvement occurs in the male.

Temporary and permanent sterility have been reported to result from long-lasting infections. However, in some cases successful therapy has enabled women to conceive and give birth to normal children.

T. hominis infections can be acquired by newborn babies by way of an infected birth canal or as a consequence of being exposed to highly unhygienic conditions. Infections of young girls have occasionally been reported.

THE TORCH COMPLEX

Infection of a fetus or of a newborn during delivery with toxoplasma (a protozoan), rubella virus, cytomegalovirus, and the herpesviruses may yield an inapparent disease. Even when the infections are clinically apparent, the associated signs and symptoms may be indistinguishable. Furthermore, all of the agents can produce long-term ill effects in the infected fetus or newborn, so that prognosis must be guarded. Because the infections are often clinically inapparent, not only in the newborn but also in the mother, specific diagnosis is dependent on special laboratory testing. Because of the serious consequence of infection and the difficulty of identifying and distinguishing the disease state, the acronym of "TORCH" was devised to focus attention on this group of microbial agents (*T*, toxoplasma; *R*, rubella virus; *C*, cytomegalovirus; *H*, herpesviruses, and *O*, others). The specific features of these disease agents have been presented in other chapters.

SUMMARY

The functions of the urinary system include eliminating waste products, regulating the chemical composition and the acid-base balance of body tissues, and maintaining the water content of the body at a constant level.

Anatomy of the Urinary System

1. The human urinary system consists of two kidneys, two ureters, the urethra, and the urinary bladder.
2. The basic unit of the kidney is the *nephron*. It is composed of a *glomerulus* (blood filter) and a long tubule (concentrator and urine collecter).
3. Blood filters through the glomeruli and is concentrated by the tubules, which empty into the ureters.

The Flora of the Normal Urinary Tract

The normal sterile kidney is highly resistant to bacteria.

Diseases of the Urinary Tract

1. Common urinary infections are caused by *coliforms*, intestinal organisms.
2. Predisposing conditions for urinary tract infections include diabetes mellitus, neurologic diseases, and lesions that interfere with urine flow.
3. The major routes of infection are by blood, lymphatics, and from the ureter.
4. Diagnostic culturing systems are used to determine the concentrations of bacteria in specimens and to detect the presence of specific medically important microbes. The presence of more than 100,000 bacteria per milliliter of urine is strongly indicative of an infection.
5. Individuals with urinary tract infections usually exhibit symptoms such as blood in the urine, accumulation of fluid in tissues, pain, kidney enlargement, and blood loss, causing anemia.

Kidney (Renal) Diseases Caused by Bacteria

1. The most common kidney infection is pyelonephritis, an inflammation of the organ's tissues. *Escherichia coli* is the major cause.
2. Other kidney infections involve the outer region, or cortex.

Diseases of the Urinary Bladder

Cystitis, or inflammation of the bladder, can be caused by various bacteria including *E. coli*, *Proteus vulgaris*, *Pseudomonas aeruginosa*, and the protozoan *Trichomonas hominis*.

Diseases of the Ureter

1. Infections of the ureter may develop independently or be a consequence of diseases involving other organs.
2. Nonspecific urethritis, an inflammation of the urethra, can be caused by various microorganisms such as *Neisseria gonorrhoeae*, hemolytic staphylococci and streptococci, the yeast *Canadida albicans*, and the protozoan *Trichomonas hominis*.
3. Chemicals and the insertion of medical devices such as a catheter can also produce urethritis.

Urinary Tract Infections Caused by Anaerobes

1. Anaerobes belonging to the genera of *Actinomyces*, *Bacteroides*, *Clostridium*, and *Streptococcus* cause infections of the kidney.
2. Organisms are introduced from other sites in the body or

by means of surgical procedures.

3. Anaerobes can complicate various clinical states.

Immunologic Kidney Injury

1. Immunologic hypersensitivity can cause severe kidney damage. Acute glomerulonephritis is an example of such injury.
2. Injury is caused either by antibodies that form against the individual's kidney tissue or by the formation of antigen-antibody complexes that are eventually trapped in glomeruli.

Anatomy of the Reproductive Systems

1. The female system includes two ovaries, two oviducts, the uterus, and the vagina. In addition to producing sex cells, the ovaries also produce several important hormones.
2. The male system includes the testes, a series of ducts or channels, auxiliary glands, and the penis. The testes also produce sex cells and male hormones.

Diseases of the Reproductive System

The reproductive organs and associated structures are susceptible to a variety of venereal and nonvenereal infectious agents.

Anaerobic Infections of the Female Genital Tract

1. Several microorganisms from the normal flora of the vaginal region as well as others can cause infections of this system.
2. Anaerobic streptococci and other bacteria can cause infections such as puerperal sepsis, which involves the genital tracts of women who have just given birth.

Selected Diseases of the Male Reproductive System

1. Several nonvenereal diseases are known to affect the penis and prostate gland.
2. *Neisseria gonorrhoeae*, *Escherichia coli*, and *Pseudomonas aeruginosa* are among the causes of prostatic infections.

The Venereal (Genitoinfectious) Diseases

1. Venereal diseases are those transmitted by sexual contact.
2. The agents of sexually transmissible diseases include bacteria, protozoans, viruses, yeast, and lice.
3. Bacterial infections include chancroid, gonorrhea, granuloma inguinale, lymphogranuloma venereum, syphilis, and other treponematoses.
4. The TORCH complex is the set of certain infectious disease agents that produce long-term ill effects in an infected fetus or newborn infant. The infections are often clinically inapparent in both the newborn and the mother.
5. The complex consists of toxoplasma (T), rubella (R), cytomegalovirus (C), herpersviruses (H), and others (O).

QUESTIONS FOR REVIEW

1. How do microorganisms gain access to the tissues of the kidney?
2. What types of urinary tract infections are associated with anaerobes?
3. Are there factors that can predispose an individual to some form of urinary tract infection? Explain.
4. Compare the venereal diseases discussed in this chapter as to causative agents, diagnosis, treatment, and prevention.
5. Can venereal diseases be transmitted by means other than sexual contact? Explain.
6. Which of the venereal diseases are known to exert harmful effects during pregnancy? Describe these manifestations and discuss preventive measures that can be taken.
7. Consider the professions of the individuals listed below in answering this question: How can these persons acquire syphilis, gonorrhea, or LGV? If there can be no professional involvement, say so:
   a. barber
   b. physical therapist
   c. nurse
   d. x-ray technician
   e. physician
   f. dictician
8. Explain how venereal diseases might be eliminated totally.

SUGGESTED READINGS

Catterall, R. D., and C. S. Nicol (eds.), *Sexually Transmitted Diseases.* New York: Academic Press, 1976. *The results of a conference on sexually transmitted diseases, approaches to control, virus diseases, and education and prevention programs are presented.*

Kunin, C. M., *Detection, Prevention and Management of Urinary Tract Infections.* 2nd ed. Philadelphia: Lea and Febiger, 1974. *An excellent short reference book. Topics include urine, evaluation of renal function, urinary bacteriology, and management of urinary tract infection.*

Morton, R. S., *Venereal Diseases.* Baltimore: Penguin Books, Ltd., 1972. *A short paperback on venereal diseases, including historical aspects, discussions of causes, and associated social problems.*

Nahias, A. J., "The TORCH Complex," *Hosp. Practice* 9:65 (1975). *An excellent summary of intrauterine infections of the fetus.*

Public Health Service, National Communicable Disease Center, Atlanta, Georgia. Public Health Service Publication No. 1660. *An excellent, well-illustrated publication dealing with the historical and clinical features of syphilis. Properties of Treponema pallidum, together with diagnostic serological tests, also are discussed.*

Microbial Diseases of the Central Nervous System and the Eye

CHAPTER **35**

Various microorganisms can invade the human central nervous system. Chapter 35 describes several nervous system diseases, including meningitis, rabies, and slow virus diseases, as well as diseases of the eye.

After reading this chapter, you should be able to:

1. **Outline the general organization of the human central nervous system and indicate the areas attacked by pathogenic microorganisms.**
2. **Discuss the general routes of microbial invasion of the central nervous system.**
3. **List and describe one each of a bacterial, mycotic, protozoan, and viral infection of the central nervous system, giving their causative agents, means of transmission, and control measures.**
4. **Explain the nature of slow virus diseases and their significance.**
5. **Compare the approaches used in the identification of bacterial, mycotic, protozoan, and viral infections of the central nervous system.**
6. **Outline the general structure of the human eye and indicate the areas attacked by pathogens.**
7. **Discuss the complications associated with infections of the eye.**

Organization of the Central Nervous System

Most of the body's systems consist of several anatomically connected organs and structures so organized that together they perform important and specific functions for the entire body. The digestion of food, for example, would be of little value without a bloodstream to distribute the products. The working together of body systems is not haphazard; the time and location of one set of activities is closely related to others. The survival of any complex organism requires the *coordination* of vital processes taking place within it. The nervous system and the hormonal systems share this important body function.

The functions of the nervous system include: (1) sensing and responding to changes that take place in the external environment; (2) regulating organ systems; and (3) maintaining several aspects of the organism's internal environment in response to conditions occurring within the organism. This system consists of a vast number of slender outgrowths of nerve cells, the ***nerve fibers,*** that connect cells sensitive to certain environmental changes ***(receptors)*** with those responsible for carrying out an organism's responses ***(effectors).***

The central nervous system (CNS) consists of the brain and spinal cord. The brain is encased within the bones of the skull. It is continuous with the spinal cord, which is surrounded by the segments of the vertebral column (Figure 35–1). The main regions of the brain are the ***cerebrum, cerebellum,*** and ***brain stem.*** It is the brain stem that serves as the relay between the brain and the spinal cord and that controls heart rate, respiration, and several other body functions. Both the brain and spinal cord are hollow, contain ***cerebrospinal fluid,*** and are covered by the three **meninges** (membranes), called the dura mater (outer), arachnoid (middle), and pia mater (inner) sheaths.

The cerebrospinal fluid fills a space between the pia mater and arachnoid known as the subarachnoid space. The fluid provides nutrients and serves as a shock absorber for the brain and cord. Normally, the skull, vertebral column, and meninges provide considerable protection to nervous system components.

A variety of microorganisms cause infections of the central nervous system. Fever, general weakness, headache, and a stiff neck are typical signs of a CNS infection. Other signs and symptoms, as well as diagnostic features and treatment for some infections, are given in Tables 35–1 and 35–3.

Diseases of the Central Nervous System

Injuries and disorders involving the parts of the nervous system produce varied but definite effects. Symptoms of such conditions are particularly distressing. Among the most severe symptoms are paralysis, uncontrolled body movements, and loss of control over body. Breathing or heart beat is sometimes affected, and the disease may produce a variety of emotional states. Injuries due to trauma, as from an automobile accident or a fall are usually quite obvious. However, other causes may produce much the same effects but often some time later. Disorders of the system can also result from birth trauma, from genetic defects, and from tumors, as well as from microbial infections (Table 35–1). Only the major microbial diseases of the brain and spinal cord, such as meningitis, encephalitis, and abscess will be described.

Bacterial Diseases of the Nervous System

BRAIN ABSCESS

Nervous tissue and the meninges respond to bacterial invasion as other tissues do. Pus-producing (pyogenic) organisms that invade brain tissue produce an inflammation with pus formation, which results in an abscess.

Several bacteria have been associated with this type of infection, including the common pyogenic organisms *Escherichia coli, Streptococcus pneumoniae,*

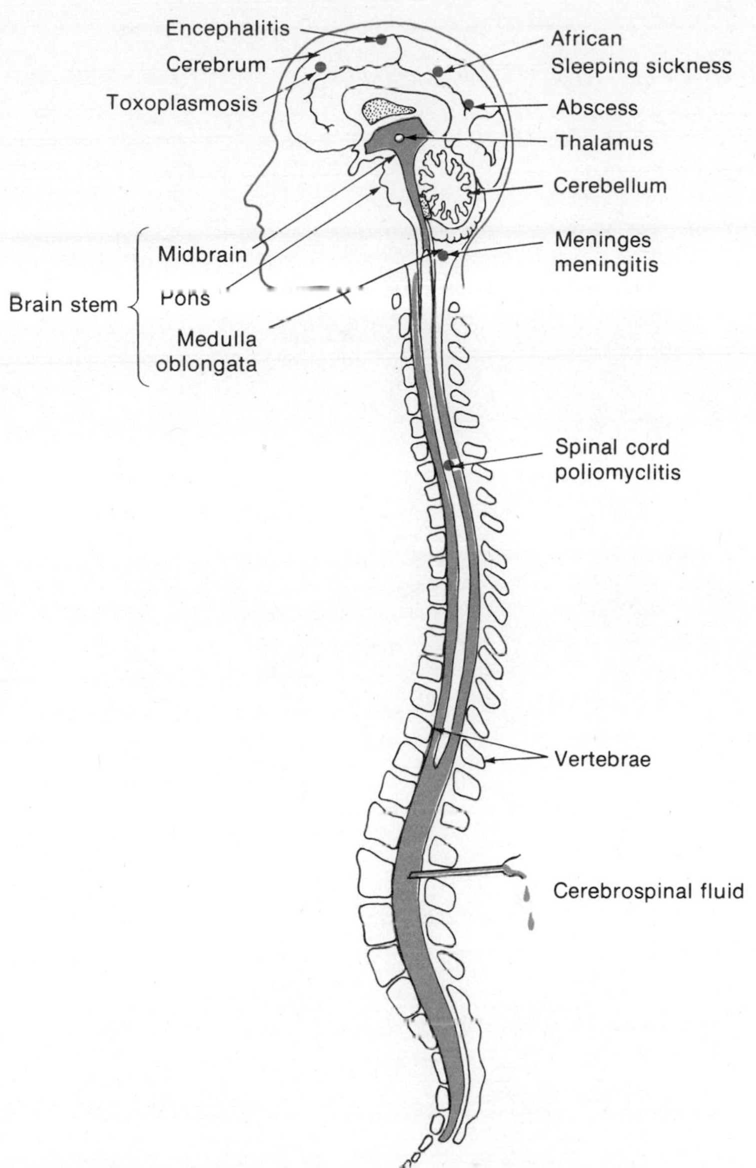

FIG. 35-1 The human central nervous system. Diseases affecting the central nervous system are also indicated.

Proteus spp., *Staphylococcus aureus*, and *Streptococcus* spp.

Anaerobic agents are believed to cause most, if not all, bacterial brain abscesses of a nontraumatic nature. The anaerobic diphtheroids and streptococci and *Bacteroides*, *Clostridium*, and *Veillonella* are involved. The anaerobic streptococci are the most frequent pathogen, followed by *Bacteroides*. Brain abscesses caused by *Clostridium* are seldom found in civilian populations.

Most brain abscesses are complications that develop from chronic (old) pus-producing sites in other portions of the body, such as the lungs, middle ear, paranasal sinuses, pelvis, and pleura. Dissemination of organisms from these foci of infection can occur (1) by direct extension through bones, (2) via the covering of the olfactory nerves, and (3) by way of the venous system. Most brain abscesses are associated with mastoiditis, middle ear infections, or tumors of the middle ear. The cerebral hemispheres are the regions of the brain in which abscesses most commonly form. This infection rarely occurs in the spinal cord.

TABLE 35-1 Representative Microbial Diseases of the Nervous System

Disease	Causative Agent	Gram Reaction	Morphology	Incubation Period	General Features of the Disease	Laboratory Diagnosis
Aseptic meningitis	Enteroviruses, mumps virus	Not applicable	Not applicable	Unknown	Fever, irritation, stiffness of the neck, and general fatigue	1. Isolation of causative agent by tissue culture or other means from spinal fluid 2. Serological tests such as complement fixation[a]
Brain abscess	*Escherichia coli*, *Proteus* spp.	−	Rods	Unknown	Fever, headache, nausea, pus formation and possible interference with vision, breathing, hearing and movement	1. Isolation and demonstration of organisms in specimens 2. Biochemical testing of isolated agent for identification
	Staphylococcus aureus,	+	Cocci			
	Streptococcus pneumoniae,	+	Cocci			
	Streptococcus spp.	+	Cocci			
Meningococcal meningitis[b]	*Neisseria meningitidis*	−	Coccus	Unknown	Fever, headache, pus formation, and infections of the bones in the skull or ear	1. Isolation and demonstration of organisms in specimens 2. Biochemical testing of isolated agent for identification
Rabies (hydrophobia)	Rabies virus	Not applicable	Not applicable	4–6 weeks or longer	Fever, general discomfort, headache, visual difficulties, painful throat spasms,[c] convulsions, delirium, respiratory paralysis, and death	1. Fluorescent antibody technique[a] 2. Demonstration of Negri bodies in brain tissue of inoculated mice
Viral encephalitis	Arbor viruses including Eastern Equine, St. Louis, and Western Equine encephalitis virus	Not applicable	Not applicable	4–21 days	Fever, chills, nausea, general fatigue, drowsiness, pain and stiffness of neck, and general disorientation; blindness, deafness, and paralysis may develop as consequence of infection	1. Serological tests such as complement fixation, hemagglutination and hemagglutination inhibition[a] 2. Isolation and identification from autopsy specimens in tissue culture of laboratory animals[d]

[a]Refer to Chapter 24 for descriptions of these procedures.
[b]Several other microorganisms can cause meningitis as a complication or secondary effect of disease states. These include the bacteria *Escherichia coli, Haemophilus influenzae, Staphylococcus aureus, Streptococcus pneumoniae*, species of *Proteus* and *Pseudomonas*, and anaerobes such as *Bacteroides, Clostridium*, and *Streptococcus*. The yeast *Cryptococcus neoformans* also is associated with meningitis.
[c]This fear of painful swallowing of fluids, which can cause attacks of convulsive choking, is responsible for naming this disease *hydrophobia*.
[d]Refer to Chapter 12 for a description of tissue cultures.

MENINGITIS

Microorganisms present in the circulatory system of the individual experience great difficulty in entering the CNS. This is largely because of the blood-brain barrier. Unless some form of injury or other condition occurs to alter the permeability of this barrier, organisms are unable to penetrate. However, once infectious agents gain entrance to the brain and the adjacent meninges, the invasion and destruction of the nervous tissue can proceed rapidly. The outcome of the disease, of course, depends upon the initial treatment of patients.

Meningitis—inflammation of the membranes around the brain and spinal cord—can result from one of several mechanisms. These include the introduction of microorganisms: (1) through penetrating injuries or primary infections involving the skull and spinal column; (2) by the direct extension of a disease process from primary foci of infection located in other parts of the body through bone via vascular channels, or along the covering of the olfactory nerves; and (3) by means of the bloodstream (hematogenous route) during the course of a septicemia.

Meningeal inflammation can be classified into two types, inflammation of the dura mater and inflammation of the pia mater and the arachnoid of the brain and spinal cord. The first of these conditions is a localized infection and almost always results from a direct extension of an infection located in the surrounding tissues. Usually inflammation of the dura mater occurs as a complication of infected skull fractures or as a related effect. The dura appears to limit the infection and prevent involvement of the leptomeninges. Although the infection may be effectively localized by the dura, it may spread to the leptomeninges or the brain by means of infected veins.

At least 50 different organisms have been incriminated in these disease states. Three bacterial species, namely *S. pneumoniae, H. influenzae,* and *N. meningitidis,* are the most commonly encountered agents. Many of these pathogens reach the meninges by the routes discussed previously. However, sometimes organisms have been introduced through the injection of contaminated solutions, such as local anaesthetics, into the cerebrospinal fluid. Certain *Pseudomonas* meningitis cases have been reported to occur in this manner.

The general clinical picture caused by many of these organisms is similar to that produced in meningococcal meningitis (Table 35–1).

MENINGOCOCCAL MENINGITIS (CEREBROSPINAL FEVER)

Neisseria meningitidis is capable of causing the death of a human faster than any other infectious agent. Death of patients has been reported to occur in less than 2 hours after the appearance of the first symptoms. Infections with meningococci frequently develop among closed populations, such as jails, military posts, schools, and ships. The causative agent is believed to be transmitted by droplets as with other respiratory diseases. *N. meningitidis*, like certain other members of the genus, is unable to withstand the adverse effects of the environment for any appreciable length of time and therefore can probably cause infections only by some form of direct contact.

Menigococcal meningitis has presented a serious problem in Africa since World War II. Group A organisms are predominant. The disease has been found in an area extending across Africa from the shores of the Atlantic Ocean to those of the Red Sea, and north of the equator to south of the Sahara. This region is referred to as the "meningitis belt."

Prevention. Preventive measures against meningococcal infections are few. The isolation of carriers during times of epidemics would be extremely difficult in view of the sheer numbers of persons involved. Prophylactic mass treatment for substantial periods of time constitutes a danger in that resistant strains would more likely emerge. Vaccines appear to be one of the few possibilities to avert epidemics. Preparations to actively immunize individuals against meningococcus have been developed.

MENINGITIS CAUSED BY ANAEROBES

Meningitis is only rarely caused by anaerobic bacteria, though several of the species associated with brain abscesses have been implicated with this disease. Included in this group of causative agents are *Actinomyces*, anaerobic streptococci, *Bacteroides*, and clostridia. Most meningitis caused by *Bacteroides* and anaerobic streptococci (Figure 35–2) has come from middle ear or sinus infections. Clostridia are usually considered the causative agents of anaerobic meningitis arising as a complication of head injuries or surgery.

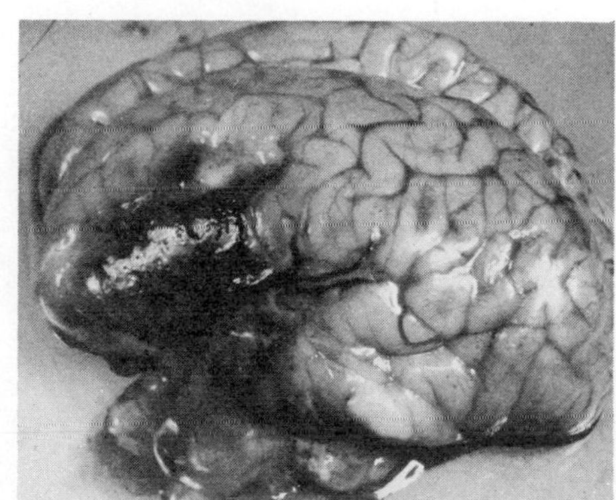

FIG. 35–2 Manifestation of anaerobic streptococci in the human brain. *Courtesy of the Armed Forces Institute of Pathology, Washington, D.C., Neg. No. 54–13308–1.*

Viral Infections of the Nervous System

Many viruses are associated with nervous system disease (Table 35–1). These pathogens are referred to as ***neurotropic***. Brief descriptions of selected diseases and the viral agents associated with them are presented in Table 35–1. Viruses may gain access to the central nervous system by several means, including cellular blood components, cerebrospinal fluid, olfactory nerve fibers, and nerves. Certain neurotropic viral infections are described in this section.

ASEPTIC (NONBACTERIAL) MENINGITIS

Aseptic meningitis is both one of the most common syndromes and also the easiest to recognize. Such infections occur world-wide in epidemic form and primarily involve children. Several viral agents have been incriminated as causes. It should be noted that a wide spectrum of clinical states can be caused by these viruses.

PICORNAVIRUSES

The picornavirus group contains several viruses that can produce infections of the human nervous system, such as coxsackieviruses, echoviruses, and polioviruses.

Poliomyelitis. This viral infection has been found in every country where it has been sought. However, within the last few years, the various types of polio vaccines have significantly reduced the incidence of the disease.

Three antigenic types are known. Poliovirus is generally (though not universally) believed to enter the body via the mouth and intestines. The organisms multiply primarily in the digestive system. The spreading of poliovirus to the nervous system occurs by way of the blood. Poliovirus is excreted in the feces before extensive involvement of the nervous system develops. Several authorities also strongly believe that poliovirus is transmitted to the central nervous system by way of the peripheral nerves (the neural route). Several effects, ranging from minor illness to paralysis, can occur as a result of poliovirus infection.

Several factors are known to either predispose or aggravate paralytic poliomyelitis. These factors include physical exertion, especially during the early phase of the disease, pregnancy near term, routine intramuscular injections, and tonsillectomy.

The effective control of poliomyelitis can be achieved by (1) adequate diagnosis, classifications, and reporting of polio cases, (2) routine immunizations, (3) control of outbreaks, and (4) mass immunization programs.

Individuals recovering from polio infection usually acquire an active state of immunity to the viral type causing the disease.

The coxsackieviruses. The first coxsackie viral agent was isolated by Dalldorf and Sickles in 1948. The virus was recovered from suckling (unweaned) mice that were inoculated with fecal matter of children from Coxsackie, New York. Two main groups of these viruses are recognized, A and B. Coxsackieviruses exhibit the general characteristics described earlier for the picornavirus group. However, their pathogenicity for suckling mice rather than for adult animals is a feature that distinguishes them from the other picornaviruses, echoviruses and polioviruses.

Diseases caused by group A coxsackieviruses include aseptic meningitis, herpangina (an ulcerative condition of the throat), minor respiratory illness, myocarditis, paralytic illness, and rubelliform rashes accompanied by fever. The diseases associated with the group B coxsackie viruses include aseptic meningitis, epidemic pleurodynia, myocarditis, neonatal encephalomyocarditis, and paralytic illness. A virus related to this group has been implicated as a

diabetes-causing agent. It was isolated from the pancreas of a 10-year-old boy who had rapidly developed symptoms of diabetes and died after a week's hospitalization.

Most often, these disease agents are spread either directly or indirectly by contact with contaminated articles **(fomites)** and aerosols.

The echoviruses. The group of viruses known as echoviruses is commonly found in the human gastrointestinal tract. They are considered to be the most common cause of aseptic meningitis, as nearly all strains comprising the group have been associated with the illness. Other disease effects caused by echoviruses include diarrhea, fever, and mild respiratory illness.

RABIES (HYDROPHOBIA)

The viral infection rabies has been a dreaded disease since the time of the ancient civilizations of Egypt, Greece, and Rome. According to the fifth report of the WHO Expert Committee on Rabies, issued in 1966, rabies exists in two "epidemiologic" varieties: (1) the urban form, characteristically associated with dogs, and (2) the wildlife variety, which occurs in animals such as bats, coyotes, foxes, jackals, mongooses, skunks, and weasels.

The principal source of rabies virus is believed to be wild mammals. Humans and domesticated animals, such as cows, goats, horses, and sheep, acquire this disease accidentally. Saliva containing the rabies virus introduced into humans by the bite of a rabid animal is the principal means of transmission. Infection through minor scratches and via the respiratory tract has also been reported. The virus responsible for the disease is called ***street virus*** or virus ***de rage de rue***. Strains of this street virus passed through rabbits are known as ***fixed virus*** or ***virus fixé***.

Rabies in lower animals. The incubation period in dogs ranges from 2 to 8 weeks. Infected animals exhibit changes in their behavioral patterns, such as stumbling and gnawing on sticks and stones. In the "furious" type of rabies, dogs characteristically snap and bite; in "dumb" rabies, they exhibit paralysis. The infection in dogs can be easily transmitted to other animals by biting. Often the saliva of infected dogs contains virus shortly before the disease symptoms appear.

Bat-transmitted rabies has been found to involve fruit-eating, insectivorous, and vampire bats. When these animals become rabid, they bite one another as well as other animals in the area.

Other important reservoirs of rabies are the wildlife populations of several countries. The infection can occur in either the furious or dumb varieties. The tendency of rabid animals, such as skunks and wolves, to enter villages, cities, and even homes poses a continuous threat to the well-being of humans and domestic animals.

Treatment. Various procedures have been used to treat individuals bitten by rabid animals. The World Health Organization Expert Committee on Rabies recommends the following:

1. Animals suspected of being rabid should be confined, if possible, observed, and examined for at least 10 days. Treatment should not await the confirmation of rabies in the animal. However, the failure to detect the virus by a thorough laboratory investigation is a sufficient basis for stopping the course of vaccine injections.
2. Local treatment of bites should be carried out. Procedures would include the thorough washing of the wound with soap and water or other appropriate materials known for their viricidal effects (e.g., quaternary ammonium

compounds). The topical administration of rabies antiserum or specific immune globulin preparations should be considered and should be conducted or supervised by a physician.

3. The injection of rabies vaccine and antiserum should be instituted.
4. Preventive measures against tetanus and other bacterial infections also should be observed.

The vaccines used in antirabies treatment are of several types. The first of these, developed by Pasteur, utilized infected rabbit spinal cord material which was suspended over a drying agent in a closed jar. The purpose of this procedure was to inactivate the viral agent. Today vaccines are prepared from the nervous tissues of various animals, such as calves, goats, horses, rabbits, and sheep. However, the method used for the inactivation of the virus is treatment with phenol at different temperatures. Vaccines prepared from duck embryos and suckling mice are inactivated by exposure to β-propriolactone and ultraviolet irradiation, respectively.

In the treatment of individuals exposed to rabies virus, the injections of vaccines are given subcutaneously in the abdominal area (but not in the stomach, as many persons believe). The number of injections is determined by the location and the severity of the wound. The most recently developed rabies treatment is Human Rabies Immune Globulin (HRIG), which produces a form of passive (temporary) immunity.

Vaccines are also available for the immunization of humans and lower animals.

Control. The control of rabies presents several problems. However, certain measures recommended by the fifth report of the WHO Expert Committee on Rabies, if properly implemented, could significantly reduce the incidence of the disease. Included in their recommendations were the following: (1) prophylactic immunization not only of dogs, but also of cats; (2) the establishment of clinics in localities where rabies prevails; (3) the elimination of stray dogs and the quarantine of dogs imported into "island communities"; and (4) the incorporation of programs to eliminate or significantly reduce "proven" wildlife vectors.

SLOW VIRUS DISEASES

The concept of slow virus infections was first introduced by Sigurdsson in 1954 in his classic descriptions of several chronic diseases of Icelandic sheep. Since then, additional slow virus infections have been described in humans and domestic animals. These disorders are characterized by a slow, almost imperceptible onset and a long-lasting and progressive course leading eventually to death. Slow virus infections may be defined as a group of disease states caused by viruses in which the incubation periods are extremely long and in which the clinical expressions or course of the infections are relatively slow to appear. The outstanding feature of these infections is the persistence of a viral agent or its genetic components in a host who ultimately experiences cellular and tissue injury from the activities of the virus.

The reason for the long incubation periods of these diseases is unknown. The viral agents may be masked or hidden as a result of either immunoglobulin activity or an integrated effect of the virus that is not fully expressed.

The agents associated with this group of disease states are classified into two major categories, conventional and nonconventional, based on the recognized characteristics of the viruses. The conventional category includes the agents of lymphocytic choriomeningitis, herpesvirus-associated persistent infections, rabies, progressive multifocal choriomeningitis, and subacute sclerosing panencephalitis (SSPE). All conventional agents show evidence of complete viral structure or substructure components. In addition, they provoke immune responses in the infected host and induce either degenerative or inflammatory changes in a variety of tissues. The unconventional group includes the agents of scrapie, kuru, Creutzfeldt-Jakob disease, and transmissible mink encephalopathy. These agents, unlike those of the conventional group, do not exhibit a virion structure or substructure, are not antigenic, and produce degenerative changes confined to the central nervous system.

THE ARBOVIRUSES (ARTHROPOD-BORNE)

To date well over 300 arboviruses have been reported. Only about 100 of these are capable of causing human infection. The first arbovirus to be identified was the causative agent of yellow fever. In 1901, Major Walter Reed and his colleagues clearly demonstrated not only the relationship of the mosquito *Aëdes aegypti* to the transmission of yellow fever but established the existence of the first human viral pathogen.

The arboviruses have the unique capability of multiplying within the tissues of vertebrates and of certain blood-sucking arthropods. Viruses of this group, following their inoculation into the tissues of a susceptible vertebrate, multiply rapidly. In cases of human and certain lower animal infections, the virus may localize in the central nervous system of the host, causing extensive viral multiplication, tissue injury, encephalitis, and eventual death.

Most arboviruses are either togaviruses or bunyaviruses. The togaviruses are divided into two genera, *Alphavirus* (previously known as group A arboviruses) and *Flavivirus* (previously known as group B arboviruses). The bunyaviruses represent about 100 arboviruses. Table 35–2 lists features of some arboviruses.

Alphaviruses. Among the alphaviruses are several pathogens that can cause severe encephalitis. A wide range of vertebrates and arthropods can be involved in their life cycles; these include domestic fowl, horses, humans, rodents, snakes, and wild birds. Humans are considered to be only incidental hosts. Horses do not appear to be significant natural reservoirs either. The primary hosts are birds, while snakes and certain rodents are probably secondary reservoirs for some alphaviruses. The majority of alphaviruses are transmitted by mosquitoes. Hibernating mosquitoes have been reported to harbor viruses for several months.

Two types of clinical disease states have been observed with these viruses. One form, which is found in Eastern, Western and Venezuelan equine encephalitis, consists of both a systemic phase with chills, fever, headache, and vomiting, and an encephalitic phase with stupor or coma, perhaps followed by slight paralysis.

Flaviviruses. The flaviviruses include at least 36 prototype strains. Most of these arboviruses are transmitted by culicine *(Culex)* mosquitoes, exhibit a host range and initial stages of pathogenesis similar to that of group A agents, and produce variable clinical syndromes. Flavivirus infections may produce three types of symptomatology: (1) acute central nervous system involvement resulting in encephalitis and death; (2) severe systemic illness affecting important visceral organs, including the kidneys and the liver; and (3) a milder form of systemic involvement characterized by fever, a rash, and severe muscle pains. Subclinical infections can also be produced by these viruses.

Bunyaviruses. The Bunyaviruses are immunologically distinct from the other arbovirus groups. Animals implicated as natural reservoirs on the basis of epidemiological investigations include monkeys, opossums, rats, and sloths. The full range of mosquito vectors has not been fully determined.

TABLE 35-2 Some Groups of the Arbovirus

Group Designation	*Disease*	*Vector (M=Mosquito; T=Tick)*	*Geographic Distribution*
Alphaviruses	Eastern equine encephalitis (EEE)	M	Argentina, Brazil, Dominican Republic, Guyana, Panama, Trinidad, United States
	Venezuelan equine encephalitis (VEE)	M	Brazil, Colombia, Ecuador, Panama, Trinidad, Venezuela
	Western equine encephalitis (WEE)	M	Argentina, Brazil, Canada, Guyana, Mexico, United States
Flaviviruses	Dengue fever	M	Australia, Greece, New Guinea, Pacific Islands, Southeast Asia
	Japanese B encephalitis	M	Eastern Asian mainland, Guam, India, Japan, Malaya
	Russian spring-summer encephalitis	T	Northern European Russia, Siberia
	St. Louis encephalitis	M	United States, Jamaica
	Yellow fever	M	Africa, Central and South America, Trinidad
Bunyavirus	Bunyamwera	M	South Africa, Uganda
	Germiston	M	South Africa
	Guaroa	M	Brazil, Colombia

Control of arthropod-transmitted diseases. The control measures used for arbovirus infections are directed against the arthropod vectors (lice, mites, mosquitoes, sandflies, and ticks). This usually involves the use of insecticides, natural predators, and other functional means. Eradication programs designed to destroy the breeding sites or structures that provide protection are necessary to reduce the reproduction rates of vectors. Measures of this type will decrease successive generations.

Control measures also involve attacks on the reservoirs of infectious agents. This can be done through the use of traps and professional hunters. Furthermore, effective vaccines can also be used as prophylactic measures against such diseases as certain rickettsial infections and yellow fever.

Protozoan Infections of the Central Nervous System

TOXOPLASMA GONDII

The causative agent of toxoplasmosis was originally discovered in 1908 by Nicolle and Manceaux, in a small North Africa rodent, the gondi *(Tenodactylus gondi)*. The organism's name is derived in part from this animal. *T. gondii* (Color Photograph 43) exhibits a wide host range. In the late 1930s it was recognized that toxoplasma are associated with a type of infection that results in brain damage of the newborn. Infants may show evidence of the infection at birth or shortly thereafter. Features of the disease, laboratory diagnosis, and possible treatment are given in Table 35-3.

Transmission. T. gondii can be transmitted through the placenta (transplacental route). Other modes of transmission have created interest among investigators, particularly because the domesticated cat was implicated as a carrier of the disease agent. Recent evidence has indicated that cat feces contain one stage of the life cycle (Figure 35-3) that has a high resistance to the environment as long as it is in the presence of moisture. Because domesticated cats bury their excreta, usually in moist soil, they are a potential link in the transmission. Cat litter and sandboxes, in particular, may be a source of infection for individuals who clean the box and inhale or ingest the cysts. Because toxoplasmosis is a disease of rodents, cats that eat infected mice can become infected in turn. A cat that is not permitted to roam or to eat raw meat is unlikely to acquire the infection.

While the cat is the main animal whose feces have been implicated in transmission, toxoplasma may be found in practically every mammal and in some birds. Therefore, ingestion of raw meat by humans or other animals can contribute to the spread of the disease agent (Figure 35–3). *T. gondii* (Figure 35–4) is also found in soil. Although the actual incidence is uncertain, it is now believed that many retarded individuals are victims of toxoplasmosis. In addition, subclinical cases of the disease are occurring in various parts of the United States.

Prevention. Infection in a pregnant woman represents the greatest public health problem by virture of transmission to the developing fetus. The following suggestions are therefore of particular importance to pregnant women.

1. Avoid eating undercooked or raw meat.
2. If a cat is already a family pet, and if a litterbox or sandbox is used, have another person clean and handle it.
3. If a cat is to be purchased and kept as a family pet, keep it indoors and don't feed it raw meat products.

It should be noted that if serological testing shows that a woman prior to becoming pregnant has antibodies against *T. gondii*, the danger to the fetus is low.

AFRICAN SLEEPING SICKNESS

The effects of African sleeping sickness (Figure 35–5) were originally recognized in two separate geographical regions and were therefore considered to be

TABLE 35–3 Selected Features of Protozoan Diseases of the Central Nervous System

Disease	*Causative Agent*	*Incubation Period*	*General Features of the Disease*	*Laboratory Diagnosis*	*Possible Treatment*
Toxoplasmosis	*Toxoplasma gondii*	Unknown	When symptoms occur in adults they include: chills, fever, headache, extreme discomfort, and muscle pain; symptoms resemble infectious mononucleosis; symptoms of newborns who contract the disease *in utero* include fever, convulsions, enlarged spleen, and serious central nervous system defects causing blindness and mental retardation	Serodiagnostic tests, e.g., fluorescent antibody procedures (Color Photograph 43) and Sabin-Feldman dye test[a]	Pyrimethamine, sulfonamides
Trypanosomiasis (African sleeping sickness)	*Trypanosoma gambiense, T. rhodesiense*	6–14 days	Disease may continue for years; symptoms include enlargement of lymph nodes, spleen, and liver; fever, chills, disturbed vision, general weakness, headache, loss of appetite, occasional rash, nausea, vomiting, and serious defects of the central nervous system, ending in death	1. Demonstration of organisms in specimens (Color Photograph 5) 2. Serodiagnostic tests, e.g., fluorescent antibody procedures[a]	For early stages, aromatic diamidine suramin; for later stages, Med b (a phenylarsonate derivative)

[a]Refer to Chapter 24 for a discussion of these techniques.

two distinctly different diseases (Table 35–3). ***Trypanosoma gambiense***, the causative agent of Gambian trypanosomiasis, was first observed in 1901. The discovery of *T.* ***rhodesiense***, the causative agent of Rhodesian trypanosomiasis, was reported some eight years later. *T.* ***gambiense*** is widely distributed in the western and central portions of Africa, while *T.* ***rhodesiense*** appears to be restricted almost entirely to the southeastern regions of the Africa continent. Neither form should be confused with the virus-induced sleeping sickness infections, Eastern and Western equine encephalitis, which are found in the United States and other parts of the world.

Transmission and life cycle. Gambian trypanosomiasis is contracted by humans through the bite of the tsetsefly, ***Glossina palpalis***. The insect vectors for *T.* ***rhodesiense***, *G.* ***morsitans***, and *G.* ***pallidipes*** are closely related tsetse fly species (Figure 35–6).

Trypanosomes are taken into the tsetse fly during a blood meal (Color Photograph 5) from an infected host. The parasites pass into the insect's intestine and other regions where they develop, mature, and eventually transform into infective units called ***metacyclic trypanosomes***. This last form is similar to the stage of the parasite as it appears in blood (Color Photograph 5). The infected tsetse fly bites a susceptible host, and the cycle is thereby perpetuated.

Rhodesian trypanosomiasis presents very much the same clinical picture as Gambian sleeping sickness. However, the infection has a much shorter incubation period and a more rapid course, with death occurring in a year's time.

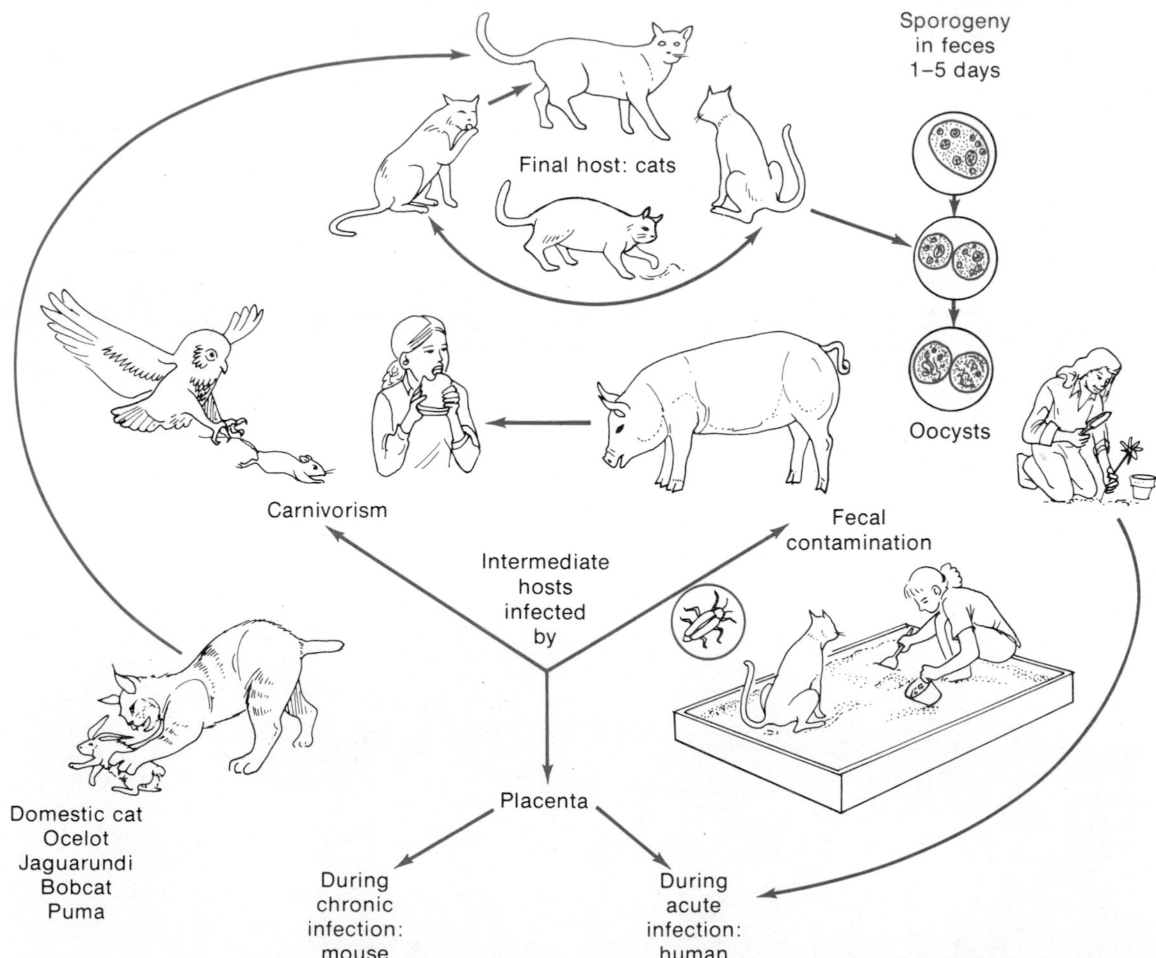

FIG. 35–3 Life cycle of *Toxoplasma gondii. After Frenkel, J. K. and J. P. Dubey,* J. Infect. Dis. *126:664–673 (1972).*

Prevention. Practical control measures for reducing the incidence of African sleeping sickness include (1) destruction of breeding sites of the tsetse flies, (2) diagnosis and treatment of the disease in patients, (3) quarantine of infected individuals, (4) wearing protective clothing against the tsetse flies, and (5) prophylactic drug administration, especially in areas where the risk of infection is great.

T. CRUZI: AMERICAN TRYPANOSOMIASIS (CHAGAS' DISEASE)

Chagas' disease, once considered rare and exotic, is now known to be a dangerous plague of the Americas. The most frequent signs of the disease involve the cardiovascular system. Involvement of the brain, liver, spleen, and spinal cord also occurs.

Trypanosoma cruzi, the causative agent of Chagas' disease, was first discovered in 1908 by Carlos Chagas in the intestines of blood-sucking, winged reduviid bugs (Color Photograph 91), common in the huts of the Brazilian hinterland. Later the parasites were found in the blood of domestic animals and of several hundred patients apparently suffering from the manifestations of *T. cruzi.* Unfortunately, it was not until much later that Chagas' disease was rediscovered and its importance recognized by Mazza and his colleagues, who recorded over 1000 acute cases by 1944. Chagas' disease is emphasized in the World Health Report of 1962, which referred to "an estimated minimum of 7 million infected individuals."

T. cruzi is known to have a geographic distribution extending from the southern United States through Mexico, Central America, and into South America to Argentina. Various wild rodents, opossums, and armadillos can harbor the parasite.

Transmission. The disease is acquired by contaminated feces of a reduviid bug (Color Photograph 91) dropped into a bite wound caused by the arthropod. After the bug has taken its blood meal, the involved area itches intensely, and scratching it moves the feces into the wound.

The parasite can also penetrate through the ocular conjuctiva. Blood transfusions from infected individuals are also an important means of the disease's transmission in endemic areas.

Infections are most common among the very young. Both sexes are equally involved.

AMOEBIC MENINGOENCEPHALITIS

A relatively "new" disease has been reported as being acquired from swimming in fresh or brackish water. Amoebic meningoencephalitis, caused by a small, free-living amoeba, *Naegleria gruberi,* has epidemiologic features that suggest a water-borne origin. In fact, in 1966 three fatal cases of primary amoebic meningoencephalitis were reported in which the evidence indicated that the disease was acquired during warm weather by swimming and diving in freshwater lakes or streams. In 1970 there was a case of meningitis reported in which a child may have acquired the disease by playing in a mud puddle.

The Eye

The eye consists of the eyeball and accessory structures, including eyebrows, eyelids, conjunctiva, and the *lacrimal* apparatus, which produces tears (Figure 35-7).

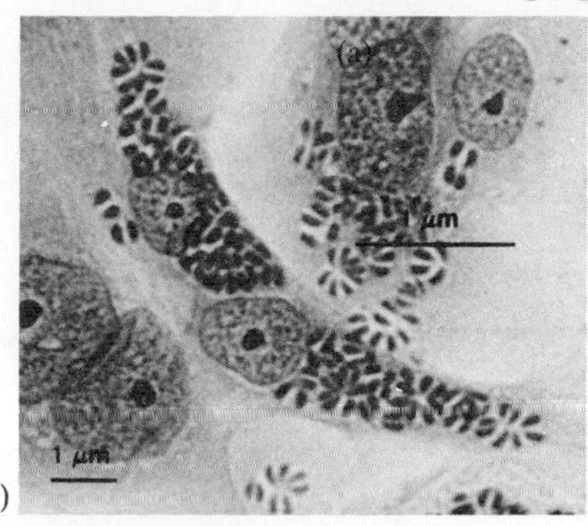

FIG. 35-4 Various stages of the parasite *Toxoplasma gondii.* The bar marker represents 10 μm. (a) A stained preparation showing an artifically excysted infective unit, or sporozoite. (b) Monkey kidney cells infected with *T. gondii* 25 days after inoculation. The infecting material was excysted sporozoites. Note the intracellular location of the parasites. *Sheffield, H. G., and M. L. Melton, National Institute of Allergy and Infectious Diseases,* Science *167:892 (1970). Copyright by the American Association for the Advancement of Science.*

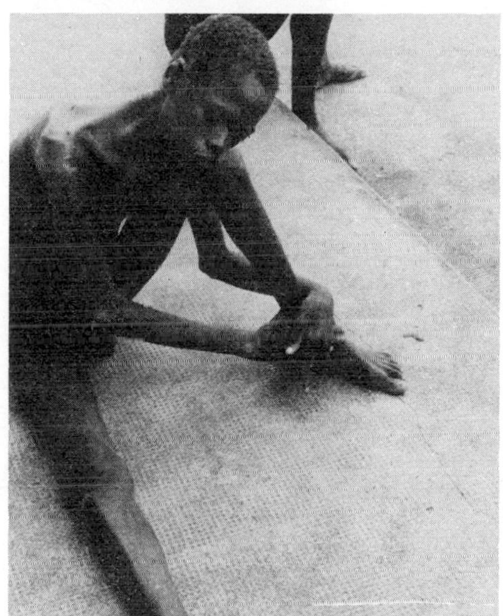

FIG. 35-5 The ravages of African sleeping sickness. *Courtesy of the World Health Organization, Geneva.*

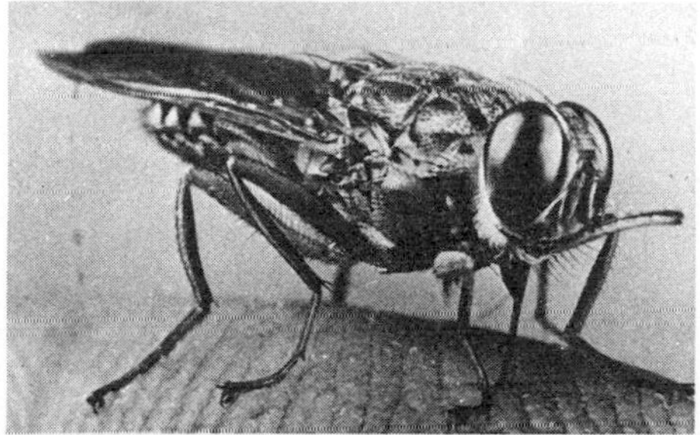

FIG. 35-6 A tsetse fly, the vector of African sleeping sickness, perched on a fingertip. *Courtesy of the World Health Organization, Geneva.*

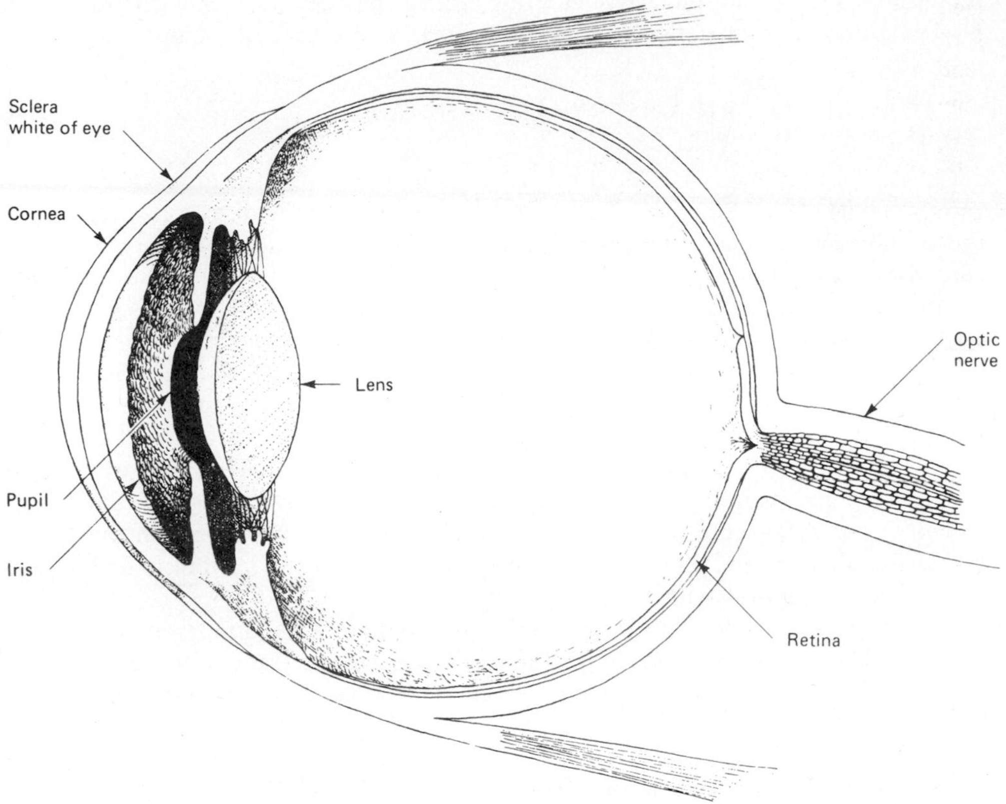

FIG. 35-7 The human eye. Diseases and associated agents of certain parts of the eye are also indicated. *Courtesy of National Institute of Neurological Diseases, Bethesda, Maryland.*

The eyeball consists of three concentric coverings, which enclose the various transparent media through which light must pass in order to reach the photosensitive retina. The outermost covering protects the inner regions and gives form to the eyeball. This coat is made up of two regions, the transparent outer ***cornea*** and the ***sclera*** (white of the eye). Light rays pass through the cornea and enter the eyeball. The sclera, behind the cornea, is opaque and mainly protective in function.

The middle vascular covering, behind the cornea, is primarily nutritive in function. It is made up of the ***chorioid proper,*** the ***ciliary body,*** and the ***iris.***

The third and innermost coat, the ***retina,*** lines the vascular covering. The retina contains several cell layers, including ***visual cells (rods*** and ***cones),*** ***ganglionic cells*** (portions of which form the optic nerve), and ***bipolar cells,*** which are involved in the visual pathway from the eye to the brain.

Figure 35-7 shows other parts of the eye, including the ***anterior chamber*** (which contains the ***aqueous humor***), the ***posterior chamber*** (which holds the ***vitreous body*** or ***humor***), and the crystalline, circular, transparent ***lens.***

The conjuctiva, a mucous membrane that lines the inner part of the eyelid, provides a thin cover for the forepart of the sclera, the inner surfaces of the eyelids, and the cornea. Tears lubricate the conjuctiva and keep it free from particulate matter.

The ***lacrimal glands*** are located above and to the side of the eyeball. Tears secreted by these glands lubricate the front of the eye and thereby prevent drying of the cornea and the development of friction between the eyelids and the eyeball. Tears have a protective function by virtue of the presence of the enzyme lysozyme. Lysozyme is bactericidal for certain saprophytic and pathogenic bacterial species.

The discussions of microbial-caused eye diseases will be limited to bacterial and viral states, since other microorganisms are rarely encountered. Tables 35–4 and 35–5 list causative agents, general disease features, laboratory diagnostic approaches, and possible treatment for microbial diseases of the eye. For discussions of treatment and of diagnostic aspects, the reader is referred to the textbooks listed in the reference section for this chapter.

Flora of the Normal Conjuctiva

A small number of microorganisms can be isolated from the normal conjuctiva, including *Corynebacterium* spp., *Branhamella catarrhalis*, staphylococci, and streptococci. Although almost any pathogenic bacterial species can cause ocular infection, such organisms may be present without producing any destructive effects. Several factors play prominent roles in protecting the human eye from infection, including the washing and bactericidal action of tears and the mechanical barrier of an intact mucous membrane.

Microbial Diseases of the Eye

Bacterial Diseases

Several bacteria are known for their specific attraction to certain ocular structures (Table 35–4). Some of them are limited only to certain regions of the eye. *Neisseria gonorrhoeae* attacks the conjuctiva, but not the lacrimal apparatus; *Hemophilus aegypticus* is associated with the conjunctiva but not with the cornea. Furthermore, several bacterial species that do not cause primary invasion of the eye or associated appendages do produce secondary infections. Examples of such pathogens include *Brucella* spp., *Escherichia coli*, and *Proteus* spp. Several organisms, such as *Bacillus anthracis*, *Clostridium* spp., and *Mycobacterium tuberculosis*, which may produce infections of the eye, rarely do so.

In several types of ocular diseases, the practice of local eye hygiene may be totally effective without the use of any other type of treatment. Local hygiene involves the removal of crusts and scales from the margins of the eyelids. The use of hot water compresses is most helpful for this purpose. Before the application of ointments, crusts and scales should always be removed.

GONOCOCCAL CONJUNCTIVITIS

Neisseria gonorrhoeae may cause two types of conjunctiva involvement—ophthalmia neonatorum (gonococcal conjunctivitis of the newborn) and conjunctivitis of the adult (Table 35–4). Complications of these infections include corneal ulceration (keratitis), scarring, and blindness.

Ophthalmia neonatorum. Ophthalmia neonatorum develops as a consequence of the passage of the fetus through the birth canal of an infected mother. Usually both eyes of the newborn infant are involved (Table 35–4).

TABLE 35-4 Diseases of the Eye Caused by Bacteria

Disease	Causative Agent	Gram Reaction	Morphology	Incubation Period	General Features of the Disease	Laboratory Diagnosis	Possible Treatment
Conjunctivitis	*Neisseria gonorrhoeae* *Staphylococcus aureus* *Streptococcus pneumoniae* *Streptococcus* spp.	– + + +	Coccus Coccus Coccus Coccus	24–27 hours	Irritation around eyelid, tearing, swelling, redness, and discharge from the involved eye	1. Demonstration of causative organisms in discharges 2. Culture and biochemical testing of isolated organisms	Erythromycin, penicillin, tetracyclines (when disease is caused by *Neisseria gonorrhoeae*); erythromycin, penicillin, cephalothin, methicillin, vancomycin (when disease is caused by *Staphylococcus aureus*, *Streptococcus pneumoniae*, or *Streptococcus* spp.)
Corneal ulcer	*Streptococcus pneumoniae*	+	Coccus	Unknown	Destruction of cornea, leading to scarring and cataract (formation of opaque area)	Diagnosis done mainly by clinical signs and symptoms	Erythromycin, penicillin
Inclusion conjunctivitis (newborn)	*Chlamydia trachomatis*	–	Rod	Within 36 hours after birth	Reddening of eyelid and pussy discharge; no scarring	1. Demonstration of organisms in scrapings or discharge from eyelid 2. Isolation by tissue culture and chick embryos 3. Immunofluorescent tests[a]	Chlortetracycline, oxytetracycline, sulfonamides
Keratitis (inflammation of the cornea)	*Moraxella lacunata* *N. meningitidis* *S. aureus* *Streptococcus mitis* *S. pneumoniae*	– – + + +	Rod Coccus Coccus Coccus Coccus	Unknown	Fever, headache, and swelling of tissues around eyes; pus formation and scarring can occur as complication; this condition can appear in combination with conjunctivitis	1. Demonstration of organisms in Gram-stained preparations of discharge 2. Culture and biochemical testing of isolated organisms	Zinc salts, antibiotics including ampicillin, kanamycin, tetracyclines (when disease is caused by *M. lacunata*); ampicillin, chloramphenicol, penicillin, tetracyclines (when disease is caused by *N. meningitidis*); cephalothin, methicillin, vancomycin (when disease is caused by *S. aureus* or *Streptococcus mitis*); erythromycin, penicillin (when disease is caused by *S. pneumoniae*)

Disease	Causative Agent	Gram Reaction	Morphology	Incubation Period	General Features of the Disease	Laboratory Diagnosis	Possible Treatment
Ophthalmia neonatorum (conjunctivitis of the newborn)	*Neisseria gonorrhoeae* *Staphylococcus aureus*	− +	Coccus Coccus	1–3 days	Effects include the involvement of both eyes, discharge consisting of blood and pus, swollen eyelids	1. Demonstration of microorganism in Gram stain of discharge 2. Culture and biochemical testing of isolated organisms	Erythromycin, penicillin, tetracyclines (when disease is caused by *N. gonorrheae*); cephalothin, lincomycin, methicillin, nafcillin (when disease is caused by *S. aureus*)
Pink eye (acute mucopurulent conjunctivitis)	*Hemophilus aegypticus*	−	Rod	1–4 days	Abundant discharge, redness, and extreme swelling of the eyelids; bleeding within the conjunctiva can occur	1. Demonstration of organisms in Gram stain of discharge 2. Culture and biochemical testing of isolated organisms	Sulfonamides, streptomycin, tetracyclines
Trachoma	*Chlamydia trachomatis*	−	Rod	5–12 days	Typical effects include accumulation of blood vessels on the surface and penetration of cornea, tumor formation, scarring, and blindness	1. Demonstration of organisms in stained scrapings of conjunctival or corneal surfaces 2. Tissue culture and embryonated egg isolation[a] 3. Immunofluorescent procedures	Chlortetracycline, oxytetracycline, sulfonamides

[a]Refer to Chapter 24 for descriptions of these procedures.

As noted in Chapter 34, preventive measures consist of the administration of a 1-percent silver nitrate solution (Crede's solution) into each thoroughly cleansed eye of the newborn infant. This procedure is given to every infant regardless of whether or not gonorrhea infection of the mother is suspected. Penicillin has also been used for prophylaxis. However, its use has not been widely accepted because instances of antibiotic sensitivity have been observed.

Gonococcal conjunctivitis in adults. In adults, gonococcal conjunctivitis is similar to that of newborns, but there is likely to be greater involvement of the conjunctiva and cornea. Adults usually contract the disease by carrying organisms to the eye from a genitourinary infection.

PINKEYE

This bacterial disease is caused by ***Hemophilus aegypticus,*** also known as Kochs-Weeks bacillus. Pinkeye is a highly contagious variety of acute catarrhal conjunctivitis. The infection occurs more commonly during the warmer months of the year.

Symptoms of pinkeye infection include a copious discharge, redness and extreme swelling of the eyelids, and subconjunctival hemmorrhages.

MORAXELLA LACUNATA (MORAX-AXENFELD DIPLOBACILLUS) INFECTIONS

Moraxella lacunata, a Gram-negative rod, has particular importance for the ophthalmologist, as it seems to cause eye diseases only involving the cornea and

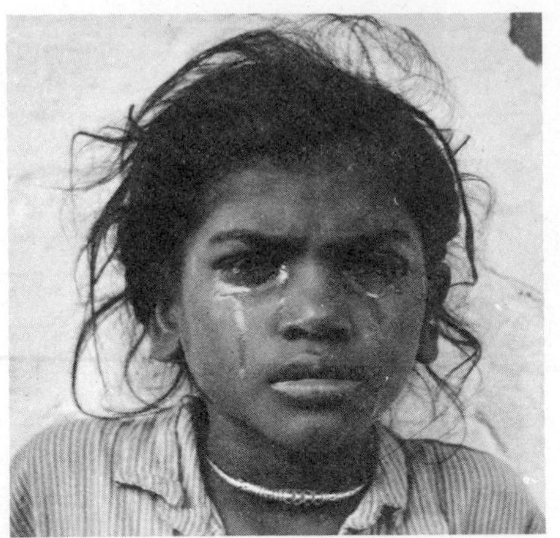

FIG. 35–8 A victim with trachoma and secondary bacterial infections. *Courtesy of World Health Organization, Geneva. Photo by Homer Page.*

conjunctiva. Infections primarily affect adults, although there have been reports of the involvement of newborns. Hot, dusty environments are closely associated with the disease states.

STREPTOCOCCAL INFECTIONS

Streptococcus pneumoniae and other species, in addition to causing upper respiratory tract infections, are known for their ability to produce severe diseases of the eye, including conjunctivitis, corneal ulcer, keratitis, and postoperative infections of the eye.

STAPHYLOCOCCAL INFECTIONS

Staphylococci are considered the most common causative agents of eye infections. Of the various eye diseases caused by staphylococci, inflammation of the eyelids and glands (blepharitis) is the most common.

In addition to blepharitis, these Gram-positive cocci cause several other diseases, including conjunctivitis in adults and newborns (staphylococcal ophthalmia neonatorum), styes, keratitis, and postoperative infections.

TRACHOMA

The contagious keratoconjunctivitis of trachoma is prevalent in various semitropical and tropical parts of the world, including Africa, the Far East, the Middle East, and South America. The disease also occurs in certain regions of North America (such as the southwest United States), as well as in certain European countries. Although trachoma does not kill, it is the largest single cause of preventable blindness (Figure 35–8). The World Health Organization has estimated that nearly 400 million people suffer from this disease. In certain rural portions of northern India, for example, the infection rate may be as high as 90 percent of the area's total population. The incidence of trachoma is closely associated with poor sanitation and heavily populated areas. Transmission of the disease agents occurs by direct contact. Flies are important mechanical vectors for *C. trachomatis*.

Immunity. Successful recovery from trachoma does not provide a guarantee against additional infections. Apparently immunity toward trachoma does not develop as a consequence of a clinical infection. The development of an effective vaccine to provide some degree of protection is now being sought.

INCLUSION CONJUNCTIVITIS

Strains of *C. trachomatis* also cause clinical diseases in the genital tract and in conjunctiva. The designation "inclusion blennorrhea" applies to genital infections, such as infections of the cervix and urethra, while "inclusion conjunctivitis" designates conjunctival inflammations caused by this organism.

Females harboring *C. trachomatis* may not exhibit any signs of infection. Mild vaginal discharges occasionally may be observed. Males acquiring the pathogenic agent usually produce a discharge, which may be a chronic or intermittent manifestation.

Inclusion conjunctivitis infection is contracted by babies on passage through the cervical canal. In the case of older individuals the disease can be acquired as a consequence of direct or indirect contact with swimming pool patrons. This type of infection, which is frequently referred to as "swimming pool conjunctivitis," is quite mild and may heal without treatment. Scarring usually does not occur.

Eye Infections Caused by Viruses

Viruses cause some of the most common and destructive eye diseases of humans (Table 35–5). Selected features of some of these pathogens and the infections they cause are included here.

TABLE 35-5 Common Eye Diseases Caused by Viruses

Disease[a]	*Causative Agent (Common Designation)*	*Possible Treatment*
Conjunctivitis	Newcastle disease virus	Symptomatic
Conjunctivitis, keratitis, or a combination of both conditions	Molluscum contagiosum virus *(Molluscovirus hominis)*	Symptomatic
Keratitis (associated with recurrent herpes); herpetic conjunctivitis (commonly found in children); purulent conjunctivitis; herpetic keratitis (corneal herpes)	*Herpesvirus hominis* (Herpes simplex virus type I)	5-iodo-2-deoxyuridine and other DNA synthesis inhibitors
Epidemic keratoconjunctivitis (EKC)	*Adenovirus*, Types 7 and 8	Symptomatic
Non-pus-forming conjunctivitis	Measles virus	Symptomatic

[a]Refer to Table 35-4 for descriptions of these conditions.

EPIDEMIC KERATOCONJUNCTIVITIS (EKC)

Human adenoviruses have a world-wide distribution. In general, these agents produce mild infections. Occasionally, involvement of the conjunctiva occurs as a consequence of direct contact with respiratory and ocular secretions. Reports have also implicated swimming pools in epidemics of conjunctivitis and sore throats with fever. Epidemic keratoconjunctivitis is commonly caused by *Adenovirus*, type 8, and appears to be the result of traumatic injury associated with dirt and dust in factories and shipyards. In addition, ophthalmologists, optometrists, and nurses may also transmit the disease agents with contaminated or improperly sterilized instruments.

Prevention. Control of keratoconjunctivitis mainly involves improvement of working conditions of factories and the incorporation of suitable measures to prevent the spread of the disease during the examination and treatment of patients. An inactivated type 8 vaccine has been effectively used in Japan to prevent this adenovirus infection.

HERPES CORNEALES

Herpesvirus hominis (herpes simplex virus) is well known for its ability to cause a wide variety of lesions in humans. One group of clinical manifestations associated with the skin or mucous membranes includes a unilateral ulcer on the conjunctiva or cornea. This ocular infection, referred to as corneal herpes, may constitute an initial (primary) infection. A recurrent type is the most commonly encountered type of eye infection caused by *H. hominis* and develops in the presence of circulating antibodies.

SUMMARY

Organization of the Central Nervous System

1. The coordination of body processes is an important function of the central nervous system (CNS).
2. The central nervous system consists of the brain and spinal cord. The brain is encased with the skull and is continuous with the spinal cord, which is surrounded by vertebrae.
3. The brain and spinal cord are hollow, contain cerebrospinal fluid, and are covered by three meninges, or membranes.

Diseases of the Central Nervous System

1. Infections and disorders of the CNS are caused by a variety of microorganisms. Typical symptoms of such infections are fever, general weakness, headache, and a stiff neck.
2. Major microbial diseases of the brain and spinal cord are abscesses, encephalitis, and meningitis.

Bacterial Diseases of the Nervous System

1. Brain abscesses are inflammations of nervous tissues caused

by pus-forming (pyogenic) aerobic and anaerobic microbes. Most brain abscesses are complications that develop from chronic (old) locations of microorganisms in other regions of the body.

2. Meningitis is an inflammation of the different protective membranes around the brain and spinal cord. The most rapidly acting form of the disease is caused by ***Neisseria meningitidis***. Infections with these meningococci frequently develop among closed populations such as jails, military posts, schools, and ships.
3. Control measures include immunization (if available) and adequate treatment.

Viral Infections of the Nervous System

1. Viruses causing infections of the CNS are called neurotropic. Examples of such infections include aseptic (nonbacterial) meningitis caused by pathogens including coxsackieviruses, echoviruses, and polioviruses; rabies (hydrophobia); and slow virus diseases.
2. Arboviruses, which replicate in and are spread by various types of arthropods, can cause extensive nervous tissue injury and encephalitis. The majority of these pathogens are known as togaviruses and bunyaviruses.
3. Most control measures for arboviruses are directed toward the elimination of arthropods and their breeding sites. Other measures involve the use of vaccines and elimination of the natural reservoirs of infectious diseases.

Protozoan Infections of the Central Nervous System

1. Protozoan infections of the CNS include toxoplasmosis, African sleeping sickness, Chagas' disease, and amoebic meningoencephalitis.
2. Toxoplasmosis, caused by ***Toxoplasma gondii***, can result in brain damage in newborns that were infected while in the uterus. Other effects include blindness and mental retardation. Sources of the disease agent include infected cats and contaminated raw meat and soil.
3. African sleeping sickness should not be confused with viral forms of encephalitis. This disease is caused by ***Trypanosoma gambiense*** and ***T. rhodesiense***, which are spread by tsetse flies.
4. Chagas' disease is caused by another trypanosome, ***T. cruzi***. Its geographic range extends from the southern portions of the United States through Mexico and into South America. Chagas' disease frequently affects part of the cardiovascular and central nervous system and is transmitted by kissing or reduviid bugs.
5. Amoebic meningoencephalitis is caused by a small, free-living amoeba, which is acquired from contaminated fresh or brackish water.

The Eye

The eye consists of the eyeball and accessory structures, including the eyebrows, eyelids, conjunctiva (inner part of the eyelid), and the lacrimal apparatus, which produces tears.

Flora of the Normal Conjunctiva

A small number of microorganisms can be isolated from the normal conjunctiva. The bactericidal action of lysozyme in tears, the flushing mechanism of tears, and the intact membranes and coverings of the eye protect against a large number of diseases.

Microbial Diseases of the Eye

Bacterial Diseases

1. Bacterial diseases of the eye include conjunctivitis, keratitis, pinkeye, and trachoma.
2. The destructive effects of these diseases can be prevented by adequate treatment with antibiotics.

Eye Infections Caused by Viruses

Examples of virus infections of the eye include epidemic keratoconjunctivitis (EKC) (caused by ***Adenovirus***, type 8) and herpes corneales (caused by herpes simplex virus).

QUESTIONS FOR REVIEW

1. Discuss the viral diseases of the central nervous system. Include in your discussion the causative agent, mode of transmission, specific structures of the system involved, diagnostic procedures used, and treatment.
2. What measures are currently available for the control of viral agents affecting the central nervous system?
3. What are slow virus infections? What significance do they have?
4. List the causative agents and the means of disease transmission for the infections given below:
   a. trachoma
   b. adult gonococcal conjunctivitis
   c. EKC
   d. angular blepharconjunctivitis
   e. pinkeye
   f. central corneal ulcers
   g. inclusion conjunctivitis
   h. stye
   i. trachoma
   j. Western equine encephalitis
5. What types of organisms comprise the normal flora of the conjunctiva? Are any of these normally pathogenic?
6. What are the distinguishing features of the arboviruses?
7. Which of the arthropod-borne diseases mentioned in this chapter are found in your immediate geographical area? What measures are utilized to control mosquito populations in your area?
8. Sleeping sickness (encephalitis) can be caused by several microbial types. Name and compare at least six causative agents as to (a) transmission, (b) geographical distribution, (c) preventive and control measures, and (d) significance as a world problem.
9. If you were planning a trip to Arabia, Egypt, Greece, Japan, and India, to which viral, bacterial, and protozoan diseases affecting the CNS would you be exposed? Refer to other chapters in this division.
10. Which of the protozoan infections mentioned in this chapter are known to occur in the United States? In your state?
11. What is toxoplasmosis? Discuss this disease from the standpoint of occurrence, life cycle, and the types of individuals susceptible to its effects.

SUGGESTED READINGS

Balows, A., R. M. DeHaan, V. R. Dowell, Jr., and L. B. Guze, *Anaerobic Bacteria: Role in Disease*. Springfield, Ill.: Charles C. Thomas, 1974. *A collection of papers on anaerobic infections, including those of the central nervous system such as meningitis and cerebral abscess. Information on the collection and handling of specimens is also provided.*

Gajdusek, D. C., "Unconventional Viruses and the Origin and Disappearance of Kuru," *Science* 197: 943–960 (1977). *An interesting description of a slow virus infection and the discovery of its mechanism of action and transmission. The article is written by a Nobel Prize recipient.*

Kaplan, C. (ed.), *Rabies, the Facts*. New York: Oxford University Press, 1977. *A collection of short articles on rabies virus, human rabies, and rabies vaccines and immunity.*

Nichols, R. L. (ed.), *Trachoma and Related Disorders Caused by Chlamydial Agents*. Assen, Netherlands: Royal Van-Gorcum, 1971. *A collection of papers, covering the molecular biology, chemistry, tissue culture, immunology, diagnostic methods, and treatment of trachoma.*

Thompson, R. A., and J. R. Green, *Advances in Neurology*. Vol. 6. *Infectious Diseases of the Central Nervous System*. New York: Raven Press, 1974. *A functional summary of infectious diseases of the fetus, children, and adults.*

CHAPTER **36**

Microorganisms and Cancer

Of all the diseases that afflict us, those labeled "cancer" produce the strongest emotions. This disease state is greatly and justifiably feared by many. What are cancers? Do microorganisms play a role in cancer causation? Chapter 36 describes the different types of malignancies and outlines the relationship of microorganisms and their products to cancer. The use of microorganisms for control and detection of cancer-causing substances is considered as well.

After reading this chapter, you should be able to:

1. **Distinguish between tumors and malignancies.**
2. **Describe the four different forms of human cancer.**
3. **Explain viral transformation.**
4. **Summarize the properties of oncogenic RNA viruses and oncogenic DNA viruses.**
5. **Discuss the role of microorganisms and their products in causing cancer.**
6. **Describe the use of microorganisms in the detection of carcinogens.**
7. **Outline and explain the current cancer virus hypotheses.**
8. **Discuss the use of microorganisms and their products in the treatment of cancerous states.**
9. **Define or explain:**
   a. **tumor antigen**
   b. **benign**
   c. **fetal proteins**
   d. **Epstein-Barr virus**

Although some animal cancers are known to be virally caused, it is widely assumed that cancers are caused by environmental factors such as chemicals and radiation, as well as certain microbial products. Despite extensive and increasingly sophisticated studies dealing with both experimentally and naturally occurring human cancers, the various causes of cancer, the role of microorganisms and their products, and the mechanisms operating in these disease states are not well understood.

General Characteristics of Cancerous States

All the tissues of the human body are composed of individual cells of varying microscopic size. These cells must be able to divide and reproduce in an exact and orderly manner for the well-being of the body to be maintained. Normal cell growth is inhibited by crowding; when sufficient cells have been produced in a given area, intercellular controls operate to stop further growth, a property called *contact inhibition*. If cellular reproduction becomes uncontrolled, growths or swellings, called *neoplasms* or *tumors*, develop. Tumors that form in a localized area and do not spread to other parts of the body are referred to as *benign*. Growths that reproduce progressively and unrestrictedly, spreading to other body regions, are called *malignant* or *cancerous*. Cancer cells spread from one part of the body to others either by invading and destroying normal tissue around the malignancy (a direct extension process) or by *metastasis*, the separation of cells from the major portion of a tumor and the movement of these cells to new sites.

Cancers have been recognized by physicians for several centuries. In ancient times they were relatively rare, and they remained a fairly insignificant cause of death until the present century. Today, however, cancers are the cause of approximately 16 percent of all deaths in the United States and more in many European countries. This great increase, especially in the past few decades, is due to improved detection procedures, environmental causes, and the increase in human life span. The effects of environmental agents on human health is currently a subject of considerable interest. Of special concern to scientists are the long-term effects of chemical, physical, and microbial agents and, more specifically, their possible *oncogenic* (tumor-causing) and *carcinogenic* (cancer-producing) effects. Many factors have been identified as modifying cellular nucleic acids and possessing carcinogenic potential.

A given tumor arises from certain normal cells of one type (its tissue of origin) that have undergone a series of changes influenced by intrinsic or extrinsic factors (Figure 36–1). *Intrinsic* factors are those within the cells or within the body as a whole. Among these are age, heredity, sex, hormonal influences, and a natural predisposition to tissue overgrowth. *Extrinsic*, or external, factors are agents that originate outside the body, such as chemicals, irradiation, and possibly viruses.

Three major characteristics seem to define cancerous states: *anaplasia*, *hyperplasia*, and metastasis. Anaplasia is a structural abnormality in which involved cells do not mature and therefore resemble primitive or embryonic cells. Hyperplasia is an uncontrolled reproduction of cells. Because malignant cells do not respond to a host's signal to stop dividing, they produce a localized accumulation of tissue. In metastasis, a malignant cell detaches itself from a tumor, moves to another anatomical site, and establishes a new tumor there.

It is interesting to note that cancers are not in themselves fatal. In general, cancerous growths do not produce toxins or otherwise kill hosts directly. Cancers create a condition of malnutrition by utilizing nutrients needed by the tissues of the host. The malnutrition state produces a generalized emaciation and poor state of health called *cachexia*.

Microbiology has had a great impact on several aspects of present-day cancer research. For example, certain microbial products have been shown to inhibit cancer. Moreover, recent progress in our understanding of the tumor growth and its prevention has come from work with microorganisms and their interactions with their hosts. This chapter describes some aspects of tumor production and malignancy with which microorganisms have been associated.

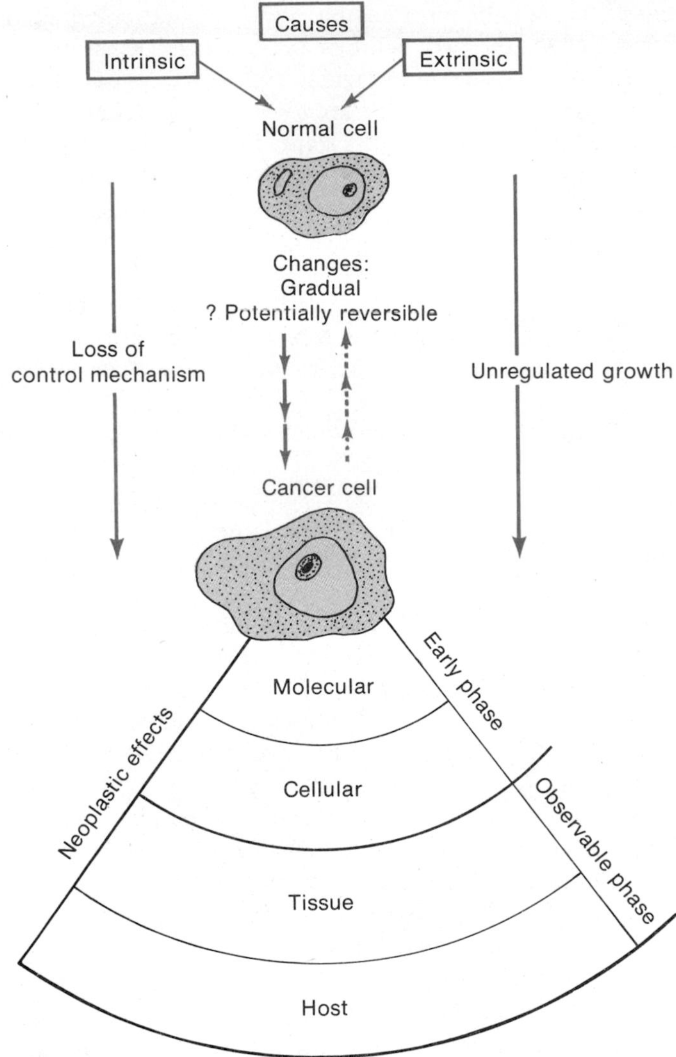

FIG. 36-1 Stages believed to take place in carcinogenesis. A normal cell interacts with the causative factors in the environment. Through a gradual process, the normal cell is transformed into a cancerous one. With the establishment of the cancerous state, the stage is set for the development of tumor cell masses and the appearance of symptoms in the host.

The Forms of Human Cancer

It is not yet clear whether the condition referred to as cancer consists of several diseases having a common pattern of general symptoms or whether it is a single disease that occurs in many forms, depending upon the tissue from which it evolves. At present, the first of these is the more widely accepted view. In any case, more than one hundred clinically distinct types of cancer are recognized, each having a unique set of specific symptoms and requiring a specific course of therapy. These types can, however, be grouped into four major categories: carcinomas, leukemias, lymphomas, and sarcomas.

Carcinomas

Carcinomas are solid tumors derived from epithelial tissues such as breasts, glands, skin, nerves, and the linings of the gastrointestinal, genital, respiratory, and urinary systems.

Leukemias

Leukemia, also called cancer of the blood, is characterized by the uncontrolled proliferation and accumulation of leukocytes, most of which do not mature into functional cells. Just as there are many different types of white cells, there are many different types of leukemia. These include (1) acute and chronic lymphocytic leukemias (lymphoblastic leukemias, Figure 36–2), which are malignancies of lymphocytes, and (2) acute and chronic myelocytic leukemias (granulocytic or myelogenous leukemias), which are disorders of granulocytes.

Acute leukemias usually appear suddenly, with symptoms similar to those of a cold, and progress rapidly. The lymph nodes, spleen, and liver may become infiltrated with leukocytes and enlarged. Symptoms frequently include bone pain, paleness, a tendency to bleed easily, and a high susceptibility to infectious diseases. The most common causes of death, which occurs if the leukemia is not treated, are hemorrhaging and uncontrolled infections.

The chronic leukemias begin much more slowly, and several years may pass before significant symptoms appear. The symptoms are similar to those of the acute leukemias. The life expectancy of an individual who goes without treatment, however, is about three years after the onset of the condition.

Although leukemias constitute one of the most common malignancies of children, persons of any age can be victims.

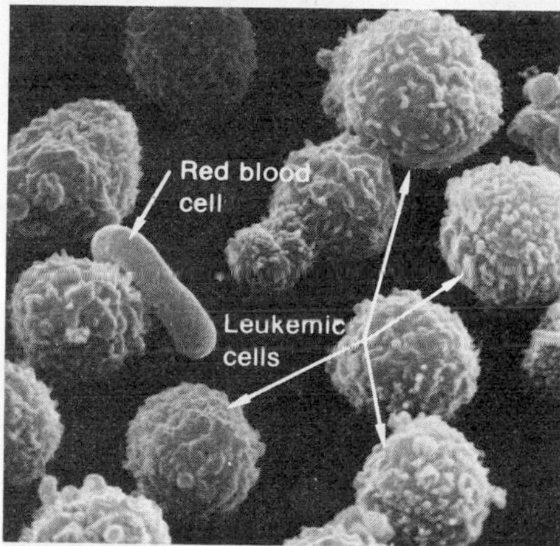

FIG. 36–2 A scanning micrograph of leukemic lymphoblasts. *Haemmerli, U., and H. Felix,* Blood Cells *2:415–430 (1976).*

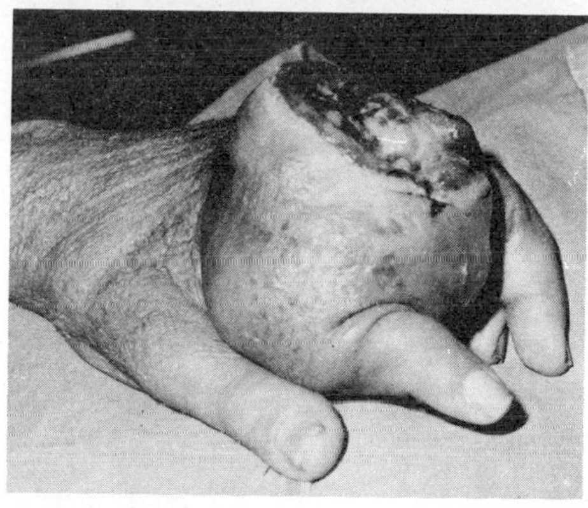

FIG. 36–3 Tumor in the bones of the hand. Because the bones of the hand are so near the surface, certain tumors of the hand extending beyond bone tend to break through the skin. *Vistnes, L. M., and W. J. Vermuelen,* J. Bone and Joint Surg. *57–A: 865–867 (1975).*

Lymphomas

In lymphomas, abnormal numbers of lymphocytes are produced by the spleen and lymph nodes. These diseases are similar to leukemia, but in some lymphomas the immature lymphocytes aggregate in the lymphoid tissues. Hodgkin's disease is the best-known form of lymphoma.

Sarcomas

Sarcomas are characterized by tumors growing from bone, cartilage, connective tissue, fat, and muscle (Figure 36–3).

Viral Transformation

Viral transformation is the process by which normal cells are altered by viral infection to become malignant. Transformed cells often undergo many changes in morphology (Figure 36–4), in metabolic functions, and in antigenicity. One of the important conclusions that some scientists have reached from animal

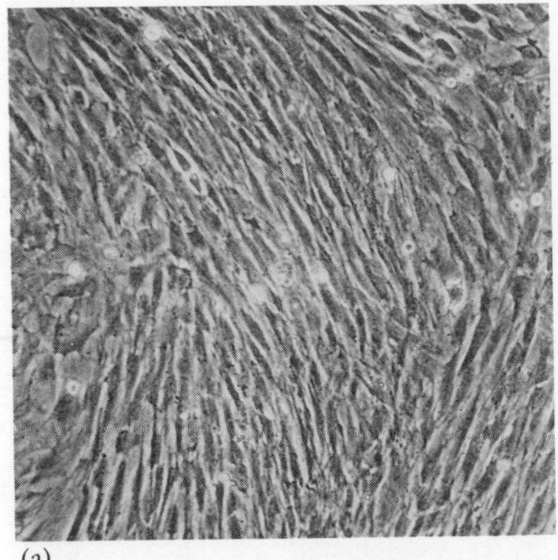

(a)

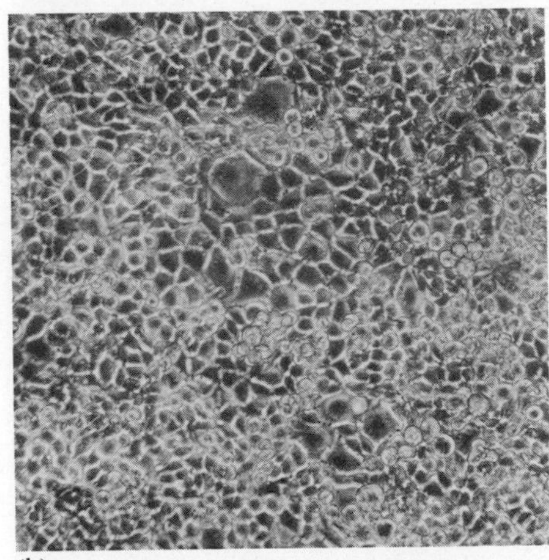

(b)

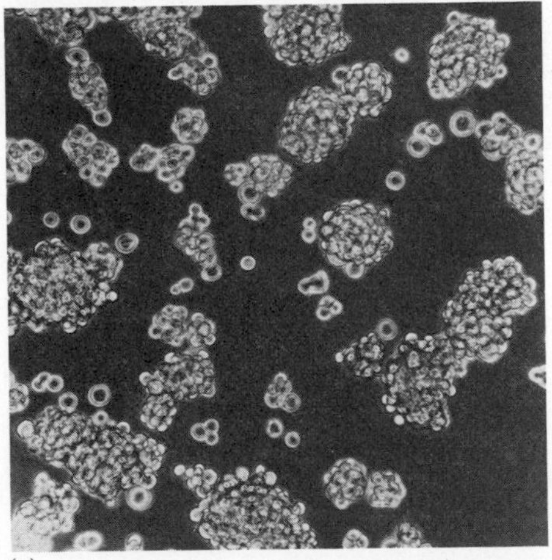

(c)

FIG. 36–4 Most viruses capable of causing tumor formation in experimental animals also transform cells to the malignant state in an *in vitro* system. Transformation results in altered cell shapes and a capacity for unregulated growth. (a) Untransformed cells. (b) The unregulated growth of transformed cells. (c) The piling up of cells over one another instead of formation of a layer such as the one shown in part (a). *Auersperg, N.* Cancer Res. *38:1872 (1978).*

experiments is that a virus must be integrated into the host cell's genome before it can transform the cell.

Certain cancer-inducing viruses readily produce cell transformation in tissue culture systems. The viral agent is often no longer recognizable in the cultures by its best-known properties, such as infectivity and antigenicity. Traces of the virus can be detected in the form of new antigens and viral DNA or RNA. Findings such as these suggest that standard procedures for the isolation and identification of viral pathogens may not be adequate for human viral cancer agents.

Early Discoveries Relating Viruses and Cancer

Acceptance of the concept that cancer can be caused by viruses has been slow despite the unequivocal and long-standing evidence from animal experiments. In 1908, V. Ellerman and O. Bang showed that leukemia in chickens could be transmitted by injecting bacteria-free filtrates from infected chickens into healthy chickens. Three years later, in 1911, Francis Peyton Rous demonstrated a similar transfer of a chicken sarcoma. But the occurrence of virus-induced tumors in chickens was generally regarded as a biological curiosity of domestic fowl. Over the next 40 years, accumulating evidence pointed to viral induction of malignancies of various types in rabbits, frogs, and mice (Figure 36–5).

The first mouse cancer viruses discovered were found to contain RNA. More recent discoveries have shown that several DNA-containing viruses also cause cancer in mice and other rodents. Virus-induced cancers in hamsters, mice, and rats by human adenoviruses were also reported. In addition, many new oncogenic viruses were discovered in the 1960s. Some of these are discussed in the next section.

Characteristics of Oncogenic RNA Viruses

Oncogenic RNA viruses are found in two of the three designated classes, A, B, and C. Type A RNA viruses, which are not infectious, are a very small group of viruslike particles that have not been found outside the confines of cells and have not been shown to be oncogenic. Type B RNA viruses have been associated primarily with certain carcinomas of the breast. Type C RNA viruses, the most important class, have been shown to infect a large number of animal species. Most type C RNA viruses are oncogenic, mainly causing leukemias, lymphomas, and sarcomas—all tumors arising in tissues such as bone, cartilage, connective tissue and lymph nodes. Table 36–1 lists RNA tumor viruses, together with their hosts and conditions produced.

Differences Among Oncogenic RNA Viruses

Distinctions among the various types of RNA tumor viruses have traditionally been based on morphology, although they can also be made on the basis of immunological differences and modes of maturation.

The type C RNA viruses consist of a roughly spherical, compact RNA core and associated proteins (nucleoid) surrounded by a lipid layer partially transpar-

TABLE 36-1 RNA Tumor Viruses

Virus	*Type*	*Host*	*Conditions Produced*
Lymphomatosis	C	Birds	Leukemias in chickens
Rous sarcoma	C	Birds, monkey, rodents	Sarcomas
Leukemia	C	Cats	Leukemia
Leukemia (MLV)	C	Mice, other rodents	Leukemia in mice (hamsters)
Mammary tumor (MTV)	B	Mice	Mammary tumors
Gibbon lymphosarcoma	C	Monkeys	Tumors
Mason-pfizer	C	Monkeys	Tumors
Wooley fibrosarcoma	C	Monkeys	Tumors

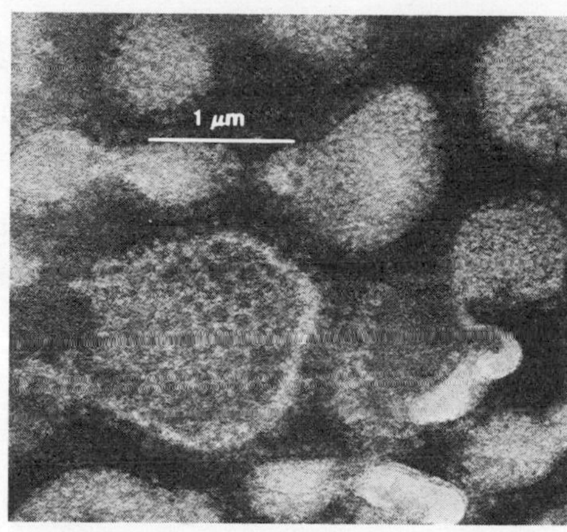

FIG. 36-5 The virion of mouse mammary tumor virus has a surface covered with spikes. The bar marker represents 0.1 μm. *Sheffield, J. B., J. Virology 12:616-624 (1973).*

ent to electrons that give electron micrographs of the virus a targetlike appearance (Figure 36-6).

The nucleoid of type B viruses is more eccentric in shape, apparently because its major internal protein is about two thirds larger than that of the type C viruses. The glycoprotein surface spikes of the type B viruses are larger and more regularly spaced than those of the type C viruses.

The type A particles occur in two subtypes, one found in cellular cytoplasm and one found in the lymph and other extracellular body fluids. Those found in the cytoplasm are believed to be immature forms of type B viruses, to which they are immunologically similar. The morphology of type A particles is similar to that of the other viruses, but the type A particles are encapsulated by a protein shell rather than by a lipid-containing membrane.

A principal difference between oncogenic RNA viruses and other animal RNA viruses lies in the size of the complete set of hereditary information contained in their genome. RNA tumor virus genomes have a mass of about 12×10^6 daltons, compared to about 6×10^6 daltons for the paramyxoviruses and about 2×10^6 daltons for the poliomyelitis virus.

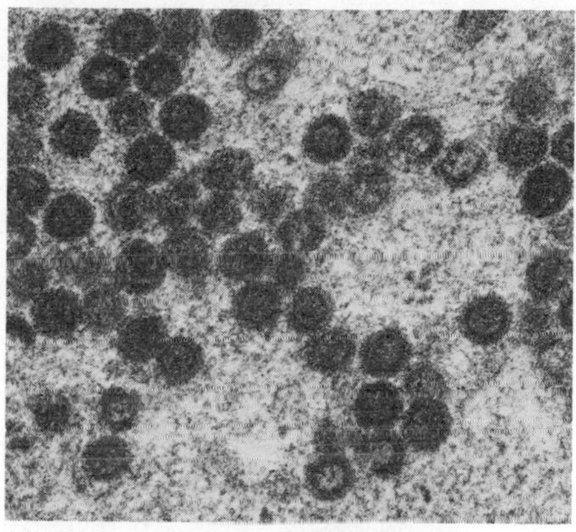

(a)

(b)

FIG. 36-6 Types B and C RNA production. Type C viruses have been implicated in causing leukemia, lymphomas, and sarcomas in a variety of avian and mammalian systems. (a) Mouse mammary tumor virus in tissue culture. This virus is a type B particle. Electron micrographs (b) through (e) show type C virions released by a mammalian cell line. *Courtesy of Dr. T. M. Murad.* (b) A budding particle from Chinese hamster tissue culture.

The Role of DNA Viruses in Carcinogenesis

Interest in the DNA viruses as possible human cancer viruses centered at first on the adenoviruses and papovaviruses. Adenoviruses, which cause respiratory infections in humans, and papova (papilloma-polyoma-vacuolating) viruses, which may be responsible for a variety of tumors, including the wart, produce tumors in experimental animals and transform animal cells in culture. Despite the fact that these viruses are widespread, there is little evidence implicating them in human cancers.

During the middle 1960s, however, the herpesviruses, a group of complex DNA viruses, attracted the attention of investigators seeking to establish a link between cancer and viruses. At least three herpesviruses may be involved in human and lower animal cancers and may thus serve as models for studying human disease. Table 36-2 lists the DNA viruses associated with cancerous states.

One of the virus diseases of lower animals, a malignant tumorous growth in the lymphoid system of chickens known as Marek's disease, has provided the first unequivocal proof that a herpesvirus is the cause of a cancer. First de-

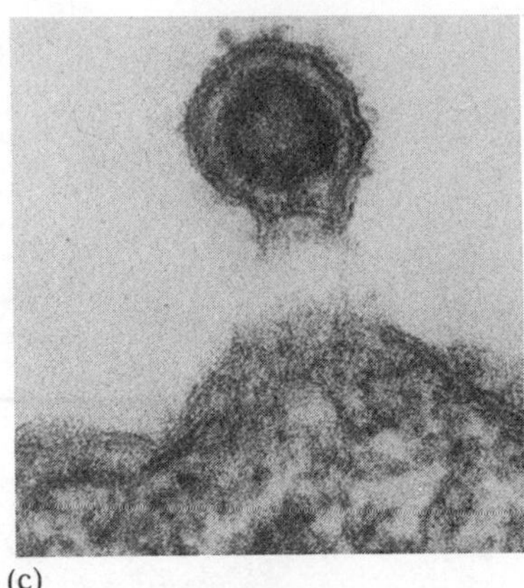

(c)

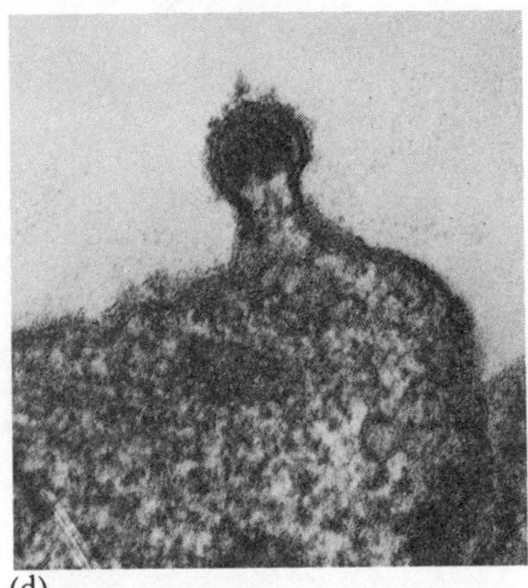

(d)

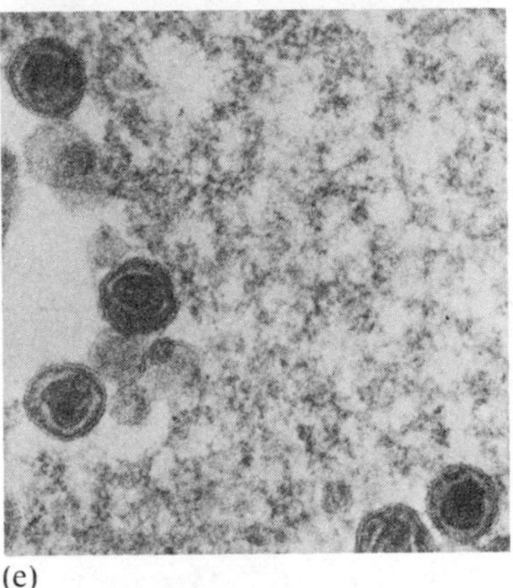

(e)

FIG. 36–6 (c) A budding particle from a rat tissue culture preparation. (d) and (e) Free and budding particles from a pig cell line. Note the similarities in particle appearance. The scale represents 100 nm. *Liever, M. M., et al.,* Science *182:56–59 (1973).*

scribed by Joseph Marek in 1901, Marek's disease remained almost unknown except among academic veterinary pathologists until the late 1960s when it became the scourge of U.S. commercial chicken flocks. In Marek's disease, cells of the lymphoid system become cancerous and invade the nerve cells, causing paralysis. As the disease progresses, other organs are invaded and the bird eventually dies. The virus that causes Marek's disease is extremely resistant to drying and may remain infectious for a long time after it has been liberated in bits of sloughed-off dead chicken skin (dander). In Marek's disease, the tumor virus is not produced in the tumor cells. The virus transforms normal cells into tumor cells without necessarily producing a new generation of viruses. The replication of the herpesvirus of Marek's disease takes place in nonmalignant skin cells that normally die in any case.

An attenuated strain of the Marek's disease virus has been used for live-virus vaccines that have effectively eradicated the disease in treated flocks. This suggests that cancer vaccines for humans may be possible.

The herpetovirus of Marek's disease is immunologically related to a herpetovirus closely associated with a human cancer: Burkitt's lymphoma. In 1958, Denis Burkitt, a missionary surgeon working in Uganda, reported that a large number of African children between the ages of 4 and 16 suffered from tumors in the connective tissue of the jaw. These jaw sarcomas were thought to be very rare in Europe and in the United States, but children of white missionaries living in Uganda sometimes acquired the disease. Although the lower jaw is the most frequent site of the tumor in Burkitt's lymphoma, tumors also arise at other sites, such as the upper jaw, the thyroid, the ovaries, the liver, and the kidneys. Intensive study of Burkitt's lymphoma began immediately after Burkitt's report was published.

Electron microscopic examinations of tumors for virus particles were fruitless, as were efforts to infect laboratory animals and tissue cultures with extracts of tumors. Efforts to establish tissue cultures with the cells from tumors also met with little success. Then M. A. Epstein and Y. M. Barr, as well as R. J. V. Pulvertaft, who worked independently of the other two investigators, undertook a series of tissue culture experiments using fresh tumor tissue flown in from Uganda. Electron microscopic examinations of some cells from these cultures clearly demonstrated the presence of herpesvirus particles (Figure 36–7). These particles have since been named Epstein-Barr virus (EBV).

The identification of a herpetovirus in Burkitt's lymphoma was a significant finding, since it is well known that certain herpetoviruses such as herpes simplex virus are widespread in the human population. In 1968, Werner and Gertrude Henle and V. Diehl reported that infectious mononucleosis not only is caused by a herpetovirus, but also is caused by an agent that cannot be distinguished from the Epstein-Barr virus. One question raised by this finding is: Do people who have had infectious mononucleosis (IM) have a greater probability of contracting cancer in later life? Thus far, it appears that a history of infectious mononucleosis is not associated with the incidence of cancer. Another interesting finding in the relationship between IM and EBV is that antibodies to Epstein-Barr virus are associated with protection against infectious mononucleosis and, conversely, IM occurs only in individuals who do not have antibodies against EBV.

Two groups of investigators have subsequently shown that EBV can induce lymphoid tumors in monkeys. Since such experiments are too hazardous to be carried out using humans, this is as far as experimentation can go in demonstrating that a virus from human cancer is in fact a cancer-causing agent. Demonstrating that a virus can induce a tumor is a different matter from finding a virus in a tumor. The prospect appears good that it will eventually be possible to show beyond a reasonable doubt that herpesviruses can cause certain forms of human cancer. However, if and when human cancers are shown to be caused by viruses, the mechanism of action will still need to be determined.

TABLE 36-2 Animal Viruses and Cancerous States

Virus Group	*Virus*	*Host*	*Conditions Produced*
Adenovirus	*Adenovirus*, type 3	Cow	Sarcomas in newborn hamsters, mice, rats
	Adenovirus (certain types)	Human	Sarcomas in newborn hamsters, mice, rats
	Adenovirus (certain types)	Monkey	Type 7 produced malignant lymphoma
Herpetovirus	Marek's	Chicken	Lymphoma
	Lucké	Frog	Adenocarcinoma frog kidney
	Herpesvirus hominis, type 2 (Herpes type 2)	Human	Suspected of producing cervical cancer
	Epstein-Barr	Human	Suspected of producing Burkitt's lymphoma
	Herpesvirus saimiri	Monkey	Lymphomas
Papovavirus	*Papillomavirus*	Cow, dog, human, rabbit	Produce warts or papillomas in their host of origin
	SV40	Monkey	Sarcomas in hamsters
	Polyomavirus	Mouse	Tumors in newborn mice and other rodents
Poxvirus	Poxvirus-Molluscum contagiosum	Human	Wartlike tumors on skin
	Yaba	Monkey	Tissue tumors
	Fibromamyxoma	Rabbit	Sarcomas

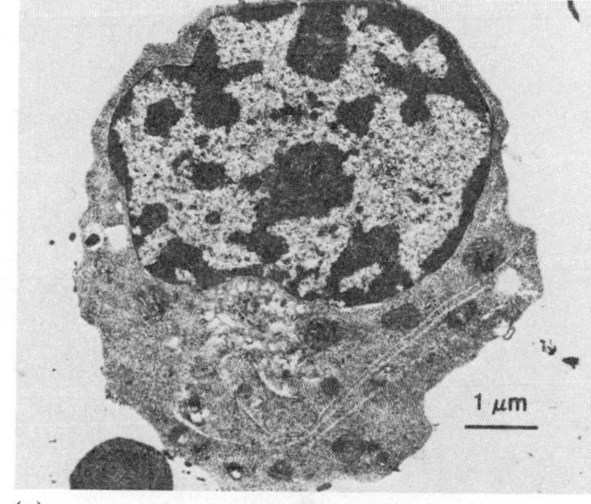

(a)

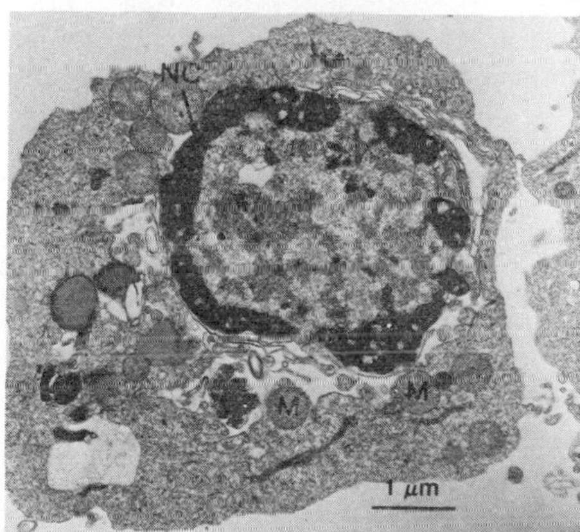

(b)

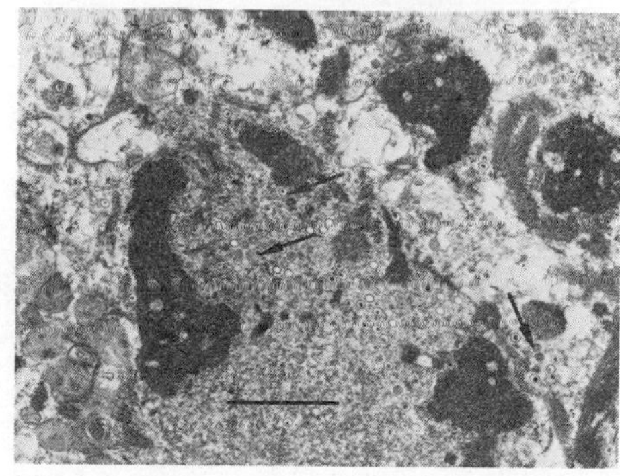
(c)

Cancer Virus Hypotheses

Reverse Transcriptase

In 1970 the surprising report was made of an enzyme that catalyzes the flow of genetic information from RNA to DNA, a reversal of the usual DNA-to-RNA direction of genetic expression. The discovery was of particular significance to cancer virus studies because viruses known to cause cancer in animals have an RNA core. The enzyme, known as ***reverse transcriptase***, provided, for the first time, a mechanism by which genetic material in the RNA of a virus might be incorporated into the DNA of a cell, where it could function like any gene (Figure 36–8). These RNA cancer viruses do not destroy cells, but if they are incorporated into a cell's genetic apparatus and then expressed, they could transform such a cell into a neoplastic one. Whether reverse transcriptase is unique to tumor cells is not totally known. However, it has been a powerful tool with which to study cancer and other biological phenomena such as the differentiation process in normal, healthy, developing cells.

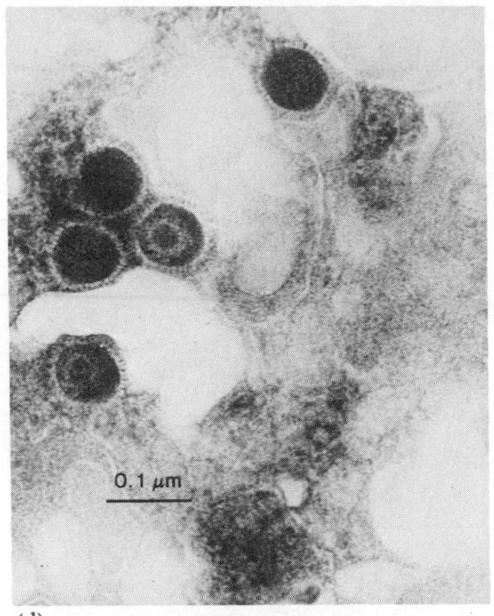

(d)

FIG. 36-7 Epstein-Barr virus (EBV) infection. (a) An ultrathin section of a non-virus-producing Burkitt lymphoma cell. The nucleus (N), cytoplasm, and organelles such as mitochondria (M) appear normal. (b) An EBV-producing cell reveals ultrastructural changes in the nucleus, margination of chromatin (NC), and production of excess nuclear membrane. The cytoplasm contains swollen mitochondria (M). (c) Virus capsids in various stages of maturation (arrows). (d) Negative staining with 2 percent phosphotungstic acid (PTA), showing a heavy concentration of viral capsids. Material is from the fluid of a tumor cell culture. The bar markers shown in photos (a), (b), and (c) represent 1 μm. The bar marker in photo (d) represents 0.1 μm. *Electron microscopy is the work of Muriel Lipman. From Miller, G.*, J. Inf. Dis. *130:187-205 (1974)*.

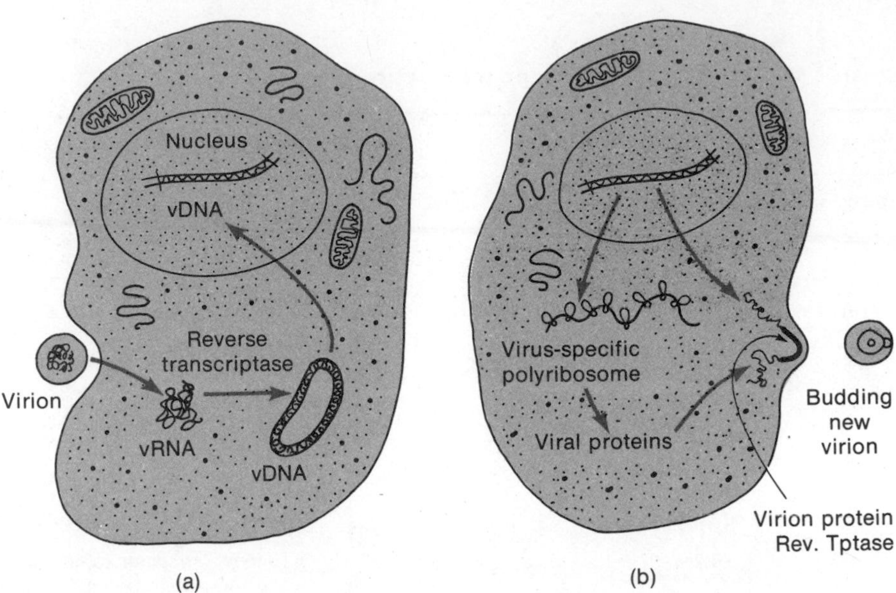

FIG. 36-8 The current understanding of the RNA tumor virus life cycle. (a) The first of two parts of a life cycle showing virion attachment and viral RNA (vRNA) and reverse transcriptase penetration and formation, respectively. The viral transcriptase initiates formation of a DNA copy (vDNA) of the RNA. This circular vDNA is thought to become integrated in the host's DNA. (b) The integrated vDNA brings about, by normal transcription, the formation of virion RNA and messenger RNA, which regulates the formation of new viral proteins. New virions are produced in this phase of the cycle. After *Baltimore, D.*, Science *192:632-636 (1976)*.

Current RNA Cancer Hypotheses

There are three current RNA virus cancer hypotheses based on the assumption that viruses do, in fact, cause human cancer. These hypotheses have been developed to account for the way in which genetic information associated with a cancerous process is expressed in cells. We should note again that cancer appears to be a number of different diseases. The demonstration of viral association with the causation of one type of cancer, or for that matter, of several types, should not be interpreted to mean that the problem of cancer will be solved. Various studies suggest that most cancers may be chemically induced.

PROVIRUS HYPOTHESIS

Of the three current RNA cancer virus hypotheses, the first was the provirus hypothesis, formulated by H. M. Temin in the early 1960s. According to the provirus concept, after infection of a cell by an RNA tumor virus, the cell makes a DNA copy of the viral RNA and incorporates this genetic information into its own DNA. This reaction gives the cell the capacity to produce oncogenic viruses and transforms it from a normal cell to a neoplastic one.

It should be emphasized that the integration of viral genetic material takes place after a viral reverse transcriptase makes a DNA copy of the viral RNA. Once this step is performed, the reverse transcriptase is no longer needed to establish the virus in the cell.

Many researchers accept the provirus hypothesis as an accurate model of oncogenesis in lower animals. The possibility also exists that a similar set of reactions can develop in humans.

ONCOGENE HYPOTHESIS

According to the oncogene hypothesis, advanced in 1969 by R. J. Huebner and G. J. Todaro, the genetic information for cancer is inherent in every cell and is transmitted from parent to child. According to this model, infection of cells by type C RNA viruses occurred millions of years ago during the course of evolution. Every cell is assumed to contain an oncogene, a region of DNA that is normally repressed (prevented from functioning). When the oncogene becomes derepressed, possibly by a virus, by a chemical carcinogen, or by radiation, it expresses itself by bringing about the formation of a transforming protein (Figure 36–9). A transforming protein of this type could change a normal cell into a malignant one even though no viruses could be recovered from it.

The oncogene is pictured as only one portion of a larger structure, the virogene (Figure 36–9). The virogene consists of several segments of genetic information, all of which must be activated in order for complete viruses to be made. This means, then, that the virogene would contain the necessary genetic information for the transforming protein, for the various components of the virus, and for the enzymes needed for making a complete virus. Thus it would not be necessary for the complete virogene to be expressed to produce a transformed cell. As a matter of fact, such complete expression could work against a virus-associated cancerous state. The body might recognize and destroy the

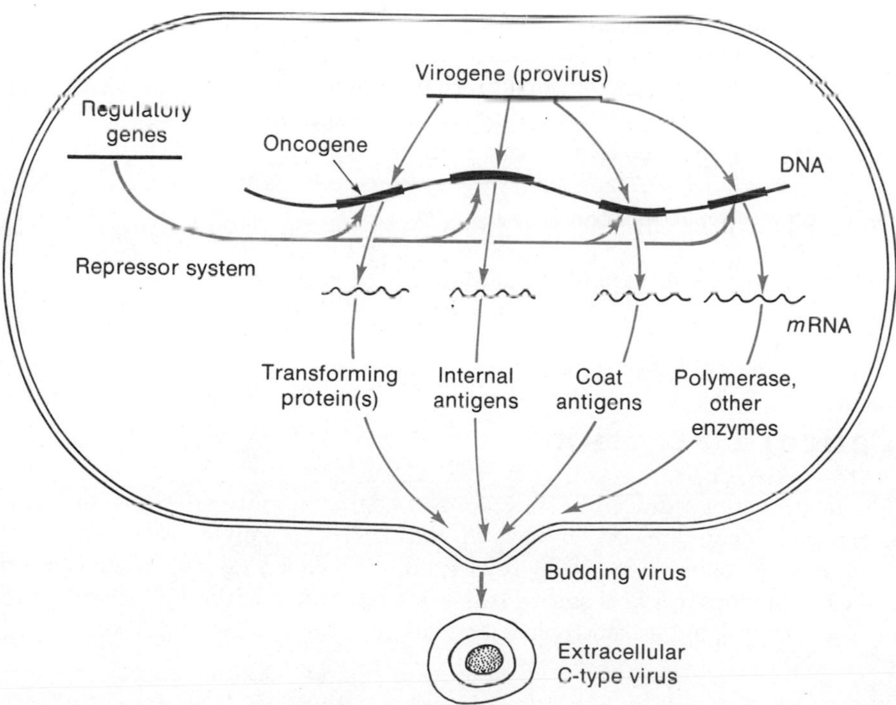

FIG. 36–9 The oncogene hypothesis proposes that tumors are induced by transforming proteins, which are the products of virogene activity. A virogene has the capacity to produce a complete tumor virus. According to this theory, in normal cells oncogens are turned off by regulatory genes that code for a repressor system. *Culliton, B. J.,* Science *177:44–47 (1972).*

antigens of the whole virus, while it would be unable to act against the transforming protein of the oncogene.

PROTOVIRUS HYPOTHESIS

Temin proposed the protovirus hypothesis in 1970. In many ways it is similar to the oncogene concept. However, there are some distinguishing points. The protovirus hypothesis holds that cancer viruses arise from segments of genetic information randomly brought together by a variety of cellular and genetic events. These segments form the protovirus. An important distinction between this and the oncogene hypothesis is that cells do not come into being with all the genetic information necessary for the development of a malignancy. What they do have, however, is the potential for assembling such information.

As more and more information about the molecular processes of normal and malignant cells accumulates, evidence in favor of each of the cancer virus hypotheses correspondingly increases. However, while evidence is increasing in support of the presumption of a viral cause of human cancers, there is still reason to be skeptical. It is possible, for example, that a virus may be a necessary, but not a sufficient, contributor to the development of a cancerous state. Other factors, such as genetic disposition, immunological deficiency, or exposure to chemicals or radiation, may also be required. The need for two or more causes acting together in the proper sequence, may help to explain why—if in fact viruses are involved—there is little evidence that cancer is contagious.

Microbial Carcinogens

Although it is known that some fungi are harmful or toxic to plants and animals, there is a common tendency to regard molds as harmless. However, in addition to the "side effects" of treatment with fungal antibiotics, both humans and lower animals can be affected by contamination of foodstuffs with mycotoxins. Evidence from field and storage studies confirms contamination of human and animal foods with carcinogenic mycotoxins such as aflatoxins. Extensive studies have shown that mycotoxins, especially aflatoxins, produce carcinogenic effects on organs such as the kidney, liver, intestines, stomach, and trachea.

Carcinogens are also known to be synthesized or activated by bacteria.

Cancer Detection

The treatment of a cancerous state can be undertaken only after the condition is detected. There are several ways to do this, but no single test will find all cases. A basic method used today involves routine screening tests, such as physical examinations, cervical smears (the Pap test) for women of childbearing age or older, x rays, and proctoscopic examination of the rectum and lower bowel.

Fetal Antigen

Recently, biochemical tests for cancer have become important. Researchers have known for several years that a protein normally present only in human fetuses shows up in cancer patients. At first the protein, named ***carcinoembryonic antigen*** (CEA), was thought to occur only in patients with cancer of the colon. Then it was discovered in patients with other types of cancers as well. Later, small amounts of CEA were found in individuals who seemed to be free of cancer. It now appears that the amount of CEA in a person's bloodstream is related to the presence or absence of cancer.

Although CEA level does not signal any specific type of cancer (and may not, by itself, indicate cancer at all), it is already proving a valuable aid in monitoring treatment and in diagnosing a tumor's recurrence. Antigens such as CEA may eventually be used to indicate specific types of cancer, just as different microorganisms indicate specific diseases.

Other fetal antigens have been associated with certain human cancers. These include α-fetoprotein, which is found in cases of liver and embryonic tumors, and γ-fetoprotein, which is found in patients having several different types of cancer.

Tumor-specific Antigens (TSAs)

Immune reactions of humans to their cancers depend on tumor-specific antigens (TSAs) that are absent from or hidden in normal cells. Because these antigens are usually present in the surface membranes of tumor cells, the host can react against his or her tumor as if it were a transplant involving genetically different members of the same species. Immunological surveillance by the host immune system probably eliminates many potentially neoplastic cells during a normal lifetime. However, individuals with certain impairments of the immune system have an increased probability of developing a tumor or related condition. Direct evidence for TSAs on human cancer cells has been provided by immunofluorescent procedures and other tests. Increasing evidence for the presence of these antigens on a wide variety of tumors and for host-associated immune responses to the TSAs has raised hopes for the development of diagnostic allergic skin tests or serological procedures for the early detection of cancers, as well as for some form of immunization against certain tumors.

Microbial Detection of Carcinogens and Mutagens

In the past, the use of laboratory animals was the only acceptable means of demonstrating the carcinogenicity and mutagenicity of chemicals. Recently, a rapid, accurate and inexpensive ***in vitro*** procedure, the Ames/*Salmonella* microsome mutagenicity test, was developed for the detection of potential chemical mutagens and carcinogens (Figure 36–10). This test, which was developed by Bruce N. Ames, has been widely adopted as an early warning system to identify and to reduce human exposure to dangerous chemicals. For example, prior to the commercial production of a new food additive or pharmaceutical product, manufacturers can utilize the Ames/*Salmonella* bioassay to determine the carcinogenic potential of the new substances. With the test results, which are obtainable in a matter of days, hazardous chemicals can be eliminated before they are introduced to the public.

The Ames test detects compounds that are capable of inducing permanent genetic changes in DNA molecules of specially developed histidine-deficient strains of *Salmonella typhimurim* and *Escherichia coli.* Since these organisms cannot produce the required amino acid histidine, they cannot grow unless the nutrient is provided or unless a genetic change occurs that restores their ability to produce histidine. Chemicals can be quickly detected if they cause mutations at levels greater than those occurring at normal (spontaneous) levels.

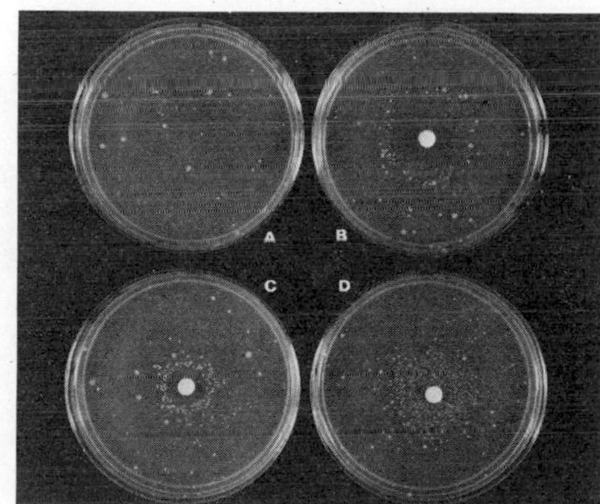

FIG. 36–10 The ames test for the detection of mutagenic or carcinogenic activity. In this "spot test," the bacterial colonies develop if mutations occur. In (b), (c), and (d), a chemical mutagenic agent was applied to the filter-paper disc seen in the center of each plate. (a) is a control and shows the amount of bacterial growth that occurred due to spontaneous mutation. ***Ames, B. N., J. McCann, and E. Yamasaki,*** Mutation Research *31:347 (1975).*

The Use of Microorganisms in Cancer Treatment

The major forms of cancer treatment used today are surgery, radiation, chemotherapy, or a combination of the three. However, for neoplastic disease there are limitations to these conventional methods, a realization that has resulted in the search for new measures of treatment. One approach is to stimulate the host's immune system to kill neoplastic cells. This method involves the use of nonspecific immunological stimulators (NISs), incorporating microorganisms such as vaccinia virus, *Corynebacterium parvum*, and the Bacillus of Calmette and Guérin (BCG). Nonspecific immunological stimulators appear to offer several advantages over the conventional approaches. Radiotherapy, hormonal therapy, and chemotherapy all reduce immunological responsiveness; they can, therefore, severely impair normal immunological function, particularly resistance to microorganisms and their products. We have seen in preceding chapters many cases in which use of these methods or of immunosuppressive drugs predisposed individuals to serious disease. The nonspecific stimulators can prevent or reverse such immunosuppression.

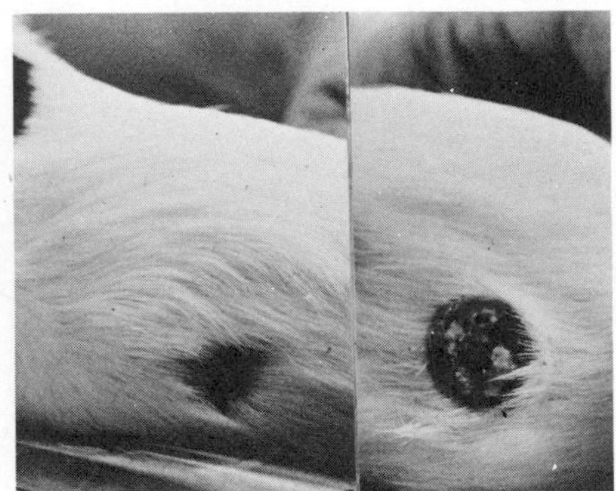

FIG. 36-11 A skin tumor (left) in guinea pigs at the site of injection of BCG *(Bacillus of Calmette and Guerin)*. The photograph on the right shows the tumor 26 days after administration of one million (10^6) tumor cells. *Bekierkunst, A., et al.* Inf. and Imm. *10:1044 (1974).*

The tumor-destructive effectiveness of BCG (Figure 36–11) serves as an example of NIS use. BCG is a live, attenuated organism derived from a bovine strain of *Mycobacterium tuberculosis*. There is a general consensus that infection with BCG bacilli causes a change in the immunological apparatus of the host. One expression of this altered state is increased immunoglobulin response to unrelated antigens. Tumor inhibition requires the host to develop and express delayed hypersensitivity reaction to BCG antigens.

The current understanding of the cellular and molecular basis for BCG-mediated tumor destruction can be summarized as follows. After injection of the host with BCG, sensitized T-lymphocytes develop that are able to recognize distinctive tubercle bacillus antigens. These lymphocytes react with the bacillus and produce a variety of potent molecules, the lymphokines. Some of these molecules immobilize or activate macrophages; others may be directly cytotoxic. If tumor cells are located close to the bacteria, they are killed by activated macrophages and lymphotoxins. As a result, immunity to specific tumor antigens may develop and in turn cause additional tumor cell death.

Living BCG has been used effectively in humans in some cases. Preparations have also proved effective in lengthening remissions in acute leukemia. Unfortunately, living BCG can cause disseminated disease in an immunosuppressed host. Although local reactions at the site of injections may be severe, they usually disappear. It seems that these adverse effects of using living BCG can be avoided by using lyophilized (freeze-dried), killed BCG alone or with other preparations having antitumor effects. One of these is the cord factor (trehalose-6,6′-dimycolate) obtained from mycobacterial cell walls.

Other bacterial sources of antitumor agents include bacterial endotoxins from *Salmonella enteritidis* and *Serratia marcescens*, both of which have been shown to inhibit tumor growth in laboratory animals.

A Future Outlook

Proving that a virus causes human cancer has been elusive because both Koch's and Rivers' postulates, which have served for years as the criteria for establishing that a disease is caused by a given infectious agent, cannot be fulfilled. The first postulate requires the isolation of the causative agent from all infected organisms. But infectious particles cannot be recovered from most fresh tumor cells. Only after careful manipulations have been performed on tumor cells (for example, culturing them, sometimes with other kinds of cells) can infectious virus be demonstrated. This raises the possibility that the virus is a contaminant and is not involved in the development of the tumor itself.

Another postulate requires induction of the disease state in question in a suitable host by a pure preparation of the suspected causative agent. However, such experiments are not normally performed on humans.

Thus investigators must rely on indirect, circumstantial evidence to prove the case for a suspected oncogenic virus. Current strategies include (1) epidemiological studies, usually done in conjunction with immunological studies, to determine whether the virus has left traces of its presence in the form of antibodies against it in the patient's blood; (2) study of tumor cells to detect the presence of viral DNA or RNA or of virus-associated antigens; (3) comparison with virus-induced animal tumors; and (4) study of the oncogenic potential of the virus both in cultured cells and in living animals, especially nonhuman primates.

If human oncogenic viruses can be isolated and obtained in sufficient quantities of pure form, there is hope that the associated forms of cancer can be eliminated, or at least reduced in frequency, through the development of effective vaccines or the discovery of ways with which to interrupt the primary routes of infection.

SUMMARY

General Characteristics of Cancerous States

1. Normal cells must be able to divide and reproduce in an exact and controlled manner for the well-being of the body.
2. Uncontrolled cellular reproduction leads to the formation of swellings called *neoplasms* or *tumors*.
3. Tumors that remain localized and do not cause destruction and death are called *benign*, while those that spread to other body areas and endanger the life of the individual are called *malignant* or *cancerous*.
4. The process by which cells separate from tumors and spread to other sites is called *metastasis*.
5. Cancers are believed to be caused by extrinsic, or environmental, factors including chemicals, radiation, certain microbial products, and viruses. Cancers are also influenced by intrinsic factors such as age, heredity, sex, and hormones.
6. Cancerous states have several major properties, which include uncontrolled cellular reproduction and an inability of the cells to mature into recognized structures.
7. While some microbial products are known to have cancer-causing (carcinogenic) capabilities, other products have been shown to inhibit the progress of cancer.

The Forms of Human Cancer

1. More than one hundred clinically distinct types of cancer are recognized, each with a unique set of specific symptoms.
2. Most cancerous conditions can be classified as being one of four general types: *carcinomas*, solid tumors from tissues covering the internal and external portions of the body; *leukemias*, uncontrolled production and accumulation of different white blood cells; *lymphomas*, abnormal production of immature lymphocytes; and *sarcomas*, tumors growing from bone, cartilage, connective tissue, fat, and muscle.

Viral Transformation

1. Viral transformation is the process by which normal cells are changed into malignant ones.
2. Such altered cells show changes in appearance, metabolism, and antigenicity.

Early Discoveries Relating Viruses and Cancer

Proof of the viral cause of human cancer has been difficult to obtain, despite long-standing evidence from experiments with lower animals.

Characteristics of Oncogenic RNA Viruses

1. Cancer-producing (oncogenic) RNA viruses are found in two of the three main classes, A, B, and C.
2. Type A viruses are not infectious or oncogenic and are found in the cytoplasm of cells.
3. Type B viruses are associated with carcinomas of the breast.
4. Type C viruses, the most important class, cause a variety of cancerous states, including leukemias, lymphomas, and sarcomas.

The Role of DNA Viruses in Carcinogenesis

Several DNA viruses are considered possible causes of human cancer. These include adenoviruses, papovaviruses, and herpesviruses.

Cancer Virus Hypotheses

Reverse Transcriptase

The enzyme *reverse transcriptase*, found in RNA cancer viruses, promotes the incorporation of viral genetic material into a susceptible host cell by transcribing DNA from the viral RNA host cell. This type of enzyme action results in a change of cellular properties.

Current RNA Cancer Hypotheses

1. Three current RNA virus cancer hypotheses are recognized: the *provirus, oncogene,* and *protovirus* hypotheses.
2. According to the provirus hypothesis, normal cells are changed into cancerous ones by infection with an RNA tumor virus. These transformed cells produce new oncogenic viruses.
3. The oncogene hypothesis assumes that the genetic information, or oncogene, for cancer exists in every cell in an inactive or repressed form. Viruses or environmental factors activate the oncogene, which changes the normal cell into a malignant one.
4. The protovirus hypothesis is similar to the oncogene concept. It differs in several ways, however, including the process for cancer virus production and the assumption that cells do *not* come into being with all of the information necessary to become malignant.

Microbial Carcinogens

Several products of microorganisms are harmful to various forms of life. Mycotoxins, which include aflatoxins, have been shown to be carcinogenic.

Cancer Detection

1. Method of cancer detection include physical examinations and various laboratory tests for the detection of tumors and other cancer-related antigens.
2. A rapid, accurate, and inexpensive procedure using bacteria known as the Ames/*Salmonella* microsome mutagenicity test exists for the detection of potential chemical mutagens and carcinogens.

The Use of Microorganisms in Cancer Treatment

1. The major forms of cancer treatment used today are surgery, radiation, chemotherapy, or a combination of these treatments.
2. New approaches involve the use of microorganisms such as the Bacillus of Calmette and Guérin (BCG) to stimulate the immune system of the host to destroy cancer cells.

A Future Outlook

If researchers can succeed in proving that a virus or viruses cause human cancer, there is hope that cancer can be eliminated or treated by the development of vaccines or the interruption of the primary routes of infection.

QUESTIONS FOR REVIEW

1. Distinguish between the following:
   a. carcinoma and leukemia
   b. sarcoma and lymphoma
2. What is reverse transcriptase? Of what significance is it to cancer virus studies?
3. Summarize the current RNA virus cancer hypotheses.
4. What is an oncogene?
5. Do oncogenic RNA viruses differ structurally from other RNA viruses? How?
6. Distinguish between a type B and type C virus particle.
7. What role do DNA viruses have in carcinogenesis?
8. What promise do microorganisms hold for the treatment of tumors?
9. How are microorganisms used to detect potential carcinogens?

SUGGESTED READINGS

Cairns, J., "The Cancer Problem," *Sci. Amer.* 233:64 (1975). *A general review of the biological aspects of cancer. Emphasis is given to possible environmental causes of this dreaded disease state.*

Griffith, A. H., and R. H. Regamey, *Biological Preparations in the Treatment of Cancer.* Basel, Switzerland: S. Karger AG, 1978. *Slightly advanced set of papers describing a few microorganisms and how they may be used in the treatment of cancer. Their mechanisms of action in laboratory animals are also presented.*

Kleen, P. A., and R. T. Smith, "The Role of Oncogenic Viruses in Neoplasia," *Ann. Rev. Medicine* 28:311 (1977). *A review of the role of viruses in causing cancer in animals and the immunological prophylaxis that may provide protection against many virus-induced cancers.*

Koprowski, C., and H. Koprowski (eds.), *Viruses and Immunity—Toward Understanding Viral Immunology and Immunopathology.* New York: Academic Press, 1975. *Immunity to viral attack, the mechanisms involved, and the "causes" of viral cancer tumor growth are topics discussed in some of the articles.*

Moloney, J. B., *The Virus Cancer Program.* Government Publications Dept., 1977. *A report of various viruses involved in cancer, their clinical studies and control.*

Nagao, M., T. Sugimura, and T. Matsushima, "Environmental Mutagens and Carcinogens," *Ann. Rev. Genet.* 12:117–159 (1978). *A rather complete, detailed review of the effects environmental mutagens and carcinogens have on humans. Attention is given to screening methods and specific industrial and natural sources of dangerous substances.*

Nicolson, G. L., "Cancer Metastasis," *Sci. Amer.* 240:66–76 (1979). *A view of current knowledge of how and which cancer cells spread throughout a tumor system (metastasis). The article stresses that metastasis, and not the initial or primary tumor, is the threat to life.*

Old, L. J., "Cancer Immunology," *Sci. Amer.* 236:62 (1977). *Tells how cancer cells, even though they have "foreign" labels, can escape destruction by the immune system. The latest studies on how cancer cells do this and how the immune system may be used for the treatment of cancer are also discussed.*

Tooze, J., *The Molecular Biology of Tumor Viruses.* Cold Spring Harbor: Cold Spring Harbor Laboratory, L.I. New York. 1973. *A clear and authoritative treatment of cancer viruses and cancer biology.*

Helminths and Disease

CHAPTER 37

Many human parasites are helminths, or worms, known to invade and cause disease in lower animals and plants as well as in humans. Chapter 37 deals with diseases caused by worms and with the transmission and control of these parasites.

After reading this chapter, you should be able to:

1. **List five structural, metabolic, or other modifications that favor the parasitism of worms.**
2. **Outline the life cycles of at least two different parasitic nematodes, cestodes, and trematodes.**
3. **Describe three characteristics of tapeworms that distinguish them from roundworms.**
4. **List three characteristics of flukes that distinguish them from roundworms and tapeworms.**
5. **List three preventive and control measures used against nematodes, cestodes, and trematodes.**
6. **Identify the basic structures of cestodes and flukes.**
7. **List two methods for the diagnosis of three nematode, cestode, and trematode infections.**
8. **Discuss the importance of parasitic worms to human welfare.**

Worms are among the most abundant animals on earth. Most are free-living and do not cause serious problems. However, some worms are parasitic, causing diseases of great importance to humans and to domestic and wild animals and plants. Parasitic worms live in varying environments and must adapt to conditions in order to survive a host's body defenses and chemical peculiarities.

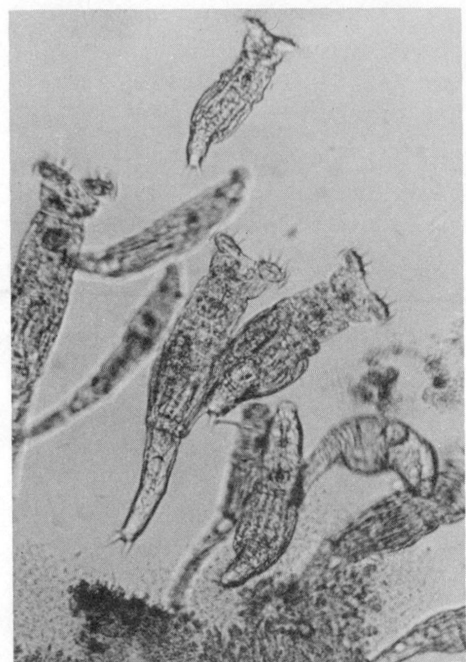

FIG. 37-1 *Rotifers.* A common rotifer, *Philodina* shows various primitive organ systems. The bilateral symmetry, cephalization (definition of head region), and organ systems familiar throughout the animal kingdom appear at this level of life. These organisms are free-living and commonly found in natural bodies of water such as ponds and streams.

One of the major subdivisions of parasitology is the study of helminths. This term, derived from the Greek word ***helmins***, meaning "worm," designates both parasitic and free-living species of worms. The helminths are a large group of animals including some of the most notorious forms of parasitic life, such as leeches and tapeworms. There are also, however, a great many free-living (Figure 37-1) and beneficial forms as well.

The worms of medical and agricultural importance discussed in this chapter include representative parasites from the phyla of Nemathelminthes (roundworms), also called Nematoda, and Platyhelminthes (flatworms, or flukes, and tapeworms). Several nematode species, as well as other parasites, are known to be damaging to plants, causing spoilage and destruction of agricultural products (Figure 37-2). These forms will also be described.

The Equipment of Parasitic Worms

Adaptation of a **helminth** to a parasitic existence is in large part determined by the development of certain structural and metabolic modifications. Many intestinal worms (and certain others) have an especially hard outer covering, or integument (Figures 37-3a and 37-3c), enabling them to resist digestion by the host. Other modifications include (1) the possession of hooks (Figure 37-3b), spines, cutting plates, suckers (Figure 37-3c), various enzyme secretions, and additional weapons for purposes of attachment or penetration and (2) the development of elaborate reproductive systems (Figure 37-3d). The latter feature is represented by hermaphroditism in cestodes (tapeworms) and a large number of trematodes (flukes), whereby the reproductive organs of both sexes occur in the same animal. More detailed descriptions of specific helminths will be provided in the sections that follow.

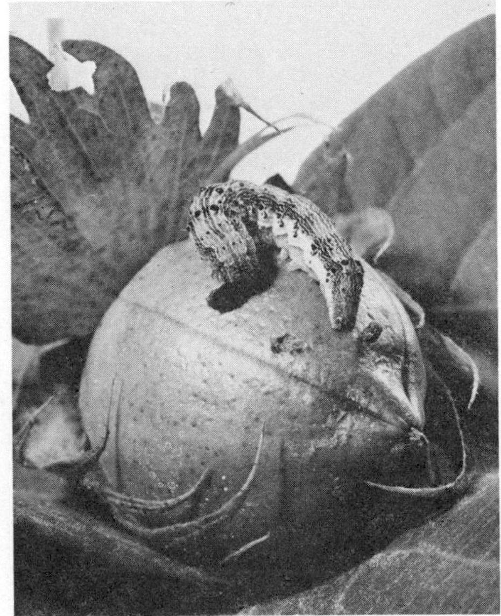

FIG. 37-2 A cotton bollworm, its damage done. This parasite is one of the serious pests of cotton. *USDA photo by Jim Strawser.*

Life Cycles and Control of Parasitic Helminths

Hosts

Some worms are capable of either a parasitic or a free-living existence. Such organisms are referred to as **facultative** parasites. Other forms, the *obligate* parasites, cannot complete their life cycles without the participation of the required host or hosts.

Many other terms denote the special functions, types of parasites or states of parasitoses encountered. The term *infection* is used to indicate the relationship of a parasite to its host. The term applies to animal species found internally **(endoparasites).** The term **infestation,** however, is used for parasites that attach to the skin or temporarily invade the superficial layers of the skin **(ectoparasites).** Thus, a state of parasitosis is caused by either an infection or infestation by an animal parasite.

Temporary parasites invade a host intermittently during their life cycles only to obtain nutrients. *Incidental* parasites may establish an infection in a host that ordinarily is not parasitized. Other types of diagnosed parasites include *coprozoic*, or *spurious*, forms (foreign organisms that pass through the

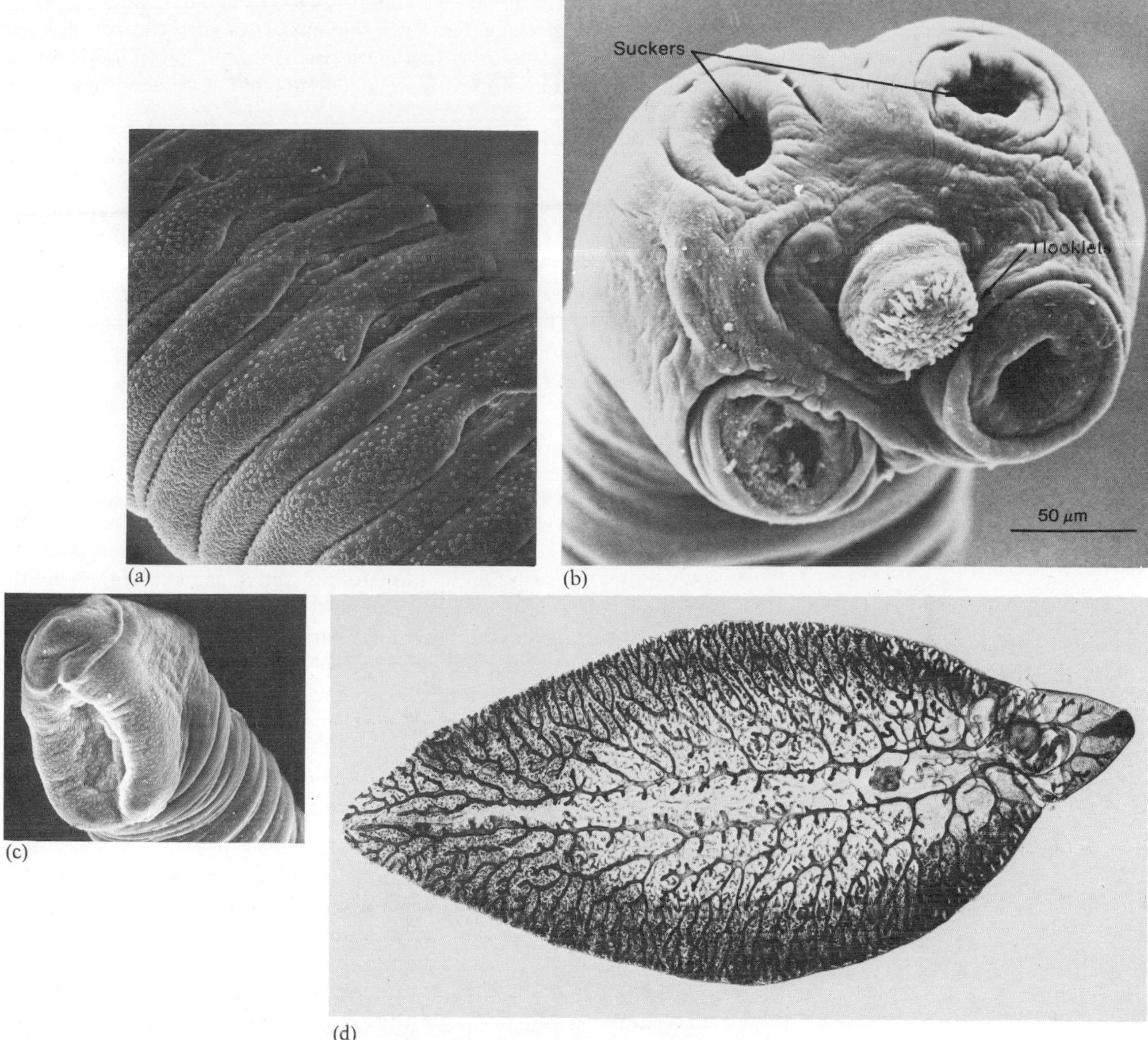

FIG. 37-3 The equipment of parasitic worms. (a) A scanning micrograph showing the surface of a tapeworm's body covered with small structures that probably function in the uptake of nutrients. *(a and c) Reproduced by permission of the National Council of Canada, from Boyce, N. P.* Can. J. Zool. *54:610–613 (1976).* (b) The head (scolex) of the mouse bile duct tapeworm *(Hymenolepis microstoma)*. The hooklets and suckers shown are used for attachment. *Pappas, P. W., and H. R. Gamble,* J. Parasitol. *64:760–762 (1978).* (c) A sucker of the cestode *Eubothrium salvelini.* (d) The reproductive network of the fluke *Fasciola hepatica*. The fluke is another type of flatworm. *Sahha, G. H., et al.,* J. Parasit. *58:712–716 (1972)*

intestinal tract without causing an infection), and ***pseudoparasites*** (particles misdiagnosed as parasites).

Several different types of host are distinguished. For example, the ***definitive***, or ***final***, host harbors the adult or sexually mature parasite; the ***intermediate*** host provides the environment for some or all of the immature or larval stages. Although human beings may be the only definitive host for several parasites, occasionally humans are accidental victims. When other animal species act as hosts for species that are parasitic for humans, such animals are called ***reservoir*** hosts.

The life cycles of parasites can be complex, sometimes involving several hosts. Apparently the more complicated life cycle greatly decreases chances for survival of the parasite. However, some parasites with complex life cycles have compensating adaptations including parthenogenesis (reproduction without a male) and "overdeveloped" reproductive organs.

Distribution and Transmission

The distribution of parasites such as worms is influenced by the habits of suitable definitive hosts and by favorable environmental conditions such as appropriate temperature and moisture and the availability of intermediate hosts. Many parasitic species are widely distributed only in the tropical regions of the world, but this condition appears to be disappearing; because of the revolutionary changes in the international transportation of cargo and passengers, opportunities for the distribution of parasites and their vectors have increased substantially.

Economic and social conditions are also important in the distribution of parasites. A low standard of living, inadequate sanitation, and ignorance of the means to control parasitic diseases favor the establishment of parasitoses.

The sources of parasitic diseases and their means of transmission include (1) domestic or wild animals in which parasites can live (domestic and sylvatic reservoirs, respectively); (2) bloodsucking insects, mosquitoes, for example; (3) various foods containing immature infective parasites; (4) contaminated soil or water; and (5) humans and any portion of their environment that has been contaminated. Even the individual harboring a parasite can cause his or her own re-exposure with the same species of parasite, a process known as **autoinfection.**

The destructive effects of parasites depend on their number, size, degree of activity, location, and toxic products. Consequently, symptoms may be absent, few, or severe. A wide range of symptoms can be encountered.

Symptoms and Pathology

The clinical effects observed in helminth infections usually depend upon the number and location of the parasites in the body and upon the general health and resistance of the host. Many infections are asymptomatic. If symptoms do occur, they may include anemia, excess numbers of eosinophils **(eosinophilia),** fever, intestinal obstruction, muscular pains, and respiratory difficulties. Tables 37–2, 37–4, and 37–6 list clinical features of the more common helminth infections.

Laboratory Diagnosis

The finding and identification of ova (eggs), larvae, or adult worms are sufficient in most cases for the diagnosis of specific helminth infections. Skin tests and other immunological procedures are used in certain cases to identify susceptible individuals, to distinguish one type of infection from another, or to follow the progress of recovery. Tables 37–2, 37–4, and 37–6 list the types of specimens and method of identification for the more common helminths.

Treatment of Parasitic Infections

Several antiparasitic medications have been developed. Because many of them are unlicensed, their use is limited in various countries, including the United States. The increase in Americans traveling or working in tropical areas where parasitic disease agents abide seems to be increasing U.S. infection rates. Therefore, it may become essential to have certain medications licensed for use and available to physicians.

This chapter emphasizes the parasitic helminth infections that have occupied the center of attention in recent years. Classification is based upon a system commonly used at the present time (see Appendix E).

The Nematodes

Parasitosis caused by roundworms, or nematodes, can involve the skin and organs of the circulatory, digestive, nervous, and respiratory systems (Table 37–1). Practically every tissue of the body is vulnerable to attack by certain nematode species. True nematodes are unsegmented, typically cylindrical and long, tapered at both ends, fundamentally bilaterally symmetrical, and without any appendages. These parasites all have digestive, nervous, and reproductive systems. The digestive system is a complete one. With relatively few exceptions, the sexes are in separate worms. Excretory systems are not found in all nematodes; adults of certain species lack such a system.

The worm's body is covered by a cuticle, which may have ridges, striations, or wartlike structures. These structures are considered in classification. The sizes of roundworms vary widely. Some species are microscopic (Color Photograph 92); others are several centimeters in length (Figure 37–4).

The mouths of primitive nematodes are surrounded by three lips (Figure 37–5). In *Ancylostoma duodenale* and *Necator americanus* (the Old and New World hookworms, respectively) these regions are equipped with cutting plates or teeth (Figure 37–5b). Such modifications, as well as others that will be mentioned, are important in nematode identification.

LIFE CYCLE

The life cycles of nematodes vary. However, there are fundamental stages involving an adult worm, egg, and **larvae.** The eggs of some roundworms are discharged in the host's feces, mature on the ground, and may either be swallowed by a host or hatch out larvae that undergo further development and consequently become infective. With infective larvae, penetration of the host's skin leads to parasitosis. In still other nematode life cycles, larvae are discharged

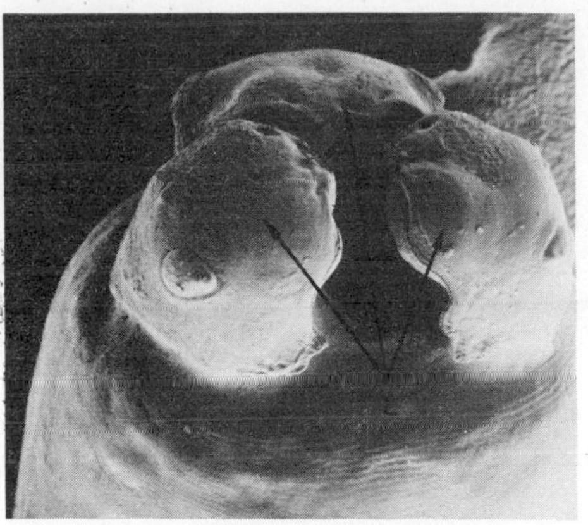

(a)

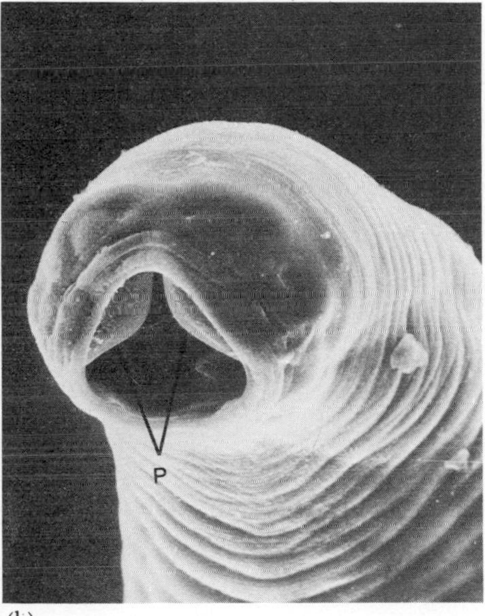

(b)

FIG. 37–5 *Ascaris suum.* (a) A scanning electron micrograph showing the attachment surface of the nematode's head with three lips. This worm infects both humans and pigs. *Dr. R. W. Weise, Department of Pathology, Wayne State University School of Medicine.* (b) The head of an adult *N. americanus,* shown by scanning electron microscopy. Note the internal biting plates. *McLaren, D. J.,* Internat. J. Parasit. *4:25–37 (1974).*

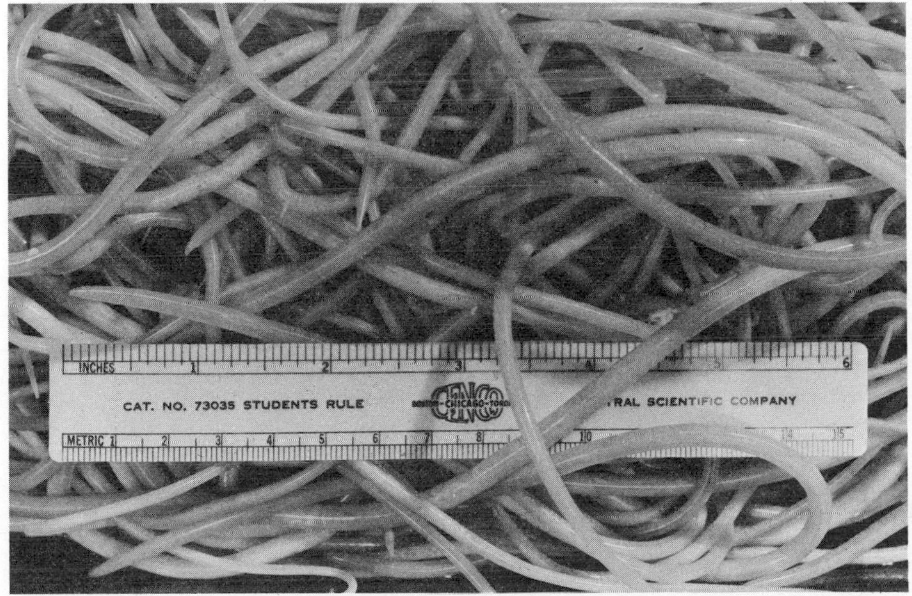

FIG. 37–4 *Ascaris lumbricoides.* Female worms range in size from 20 to 35 cm in length; male specimens measure approximately 30 cm (see Table 37–1). *Courtesy of the Dow Chemical Company.*

in the fecal matter, and the infective forms that develop are capable of penetrating the host.

Some parasites utilize two hosts. ***Trichinella spiralis,*** the causative agent of pork roundworm infection, or trichinosis, is one such worm. All the stages of its life cycle can be completed in the pig. Human infection depends on ingestion of encapsulated larvae in the striated muscles of this host as inadequately cooked pork.

These and other examples of life cycles will be described along with the features of specific roundworms and the infections they cause.

LARVAL FORMS

Frequently, in describing the life cycles of these worms, references are made to ***filariform*** and ***rhabditiform*** larvae. These terms reflect the type of esophagus of the larval forms. The esophagus of filariform larvae is a tube with a uniform diameter throughout. The esophagus of rhabditiform larvae expands toward the rear of the worm, forming a bulb that has a valve mechanism.

The geographical distribution of medically important roundworms is shown in Table 37–1.

TABLE 37–1 Representative Medically Important Nematodes

Organism	*Disease*	*Host Range*	*Location of Adult Forms in the Body*	*Geographical Distribution*
Ancylostoma duodenale	Old World hookworm infestation	Primarily humans	Duodenum and jejunum	Chiefly found in Africa, Europe, the Orient
Anisakis species	Anisakiasis	Humans and marine mammals	Small intestine	Europe and the Orient
Ascaris lumbricoides	Ascariasis	Humans and other vertebrates	Small intestine	World
Brugia malayi	Malayan filariasis	Humans, other primates, cats	Lymphatics	Far East
Dracunculus medinensis	Dracunculiasis (guinea worm infestation)	Humans, dogs, cats, several wild mammals	Skin, connective tissue	Certain areas of Africa and Asia, and rarely in South America
Enterobius vermicularis	Enterobiasis or oxyuriasis (pin- or seatworm infestation)	Humans, especially children	Large quantities occur in cecum and appendix. Female worm is especially found in the rectum	Widespread
Loa loa	Loiasis (eye worm infection)	Humans, monkeys	Connective tissue, eyes	Central and west Africa
Necator americanus	New World or American hookworm	Humans	Small intestine	Generally in southern United States, Central and South America
Onchocerca volvulus	Onchocerciasis	Humans	Skin, subcutaneous connective tissue, eyes	Africa, tropical America
Strongyloides stercoralis	Strongyloidiasis	Humans, dogs, cats	Intestinal mucosa, lungs	World, but more commonly encountered in tropical areas
Trichinella spiralis	Trichinosis	Humans and several other mammals, including rats, rabbits, dogs, wolves	Small intestine	World, encountered in areas where pork is eaten
Trichuris trichiura	Whipworm infestation	Humans	Caecum	World
Wuchereria bancrofti	Bancroft's filariasis (elephantiasis)	Humans	Lymphatics	Australia, East Europe, Near East, Orient, Central and South America, Mediterranean, and central Africa

Representative Animal Roundworm Infections

The effects of roundworm infections and their laboratory diagnoses are listed in Table 37–2.

TABLE 37–2 Characteristics of Nematode (Roundworm) Infections

Disease	*Clinical Features*	*Location of Adult Worm*	*Specimen of Choice for Diagnosis*	*Laboratory Diagnosis*
Filariasis (elephantiasis)	Lymphatic inflammation, chills, fever, inflammation of testes with sudden enlargement, obstruction of lymphatics, thickened and cracked skin[a]	Blood, lymphatics	Blood	Microscopic identification of larvae
Hookworm	Iron-deficiency anemia, abdominal pain, protein deficiency, delayed puberty, lowered antibody response, "potbelly" in children[b]	Small intestine	Feces	Microscopic identification of ova or adult worms
Pinworm	Tickling or intense itching in perianal area	Intestine, anus	Scotch tape swab[c]	Microscopic identification of ova
Trichinosis	Diarrhea, muscular pain, nervous disorders, eosinophilia, respiratory complications[b]	Intestine	Muscle	Microscopic identification of larvae

[a]Most symptoms here are caused by wandering larvae.
[b]Most light infections are asymptomatic.
[c]A short piece of Scotch tape, held against a flat, wooden applicator, with the sticky surface out. This device is pressed against the perianal area to obtain a specimen. The tape is reversed on a slide for examination.

FILARIASIS

The filaria are long, slender nematodes that invade portions of the lymphatic system and various other tissues of the human body (Figure 37–6). As a group, these helminths undergo a unique stage in their life cycle, the production of motile laval forms called **microfilaria** (Color Photograph 92). Although there are at least six species of filarias for which human beings are believed to be the definitive host, the discussion here is limited to the two most important forms of infection, Bancroftian and Malayan filariasis.

Bancroftian filariasis has been known since 600 B.C. The causative agent, ***Wuchereria bancrofti,*** is transmitted by the bite of mosquitoes, specifically ***Culex fatigans. Brugia malayi*** is the causative agent of Malayan filariasis. Selected characteristics of other filarian worms (e.g., *Loa loa* and *Onchocerca volvulus*) can be found in Table 37–1.

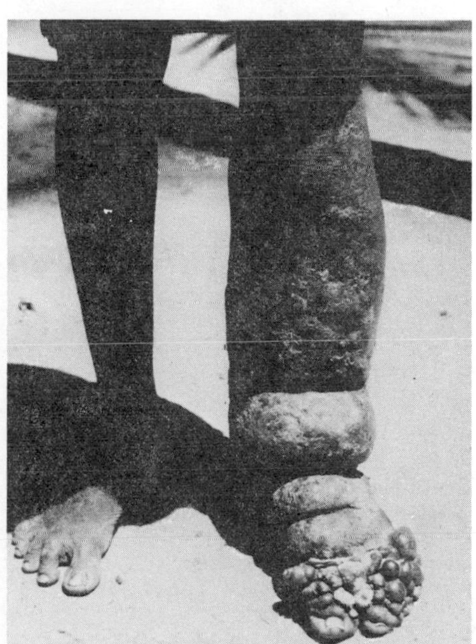

FIG. 37–6 A victim of elephantiasis. *Courtesy of World Health Organization.*

Transmission and life cycle. The filarias capable of infecting humans have similar life cycles. Mosquito vectors include species of *Aëdes, Anopheles, Culex,* and *Mansonia.* Microfilaria are introduced into humans by the bite of an infected mosquito. The human host provides a suitable environment for the further development of the parasite.

The microfilaria of *W. bancrofti* (Color Photograph 92) appear in the peripheral circulation of the human host only at night ("nocturnal periodicity"). They

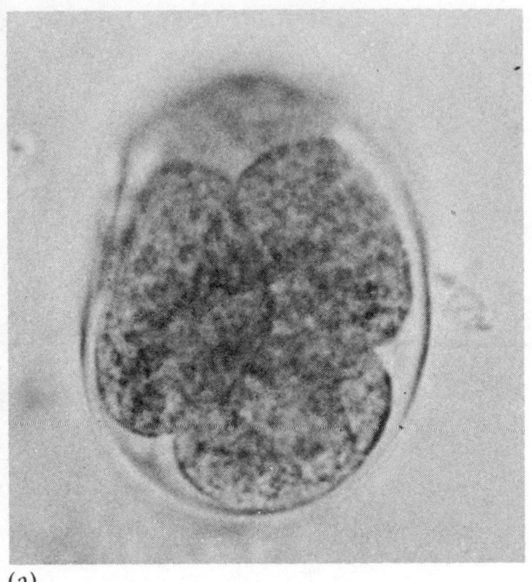

(a)

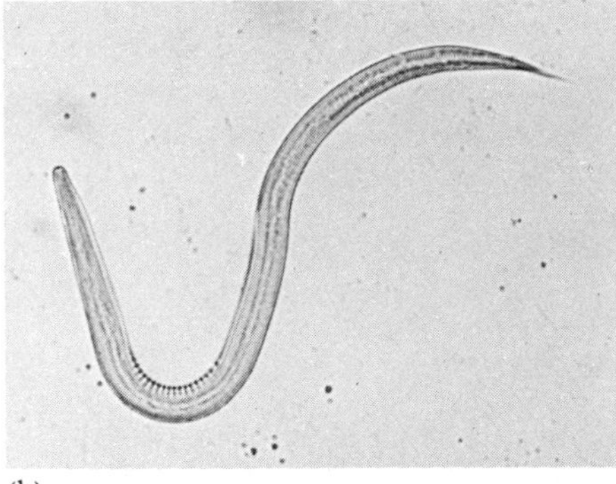

(b)

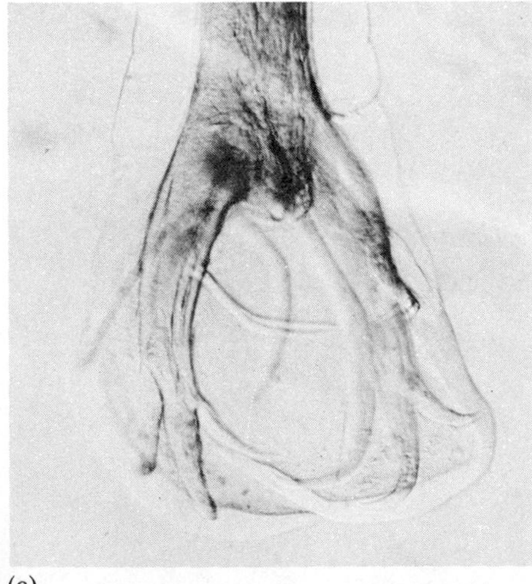

(c)

FIG. 37–7 Stages in the life cycle of hookworms. (a) The ovum of *Necator americanus*. Hookworms range from 56 to 76 μm in length and 36 to 49 μm in width. (b) An infective larva of *N. americanus*. These forms average 700 μm in length. (c) The bursa of the male worm.

are ingested by the appropriate species of mosquito during the course of a blood meal from an infected individual.

Once in the body, the microfilaria usually pass into the lymphatics and occasionally into subcutaneous tissues, where they mature into adult male and female worms. After mating, the female releases her offspring into the lymphatic system of the host. The larvae become widely distributed in the bloodstream and exhibit the "nocturnal" pattern described. If suitable vectors do not ingest the microfilaria, the parasites die and disappear from the circulation. If ingested by mosquitoes, the larva develop into active, elongated infective forms. These larvae migrate to the mosquito's mouth parts from where they can be introduced into the human host at the time of the next blood meal.

The life cycle of *B. malayi*—also known as *Wuchereria malayi* or *Filaria malayi*—is similar to that of *W. bancrofti*, except that these filaria are present in the peripheral blood for approximately 20 hours a day.

Prevention. Measures taken to prevent or control filariasis are similar to those for other arthropod-borne diseases.

HOOKWORM INFECTION

The term ***hookworm*** was coined either on the basis of the curved or bent front end of the worm or on the basis of the hooklike supporting structures found in the posterior extremity of male worms (Figure 37–7c shows a copulatory structure, the bursa).

Transmission and life cycle. The two hookworm species most important for humans are *Ancylostoma duodenale* (the Old World hookworm) and *Necator americanus* (the American or New World hookworm). Both have the same general life cycle. The ova of hookworms (Figure 37–7a) are passed in the fecal matter of an infected person. These eggs develop in the soil and give rise to rhabditiform larvae. They further develop into infective filariform larvae (Figure 37–7b). Under favorable conditions, the larvae may live for several months in the soil. A hookworm infection is acquired when these larvae penetrate the skin, often through the soles of the feet. Once in the body, the parasites are carried to the heart and lungs by the bloodstream. After further growth and development, the larvae penetrate the lung air sacs, ascend the respiratory tree, and are swallowed. Thus the parasites reach the small intestine, where they mature into adult male and female worms. Mating takes place in this area, the female lays eggs (which are passed out with the host's feces), and the cycle begins again.

Prevention. Measures to prevent hookworm infections include (1) the use of footwear in endemic areas, (2) improvement of general sanitation (especially disposal of human fecal matter), (3) mass treatment of infected persons, and (4) public education as to the parasite and its effects.

ENTEROBIUS VERMICULARIS INFECTION (PINWORM, SEATWORM)

Enterobiasis (oxyuriasis) has been known since ancient times. Its incidence is higher in temperate and colder climates than in tropical regions. Infections are more prevalent where large groups congregate, as in schools, mental institutions, and even large families. Children appear to have higher rates of enterobiasis than adults.

Transmission and life cycle. Infection results from the ingestion of ova containing infective larvae. Such infections can be acquired through the handling of fomites, inhalation of eggs (Figure 37–8), or a transfer of ova to the mouth from the perianal region via the fingers.

Ingested ova hatch in the small intestine, forming infective larvae that migrate to the first portion of the large intestine. Here maturation and mating of the parasites occur. The female worm carrying fertilized eggs migrates to the perianal region, releasing masses of eggs as it crawls. The deposited eggs are fully embryonated and infective. Eventually the female's body ruptures.

The migration of worms produces a tickling or intense itching, which causes the individual to scratch the area, often contaminating the fingers. Infection of other individuals by means of contaminated bedding or clothing is frequently encountered. Larvae that hatch in the perianal region eventually may migrate back into the large bowel. This type of infection is referred to as "retrofection."

Prevention. Preventive measures include treatment of all infected individuals and the development of good habits of personal hygiene.

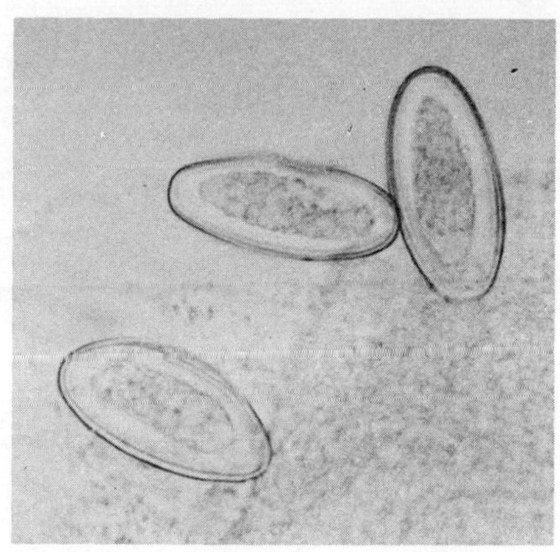

FIG. 37–8 *Enterobius vermicularis* ova. These eggs range in width from 20 to 32 μm and are approximately 50 to 60 μm in length.

TRICHINOSIS

Trichinella spiralis was first observed in encapsulated larval form in the early 1800s. The pathologic significance of trichinosis in humans was not truly recognized until 1860 when Friedrich Albert von Zenker showed the serious and often fatal consequences of the disease.

Trichinella spiralis infection was first found to be a public health problem in the pork-consuming populations of Europe. However, trichinosis has a much wider distribution today, especially in the United States.

Transmission and life cycle. T. spiralis infection generally results from consumption of improperly cooked or inadequately processed pork (Color Photograph 93). The parasite exhibits very little host specificity, as evidenced by trichinal infections associated with bear meat and walrus flesh. The life cycle of this parasite is shown in Figure 37–9.

Prevention. The proper cooking of pork and related products and the freezing of pork at −10° C or lower for more than 24 hours are relatively effective procedures in preventing *Trichinella spiralis* infection.

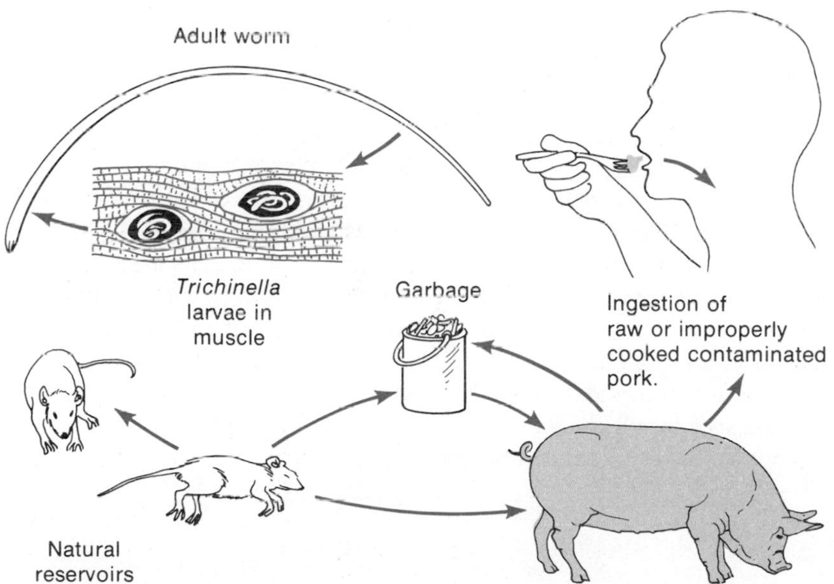

FIG. 37–9 The life cycle of *Trichinella spiralis.* In the case of human infections, the full life cycle of the parasite usually involves two omnivorous mammals. *T. spiralis* is commonly found in rats and in swine raised on uncooked garbage. The ingestion of meat containing encepted larvae begins the parasite's life cycle in the host. The ingested larvae excyst, invade the intestinal mucosa, and soon develop into adult female and male worms. Mating occurs and the female releases larvae, which eventually enter the host's bloodstream and are distributed throughout the body. These parasites are often filtered out in striated muscle where they attain full size, embed in the host's muscle tissue (Color Photograph 93) and eventually become calcified.

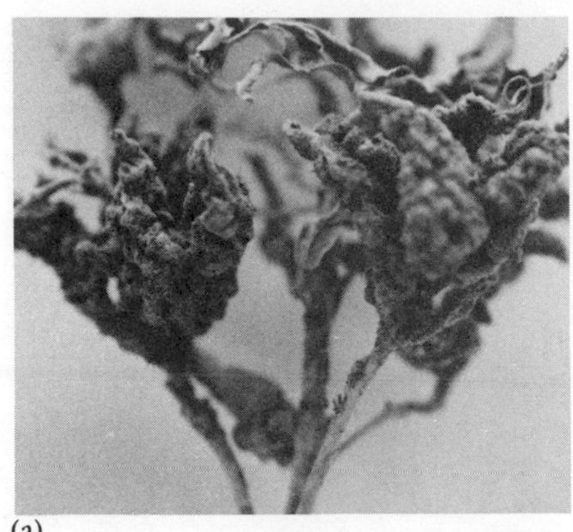

(a)

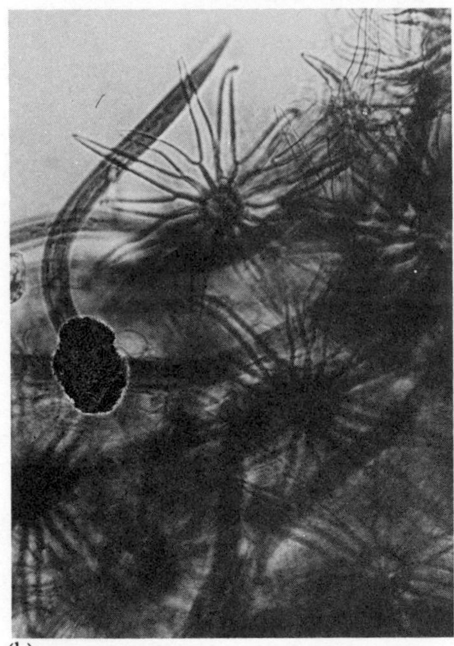

(b)

FIG. 37-10 A potential biological control agent for weeds. (a) The nematode ***Nothanguina phyllobia*** causes lethal infections of the weed silverleaf nightshade ***(Solanum elaegnifolum)***. This weed interferes with cotton production in the southwestern United States. The leaf-damaging effects caused by the nematode are evident. (b) Larvae of the roundworm on the weed's leaf surface before penetration. *Orr, C. C., J. R. Abernathy, and E. B. Hudsepth,* Plant. Dis. Rep. *59:416–418 (1975).*

Parasitic Nematodes of Plants

The roundworm parasites of plants are often called ***eelworms***. The enormous damage they cause cultivated plants is responsible for agricultural losses amounting to millions of dollars per year (Color Photograph 6B). Free-living and parasitic plant nematodes occur in great numbers in all types of soil capable of supporting plant growth. Nematodes may either damage susceptible plants directly or introduce microorganisms such as viruses, which in turn cause plant destruction and death.

Damage to plants attacked by nematodes is due primarily to the feeding of the nematodes on the plant tissues (Figure 37–10a). The survival of the worms depends on the availability of suitable hosts. Some nematodes attack the root surfaccs of plants as well as those parts that are above ground. These worms are ectoparasitic (Figure 37–10b). Other worms enter and attack the internal parts of plants. Such roundworms are referred to as endoparasitic. Formation of a **gall** (a type of tumor) is one of the plant responses to endoparasitic activity.

Parasitic plant roundworms have a special feeding organ known as a stylet or spear. Its hollow form enables the worm to pierce plant tissue or cell walls and to suck out cellular contents. Nematodes may enter a plant to feed, may feed from the outside, or may be only partially embedded. The most common effects of roundworm infections are the rotting of the attacked plant parts and adjacent tissue and the development of galls (knots) and other abnormal growths (Color Photograph 6B). Either of these effects can interfere with the development of a plant and cause shortening of roots and stems, twisting, crinkling, or death of parts of stems and leaves, and other abnormalities.

Root knot galls distort plant tissue that conducts nutrients to the upper portions of the plant. Injuries to stems and leaves also interfere with normal growth. The effects of plant nematode parasites may not be evident soon after the organisms are introduced into a field. However, once the parasites have had sufficient time to multiply, their effects become obvious. For example, crops attacked by root-damaging nematodes give the impression of a deficiency of water and fertilizer even though abundant quantities of these materials are available in the soil. Heavily infected plants may also exhibit lighter coloration and die prematurely.

In physical appearance, plant nematodes are similar to the ascarid worms associated with vertebrates (Figure 37–4), only they are much smaller. The life cycles of the worms consist of eggs, larval stages, and adults. Details of the life cycle vary considerably according to species and environment.

Plant parasitic nematodes have several enemies in the soil. At any stage of their life cycle they may be captured and eaten by other soil animals, such as insects or predatory, free-living roundworms. Certain soil fungi almost seem designed to catch nematodes. Some of these traps are hyphal loops (Figure 8–1) that close when roundworms start to crawl through them. Other fungal traps have surfaces to which nematodes stick. In either case, the fungus penetrates the body of the worm and subsequently kills it.

The Platyhelminthes

The platyhelminthes, or flatworms, are among the most primitive groups of animals to have bilateral symmetry, the basic body plan exhibited by all higher forms of animal life. Flatworms range in size from less than a millimeter to several meters in length. Tapeworms have been reported to measure 75 meters.

The flattened bodies of these worms may be slender, broadly leaflike, or long and resembling a ribbon.

The platyhelminthes include both free-living and parasitic forms. Most free-living worms are bottom dwellers in marine or fresh water or live in moist areas on land; they are found under stones and other hard objects in freshwater streams. The common planaria are found in such environments.

The true parasitic flatworms include the classes Cestoda (tapeworms) and Trematoda (flukes). The members of both groups have undergone several adaptive changes that make them well equipped for their parasitic existence. For example, they possess adhesive organs such as suckers, excessive reproductive capacity, and no digestive system. (Additional details are given in the following sections.)

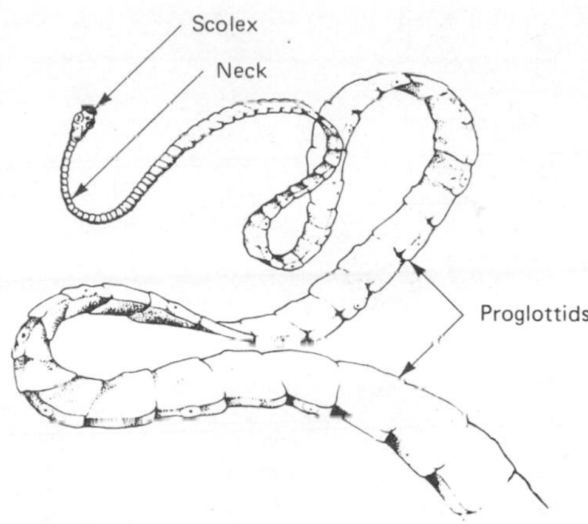

FIG. 37-11 A typical tapeworm.

The Cestodes

The cestodes are endoparasites, which as adults live in the intestines of vertebrate hosts. Several species are capable of parasitizing humans (Table 37-3).

The bodies of cestodes are flattened front-to-back and consist of (1) a head or attachment organ (**scolex,** plural *scolices*), which, depending on the particular species, may or may not have hooks or suckers (Figures 37-3b and 37-3c); (2) a neck region (the region where new body segments, or **proglottids,** grow); and (3) the body, properly called the *strobila.* Figure 37-12 shows the relationship of these tapeworm parts to one another.

The hooks of the armed scolices of tapeworms are attached to a fleshy elevation region, or rostellum (Figure 37-3b), which may or may not be retractable. The armed scolex is characteristic of the pork tapeworm *(Taenia solium)*; the unarmed structure is found in the beef tapeworm *(T. saginata)*. Still other tapeworm species such as the fish tapeworm *(Dibothriocephalus latus)* have heads in the form of a trenchlike groove (Figure 37-12). Usually scolices of this type have weak suction power.

The strobila is composed of a series of *proglottids,* which, proceeding from the neck of the tapeworm, include first sexually immature units, then sexually mature segments (Figure 37-13), and finally gravid structures filled with eggs. These body segments account for the ribbonlike appearance of tapeworms (Figure 37-11). Usually each proglottid has a complete set of female and male reproductive organs, making tapeworms **hermaphroditic.** Fertilization may occur between proglottids of the same or different worms *(reciprocal fertilization)* or between the sexual organs of a single body segment *(self-fertilization)*.

Cestodes do not have circulatory, digestive, respiratory, or skeletal organs. They have no special sense organs, but do have free sensory nerve endings.

The life cycles of cestodes are complex. Most utilize a nonhuman host for the development of infective larvae. The eggs of the cestodes, with one exception (Figure 37-14b), do contain lids (operculated) (Figure 37-14a). They vary in appearance, as well as in the protective coverings of embryos (embryonic membranes). The embryo is referred to as the *oncosphere.* Cestodes, with few exceptions, involve at least two hosts of different species. The adult worms are found only in vertebrates. Other stages may be found in either invertebrates or vertebrates. The life cycle of the beef tapeworm is shown in Figure 37-15. Table 37-4 lists the signs and symptoms and features of laboratory diagnosis of several tapeworms that affect humans.

FIG. 37-12 The fish tapeworm *Diphyllobothrium ditremum.* (a) The scolex. (b) The parasite attached to the intestinal lining of a host. *Anderson, K.,* Internat. J. Parasit. *5:487-493 (1975).*

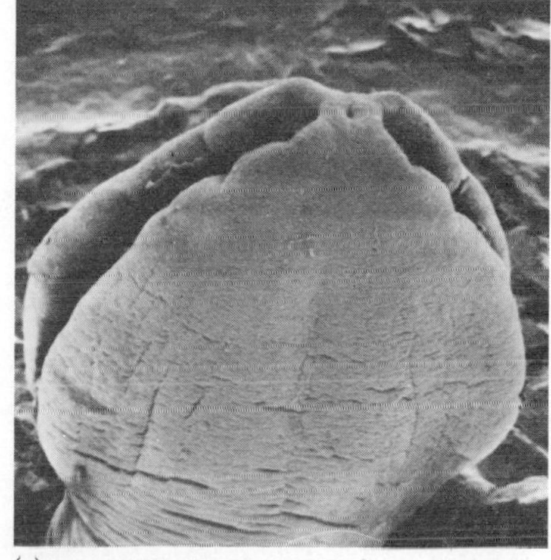

(a)

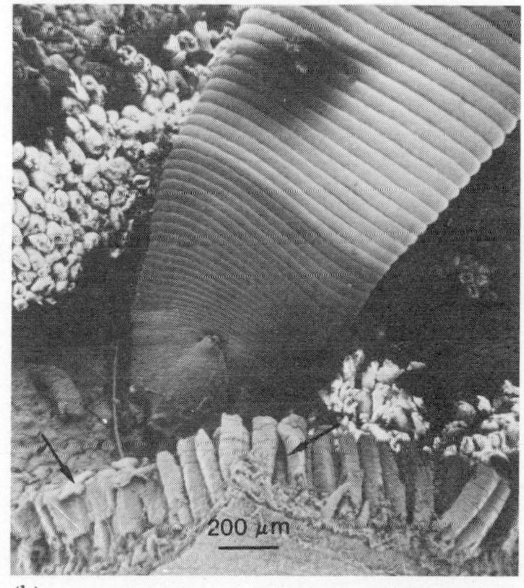

(b)

The Trematodes

The Trematoda, or flukes, are another parasitic class of Platyhelminthes. Although thousands of species are known today, not all flukes are of medical

TABLE 37-3 Representative Medically Important Cestodes

Organism	Disease	Host Range	Location in the Body	Geographical Distribution
Dibothriocephalus latus (also known as *Diphyllobothrium latum*)	Dibothriocephaliasis (Diphyllobothriasis)	Humans, dogs, cats, bears, other fish-consuming mammals	Intestine	Orient, Europe, United States, most of the great lakes of the world
Echinococcus granulosis	Hydatid disease	Cattle, deer, dogs, foxes, horses, humans, jackals, pigs, rabbits, sheep, and wolves	Bone, brain, heart, kidney, liver, lungs, and spleen	Australia, Middle East, portions of South America, and United States
Hymenolepsis diminuta	Hymenolepiasis diminuta	Rats, mice, humans, dogs	Intestine	Widespread; sporadic in most instances
Hymenolepsis nana	Hymenolepiasis nana	Rats, mice, humans	Intestine	United States, Asia, Europe; sporadic in many instances
Taenia saginata	Taeniasis saginata	Cysticercus in cows, adult worms in humans	Small intestine	Areas in which beef is consumed
Taenia solium	Taeniasis solium	Cysticercus in pigs, adult worms in humans	Small intestine	Areas in which beef is consumed

TABLE 37-4 Characteristics of Tapeworm Infections

Disease	Clinical Features	Location of Adult Worm	Specimen of Choice	Laboratory Diagnosis
Diphyllobothriasis (fish tapeworm)	Abdominal discomfort, diarrhea, nausea, vitamin B_{12} deficiency (pernicious anemia), general weakness	Intestines	Feces	Microscopic demonstration of ova or proglottids
Hydatid disease (sheep tapeworm)	Dependent on body location	Various locations, including nervous system and bone marrow	Surgical specimens	1. Intradermal skin test (Casoni) 2. Medical x-ray examination 3. Complement fixation, fluorescent antibody, etc.
Beef tapeworm	Abdominal pain, headache, loss of appetite, localized sensitivity to touch, nausea[a]	Intestines	Feces	Microscopic identification of scolex or gravid proglottid
Pork tapeworm	Mild symptoms, if any[a]	Intestines	Feces	Same as for beef tapeworm

[a]Most cases are asymptomatic or have poorly defined distinctive symptoms.

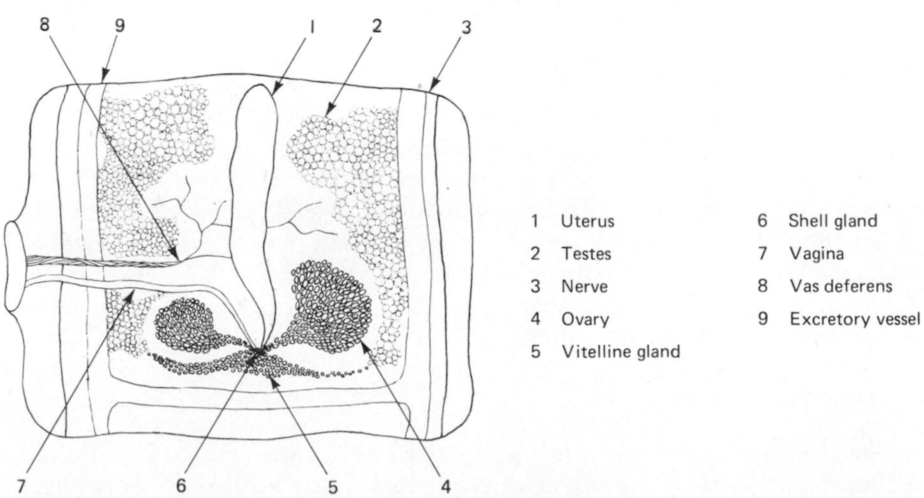

FIG. 37-13 A mature proglottid from *Taenia solium*.

TABLE 37-5 Representative Medically Important Trematodes

Organism	*Disease*	*Host Range*	*Location in the Body*	*Geographical Distribution*
Opisthorchis (Clonorchis) sinensis (Chinese liver fluke)	Clonorchiasis	Humans, dogs, cats	Liver, bile ducts	China, Japan, Korea, Indochina
Fasciola hepatica (sheep liver fluke)	Fascioliasis	Humans, sheep, goats, cattle	Liver, bile ducts	Sheep-raising regions
Fasciolopsis buski	Fasciolopsiasis	Humans, pigs	Small intestine (duodenum, jejunum)	Orient
Heterophyes heterophyes	Heterophyiasis	Humans, cats, dogs	Small intestine	Near East, Far East
Metagonimus yokogawai	Metagonimiasis	Humans, cats, dogs, pigs	Small intestine	Far East, Siberia, Balkan states
Opisthorchis felineus	Opisthorchiasis	Cats, occasionally humans	Biliary and pancreatic ducts	Mainly in central and eastern Europe, U.S.S.R.
Paragonimus westermani	Paragonimiasis	Humans, cats	Lungs	Far East, Nigeria, Belgian Congo, Central America
Schistosoma haematobium	Schistosomiasis	Humans, monkeys	Blood vessels, urinary bladder	Mainly Africa and Madagascar
Schistosoma japonicum	Schistosomiasis	Humans, domestic animals	Blood vessels	Japan, China, Formosa, Philippines
Schistosoma mansoni	Schistosomiasis	Humans	Blood vessels, intestines	Africa, South America, including Puerto Rico and the Lesser Antilles

significance. Table 37-5 lists some of the parasites belonging to this group that cause disease in humans (Figure 37-16).

Generally speaking, flukes are flattened (somewhat in the form of a leaf or pear), lack a distinct and segmented body, and are covered by an external cuticular layer. They range in size from less than one millimeter to several centimeters, depending on the species.

As shown in Figure 37-17, these worms possess suckers and excretory, digestive, and reproductive systems. The digestive systems of the medically important parasites are incomplete. With one exception—the schistosomes, or blood flukes—all trematodes are hermaphroditic. Sexual reproduction is by self-fertilization or cross-fertilization between two individual parasites.

LIFE CYCLES

Most human-associated flukes produce operculated eggs (Figure 37-18a) and pass through four larval stages. The one exception is the schistosomes, which have nonoperculated eggs and only three larval stages (Figure 36-19b).

The eggs of trematodes can be found in sputum, urine, or feces, depending upon the location of the parasite in the host (such as *Paragonimus westermani* in the lungs, *Schistosoma haematobium* in the urinary bladder). By contrast, among human-associated cestodes, the eggs of adult worms are encountered only in the feces.

The individual larval stages of flukes are (1) ***miracidium***, (2) ***sporocyst***, (3) ***redia***, and (4) ***cercariae*** (Figure 37-19). The last three stages are found in freshwater snails. In certain trematode species, such as ***Opisthorchis (Clonorchis) sinensis, Fasciola hepatica,*** and ***Paragonimus westermani***, the last infective stage (known as ***metacercariae***) can be found in crustaceans, in fishes, or on vegetation. The life cycle of a blood fluke can be used to show the relationships of these larval stages (Figure 37-20).

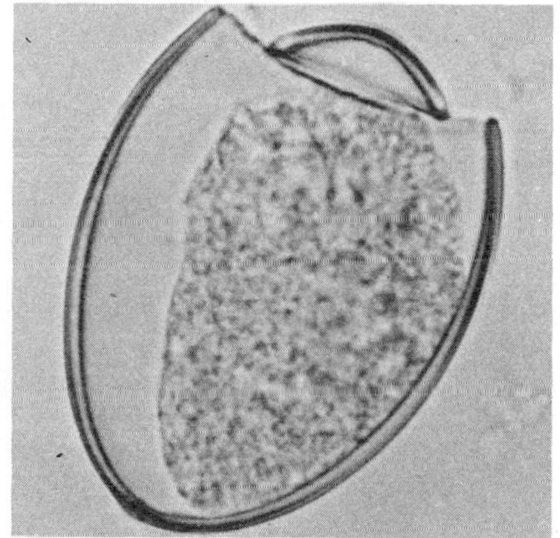

(a)

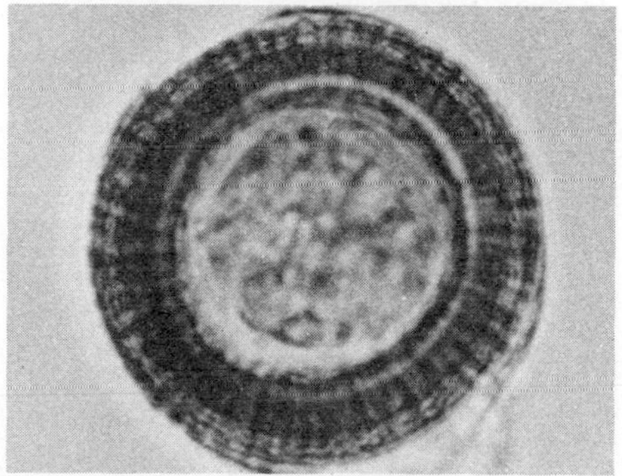

(b)

FIG. 37-14 Representative cestode eggs. (a) An operculated egg. (b) A non-operculated egg.

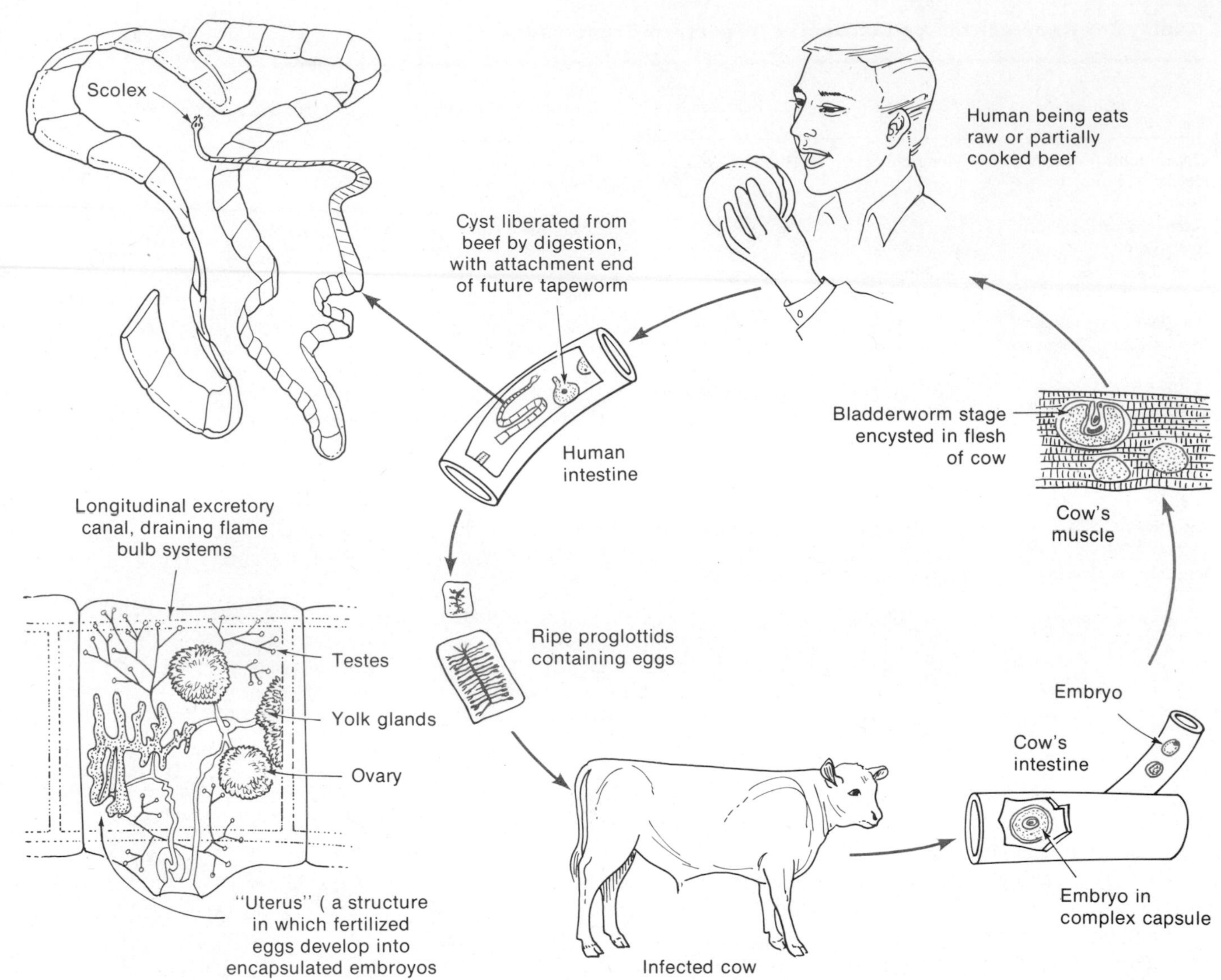

FIG. 37-15 The beef tapeworm *Taenia saginata* and its life cycle. Several important structures of the helminth are shown, including those of a typical adult tapeworm and a mature proglottid.

The life cycle of a schistosome begins when ova containing fully developed miracidia are passed by human infected feces. If the fecal matter comes into contact with water, the miracidium becomes active, ruptures the egg, and escapes into the watery surroundings. The miracidium swims about in search of an appropriate snail host. Upon penetrating the intermediate host, these larval forms lose their ciliated covering, develop into sporocysts, and migrate to the visceral mass of the mollusc. The sporocysts multiply rapidly, and within two weeks large numbers of minute daughter sporocysts develop.

Unlike other flukes of medical importance, schistosomes do not produce rediae at any time during their life cycles. The final larval stage, cercariae, arise from sporocysts. Once formed, these fork-tailed cercariae escape from the snail and swim freely in a water environment, looking for an appropriate host. In penetrating the unbroken skin of a mammalian host, the fork-tails of the cercariae are discarded. The schistosomes develop into male and female worms, mate, and deposit eggs within the tissues of the new host.

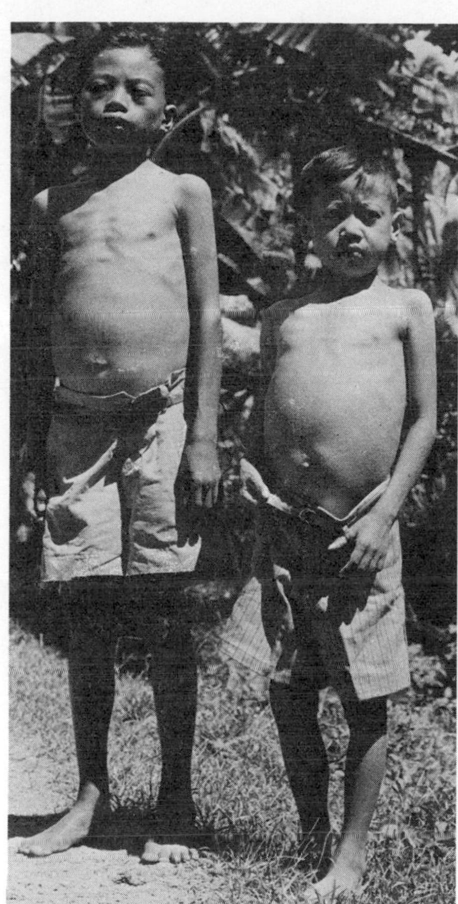

FIG. 37-16 Victims of blood fluke infection. Note the enlarged abdomens and puffy faces. *Courtesy of the World Health Organization.*

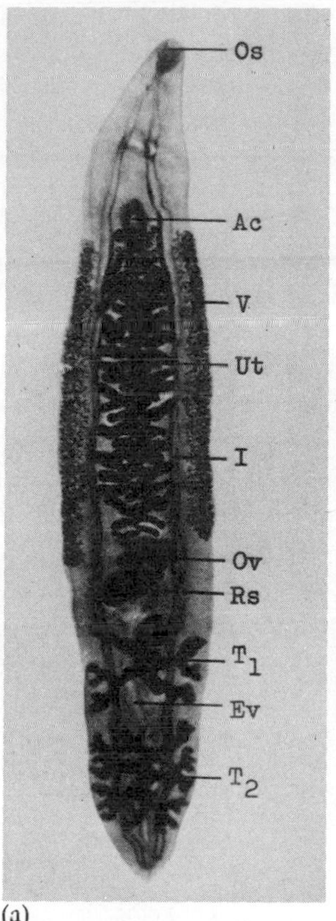

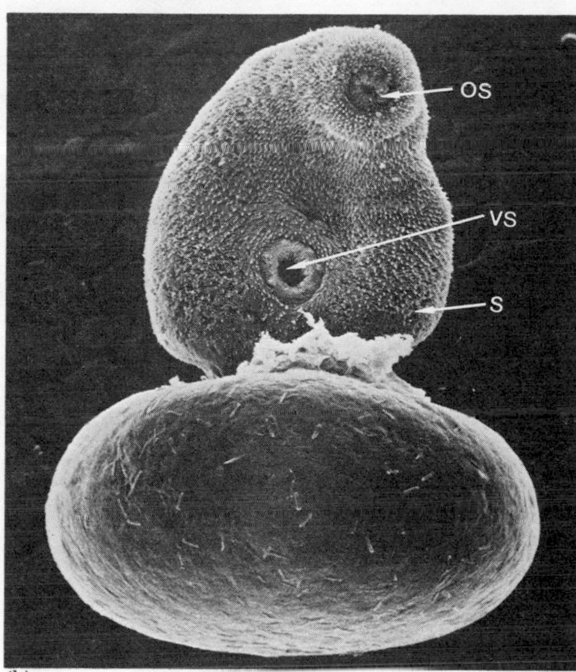

(a) (b)

FIG. 37-17 Characteristics of flukes. (a) The anatomy of a sexually mature *Clonorchis sinensis* (Chinese liver fluke). This morphological type, the ***distome*** (possessing two suckers), is one of the most frequently encountered. Shown here are the oral sucker (Os); ventral sucker (Vs); viterleria (V); uterus (Ut); intestines (I); ovary (Ov); seminal receptacle (Sr); testes (T_1 and T_2); excretory bladder (E). *Courtesy of Dr. Y. Komiya, Director, National Institute of Health, Tokyo, Japan.* (b) A newly emerging fluke, *Fasciola hepatica* showing its oral sucker (OS), ventral sucker (VS), and an outer covering of spines. *Bennet, C. E.,* J. Parasit. *61:886–891 (1975).*

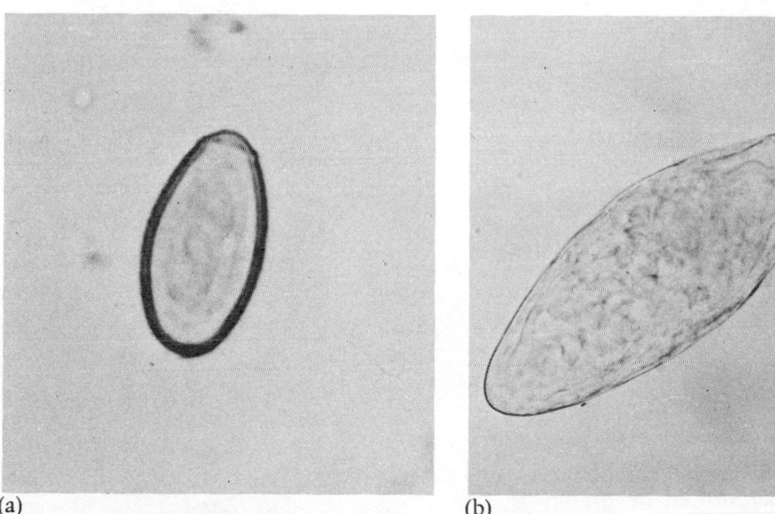

(a) (b)

FIG. 37-18 A comparison of operculated and nonoperculated ova of flukes. (a) *Clonorchis sinensis.* Eggs of this parasite are approximately 29 μm long and 16 μm wide. Notice the thin operculum (O). (b) *Schistosoma haematobium.* These ova have dimensions of 110 to 175 μm in length and 40 to 70 μm in width. Note the terminal spine.

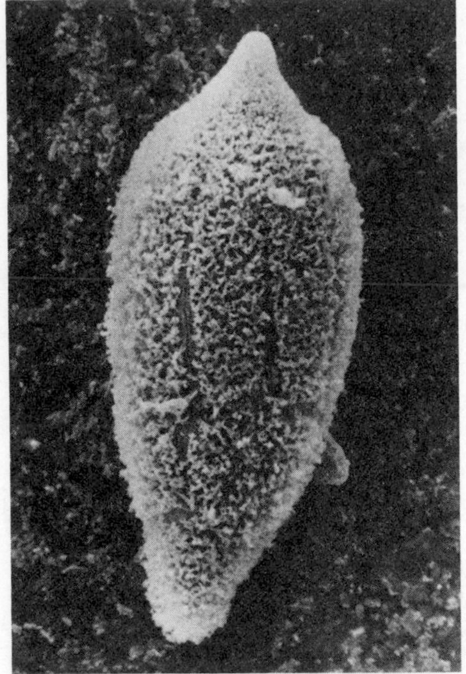

(a)

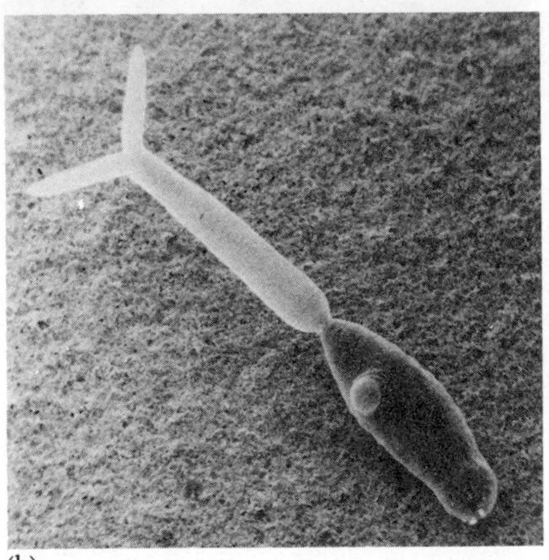

(b)

FIG. 37-19 Two larval stages of flukes as shown by scanning electron microscopy. (a) The miracidium. Note its highly ciliated surfaces. (b) The fork-tailed cercarium of the schistosome. This form penetrates the skin surfaces of a susceptible host immersed in contaminated water. *Courtesy of Dr. H. D. Blankespoor, the University of Michigan.*

The effects and laboratory diagnosis of fluke infections are given in Table 37-6.

TABLE 37-6 Characteristics of Fluke Infections

Disease	*Clinical Features*	*Location of Adult Worm*	*Specimen of Choice*	*Laboratory Diagnosis*
Clonorchiasis	Abdominal pains, diarrhea, enlarged spleen and liver, increases in eosinophils	Liver and bile duct	Feces	Microscopic demonstration of ova
Paragonimiasis (lung fluke)	Chronic cough, respiratory difficulties, sputum with brownish streaks	Lungs	Sputum, surgical specimens	1. Microscopic identification of adults in surgical specimens or ova in sputum 2. Skin test and immunological laboratory tests
Schistosomiasis (bilharziasis)	Abdominal pain, fever, allergic reactions, inflammation of urinary bladder *(S. haematobium)*, neurological destruction, spleen and liver enlargement	Urinary bladder, liver, mesenteric vein in large intestine	Feces, urine,[a] biopsy	1. Microscopic demonstration of ova 2. Intradermal tests 3. Complement fixation 4. Circumoval precipitin test[b]

[a] *S. haematobium* only.
[b] Test depends on the formation of a precipitate around preserved eggs incubated in immune serum.

PREVENTION

Preventive measures for many helminthic infestations involve interrupting the life cycle of the parasite, the destruction of the adult flukes and ova, and the control of intermediate hosts (Figure 37-21). More public health education is needed to improve sanitation and persuade individuals in endemic areas to stop eating raw or improperly cooked fecal-contaminated foods.

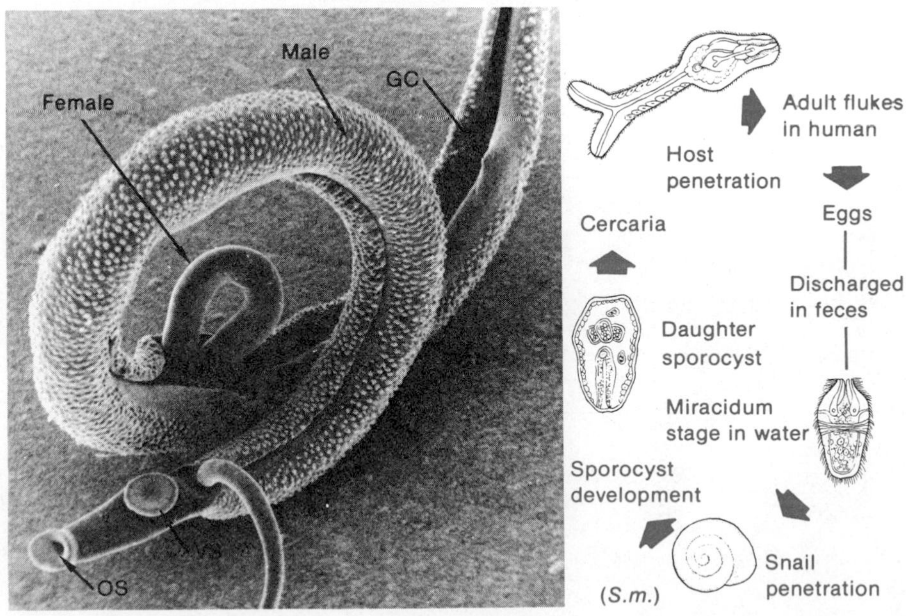

FIG. 37-20 A schistosome life cycle. Male and female *Schistosoma mansoni* (scanning EM) are shown in the upper left portion of the cycle. Note the following anatomical parts: gynecophoric canal (GC); oral sucker (OS); and ventral sucker (VS). *Scanning micrograph through the courtesy of Dr. H. D. Blankespoor, the University of Michigan.*

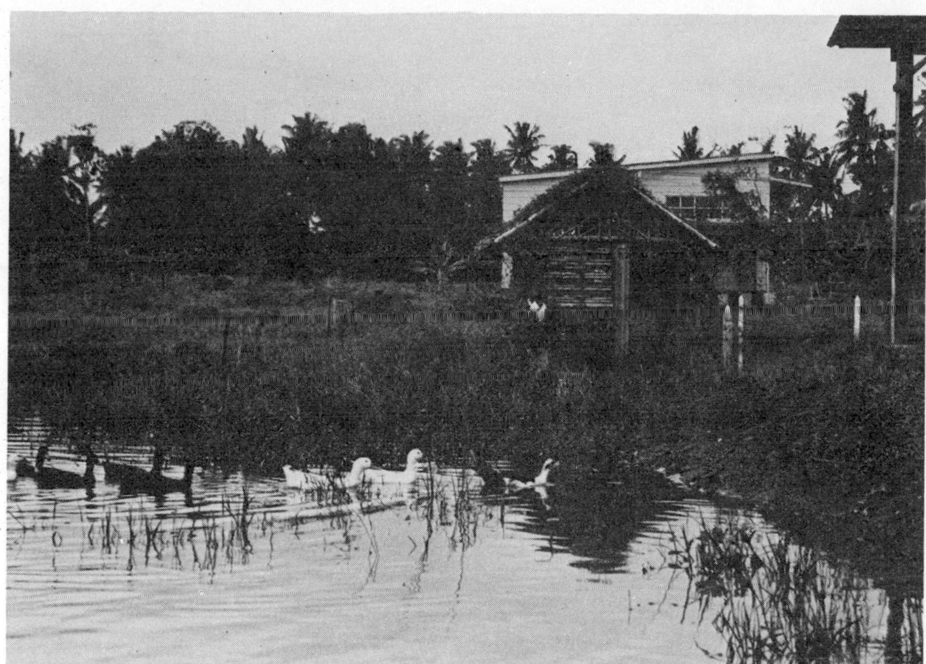

FIG. 37–21 An experiment is being conducted in the Philippines to determine whether ducks can effectively reduce the population of snails living in sluggish water environments. *Courtesy of World Health Organization.*

SUMMARY

1. Most helminths, or worms, are free-living, but some are parasitic and can cause diseases in humans and in domestic and wild animals and plants.
2. Helminths of medical and economic importance include roundworms (nematodes), tapeworms (cestodes), and flukes (trematodes).

The Equipment of Parasitic Worms

Various worms have several modifications that favor their survival as parasites; these include hardened outer surface coverings, the possession of hooks, spines, cutting plates, suckers, and enzymes for attachment to host tissues, and elaborate reproductive systems.

Life Cycles and Control of Parasitic Helminths

1. Worms capable of either a parasitic or free-living existence are *facultative* parasites. Those incapable of completing their life cycles without a host are *obligate* parasites.
2. *Endoparasites* are found internally in hosts; *ectoparasites* are found attached to the skin or in the outer layers of skin.
3. *Definitive hosts* harbor the adult, or sexually mature, form of the parasite; *intermediate hosts* provide the environment for the development of some or all larval stages.

Distribution and Transmission

1. The distribution of parasitic worms is influenced by the habits of suitable hosts and by environmental conditions such as appropriate temperature and moisture.
2. The sources and transmission of parasitic diseases involve susceptible domestic and wild hosts, bloodsucking insects, foods containing immature infective parasites, and contaminated soil, water, or other portions of the environment.
3. Destructive effects of parasitic worms depend on their number, size, location, degree of activity, and toxic products.

Symptoms and Pathology

Symptoms of helminth infections may be absent, few, or severe.

Laboratory Diagnosis

1. The finding and identification of ova, larvae, and adult worms are sufficient for diagnosis.
2. Skin tests and other immunological procedures are used to identify susceptible individuals, to distinguish one type of infection from another, or to follow the progress of recovery.

The Nematodes

1. Practically every tissue of the human body is vulnerable to attack by certain roundworms.
2. Roundworms are unsegmented, cylindrical, tapered at both ends, bilaterally symmetrical, and do not have any appendages.
3. These worms have digestive, nervous, and reproductive systems. The sexes, with few exceptions, are in separate worms.
4. The life cycles of nematodes vary and usually include the adult worm, egg, and larvae.

Representative Animal Roundworm Infections

1. Examples of human nematode infections include filariasis (elephantiasis), hookworm, pinworm, and trichinosis (pork roundworm).
2. Examples of measures for the prevention and control of these and other helminth infections are mass treatment of infected persons, improved general sanitation, and education of individuals as to the parasite, its mode of transmission and effects.

Parasitic Nematodes of Plants

1. Roundworm plant parasites cause enormous damage to cultivated plants and are responsible for major agricultural losses.
2. Both internal and external plant parts are subject to attack. Examples of the most common effects include tumors (galls), rotting of plant tissue, and interference with normal plant growth and development.
3. Several species of soil fungi are natural enemies of nematodes.

The Platyhelminthes

1. The Platyhelminthes, or flatworms, include both free-living and parasitic forms.
2. The true parasitic flatworms are the tapeworms (cestodes) and the flukes (trematodes). Both of these groups have undergone several adaptive changes that equip them for a parasitic existence. These changes include the possession of structures for attachment, excessive reproductive capacity, and the loss of a digestive system.

The Cestodes

1. Adult cestodes, or tapeworms, live in the intestines of vertebrate hosts.
2. These worms consist of a head, or *scolex*, a neck region, and a main body composed of segments called *proglottids*. The proglottids contain the reproductive organs and are responsible for the ribbonlike appearance of tapeworms.
3. The life cycles of cestodes are complex and involve eggs, larval forms, and adult worms.
4. Human tapeworm infections can be acquired by ingestion of contaminated, inadequately cooked fish, beef, pork, or lamb.

The Trematodes

1. Most flukes are flat, are covered by an external resistant layer, have suckers for attachment, and have excretory, digestive, and reproductive systems. These worms lack a head and a segmented body.
2. Except for the schistosomes, all individual trematodes are hermaphroditic.
3. The life cycles of most flukes include eggs, four larval stages, and adults.
4. Flukes can be acquired through the ingestion of inadequately cooked, contaminated fish, vegetation, or crayfish, as well as by swimming or working in contaminated waters.
5. Preventive and control measures are similar to those for other worm diseases.

QUESTIONS FOR REVIEW

1. Define or explain the following terms:
   a. scolex
   b. proglottid
   c. cercaria
   d. ova
2. What types of structural and functional modifications favor the parasitic existence of helminths? List at least four.
3. List the type of parasitic worms one might find if the following food sources were contaminated:
   a. beef and beef products
   b. pork
   c. fish
   d. crayfish
   e. lamb
   f. vegetation
4. What role do arthropods play in the transmission of parasitic helminths?
5. By what methods are helminthic infections controlled?
6. How are the following worm infections acquired?
   a. hookworm
   b. pinworm
   c. elephantiasis
   d. pork roundworm

SUGGESTED READINGS

Ansari, N. (ed.), *Epidemiology and Control of Schistosomiasis (Bilharziasis)*. Baltimore: University Park Press, 1973. *A detailed consideration of this most important fluke infection. The life cycle, distribution, and approaches to prevention and control are major topics.*

Brown, H. W., *Basic Clinical Parasitology*. 4th ed. New York: Appleton-Century-Crofts, 1975. *An excellent text with many illustrations. Descriptions of human parasitic diseases, especially those caused by roundworms, tapeworms, and flukes, and arthropods are included.*

Lobel, H. O., and I. G. Kagan, "Seroepidemiology of Parasitic Diseases," *Ann. Rev. Microbiol.* 32:329 (1978). *This review describes the use of immunological tests in investigations concerned with measuring the intensity and geographic distribution of infection. Also describes disease surveillance and control.*

Noble, E. R., and G. A. Noble, *Parasitology*. 4th ed. Philadelphia: Lea and Febiger, 1976. *Describes parasites according to individual phyla. Diseases, epidemiology, means of transmission, and life cycles are presented in a readable manner.*

Olsen, O. W., *Animal Parasites: Their Life Cycles and Ecology*. 3rd ed. Baltimore: University Park Press, 1974. *An excellent atlas of tapeworm life cycle.*

Smyth, J. D., *Introduction to Animal Parasitology*. 2nd ed. New York: John Wiley and Sons, 1976. *A nicely written basic text, describing the parasites of medical importance together with their treatment, control, and diagnosis. Many illustrations.*

PART SIX

Microorganisms and Industrial Processes

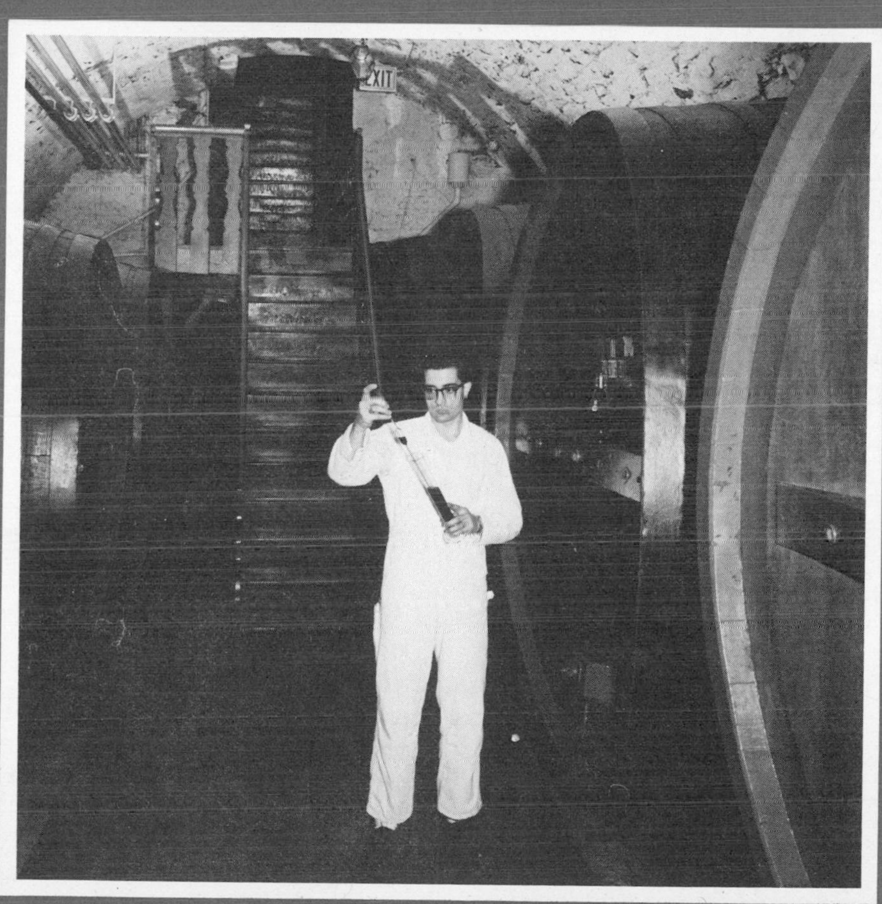

CHAPTER **38**

Industrial Microbiology

Human beings have used a great variety of microorganisms for economic gain or for prevention of economic loss. The utilization of microbes is an indisputable factor in the economic livelihood of the world, in meeting individual needs, as an environmental consideration, and for food production. Modern industrial microbiology seeks to manipulate and control microorganisms in the large-scale production of foods, antibiotics, and other microbial products. This chapter presents several aspects of industrial microbiology. In so doing, we shall also survey the increasing automation of routine manual techniques of microbiology.

After reading this chapter, you should be able to:

1. **Describe at least three microbial processes that are of commercial interest.**
2. **Discuss the basic similarities and differences in the making of beers, wines, and spirits.**
3. **Outline the processes by which the following microbial products are made: antibiotics, vinegar, amino acids, vitamins, lactic acid, citric acid, butanol, and isopropanol.**
4. **List six enzymes, their microbial origins, and their uses.**
5. **Describe the basic difference between most microbial processes and steroid transformation.**
6. **Discuss the use of microorganisms as pesticides.**
7. **Discuss the importance of automation to industrial microbiology.**

Many household substances are products of microbial activity. Several of these substances have been used since antiquity. Through the combined efforts of chemists, engineers, and microbiologists, modern technology can direct microorganisms to do the bidding of human beings.

An Introduction to Industrial Microbiology

Industrial microbiology is the use of microorganisms or a microbiological technique in a commercial enterprise. Beneficial microbial activities range from the production of foods, antibiotics, enzymes, and various organic chemicals to the preparation of alcoholic beverages, blood plasma substitutes, and **steroids** such as **hormones.** Important microbiological techniques are used for microbial contamination control, sterilization, and vitamin assays. Clinical microbiology is not usually considered part of industrial microbiology. However, the advent of many highly profitable laboratories concerned with medical microbiology and chemistry suggests that these clinical testing laboratories should be added to the roster. Automation and associated approaches have also influenced several of these industries.

This chapter will deal with a group of important and representative processes: the manufacture of alcoholic beverages, antibiotics, selected organic acids, alcohols, enzymes, and steroids; the use of microorganisms as pesticides; and automated techniques of industrial microbiology. Chapter 39 surveys food and dairy microbiology, and Chapter 40 presents a general view of the microbiology of soil, water, and waste treatment. The preparation of vaccines has been discussed in Chapter 26.

Aerobic versus Anaerobic Processes

The common reference to industrial fermentation is often mistaken. The term **fermentation** applies only to microbial processes performed under anaerobic conditions. Fermentation refers to the anaerobic reduction of organic substrates. A classic example of fermentation is the reduction of pyruvic acid to lactic acid, a reaction particularly important in the food and dairy industries. Many industrial processes are performed as ***submerged cultures*** resembling fermentation vats. However, the similarity ends there. These industrial processes are aerobic and require large quantities of air to be maintained. A major example of a submerged culture process involves the production of antibiotics. Many of the following processes are also aerobic in nature.

Alcoholic Beverages

The production of alcoholic beverages is an industry of enormous economic significance in many countries. The manufacture of all three major types of these products—beer, wine, and spirits (distilled alcoholic beverages)—is an application of industrial microbiology.

Historically, there is evidence that professional wine and beer making was well established by 3000 B.C. An Assyrian tablet dating back to 2000 B.C. states that Noah took beer with him aboard the ark. Egyptian and Chinese documents describe the production and use of beer in 2500 and 2300 B.C., respectively.

Beer

Beer is the product of a yeast fermentation process that uses barley or other grains as the source of sugars and various nitrogen-containing compounds. Because yeasts cannot ferment starch (the complex form of sugars contained in grains), a preliminary step, called ***malting,*** is required to break down the starches. In this process, the grain is kept moist, causing it to sprout, and initiating the production of the enzyme amylase. The enzyme breaks starch down into various simpler sugars that can be fermented by yeast. The sprouting malt grains are readied for fermentation by drying, and then mashing with water. Before the introduction of yeast, the fermentation medium is heated to eliminate undesirable microorganisms. Hops, dried petals of the vine ***Humulus lupulus,*** are added to enhance the color and flavor of the final product and to stabilize it. Hops contain, among other chemical compounds, two antibacterial substances, ***humulon*** and ***lupulon,*** which prevent bacterial contaminants from spoiling the beer. The fermentation process is complete when the desired alcohol concentration is reached. The beer is then filtered and pasteurized, or filtered through a very fine screen to remove bacteria. It may also be chillproofed to prevent formation of a haze or cloudiness when refrigerated.

There are two general types of beer, ***ales*** and ***lagers.*** Ales are fermented by ***Saccharomyces cerevesiae*** strains, which are called ***top yeasts.*** This terminology refers to the fact that the yeast cells produce uniform cloudiness (turbidity) and are carried up in containers to form foams by carbon dioxide. Ales are incubated at 14° to 23° C for 5 to 7 days and have higher alcohol concentrations than lagers. Lagers are fermented by strains of ***Saccharomyces carlsbergensis,*** also known as ***bottom yeasts*** because they tend to form sediments. Lagers are incubated at lower temperatures, 6° to 12° C, for a slightly longer time, 8 to 10 days. They contain more unfermented carbohydrates that are not converted into ethanol.

Wine

Wine is made by the fermentation of almost any ripe fruit juice or from extracts from certain vegetable products, such as dandelions. Because these starting materials contain a high concentration of sugar (up to 30 percent), as much as 15 percent alcohol may be obtained with certain yeast strains. The grapes used for wine usually range in sugar content from 12 to 30 percent and in water content from 70 to 85 percent. The other constitutents in grapes, including acids and minerals (Color Photograph 98), account for the different color, taste, and sometimes bouquet of wines.

As soon as the skin of the grape is broken, the fermentation begins. Commercially, the fruit is crushed and pressed mechanically (Figure 38–1 and Color Photograph 99). The resulting pressed grape juice, called **must,** can be fermented naturally by the enzymatic activity of wild yeasts that grow on the grapes. In Europe, the yeasts normally on the grapes are used to perform the fermentation. In the United States, grape juice and other fermentable substances are usually sterilized to prevent the growth of undesirable microorganisms. Specific yeast cultures, strains of ***Saccharomyces ellipsoideus,*** are then introduced, and the mixture of fruit juice and microorganisms is aerated to promote yeast growth. Anaerobic conditions are instituted when yeasts are present in sufficient numbers to carry out the fermentation.

When the fermentation is complete, as determined by the alcohol content of a sample, the wine is placed in vats to clarify and age. Aging involves continuing the enzymatic activities under anaerobic conditions until the flavor and aroma for that particular wine have developed. While aging takes place, the wine slowly clears and the suspended solid material settles to the bottom of the container in the form of a sediment. Normally, the product is separated from its sediment and transferred several times to smaller containers. This procedure, called *racking*, is continued until the aging process reaches its limit in the tanks. To prevent spoilage, the resulting product is pasteurized or filtered and then bottled.

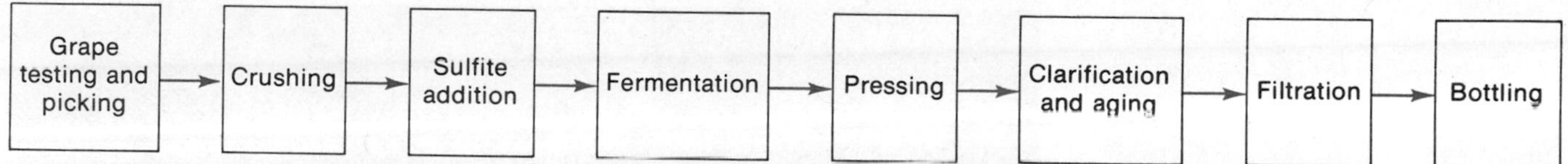

FIG. 38-1 A summary of the basic steps involved in red wine making. The sulfite is added to control spoilage microorganisms. For white wines, pressing precedes fermentation.

Sake

Although sake is called a rice wine, it is actually manufactured more like beer. A mixed culture of the mold ***Aspergillus oryzae*** and a species of ***Saccharomyces*** is used to inoculate steamed rice. The mold grows throughout the rice, producing a partially fermented material called koji, which is then mixed with water and more steamed rice and incubated. As the ***Aspergillus*** digests the starch in the rice to form maltose and glucose, the ***Saccharomyces*** uses the sugars to produce ethyl alcohol to the extent of about 14 percent.

Distilled Beverages

Beverages obtained through distillation include whiskey, brandy, and rum. The product is dependent upon the material used in the fermentation. The whiskeys are prepared from different types of grains, brandy from fruit juices, and rum from molasses. Rye whiskey is produced from distilled fermented rye grains, bourbon from corn, and scotch from barley malt. The various flavors of whiskeys result from the presence of minor ingredients known as congenerics. These substances include aldehydes, esters, ethers, higher alcohols, and volatile acids.

Whiskey can be distilled by the use of vacuum and heat. This separates the volatile products from most of the water and solids. The resulting distillate has an alcohol content of 90 to 96 percent. Distilled products are labeled according to their alcohol content in terms of ***proof levels.*** Proof is twice the value of the percent alcohol. Thus, in beverages containing 90 to 96 percent alcohol the proof is between 180 and 192. The raw product is then aged, or matured, in wooden casks or barrels. The distillate is also diluted with water to reduce the alcohol content to approximately 51.5 percent, or 103 proof. During storage, the concentration will vary due to evaporation. When ready for bottling, the product is usually standardized to a particular value, commonly 80 proof.

Antibiotics

The discovery of penicillin was reported by Alexander Fleming in 1929, and the subsequent development of this compound in the early 1940s by Ernst Boris Chain and Sir Howard Walter Florey was the basis for today's multi-billion-dollar antibiotics industry. **Antibiotics** are usually produced by growing a specific bacterial or fungal species in a submerged culture in large, well-aerated tanks (Figure 38–2). In the case of penicillin production, for example, a suitable medium (which usually contains by-products of the distilling industry) is aseptically inoculated with fungi such as ***Penicillium chrysogenum*** or *P. notatum* (Color Photograph 34). After one or two weeks of growth, conditions develop that interfere with the production of penicillin. At this time the fungal growth is removed by centrifugation, sometimes with filtration, followed by the complex extraction and purification of the antibiotic.

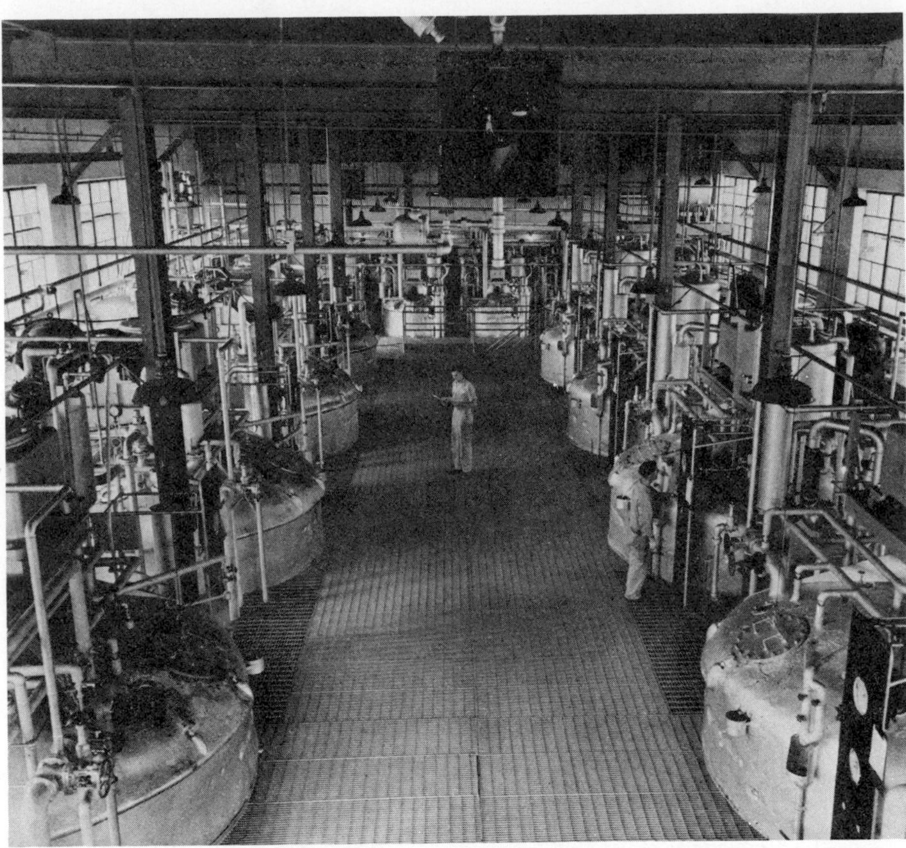

FIG. 38–2 A portion of the fermentation unit used for streptomycin production. *Streptomyces griseus,* the microorganism, from which the antibiotic is produced, is grown from test tube quantities through increasingly larger tanks. When it has multiplied itself billions of times, the living material is transferred to the huge tanks shown for final fermentation. *Courtesy of Merck and Co., Inc.*

Other commercial antibiotics have been obtained from similar activities of bacteria (such as *Bacillus polymyxa, B. subtilis,* and *Actinomyces* spp.) and fungi (such as *Aspergillus fumigatus).* The antibiotics produced by these and other microorganisms are largely responsible for the successful treatment of many dread bacterial diseases, including anthrax, gonorrhea, meningitis, strep throat, syphilis, and tuberculosis. Research by the pharmaceutical industry is constantly developing new and modified antibiotics that have already broadened the application of these "wonder drugs."

Acids, Vitamins, and Alcohols

Vinegar

Commercial vinegar is usually made from wine or cider. It contains 3 to 5 percent acetic acid, which is responsible for its sour taste. In one process, fruit juice is fermented by brewer's yeast, *Saccharomyces cervisiae,* until it contains

TABLE 38-1 Selected Amino Acids and Vitamins Produced by Microorganisms

Products	Microorganisms
Amino Acids	
Glutamic acid	*Micrococcus glutamicus, Arthrobacter* sp., *Brevibacterium* sp.
Lysine	*Escherichia coli, Enterobacter aerogenes*[a]
Valine	*Escherichia coli*
Vitamins	
Cyanocobalamine (B_{12})	*Streptomyces olivaceus, Propionibacterium freundenreichii*
Riboflavin (B_2)	*Ashbya gossypii*[b]

[a]Both of these organisms are required for the process.
[b]This organism is a mold; all others are bacteria.

10 to 12 percent alcohol. This alcoholic solution is then sprayed into a tank that contains aerated wood shavings, coke, or gravel. These materials provide the surfaces on which species of *Acetobacter* can grow and oxidize the alcohol to acetic acid. The overall reaction is

$$\underset{\text{ethanol}}{CH_3CH_2OH} \rightarrow \underset{\text{acetaldehyde}}{CH_3CHO} \rightarrow \underset{\text{acetic acid}}{CH_3COOH}$$

Acetobacter aceti, which was first studied by Pasteur in 1862, is one of the more common species involved in the reaction. Another organism, *A. xylinum,* has been observed to produce its own supporting material by forming a meshwork of cellulose fibers. This enables the organism to have intimate contact with the alcohol solution and permits air to circulate around participating cells. The entire process must be carefully controlled, especially as regards aeration and temperature. The oxidation of the alcoholic fluid produces so much heat that bacterial growth may be stopped if the system is not cooled. The vinegar is collected at the bottom of the tank and may be recirculated to produce more oxidation and a higher-strength product. Residual alcohol evaporates in the process, leaving none to be bottled with the vinegar.

Amino Acids

Although amino acids are obtained through the consumption of foods, some plant proteins lack amino acids essential for human nutrition and well-being. If foodstuffs prepared from plant products are supplemented with the amino acids for which they are deficient, their nutritional value is substantially improved. A variety of microorganisms can be used to synthesize amino acids for use as supplements and food flavorings for humans and other animals. Table 38–1 lists several products and the microorganisms involved with their formation.

In the glutamic acid process, bacteria such as *Micrococcus glutamicus* or species of *Arthrobacter* or *Brevibacterium* are able to add ammonia to alpha-ketoglutaric acid (Figure 14–13), one of the intermediate compounds of the citric acid cycle. This process produces glutamic acid in yields much greater than needed by the bacteria. The surplus can be recovered from the medium. The usual substrates in the glutamic acid process are molasses, fish meal, soybean cake, and ammonium compounds. In addition to being a potential food supplement, glutamic acid is used in flavoring as monsodium glutamate (MSG).

The lysine process requires two different bacteria, each for a different step. *Escherichia coli* is inoculated into glycerol, corn steep liquor, and ammonium compounds to produce diaminopimalic acid. This chemical is then modified by *Enterobacter aerogenes* to produce lysine.

Other amino acids produced by microorganisms and fermentation include methionine, threonine, tryptophan and valine.

Vitamin Production

Vitamins can be made commercially by synthetic processes. However, some vitamins are rather complicated and expensive to produce by such means and can be more economically made by microbial fermentation. Vitamin B_2 (riboflavin) and vitamin B_{12} (cyanocobalaminc) are two such products of microbial activity. To produce riboflavin, the mold *Ashbya gossypii* is grown in corn steep liquors. The process for cyanocobalamine utilizes either *Streptomyces olivaceus* or *Propionibacterium freundenreichii*, grown in malt extract and corn steep liquor and supplemented with cobalt, an essential part of the vitamin's structure.

Other Products of Fermentation

A wide variety of other chemicals can be produced by microorganisms in sufficient quantities to make such activities commercially profitable. Table 38–2 lists examples of organic acids and alcohols other than ethanol together with the responsible microorganisms. Two interesting organic acids manufactured commercially by fermentation are citric and lactic acids.

TABLE 38–2 Selected Organic Acids and Alcohols Produced by Microorganisms

Product	Microorganisms	Uses
Citric acid[a]	*Aspergillus niger,*[b] *A. wentii*	Anticoagulant; flavoring of foods, etc.; manufacture of ink and dyes; engraving
Lactic acid	*Lactobacillus delbrueckii, L. bulgaricus*	Calcium lactate, and iron lactate for nutritional deficiency conditions; solvent in lacquers; leather manufacture
Butanol[c]	*Clostridium butylicum* *C. acetobutylicum*	Solvent; perfume manufacture
Isopropanol[c]	*C. butylicum*	Solvent; perfume manufacture; rubbing alcohol

[a]The citric acid process is aerobic.
[b]Molds.
[c]Now made primarily as by-products of gasoline manufacturing.

Citric acid is produced as a surplus, an intermediate compound of the citric acid cycle. The molds *Aspergillus niger* and *A. wentii* are grown in cornstarch, corn meal, beets, molasses, sugar cane juice, and raw sugar. The process is an aerobic one carried out in large, aerated fermentors. Once the citric acid is formed, it can be recovered from the growth medium.

Lactic acid is produced by a fermentation process carried out by *Lactobacillus delbrueckeii* or *L. bulgaricus*. These bacteria are grown in acid-hydrolized corn or potato starch, molasses, or whey from cheese making. In the process, the lactic acid is usually neutralized with lime (CaO) to form calcium lactate. This compound can be used as a food supplement or it can be converted back to lactic acid for other uses.

TABLE 38-3 Microbial Enzymes and Selected Uses

Enzyme	*Microorganisms*	*Uses*
Amylase	*Aspergillus oryzae*[a]	Adhesives; baking; brewing; laundry presoak products; spot remover; syrups
Asparaginase	*Azotobacter vinelandii, Bacillus coagulans, Bacterium cadaveris, Escherichia coli* B, *Pseudomonas* sp., *Serratia marcescens*	Antitumor activity
Lipase	*Bacillus licheniformis*	Leather manufacture
Pectinase	*Aspergillus aureus,*[a] *A. wentii*[a]	Clarifying fruit juices and wines; rett flax for linen
Protease	*Aspergillus oryzae*[a] *Bacillus* spp.	Baking and brewing; chillproofing beer; degum silk goods; glue; laundry presoak; leather manufacture; meat tenderizer; cheese ripener; spot remover; wound cleaning
Streptodornase	*Streptococcus hemolyticus*	Dissolving blood clots
Streptokinase	*Streptococcus hemolyticus*	Wound cleaning

[a]Molds.

The industrial need for large amounts of alcohol can be met by such compounds as butanol and isopropanol. Both compounds are produced primarily as by-products of the nonbiological process for making gasoline from crude petroleum. However, as petroleum becomes more scarce, it is entirely likely that the microbial fermentation processes will replace this source. Butanol and isopropanol can be produced together by certain species of ***Clostridium butylicum***. Butanol alone can be produced by ***C. acetobutylicum***. The products are produced from fruit cannery wastes or molasses.

Microbial Enzymes

Enzymes of fungi and bacteria have a wide variety of industrial applications, including alcoholic beverages, food, detergents and pharmaceuticals. Table 38–3 lists some of these enzymes, along with their microbial origins and selected uses.

In the production of alcoholic beverages, microbial amylase and protease may be used instead of the enzymes from barley malt to prepare grains for fermentation. These enzymes can also chillproof beer by degrading the proteins that cause cloudiness in such beverages upon refrigeration.

Proteases and lipases are used in cleaning animal hides, a necessary step in leather production. Proteases are also used commercially for meat tenderizing, as they are capable of breaking down some of the tough meat protein.

One commercial application of microbial enzymes has been the removal of stains from clothing. Many substances that stain clothes either are made of lipids, proteins, or starches or are held in a fabric by these types of compounds. Certain enzymes, under suitable conditions, can decompose stains or the cementing substances associated with them, thereby helping to clean the soiled fabric. Needless to say, stains can be caused by a large variety of substances, and appropriate enzymes may not be available or, if available, may not be incorporated into detergent or presoak compounds used in laundering. Thus it is not so surprising that all stains are not removed by commercial products. Moreover, such enzyme-containing products have been associated with the development of **allergies.**

Microbial enzymes are obtained by processes carried out either in shallow pans for optimum aeration by diffusion or in tanks where aeration is produced by bubbling air through the growth medium. Usually rich organic wastes from dairy or canning plants are used as the growth medium. When microbial growth is judged complete on the basis of an analysis for the desired enzyme, the microorganisms are removed by filtration, leaving the culture filtrate, which can be processed for the desired enzyme.

Immobilized Enzymes

We noted in Chapter 19 the development of filters coated with certain enzymes to improve the efficiency of filtration. Such immobilized (stationary) enzymes within polyacrylamide gel columns are used in certain commercial processes, such as the conversion of starch to simpler sugars (glucose to fructose and sucrose to glucose and fructose). Other applications of enzymes are being developed: the use of lactase for the processing of whey during the manufacture of cheese; urease for treatment of certain waste waters; phenol oxidase for the processing of phenolic wastes; and pesticide-hydrolyzing enzymes for various pesticides. The advantage of immobilizing the enzymes wherever possible is that it provides a means of removing them once the process is complete.

Steroid Transformations

Steroid hormones are extremely important in contraception and in the treatment and management of various conditions, including arthritis and shock. Corticosterone, an adrenal cortex hormone, has been very useful in the treatment of shock. Supplies of this compound were obtained from cattle and were in limited supply until studies showed that microorganisms could transform other steroids into corticosterone. Investigations also showed that a combination of chemical and microbial reactions could be used to produce another steroid hormone, cortisone, widely applied in the treatment of **arthritis** and in control of other types of inflammatory states.

Industrial fermentative processes, such as the production of beer, wine, and rum, involve many enzymes in the conversion of the sugar substrate to the alcohol product desired. Steroid transformations are quite different: a single specific enzyme changes one particular chemical component on a steroid molecule, thus creating a new compound. Such an enzyme may be associated with only one microbial species. Table 38–4 gives several examples of microorganisms and the particular steroid each can produce from progesterone (Figure 38–3). These and related microorganisms are the only practical means available for the large-scale production of selected steroids. These compounds are used to correct or lessen the effects of hormonal and related disorders.

TABLE 38–4 Microbial Steroid Transformations

Microorganism	*Transformation*
Aspergillus ochraceus	Progesterone $\rightarrow$ 11 α hydroxyprogesterone
Curvuloria lunata	Progesterone $\rightarrow$ 4 pregnene-11β, 21-diol-3, 20-dione
Dactylium dendroides	Progesterone $\rightarrow$ 11 α hydroxyprogesterone
Streptomyces lavendulae[a]	Progesterone $\rightarrow$ 20 β hydroxyprogesterone

[a]This organism is a bacterium; all the others are fungi.

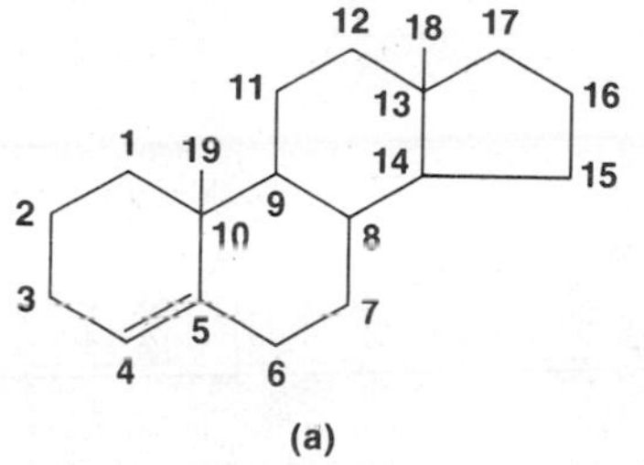

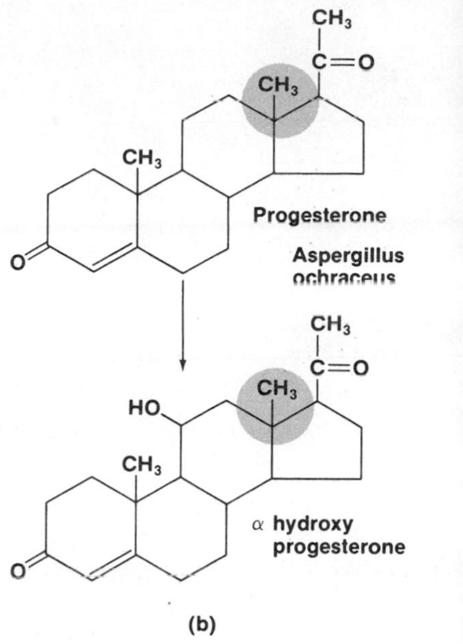

FIG. 38-3 The microbial transformation of progesterone. (a) The basic steroid structure. The numbers designate the location of particular carbon atoms. (b) The microbial transformation by the mold *Aspergillus ochraceus* of progesterone into 11 α (alpha) hydroxyprogesterone. This product can be modified further to produce cortisone.

Microbial Insecticides

Many insects associated with the destruction of agricultural products (Figure 38–4) or with the transmission of various disease agents to humans, other animals, and plants appear to be susceptible to the effects of certain microorganisms. Agostino Bassi in 1838 first proposed the use of microorganisms to control insect pests. In order for a prospective insect pathogen to be an effective "microbial insecticide," it should meet certain requirements, including (1) ability to injure the specific insect host enough so that its "competitive" activities are inhibited; (2) fast action; (3) specificity for a particular insect pest (the insect pathogen should be harmless to useful insects and invertebrates); (4) relative stability to environmental factors, such as drying and sunlight, and to the manner in which it is dispensed in the field (dust or spray); and (5) economically feasible manufacture. Unfortunately, taken as a whole, the majority of microorganisms isolated from diseased insects do not seem to fulfill these requirements, making microbial control of agricultural pests a difficult task. The microorganisms that have proven particularly effective as pesticides are listed in Table 38–5 with the pests they control. These organisms either infect the insect pests and produce a disease that spreads to other insects (*Bacillus popillae, B. lentimorbus, Beuveria bassiana,* for example) or produce a toxin effective when applied to the insects but do not reproduce in the field.

Bacillus popillae and *B. lentimorbus* produce milky white disease. The name refers to the massive whitish growth of the bacteria in the insect's body fluids. *B. popillae* (Figure 7–24d) and *B. thuringiensis* produce crystalline structures during their sporulation. Such crystals are called *parasporal bodies* due to their location. In the case of *B. popillae,* they do not appear to be related to the disease process. On the other hand, for *B. thuringiensis,* the significance of these crystals lies in the fact that the protein of which they are made functions as a toxin capable of injuring the mid-gut cells of susceptible insects. The activity of these crystals may inhibit the feeding of the pest or may cause other harmful effects.

Another bacterium, *Pseudomonas aeruginosa,* has also been shown effective in controlling adult grasshoppers, locusts, some caterpillars, and the wax moth. However, because of its known ability to cause infections in humans and other animals, its potential as a microbial insecticide is questionable.

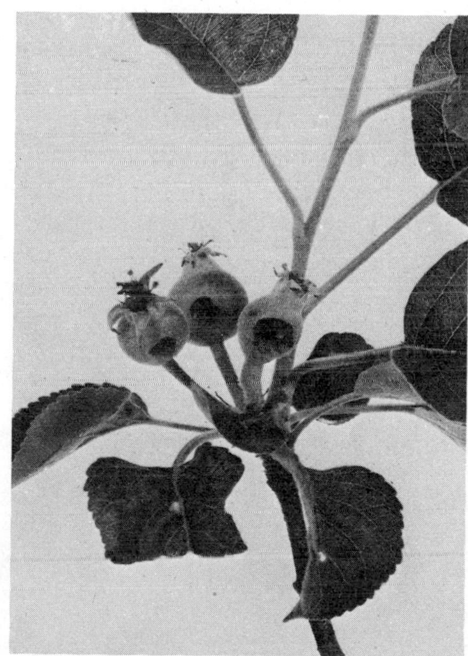

FIG. 38-4 Feeding injury to developing apples caused by green fruitworms *(Orthosia hibisci)*. Fruitworms are the larval stages of certain insects (lepidoptera). These larvae have been given this name because of their habit of eating holes in the fruits of apple, cherry, peach, pear, and plum trees. *Courtesy of Dr. R. W. Rings and the Ohio Agricultural Research and Development Center. From* J. Econ. Entomol. *63:1562–1568 (1970).*

TABLE 38-5 Microorganisms Used As Pesticides

Microorganism	*Insect Pests*
Bacillus popillae	Japanese beetle European chafer
B. lentimorbus	European chafer
B. thuringiensis	Chicken louse Tobacco hornworm Fall and spring cauberworm
B. thuringiensis and nuclear polyhedrosis virus[a]	Cotton bollworm Cabbage looper Alfalfa caterpillar Western test caterpillar
B. thuringiensis and granulosis virus[a]	Cabbage worm
B. thuringiensis and *Beuveria bassiana*[b]	European cabbage worm

[a]These combinations are required for effective control.
[b]*B. bassiana* is a fungus.

Automation for Microbiology

Automation has touched many areas of science and technology, and microbiology is no exception. The development and application of automated instruments (Figure 38-5) are gaining importance in various applied and industrial areas of microbiology. For example, a variety of automated procedures are used in antibiotic testing, food microbiological analysis, and immunology. The development of automated microbiology technology has been accompanied by many rapid methods for the detection, counting, and identification of microorganisms and their products (Color Photographs 94, 95, and 96).

Several miniaturized systems for the biochemical identification of pure bacterial cultures have become available in recent years. Although these systems differ in many respects, they all represent prepacked combinations of tests based upon fairly conventional biochemical identification schemes. Some are integrated with a computerized data base to speed microbial identification. Most systems on the market today were originally designed to identify gastrointestinal and related bacterial pathogens. However, other wider applications have been developed, and rapid methods will continue to have practical application and value in microbiology.

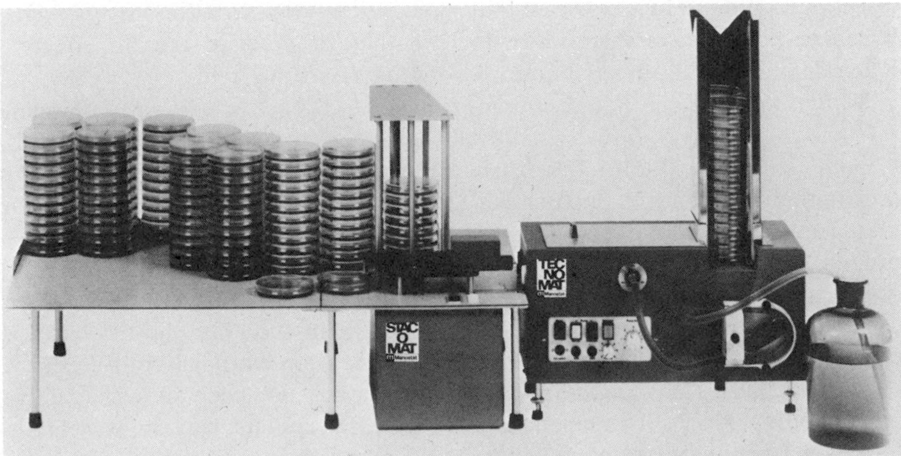

(a)

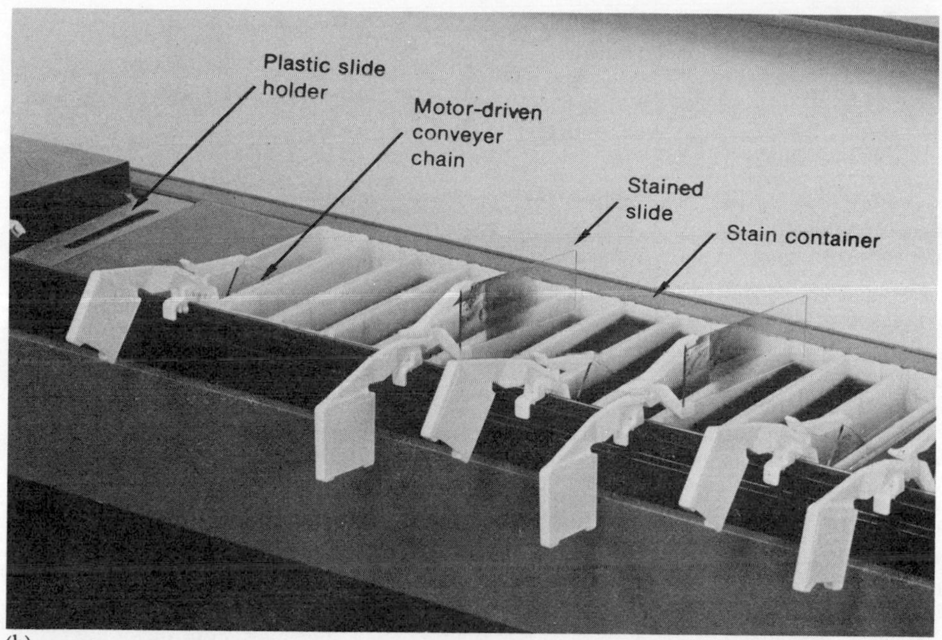

(b)

(c)

FIG. 38-5 Automation in microbiology. Various routine procedures and manual methods in microbiology can be automated. Left (a) Equipment used to help prepare plate media. This device pours and stacks filled Petri plates for immediate use in a much shorter time than manual preparation takes. Above (b) Automatic stainers are also appearing in laboratories. Machines of this type can perform Gram stains, acid-fast stains, and other procedures seven or eight times faster than manual operations. *Courtesy Honeywell, Inc.* (c) This instrument, the AutoMicrobic System (AMS), combines detection and identification without the use of pure cultures. *Courtesy Vitek Systems, Inc., Sub. McDonnell Douglas Corp.*

SUMMARY

An Introduction to Industrial Microbiology

1. Industrial microbiology refers to the use of microbes, or microbiological techniques, in a commercial enterprise.
2. Examples of beneficial industrial application include the production of antibiotics, enzymes, and certain steroid hormones.

Aerobic versus Anaerobic Processes

Fermentation is the anaerobic reduction of organic substrates. Products of fermentation reactions include ethyl alcohol, butanol, isopropyl alcohol, acetone, and glycerol.

Alcoholic Beverages

1. The production of beer, wine and spirits is a significant division of industrial microbiology in many countries.
2. Beer is produced by a yeast fermentation process that uses barley or other grains as sources of sugars and nitrogen-containing compounds. Beer production also incorporates the addition of hops for color and flavor and antibacterial substances.
3. Wine is made by the fermentation of almost any ripe fruit juice or of certain extracts from vegetable products. The presence of other substances such as acids and minerals accounts for the different color, taste, and sometimes bouquet of wines. The general wine-making process includes grape testing and picking, crushing, fermentation, pressing, clarification, aging, filtration, and bottling.
4. Distilled beverages include whiskey, brandy, and rum. The type of product depends upon the material used in the fermentation.

Antibiotics

Antibiotics are usually produced by growing a specific bacterial or fungal species in a submerged culture in large, well-aerated tanks.

Acids, Vitamins, and Alcohols

1. Vinegar, or acetic acid, is usually made from wine or cider. Species of the bacterial genus *Acetobacter* perform the overall reaction.
2. A variety of microorganisms can be used to synthesize amino acids and vitamins. Such products are used as food supplements and flavorings.

Other Products of Fermentation

Other products of microbial fermentations include citric and lactic acids, butanol, and isopropanol.

Microbial Enzymes

Commercially produced microbial enzymes have applications in a variety of industrial areas including the manufacture of alcoholic beverages, foods, detergents, and pharmaceuticals.

Steroid Transformations

A combination of chemical and microbial reactions can be used to produce various steroid hormones such as cortisone.

Microbial Insecticides

1. Many microorganisms destroy agricultural products and cause diseases in humans, lower animals, and plants.
2. Some of these organisms are susceptible to the effects of certain microorganisms or their products. The effective microorganisms are referred to as *microbial insecticides*.

Automation for Microbiology

Various routine procedures and methods in microbiology can be automated. These include the preparation of agar plates and several staining procedures.

QUESTIONS FOR REVIEW

1. What is industrial microbiology?
2. a. Describe the processes involved in making beer, wine, and spirits.
   b. What microorganisms are involved?
   c. What is a top yeast?
   d. What is a bottom yeast?
3. For each of the following, give a brief outline of the manufacturing process, including the types of microorganisms involved:
   a. antibiotics
   b. lactic acid
   c. isopropanol
   d. vinegar
   e. citric acid
   f. amino acids
   g. vitamins
   h. butanol
4. For each of the following, give the microbial origin and uses:
   a. amylase
   b. asparaginase
   c. lipase
   d. pectinase
   e. protease
5. a. How do steroid transformations differ from most other microbial processes?
   b. Describe one transformation.
6. a. What two categories of microbial insecticides are recognized?
   b. What are the advantages and disadvantages of each?
7. Of what value is automation to industrial and other areas of microbiology?

SUGGESTED READINGS

Casida, L. E., Jr., *Industrial Microbiology.* New York: John Wiley and Sons, 1968. *A basic text on industrial microbiology, describing industrial fermentation processes involved in the production of antibiotics, vitamins, enzymes, and organic acid.*

Irons, E. S., and M. H. Sears, "Patents in Relation to Microbiology," *Ann. Rev. Microbiol.* 29:319 (1975). *This review describes the pros and cons of patenting microorganisms for industrial purposes. It also presents the legislation now governing such patents.*

Porter, J., *All About Beer.* Garden City, New York: Doubleday &

Company, 1975. *A rather complete, easy-to-read book about all aspects of beer, from ingredients and the brewing process to the unusual ways beer can be used with food.*

Riviere, J., *Industrial Applications of Microbiology.* New York: John Wiley and Sons, 1977. *Explains many microorganism-mediated processes such as fermentation, antibiotic production, and the formation of many types of alcoholic beverages.*

Rossmoore, H. W., *The Microbes, Our Unseen Friends.* Detroit: Wayne State University Press, 1976. *An enjoyable, easy-to-read book explaining many of the industrial applications of microbiology such as clothing, antibiotic, enzyme, vitamin, hormone, and amino acid production.*

Sichel, P. M. F., and J. Ley, *Which Wine? The Wine Drinker's Buying Guide.* New York: Harper & Row, 1975. *A clearly indexed, at-a-glance guide to wines. While the emphasis appears to be on wine purchases, this book contains interesting and functional information about wine making and features of wines known the world over.*

Slodki, M. E., and M. C. Cadmus, "Production of Microbial Polysaccharides," *Adv. Appl. Microbiol.* 23:19 (1978). *Many of the polysaccharides used today produced by bacteria are described. Examples of such compounds include xanthan gum, mannans, n-alkanes, and pullulan.*

CHAPTER **39**

Food and Dairy Microbiology

Fermentation is a valuable process in the preparation and preservation of foods other than beer, wine, and spirits. For centuries, people have used such foods as fermented milk products, cheeses, sauerkraut, pickles, and many other substances produced partly or wholly by microorganisms. This chapter describes several types of food and dairy products and the different fermenting organisms involved with their production. Some consideration will also be given to food spoilage caused by microorganisms and ways with which to control it.

After reading this chapter, you should be able to:

1. **Discuss the types, sources, and importance of microorganisms in foods.**
2. **List five fermented foods or related products of fermentation and name the microorganisms and the starting material involved in their production.**
3. **Discuss three factors that influence the fermenting activities of microorganisms used in food and dairy products.**
4. **Describe the general sequence of events involved with the production of a fermented food such as pickles or sauerkraut.**
5. **Select one dairy product and describe the process by which it is produced.**
6. **List four microbial disease agents and/or their products that can be spread by food.**

7. **Discuss the sanitary quality of food and food preservation.**
8. **List the types of microorganisms involved in food spoilage.**
9. **Explain how microorganisms cause food spoilage.**
10. **List and describe at least four methods of preventing microbial food spoilage.**
11. **Define the term *single cell protein*, and discuss its potential role in solving the world's food shortage.**

Many foods and dairy products owe their production and characteristics to the activities of microorganisms (Color Photograph 97). Fermented milk products, innumerable varieties of cheese, pickles, sauerkraut, and fermented sausages all have unique aromas and flavors that result directly or indirectly from the enzymatic actions of specific fermenting organisms. In some cases, microbial activity even increases the vitamin content of the fermented foods, as well as their digestibility. No other single group of foods and food products has been so important for human well-being throughout the world and throughout history.

This chapter describes various aspects of the microbial ecology of food and dairy products. The types of microorganisms in food, the factors upon which the activities of fermenting organisms depend, the causative agents of microbial food spoilage, and approaches to food preservation are also discussed in this chapter.

Fermented Foods

The microorganisms that grow in or on a food and the changes they cause in flavor, texture, and general appearance are influenced by factors such as acidity, available carbohydrates, oxygen, temperature, and water. Fermented foods and food products used all over the world are the result of microbial activities (Table 39–1). The commercial manufacture and sometimes the home production of many of these fermented foods is begun by appropriate microbial **starter cultures.**

Fermented Vegetables

Foods such as sauerkraut and pickles result from the microbial fermentation of carbohydrates in plant tissues into acids. The addition of salt controls undesirable microbial activities, establishing a favorable environment for the desired fermentation. The organic acids and related compounds formed during the process act as preservatives and contribute to the characteristic flavor and aroma of fermented products. Foods of this type are less likely to spoil or to harbor pathogenic microbes. In addition, they lose very little of their nutritive value during fermentation. Most green vegetables and fruits can be preserved by this type of *pickling* process (Table 39–1).

SAUKERKRAUT

The origins of sauerkraut are not known, but they are believed to derive from central Europe where this fermented product of cabbage is still used as a main course vegetable. Sauerkraut is the product of lactic acid fermentation, usually carried out by the normal mixed bacterial flora of cabbage and

TABLE 39-1 **Fermented Foods and Products Produced by Microorganisms**[a]

Food or Product	Raw Starting Material	Fermenting Microorganisms: Bacteria	Fungi
Breads			
Cakes, rolls, etc.	Wheat flours		*Saccharomyces cerevisiae*
San Francisco sourdough bread	Wheat flours	*Lactobacillus sanfrancisco*	*S. exiguus*
Dairy Products			
Acidophilus milk	Milk	*L. acidophilus*	
Cheeses (ripened)	Milk curd	Lactic acid bacteria	
Yogurt	Milk and milk solids	*L. bulgaricus, S. thermophilus*	
Meat Products			
Country cured hams	Pork hams		*Aspergillus* spp. *Penicillium* spp.
Dry sausages (salami, etc.)	Pork, beef	*Pedicoccus cerevisiae*	
Nonbeverage Plant Products			
Olives	Green olives	*Leuconostoc mesenteroides Lactobacillus plantarum*	
Pickles	Cucumbers	*L. plantarum, P. cerevisiae*	
Poi	Taro roots	Lactic acid bacilli	
Sauerkraut	Cabbage	*L. mesenteroides L. plantarum*	
Soy sauce (shoyu)	Soybeans, wheat, rice	*Lactobacillus delbrueckii*	*A. oryzae* or *A. soyae, S. rouxii*

[a]Alcoholic beverages and related products, including beer, vinegar, and wines, are described in Chapter 38.

lactobacilli. Its manufacture is simple and inexpensive and requires very little equipment. Cabbage is shredded and layered in large vats. The layers are pressed down to produce anaerobic conditions. Salt is added between the layers to restrict the actions of undesirable bacteria while favoring the two most desirable lactic acid bacteria, ***Leuconostoc mesenteroides*** and ***Lactobacillus plantarum***. Kept at room temperature, these organisms produce large quantities of lactic acid from the cabbage juices within the first week of the fermentation. As acidity increases the ***L. mesenteroides*** decrease in numbers and are replaced by various species belonging to the genus ***Lactobacillus***. In most cases the extremely acid-tolerant ***L. brevis*** predominates and carries on the fermentation, producing-acetic and lactic acids and alcohol. A variety of other organic acids and related compounds are also formed, giving sauerkraut its distinctive flavor. The entire process requires about 3 to 6 weeks for completion.

PICKLES

Pickles, which are the fermentation products of fresh cucumbers, involve the microorganisms in the normal mixed flora of cucumbers to start the process. ***L. plantarum*** is the most essential microbial species in pickle production. In general, the fermentations are the same for most types of pickles, dill, sour, and sweet. The differences among the pickles result from differences in the spices and other ingredients used or in the post-pickling procedure. The keeping quality of various pickles is assured by heat pasteurization or the addition of vinegar. Other details of pickle production as well as related fermented foods can be found in the references given at the end of this chapter.

Dairy Products

Milk acquires microorganisms at the time it is drawn from the cow or other milk-producing animals, and it may be further contaminated as it is handled and processed. Since milk contains a variety of nutrients including fat, minerals, protein, the sugar lactose, vitamins, and water, it can serve as an excellent medium for numerous microorganisms. Unless measures are taken to eliminate spoilage organisms, souring occurs. To prevent such spoilage and to make milk commercially marketable in the United States, it is usually pasteurized. Samples of products are routinely checked for bacterial content by direct microscopic count and standard plate count techniques. Recommended grading standards for dairy products have been developed and maintained by the United States Public Health Service based on the results of such procedures.

Milk is the starting material for a variety of products that both increase its appeal and serve to preserve it (Tables 39–1 and 39–2). The fermentation of milk sugar (lactose) is the basis for a variety of these food products. Milk usually contains a wide variety and number of microorganisms. In order to ensure a high-quality dairy food, such organisms must be eliminated. After this step, pure cultures of reliable microorganisms, called lactic ***starter cultures***, are introduced into the starting material. Lactic starters always include bacteria such as *Streptococcus cremoris, S. diacetilactus,* or *S. lactis,* which convert lactose to lactic acid. The characteristic flavors and textures of butter, buttermilk, cheeses (Figures 39–1 and 39–2), yogurt, and related foods are due to the types of microorganisms (bacterium or fungus) used in the fermentation and subsequent processes.

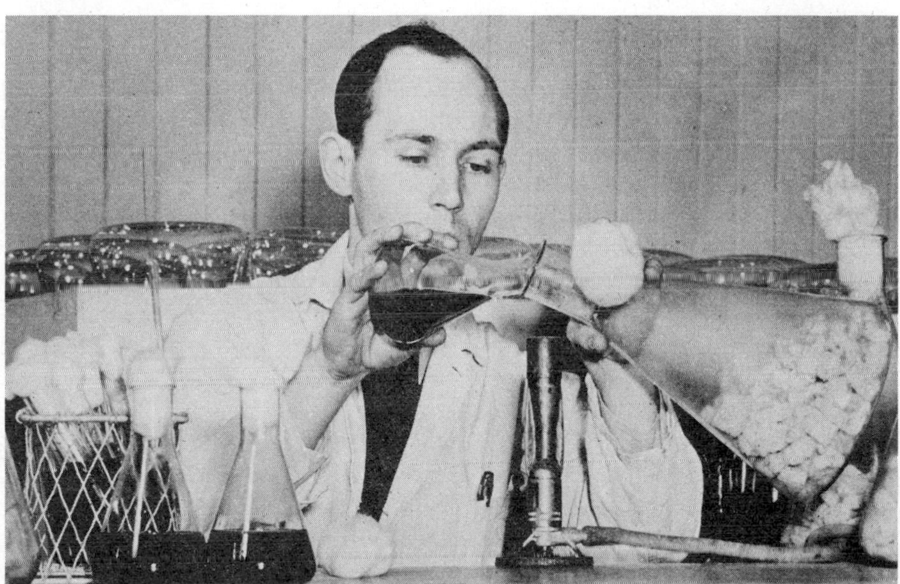

FIG. 39–1 Microorganisms and dairy products. (a) Cubes of sterilized whole wheat bread are inoculated with *Penicillium roqueforti* by a laboratory technician. Eventually the cubes will be removed from the flasks, dried, and powdered for use in making blue cheese. *Courtesy of Borden, Inc.*

BUTTER, BUTTERMILK, AND SOUR CREAM

Butter, buttermilk and sour cream are produced by inoculating pasteurized cream or milk with a specific lactic starter culture and holding it until the necessary amount of acidity is obtained. In the case of butter, acidified cream is churned until the thick butter forms. It is then worked to remove excess liquid, washed, salted, and packaged. The characteristic aroma and taste of butter is due to the compound diacetyl, which is formed by bacteria such as *Streptococcus diacetilactis.*

Buttermilk is the liquid remaining after cream is churned for butter production. Commercially, it is usually prepared without churning by inoculating skim milk with a starter culture and holding until sufficient souring typical of the final product occurs.

Cultured sour cream is prepared by fermenting pasteurized light cream with a lactic starter.

The starting materials and cultures used for the production of other fermented dairy products are listed in Table 39–1.

TABLE 39–2 Categories and Examples of Cheese

Texture Category	*Unripened*	*Ripened by Bacterial Action*	*Ripened by Mold Action*
Soft	Cottage cheese, cream cheese, Neufchatel, Ricotta	Limburger	Brie, Camembert
Semihard		Brick, Gouda, Jack, Muenster, Port du Salut	Bleu, Gorgonzola, Roquefort, Stilton
Hard		American, Cheddar,[a] Edam,[a] Gruyere,[b] Parmesan,[b] Provolone,[a] Swiss[b]	

[a]Final product does not have holes.
[b]Final product characteristically has holes.

CHEESE PRODUCTION

The production of most cheeses is the result of microbial activity. A great number and variety of cheeses are manufactured throughout the world (Table 39–2). Basically, they can be divided into three texture types: *soft* (such as cottage cheese or cream cheese); ***hard*** (such as Cheddar or Swiss); and ***semisoft*** (such as Camembert).

Most cheese-making processes start with cow's milk, either whole or skimmed. The customary first step is to curdle the milk (Figure 39–2a). Adding an appropriate bacterial culture to the starter material causes a firm ***curd*** and a watery fluid portion (called ***whey***) to form. Addition of the enzyme rennin (which is obtained from butchered calves) hastens the process. The best curds for cheese making are obtained with the combined actions of lactic acid bacteria and rennin.

Moisture removal is the second step in cheese production. The extent to which moisture is reduced depends upon the type of cheese to be produced. Heat, pressure, or cutting and compression of the curd are used for this purpose. When suitable amounts of whey have been removed, the curds are molded into characteristic shapes. Salt is sometimes added during cheese production to reduce moisture, prevent the growth of unwanted microbes, and contribute to the flavor of particular cheeses (Figure 39–2b).

Another important step in cheese production is ripening. Certain cheeses are obtained after milk curdles without any further curing. These are called unripened cheeses. A good example of this type of product is cottage cheese. When cheeses undergo ***ripening*** by bacteria or fungi, protein or fat is usually degraded, depending upon the dairy product desired. For instance, in the case of Camembert and Limburger cheeses, proteins are broken down during the ripening process. In the case of Roquefort and blue cheese, fat is degraded. Swiss cheese presents another situation. The activity of bacteria in Swiss cheese causes fermentation of lactic acid, which results in the characteristic holes in the cheese.

Ripening can be conducted in one of two ways. The particular procedure depends, again, on the type of cheese desired. In the case of hard cheeses, such as Cheddar and Swiss, the microorganisms are introduced and distributed into the interior of the cheese. In the case of soft cheeses (Camembert and Limburger, for example), the microorganisms are encouraged to grow on the surface and not in the interior of the product. These ripening methods also affect the sizes and shapes of cheese bricks or other units. Hard cheeses can be prepared in rather large dimensions, while soft ones are usually found in small sizes with relatively large surface area so that microbial products can spread through the cheese rapidly.

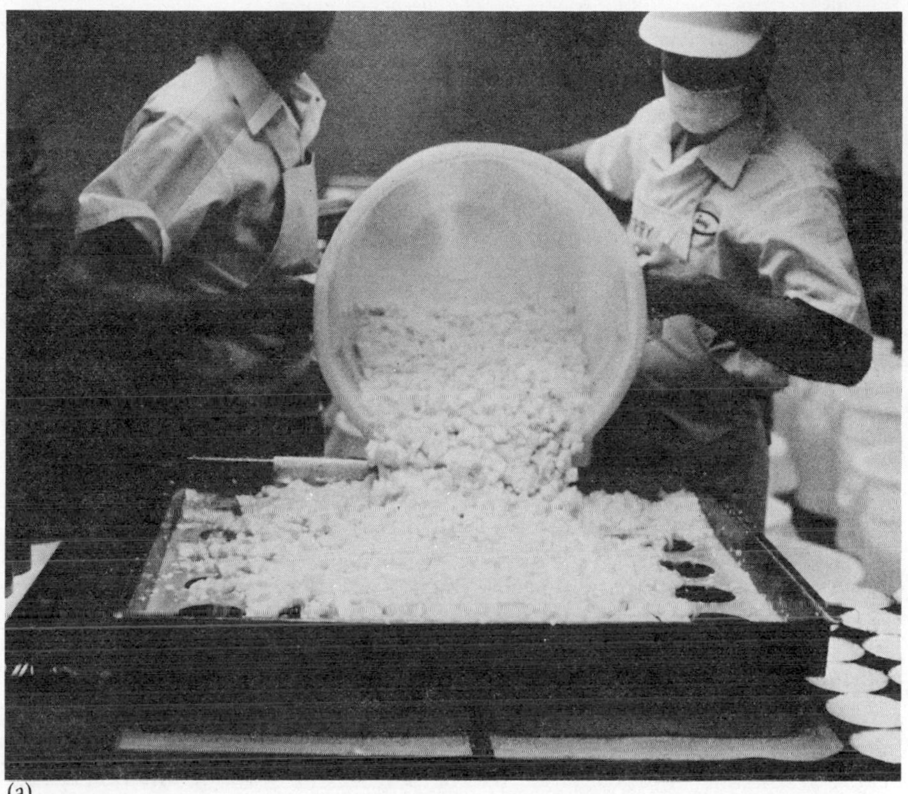

(a)

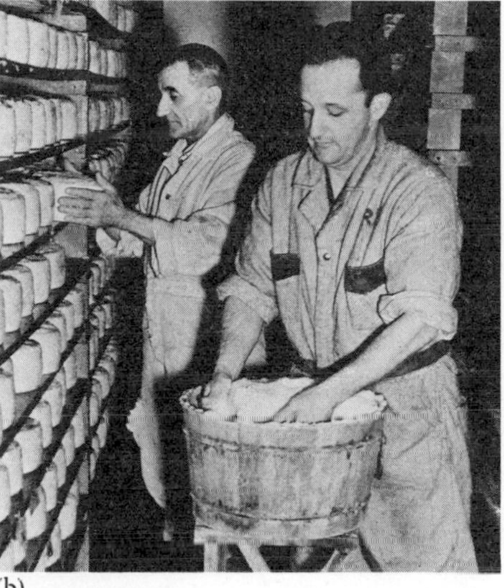

(b)

FIG. 39–2 Selected aspects of cheese making. (a) Curd is poured into containers or forms to allow for drainage and to separate it from whey. *Courtesy of Fisher Cheese Co., Wapukoneta, Ohio.* (b) To give flavor and start the formation of a crust, a product such as blue cheese is taken from its cold, dry storage room and punctured so that the mold can get air in order to grow and develop. Next it is placed in curing cellars where the temperature and humidity encourage mold growth. *Courtesy Borden, Inc.*

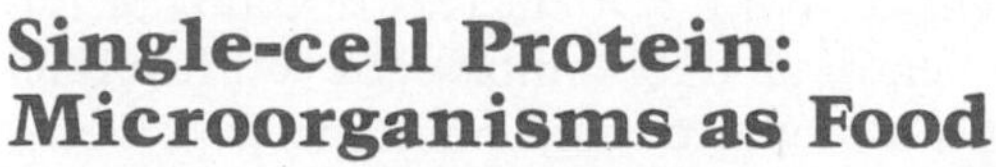

Single-cell Protein: Microorganisms as Food

Two thirds of the world's people suffer from inadequate nutrition. Furthermore, the production of traditional agricultural foodstuffs by existing methods cannot possibly meet the protein demands of a human population that continues to grow in an uncontrolled manner. Attempts to solve problems of protein nutrition are usually directed at increasing productivity of agriculture, animal breeding, and fishery. However, attention is shifting to the wider use of nonconventional proteins such as protein concentrates of low-quality fish; protein products of oil-producing crops such as cotton seeds, soybean, and sunflowers; and protein provided by single-cell microbes.

As difficult as it may be to believe, milligram for milligram, bacteria and many other microorganisms contain as much protein as steak. The protein

TABLE 39-3 Examples of Microorganisms and Materials Used In the Production of SCP

Materials Utilized (Substrates)	*Microorganisms*		
	Algae	*Bacteria*	*Fungi*
Cellulose		*Cellulomonas* sp.	*Trichoderma viride*
CO_2 (and photosynthesis)	*Chlorella pyrenoidosa* *Scenedesmus quadricauda*		
Ethanol		*Acinetobacter calcoaceticus*	*Candida utilis*[a]
Gas oil		*A. calcoaceticus*	
H_2 and CO_2		*Alcaligenes eutrophus*	
Kerosene and related substances		*Nocardia* sp.	*Candida intermedia*,[a] *C. lipolytica*, *C. tropicalis*
Methane		*Methylococcus capsulatus*, *Methylomonas* sp.	*Trichoderma* sp.
Methanol		*Methylomonas methanica*	
Simple sugars			*Candida utilis*,[a] *Kluyveromyces fragilis*,[a] *S. cerevisiae*
Starches			*Endomycopsis fibuligera*

[a]Yeast

content of these one-celled forms of life is high (Table 39-3), as much as 40 to 60 percent or more of their weight. Although it may be some time before this source of protein, called single-cell protein (SCP), is used to replace conventional human foods, more and more attention is being directed toward the ability of microorganisms to grow rapidly on materials previously not considered food sources or on substances that are edible but not nutritious, such as cellulose. Bacteria and fungi can be utilized to exploit nuisance plants such as various weeds, urban solid waste, oil, and almost anything containing carbon (Table 39-3). The substances used by microorganisms in the production of SCP are supplemented with other nutrients such as inorganic nitrogen compounds. By microbial enzymatic activity the energy in the carbon source is converted into biomass, that is, the total weight of living matter. This resulting SCP is harvested, usually dried, and subsequently used for animal feed. With further processing, most SCP can be used as a source of food for humans. The by-products of the generation of SCP are largely carbon dioxide, heat, and some waste water.

In an overpopulated world, there is not enough animal protein to go around. Animal protein has the best nutritional value because it contains more of the essential amino acids than does plant protein. The burgeoning demand for animal protein in the United States and other affluent nations is going to require some type of livestock population explosion. It will also require gigantic quantities of feed to fatten all of these animals.

Various animals, such as cattle and hogs, although excellent sources of amino acids, must consume an extremely large amount of plant mass to produce their own smaller mass. The fattening of livestock requires unbelievable quantities of human edible plant material. This often involves feeding such animals one of the best protein sources known, namely soybean meal, while the people in poor and developing countries may have to subsist on a protein-deficient plant diet. SCP has the potential to correct this situation by replacing the human edible feeds used in the livestock industry, thereby making these feeds available for human consumption.

A safe single-cell protein product can also be a direct source of protein for humans. It would probably first have to be fortified with certain essential amino acids. Single-cell protein preparations are often deficient in lysine or methionine.

SCP may sound unappealing to people who only associate microorganisms with disease and spoilage. Nonetheless, as we have seen, microbes already exist in several types of food and beverages consumed by humans.

Microbial Food Spoilage

Major Sources of Microorganisms

Most food for humans is of animal or plant origin. Most of these foods, including market fruits and vegetables, may be expected to normally contain a wide variety and a varying number of bacteria and fungi. Most of these organisms are occupying their normal ecological habitats and do not cause any problems, but some can be destructive and produce significant food spoilage (Figure 39–3 and Color Photographs 3B and 39). The sources of microorganisms in foods include air, dust, soil, water, utensils, food handlers, and the intestinal tracts of humans and other animals.

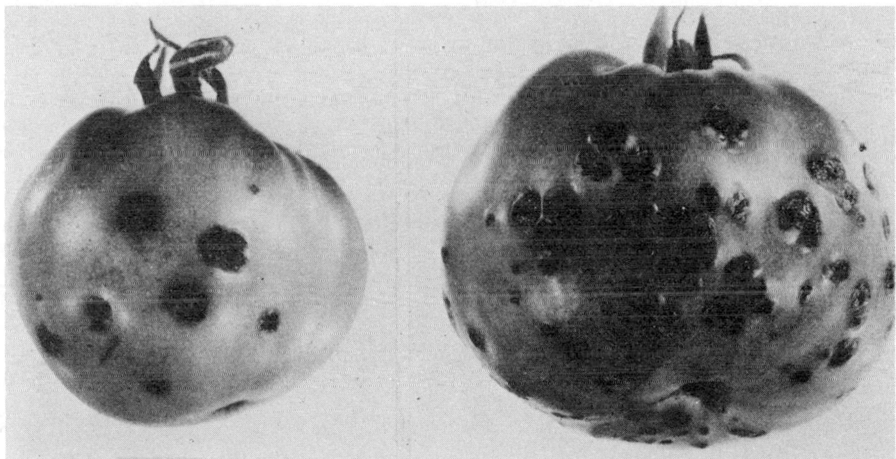

FIG. 39–3 The nutrient content of fruits and vegetables can support the growth of bacteria, mold, and yeasts. Their high water content also contributes to the growth of many spoilage bacteria. These tomatoes have bacterial spot disease. *Courtesy USDA.*

Various factors influence the numbers and types of microorganisms in fruits and vegetables or a finished food product. Among these factors are the properties of the food itself—its pH, moisture, and nutrient content—as well as the general environment from which the food was obtained and the conditions of handling, processing, and storage to which it was exposed. The number of microorganisms should be kept as low as possible. Excessively high numbers of microbes, some of which may cause food spoilage (Table 39–4), or the presence of pathogens or their products (Table 39–5) are cause for alarm.

TABLE 39-4 Examples of Microorganisms and Effects Associated with Food Spoilage

Food	Spoilage Effects	Microorganisms Involved	
		Bacteria	*Fungi*
Canned Food			
Fruits	Mold growth		*Byssochlamys fulva*
Cereal Products			
Bread	Ropiness texture	*Bacillus subtilis var. mesentericus*	
	Mold growth		*Aspergillus niger, Mucor* sp., *Penicillium* spp., *Rhizopus nigricans*
Dairy Products			
Pasteurized milk	Gas formation	*Bacillus* spp., *Clostridium* spp.	
	Lactic acid souring	*Lactobacillus thermophilus, Microbacterium lacticum, Streptococcus thermophilus*	
	Proteolysis (protein breakdown)	*Bacillus* spp., *Clostridium* spp., *Micrococcus* spp.	
Fish			
Fresh fish	Discoloration	*Micrococcus* spp., *Pseudomonas fluorescens, Sarcina* spp.	Various fungi (both molds and yeast)
	Pronounced fishiness of flavor	*Flavobacterium* spp., *Micrococcus* spp., *Pseudomonas* spp., *Serratia* spp.	
Jellies and Jams	Mold growth		*Aspergillus* spp. *Penicillium* spp.
Meat			
Fresh meats	Slime formation in cold environments	*Flavobacterium* spp., *Micrococcus* spp., *Pseudomonas* spp.	Yeasts
Cured and smoked bacon, sausage	Greening	*Lactobacillus* spp. *Leuconostoc* spp.	
	Mold growth		*Alternaria* spp., *Aspergillus* spp., *Mucor* spp., *Rhizopus stolonifer*
Eggs	Green discoloration and rot	*Pseudomonas fluorescens, Proteus* spp.	

Various techniques are used to determine the numbers and kinds of microorganisms and their products in foods. These include direct microscopic counts for both living and dead cells, standard plate counts, specific staining procedures, immunological tests for enzymes and other microbial products, isolation and biochemical identification, and statistical determinations for living cells.

TABLE 39-5 Some Biological Hazards Associated with Contaminated Foods[a]

Food-Poisoning Bacteria	*Other Bacteria*	*Fungal and Algal Toxins*
Bacillus cereus, Clostridium botulinum, C. perfringens, Escherichia coli (EPEC), *Salmonella* spp., *Staphylococcus aureus, Streptococcus faecalis, Vibrio parahemolyticus*	*Brucella* spp., *Leptospira, Mycobacterium tuberculosis, Vibrio cholerae, Yersinia enterocolitica*	Aflatoxins, other mycotoxins, saxitoxin (red tide product)
Protozoa	*Viruses*	*Worms*
Entamoeba histolytica, Toxoplasma gondii	Enteroviruses, hepatitis A virus, Newcastle disease virus	Chinese liver fluke; beef, fish, and sheep tapeworms; pork roundworm

[a]Refer to earlier chapters for details concerning these and other microorganisms and the disease states associated with them.

How Microorganisms Affect Food

Not only can foods spoil, but they can also contain a variety of other biological hazards (Tables 39–4 and 39–5). Microbial pathogens, their products, and the diseases they can cause were presented in several earlier chapters. Here, we will deal with microbial food spoilage.

Spoiled food can be defined as food that has been so damaged or altered as to make it unfit for human consumption. The principal causes of such spoilage are dehydration, enzymatic action, microbial growth, and oxidation. The type of spoilage is influenced by such factors as the composition of the food, the types of microorganisms present and the degree of microbial contamination, the presence of microbial growth inhibitors, and conditions of storage, including temperature (Figure 39–4) and moisture. Spoilage microorganisms are affected by these same factors. Examples of foods, spoilage effects, and the microorganisms causing these effects are listed in Table 39–4. Control of one or several of the factors mentioned usually reduces microbial spoilage of foods.

Food Preservation

Drying

Among the oldest methods to prevent or control food spoilage are fermentation, refrigeration, and drying (Table 39–6). The preservation of foods by drying is based upon the fact that microorganisms and enzymes need water to be active. The term **water activity** (a_w) is used to indicate the water content of foods. In preserving foods by drying, the water activity is lowered to a point where the activities of food-spoiling and food-poisoning microbes are inhibited. Examples of foods so preserved include dried fruits (apricots, figs, prunes, raisins) and powdered eggs and milk. Frozen dried foods are also in this category. Organisms including molds, yeasts, and salt-tolerant bacteria can grow in foods with a low water activity.

Canning

The development of canning as a process to prevent food spoilage had its beginnings in Napoleonic France in 1795, when the French government offered

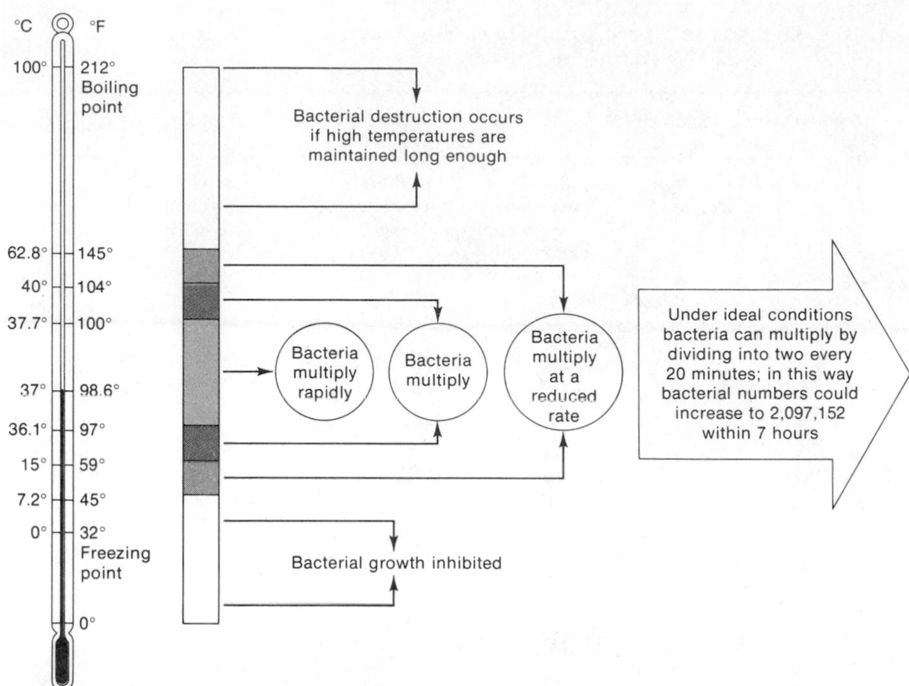

FIG. **39–4** Microorganisms grow over a wide range of temperatures. Knowing the temperature growth ranges for organisms such as those capable of causing spoilage or disease is important to selecting the proper temperature for the storage of different foods. This diagram shows the effect of temperature on the growth of bacteria in foods. The safe and growth supportive temperatures for bacteria are indicated. *After Hobbs, B. C.,* Food poisoning and Food Hygiene. *London: Edward Arnold Publishers, Ltd. (1968).*

a cash prize for the development of a practical method of food preservation. In 1809, a French confectioner, Francois Appert, succeeded in preserving meat in stoppered glass bottles that were kept in boiling water for varying periods of time. Appert probably was unaware not only of microorganisms but also of the long-term significance of his heating process. Interestingly enough, this beginning of canning as it is known and used today preceded by some 50 years Pasteur's demonstration of the role of microbes in the spoilage of wine.

Both canning and pasteurization are high-temperature treatments used in the processing of foods. Pasteurization, however, destroys only non-spore-forming pathogens. It is not a method for sterilization. In the canning process, foods are sterilized by heating in cans or jars that can be sealed in such a way that no microorganisms can enter. Commercial cans are made of 98.5 percent sheet steel with a thin coating of tin. The time and temperature for heating vary with the type of food, acid content, and the ease with which sterilization can be achieved. Acid foods such as lemon juice, sauerkraut, and tomatoes, for example, require shorter heat processing times than do low-acid foods such as milk, ripe olives, and sardines. Commercial canning operations are adjusted to prevent the destruction of vitamins and other important food components.

A wide variety of foods are canned, including fruits, vegetables, meats, and fish. There are many steps involved with the commercial canning operations for such foods. Preparatory operations include cleaning, washing, and ***blanching***. Blanching involves treatment of raw food products such as fruits or vegetables with hot water or live steam to soften the plant tissues, making the filling of cans easier, and destroying any enzymes that may change the color, flavor, or texture of the final product. Depending on the food, peeling, slicing, or dicing may also be necessary during the early operation. Cans are then filled, heated for a short time and exposed to a vacuum system to remove any excess air

TABLE 39-6 Food Preservation Approaches and Examples of Methods

Method	*Examples*
Killing microorganisms	1. Heating, e.g., canning 2. Ionizing radiation, e.g., gamma radiation 3. Mechanical disruption 4. Nonionizing radiation, e.g., microwave and ultraviolet light
Growth inhibition	1. Drying by dehydration and freeze-drying 2. Chemical preservatives 3. Refrigeration or freezing 4. High osmotic pressure by use of salt brines and sugar syrups 5. Low pH with acidulants 6. Anaerobic conditions
Removal of microorganisms	1. Centrifugation 2. Filtration
Prevention of contamination	1. Observing and maintaining aseptic conditions

(thermal exhaustion), and sealed. The finished, sealed cans are subjected to heat sterilization for thermal processing. Established time and temperature exposure schedules are followed here to ensure the destruction of spoilage and pathogenic microorganisms that may be in or on the raw food product. The heat-treated cans are usually cooled in cold-water tanks or by cold-water sprays. Home canning follows the same general steps except that the glass jars most often used do not undergo a separate evacuation and sealing process. They are sealed by cooling after heat processing. Because it is not usually feasible to check for complete sterilization of home canned foods, the prescribed times and temperatures should be followed scrupulously.

SPOILAGE OF COMMERCIAL CANNED FOODS

The microbial spoilage of various commercial canned foods can be divided into five categories: ***incipient spoilage, gross underprocessing, leaker spoilage, thermophilic spoilage,*** and ***insufficient heat treatment.***

Incipient spoilage is caused by keeping products, prior to canning, under conditions favoring microbial growth, and using highly contaminated foods or ingredients. Gross underprocessing is brought about by ineffective sterilization procedures. Poorly constructed containers, defects in the canning operation, or contamination of foods after processing result in leaker spoilage. Storage of foods at temperatures favorable for microbial growth or contamination by thermophilic sporeformers is responsible for thermophilic spoilage. Reduced exposure to heat, insufficient heat treatment, will favor the growth of spoilage-causing and toxin-producing microorganisms.

Chemical Preservatives

Several chemical additives are used to prevent microbial spoilage of foods. Examples are citric acid used in jams, jellies, and soft drinks; the mold inhibitor sodium propionate, used in bakery goods and processed cheese; and the bacterial inhibitors sodium nitrate and sodium nitrite, used in the curing of meat and fish. These substances are classified as food additives under the Federal Food, Drug and Cosmetic Act, indicating that they have been tested and found safe for human consumption by the Food and Drug Administration. This agency is currently reviewing all food additives as to levels of safety and effectiveness for food preservation. The levels of substances such as nitrates and nitrites may be reduced considerably in the near future as a result of such studies.

Chemical preservatives include both inorganic and organic compounds. These compounds either kill microorganisms or inhibit their growth, enzymatic activities, or reproduction. Some are also used to destroy or reduce the number of microorganisms on food processing equipment and food utensils or to treat water used in the processing of foods.

SUMMARY

1. Fermentation is a valuable process for preparation and preservation of various foods and dairy products.
2. The unique aromas and flavors of fermented foods result directly or indirectly from the enzymatic action of specific microorganisms.

Fermented Foods

1. Microorganisms used in the fermentation of foods are influenced by factors such as acidity, available carbohydrates, oxygen, temperature, and water.
2. Microbial starter cultures contain the specific organisms necessary to begin fermentation processes.

Fermented Vegetables

Fermented vegetables such as sauerkraut and pickles result from the fermentation of carbohydrates present in the plant tissues. Such fermentations are started by the microorganisms in the normal mixed flora of the vegetables.

Dairy Products

1. Milk contains a variety of nutrients, which make it an excellent medium for many microorganisms.
2. Unless measures are taken to eliminate unwanted spoilage organisms, milk quickly sours.
3. In the United States, milk and related products are tested by procedures such as standard plate counts and direct microscopic examinations to determine their safety for human consumption.
4. The fermentation of lactose (milk sugar) is the basis for the production of various dairy products including butter, buttermilk, sour cream, and numerous cheeses.
5. The particular microorganisms and their enzymatic actions in starter cultures are responsible for the characteristic flavors, texture, and aromas of dairy products.
6. The first step in most cheese-making processes is the curdling of milk, which results in the formation of a solid portion, or *curd*, and the liquid *whey*. Other steps include moisture removal and further enzymatic action by microorganisms, called *ripening*. Based on their texture and method of production, cheeses are classified as soft, semihard, and hard.

Single-Cell Protein: Microorganisms as Food

The product obtained through the use of microorganisms as a source of protein is known as single-cell protein (SCP). In their ability to produce protein, microorganisms offer a potential solution to meeting the world's demands for protein. They have several advantages as sources of protein: they can utilize a variety of substrates as carbon sources, they are easily harvested, and they contain milligram for milligram as much protein as steak. For human consumption, SCP preparations must be fortified with certain essential amino acids.

Microbial Food Spoilage

Major Sources of Microorganisms

1. Most foods used for human consumption contain a variety and a varying number of bacteria and fungi. Some of these microorganisms can be destructive and cause food spoilage.
2. Sources of microorganisms in foods include air, dust, soil, water, utensils, food handlers, and the intestinal tracts of humans and other animals.
3. Factors such as pH, moisture, nutrient content, and conditions of processing and storage influence the numbers and types of microorganisms in finished food products.
4. Techniques used to determine the numbers and kinds of microorganisms in food are similar to those used with various types of medically important specimens. They include direct microscopic counts, standard plate counts, staining procedures, immunological tests for enzymes and other microbial products, and isolation and biochemical identification.

How Microorganisms Affect Food

1. Spoiled foods have been damaged or changed so as to make them unfit for human consumption.
2. The type of spoilage is influenced by factors such as the composition of the food, numbers and kinds of microbes present, the absence or presence of microbial growth inhibitors, and conditions of storage.

Food Preservation

1. Food preservation methods are used to prevent and control food spoilage.
2. Examples of such methods include fermentation, refrigeration, drying, canning, and the use of chemical preservatives.
3. Canning and pasteurization are examples of high-temperature methods used in the processing of foods to control microbial numbers. Only canning is a method for sterilization.
4. Chemicals added to foods to prevent microbial spoilage are classified as food additives. Such substances must be determined as safe for human well-being by the Food and Drug Administration. Chemical preservatives can also be used to destroy or reduce the number of microorganisms on food processing equipment and utensils and to treat water to be used in the processing of foods.

QUESTIONS FOR REVIEW

1. List the types of microorganisms and starting materials needed for the production of the following foods:

a. butter
b. pickles
c. yogurt
d. ripened cheese

2. What is lactic acid fermentation?
3. a. Outline the general procedure for sauerkraut production.
   b. What is the source of the microorganisms responsible for the reaction?
4. Do fermented foods harbor pathogens? Explain.
5. List four factors that influence the activities of microbes involved with fermented food production.
6. a. Describe the general process of cheese making.
   b. Distinguish between curd and whey.
7. Give the categories of cheeses and an example of each one.
8. a. What is single-cell protein (SCP)?
   b. What types of microorganisms can be used for its production?
   c. Why are microorganisms good sources for single cell protein?
9. Why is milk an extremely good medium for microbes?
10. Distinguish between pasteurization and sterilization.
11. a. Is milk sterile when it is drawn from a cow? Explain.
    b. How is the safety of milk and related products for human consumption determined?
12. Are fermented foods less nutritious than other types of food products?
13. List four sources of microbes found in market fruits and finished food products.
14. What techniques are used to determine the numbers and kinds of microorganisms in foods? List three.
15. List four principal causes of food spoilage.
16. a. What is a spoiled food?
    b. What factors influence the growth and effects of spoilage microorganisms?
17. a. List three different categories of food, and give two examples of spoilage effects and the types of microorganisms associated with each.
    b. How is food spoilage prevented?
18. List four different types of biological hazards associated with contaminated foods.
19. List four general approaches to food preservation and two methods for each of them.
20. a. List two chemical preservatives and the types of food for which each is used.
    b. Examine the label of two food products and find the food preservatives they contain.
    c. Do you know of any food preservatives that are unsafe for human consumption? Explain.

SUGGESTED READINGS

Beuchat, L. R., *Food and Beverage Mycology.* Westport, Conn.: Avi Publishing Co., Inc., 1978. *Molds and yeasts and their relationships to food and beverage spoilage and processing are the subjects of this excellent book.*

International Commission on Microbiological Specifications for Foods, *Microorganisms in Foods,* vols. 1 and 2. Toronto: University of Toronto Press, 1978. *These two volumes describe the significance of microorganisms and their toxins in foods. Microbiological examination methods and techniques for the sampling of many types of foods are also well described.*

Kharatyan, S. G., "Microbes as Food for Humans," *Ann. Rev. Microbiol.* 32:301 (1978). *The use of biomass of various microorganisms for human consumption and single-cell protein substrates and their nutritional value and safety are discussed.*

Proceedings of the Sixth International Sympsoium, *Conversion and Manufacture of Foodstuffs by Microorganisms.* Japan: Saikon Publishing Co., Ltd., 1972. *An excellent collection of articles on many aspects of food microbiology, including applications of microbial enzymes to food processing, microorganisms in wine, beer, cheese, and sake making, single-cell protein, and edible mushrooms.*

Rossmore, H. W., *The Microbes, Our Unseen Friends.* Detroit: Wayne State University Press, 1976. *A well-written and enjoyable book that emphasizes the beneficial importance of microorganisms, especially in food production. The author combines technical information with touches of humor.*

Ryther, J. H., and J. C. Goldman, "Microbes as Food in Mariculture." *Ann. Rev. Microbiol.* 29:429 (1975). *The use of microorganisms in sea farming as a source of food directly or indirectly for cultured organisms and as causative agents of disease are discussed.*

Shipman, R. H., L. T. Fan, and I. C. Kao, "Single-cell Protein Production by Photosynthetic Bacteria," *Adv. Appl. Microbiol.* 21:161 (1977). *This article describes the possibilities of using photosynthetic bacteria as a food source for aquaculture and livestock.*

CHAPTER 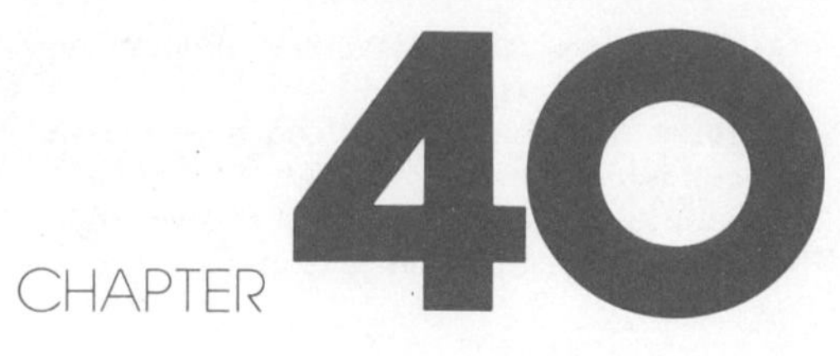

The Microbiology of Soil and Water and Waste Treatment

Through the years, various practices associated with agriculture, industry, and construction have contributed to incredible accumulations of wastes in the general environment. Frequently microorganisms are intricately involved with the processing and ultimate decomposition of such wastes. This chapter is concerned with the involvement of microorganisms in a variety of processes, including soil formation, water purification, waste treatment, and some of the problems associated with waste disposal.

After reading this chapter, you should be able to:

1. **Discuss soil formation and associated microbial activities.**
2. **Describe the water, or hydrologic, cycle in terms of natural water purification and the distribution of microorganisms in aquatic environments.**
3. **List the types of materials found in domestic waste water.**
4. **List at least five microbial pathogens associated with waste water.**
5. **Describe the basic features of the following procedures used to determine water quality: most probable number (MPN), membrane filter technique (MF) and standard plate count (SPC).**
6. **Discuss biological oxygen demand (BOD) and the way it is measured.**
7. **Outline the steps involved in waste water treatment and**

list potential products and problems associated with waste disposal.

8. **List and describe two general procedures for solid waste disposal.**
9. **Define or explain the following:**
   a. **humus**
   b. **trickling filter**
   c. **compost**
   d. **sludge**
   e. **floc**
   f. **reclamation of waste water**

Many diverse microorganisms and other forms of life are found in soil and contribute to its formation and fertility. Microbial contributions include the decomposition of organic matter to produce better soil texture and water-binding capacity, release of minerals important for plant growth from soil particles, and the transformation of various chemical compounds into substances useful for plants and other forms of life. Soil also serves as the habitat for antibiotic-producing microbes and pathogens of lower animals, humans, and plants.

The significance of microorganisms in aquatic environments is also well recognized. Some of these microorganisms play vital roles in aquatic ecosystems and contribute to the operation of biogeochemical cycles. Others are of interest and importance because of their association with waste treatment and their potential dangers to safe water supplies.

Environmental reservoirs of infectious disease agents for humans include soil, water supplies, sewage, and some foods. Thousands of other substances used or produced by human society are introduced into various bodies of water through natural means as well as by industrial and domestic processes. Through the years several areas of the world have been declared unsafe because of potentially toxic levels of biological and chemical pollutants. Raw sewage, with its vast numbers of potentially pathogenic bacteria and viruses, is the most dangerous threat to water supplies. Indeed, it may have disastrous consequences for fish, wildlife, and humans.

Soil and Its Formation

The general ability of soil to support life varies considerably, as does its chemical and microbial composition. Soil consists of solids, both minerals and organic compounds, water, and air. The minerals in soil range from the larger particles of gravel and sand to the smaller silt and finest of clay. The variety and proportion of such materials affect the suitability of soil for agricultural and other purposes.

Steps in Soil Formation

Soil, which is formed by the breakdown of rock, usually contains a combination of minerals and organic compounds in various stages of decomposition, water, and dissolved organic and inorganic materials and gases. The disintegration of rocks is caused by a variety of mechanical, chemical, and biological processes collectively called *weathering* (Figure 40–1).

Mechanical weathering includes the breaking of rock by forces such as glaciers and avalanches, as well as the effects of wind, blown sand, and cracking by

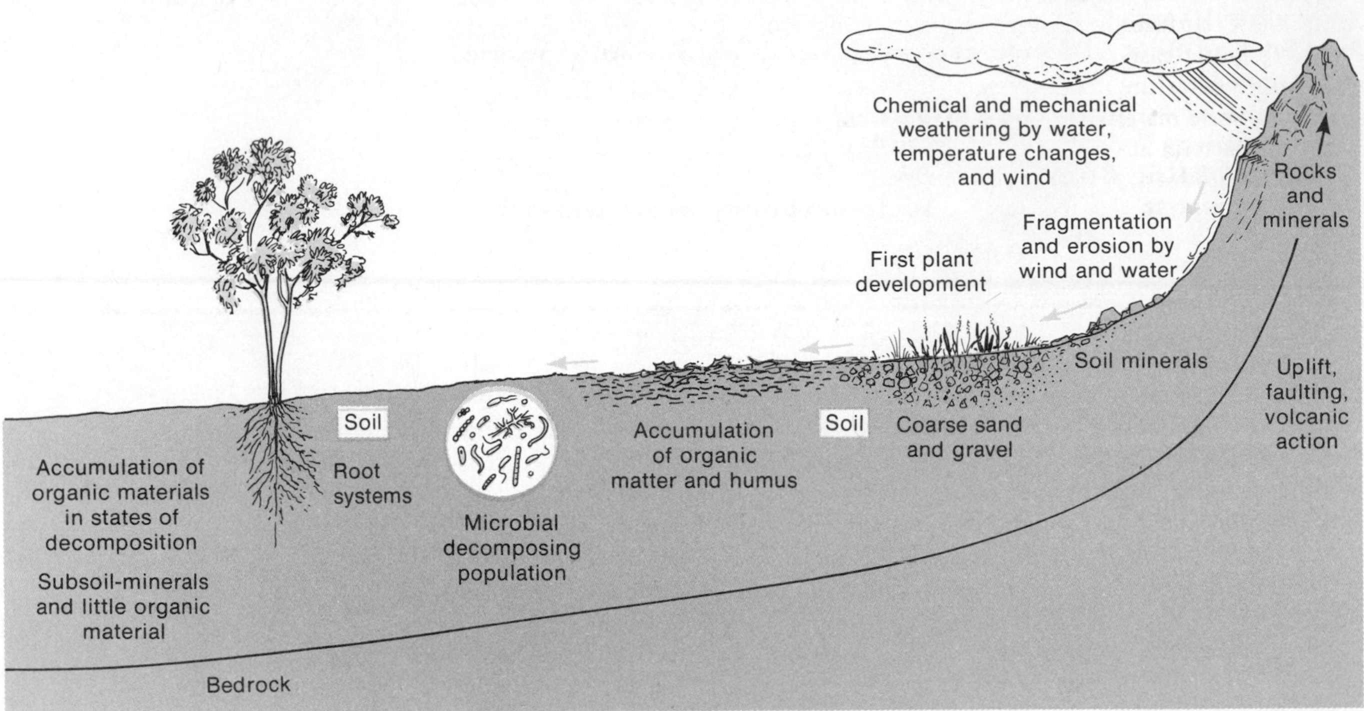

FIG. 40–1 Soil formation. The various components of rocks and mountains become disintegrated into soil particles. Soil particles are produced by erosion, water, and wind.

freezing and thawing. ***Chemical weathering*** involves the dissolving of rock materials by rain, streams, or groundwater. ***Biological processes*** include the cracking of rock by root growth and the action of metabolic by-products of microbial growth, such as acids, to dissolve and disintegrate rocks. Organisms associated with rocks are algae (Color Photograph 47), lichens (Color Photograph 51), and higher plants such as mosses.

The type of soil in a particular region depends on the chemical make-up of the parent rock, the climate, and all the life forms in or on the soil. Another important component of soil is **humus.** Humus is a mixture of slowly decaying remains of vegetation and animal life, finely ground, and includes various organic and inorganic materials. Humus increases the water-holding capacity of the soil. It is also a source of food for microorganisms and various other forms of life such as insect larvae, earthworms, and plants.

As the weathering processes continue, the soil levels increase in depth, providing better conditions for the establishment of the root systems of larger plant life (Figure 40–1). The movement of soil animals such as earthworms contributes to the weathering processes. Water moving down through the soil dissolves minerals and carries them deeper into lower regions of the area. The depositing of various materials frequently results in the formation of soil layers with different compositions.

The best soil structure for plant growth is *loam*. Loam contains both large and small particles, which provide good water retention, drainage, and aeration. In loam, root penetration proceeds easily and rapidly. In addition, the environment is well suited for the activities of soil microorganisms and other forms of life. Particle size is determined by the dimensions of inorganic materials and by smaller particles that are literally glued together. Such adhesion is caused by polysaccharides and other gummy substances produced by cyanobacteria, other bacteria, fungi, and other substances formed by higher forms of life. Soil particles are particularly important, since they serve as the surfaces on which microorganisms live and perform their life functions. Food substances tend to adsorb onto these surfaces, providing high concentrations of organic compounds. Many bacteria easily adsorb to such substances by means of their pili. This appears to be a functional mechanism by which decomposing microbes gain access to waste materials in soil. Microbial actions of this type contribute to soil fertility. Bacteria are by far the most numerous soil microorganisms, followed by molds, protozoa, and yeasts.

The Aquatic Environment

The Water (Hydrologic) Cycle

By means of the *water cycle* (Figure 40–2), there is a constant interchange of water among air, land, and sea and between different forms of life and their environments. Moreover, water greatly influences such environments. The water cycle involves *evaporation, cloud formation, precipitation, surface water runoff*, and *percolation through the soil.*

Evaporation from bodies of water provides some of the moisture that forms clouds. Additional atmospheric moisture results from a plant process known as *transpiration*, through which water vapor is released from leaves as water and minerals are drawn up stems from the roots. Under the proper meteorological conditions, the clouds lose their water as precipitation in the form of rain, snow, or hail. Some water from precipitation seeps into the ground and filters, or percolates, through dirt and sand to enter the underground water, known as an *aquifer*. This *groundwater* is usually of good overall quality. Though it may be high in dissolved minerals, such water has little color and turbidity (cloudiness) and relatively low levels of microorganisms.

Some of the precipitation enters streams of various sizes as runoff and may enter lakes or ponds or flow into the oceans. Often water from soil runoff and

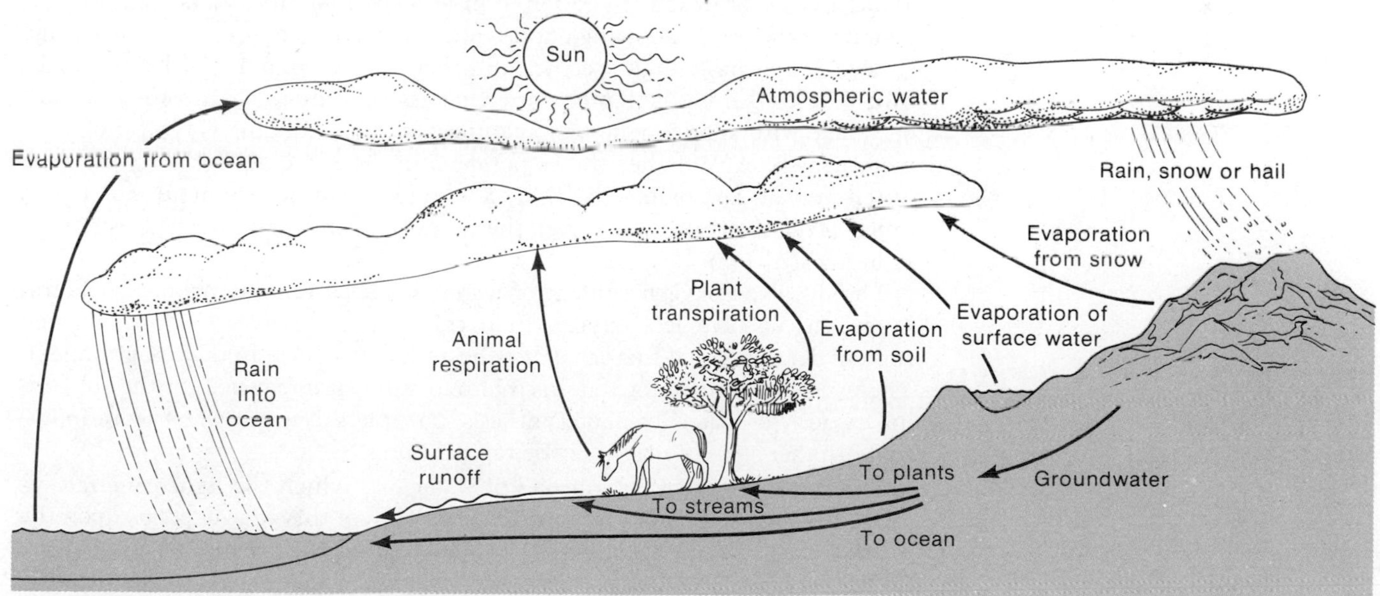

FIG. 40–2 The water cycle provides the mechanisms by which constant interchanges of water take place among air, sea, and land and between different forms of life and their environments. Such interchanges produce daily and seasonal changes in the environments of animals, plants, and microorganisms.

streams filters into sandy soil. If this occurs over a period of time, the filtration capability of the sand is improved by the formation of a slimy film of microorganisms on them. This material is known as *schmutzdecke*, meaning "dirt layer." It not only improves filtration by decreasing the size of spaces between grains of sand, but also serves to oxidize dissolved organic compounds and some inorganic waste materials. Water that does not filter into the soil is usually of fair overall quality. However, it may be colored from plant materials, cloudy from silt or small pieces of organic matter *(detritus)*, and have high counts of microorganisms. When this water is also used for domestic and industrial purposes, it is treated to improve the quality to meet federal standards. This is usually accomplished by some combination of chemical treatment, flocculating sedimentation, and aeration process for oxidation. Some water purification plants use aeration and a slow sand system, which provides good filtration.

Whether from aquifers or reservoirs, the water is used for many domestic and industrial purposes. It must then be treated before it can be released into the environment for eventual return to the atmosphere by evaporation. Water treatment is discussed later in this chapter.

Aquatic Microorganisms

Various microorganisms are found naturally in fresh and salt waters. Others gain entrance to these waters from natural sources such as air or soil or from industrial or domestic processes. The microbial populations of water environments are influenced by several chemical and physical factors, including hydrostatic pressure, light, pH, salinity, and temperature. Water with less than about 0.2 percent salt is fresh water. Marine water may contain 3.5 percent salt or more. Aquatic microbiology, the study of microorganisms in aquatic environments, includes the distribution and activities of these organisms and the various factors affecting such activities.

Properties of the Aquatic Environment

Water environments have two rather unique properties: (1) temperature variations are not as great as those found in terrestrial environments, and (2) light penetrates the water, allowing photosynthetic activities to occur well below the surface. Water has a high specific heat; that is, large amounts of heat must be gained or lost before the temperature changes very much. Figure 40–3 shows a deep lake with approximate temperatures and other conditions typical of summer and winter. Whether the air temperature is 32° C or −12° C, the deep waters remain approximately 4° C. The middle area varies more, but not as much as the air temperature. Even the water just below the surface doesn't vary as much as the air.

The dissolved oxygen content of water is related to its temperature. Warm water can dissolve less oxygen than cold water. As water warms, oxygen content decreases, and this can affect the animals thriving in that environment. The usual heat source for water is solar radiation, also required for the supporting capacity of water for photosynthesis, but inlets of warm water from industrial or other sources may increase temperatures.

The upper region of large bodies of water into which the light penetrates is called the ***photic*** or ***trophogenic*** zone. The depth of this zone depends upon the relative clarity of the water. Light, particularly red light required in photosynthesis, penetrates to approximately 6.5 meters in clear water, to significantly less in turbid water. In especially clear ocean waters, the depth at which photosynthesis can occur may extend to 200 meters. Below the photic zone no photosynthesis occurs, and therefore no oxygen is produced. At these depths aerobic organisms must rely on the oxygen dissolved in the water. Facultative anaero-

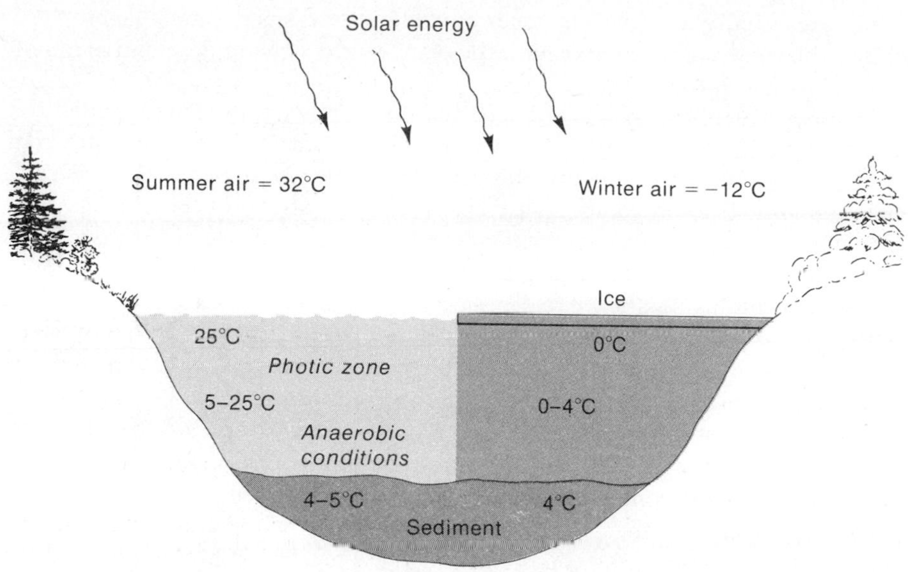

FIG. 40–3 Typical temperature distribution in deep water in summer and winter.

bic and obligate anaerobic organisms abound in the depths of freshwater and saltwater systems.

As in terrestrial habitats, fresh and salt waters contain nutrients in the form of waste organic materials. In water habitats this detritus consists of plant and animal wastes and remains as well as dead microorganisms. The microscopic forms of life in the water include ***zooplankton***, minute animal life, and ***phytoplankton***, plant life and algae such as diatoms and dinoflagellates.

BLOOMS

When nutrients are available in excess, they may cause ***blooms***, rapid growth of algae or cyanobacteria that discolor the water (Color Photograph 4A). Initially these photosynthetic organisms release increased quantities of oxygen, but as they die, aerobic and facultative anaerobic microorganisms consume the dissolved oxygen in decomposing the photosynthesizers. This oxygen depletion leads to fish kills and the development of anaerobic digestion, which ultimately produces a considerable stench (Figure 40–4). The blooms usually occur because of increased nutrients in the water from sewage, rain-dissolved fertilizers from agricultural land, phosphate detergents, or similar sources. The nutrients may be organic or inorganic. Freshwater blooms are often due to blue-green bacteria, and saltwater blooms are commonly dinoflagellates. The dinoflagellates have a reddish pigment, giving rise to the name "red tide," which describes blooms that occur in summer months along the shores of California and Florida.

FIG. 40–4 One consequence of the development of anaerobic conditions in a river. This fish kill was caused by excessive pollution. The remains of such animals putrefy, not only producing foul odors but adding significant amounts of organic matter to natural water systems. *Courtesy of USDA.*

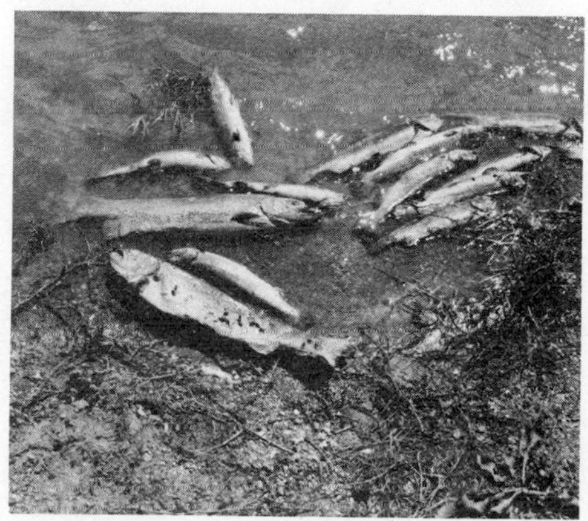

FRESHWATER HABITATS

Fresh water makes up only about 2 percent of the water on this planet; much less than that is readily available for domestic and industrial uses. The science of fresh water, called ***limnology***, deals with the physical, chemical, and biological factors influencing the role of fresh water in nature. There are two types of natural freshwater habitats, standing and flowing bodies of water.

STANDING FRESH WATER

A large, often deep depression of land that retains water is called a *lake*. A small shallow lake is considered a ***pond***, and a shallow pond that has vegetation of a particular type, that is, large, floating leaves or cattails, is called a *marsh*. Lakes are usually divided into zones of shallow or deeper waters. Figure 40–5 shows the conditions that prevail in these zones and some representative microorganisms found there.

Shallow water around a lake often has rooted vegetation. This is called the *littoral* zone. The sediment in this area is richer in nutrients than the *profundal* zone, or bottom, situated below the open water, the *limnetic* zone. As vegetation and animal life decompose in the littoral zone, sediment tends to accumulate, and slowly this zone may extend out toward the middle of the lake. This process continues, often leading to the development of a pond as the lake shrinks, becoming shallower, and perhaps eventually becoming a marsh. This natural process is called **eutrophication,** the aging process whereby lakes may eventually become dry land through sediment accumulation and increased growth of vegetation. In nature this happens very slowly, over thousands or hundreds of thousands of years. Sewage and other pollution can hasten eutrophication by producing algal and blue-green bacterial blooms. As detritus accumulates, the decomposers do their job and sedimentation occurs. The decomposition leads to the production of anaerobic conditions in the sediment (Figure 40–5). Under these conditions, methane-producing bacteria yield sufficient gas to form bubbles that rise to the surface (Color Photograph 66). This so-called *marsh gas* is a natural gas and will burn if ignited.

FLOWING FRESH WATER

Any flowing fresh water is a *stream*. The stream is called a *creek* or *brook* if it is less than 3 meters in width or a *river* if wider than 3 meters. Two types of habitats in a stream are *rapids* and *pools*.

Rapids are swiftly moving waters, aerated by their turbulent flow over rocks. Their high oxygen content supports abundant animal life. The rapid flow is often too brisk for much sediment accumulation or development of a diverse community of microorganisms. Nutrients enter the water as soil runoff, leaves, branches, animal wastes, and the remains of animals. Some decomposition occurs, but most of it in pools where current is reduced, allowing sedimentation

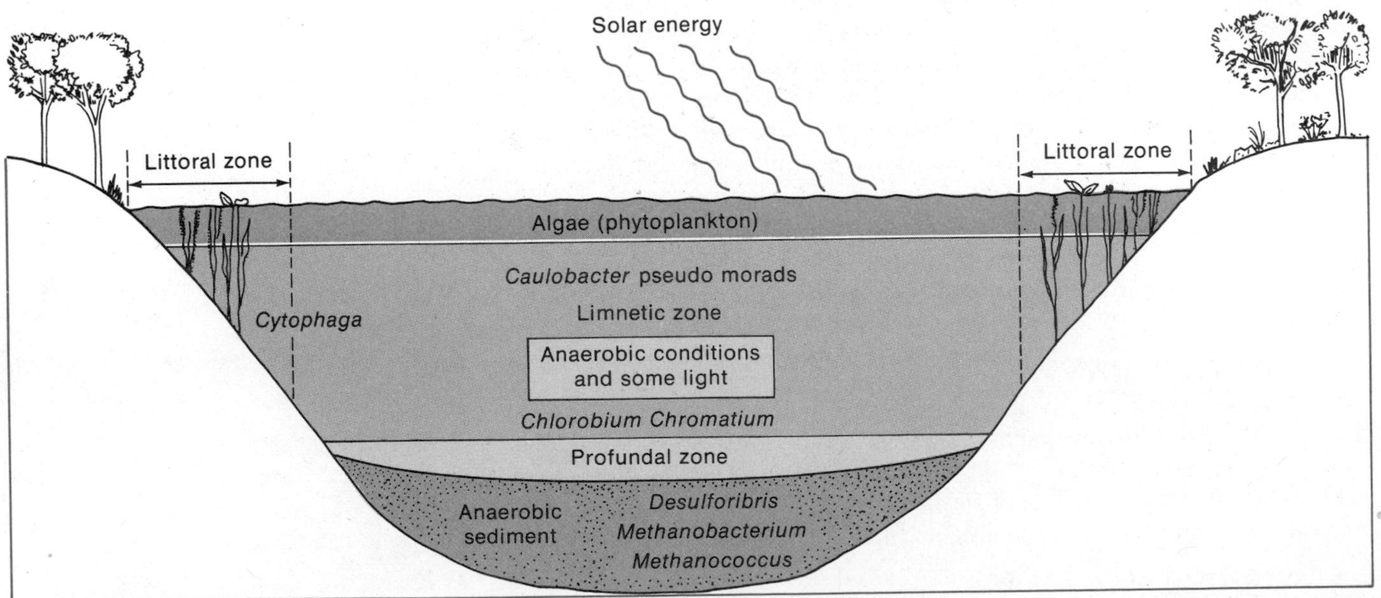

FIG. 40–5 Three regions, or zones, commonly identified in lakes. General conditions and some representative microbial genera are also indicated.

of sand or dirt carried by the water. Detritus accumulates as well, and decomposition occurs. Marsh plants may also grow in pools.

The source of water for some streams are *springs*, water flowing from the ground. This water is often of excellent quality, meeting all the standards set by the federal government. Such water is called *potable* (drinkable). Some springs, however, contain high concentrations of sulfur or iron and may even be heated in volcanic areas. These waters have their own peculiar communities of microorganisms. Sulfur-oxidizing bacteria of hot springs have been discussed earlier.

MARINE ENVIRONMENTS

Oceanography is the study of the seas—the waters with a salt content of about 3.5 percent and higher. Approximately 70 percent of the earth's surface is salt water, made up of the oceans, seas, and inland lakes, such as Great Salt Lake in Utah. Most of this water is 3.5 percent salt, but the Great Salt Lake and Dead Sea have salt concentrations of approximately 30 percent. Sodium and chloride ions constitute about 85 percent of the salt in seawater. The next five elements, in order of concentration, are magnesium, sulfur, calcium, potassium, and bromine. Commercial processes are being developed to extract magnesium, bromine, and sodium chloride from seawater in significant quantities.

Unlike the deep water and profundal zone in lakes where anaerobic conditions are expected, aerobic or at least **microaerophilic** conditions can occur in deep seawater. Extensive currents circulate the water and keep the concentration of dissolved oxygen at reasonable levels. Offshore currents, such as riptides or other tidal circulation, cause what is commonly known as *upswelling*. This refers to the movement of nutrient-rich waters from the sediments to the surface while the oxygen-rich waters travel down. This upswelling of some major ocean currents contributes significantly to the productivity in associated areas of the oceans, literally creating areas of extensive fish farms. Figure 40–6 shows the major zones in marine environments: *estuary*, *littoral* zone, *neritic* zone, and *pelagic* zone.

ESTUARIES

An estuary is a coastal area where seawater mixes with fresh water. It may be a marsh or the mouth of a river. The relative content of salt varies with the

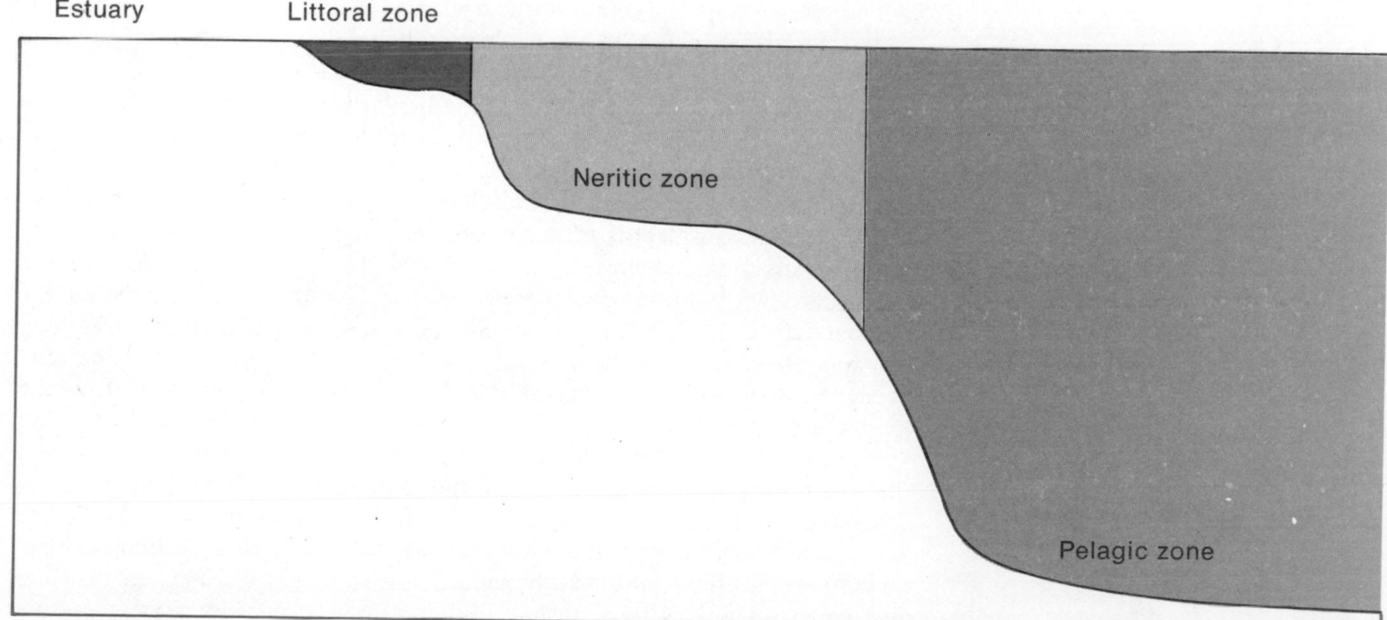

FIG. 40–6 Major zones in marine environments.

tides and the flow of fresh water in the area. Thus all organisms living in estuaries must be able to tolerate significant shifts in the salt content of their habitats. Estuaries, particularly marshes, tend to be rich in nutrients from land runoffs and detritus. As to the capacity of various areas to produce vegetation, estuarine habitats are considered the most productive, being at least two and one half times as productive as agricultural land areas and as much as 30 times as productive as the open ocean. Estuaries produce large quantities of marsh grasses adapted to a fluctuating saline environment. In one particular estuarine marsh studied on the southeast coast of the United States, heterotrophic bacteria included species of *Bacillus, Serratia, Flavobacterium, Achromobacter,* and *Pseudomonas.* In addition to these bacteria, many fungi and protozoans were found associated with the marsh grasses and detritus.

LITTORAL ZONE

Unlike the freshwater littoral zone of lakes, which contain rooted vegetation in shallow waters, the littoral zone in the oceans refers to the shoreline between extremes of high and low tides. The only similarity of marine and freshwater littoral zones is that both are shallow. Because the zone is marked by the tides, physical conditions of temperature and water loss by evaporation occur regularly. These are harsh conditions for most organisms, probably more harsh than salinity changes in estuaries. Rocky beaches tend to have some plant and algal production for food chains. Sandy beaches, on the other hand, produce little plant or algal material directly. Thus food chains are based primarily on detritus decomposition from plant and animal materials cast on to the shore and beaten by the waves.

NERITIC AND PELAGIC ZONES

The *neritic zone* is the water located over the continental shelf. The depths in this region go to about 200 meters. Populations of life forms there are not as great as those in the littoral zone or estuaries. The greater depths create regions of different light penetration, so that photic and aphotic areas are established. The productivity in neritic zones is related primarily to diatoms, dinoflagellates, and microflagellates. Seaweeds are restricted more to the shallower portions. The cloudiness of neritic water due to upswelling and land runoff limits the photic zone to no more than 30 meters as a rule.

The *pelagic zone* is essentially the open waters, with depths averaging 4000 meters to 10,000 meters in the deepest trenches. Light penetration in these clearer waters may allow photosynthesis to occur down to about 200 meters. The organisms below the photic zone, particularly in the pelagic area, rely on the "rain" of wastes—plant and animal detritus and sedimenting phytoplankton, zooplankton, and other microorganisms. The process of decomposition proceeds as the material descends, feeding various organisms in the process.

Life in the ocean depths must tolerate very high pressure as well as nearly complete darkness. Various forms of animal life have adapted by forming associations with luminescent bacteria (Color Photograph 67) in which the microorganisms produce light in specific animal organs. This light serves several functions, including luring prey and acting as a sex attractant. The temperature in the deepest portions of the ocean is approximately 0° C; thus the most abundant forms of bacteria here are marine psychrophiles (lovers of cold).

It is commonly believed that tropical waters are very rich in life forms and that the oceans are highly productive and extremely useful for potential food production. In fact, the open ocean has about the same productivity as the dry desert, far less than the productivity of the neritic zone, which is almost comparable to some agricultural land. In addition, warm tropical waters are less productive than colder waters because dissolved oxygen concentrations decrease with increased temperature. This directly influences development of aerobic life. Some ocean waters have so little dissolved organic materials that heterotrophic organisms would not be expected to exist. However, the marine psychrophilic *Vibrio* sp. was found to be able to survive extended periods of starvation without being a sporeformer.

Waste Treatment

Each village, town, municipality, or region must deal with its liquid and solid waste materials. Very small communities can run their waste waters into shallow ponds or streams for biological decomposition and bury the solids. Natural cycles such as those associated with carbon, sulfur, and phosphorus can process considerable amounts of these materials and do so with or without human input. The breakdown of much litter results in the formation of humus and the decomposition of detritus in fresh- and marine-water sediments. Large communities produce far too much wastes for environmental processes to handle. Thus, specialized ponds, or lagoons (Figure 40–17), have been developed for handling some wastes, and treatment facilities are built and maintained for many domestic and industrial wastes (Figure 40–7). Solid waste materials are still largely buried, but in a manner that should not prove harmful to the environment. Consolidating treatment processes in larger facilities reclaims valuable by-products in a way that might otherwise not be practical. Some materials are converted into fertilizer, compost, and methane. Certain residual substances can be partially pyrolized (decomposed by heating) to produce activated carbon for water purification or more completely pyrolized to ashes for the recovery of various heavy metals.

Waste Water

Waste water, or sewage, contains about 99 percent water and is therefore easily pumped through sewage pipes to a treatment plant (Figure 40–7). The remainder of the material consists of suspended, relatively insoluble solids such as starch granules, cellulosic (plant) remains, lignins, and proteins. Dissolved substances in sewage include sugars, fatty acids, alcohols, amino acids, and many inorganic compounds. Sewage also contains litter, paper, gravel, and many varied materials from garbage disposal units and community industrial processing facilities (Figure 40–7).

Domestic waste water is largely human fecal matter and urine diluted with laundry and wash water. One estimate is that each person in the United States produces more than 100 gallons of waste water per day. A treatment facility serving an area of one million people must therefore process 100 million or more gallons of domestic water daily. Industrial and commercial waste waters include materials from food canning processes, dairies, slaughterhouses, and cattle or hog feedlots, as well as from many chemical and pharmaceutical industrial plants. The food- or animal-related enterprises and pharmaceutical companies produce waste waters of considerably higher organic content than that of domestic wastes. The chemical industries vary considerably in their organic contributions to waste water. Unfortunately, chemical wastes often contain toxic materials, such as heavy metals or pesticides, that may reduce the effectiveness of a treatment facility.

Microorganisms commonly found in waste waters include bacteria of intes-

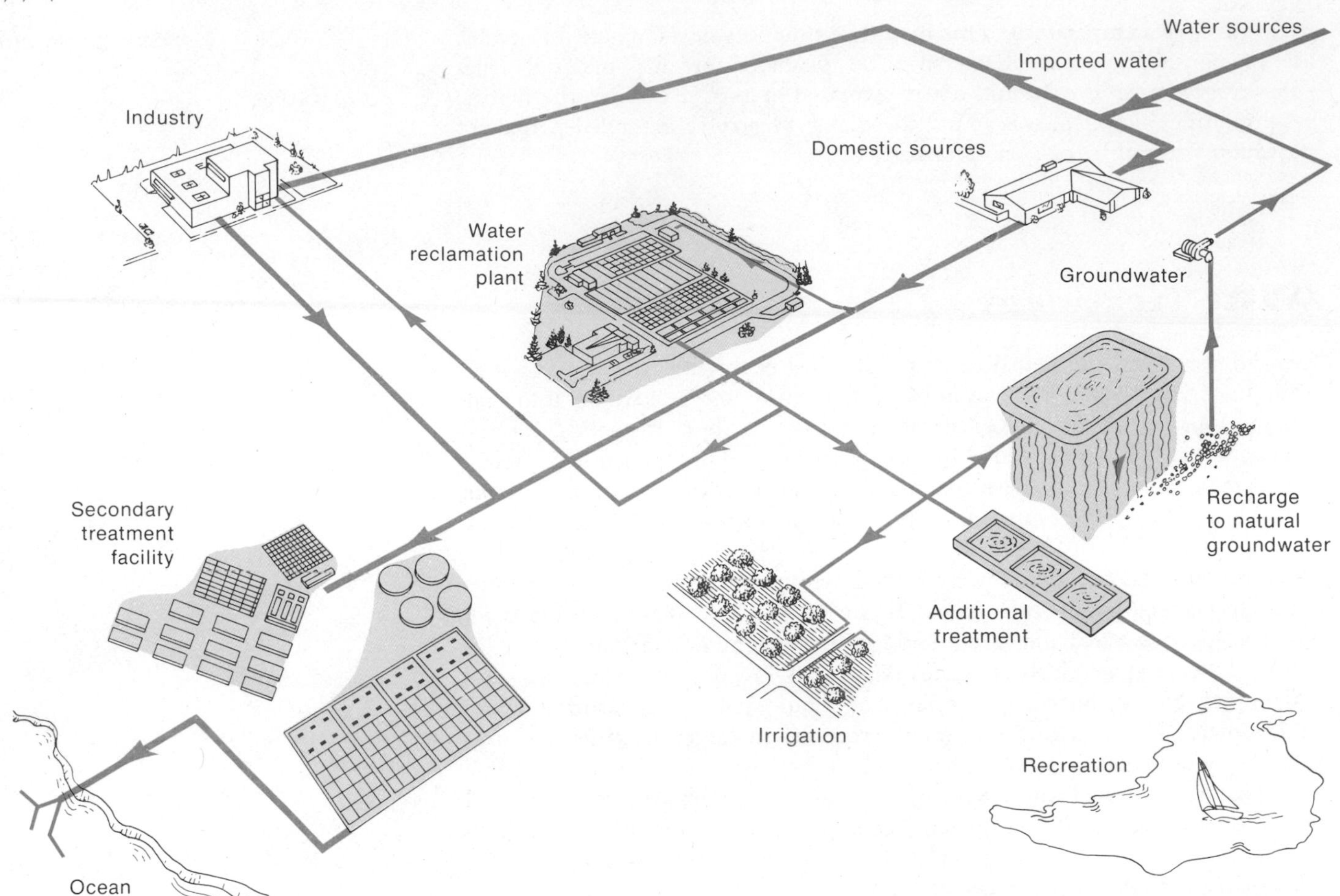

FIG. 40–7 A collection system for sewage and waste water, showing the treatment of water to render it reusable. Note that treated water can be used for recreational activities, but additional treatment is needed first. *Courtesy of the Sanitation Districts of Los Angeles County.*

tinal origin such as *Bacteroides* spp., *Bifidobacterium* spp., *Clostridium perfringens, Enterobacter aerogenes, Escherichia coli, Lactobacillus* spp., and *Streptococcus faecalis.* Because of the origin of some of the wastes, many human pathogens are sometimes found in sewage. Table 40–1 lists some of these microorganisms. One of the major purposes of waste water treatment is to eliminate such potential hazards to public health.

Some microorganisms found in waste water are primarily from soil and water. These include species of bacteria including *Sphaerotilus, Crenothrix,* and *Beggiotoa* and fungi such as *Saprolegnia* and *Leptomitus.* All of these organisms can form slimy growths in pipes and ditches. Some can also produce iron, sulfur, or manganese deposits, which clog pipes, or hydrogen sulfide, which is noted for its offensive rotten-egg odor. Other bacteria found in waste water include species of *Cytophaga, Micrococcus, Pseudomonas, Bdellovibrio, Chromobacterium, Aeromonas, Rhodospirillum,* and various methanogenic organisms.

Environmental Effects

A wide variety of microorganisms may be present in drinking water. If water supplies are contaminated by waste waters, a number of infectious disease

TABLE 40-1 Examples of Principal Human Pathogens Associated With Waste Waters

Bacteria	Protozoans	Viruses
Leptospira spp.	*Entamoeba histolytica*	Adenoviruses
Salmonella paratyphi	*Giardia (lamblia) intestinalis*	Enteroviruses (Coxsackie-, echo- and polioviruses)
S. typhi		Parvoviruses (hepatitis A virus)
S. typhimurium		Reoviruses
Shigella dysenteriae		
Vibrio cholerae		

agents could be transmitted (Table 40–1). Asiatic cholera, bacillary and amebic dysenteries, leptospirosis, and several viral and protozoan diseases are some of the diseases transmitted by contaminated drinking water. Even water that looks clear and pure may be sufficiently contaminated with pathogens to pose a considerable health hazard.

CONTAMINATION DETECTION

It is neither practical nor possible to test drinking water for all the possible microbial pathogens that may be present. Fortunately, it is also unnecessary. There are several microorganisms commonly found in human and other animal intestinal tracts that can be used as indicators of fecal pollution. Their presence in water supplies in sufficient numbers signals contamination of an intestinal source. The most common of these indicator organisms are the ***coliforms***. These microbes are facultatively anaerobic, Gram-negative, non-spore-forming rods, that ferment lactose with the production of acid and gas in 24 to 48 hours when grown at 35° C. The group includes various strains of ***Escherichia coli, Enterobacter aerogenes***, and ***Klebsiella pneumoniae***. These microbes populate the intestine in large numbers and survive longer in water than do the pathogenic bacteria. *Salmonella typhi*, the causative agent of typhoid fever, has been shown to be outnumbered in feces by the coliforms in the ratio of one million to one. *S. typhi* survives in water for only about one week, but the coliforms survive for weeks and even months. A large number of coliforms in water usually indicates recent pollution; relatively low numbers reflect a past contamination problem.

Procedures for testing water for coliforms and other indicator organisms are published regularly by the American Public Health Association in ***Standard Methods for the Examination of Water and Wastewater***. Two procedures used for coliforms are the ***most probable number (MPN) method*** and ***membrane filtration (MF)***. A general count of microorganisms in the water is also performed.

Most probable number. One means of the MPN procedure uses 15 lactose fermentation tubes, 5 of which are inoculated with 10 ml of the water sample. A second set of 5 tubes receives 1 ml each, and a third set of 5 tubes is inoculated with 0.1 ml of the sample. The lactose tubes are incubated for 24 to 48 hours at 37° C. The number of coliform organisms per 100 ml of the water is determined by recording the number of fermentation tubes showing the presence of acid and gas for each sample size and comparing these data with a statistical table, part of which is presented in Table 40–2.

Consider a complete procedure for bacteriological examination of water. A water sample that is estimated to have greater than 2.2 coliforms per 100 ml is presumed to be contaminated. This, then, is known as the ***presumptive test*** for total coliforms (Figure 40–8). The ***confirmed test*** involves plating an inoculum from the lactose tubes positive for gas production onto an eosin-methylene blue

TABLE 40–2 The Application of the Most Probable Number Technique to Water Bacteriology

Number of Positive Lactose Broth Tubes			*An Estimate of the Number of Coliform Organisms per 100 ml of Water*
10 ml	*1 ml*	*0.1 ml*	
0	0	0	0
0	0	1	2
0	1	0	2
0	1	1	4
1	0	0	2.2
1	0	1	4.4
1	1	0	4.4
1	1	1	6.7

agar plate or other comparable selective and differential medium. Coliform bacteria typically produce deep purple colonies, often with a green metallic surface. The dark colonies indicate lactose fermentation. Appearance of such colonies confirms the presumptive test. Isolated positive cultures are then subjected to the *completed test*. This involves their inoculation into lactose broth fermentation tubes and nutrient agar slants. If when the medium is fermented and stained, smears of the organisms from the slant are Gram-negative, non-spore-forming rods, the proof for coliform contamination is complete. By incubating cultures at 44.5 ± 0.2° C, coliforms of enteric or fecal origin can be distinguished from those normally present in soil or water. Only fecal coliforms grow at this temperature.

Membrane filter technique. Membrane filters can be used in a more rapid procedure for the isolation and identification of various types of microorganisms including coliforms (Figure 40–8). Total and fecal coliform tests can be performed using these filters. In this method, a specified volume of water is filtered to trap any bacteria present. The filter is then removed and incubated at 35° C or 44.5° C on a pad soaked with an appropriate selective and differential medium, such as EMB or Endo agar. Suspect colonies of coliforms appear on the filter within 24 hours.

A cloudy water sample cannot be tested by this method, since the suspended materials will clog the pores of the filter. Even with this limitation, the membrane filter method has significant advantages in terms of the amount of suspect water that can be tested and the time involved in obtaining completed tests for water quality.

WATER STANDARDS AND OTHER INDICATOR MICROORGANISMS

Standards for water quality usually refer to coliform counts such as the ones described. They are based on the general assumption that the possibility that pathogens are present increases with the pollution of water by feces and urine. When the results of bacteriologic examinations of water show unacceptable levels of fecal contamination, the search is made for pollution sources or for failures in the water purification system.

Other than coliforms, the most common indicator organisms for fecal contamination in the United States are strains of *Streptococcus faecalis*. Membrane filtration and MPN procedures are performed for these organisms using

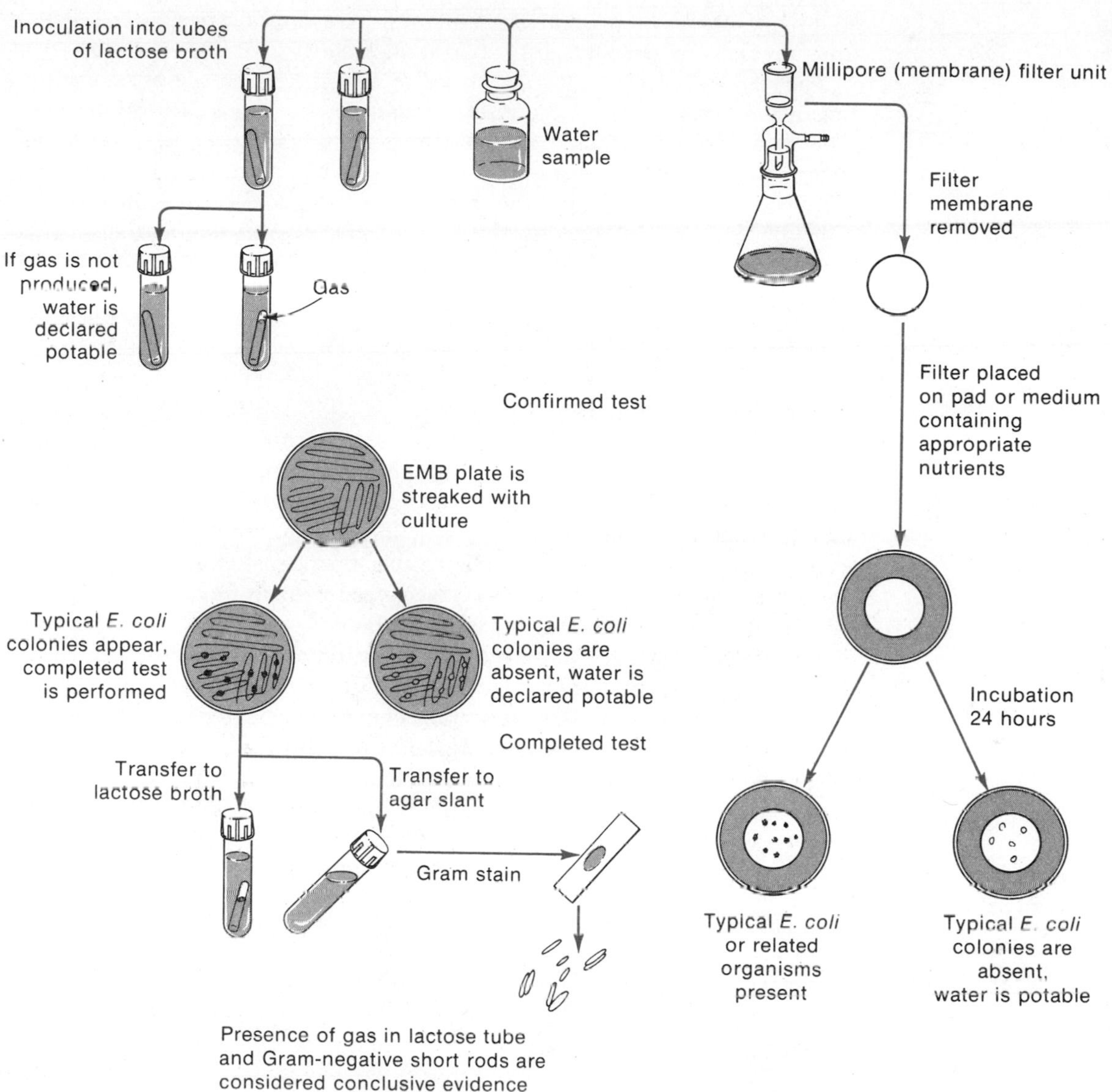

FIG. 40-8 The steps in the standard bacteriological analysis of a water sample. The presumptive, confirmed, and completed tests are represented. The use of a membrane filter is also shown.

selective media with sodium azide as the selective ingredient. *S. faecalis* does not survive well in water, so its presence indicates recent pollution. Two other test organisms are *Bifidobacterium bifidus* and *Clostridium perfringens*. *B. bifidus* is unable to reproduce in waste water and is therefore an indicator of recent pollution. *C. perfringens* may survive indefinitely due to its spore-forming capability. The presence of *C. perfringens* therefore indicates any contamination by feces or waste water over an extended period of time.

Standard plate count. Although there are no specific regulations concerning water quality in terms of total aerobic colony count, the periodic use of the assay procedure known as the *standard plate count* can be used to find unusual changes in bacterial counts of water samples. The procedure involves the preparation of agar pour plates, incorporating 1-ml samples of water or dilutions of samples. After incubation at 35° C for 24 hours, colony counts are made. A finding of 100 or fewer colony-forming units per milliliter of sample is considered a reasonably safe standard for drinking water.

The standard plate count can be used to detect the presence of noncoliform organisms that may affect the results obtained with assays of drinking water. The procedure is also used in evaluating the efficiency of water treatment processes. Plate counts on samples of raw water and on samples of water at various purification steps indicate how effectively the bacterial contamination is being reduced. Different incubation temperatures are frequently necessary to allow for the growth of a greater number of organisms present in the water samples.

NUTRIENT CONTAMINATION

The quantity of organic and inorganic materials in the waste waters is the second critical problem in water treatment. Organisms in the soil and water often cannot metabolize such materials fast enough, so they accumulate and establish anaerobic conditions. The depletion of dissolved oxygen in water, for example, is due to the bacteria oxidizing the organic matter and consuming the oxygen in the process. The decrease in oxygen content has several important and usually obvious effects as already noted.

The *biological* or **biochemical oxygen demand** (BOD) is the amount of oxygen consumed by microorganisms during their decomposition of organic materials. BOD is used as an indication of the extent of organic pollution in bodies of water. From the BOD, the level of pollution or nutrient load, as well as the efficiency in correcting unfavorable situations, can be determined. To make this determination, several water samples are obtained in sterile, glass-stoppered bottles. In one sample, the initial concentration of dissolved oxygen is measured in milligrams per liter. The other samples are incubated at 20° C for 5 days before the final dissolved oxygen in these samples is measured. The difference between the initial value and the later ones represents the BOD.

Waste Water Treatment

PRELIMINARY AND PRIMARY TREATMENT

Most waste waters are processed for disposal by one or more of the steps outlined for waste water treatment in Figure 40–9. Step A represents what is called *preliminary treatment* in which waste water enters a tank or settling chamber for the physical removal of some wastes.

This stage of sewage treatment relies on the force of gravity and a few screens to take out the heavier materials; thus it begins with the removal of solids, including cardboard, plastics, glass, wood, and gravel, from the more readily digestible components. The large solids, grease, and scum caught in this manner are raked off. Some plants use a shredding device in place of screens to chop up the heavier items, which then stay in the sewage water until the next stage of treatment.

Screened or shredded sewage passes next through a grit chamber, which removes cinders, sand, and small stones. This serves a protective function in that pumps and other equipment used in later stages are protected from damage. The effluent (liquid material) from the preliminary treatment is then pumped to the primary settling tank (step B). In this *primary treatment*, suspended solids of plant, animal, and mineral material settle slowly. In some systems such settling requires 1½ to 2 hours. The settled solids are collected by

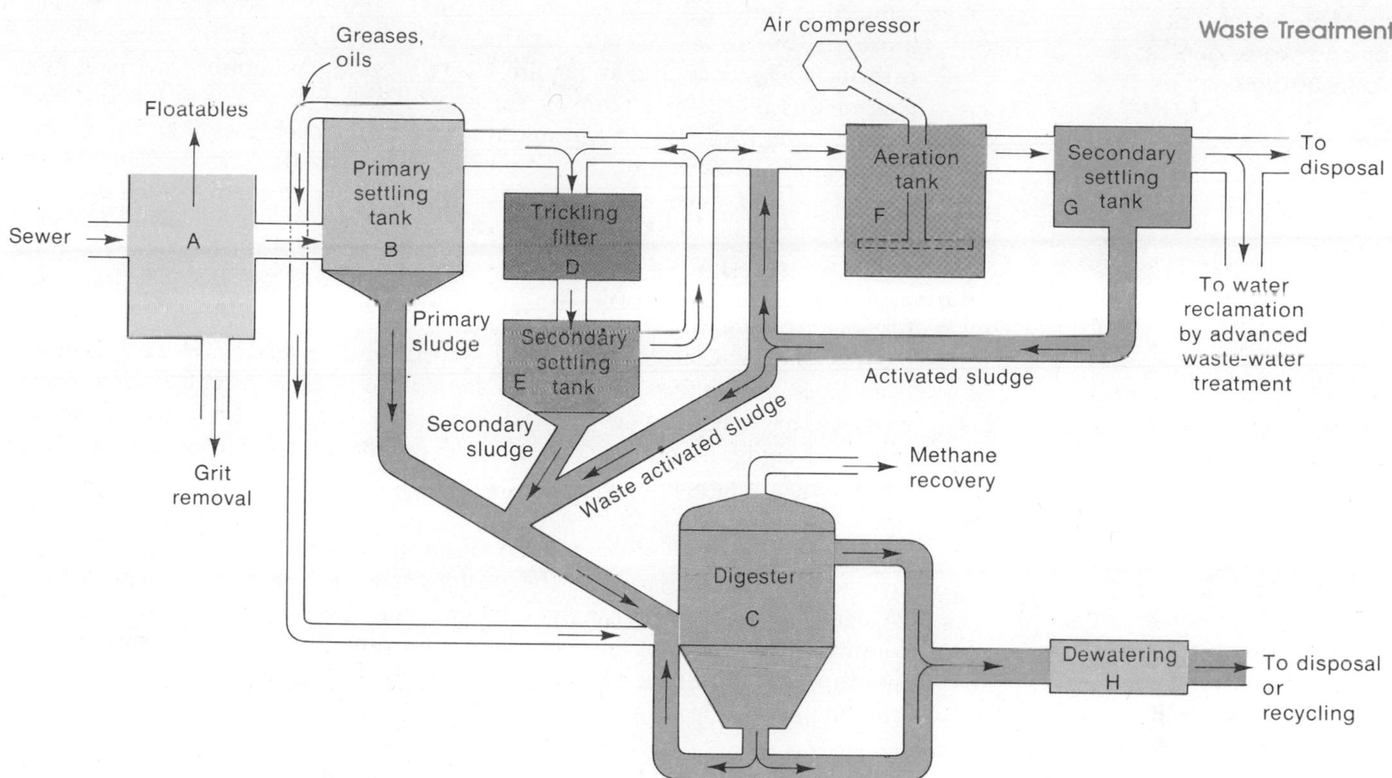

FIG. 40–9 A general procedure used in waste water treatment.

a wiper blade and pushed to a pit in the center of the tank. There solids collectively form ***sludge*** that is pumped to the next station in the process, the ***digester*** (step C). Any material, such as grease or oil, that floats in primary settling, is removed and also pumped to the digesters. This ends primary treatment. Like the preliminary treatment, primary treatment involves only physical activities: floating, settling, scraping, and pumping. If treatment ends at the primary stage, the settled material, known as sludge, may be removed either manually or by mechanical means. Sometimes sludge is dried in beds and disposed of on land. However, because sludge itself can be a pollutant, it is preferable to initiate microbial decomposition in sludge digestion tanks before drying. This is an aspect of secondary treatment.

The effluent in the sedimentation tank is usually treated with chlorine to kill microorganisms and reduce objectionable odors. Once this occurs, primary treatment is complete and the effluent can be released into some natural water environment. Today approximately 30 percent of the cities in the United States do not go beyond primary treatment of their sewage. By federal law, all municipalities that dispose of treated waste waters into navigable waters are required to install secondary treatment facilities by the end of 1983 (Figure 40–7).

SECONDARY TREATMENT

Because of the objectionable properties of the effluent from primary treatment, secondary treatment is usually employed.

This type of operation involves the biological degradation of organic material by microorganisms under controlled conditions. It is performed in two phases, anaerobic and aerobic digestion.

Anaerobic digestion. The digester labeled step C in Figure 40–9 represents anaerobic decomposition of the wastes. The primary sludge, greases, and oils are pumped to the digester. Anaerobic digestion is much slower than the aerobic processes, but it can tolerate materials of much higher BOD values. A 90-percent BOD reduction may require several weeks to a month. The main purpose of this process is to convert some organic carbon to carbon dioxide and methane and convert some organic nitrogen to nitrogen gas. Note the gas removal pipes at the top of the digester in Figure 40–10. The methanogenesis process often produces a gas mixture of 70 to 77 percent methane and 23 to 30 percent carbon dioxide. The mixture can fire boilers or run motors, or it can be stored in a gas sphere for future use. Methanogenic bacteria isolated from digesters include *Methanococcus vannielli*, *Methanobacterium ruminafum*, *M. formicicum*, and a *Methanospirillum* sp. Many other anaerobic and facultatively anaerobic heterotrophic and denitrifying bacteria have been isolated from digesters. The few fungi found show little or no apparent activity. Some protozoa have been observed and apparently are predators. Some of the processed sludge is returned to the inlet of the digester to ensure that the correct inoculum is present for digestion of the new material.

Aerobic stabilization. Waste decomposition by aerobic processes is often called *aerobic stabilization* because of the greater degree of BOD removal. About 85 to 95 percent of the BOD can be removed from the primary effluent by two common processes in a matter of hours. The same result might require up to a month in the anaerobic digester (Figure 40–9). These aerobic processes are the *trickling filter* (step D) and *activated sludge* (step F).

Trickling filter. Suspended solids may be sprayed onto the surfaces of artificial beds of a trickling filter made up of broken stone, cork, plastic balls, or another supporting matrix contained in tanks. Microorganisms form a living film on the components of the matrix and digest the organic matter of the sewage as it filters through the bed (Figure 40–11). Figure 40–11 shows a typical trickling filter equipped with spraying arms. Fungi and algae appear to be the primary agents in the aerobic stabilization process, but a number of bacteria are also involved. The microorganisms commonly isolated from trickling filters are listed in Table 40–3. The film averages about 2 mm in thickness and consists of three distinct layers. The outer layer is primarily fungi. The middle layer is primarily fungi and algae. The inner layer consists of fungi, algae, and bacteria. In addition to being quite efficient for BOD removal, the process also removes 90 to 98 percent of viruses present in the initial waste water. The effluent of the trickling filter is usually pumped to a settling tank (step E, in Figure 40–9),

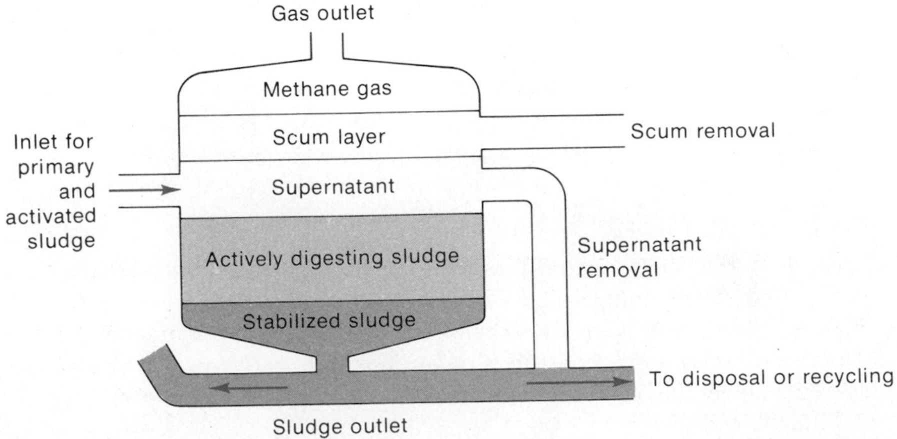

FIG. 40–10 An anaerobic sludge digester. Note the presence of the methane gas close to the gas outlet or removal pipes.

TABLE 40–3 Common Microorganisms Found in Films on Rock Supports in Trickling Filter Systems

Algae	*Bacteria*	*Fungi*
Anacystis *Euglena* *Ulothrix*	*Alcaligenes* sp. *Flavobacterium* *Pseudomonas* sp. *Zoogleoa*	*Aureobasidium pullulans* *Fusarium* sp. *Subboromyces splendeus*

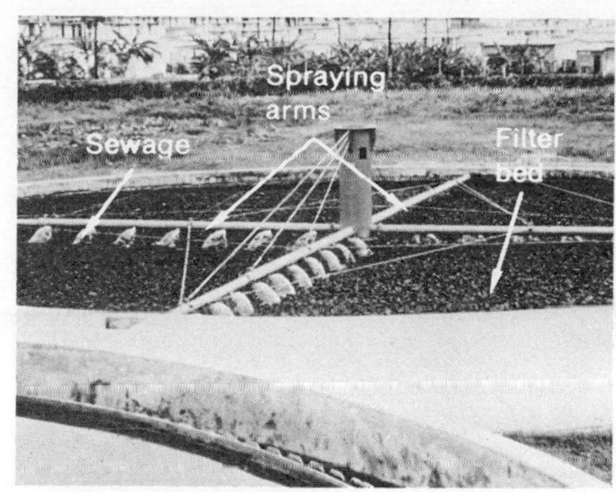

FIG. 40–11 A trickling filter with a spraying or distributing device. This type of filter is commonly used in sewage treatment plants. *Courtesy of the National Medical Audiovisual Center, Atlanta.*

where the fluid is separated from any portions of the film that may have dislodged from the supporting materials. Such settled solids are pumped to digesters. The effluent of the secondary settling process can be diverted to the second aerobic stabilization process.

The effluent from primary or secondary settling tanks is pumped into aeration tanks or rectangular chambers for the activated sludge process (Figure 40–13). Previously digested material is mixed in with the effluents to ensure the proper inoculum (Figure 40–9), and air compressors provide oxygen for stabilization and mix the digesting materials. Some foamy material is caused by the formation of masses of microbial growth known as *floc* (Figure 40–14) or *zoogloeal masses.* This floc exists as a branched system or as a formless gel containing a celluloselike polymer and a polymer of hydroxybutyric acid. This mass is thought to be due to the activities of the bacterium *Zoogloea ramigera,* which forms fingerlike colonies almost resembling multiple pseudopods on an amoeba. The name *zoogloea* means "living glue" and is quite appropriate. Other bacteria identified in floc include species of *Pseudomonas, Alcaligenes, Achromobacter, Microbacterium,* and *Brevitbacterium.* Slime and capsule formation by these organisms may contribute to the floc formation. Ciliated protozoa, such as the *Vorticella* sp. shown in Figure 40–15, control the overgrowth of bacteria by predation and contribute to floc formation. As many as 67 species of protozoa have been reported in activated sludge. The formation of floc is important for two reasons: (1) it speeds the adsorption and absorption of nutrients and (2) the floc settles out in the secondary settling tank (step G, Figure 40–9), leaving a clear supernatant liquid. Some of the floc is returned to inoculate incoming waste water, and most of it is pumped to the digesters. The effluent of the activated sludge system has been reduced in its BOD by about 85 to 95 percent. This fluid may be chlorinated and disposed of in streams and lakes or it may be pumped for reclamation by an advanced waste-water treatment as shown in Figure 40–16. It may also be used to water lawns and trees, as well as for irrigation. The final step in secondary treatment is the disposal or reuse of digested sludge from the digester (step H, Figure 40–9). In this step much of the water is removed and the thickened sludge is dried. This material is dumped as landfill or processed for sale as fertilizers and soil conditioners.

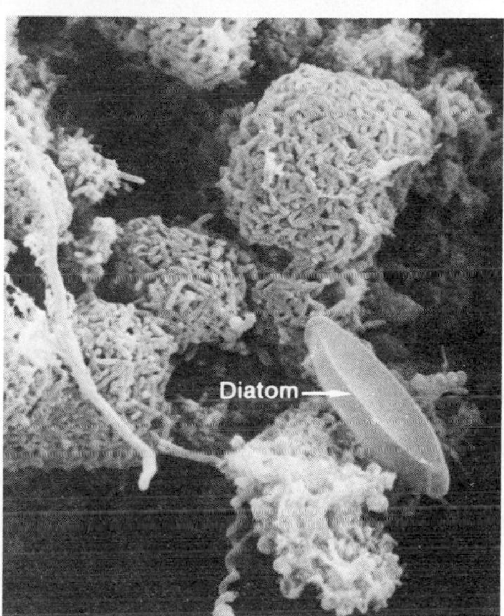

FIG. 40–12 Microbial films develop upon all objects submerged in natural waters. Microbial growth is especially plentiful when the water environment is rich in organic material and oxygen. Algae, bacteria, fungi, and protozoa are among the forms of life in such growth. These bacterial colonies were found 30.48 cm below the surface of a trickling filter. A diatom can also be seen. *From Mack, W. N., J. P. Mack, and A. O. Ackerson,* Microbial Ecol. *2:215–226 (1975).*

ADVANCED WASTE-WATER TREATMENT

Figure 40–16 represents one approach to the further purification of the treated waste water to provide a high-quality product. In advanced waste-water treatment, lime is mixed with the effluent to produce accumulations of impurities and settling of the limed sludge. The lime is recovered by pyrolysis and the liquid is aerated to remove ammonia and other gases. The liquid is then filtered first in a separation bed and finally in activated carbon. The resultant water has been used by some communities for the development of recreational lakes or for injection into groundwater for storage, as well as to prevent salt-water intrusion in coastal communities (Figure 40–6).

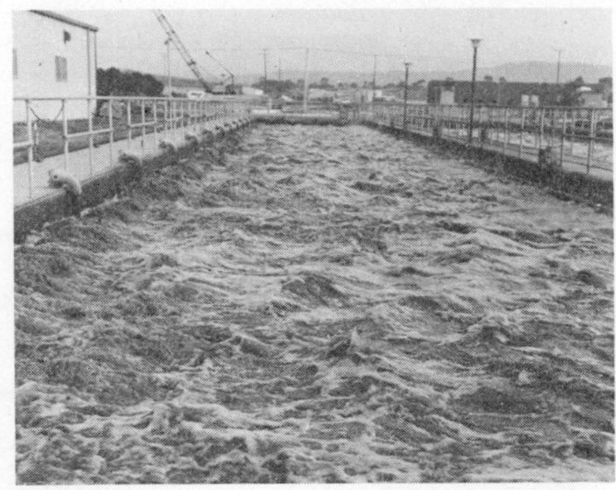

FIG. 40–13 An activated sludge system demonstrating the foaming and agitation caused by the compressed air. *Courtesy of the Orange County Sanitation District, Fountain Valley, CA.*

Lagooning. Aerobic waste stabilization does not have to be performed in large buildings and concrete reservoirs, but is also being done in so-called "algae lagoons." These are actually very shallow ponds into which wastes are pumped for treatment. If the proper slime- or floc-forming bacteria are present, along with other microbes necessary for aerobic stabilization, one requirement for suitable treatment is present, namely, suitable flora. Since mixing and spraying are impractical in a situation of this type, algae are used as a source of oxygen for the organisms. Together these components form a sound ecological system, with groups of different organisms working for mutual benefit. The algae require carbon dioxide, water, and other compounds that the bacteria supply by the digestion of the sewage. The bacteria require the oxygen that the algae now are able to produce. This concept of combining algae and other microorganisms in waste treatment has been considered both for the production of food and oxygen for astronauts and as a means of disposing of their waste materials. It has also been applied to the problem of disposing of unusual industrial waste (Figure 40–17).

Algae and bacteria appear to predominate in these lagoons. The algae usually must be harvested to prevent the development of anaerobic conditions, but in some systems brine shrimp are used to graze on the algae. These shrimp subsequently are used as food by fish.

Waste waters of particularly high BOD may be forcibly aerated to speed up the process.

Anaerobic waste digestion can also be performed in lagoons when the BOD loading is too great for an aerobic process. The lagoons are made anaerobic by their being at least four feet deep and containing the high BOD waste water. As the aerobic and facultatively anaerobic microorganisms grow in the system, the oxygen is depleted. Subsequently, the bubbling of generated methane helps carry more oxygen out from the water. Photosynthetic bacteria, such as *Rhodospirillum* spp., play an important role in odor control in these anaerobic lagoons. Hydrogen sulfide is produced during anaerobic decomposition of proteins containing the amino acids methionine, cysteine, and cystine. If allowed to accumulate, the H_2S would become offensive. Since the bacteria use the hydrogen sulfide as a hydrogen donor, they prevent the condition from happening.

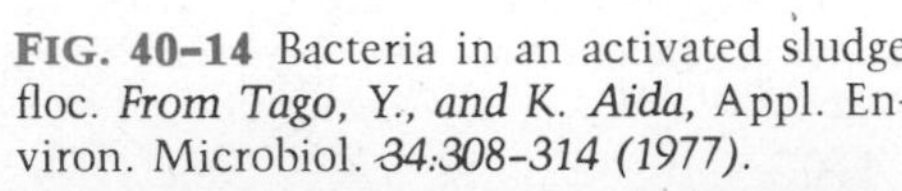

FIG. 40–14 Bacteria in an activated sludge floc. *From Tago, Y., and K. Aida,* Appl. Environ. Microbiol. *34:308–314 (1977).*

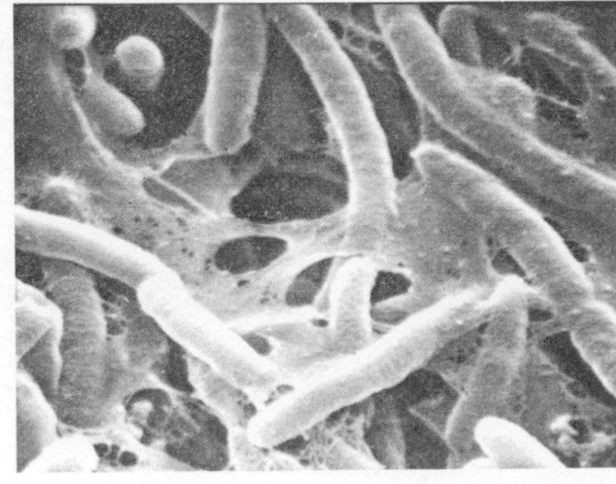

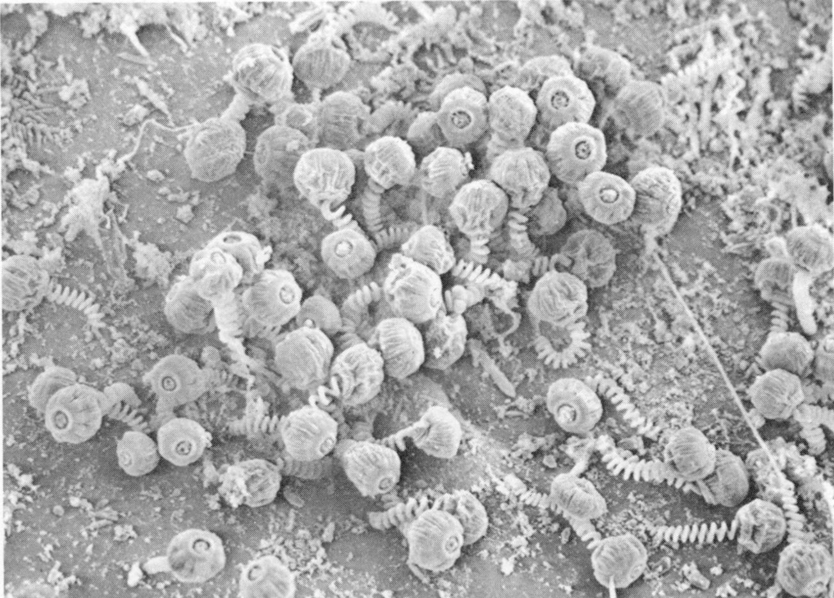

FIG. 40–15 One of the many types of protozoans *vorticella* sp. found in sludge systems as well as trickling systems. *Courtesy W. N. Mack and J. P. Mack.*

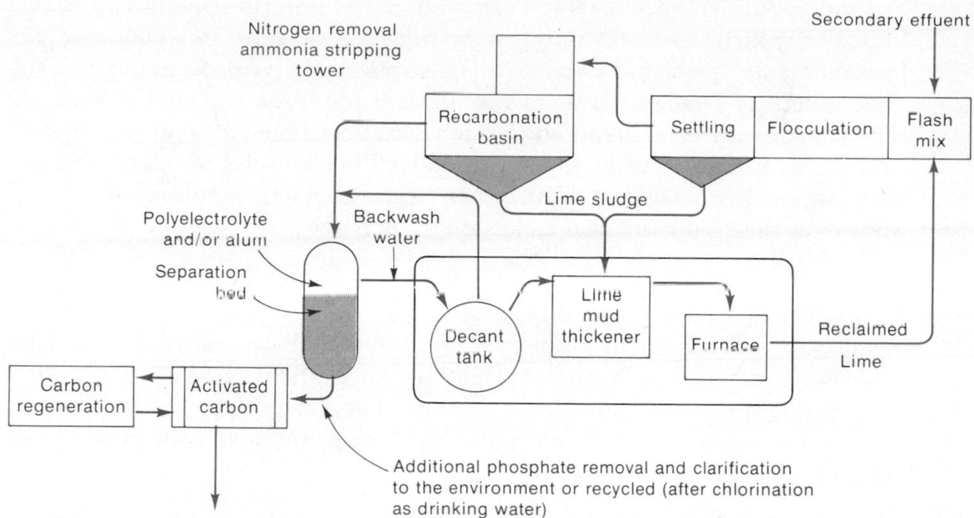

FIG. 40-16 Advanced waste water treatment. *After Odum, Fundamentals of Ecology, Philadelphia: W. B. Saunders, 1971.*

Solid Waste Disposal

Solid waste materials probably pose a greater and more complex problem than does waste water. This is because of their higher BOD loading. In addition, solid wastes cannot be pumped and may contain considerable material that is either not biodegradable or that degrades very slowly. Solid wastes from urban areas include garbage, glass, metals, ceramics, ashes, paper, dried sewage sludge, plant and tree trimmings, plastics, and other miscellaneous ingredients. The processes used for solid waste disposal are directed toward the reduction of its volume and weight and its conversion into a less troublesome and offensive form.

Solid wastes have traditionally been dumped into pits or gullies, and allowed to contaminate the air and water in the environment. Burning dumps were sources of pollution. More modern approaches involve controlled dumping and the establishment of sanitary landfills. In such systems, solid wastes are spread and compacted by machines into layers. After 2 to 3 meters of such material has been deposited, a layer of clean earth is applied and compacted. When the physical capacity for solid wastes of a sanitary landfill has been reached, it is sealed with an appropriate amount of compacted earth. This approach to solid-waste disposal controls the usual problems of odor, pests, and air and water pollution.

Since a large portion of a city's wastes is organic in nature, microorganisms are also involved in the decomposition of such material. Microbial decomposition activities in landfills are ***primarily anaerobic digestion.***

Initially aerobic and facultative anaerobic microorganisms are involved with the decomposition process. Because of the compacted layers in a sanitary landfill, the free movement of air into the system is prevented. Soon the oxygen is depleted and the activities of anaerobes dominate the digestion of the organic matter in the landfill. The heat that accompanies decomposition may raise the temperature to over 65° C within the landfill.

The decomposition processes in the landfill are similar to those in anaerobic sludge digestion and in the digestive systems of ruminants. Cellulose and other insoluble organic substances undergo digestion, and the resulting products are fermented. Methane and carbon dioxide are slowly released by these activities. While the release of methane is slow and does not appear to cause problems, accidental ignition of the escaping gas can occur. Studies are underway in Los Angeles and San Francisco to determine the commercial value of collecting this

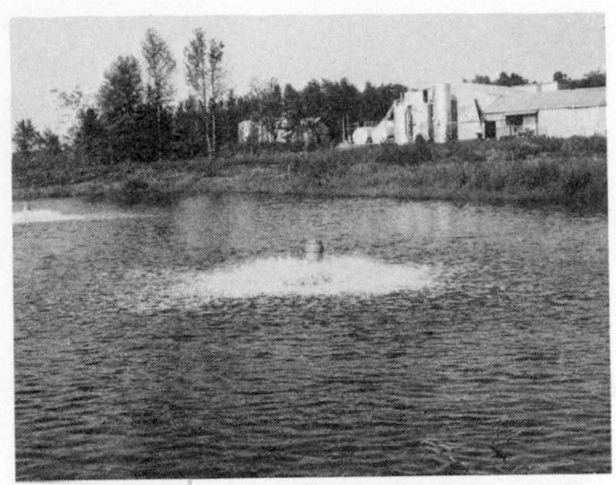

FIG. 40–17 One of two lagoons for a standard rendering plant. Waste material is processed before being released into a neighboring creek. Here waste material from poultry preparation facilities (which includes intestines, head, feet, and dead animals) are processed. Three agitator aerators can be seen in this lagoon. A major portion of the resulting clear water is recycled into the waste treatment plant and reused. *Courtesy USDA-Soil Conservation Service.*

natural gas to help meet energy needs. The carbon dioxide produced dissolves in water, which percolates through the fill. In general, it does not cause any environmental problem. The landfill areas are usually made into parks and other types of recreational areas not affected by small amounts of escaping methane or substances produced through decomposition and compaction. Studies are also underway to develop digestion facilities for solid wastes comparable to those used in secondary waste-water treatment. This would permit better control of the production and collection of methane.

COMPOSTING

Another approach to the disposal of solid wastes is the aerobic process of *composting*. In this microbial process, waste materials are mixed with soil for an inoculum. With an appropriate mixture of nutrients for microorganisms, the organic wastes are converted to humus. This material is rich in nitrogen, has good water-holding capacity, and is used for planting as a soil conditioner. The establishment of a compost heap on a small individual basis is quite feasible.

Some Products and Problems of Waste Treatment

Throughout this discussion on waste-water and solid-waste treatment, a number of potentially valuable products have been discussed—among them methane, humus, fertilizer, and good quality water. Other beneficial substances have been found in waste treatment. For example, activated sludge may contain from 1 to 10 mg per kg dry weight of vitamin B_{12}, cyanocobalamin. Sludge can also be pyrolized to produce activated carbon necessary for the advanced water treatment process described.

Unfortunately, problems that may limit the use of some of these products have surfaced. The use of treated water is regulated because of its potential to harbor viruses. In areas where digested sludge has been used as fertilizer, vegetables have been found to be contaminated with viruses originally found in raw sewage. The composting process can also pose problems. Humus has been found to contain the fungal pathogen *Aspergillus fumigatus*, which is often associated with composting of sewage sludge, municipal refuse, and wood chips. This organism can cause severe infection of individuals who are otherwise ill or who have diminished immunological capacity due to age, physical condition, or use of drugs such as steroids. Many people are allergic to this mold, and asthma can be a common complication of exposure.

SUMMARY

1. Numerous and various types of microorganisms and other forms of life contribute to soil formation and fertility.
2. The decomposition of organic matter by microorganisms results in better soil texture and water-binding capacity, releases important minerals for plant growth from soil particles, and transforms various chemicals into forms used by plants and other organisms.
3. Environmental reservoirs of infectious disease agents for humans include soil, water supplies, sewage, and some foods.

Soil and Its Formation

1. The chemical and microbial composition of soil, as well as its general suitability to support life, varies considerably.
2. Soil consists of solids (both minerals and organic compounds), water, and air.
3. Soil is formed from the breakdown of rock by mechanical, chemical, and biological processes collectively called *weathering*.
4. The type of soil in a particular region depends on the chemical make-up of the parent rock, the climate, and all forms of life on or in the soil.

The Aquatic Environment

The Water (Hydrologic) Cycle

1. The water cycle provides for a constant interchange of water among air, land, sea, and different life forms.

2. The water cycle involves evaporation, cloud formation, precipitation, surface water runoff, and percolation through the soil.

Aquatic Microorganisms

1. Various microorganisms are found regularly in natural waters. Their presence within such environments is influenced by both chemical and physical factors including hydrostatic pressure, light, pH, salinity and temperature.
2. Aquatic microbiology is the study of microorganisms and their distribution and activities in aquatic environments.

Properties of the Environment

1. Water environments have two unique properties that make them suitable for microbial and related activities: temperature variations in water are not as great as those found in adjacent terrestrial environments; and light penetrates the water, allowing photosynthetic activities to occur well below the surface.
2. Facultative anaerobic and obligate anaerobic organisms abound in the depths of freshwater and salt-water systems. Other microscopic forms of life in water include zooplankton and phytoplankton.
3. The presence of high concentrations of nutrients can lead to the rapid growth of algae or cyanobacteria called *blooms*. Such conditions cause a discoloration of the water and a depletion of oxygen used by fish and other forms of life.
4. Freshwater habitats amount to about 2 percent of the water on earth. Two categories of such habitats are standing and flowing bodies of water. Lakes, examples of standing bodies of water, may eventually become dry land through sediment accumulation and increased growth of vegetation. This process is known as *eutrophication*.
5. Flowing fresh waters are represented by streams.
6. Estuaries are coastal areas where seawater mixes with fresh water. Organisms living in such regions must be able to tolerate significant shifts in the salt content of their habitats.

Waste Treatment

Large communities produce too much wastes for environmental processes to handle. They have developed a variety of methods for dealing with disposal of waste water and solid wastes.

Waste Water

1. Waste water or sewage contains about 99 percent water and is easily pumped through sewage pipes to treatment plants. The remainder of the material consists of suspended insoluble solids.
2. Domestic waste is largely human excrement diluted with laundry and wash water.
3. Industrial and commercial waste waters include materials from canning processes, dairies, slaughterhouses, cattle feedlots, and chemical and pharmaceutical plants. Chemical wastes often contain toxic components, such as heavy metals or pesticides.
4. One of the major purposes of waste-water treatment is to eliminate such potential hazards to public health.
5. Some microorganisms found in waste water are from soil and water sources. Many of them form slimy growths in pipes and ditches. Others produce metal deposits, which clog pipes, or the highly odorous hydrogen sulfide.

Environmental Effects

1. A wide variety of microorganisms may be present in drinking water, some of which may be pathogenic.
2. The presence of coliforms, which include *Escherichia coli, Enterobacter aerogenes,* and *Klebsiella pneumoniae,* serve as indicators of fecal pollution.
3. Two procedures used to detect coliforms in water are the most probable number (MPN) method and membrane filtration. *Presumptive, confirmed* and *completed tests* are used.
4. Indicator microorganisms for fecal contamination other than coliforms include *Bifidobacterium bifidus, Clostridium perfringens* and *Streptococcus faecalis.*
5. Noncoliform organisms can be detected by the standard plate count procedure.
6. The depletion of dissolved oxygen in water through the addition of considerable quantities of organic and inorganic materials creates severe environmental conditions.
7. The consumption of oxygen by microbes is known as the *biological* or *biochemical oxygen demand* (BOD). It refers to the amount of oxygen consumed by microorganisms during their decomposition of organic materials.

Waste Water Treatment

1. The vast bulk of waste waters are processed for disposal by one or more steps, which include *preliminary treatment, secondary treatment*, and *advanced treatment*.
2. Preliminary treatment is directed toward the removal of solids from plant, animal, and mineral materials. Solid material known as *sludge* is removed during this process. The liquid portion obtained is usually exposed to chlorine to kill microbes and to reduce objectionable odors.
3. Secondary treatment involves the biological degradation of organic material by microorganisms, and is performed in two phases: *anaerobic* and *aerobic digestion*.
4. The main purposes of anaerobic digestion are to convert some organic carbon compounds to carbon dioxide and methane, and to convert some organic nitrogen compounds to nitrogen gas.
5. Aerobic digestion results in a greater degree of BOD removal. Two processes used are the *trickling filter* and activated sludge.
6. Advanced waste-water treatment represents one approach to the further purification of treated waste water to provide a high quality product.

Solid Waste Disposal

1. Solid waste materials probably pose a greater and more complex problem that does waste water. This is because of their higher BOD loading, inability to be pumped, and inclusion of materials that are either not biodegradable or degrade very slowly.
2. Solid-waste disposal is directed toward reduction in volume and weight and conversion into a less troublesome and offensive form.
3. Traditionally solid wastes have been dumped in pits or similar depressions. Modern approaches involve controlled dumping and the establishment of sanitary landfills, where solid wastes are spread and compacted by machines into layers. Microbial activities in landfills primarily consist of *anaerobic digestion*.

QUESTIONS FOR REVIEW

1. List the various types of materials found in waste water.

2. Name five water-borne infectious diseases and their specific causative agents.
3. a. Describe a water-quality testing procedure for indicator microorganisms.
   b. What are the common indicator organisms?
4. How does the nutrient load in waste water affect the environment?
5. Define BOD, and describe how it is determined.
6. What is the role of the water cycle in water purification?
7. Describe each of the following waste-water treatment processes:
   a. preliminary
   b. primary
   c. secondary anaerobic
   d. secondary aerobic
8. What is the basis for efficient aerobic digestion of wastes in the trickling filter process and in the activated sludge process?
9. Compare the effectiveness of aerobic and anaerobic waste-water processes.
10. How does advanced water treatment work?
11. How can solid wastes be processed?
12. List both the potential products and problems associated with waste treatment.
13. a. What is soil?
    b. What types of microbial activities contribute to soil fertility?
14. a. Describe the water cycle.
    b. Why is this cycle important?
    c. What factors influence the presence of microorganisms in bodies of water?
15. Distinguish between the following pairs:
    a. zooplankton and phytoplankton
    b. algal bloom and eutrophication
    c. littoral zone and profundal zone
16. a. What is a lake?
    b. What types of microorganisms would you expect to find at different depths of a lake?

SUGGESTED READINGS

Berg, G. (ed.), *Indicators of Viruses in Water and Food.* Ann Arbor, Mich.: Ann Arbor Science Publishers, 1978. *Articles covering the types of indicators and media used in the detection of viruses in water and food.*

Jannasch, H. W., "Experiments in Deep-sea Microbiology," *Oceanus* 21:50 (1978). *An interesting article dealing with the study of microorganisms in deep-sea environments and how decomposition of organic materials occurs under conditions of high pressure and low temperature.*

Johnson, J. D. (ed.), *Disinfection of Water and Wastewater.* Ann Arbor, Michigan: Ann Arbor Science Publishers, 1975. *Details are given of the chemical and microbiological basis of the treatment of drinking, swimming, and waste water with chlorine bromine, iodine, and ozone.*

Rangaswami, G., *Agricultural Microbiology.* New York: Asia Publishing House, 1966. *A good, general book on historical aspects of agricultural microbiology, the organisms involved, and the methods used to study them. Pathogenic organisms in the soil and on plants, and organisms in food and dairy microbiology are also discussed.*

Taber, W. A., "Wastewater Microbiology," *Ann. Rev. Microbiol* 30:263 (1976). *Describes the uses of microorganisms in the treatment of many types of waste water.*

Tippo, O., and W. L. Stern, *Humanistic Botany.* New York: W. W. Norton & Co., 1977. *An easy-to-read text that provides functional up-to-date information on the various uses of plants in everyday life. Chapter 13 presents a well-illustrated description of algae and their impact on humans.*

Appendices

Appendix A Classification Outline of Division II, The Bacteria

This table has been prepared in accordance with the information contained in *Bergey's Manual of Determinative Bacteriology*, 8th ed., E. Buchanan and N. E. Gibbons, eds. (Baltimore: Williams and Wilkins, 1974).

Part	*Order*	*Family*	*Tribe*	*Genus*
1. Phototrophic bacteria	Rhodospirillales	I. Rhodospirillaceae		I. *Rhodospirillum*
				II. *Rhodopseudomonas*
				III. *Rhodomicrobium*
		II. Chromatiaceae		I. *Chromatium*
				II. *Thiocystis*
				III. *Thiosarcina*
				IV. *Thiospirillum*
				V. *Thiocapsa*
				VI. *Lamprocystis*
				VII. *Thiodictyon*
				VIII. *Thiopedia*
				IX. *Amoebobacter*
				X. *Ectothiorhodospira*
		III. Chlorobiaceae		I. *Chlorobium*
				II. *Prosthecochloris*
				III. *Chloropseudomonas*
				IV. *Pelodictyon*
				V. *Clathrochloris*
2. Gliding bacteria	I. Myxobacterales	I. Myxococcaceae		I. *Myxococcus*
		II. Archangiaceae		I. *Archangium*
		III. Cystobacteraceae		I. *Cystobacter*
				II. *Melittangium*
				III. *Stigmatella*
		IV. Polyangiaceae		I. *Polyangium*
				II. *Nannocystis*
				III. *Chondromyces*
	II. Cytophagales	I. Cytophagaceae		I. *Cytophaga*
				II. *Flexibacter*
				III. *Herpetosiphon*
				IV. *Flexithrix*
				V. *Saprospira*
				VI. *Sporocytophaga*
		II. Beggiatoaceae		I. *Beggiatoa*
				II. *Vitreoscilla*
				III. *Thioploca*
		III. Simonsiellaceae		I. *Simonsiella*
				II. *Alysiella*
		IV. Leucothrichaceae		I. *Leucothrix*
				II. *Thiothrix*
				Toxothrix[a]
		Achromatiaceae[b]		*Achromatium*[a]
		Pelonemataceae[b]		*Pelonema*[a]
				Achroonema[a]
				Peloploca[a]
				Desmanthos[a]
3. Sheathed bacteria				*Sphaerotilus*
				Leptothrix
				Streptothrix
				Lieskeella
				Phragmidiothrix
				Crenothrix
				Clonothrix
4. Budding and/or appendaged bacteria				*Hyphomicrobium*
				Hyphomonas
				Pedomicrobium
				Caulobacter
				Astic acaulis
				Ancalomicrobium

Part	Order	Family	Tribe	Genus
				Prosthecomicrobium
				Thiodendron
				Pasteuria
				Blastobacter
				Seliberia
				Gallionella
				Nevskia
				Planctomyces
				Metallogenium
				Caulococcus
				Kusnezovia
5. Spirochetes	I. Spirochaetales	I. Spirochaetaceae		I. *Spirochaeta*
				II. *Cristispira*
				III. *Treponema*
				IV. *Borrelia*
				V. *Leptospira*
6. Spiral and curved bacteria		I. Spirillaceae		I. *Spirillum*
				II. *Campylobacter*
				Bdellovibrio[a]
				Microcyclus[a]
				Pelosigma[a]
				Brachyarcus[a]
7. Gram-negative, aerobic rods and cocci		I. Pseudomonadaceae		I. *Pseudomonas*
				II. *Xanthomonas*
				III. *Zoogloea*
				IV. *Gluconobacter*
		II. Azotobacteraceae		I. *Azotobacter*
				II. *Azomonas*
				III. *Beijerinckia*
				IV. *Derxia*
		III. Rhizobiaceae		I. *Rhizobium*
				II. *Agrobacterium*
		IV. Methylomonadaceae		I. *Methylomonas*
				II. *Methylococcus*
		V. Halobacteriaceae		I. *Halobacterium*
				II. *Halococcus*
				Alcaligenes[a]
				Acetobacter[a]
				Brucella[a]
				Bordetella[a]
				Francisella[a]
				Thermus[a]
8. Gram-negative facultatively anaerobic rods		I. Enterobacteriaceae		I. *Escherichia*
				II. *Edwardsiella*
				III. *Citrobacter*
				IV. *Salmonella*
				V. *Shigella*
				VI. *Klebsiella*
				VII. *Enterobacter*
				VIII. *Hafnia*
				IX. *Serratia*
				X. *Proteus*
				XI. *Yersinia*
				XII. *Erwinia*
		II. Vibrionaceae		I. *Vibrio*
				II. *Aeromonas*
				III. *Plesiomonas*
				IV. *Photobacterium*
				V. *Lucibacterium*

Part	Order	Family	Tribe	Genus
9. Gram-negative, anaerobic bacteria		I. Bacteroidaceae		I. *Bacteroides* II. *Fusobacterium* III. *Lepotrichia* *Desulfovibrio*[a] *Butyrivibrio*[a] *Succinovibrio*[a] *Succinomonas*[a] *Lachnospira*[a] *Selenomonas*[a]
10. Gram-negative cocci and coccobacilli (aerobes)		I. Neisseriaceae		I. *Neisseria* II. *Branhamella* III. *Moraxella* IV. *Acinetobacter* *Paracoccus*[a] *Lampropedia*[a]
11. Gram-negative anaerobic cocci		I. Veillonellaceae		I. *Veillonella* II. *Acidaminococcus* III. *Megasphaera*
12. Gram-negative chemolithotrophic bacteria a. Ammonia- or nitrite-oxidizing organisms		I. Nitrobacteraceae		I. *Nitrobacter* II. *Nitrospina* III. *Nitrococcus* IV. *Nitrosomonas* V. *Nitrosospira* VI. *Nitrosococcus* VII. *Nitrosolobus*
b. Sulfur-metabolizing organisms				*Thiobacillus* *Sulfolobus* *Thiobacterium* *Macromonas* *Thiovulum* *Thiospira*
c. Iron- or manganese-oxide-depositing organisms		I. Siderocapsaceae		I. *Siderocapsa* II. *Naumanniella* III. *Ochrobium* IV. *Siderococcus*
13. Methane-producing bacteria		I. Methanobacteriaceae		I. *Methanobacterium* II. *Methanosarcina* III. *Methanococcus*
14. Gram-positive cocci a. Aerobic and/or facultatively anaerobic		I. Microciccaceae		I. *Micrococcus* II. *Staphylococcus* III. *Planococcus*
		II. Streptococcaceae		I. *Streptococcus* II. *Leuconstoc* III. *Pediococcus* IV. *Aerococcus* V. *Gemella*
b. Anaerobic		III. Peptococcaceae		I. *Peptococcus* II. *Peptostreptococcus* III. *Ruminococcus* IV. *Sarcina*
15. Endospore-forming rods and cocci		I. Bacillaceae		I. *Bacillus* II. *Sporolactobacillus* III. *Clostridium* IV. *Desulfotomaculum* V. *Sporosarcina* *Oscillospira*[a]
16. Gram-positive non-spore-forming rods		I. Lactobacillaceae		*Lactobacillus* *Listeria* *Erysipelothrix* *Caryophanon*

Part	Order	Family	Tribe	Genus
17. *Actinomycetes and related organisms*				I. *Corynebacterium*
				II. *Arthrobacter*
				Brevibacterium[c]
				Microbacterium[c]
				III. *Cellulomonas*
				IV. *Kurthia*
		I. Propionibacteriaceae		I. *Propionibacterium*
				II. *Eubacterium*
	I. Actinomycetales	I. Actinomycetaceae		I. *Actinomyces*
				II. *Arachnia*
				III. *Bifidobacterium*
				IV. *Bacterionema*
				V. *Rothia*
		II. Mycobacteriaceae		I. *Mycobacterium*
		III. Frankiaceae		I. *Frankia*
		IV. Actinoplanaceae		
		V. Dermatophilaceae		I. *Dermatophilus*
				II. *Geodermatophilus*
		VI. Nocardiaceae		I. *Nocardia*
				II. *Pseudocardia*
		VII. Streptomycetaceae		I. *Streptomyces*
				II. *Streptoverticillium*
				III. *Sporichthya*
				IV. *Microellobosporia*
		VIII. Micromonosporaceae		I. *Micromonospora*
				II. *Thermoactinomyces*
				III. *Actinobifida*
				IV. *Thermomonospora*
				V. *Microbispora*
				VI. *Micropolyspora*
18. The rickettsia	I. Rickettsiales	I. Rickettsiaceae	I. Rickettsieae	I. *Rickettsia*
				II. *Rochalimeae*
				III. *Coxiella*
			II. Ehrlichieae	IV. *Ehrlichia*
				V. *Cowdria*
				VI. *Neorickettsia*
			III. Wolbachieae	VII. *Wolbachia*
				VIII. *Symbiotes*
				IX. *Blattabacterium*
				X. *Rickettsiella*
		II. Bartonellaceae		I. *Bartonella*
				II. *Grahamella*
		III. Anaplasmataceae		I. *Anaplasma*
				II. *Paranaplasma*
				III. *Aegyptionella*
				IV. *Haemobartonella*
				V. *Eperythrozoon*
19. Mycoplasma[d]	I. Mycoplasmatales	I. Mycoplasmataceae		I. *Mycoplasma*
	II. Chlamydiales	II. Chlamydiaceae		I. *Chlamydia*
		III. Acholeplasmataceae		I. *Acholeplasma*
				Spiroplasma[a]
				Thermoplasma[a]

[a]Genus of uncertain affiliation within the classification system.
[b]Family of uncertain affiliation within the classification system.
[c]*Genera incertae sedis.*
[d]Various changes have occurred in the classification of this microbial group in recent years. These are described in Chapter 8.

Appendix B Classification Outline of True Fungi[a]

Class	*Series*[b]	*Order*	*Family*	*Representative Genera*
Chytridiomycetes[c]		Blastocladiales	Blastocladiaceae	*Allomyces, Blastocladia, Blastocladiella*
			Coelomomycetaceae	*Coelomomyces*
		Chyridiales	Megachytriaceae	*Nowakowskiella*
			Olipidiaceae	*Entophyctis, Olpidium*
			Phylctidiaceae	*Rhizophydium*
			Synchytriaceae	*Synchytrium*
		Monoblepharidiales		*Monoblepharis*
Hyphochytridiomycetes		Hyphochytriales	Rhizidiomycetaceae	*Rhizidiomyces*
Oomycetes		Lagenidiales		*Lagenidium, Olpidiopsis*
		Leptomitales		*Sapromyces*
		Peronosporales		*Albugo, Pythium, Phytophthora*
		Saprolegniales		*Saprolegnia*
Trichomycetes	Eccrinales[d]			
Zygomycetes	Entomophthorales			*Basidiobolus, Entomophthora*
	Mucorales			*Blakeslea, Cunninghamella, Mortierella, Mucor, Rhizopus, Thamnidium*
	Zoopagales[d]			
Ascomycetes	Discomycetes	Helotiales	Phacidiaceae	*Rhytisma*
			Sclerotiniaceae	*Monilia*
		Ostropales[d]		
		Pezizales		*Anthracobia, Gyromitra, Morchella, Sarcosoma*
		Tuberules		*Elaphomyces, Tuber*
	Hemiascomycetes	Endomycetales	Ascoideaceae	*Dipodascus,*
			Endomycetaceae	*Eremascus*
			Saccharomycetaceae	*Cryptoccus, Hansenula, Saccharomyces*
		Taphrinales		*Taphrina*
		Protomycetales[d]		
	Laboulbeniomycetes			*Diplomyces, Stigmatomyces*
	Loculascomycetes	Myriangiales		*Elsinoe, Piedraia*
		Pleosporales	Venturiaceae	*Ventura*
	Plectomycetes	Eurotiales	Ascophaeriaceae	*Ascophaera*
			Eurotiaceae	*Eurotium*
			Gymnoascaceae	*Arthroderma, Ctenomyces*

Class	*Series*[b]	*Order*	*Family*	*Representative Genera*
	Pyrenomycetes	Chaetomiales[a]		
		Clavicipitales		*Claviceps*
		Erysiphales	Erysiphaceae	*Erysiphe, Podosphaera*
		Sphaeriales	Sordariaceae	*Cordyceps, Daldinia, Gelasinospora, Neurospora, Podospora, Sordaria*
Basidiomycetes	Gastromycetes	Lycoperdales		*Geastrum*
		Nidulariales[d]		
		Phallales		*Dictyophora, Phallus*
	Hymenomycetes	Auriculariales	Auriculariaceae	*Auricularia, Eocronartium, Herpobasidium*
		Septobasidiales	Septobasidiaceae	*Septobasidium*
		Tremellales		
		Agaricales		*Agaricus, Amanita, Mycena, Pleurotus, Russula*
		Aphyllophorales		*Clavaria, Fomes, Stereum*
		Dacrymycetales		*Calocera*
		Tulasnellales[d]		
	Teliomycetes	Uredinales	Melampsoraceae Pucciniaceae	*Conartium, Puccinia*
		Ustilaginales	Tilletiaceae Ustilaginaceae	*Tilletia, Ustilago*

[a]Prepared from information contained in the following publications: Nouhul, M. *Botany.* Santa Barbara, Calif.: Hamilton Publishing Company, 1974; Ross, I. K. *Biology of the Fungi, Their Development, Regulation, and Associations.* New York: McGraw-Hill Book Company, 1978. The Deuteromycetes are not included in this classification.
[b]Depending on the reference authority used, this category may be given a Class designation.
[c]The organisms in classes Chyridiomycetes, Hyphochytridiomycetes, Oomycetes, Trichomycetes, and Zygomycetes are considered lower fungi in comparison to the higher fungi belonging to Ascomycetes, Basidiomycetes and Deuteromycetes.
[d]Subdivisions into orders, families, or genera were not specified.

Appendix C Classification Outline of Medically Important Protozoa[a]

Subphylum	*Superclass*	*Class*	*Order*	*Family*	*Genus*
Sarcomastigophora	Mastigophora	Phytomastigophorea	Chrysomonadorida	Chromulinidae	*Caviomonas* *Oikomonas* *Sphaeromonas*
				Ochromonadidae	*Monas*
				Prymnesiidae	*Pyrmnesium*
			Dinoflagellorida	Gymnodiniidae	*Gymnodinium*[b]
				Gonyaulacidae	*Gonyaulax*[b]
			Euglenorida	Astasiidae	*Copromonas*[b]
			Phytomonadorida	Chlamydonomadiae	*Polytoma*[b]
		Zoomastigophorea	Rhizomastigorida	Tetramitidae	*Tetramitus*
			Kinetoplastorida	Bodonidae	*Bodo* *Cercomonas* *Pleuromonas* *Proteromonas* *Spiromonas*
				Trypanosomatidae	*Blastocithidia* *Crithidia* *Endotrypanum* *Herpetomonas* *Leishmania* *Leptomonas* *Rhynchoidomonas* *Trypanosoma*
			Retortamonadorida	Retortamonadidae	*Chilomastix* *Retortamonas*
				Cochlosomatidae	*Cochlosoma*
				Hexamitidae	*Giardia* *Hexamita* *Octomitus* *Trepomonas*
			Oxymonadoriada	Monocercomonoididae	*Monocercomonoides*
			Trichomonadorida	Trimastigidae	*Trimastix*
				Monocercomonadidae	*Chilomitus* *Hexamastix* *Histomonas* *Hypotrichomonas* *Monocercomonas* *Parahistomonas* *Pseudotrichomonas* *Tetratrichomastix* *Triceromitus*
				Trichomonadidae	*Pentatrichomonas* *Pentatrichomonoides* *Pseudotrypanosoma* *Tetratrichomonas* *Trichomitopsis* *Trichomitus* *Trichomonas* *Tritrichomonas*
			Hypermastigorida	Callimastigidae	*Trichonympha* *Callimastix* *Selenomonas* *Enteromonas*
	Opalinata		Opalinida		*Opalina*
	Sarcodina	Rhizopodasea	Amoebida	Vahlkampfiidae	*Naegleria* *Trimastigamoeba* *Vahlkampfia*

Subphylum	Superclass	Class	Order	Family	Genus
				Hartmannellidae	*Acanthamoeba* *Hartmannella*
				Amoebidae	*Sappinia*
				Endamoebidae	*Dientamoeba* *Endamoeba* *Endolimax* *Entamoeba* *Iodamoeba*
			Arcellorida	Arcellidae	*Chlamydophrys*
Apicomplexa		Sporozoa	Eucoccida	Adeleidae	*Klossia*
				Klossiellidae	*Klossiella*
				Haemogregarinidae	*Hemogregarina* *Hepatozoon* *Karyolysus*
				Aggregatidae	*Merocystis*
				Lankesterellidae	*Lankesterella* *Schellackia*
				Eimeriidae	*Dorisiella* *Eimeria* *Isospora* *Tyzzeria* *Wenyonella*
				Plasmodiidae	*Haemoproteus* *Hepatocystis* *Leucocytozoon* *Plasmodium*
				Toxoplasmatidae	*Frenkelia* *Toxoplasma*
				Besnoittiidae	*Besonitia*
				Sarcocystidae	*Arthrocystis* *Sarcocystis*
		Piroplasmasea	Piroplasmorida	Babesiidae	*Babesia* *Echinozoon* *Entopolypoides*
				Theileriidae	*Haematoxenus* *Theileria*
	Microspora		Microsporida		*Nosema* *Thelohania*
	Ciliophora	Ciliata	Gymnostomorida	Buetschliidae	
				Pycnotrichidae	*Buxtonella* *Infundibulorium*
			Trichostomorida	Blepharocrythidae	*Blepharocorys* *Charonima* *Ochoterenaia*
				Cyathodiniidea	*Cyathodinium*
				Isotrichidae	*Dasytricha* *Isotrichia*
				Paraisotrichiidae	*Paraisotricha*
				Balantidiidae	*Balantidium*
	Suctorida		Hymenostomorida	Ophryoglenidae	*Ichthyophthirius*
				Tetrahymenidae	*Tetrahymena*
				Parameciidae	*Paramecium*
				Acinetidae	*Allantosoma*
			Heterotrichorida	Plagiotomidae	*Nyctotherus*
			Entodiniomorphida	Ophryosocolecidae	*Amphacanthus*

Subphylum	Superclass	Class	Order	Family	Genus
					Caloscolex
					Cunhaia
					Diplodinium
					Diploplastron
					Elytroplastron
					Enoploplastron
					Entodinium
					Eodinium
					Epidinium
					Epiplastron
					Eremoplastron
					Eudiplodinium
					Metadinium
					Ophryoscolex
					Opisthotrichum
					Ostracodinium
					Polyplastron
				Cycloposthiidae	*Cochliatoxum*
					Cycloposthium
					Ditoxum
					Elephantophilus
					Polydiniella
					Prototapirella
					Spirodinium
					Tetratoxum
					Thoracodinium
					Triadinium
					Trifascicularia
					Tripalmaria
					Triplumaria
					Troglodytella

[a]Some current modifications have been made from the classification proposed by a Committee of the Society of Protozoologists. The uniform endings that were proposed by N. Levine in 1959 have been added to Class and Order taxonomic ranks.

[b]According to some authorities this microorganism also is considered to be an alga.

Appendix D Classification Outline of the Algae[a]

Division	Class	Representative Genera
Chlorophycophyta	Chlorophyceae	*Chlamydomonas, Chlorococcum, Chlorogonium, Closterium, Cosmarium, Eudorina, Gonium, Haematococcus, Oedogonium, Scenedesmus, Spirogyra, Ulothrix, Volvox*
	Charophyceae	*Chara, Nitella, Tolypella*
Chyptophycophta[b]	Cryptophyceae	*Chilomonas, Chroomonas, Cryptomonas, Tetragonidium*
Chrysophycophyta	Bacillariophyceae	*Asterionella, Cymbella, Diatoma, Navicula, Pinnularia, Tabellaria, Thalassiothrix*
	Chrysophyceae	*Chysamoeba, Chryosococcus, Dinobryon, Lagynion, Mallomonas, Synura*
	Eustigmatophyceae	*Ellipsoion, Pleurochloris, Polyedriella, Vischeria*
	Haptophyceae	*Apistonema, Chrysochromulina, Coccolithus, Hymenomonas, Phaeocyctis, Prymnesium*
	Xanthophyceae	*Botrydium, Tribonema, Vaucheria*
Euglenophycophyta	Euglenophyceae	*Astasia, Euglena, Phacus, Trachelomonas*
Phaeophycophyta	Phaeophyceae	*Agarum, Desmarestia, Dictyota, Ectocarpus, Elachistea, Fucus, Giffordia, Laminaria, Scytosiphon*
Pyrrophycophyta	Dinophyceae	*Ceratium, Gonyaulax, Gymnodinium, Ornithocercus, Peridinium, Prorcentrum, Pyrocystis*
Rhodophycophyta	Rhodophyceae	*Ceramium, Polysiphonia, Porhyridium, Rhodella, Rhodosorus*

[a]Developed from information contained in Trainor, F. R., *Introductory Phycology*. New York: John Wiley & Sons, 1978.
[b]A relatively new algal grouping.

Appendix E Classification Outline of the Pathogenic Helminths[a]

Phylum	Class	Order	Family	Genus	Species
Platyhelminthes (flatworms)	Trematoda (flukes)	Strigeata	Schistosomatidae	*Schistosoma* *S.* *S.*	*haematobium* *japonicum* *mansoni*
		Echinostomata	Fasciolidae	*Fasciola* *Fasciolopsis*	*hepatica* *buski*
		Plagiorchiata	Troglotrematidae	*Paragonimus*	*Westermani*
		Opisthorchioidea	Opisthorchiidae	*Clonorchis*	*sinensis*
	Cestoidea (tapeworms)	Cyclophyllidea	Taeniidae	*Taenia* *T.* *Echinococcus*	*saginata* *solium* *granulosus*
			Hymenolepididae	*Hymenolepsis* *H.*	*diminuta* *nana*
		Pseudophyllidea	Diphyllobothriidae	*Diphyllobothrium*	*latum*
Nematoda (roundworms)	Aphasmidea	Trichurata	Trichinellidae	*Trichinella*	*spiralis*
			Trichuridae	*Trichuris*	*trichiura*
	Phasmidia	Ascaridata	Ascaridae	*Ascaris*	*lumbricoides*
		Strongylata	Ancylostomidae	*Ancylostoma* *Necator*	*duodenale* *americanus*
		Rhabditata	Strongyloididae	*Strongyloides*	*stercoralis*
		Oxyurata	Oxyuridae	*Enterobius*	*vermicularis*
		Filariata	Filariidae	*Brugia* *Wuchereria* *Onchocerca* *Loa*	*malayi* *bancrofti* *volvulus* *loa*

[a]Modified from Faust, E. C., P. F. Russell, and R. C. Jung. *Craig and Faust's Clinical Parasitology*. 8th ed. Philadelphia: Lea & Febiger, 1970.

Glossary

Important and widely used terms and concepts are included in this glossary. Other terms defined in the text are referred to by page number in the index.

A

abscess: A localized collection of pus.

acid: A compound that releases hydrogen (H^+) ions when dissolved in water.

acid-fast staining technique: One type of differential stain procedure. It is used to determine a particular property of certain bacteria to retain the primary stain, carbol fuchsin, and resist decolorization with acid alcohol.

acquired immunity: Resistance obtained after birth.

active immunization: The production of immunoglobulins (antibodies) in response to a direct immunogenic stimulus.

active transport: A process occurring at the cell membrane in which a cell expends energy to move materials through the membrane, often against a concentration gradient.

adenosine triphosphate (ATP): The macromolecule that functions as an energy carrier in cells. The energy is stored in a high-energy bond between the second and third phosphates.

aerobe: A microorganisms whose growth requires the presence of air or free oxygen.

aerobic respiration: The process by which a cell releases the energy in glucose, producing adenosine triphosphate (ATP). Aerobic respiration includes glycolysis, the Krebs (citric acid) cycle, and electron and hydrogen transport.

aerosol: A fine suspension of particles or liquid droplets sprayed into the air.

Aflatoxin: One type of mycotoxin produced by some strains of the fungus *Aspergillus flavus.*

agar: A dried polysaccharide (galactan), extract of red algae, used as the solidifying agent in various microbiological media.

agglutination: The visible clumping of cellular or particle-like antigens by homologous antibodies; e.g., blood typing.

Agranulocyte: White blood cells lacking cytoplasmic granules; e.g., lymphocytes, monocytes.

akinete: A resting spore of cyanobacteria.

alkaline: A condition in which hydroxyl (OH^-) ions are in abundance. Solutions with a pH of 7.1 or higher are alkaline or basic.

allergen: A substance capable of bringing about an allergic state when introduced into the body.

allergy: Any altered activity of an individual caused by contact with animate or inanimate substances in the environment; e.g., hay fever, penicillin reaction.

amino acid: A nitrogenous organic compound that serves as a basic unit of a protein molecule.

ammonification: The microbial decomposition of organic nitrogen-containing compounds such as proteins, with the formation of ammonia.

amphibionts: Obligately parasitic, but not pathogenic, organisms found on humans and lower animals.

anabolism: Metabolic processes that are synthetic in nature and result in the formation of cell materials, e.g., protein nucleic acids and lipids.

anaerobe: A microorganism that grows only or best in the absence of free oxygen. Organisms utilize bound oxygen.

anaerobic respiration: Reduction of inorganic substances for energy production in the absence of oxygen.

anamnestic response: The sudden secondary rise in immunoglobulin (antibody) concentration produced by a second exposure to an immunogen some time after the initial exposure.

anemia: A deficiency of red blood cells, hemoglobin or both.

Angstrom unit (Å): A unit of length measuring 10^{-8} cm (1/100,000,000 cm).

Animalia: The animal kingdom.

anoxygenic photosynthesis: A form of phytosynthesis in which oxygen is not produced.

antibiogram: The results obtained from tests to determine the sensitivity of an organism to a series of antimicrobial agents.

antiobiotic: A microbial metabolic or laboratory-synthesized product with the capacity to inhibit or kill bacteria and other microorganisms. Antibiotics are used in the treatment and control of various infectious diseases.

antibody (immunoglobulin): A protein molecule formed in response to a foreign substance (immunogen). Antibodies react with and/or inactivate the foreign matter causing their formation.

anticoagulant: A substance that prevents coagulation, e.g., heparin, sodium citrate.

anticodon: A sequence of three nucleotides in transfer RNA (tRNA) that is complementary to and combines with the three-nucleotide codon of messenger RNA (mRNA). This reaction binds the activated amino acid—tRNA combination to mRNA.

antigen determinant: The portion of a molecule that determines the specificity of an antigen-antibody reaction.

antiseptic: Against or opposing sepsis (infection), putrefaction, or decay. An antimicrobial agent used to prevent or arrest microbial growth.

antiserum: Serum containing specific antibodies.

antitoxin: An antibody (immunoglobulin) capable of neutralizing the toxin or toxoid that stimulated its production.

aplanospore: A nonmotile asexual spore.

arthritis: Inflammation of the joints.

arthropod: An animal lacking a backbone (invertebrate) and having jointed legs; e.g., insects, crustaceans.

arthrospore: An asexual spore of fungi formed by the fragmentation of hyphae.

Ascomycetes: The class of fungi known for the formation of a saclike structure, the ascus.

ascospore: A sexual spore found in the Ascomycetes.

ascus: A saclike structure found in Ascomycete fungi within which ascospores are formed.

aseptic technique: A procedure in which precautions against microbial contamination are taken.

asexual: Not involving sex cells or union of nuclear material.

asexual reproduction: A form of reproduction not involving sex cells or fusion of their nuclei.

atrium: A chamber affording entrance to another structure or organ; a chamber of the heart receiving blood from a vein.

attenuated: Weakened; reduced in virulence.

autoantigens: Body components that provoke antibody production against themselves.

autoclave: An apparatus utilizing pressurized steam for sterilization.

autogamy: A modified form of conjugation that occurs within one protozoan.

autoinfection: An infection of one part of the body caused by organisms derived from another region of the body.

autolysis: Cellular disintegration caused by the organism's own enzymes.

autotroph: An organism that can synthesize all of its organic components from inorganic sources.

auxotrophic mutant: An organism that requires one or more specific growth factors not needed by the parental (wild type) strain.

avirulent: Unable to produce disease.

B

bactericidal: Lethal to bacteria.

bacteriophage: A virus that infects bacteria.

bacteriostatic: Inhibiting bacterial growth without killing organisms.

Basidiomycetes: A class of fungi that includes molds, rusts, mushrooms, and yeasts. Members of the class form a special structure called a basidium, which bears basidiospores.

binary fission: An asexual reproductive process in which one cell splits into two independent daughter cells.

binomial system of nomenclature: The method of naming organisms devised by Carolus Linnaeus. Each organism is given two names designating genus and species, such as *Staphylococcus aureus*.

bioassay: Determination of the activity or amount of a biologically active material by measuring its effect on living organisms.

biochemical oxygen demand (BOD): A measure of the amount of oxygen consumed in biological processes associated with the decomposition of organic matter in water. An index of water pollution.

bioconcentration: The reactions during natural cycles that lead to the storage of particular materials, e.g., sulfur, nitrate.

bioconversion: The enzymatic modification of chemicals.

biosphere: The portion of the earth in which all life exists, including the upper layers of soil and water and the lower atmosphere.

Brownian movement: A type of jiggling motion of particles and bacteria in suspension caused by the bombardment of molecules in the suspending fluid.

B-type lymphocyte: Immunoglobulin-forming lymphocyte.

bubo: An enlarged regional lymph node usually found in cases of bubonic plaque.

buffer: Any substance present in a preparation or body fluid that tends to control the change in pH when either an acid or base is added.

bursa of Fabricius: A cloacal organ in fowl from which the immunoglobulin-forming B-type lymphocytes originate.

C

capsid: The symmetrical protein coat that surrounds the nucleic acid core of viruses.

capsomere: The smallest unit of a viral protein coat (capsid).

capsule: A thick, sticky structure surrounding the cell walls of certain bacterial and yeast cells. Usually composed of polysaccharide or polypeptide.

carbohydrate: A class of organic compounds made of carbon, hydrogen, and oxygen, with the latter two elements in a ratio of 2 to 1; e.g., sugars, starches, cellulose.

carbon cycle: A geochemical cycle in which carbon is recycled by natural processes. Carbon in the form of a gas (CO_2) is converted into food by producers; consumer organisms obtain their carbon by eating producers; carbon leaves producers and consumers in the form of wastes and dead material, which are broken down by decomposers.

caries: Gradual decay of a bone or tooth associated with the inflammation of bone or progressive decalcification of teeth.

carrier: An individual harboring a disease agent without apparent symptoms.

catabolism: The chemical reactions by which food materials or nutrients are converted into simpler substances for the production of energy and cell materials.

catalyst: A substance that can speed up a reaction or cause a reaction to occur without itself being altered permanently.

catheter: A tubular surgical device used for the withdrawal of fluids from a body cavity or structure.

cell wall: The cell structure exterior to the cell membrane of typical plants, algae, bacteria, and fungi. It provides form and shape to cells.

chemoautrotroph: An organism that obtains its energy from the oxidation of inorganic chemical compounds.

chemolitotroph: An organism that utilizes inorganic compounds as energy sources.

chemotherapy: The treatment of disease by the use of chemicals that inhibit or kill the causative agents but ideally do not injure the cells or tissues of the host.

chitin: A complex polysaccharide that is the main component of the exoskeleton of certain shellfish and arthropods and of the cell walls of some fungi.

chloroplast: A chlorophyll-containing intracellular organelle of eucaryotic organisms such as algae, plants, and certain protozoans.

chronic: Of long duration.

cisterna: The space between two unit membranes, characteristically found in mitochondria and golgi bodies.

class: A major taxonomic subdivision of a phylum. Each class is composed of one or more related orders.

coccus: A spherical bacterium.

codon: Nucleotide triplet containing the information needed to specify a particular amino acid to be used in the formation of proteins and related compounds.

coenzyme: The simpler portion of an enzyme, which is necessary for the enzyme's activation and reaction with a substrate.

coliform: Gram-negative rods, including *Escherichia coli* and similar species that normally inhabit the colon (large intestine). Commonly included in the coliform group are *Enterobacter aerogenes, Klebsiella* sp., and other related bacteria.

commensalism: The association between two organisms in which one is benefited and the other is neither harmed nor benefited.

community: All organisms that occupy the same habitat and interact with one another.

competition: An association between two species, both of which need some limited environmental factor such as a nutrient for survival.

complement: A complex protein found in the blood of most warm-blooded animals, which participates in the destruction of bacteria and certain other cells when it is combined with an antigen-antibody complex.

conjugation: A form of sexual reproduction in which there is a temporary fusion of mating partners for the exchange of nuclear material.

contact dermatitis: A particular form of delayed hypersensitivity (Type IV), which may be associated with simple chemicals, metals, certain drugs, cosmetics, insecticides, or the active components of plants such as poison ivy and poison oak.

contractile vacuole: A pulsating vacuole found in certain protozoa and used for the excretion of wastes and the maintenance of proper osmotic balance.

culture: Any growth or cultivation of microorganisms.

cyst: A walled sac or pouch that contains fluid, semisolid, or solid material. Also, a resting structure formed by certain microorganisms.

cytopathic effect (CPE): Morphological changes in tissue culture cells caused by a pathogen such as a virus.

cytoplasm: The substance of a cell exclusive of the nuclear area.

D

deamination: The removal of an amino (NH_2) group from a compound.

delayed hypersensitivity: A form of allergy characterized by several factors including the absence of circulating antibodies (immunoglobulins), reactions taking place from 24 to 48 hours after exposure to antigen, possible transfer in humans by a nonantibody 'active' transfer factor, and lack of an inhibition of the reaction by antihistamines.

denaturation: A change in the secondary or tertiary structure of a macromolecule, such as protein or nucleic acid, that affects solubility and various biological activities.

denitrification: The microbial process whereby nitrates (NO^{-3}) are transformed into nitrogen (N_3) or ammonia (NH_3), which then reenters the atmosphere as a gas.

deoxyribonucleic acid (DNA): A macromolecule that contains genetic information coded in specific sequences of its constituent nucleotides.

densensitization: The elimination or reduction of an allergic sensitivity, usually by means of a programmed course of allergen injections.

Deuteromycetes: A class of fungi that have not been observed to form sexual reproductive structures.

diabetes mellitus: A disease state caused by an inability of the pancreas to produce a functional form of the hormone insulin. As a result, carbohydrates are improperly metabolized.

diaminopimelic acid: A compound found in nature only in procaryotic organisms, particularly in the cell-wall mucocomplex of bacteria.

diatomaceous earth: The remains of diatoms, often used as filtering material.

differential medium: A growth medium for most bacteria on which the appearance of growth exhibited by certain organisms is sufficient to distinguish them from others growing on the same medium.

differential staining methods: Procedures used to distinguish among bacterial species and in some cases between the bactertial cell and its parts; e.g., Gram stain, acid-fast stain, spore stain.

diluting: The procedure of increasing the proportion of liquid diluent to particular matter or other material being diluted.

dimorphic: Exhibiting two forms in two different environments.

***dipicolinic acid*:** A compound of bacterial spores that contributes to their heat resistance.

***disaccharide*:** A sugar consisting of two monosaccharides.

***disinfection*:** The treatment of certain inanimate materials to reduce the level of microbial contamination.

***disseminated*:** Spread.

***division*:** A major taxonomic subdivision, usually of the plant kingdom. Each division is composed of one or more classes. This subdivision is equivalent to the taxonomic rank of phylum.

***dormancy*:** A state of inactivity.

E

***ecology*:** The study of the interrelationship of an organism and its environment.

***ecosystem*:** All of the organisms in a habitat plus all of the factors in the environment with which the organisms interact.

***ectoparasite*:** A parasite that lives or feeds on the outer surface of the host's body.

***ectosymbiont*:** An organism living on the surface of a host.

***electron transport system*:** A series of oxidation-reduction reactions in which electrons are transported from a substrate to a final acceptor, usually O_2, and ATP is formed.

***encephalitis*:** Inflammation of the brain.

***endemic*:** Present more or less continuously in a community.

***endocarditis*:** Inflammation of the inner portions of the heart.

***endoparasite*:** A parasite found within host tissues and cells.

***endoplasmic reticulum*:** Interconnected membranes within the cytoplasm of a eucaryotic cell.

***endospore*:** A resistant body formed within certain bacterial cells.

***endotoxin*:** A poisonous substance usually released after an organism disintegrates.

***envelope (bacterial)*:** The cellular component that encloses the cytoplasm, including the cytoplasmic membrane, cell wall, and capsule.

***envelope (viral)*:** The outer lipid-containing layer possessed by some virions, obtained from modified host cell membranes upon the release of the virus particle.

***enzyme*:** An organic (protein) catalyst that causes changes in other substances without undergoing any alteration itself.

***eosinophilia*:** An increase in the number of eosinophiles.

***epidemic*:** An outbreak of a disease that appears rapidly and attacks a large number of persons in a community at approximately the same time.

***etiology*:** Cause.

***eucaryote*:** An organism characterized by a cellular organization that includes a nuclear membrane and other internal membrane organelles such as mitochondria and mitotic apparatus.

***eutrophication*:** Nutrient increase and enrichment in lakes and other bodies of waters, leading to an overproduction of algae and a decrease in dissolved oxygen levels.

***exocytosis*:** The cellular elimination of a vacuole's contents, the reverse of pinocytosis.

***exoenyzme*:** An enzyme secreted by the cell to the environment.

***exotonix*:** A poisonous protein product released during the lifetime of an organism or on its disintegration.

F

***facultative*:** Adjustable.

***fastidious organism*:** An organism that has complex nutritional and environmental requirements.

***fat*:** One of the several classes of lipids, composed of glycerol and fatty acids.

***fatty acid*:** A straight chain of carbon atoms with a COOH at one end in which most of the carbons are attached to hydrogen atoms.

***F^+ cell*:** A bacterial cell that can transfer the extrachromosomal F (fertility) particle to a recipient (F^-) cell.

***F^- cell*:** A bacterial cell that does not contain an F particle but can act as a recipient and receive one from an F^+ cell.

***fermentation*:** The enzymatic breakdown of complex organic compounds under anaerobic conditions in which the final hydrogen acceptor is an organic compound.

***fetus*:** The unborn offspring after it has largely completed its embryonic development.

***filtration*:** Passage of a liquid through a porous membrane for the removal of particles. Also, the use of certain types of glass to remove particular wavelengths of light.

***fission*:** A form of splitting asexual reproduction in which a unicellular organism divides into two new cells.

***five-kingdom system*:** The arrangement of eucaryotic and procaryotic forms of life into five kingdoms of Animalia, Plantae, Fungi, Protista, and Monera.

***fixation*:** The process of preserving a specimen.

***flagellum*:** A long, whiplike organelle used in the movement of certain organisms and cells; it is structurally similar to a cilium.

***floc*:** A mass of microorganisms caught together in a slime produced by certain bacteria; usually found in waste treatment plants.

***fluorescence*:** Unused potential energy released as light by a substance that has absorbed radiation from another source.

***focal infection*:** A local infection from which microorganisms continuously or intermittently spread to other areas.

***fomite*:** Inanimate contaminated object.

***food chain*:** A sequence of organisms by which food energy is transferred from autotrophs to heterotrophs; each organism consumes the preceding one and in turn is eaten by the following member of the sequence.

***freeze-fracture*:** A special preparative procedure used in electron microscopy in which the exposed surface of a supercooled specimen is used for a metal impression (replica).

***frustule*:** The characteristic cell wall of diatoms.

***fungus*:** Eucaryotic unicellular and sometimes multicellular organism with rigid cell walls and an absorptive type of nutrition; e.g., molds, mushrooms, puffballs, yeasts.

G

***gall (plant)*:** A tumor produced on various plant parts due to infections caused by certain bacterial species.

***genetic code*:** The composition and sequence of all the sets of three nucleotides that code for the amino acids in a protein molecule. The sequence of three nucleotides that codes for one amino acid is referred to as a code word.

***genome*:** The entire set of genetic information in an organism.

***genus (pl. genera)*:** A taxonomic category of related organisms, usually containing several species; the first name of an organism in the binomial system of nomenclature.

***germination*:** The sprouting of a spore.

***Giemsa stain*:** A stain (composed of the dyes azure and eosin) used for the demonstration of chlamydia, rickettsia, and protozoa.

***glucoside*:** A compound resulting from the combination of glucose and another compound containing an alcohol group; a glycoside.

***glycolysis*:** The anaerobic process of glucose breakdown with the formation of pyruvic acid or lactic acid and the production of energy.

***gnotobiotics*:** The study of animals that have been born and raised in a germ-free environment.

***golgi apparatus*:** A cytoplasmic organelle of eucaryotic cells consisting of unit membrane foldings. The golgi apparatus serves as a collecting and processing center for lipids and proteins, changing these macromolecules to meet the needs of the cell.

***Gram stain*:** A differential staining procedure by which bacteria are categorized as either Gram-positive or Gram-negative based on their retention of a primary dye (usually crystal violet) after treatment with a decolorizing agent such as acetone alcohol.

***granulocytes*:** One group of white blood cells containing cytoplasmic granules that stain differently; e.g., basophile, eosinophile, neutrophile.

***gumma*:** A tumorlike fleshy mass of tissue (granuloma) found in the late stages of syphilis.

H

***habitat*:** The specific location where a particular organism lives.

***helminth*:** Worm.

***hemagglutination*:** The clumping of red blood cells.

***hemagglutination inhibition*:** The prevention of hemagglutination, usually by means of specific immunoglobulins or specific enzymes.

***hemolysis*:** The disruption of red blood cells with the leakage of hemoglobin.

***hepatitis*:** Inflammation of the liver.

***hermaphroditic*:** Having both female and male sex cell–producing organs.

***heterophile antigen*:** A substance present in various tissues that causes the production of immunoglobulins, which react with the tissues of several mammals, fish, and plants.

***heterotroph*:** An organism incapable of utilizing CO_2 as its sole source of carbon and requiring one or more organic compounds for its nutrition.

***holozoic*:** A form of nutrition exhibited by an organism capable of existing only by ingesting entire organisms or solid or particulate matter.

***homo*:** A prefix meaning "same."

***homologous*:** Derived from the same system or species.

***hormogonium*:** A motile section of a filamentous cyanobacterium, usually located between heterocysts.

***hormone*:** A substance produced in minute amounts in one part of the body and transported to another region where it produces its effects; e.g., insulin, gonadotropin.

***host*:** The particular animal, plant, or microorganism harboring another form of life as an parasite.

***humus*:** A dark mass of decayed animal and plant matter remaining after microbial decomposition that gives soil a loose texture and brown or black color.

***hyphae*:** The filaments or threads that form a mycelium.

***hypotroph*:** An obligate intracellular parasite, including viruses and other forms of microorganisms requiring living cells for their nutrition.

I

***immunofluorescence*:** Fluorescence resulting from a reaction between a substance and specific immunoglobulins that are bound to a fluorescent dye.

***immunogen*:** A substance that provokes immunoglobulin (antibody) production.

***immunogenicity*:** The capacity to stimulate the formation of specific immunoglobulins (antibodies).

***immunoglobulin*:** In general, any protein exhibiting antibody activity.

***immunology*:** The study of immunity to disease.

***immunopoietic*:** Immunoglobulin (antibody)-forming.

***infestation*:** The attachment to or temporary invasion of the superficial skin layers by a parasite.

***inflammation*:** Tissue reaction to injury; a defensive response to irritation.

***innate immunity*:** The various factors providing resistance to disease determined by the genetic make-up of the individual.

***inoculum*:** The microorganism-containing specimen used to start cultures.

***inorganic*:** Not containing long chains of carbon atoms; e.g., phosphates, nitrates, sulfates and carbon dioxide.

***interferon*:** Antiviral substance produced by animal tissues.

***in vitro*:** In glass; in essence, experiments performed under artificial conditions.

***in vivo*:** In the living body or organism.

***isoantigens*:** Antigens (immunogenic substances) of the same species.

J

***jaundice*:** Yellowing of body tissues.

K

***kingdom*:** A major taxonomic category, consisting of several phyla or divisions.

***Koch's postulates*:** A definite sequence of experimental steps that shows the causal relationship between a specific organism and a specific disease.

Krebs (citric acid) cycle: A series of aerobic enzymatic reactions by which pyruvic acid produced in glycolysis is converted into energy, CO_2, and H_2O.

L

larva: An immature form of certain animals that differs morphologically from the adult form.

L-forms: A procaryotic form lacking a cell wall, developing from a normally wall-containing organism.

lichen: A mutualistic association of a fungus and either algae or cyanobacteria, resulting in a new structural form. The new formation is morphologically distinct from either of its microbial components and possesses separate chemical and physiological properties.

lipids: A group of organic compounds composed of carbon and hydrogen; e.g., fats, phospholipids, waxes, steroids.

lymphokines: A variety of lymphocyte products associated with cellular hypersensitivities.

lysogeny: The state in which the bacteriophage genome (prophage) persists in direct association with the bacterial genome.

lysosome: A eucaryotic saclike organelle containing digestive enzymes.

M

malaise: General discomfort, uneasiness.

medium: A liquid or solid nutrient preparation used for the cultivation of microorganisms.

meiosis: Nuclear division, characteristic of sex cell formation, in which the number of chromosomes in daughter (newly formed) cells is half the number in the original cell.

meninges: Protective coverings of the brain and spinal cord.

meningitis: Inflammation of the membranes covering the brain and spinal cord.

mesosome: A membranous in-folding (involution) of the cytoplasmic membrane of procaryotes found mainly with Gram-positive cells.

messenger RNA (mRNA): Ribonucleic acid (RNA) that serves as a pattern, or template, for protein synthesis.

metabolism: The sum total of cellular chemical reactions by which energy is provided for vital processes and new cell substances are assimilated.

metastasis: Spreading of a disease.

methanogen: A methane-utilizing procaryote.

metric system: Standardized decimal measurement based upon the meter as a unit of length, the gram as a unit of weight, and the liter as a unit of liquid measure.

microaerophilic: Growing best in the presence of low concentrations of oxygen.

microfibril: Threadlike structure found in the cell walls of filamentous fungi. Chemically, microfibrils consist of chitin.

microfilaria: Microscopic larvae of certain nematodes, e.g., *Wuchereria bancrofti*, the causative agent of elephantiasis.

micrometer (μm): One millionth (10^{-6}) part of a meter, or 10^{-3} of a millimeter.

microtubule: A microscopic structural unit of eucaryotic cilia and flagella. Microtubules aid in maintaining cell shape and serve as spindle fibers in mitosis.

minimal inhibitory concentration (MIC): The lowest concentration of a drug that will prevent growth of a standard microbial suspension.

mitochondrion: A eucaryotic cellular organelle consisting of an outer membrane and an inner one folded into cristae.

mitosis: The asexual process in which genetic material is duplicated and equally distributed in newly formed cells.

mold: A type of fungus having a filamentous (hyphal) structure.

Monera: The kingdom of procaryotic organisms with unicellular and simple colonial organization.

monosaccharide: A category of six-carbon sugars having the molecular formula $C_6H_{12}O_6$; e.g., glucose.

morbidity: The number of cases of a disease per unit of the population within a given time period.

morphology: The study of shape and structure.

must: Pressed grape juice used for wine-making.

mutation: A sudden change in the genetic code of an organism, resulting in a hereditable property differing from the parent cell.

mutualism: A symbiotic association in which two different organisms are obligately dependent upon each other.

mycelium (pl. mycelia): An interwoven mat of hyphae, i.e., mass of fungal filaments.

mycology: The study of fungi.

mycoplasma: A group of bacteria composed of cells lacking cell walls and exhibiting a variety of shapes (pleomorphism).

mycosis: A fungus infection of animals.

mycotoxicosis: Poisoning caused by fungal toxins (mycotoxins).

mycotoxin: A poison (toxin) produced by and associated with fungi.

N

nanometer (nm): 10^{-6} millimeter or 10^{-9} meter. This designation has in most cases replaced the millimicron.

native immunity: A state of resistance conferred by one's genetic make-up, not acquired by exposure to infectious disease agents.

niche: The biological role of an organism in its community, which includes its location and its activities.

nitrogen cycle: A geochemical cycle in which atmospheric nitrogen gas is converted into a usable form for plants by microbial enzymatic reactions.

nitrogen fixation: The formation of nitrogen compounds (NO_2^-, NO_3^-) from free atmospheric nitrogen (N_2).

nosocomial infection: Hospital-acquired infection.

nucleic acid: One of a class of macromolecules consisting of a series of nucleotides; e.g., deoxyribonucleic acid (DNA), ribonucleic acid (RNA).

nucleocapsid: The capsid and the enclosed nucleic acid core of a virus particle.

nucleolus: A dense oval to round organelle found in the nucleus of eucaryotic cells. It is largely composed of RNA and thought to be the site for RNA formation.

***nucleoplasm*:** Cellular material contained within the nucleus.

***nucleus*:** The eucaryotic cellular organelle enclosed by a nuclear membrane and containing the cell's chromosomes. Also, the center, or core, of an atom.

***numerical taxonomy*:** A technique for determining the relationships among organisms by determining the number of properties the organisms have in common.

O

***Oomyetes*:** A class of fungi that includes organisms noted for causing "downy mildew of grapes" and parasitizing green algae.

***operon*:** A group of structural genes and the operator gene that controls them.

***opportunist*:** A microorganism that causes infection only under especially favorable conditions (e.g., when defense host mechanisms are not fully functioning).

***opsonization*:** A form of phagocytosis enhanced by specific immunoglobulins and complement.

***order*:** In taxonomy, a major subdivision of a class. Each order consists of one or more related families.

***organelle*:** A specialized part of a cell that performs a specific function; e.g., mitochondrion, ribosome.

***organic compound*:** A substance primarily composed of carbon, hydrogen, oxygen, and nitrogen and that in nature is produced only by various forms of life.

***oxidation*:** The loss of electrons or hydrogen.

***oxidative phosphorylation*:** The generation of energy in the form of adenosine triphosphate (ATP) that results from the passage of electrons through the electron transport chain to the final electron acceptor, oxygen.

***oxygen cycle*:** The general cycle by which oxygen is exchanged and distributed within the biosphere.

P

***pandemic*:** Affecting the majority of the population of a large region, or epidemic concurrently in many different parts of the word.

***papule*:** Pimple.

***parasite*:** An organism that lives within or upon another form of life.

***passive immunization*:** The transfer of antibodies from an immunized donor to a nonimmune recipient.

***pasteurization*:** The processes of heating food or other substances under controlled conditions of time and temperature, 63°C for 30 minutes.

***pathogenic*:** Capable of producing disease.

***pathogenicity*:** The ability of an organism to produce disease.

***pellicle*:** A thin membranelike film formed on the surface of microbial broth culture. Also, the thickened, outer surface of certain protozoans.

***peptide bond*:** The covalent bond that joins an amino group of one amino acid to the carboxyl group of another amino acid, with the formation of water.

***peroxisome*:** The microbody in which photorespiration takes place.

***Petri dish*:** A commonly used container in the cultivation of various microorganisms.

***phage*:** A bacterial virus (bacteriophage).

***phagocytosis*:** Cellular engulfment of foreign particles.

***phosphorus cycle*:** A geochemical cycle by which phosphorus is exchanged and distributed within the biosphere.

***phosphorylation*:** The introduction of a phosphate (PO_4^{-3}) group into an organic molecule.

***phycology*:** The study of algae.

***phylum (pl. phyla)*:** A large taxonomic rank of related families in the classification of living organisms. The classification system is subdivided progressively from World → kingdoms → subkingdoms → phyla → classes → orders → families → genera → species.

***phytotoxin*:** Bacterial toxins that affect plants.

***pilus (pl. pili)*:** Surface-associated structures found on certain bacterial cells and some yeasts that are not organelles of locomotion. Depending on the pilus type, activities such as attachment and transfer of genetic material are associated with them.

***pinocytosis*:** The process performed by a cell in which liquid or small particles are enveloped in a vacuole and brought into the cell.

***plankton*:** Microscopic, floating animal, microbial, and plant-life distributed throughout various bodies of water.

***Plantae*:** The kingdom of plants.

***plaque (dental)*:** A collection of bacteria tightly adhering to a tooth surface, involved in the production of dental caries.

***plaque (viral)*:** A clear area in a single layer or monolayer of cells created by viral lysis of infected cells.

***plasma*:** The liquid portion of lymph and blood.

***plasmid*:** The eucaryotic organelle found in plant cells that is the center of chemical activity involved in cell metabolism.

***plasmolysis*:** Contraction or shrinking of a cell's cytoplasm due to the loss of water by osmotic action; i.e., a loss of water molecules.

***PMNL*:** Polymorphonuclear leukocyte.

***polyhedron*:** Many-sided figure.

***polysaccharide*:** A carbohydrate composed of more than three molecules of monosaccharides.

***polysome*:** A chain of ribosomes held together temporarily by messenger RNA.

***population*:** The group of individuals of a given species inhabiting a specified location or area.

***precipitin reaction*:** The visible interaction of soluble antigens with homologous antibodies.

***predation*:** A relationship between two forms of life in which one species unfavorably affects the other but cannot live without it; the first species (the predator) kills and devours the second (the prey).

***primary immunodeficiency*:** Conditions developing from an inherited failure of one or more immune-system components to develop.

***procaryote*:** An organism exhibiting a cellular organization characterized by an absence of a true nucleus and other internally membrane-bound organelles.

***proglottid*:** Tapeworm segment.

***protein*:** A macromolecule containing carbon, hydrogen, oxygen, nitrogen, and at times sulfur and phosphorus, composed of chains of amino acids joined by peptide bonds.

Protista: The kingdom of living microorganisms including protozoans and certain algae.

protoplasm: The living substance of a cell.

prototroph: The "normal" or usually encountered form of an organism (wild type).

protozoology: The study of protozoans.

pseudopod: A temporary cytoplasmic protrusion of amoeba, or amoeboid cells, which functions in cellular feeding and movement.

psychrophile: Microorganisms that grow well between 0° and 30°C. The optimum is usually above 25°C.

purified protein derivative (PPD): Substance obtained from cultures of *Mycobacterium tuberculosis* or related organisms and used in skin testing.

purines: Organic bases with carbon and nitrogen atoms in two interlocking rings; components of nucleic acids, adenosine triphosphate (ATP), and other biologically active substances.

pustule: Small elevated skin lesion containing pus.

putrefaction: The anaerobic decomposition of protein resulting in foul odors.

pyogenic: Pus-producing.

pyrimidines: Nitrogenous bases consisting of a single ring of carbon and nitrogen; components of nucleic acids and certain antimicrobial drugs.

R

recombination: A process in which the transfer of genetic material occurs between two organisms.

reduction: The addition of electrons to an atom or molecule; opposite of oxidation.

resistance transfer factors (RTF): A set of genes that are associated with antibiotic resistance and that carry the genetic information for the transfer of such resistant (R) factors.

reverse transcriptase: An enzyme involved in the formation of DNA complementary to an RNA pattern or template.

R factor: A transferable plasmid found in many enteric bacteria, which carries genetic information for resistance to one or more chemotherapeutic agents; often associated with a transfer factor that is responsible for conjugation with another bacterium and for transfer of the R factor.

S

saprophyte: Any organism that derives its nutrition from dead or decaying organic matter.

schizogony: The asexual phase of sporozoans, e.g., malarial parasites.

scolex: The head of a tapeworm.

secondary immunodeficiency: Immunodeficiency caused by such factors as malnutrition, malignancies, radiation exposure, burns, and various drugs that interfere with the functions of the lymphatic system.

selective medium: A growth medium containing a component that will inhibit the growth of certain microorganisms and either enhance or not affect the growth of other organisms.

sequelae: Conditions following or resulting from a disease.

serum: The light yellow fluid left after the clotting of blood has occurred.

sexual reproduction: The formation of an organism from the union of two different sex cells (gametes).

sheath: A tubular structure surrounding certain microbial cells.

simple staining: A procedure using only one dye.

sinus: Any cavity having a relatively narrow opening.

SI system: Système International d' Unités. An international system of units for the measurement of length, volume, and mass. It is based on the metric system.

sludge: The precipitated solid matter produced by water and sewage treatment.

smear: A thin film of material spread on a clean glass.

species: The unit of taxonomic classification for most forms of life; a population of similar individuals, alike in their structural and functional properties and able to reproduce sexually with each other but with no other types of organisms.

spontaneous generation: A theory that certain forms of life arose spontaneously from nonliving matter.

sporadic: Irregular in occurrence.

spore: A resistant structure or stage formed by procaryotes. Also, the reproductive cell of certain types of organisms.

sporogony: The sexual phase of sporozoans such as *Plasmodium* spp., which cause malaria.

sporozoite: An elongated, sickle-shaped body formed in an oöcyst as the result of the sexual reproduction phase of sporozoans such as *Plasmodium* spp.

starter culture: A pure or mixed culture of microorganisms used to initiate a desired fermentation process, as in cheese manufacture.

sterile: Free from all living organisms.

sterilization: The destruction of all living forms.

steroid: A complex macromolecule containing carbon atoms arranged in four interlocking rings, three of which contain six carbon atoms each and the fourth of which contains five.

STS: Standard tests for syphilis.

subclinical infection: A state in which the individual does not experience all of the characteristic symptoms of a particular disease, or such effects are less severe.

substrate: A substance acted upon, as by an enzyme.

sulfur cycle: A geochemical cycle by which sulfur is utilized and distributed through the biosphere.

symbiosis: The living together of two dissimilar organisms; such associations may be commensal, mutualistic, or

symptomatic treatment: Treatment of existing or expected symptoms.

syngamy: Sexual reproduction, the union of the two haploid chromosome complements in fertilization.

synthetic medium: A medium of known composition.

syntropism: Feeding together.

T

taxonomy: The description, classification, and naming of organisms.

template: The molecule that serves as the pattern for processes such as the formation of another molecule; a pattern or mold that guides the formation of a duplicate.

test: An outer protective covering or shell formed by certain protozoans, e.g., foraminfera.

thallus: The vegetative body of certain microorganisms and plants that does not show differentiation into roots, stems, or leaves.

thermophile: An organism that grows best at high temperatures, e.g., 45° to 75°+C; its optimum growth temperature is about 55°C.

thylakoid: An organelle consisting of layers in the cytoplasm; the site of photosynthesis.

titer: The potency of a biological reactant expressed in units per milliliter. The level of immunoglobulins is frequently given in this way.

toxin: A poisonous substance.

toxoid: A converted toxin; the resulting preparation is nontoxic but still capable of provoking immunoglobulin production.

transcriptase: An enzyme that catalyzes the flow of genetic information from DNA to RNA.

transcription: Formation of messenger RNA (mRNA), the nucleotide sequence of which is dictated by that of deoxyribonucleic acid (DNA).

transduction: A recipient bacterium's incorporation into its chromosome of genetic material obtained from a donor bacterium. The transfer of such material is performed by a bacterial virus.

transformation: The conversion of a bacterial type by means of free, extracellular, bacterial DNA.

translation: Formation of proteins or related macromolecules containing amino acids in the sequence dictated by the information in messenger RNA.

trichocyst: An organelle in the cytoplasm of ciliated protozoans, such as *Paramecium* spp., which can discharge a filament for defense or for trapping prey.

trichome: A single row of cells of a multicellular organism in which the multicellular nature is evident without staining.

trophozoite: The vegetative cell of a protozoan, i.e., active feeding stage.

T-type lymphocyte: A thymus-derived lymphocyte that is responsible for cell-mediated immunity (CMI).

tubercle: A nodule, a specific lesion in certain diseases such as tuberculosis.

tumor: An accumulation of cells resulting in the appearance of an observable lump.

U

ulcer: A rounded or irregularly shaped area of inflammatory tissue destruction in the epithelial lining of a surface.

ulceration: The process of ulcer formation.

V

vacuole: A clear area in a cell's cytoplasm.

V.D.R.L. (Venereal Disease Research Laboratory) test: A precipitin test for the diagnosis of syphilis.

vector: A carrier of pathogenic agents, especially an arthropod.

venereal disease: A disease, such as gonorrhea and syphilis, that is spread by sexual contact and involve parts of the genitourinary system.

virion: A complete, fully infectious virus particle.

viroid: Short strands of RNA capable of causing diseases in plants.

virology: The study of viruses.

virulence: The capacity to produce disease, it is a function of microbial invasiveness and toxigenicity and is measured with reference to a particular host.

W

water activity: The ratio of the water pressure of a food substance to the vapor pressure of pure water at the same temperature.

wheal and flare: A circumscribed, reddened elevation of the skin.

Y

yeast: A type of unicellular fungus that characteristically does not form typical mycelia.

Z

zoonosis: An animal disease that is transmitted to humans by natural means.

zoospore: An asexual, flagellated, motile spore.

Zygomycetes: The smallest class of fungi, including organisms such as the common bread mold.

Index

Explanation of symbols: f, figure; t, table

A

Abbé condenser, 56
Abiotic factors, 325
ABO system, 482–483
  blood typing for, 484
  genetic factors in, 484–485
  subgroups of, 484
  universal donor, 483
  universal recipient, 483–484
Abscess, 425
Acariasis, 536
Acetobacter, 146t
  in vinegar production, 741
Acholeplasma, 147–149
Acid-fast bacteria:
  chemotherapy against, 391t
  identification of, 556–557
Acid-fast stain, 62–63
Acidity:
  in fermentation, 16
  importance in cell reactions, 81
    See also pH
Acids, 81
Acinetobacter, 146t
  opportunistic infections of, 440t
Acriflavine, 362
Actinomyces, 147t
  chemotherapy of, 391t
  conidia of, 138
  spore of, 138
Actinomycosis:
  chemotherapy of, 391t
  of oral cavity, 590t
  specimen collection in, 548t
Active immunity:
  artificially acquired, 464
  naturally acquired, 462–463
Active transport, 103, 128
Acute glomerulonephritis, 667
Acute pyelonephritis, 663t, 665–666
Acute radiation injury, 430t
Adaptability, 4
Adenine, 86–87
Adenosine triphosphate (ATP), 87–89
  in energy mobilization, 88–89
  glycolysis and formation of, 274–275
  production of, 273–274
Adenovirus, 228t
  in epidemic keratoconjunctivitis, 699
  role in cancer, 707, 709t
  vaccine against, 512t
Adjuvant, 450
Adoptive immunity, 464–465
Aëdes mosquitoes:
  in filariasis, 723
  life cycle of, 538–539
  in viral diseases, 538t
Aerobes, 3, 147
  culturing, 243, 251
  Pasteur's discovery of, 17
Aerobic incubation, 256
Aerobic respiration, 276–277
Aerobic stabilization:
  of solid waste, 783
  of waste water, 780
Aerococcus, 147t
Aeromonas hydrophilia infections, 440t
Aflatoxins:
  carcinogenic properties of, 443, 712
  danger of, 173
  presence in foods, 443
African sleeping sickness, 691–692
  life cycle in, 692
  organism causing, 181, 189
  prevention of, 693
  transmission of, 692
  See also Trypanosomiasis
Agammaglobulinemia, 493
Agar, 25–26
  See also Media
Agar-overlay method, 402
Agglutination reactions, 470
  cold, 471
  hemagglutination inhibition, 472
  passive, 471–472
  in serologic diagnosis, 469t
  Weil-Felix test, 471
  Widal test, 471
Agranulocytes, 418–419
Agranulocytosis, 430t
Agrobacterium, 146t
  pH and growth of, 325t, 326
Akinetes, 132, 138, 157
Alcohol:
  as disinfectant, 359–361
  industrial production of beverages containing, 737, 742t, 743
    beer, 738
    distilled, 739
    sake, 739
    wine, 738–739
Alcoholism:
  immunity and, 430t
  opportunistic infections due to, 440t
Aldehydes, 360t, 364
Algae, 194
  activities of, 5–6
  agar extracted from, 25
  blooms of, 195, 769
  blue-green, 147
  brown, 202–203
  classification of, 196–197, 199t
  cultivation of, 196
  diatoms, 198–201
  dinoflagellates, 203
  distribution of, 195
  ecologic importance of, 197
  economic importance of, 197–198
  euglenoids, 201–202
  golden brown, 198–201
  green, 197–198
  harmful effects of, 198
  importance of, 202, 203, 206
  lichens, 205–206
  metachromatic granules in, 130
  phosphorus cycle and, 346
  radioactivity concentrated in, 353
  red, 204–205
  reproduction in, 196
  structure of, 196
  toxins of, 442
  in waste treatment, 782
Algicide, 357t
Alkaligenes, 146t
  identification of, 555
Alkalinity, 81
  in fermentation, 16
  importance in cell reactions, 81
  See also pH
Alkylating agents, 301
Allergen, 494
Allergic contact dermatitis, 503
Allergic reactions in infections, 435t
Allergic rhinitis, 496
Allergy, 494
  of infection, 502–503
  penicillin, 503–504
  See also Hypersensitivity
Allodermanyssus sanguineus, 653
Allograft, 504
Alpha-hemolysis, 249
Alpha-hemolytic streptococci, 249, 569
Alphaviruses, 689, 690t
Alternaria, 327
Amanita, 171
Amantadine, 405–407
Amblyomma, 653
Amebiasis. *See* Amoebic dysentery
Ames/*Salmonella* test, 713
Amino acids:
  fermentation with, 275
  production of, 741–742
  structure of, 90–92
Aminoglycosides, 395–396
Ammonification, 344–345

Amoebae:
cultivation of, 187
disease caused by, 189
excretion by, 183
movement of, 181
Amoebic dysentery, 181
cyst role in, 185
features of, 641t
life cycle of parasite in, 640
organism causing, 189
prevention of, 640
transmission of, 533, 640
Amoebic meningoencephalitis, 693
Amphibionts, 413–415
Amphotericin B, 405t
Ampicillin, 393–394
Amylase, 743
Amyloplasts, 110
Amylose, 85
Anabolism, 3, 246, 272
Anaerobic digestion:
of solid waste, 783
of waste water, 779–780, 782
Anaerobic incubation, 257–258
Anaerobic indicators, 257–258
Anaerobic organisms, 3, 147
aerotolerant, 244
in brain abscess, 683
characteristics of, 146–147t
culturing, 243–244, 250–251
facultative, 244
female genital tract infections by, 669–670
identification of, 556
in meningitis, 685
obligate, 243
Pasteur's discovery of, 17
in urinary tract infections, 667
Anaerobic respiration, 279
Anaerobic transfer, 255–256
Anaeroplasma, 148–149
Anamnestic response, 456
Anaphylaxis, 496–497
cutaneous, 497–498
generalized, 497
as immunization complication, 519t
mechanism of, 498
Anaplasia, 703
Ancylostoma duodenale, 721, 722t
Anemia, 418
Angstrom, 51
Animal viruses:
cultivation of
embryonated eggs in, 230–231
tissue culture in, 231–234
diseases caused by, 227
replication of, 227, 229
Animalcules, 18
Animal-protection test, 517
Animals, 37, 38t
Anisakis, 722t
Anopheles mosquitoes:
in filariasis, 723
life cycle of, 538–539
in malaria, 655
in viral diseases, 538t
Anthrax, 562, 565
in animals, 531t
chemotherapy in, 390t
control of, 566
features of skin infection, 564t
Koch's postulates applied to, 23
mechanism of disease by causative agent, 435t
organism causing, 60t
species resistance to, 411
transmission of, 531t, 532, 566
See also Bacillus anthracis
Antibiotics, 387
agricultural use of, 387
choice of, 388
discovery of, 26
dosage of, 388
factors affecting administration of, 388
as feed additives, 387
indiscriminate use of, 430t
industrial production of, 739–740
microbial sources of, 388
minimal active concentrations of, 389
minimal inhibitory concentrations of, 388
overuse of, 399
plasmids acting like, 310–311
polyene, 403–404
properties of, 389
research in development of, 387–388
resistance developing to, 398–400
sensitivity testing of, 400–402
specific mechanisms of action, 390
spectrum of activity of, 390
transfer of resistance to, 311, 399–400
See also Antimicrobial agents
Antibodies:
anamnestic response of, 456
antisera, 470
in Arthus reaction, 500–501
in atopy, 499
factors affecting production of, 456
ferritin-conjugated, 469t, 480–481
fluorescent, 478–480
immunoelectrophoresis to detect, 452
immunofluorescence and, 64
importance of measurement of, 468–469
mechanism of formation of, 460–461
normal flora and production of, 415
opsonizing, 422
properties of, 452
selective hypotheses for formation of, 460–461
significance of rising titers of, 470
template hypothesis for formation of, 460
transplacental transfer of, 458
use in passive immunization, 517–518
See also Immunity; Immunoglobulins
Antigens, 64, 449
Australia, 639
auto-, 451
carcinoembryonic, 713
classes of, 450–452
competition of, 462
determinant sites on, 450
excess in serum sickness, 501
fetal, 712–713
Forssmann, 451–452
haptens, 450
hepatitis B surface, 639, 640
heterophile, 451–452
histocompatibility of, 504
iso-, 451
salmonella, 631
somatic (O), 438
tumor-specific, 713
See also Immunity
Antimicrobial agents:
aminoglycosides, 395–396
antimycobacterial drugs, 397
blood levels of, 403
cephalosporins, 393–394
chloramphenicol, 395
clindamycin, 395
mechanism of action of, 389–390, 392t
opportunistic infections due to, 440t
penicillins, 393–395
polypeptides, 397
rifampin, 398
sulfa, 390, 392
terms describing, 357
tetracyclines, 395
See also Antibiotics
Antimycotic agents:
5-fluorocytosine, 404, 405t
griseofulvin, 404, 405t
limited number of, 403
polyenes, 403–404
Antiseptic surgery, 22, 358
Antiseptics, 357
chemical, 359
dyes, 362
iodine, 360
peroxides, 362
testing methods for, 365–367
Antisera, 470
Antistreptolysin test, 477–478
Antitoxins, 516–517
Antiviral agents, 405–407
sensitivity testing of, 406
structure of, 405f
Aphthous pharyngitis, 593
Aplanospores, 196, 203
Apoenzyme, 94
Arachnia, 147t
Arenavirus, 228t
Aristotle, 17
Arizona:
in food poisoning, 634
opportunistic infections of, 440t
Arsenic in syphilis therapy, 363
Arteries, 646–647
Arthrobacter, 147t
glutamic acid production by, 741
manganese metabolism in, 352
Arthropod-borne diseases, 534–535
cockroaches in, 539
fleas in, 537–538
housefly in, 535
lice in, 536–537
mites in, 535–536
mosquitoes in, 538–539
ticks in, 535–536
Arthropod-borne viruses, 228t
characteristics of, 689, 690t
control of, 690
Arthus reaction, 500–501
Ascariasis, 722t
Ascaris lumbricoides, 722t
Ascomycetes, 169–171
harmful effects of, 171
in lichen, 206
virus found in, 236
Ascospore, 170–171
Ascus, 171
Aseptic meningitis, 684t, 686
Aseptic technique, 253
Asexual reproduction, 3, 186
Asparaginase, 743t
Aspergillus flavus, 173
Aspergillus fumigatus, 784
Aspergillus oryzae, 739
Aspergillus species:
antimycotic agents for, 405t
in citrus acid production, 742
contaminating humus, 784
mechanism of disease caused by, 435t
mycotoxin of, 173, 443
in sake production, 739
survival in distilled water, 327
Assays, 314–315
Asthma, 496
Atmosphere, 328
Atoms, 78
Atopy, 498–499
immunotherapy of, 499–500
passive transfer of, 499
skin testing for, 499
ATP. *See* Adenosine triphosphate
Australia antigen, 639
Autoantibodies, 451
Autoantigens, 451
Autoclaving, 370t, 373–375
Autogamy, 186–187
Autograft, 504
Autoimmune diseases, 451t
Autoimmunity, 506–507
Autoimmunization, 451
Autoinfection, 720
Automated microbiology technology, 746
Autotrophs, 147, 155–157, 281, 282t
and bacterial cultures, 243
chemosynthetic, 284
in ecosystem, 324
photosynthetic, 155–157, 283
protozoa, 182
Auxospore, 200
Auxotrophs, 302
Axial filaments, 128
Axopodia, 181
Azotobacter, 146t
cysts of, 137–138
lipid inclusions in, 131

B

Babes-Ernst granules, 130
Babesia bigemina, 535
Bacillary dysentery, 61t, 626t, 631
causative agents of, 631
chemotherapy of, 391t
exotoxin involved in, 439t
prevention of, 632

Bacillary dysentery (*continued*)
transmission of, 533, 631–632
See also Shigella dysenteriae
Bacilli, 116, 118
Bacillus anthracis:
anthrax caused by, 566
capsule and invasiveness of, 124, 436
chemotherapy of, 390t
endospores of, 134
Forssmann antigen associated with, 451–452
Koch's postulates applied to, 23
leukins effect on, 427
See also Anthrax
Bacillus cereus, 634
Bacillus circulans, 134
Bacillus globisporus, 325t
Bacillus lentimorbus, 745, 746t
Bacillus megaterium:
bacteriocin in, 310–311
thermal kill in, 374
Bacillus of Calmette and Guerin. See BCG
Bacillus pasteurii, 325t, 326
Bacillus populliae, 745, 746t
Bacillus species, 147t
antimicrobials produced by, 397
denitrification in, 279
endospores of, 132, 134
fermentation in, 275
in food poisoning, 634
identification of, 554–555
lipid inclusions in, 131
manganese metabolism in, 352
in monitoring sterilization, 373
nitrogen requirements of culture media for, 246
in pesticide production, 745, 746t
pH and growth of, 325t, 326
smear used as quality control, 557
spore staining of, 63
temperature and growth of, 244, 325t
Bacillus subtilis:
culture media for, 246
transformation in, 306
Bacillus thuringiensis:
in pesticide production, 745, 746t
sporulation in, 136
Backbone layer, 125–126
BACTEC system, 552
Bacteremia, 436, 551
Bacteria, 116
amino acid synthesis by, 741
appendaged, 146t
autotrophs, 155–157
bacilli, 116, 118
biochemical testing in identification of, 550–551
blue-green, 155–157
budding, 146t
capsule effect on invasiveness, 124, 436
in carbon cycle, 340–342
carcinogens synthesized by, 712
cell immunity of, 223
cell mass determination of, 262–263
cell wall of, 124–126
chemotaxis to, 423
chemotherapy of, 390–391t
chimeras, 316–317
in circulatory system infections, 647–654
classification of, 33–34, 145–147
cocci, 116, 118f
cocco-bacilli, 116, 118
complement-fixation tests for, 478t
conidia in, 138
conjugation in, 306–307
counting chamber for, 267
cultivation of, 145
cell mass determinations in, 262–263
colony counts in, 264–265
conditions for growth and, 243–245
different categories of media for, 249–251
incubation conditions for, 256–258
inoculation and transfer techniques in, 251–254
isolation techniques in, 254–256
media for, 245–248
preparation of media for, 248
protection of personnel in, 259
purposes of, 248–249
curved, 146t, 152
cysts in, 132, 137–138
cytoplasmic inclusions in, 130–132
as decomposers in ecosystem, 324
in dental plaque, 588
direct microscopic count of, 266
discovery by Leeuwenhoek, 18
DNA in, 129
dormant structures in, 132–139
endospores in, 132–137
endotoxins of, 437–438
in estuaries, 772
evolution of, 44
exotoxins of, 439–442
eye infections due to, 695–698
female genital tract infections due to, 669
fertility determinants in, 307–308, 313
as food source, 756
food spoilage associated with, 758t, 759
functions favorable to man, 145
in gastrointestinal flora, 625
gastrointestinal infections due to, 625–635
gliding, 146t, 149
green, 155, 156t
growth of:
continuous cultures and, 261–262
lag phase, 259–260
logarithmic death rate, 261
logarithmic phase, 260
measurement of, 262–267
on solid media, 262
stationary growth phase, 261
heterotrophic, 148–155
hydrocarbon degradation by, 349–350
identification of, 547
immunogenic components of, 449
invasiveness of, 436–437
as kappa particles in protozoa, 312–313
L-forms, 127
lower respiratory infections due to, 606–614
lower urinary tract infections due to, 663
lysogenic, 223, 310
manganese metabolism in, 352
mapping genomes of, 313–314
media in identification of, 550–551
mercury methylation by, 351–352
mesosomes in, 128–129
metachromatic granules in, 130
methane-producing, 147t, 349
in mouth flora, 584, 585t
nervous system infections due to, 682–685
nitrogen assimilation by, 344–345
nitrogen fixation by, 343–344
in normal flora, 414t
obligate intracellular, 145, 152–155
opportunistic infections of, 440t
oral infections due to, 590
pesticide metabolism by, 351
in pesticide production, 745, 746t
phagocytosis of, 423–424
photosynthesis in, 130, 155, 283–285
phototropic, 146t
phytotoxins of, 442
pili found in, 122
in plant diseases, 543
plasma membrane of, 127–128
in prostatitis, 670
prosthecate, 150–151
protein content of, 755–756
purple, 155, 156t
reproduction of, 259, 260f
resistance to antibiotics developed in, 302
ribosomes in, 130
in sewage, 773–775
sexduction in, 307–309
shape of, 116, 118
sheathed, 146t, 150
size of, 116, 117f
skin diseases caused by, 562–571
skin tests for, 482t
in soil fertility, 766–767
specimen collection for, 548t
spiral, 146t, 152
spirilla, 118
spirochetes, 146t
staining of:
acid-fast, 62–63
differential, 59
gram, 59–62
simple, 58–59
in subacute endocarditis, 648
sulfur metabolism in, 346
surfaces of, 119–120
capsule, 123–124
cell wall, 124–126
flagella, 120–122
pili, 122–123
protoplast, 126–127
slime layers, 123
spheroplast, 126–127
spine, 123
in tooth decay, 589
transduction in, 309
transformation in, 304–306
transmission in food, 533
in trickling filter system, 781
upper respiratory infections due to, 601–604
urinary tract infections due to, 663t, 665–667
use in testing disinfectant, 365–367
vaccines of, 511–513
vibrios, 118
viruses attacking. *See* Bacteriophages
in waste treatment, 782
zoonoses of, 531t
See also Antibiotics; Antimicrobial agents; Blue-green bacteria; Gram-negative bacteria; Gram-positive bacteria; Procaryotes
Bacterial dysentery. *See* Bacillary dysentery
Bactericidal, 357t, 389–390
detergents as, 363
Bacteriocins, 310–311
Bacteriology, 4
Bacteriophages, 8f, 218
adsorption of, 224
basic structure of, 218–220
characterization of, 221–222
cultivation of, 221–222
exotoxin production associated with, 439
filamentous, 221
growth curve of, 225–226
in lysogenic conversion, 223, 310
lysozyme in infections with, 224, 225
lytic cycle of infections with, 223–225
natural occurrence of, 221
penetration into cell host, 224–225
replication cycle of, 222–226
resistance to infection by, 223
role in transduction, 309
typing of, 222
Bacteriostatic, 357t, 362, 390
dyes, 362
Bacteroides, 146t
in checking anaerobic systems, 258
chemotherapy of, 391t
culture requirements of, 243–244
female genital tract infections by, 669
identification of, 556
meningitis caused by, 685
opportunistic infections of, 440t
Bacteroides fragilis, 391t
Bactrachopermum, 204
Baeocytes, 156
Balanitis, 670
Balantidiasis, 641–642
Balantidium coli, 641
Bang, O., 706

Bar marker, 51
Barophiles, 327
Barr, Y. M., 708
Basal hook, 120, 121f
Bases, 81
  See also Alkalinity; pH
Basidiomycetes, 169t, 171–172
  harmful effects of, 171–172
Basophils, 419
  role in anaphylaxis, 497
Bassi, Agostino, 22–23
Bats involvement in rabies, 530
BCG, 51, 512t
  complications of, 520t
  as immunological stimulator for cancer, 714
  in tuberculosis prevention, 515–516, 609, 613
Bdellovibrio, 146t, 153
Beadle, George, 301–302
Beer production, 738
Beggiatoa, 146t
Bejel, 678
Bentonite flocculation test, 472
Berzelius, Jöns Jakob, 15
Beta-hemolysis, 249
Beta-hemolytic streptococci, 569
  identification of, 554
  in Ludwig's angina, 589
  role in rheumatic fever, 647
  skin infections of, 564–565t
Beta-propiolactone disinfection, 365
Bifidobacterium, 147t
  in infant gastrointestinal flora, 625
  in water quality determination, 777
Bile solubility test, 554
Binary fission, 186
Biochemical oxygen demand, 778
Biochemistry, 8
  microbiology and, 77–78
Bioconcentration, 348, 352
  of manganese, 352
  of pesticides, 352
  of radioisotopes, 352–353
  of sulfur, 352
Bioconversion, 348
  hydrocarbon degradation, 349–350
  mercury methylation, 351–352
  methanogenesis, 348–349
  pesticide metabolism, 351
Biogeochemical cycles:
  carbon cycle, 340–342
  nitrogen cycle, 342–345
  oxygen cycle, 346–347
  phosphorus cycle, 345–346
  sulfur cycle, 346
Biogeochemistry, 340
Biophysics, 8
Biosphere, 323
  organization of, 323–328
    See also Ecosystem
Biotic factors, 325
Biphasic system, 261
Black Death, 648–649
Bladder infections, 663t, 666
Blastomyces dermatitidis, 616
Blastomycosis, 615–617
  in oral cavity, 592t
  specimen collection in, 549t
Blood:
  components of, 416–419
  role in immune system, 416–419
Blood compatibility testing, 487–488
Blood cultures, 551–552
Blood poisoning. *See* Septicemia
Blood types, 469t, 482–485
  major, 483
Blooms, algal, 195, 769
Blue-green bacteria:
  blooms of, 769
  cellular properties of, 156
  heterocysts in, 132
  and lichens, 205–206
  properties of, 155–157
  reproduction in, 138, 156–157
  temperature and growth of, 325t, 326
  toxins of, 442
  trichomes in, 138
  virus infections of, 218, 226–227
  See also Cyanobacteria
B-lymphocytes, 458–460
Boiling, 374
Boils, 564t
  See also Staphylococci; *Staphylococcus aureus*
Bone marrow stem-cell deficiency, 493
Bordeaux mixture, 174
Bordet, Jules, 614
Bordetella, 146t
Bordetella pertussis:
  chemotherapy of, 391t
  exotoxin producing disease, 439t
  in whooping cough, 614
Borrelia, 146t
  characteristics of, 152t
  in relapsing fever, 651–652
Botulism, 634
  antitoxin for, 517
  causative agent of, 634
  exotoxin in, 439t, 440, 634
  features of, 565t
  mechanism of disease by causative agent, 435t
  organism causing, 61t
  passive immunization against, 464
  wound, 571
  See also Clostridium botulinum
Brain abscess, 682–684
Branhamella, 146t
Bread mold, 174–175
Breed smear technique, 266
Brevibacterium, 741
Brewer jar, 257, 556
Brill's disease, 652
Brochothrix thermosphactum, 262
Brown, Robert, 101
Brown algae, 202–203
Brownian movement, 120
Brucella, 146t
  in brucellosis, 629
  capneic incubation of, 256
  chemotherapy of, 391t
  culture requirements of, 243
  interferon stimulation by, 428
Brucella abortus, 391t, 428
Brucellosis, 626t, 629
  in animals, 531t
  causative agents of, 626t, 629
  chemotherapy of, 391t
  mechanism of disease by causative agent, 435t
  organism causing, 61t
  prevention of, 629
  skin test for, 482t
  transmission of, 531t, 533, 629
Brugia malayi, 722t, 724
Bubo, 651
Bubonic plague, 651
Budding:
  in bacteria, 146t, 150–151
  in protozoa, 186
  in yeasts, 164f, 171
Buffers, 81
Bunyaviruses, 228t, 689, 690t
Burkitt's lymphoma, 708
Burst size, 226
Butter production, 753–754
Buttermilk production, 754

C

Cachexia, 703
Calculus, 588
Calymmatobacterium granulomatis, 674
Campylobacter, 146t, 152
Cancer:
  aflatoxins implicated in, 443
  carcinoembryonic antigen in, 713
  carcinomas, 705
  causation of, 702–703
  characteristics of, 703–704
  detection of, 712–713
  DNA viruses in, 707–709
  forms of, 704–705
  immunoglobulin abnormalities in, 493–494
  immunological stimulators in treatment of, 714
  infectious mononucleosis and, 708
  leukemias, 705
  lymphomas, 705
  microbiology impact on, 703–704
  oncogene hypothesis for, 711–712
  opportunistic infections due to, 440t
  protovirus hypothesis for, 712
  provirus hypothesis for, 710–711
  reverse transcriptase and, 709
  RNA viruses in, 706–707
  sarcomas, 705
  treatment of, 714
  tumor-specific antigens in, 713
  vaccine for, 708
  viral transformation in, 705–706
  viruses in:
    current strategies to determine, 715
    DNA-containing, 707–709
    hypotheses of mechanisms for, 709–712
    RNA-containing, 706–707
Candida albicans:
  after antibiotic therapy, 415
  crystal violet effect on, 362
  infections due to, 575
  vaginitis due to, 672t
Candida species:
  chemotherapy of, 405t
  identification of, 547
  in mouth flora, 584, 585t
  osmotic pressure and growth of, 325t
  survival in distilled water, 325
Candidiasis, 575
  mechanism of disease by causative agent, 435t
  of oral cavity, 590–592
Candle jar technique, 256
Canker sore, 594
Canning, 759–761
Capillaries, 646
Capneic incubation, 256
Capneic organisms, 243
Capsid, 212, 216
Capsomeres, 213
Capsule:
  bacterial, 123–124
  and invasiveness, 436
  in yeast, 162
Carbenicillin, 393–394
Carbohydrates, 84
  in cells, 80
  disaccharides, 85
  glycosides, 84–85
  metabolism of, 272–273
    anaerobic, 274–276
    electron transport system in, 278–279
    energy metabolism in, 273–274, 279–280
    fat metabolism interrelated with, 280
    glycolysis, 274–276
    Krebs cycle, 276–278
    protein metabolism interrelated with, 280–281
  monosaccharides, 85
  polysaccharides, 85–86
Carbon cycle, 340–342
Carbon dioxide:
  in carbon cycle, 340–341
  incubation with, 256
  requirements by bacteria for growth, 243
Carbon monoxide metabolism, 341
Carboxysomes, 131
Carbuncle, 425, 564t, 569
Carcinoembryonic antigen (CEA), 713
Carcinogenesis, 703
  DNA viruses in, 707–709
  stages in, 704f
Carcinogens:
  Ames/*Salmonella* test for, 713
  bacteria synthesis of, 712
  microbial, 712
Carcinoma, 705
Cardinal temperatures, 244
Carotenoids, 110
Carrier, 529
  convalescent, 529
  diphtheria, 602
  in food handler, 533
  incubatory, 529
  shigella, 632
Catabolism, 3, 272
  end products of, 246
  energy production during, 279–280
Catalase, 553

Catalyst, 94
Cationic detergents, 363
Caulobacter, 146t
  division cycle of, 151
  prostheca in, 150–151
Cauterization, 357
Cefazolin, 394
Cell mass determination, 262–263
Cell membrane, 103–104
Cell theory, 101–102
Cell wall:
  in classification of microorganisms, 33
  functions of, 124
  L-forms and, 127
  penicillin effect on, 394–395
  structure of, 109, 124–126
Cell-mediated immunity, 458, 460, 495, 501–507
Cells, 101
  anatomy of:
    animal, 103–108
    plant, 109–112
  bacterial:
    dormant structures produced by, 132–139
    as model, 145
    shape of, 116, 118
    size of, 116, 117f
    structures interior to cell wall in, 127–132
    surfaces of, 119–127
  cancerous, 703
  contact inhibition of, 703
  differentiation of, 132
  eucaryotic, 102, 103f, 112
  inclusions in, 112
  internal membrane-associated structures in:
    endoplasmic reticulum, 105–106
    golgi complex, 107
    lysosomes, 107
    microbodies, 107
    mitochondria, 105
    ribosomes, 106–107
  mechanical disintegration of, 119
  nucleolus of, 101, 102f, 105
  nucleus of, 101, 104–105
  organelles in, 102–103
  organization of, 102
  plant, 109–112
  procaryotic, 102
  stalk, 177
  viral transformation of, 705–706
Cellulose, 86
  decomposition as energy source, 342
Celsius degree, 50
Central nervous system:
  functions of, 682
  infections of, 682
    brain abscess, 682–684
    meningitis, 684–685
    protozoan, 690–693
    viral, 686–690
  organization of, 681–682
Cephalexin, 394
Cephaloridine, 394
Cephalosporins, 393–394
Cephalosporium, 394
Cephalothin, 394
Cerceriae, fork-tailed, 730
Cerebrospinal fluid, 682
Cervical smear, 712
Cestodes:
  infestations by, 727, 728t
  life cycle of, 727
Chagas' disease, 693
  in animals, 531t
  causative agent of, 693
  insects involvement in, 538
  transmission of, 531t, 693
Chancre:
  hard, 676
  soft, 670–671
Chancroid, 670–672
  causative agent of, 670
  diagnosis of, 671
Chediak-Higashi syndrome, 424
Cheese production, 754–755
Chemical preservatives, 761–762
Chemoautotrophs, 155
Chemolitotrophs, 155
Chemotaxis, 423
Chemotherapy:
  of fungi, 403–405
  history of, 26, 387
  principles of, 388–390
  of protozoa, 404
  upset in normal flora by, 415
  of viruses, 405–407
  See also Antibiotics; Antimicrobial agents
Chickenpox:
  chemotherapy of, 406t
  control of, 577
  identity to virus causing shingles, 577
  immune serum globulin to prevent, 517
  immunity after, 462, 577
  in oral cavity, 593t
  virus causing, 228t
Chigger, 538
Chitin, 168
Chlamydia, 147t
  differences from viruses, 154
  diseases caused by, 154, 608, 674, 698
  lymphogranuloma venereum caused by, 674
  properties of, 154
Chlamydia psittaci:
  chemotherapy of, 391t
  in psittacosis, 608
Chlamydia trachomatis:
  chemotherapy of, 391t
  in trachoma, 698
Chlonothrix, 150
Chloramphenicol:
  effect on spore germination, 137
  range of activity of, 395
Chlorine, 360t, 361
Chlorobium vesicles, 130
Chlorophycophyta, 197–198
Chlorophyll, 110
  in bacteria, 283
  in photosynthesis, 111
Chloroplasts, 101
  duplication of, 311
  function of, 110–111
  structure of, 110
Cholera, 626, 628
  lice in transmission of, 537
  mechanism of disease by causative agent, 435t
  organism causing, 61t, 245
  prevention of, 629
  recommended immunization for, 521t
  transmission of, 533, 537, 628
  vaccine for, 512t, 521t
  See also Vibrio cholerae
Chromatium, 146t
Chromatography, 293–294
Chromoplastids, 109
Chromosomes:
  DNA and, 299
  location in nucleus, 104
Chrysanthemum stunt, 236
Chrysophycophyta, 198–201
Chylomicrons, 416
Cidal effect, 389
Cilia:
  of protozoa, 182, 187
  role in immunity, 412
Ciliata, 187–188
Circulatory system:
  bacterial infections of:
    plague, 648–651
    relapsing fever, 650–652
    rheumatic fever, 647
    subacute bacterial endocarditis, 648
    tularemia, 650t, 653–654
    typhoid fever, 650t, 654
  components of, 646–647
  in pathogenesis of infectious diseases, 644–645
  protozoan infections of, 654–656
    kala azar, 654–655, 658t
    malaria, 655–656, 658t
  rickettsial diseases of, 651t, 652
    epidemic typhus, 650–653
    flea-borne typhus, 650t, 651, 653
    rickettsialpox, 650–651t, 653
    Rocky Mountain spotted fever, 650–651t, 653
    scrub typhus, 650–651t, 653
Cirrhosis, 624
Cirri, 182
Cisternae in golgi complex, 107
Citric acid cycle, 276–278
Citric acid production, 742
Citrobacter, 146t
  antibiotic resistance in, 399
  opportunistic infections by, 440t
Citrobacter freundii, 399
Citrus exocortis, 236
Classes, 32
Classification:
  of all life forms, 31–32
  bacterial, 33–34
  computer analysis in, 40
  five-kingdom approach, 34, 37–38
  genetic characteristics in, 41
  Linnaean system, 32
  natural versus artificial, 31
  phylogenetic, 31
  trends in, 40–41
  of viruses, 39–40
Claviceps purpurea, 171
Clindamycin, 395
Clock plate technique, 255
Clones, 32
  in antibody formation, 461
Clonorchiasis, 729t, 732t
Clostridium, 147t
  in checking anaerobic systems, 258
  exotoxins producing disease, 439t
  female genital tract infections by, 669
  fermentation in, 275
  in gas gangrene, 564t, 566
  hyaluronidase and invasiveness of, 437
  identification of, 556
  infections of, 571
    tetanus, 571
    wound botulism, 571
  meningitis caused by, 685
  mercury methylation in, 351
  opportunistic infections of, 440t
  in organic alcohol production, 742t, 743
  spore germination in, 137
  spore staining of, 63
  spores in, 132, 134
  streptokinase and invasiveness, 437
  See also Botulism; Gas gangrene; Tetanus
Clostridium bifermentans, 137
Clostridium botulinum:
  bacteriophage influence on exotoxin, 439
  as cause of botulism, 634
  disease potential of, 316–317
  exotoxin of, 439t, 440
  heat-resistance of spores of, 372
  in wound botulism, 571
Clostridium cochlearium, 351
Clostridium novyi, 439t
Clostridium perfringens:
  exotoxin producing disease, 439t, 441
  occurrence of poisoning by, 635
  virulence and capsule of, 124
  in water quality determination, 777
Clostridium tetani:
  chemotherapy of, 390t
  disease caused by, 571
  exotoxin of, 439t, 441
Clotrimazole, 405t
Coagulase, 436–437
Cocci:
  pathogenic, 553–554
  variety of arrangements of, 116, 118f
Coccidioides immitis, 615
Coccidioidomycosis, 614–615, 617t
  antimycotic agents for, 405t
  immunity after, 615
  in oral cavity, 592t
  skin test for, 482t
  specimen collection in, 549t
  transmission of, 615
Cocco-bacilli, 116, 118
Cockroaches, 539
Coenzyme, 94, 247
Cofactor, 94
Cohn, Ferdinand, 33
Cold hemagglutination, 471
Cold sore, 576t
Cold sterilization, 359
Colicin, 310
Coliforms:
  in detecting water contamination, 775–776

in urinary tract infections, 663
See also Escherichia coli
Colistin, 397
Colon, 624
Colony, 145
Colony counts, 264–265
Colony-forming units, 264–265
Colorimeter, 263
Colostrum, 463–464
Commensalism, 187, 335
Common cold, 606t
control of, 605
rhinoviruses in, 605
virus causing, 228t
Communicable diseases, 527
See also Infectious diseases
Compatibility testing, 487–488
Competence factor, 305
Competition in ecosystem, 330
Complement:
deficiencies of, 430t
role in immunity, 426–427
Complement fixation, 475–477
mechanism of, 477
procedure for, 475–477
in serologic diagnosis, 469t, 477
Compost, 326, 784
Compound, 78
Condenser, 56
in phase microscopy, 65
Congenital infections, 679
Congenital syphilis, 677–678
Congenital toxoplasmosis, 691
Conidia:
bacterial, 132
endospore differentiated from, 398
Conjugation, 304
in bacteria, 306–307
in protozoa, 186
Conjunctiva, 694
normal flora of, 695
Conjunctivitis:
gonococcal, 695–597
inclusion, 696t, 698
Contact dermatitis, 503–504
Contact inhibition, 703
Contact skin sensitivity, 503
Contagion, 22
Contagious diseases, 532
See also Infectious diseases
Convalescent carrier, 529
Coombs test:
direct, 488
indirect, 488
Coprozoic parasites, 718–719
Cornea, 694
infections involving, 697–699
Coronavirus, 228t
Corynebacteria, 147t
hydrocarbon degradation by, 349
identification of, 554
as immunological stimulator for cancer, 714
lipid inclusions in, 131
opportunistic infections of, 440t
phytotoxins of, 442
pili in, 122
Corynebacterium diphtheriae:
arrangement of cells of, 118
bacteriophage influence on exotoxin of, 439
as cause of diphtheria, 602
culture medium for, 250
exotoxin producing disease, 439t
identification of, 554
lysogenic conversion in, 310
metachromatic granules in, 130
See also Diphtheria
Corynebacterium parvum, 714
Coulter counter, 267
Counting chamber, 267
Cowdria, 147t
pathogenicity, 154
Coxiella burnetti, 147t
chemotherapy of, 391t
pasteurization in control of, 375
in Q fever, 608
Coxsackievirus, 637, 686–687
Crenothrix, 146t
sheath-forming ability of, 150
Cresylacetate, 362
Cristae, 105
Cristispira, 146t, 152
Cross matching, 487–488
Cross-reactions, 475
Croup, 606
Cryoduric, 244
Cryptococcosis:
antimycotic agents for, 405t
in oral cavity, 592t
pathogenesis of, 435t
survival in distilled water, 327
Cryptococcus neoformans:
capsule of, 162
destructive effects of, 162f
identification of, 547
Crystal violet, 362
Culex mosquitoes, 538
in filariasis, 723
Cultivation:
of algae, 196
of animal viruses, 230–234
of bacteria, 145
acidity or alkalinity and, 244–245
aerobic incubation in, 256
anaerobic incubation in, 256–258
anaerobic transfer in, 255–256
biphasic system, 261
capneic incubation in, 256
cell mass determination and, 262–263
chemical analyses in, 263
colony counts in, 264–265
continuous cultures in, 261–262
dialysis bag technique, 261
different categories of media in, 249–251
dry weight measures in, 262–263
gaseous requirements and, 243–244
inoculation and transfer techniques in, 251–254
media properties for, 245–248
nutritional conditions in, 243
oxidation-reduction potential and, 244
pour-plate technique in, 254
preparation of media for, 248
protection of personnel in, 259
purposes of, 248–249
on solid media, 262
streak-plate technique in, 254–255
thermal conditions and, 244
turbidity in, 264
vessels used in, 242
viable counts and, 264–267
in vitro, 242
in vivo, 242
of bacteriophages, 221–222
of cyanophages, 227
early techniques of, 25–26
of fungi, 168–169
of plant viruses, 234–235
of protozoa, 187
of viruses, 264–265
Cultures:
blood, 551–552
starter, 751, 753
See also Cultivation
Cyanobacteria:
carboxysomes in, 131
in ecosystem, 324
endospores in, 132
nitrogen fixation by, 343–344
phosphorus cycle and, 346
See also Blue-green bacteria
Cyanocobalamine synthesis, 741t
Cyanophages, 226–227
Cystitis, 663t, 666
Cysts:
bacterial, 132, 137–138
protozoan, 185
Cytology, 7, 101
Cytomegalovirus inclusion disease, 636t, 637, 679
Cytopathic effect, 232–233, 445
Cytophaga, 146t
cellulose decomposition by, 330
Cytoplasm, 102
anatomy of, 103–104
genetic activity in, 311–313
Cytoplasmic membrane, 103–104
Cytopyge, 183
Cytosine, 86
Cytosine arabinoside, 405–407
Cytotoxic hypersensitivity, 500

D

D value, 371–372
Dairy products production, 753–755
Dane particle, 639
Dark reaction, 111
Dark reactivation, 378
Dark-field microscopy, 63
Darwin, Charles, 43, 298
Deamination, 301
Deer-fly fever. *See* Tularemia
Degranulation, 424
deLamarck, Jean Baptiste, 298
Delayed hypersensitivity, 495, 501–502
allergy of infection, 502–503
Delbrück, M., 302–303
Denaturation, 93
Dengue fever, 538t
Denitrification, 279, 345
Dental caries, 589
Dental plaque, 583
in periodontal disease, 588
and tooth decay, 589
Deoxyribonucleic acid. *See* DNA
Deoxyribose, 85
Dermacentor, 653
Dermatophytes, 572–573
Desensitization, 499–500
Desulfotomaculum, 346
Desulfovibrio, 146t
anaerobic respiration in, 279
sulfur metabolism by, 346
Detergents, 360t, 363
Deuteromycetes, 169t
harmful effects of, 172–173
reproduction by, 172
Diabetes:
coxsackieviruses implicated in cause of, 686–687
opportunistic infections in, 440t
Diagnosis. *See* Identification of disease agent
Dialysis bag technique, 261
Diatomaceous earth, 198
Diatoms:
importance of, 200–201
properties of, 198–201
reproduction of, 200, 204f
silicon requirement of, 247
structure of, 198
use in filtration sterilization, 379–380
Dick test, 482
Didinium, 187
Differential count, 419
Differential media, 249–250
Differentiation, 132
DiGeorge's syndrome, 493
Dimorphic fungi, 165
Dinoflagellates, 203
Diphtheria:
antibody production to toxin of, 452, 516–517
exotoxin involved in, 439t, 441
immunity after, 603
lysogenic conversion in toxin production in, 310
mechanism of disease by causative agent, 435t
membrane in, 602
organism causing, 61t
passive agglutination in detection of, 471
passive immunization against, 464
prevention of, 603
Schick test for, 603
skin test for, 482
specimen collection in, 548t
toxoid preparation for, 513
transmission of, 602
of upper respiratory tract, 601–603
vaccine for, 512t
See also Corynebacterium diphtheriae
Diphtheria-pertussis-tetanus (DPT), 515, 603
complications of, 520t
Diphtheroids, 555
Diplococci, 116, 118f
See also Neisseria gonorrhoeae; Streptococcus pneumoniae
Disaccharides, 85
Disease:
chemotherapy for, 26
germ theory of, 22–24

Disinfectants, 357
alcohol, 359–361
aldehydes, 360t, 364
bacteriostatic-bactericidal test, 366–367
beta-propiolactone, 365
chemical, 358–359
chlorine, 361t
detergents, 363
ethyl alcohol, 365
formaldehyde vapor, 364–365
gaseous, 364–365
heavy metals, 360t, 363–364
mercury, 363
methyl bromide vapor, 365
phenol-coefficient test on, 365–366
phenols, 361–362
testing methods for, 365–367
tissue toxicity test, 367
use-dilution test on, 366
viral, 367
See also Sterilization
Disodium carbenicillin, 393
Distilled alcoholic beverages, 739
Divisions, 32
DNA, 86
in bacterial cells, 129
in bacterial endospores, 135
in bacteriophage, 8f
in chromosomes, 104, 299
composition of, 300
in F particles, 307–308
genetic code and, 90, 285–286
genetic function of, 90, 299
hybridization of, 316
implicated in autoimmune disease, 451t
ionizing radiation effect on, 378
manipulation of, 316–319
mutagenic agents on, 90, 301
in oncogenic viruses, 707–709
in plant viruses, 234
in plasmids, 310
recombinant, 316–319
potential benefits of, 316
potential hazards of, 316–317
techniques for, 317–319
replication in bacteriophage infections, 225
restriction endonuclease effect on, 317–318
structure of, 89–90
in transduction, 309
transformation by, 304–306
ultraviolet radiation effect on, 377–378
in viruses, 212–213, 218t, 228t
and carcinogenesis, 707–709
Domagk, Gerhard, 390
Dormancy, 132–134
Double diffusion test, 473
DPT. *See* Diphtheria-pertussis-tetanus
Dracunculus medinensis, 722t
Droplet nucleus airborne infections, 534
Drug diffusion method, 400–402
Drug resistance:
mechanisms of, 398–400
transferable, 399–401
Dry heat. *See* Sterilization, heat
Dry socket infections, 586
Drying foods, 759
Duodenum, 623
Durham tube, 290–291
Dyes:
fluorescent, 64
in staining, 58
Dysentery. *See* Amoebic dysentery; Bacillary dysentery

E

Ear infections, 603, 604t
Echinococcus, 728t
skin test for, 482t
Echoviruses, 637
Ecology, 323
of gastrointestinal tract, 624–625
microbial, 7
oral, 583–584
water cycle in, 767–768
Ecosystem, 323–324
abiotic factors in, 325–327
action in, 329–330
bioconcentration in, 352–353
bioconversion reactions in, 348–352
biogeochemical cycles in, 340–347
biotic factors in, 325
carbon cycle in, 340–342
categories of living organisms in, 324
coaction in, 329–330
competition in, 325, 330
components of, 325–328
consumers in, 324
decomposers in, 324
food chain in, 324
hydrocarbon degradation in, 349–350
manganese metabolism in, 352
mercury methylation in, 351–352
methanogenesis in, 348–349
microbial interactions in, 329–336
natural habitats of microorganisms in, 328–329
nitrogen assimilation in, 344–345
nitrogen cycle in, 342–345
nitrogen fixation in, 342–344
nitrogen recovery in, 345
oxygen cycle in, 346–347
pesticide metabolism in, 351–352
phosphorus cycle in, 345–346
pollutants effect on, 328
predation in, 330
producers in, 324
radioisotope accumulation in, 352–353
reactions of concern in, 329–330, 347–353
sulfur cycle in, 346
symbiosis in, 330–336
syntropism in, 330
Ectoparasites, 718
Ectosymbiotic, 330–331
Ectothrix infection, 574
Edema, 425
Edwardsiella, 146t
Eelworms, 726
Ehrlich, Paul, 26, 62, 387
Ehrlichia, 147t
disease in dogs caused by, 154
pathogenicity of, 154
Electron microscope, 49
high-voltage, 72
immune, 480
immunological procedure using, 469t
light microscope compared with, 67t
scanning, 73
specimen preparation for, 69–72
transmission, 65–68
Electron staining, 70
Electron transport system, 278–279
Electronic counting, 267
Electrons, 78
Elementary bodies, 154
Elements, 78
Ellerman, V., 706
Embryonated eggs:
in animal virus cultures, 230–231
candled, 231
Encephalitis:
alphavirus, 689, 690t
in animals, 531t
arthropod-borne, 684t, 689–690
flavivirus, 689, 690t
mode of transmission of, 531t, 538t
Endemic, 527
Endocarditis, 647
subacute bacterial, 648
Endocardium, 646
Endoparasites, 718
Endoplasmic reticulum, 105–106
Endospores:
activation of, 136
bacterial, 132–134, 147t
baeocytes, 156
characteristics of, 134–135
chemical makeup of, 135–136
conidia differentiated from, 138
dormancy of, 134
formation of, 134–136
germination of, 136–137
outgrowth of, 137
thermal resistance of, 136
See also Spores
Endosymbionts, 235
Endosymbiotic, 330–331
Endotoxin, 437–438
as antitumor agent, 714
detection of, 438
exotoxin compared to, 438t
interferon stimulation by, 428
modes of action of, 438, 439
in Shwartzman reaction, 501
Endozoic, 197
Energy metabolism, 273–274
Energy production, 279–280
English system, 50
Entamoeba coli, 335
Entamoeba histolytica, 185, 189, 640
See also Amoebae; Amoebic dysentery
Enterobacter, 146t
development of antibiotic resistance in, 399
Enterobacter aerogenes:
in amino acid synthesis, 741t, 742
inhibition of *Candida* by, 415
Enterobiasis. *See* Pinworms
Enterobius vermicularis, 722t
Enteropathic *Escherichia coli*, 633
Enterotoxin, 441
Enteroviruses. *See* Picornaviruses
Enveloped viruses, 215
Environment, 323
aquatic, 767–773
marine, 771–773
See also Ecosystem
Enzymes:
conjugated, 94–95
factors affecting activity of, 95–96
functions of, 93–95
immobilized, 744
industrial production of, 743–744
mechanism of action, 95–96
pH effect on, 81
simple, 94
use in filtration sterilization, 382
Eosin Methylene Blue (EMB) agar, 254
Eosinophilia, 720
Eosinophils, 419
Epidemic, 527
Epidemic keratoconjunctivitis, 700
Epidemic typhus:
features of, 650–653
transmission of, 652–653
See also Typhus
Epidemiology, 527
Episomes, 310
in eucaryotes, 312
in *Staphylococcus aureus*, 311
Epstein, M. A., 708
Epstein-Barr virus:
in infectious mononucleosis, 708
in liver disease, 639
in lymphoma, 708
Ergot production by fungi, 171
Ergotism, 443
Erwinia, 442
Erysipelas, 564t, 570
Erysipelothrix, 147t
Erythroblastosis fetalis, 486–487
Erythrocytes, 418
Erythrogenic toxin, 439, 441
Escherichia coli, 146t
in amino acid synthesis, 741t, 742
antibiotic resistance development in, 399
autoradiograph of, 293
bacteriocin in, 310
bacteriophages attacking, 219, 221, 223–224
in carcinogen detection test, 713
chemotherapy of, 391t
as commensal, 335
conjugation in, 306
continuous culture of, 262
culture requirements of, 244
DNA hybridization in, 316
enteropathogenic, 633
in food poisoning, 634
in gastrointestinal tract, 625
genetic mapping in, 313–314

heat-resistance of, 372
immunizing properties of, 513
inhibition of *Candida* by, 415
isoleucine synthesis by, 288
in kidney infections, 665, 666
manometry to measure metabolism in, 291
mutation to bacteriophage resistance, 302
mutational research with, 302
opportunistic infections of, 440t
recombinant DNA studies in, 317–319
resistance transfer factor plasmids in, 318–319
restriction endonuclease in, 317–318
survival after ultraviolet radiation, 378
turbidity measurement in cultures of, 263
Ester formation, 80
Estuaries, 771–772
Ethyl alcohol, 365
Ethylene oxide, 360t, 364
Ethylhydrocupreine hydrochloride, 554
Eucaryotes, 102, 103f
cellular organization in, 34–36
cytoplasmic inheritance in, 311–313
organelles in, 112t
procaryotes compared with, 36t
viruses associated with, 235–236
See also Algae; Fungi; Protozoa
Euglenoids, 201–202
Eustachian tube, 597
Eutrophication, 770
Evaporation, 767
Evolution, 41–45, 298
Exocytosis, 103
Exoenzymes, 128
Exospore, 133, 135
Exotoxin, 437
algal, 442
association with bacterial viruses, 439
bacterial pathogens producing, 439t
of blue-green bacteria, 442
in botulism, 440, 634
in cholera, 628
in diphtheria, 441
endotoxin compared to, 438t, 439
in *Escherichia coli* infections, 633
in food poisoning, 633–635
fungal, 443
in gas gangrene, 441
inactivation as toxoids, 464
of major clinical significance, 440–442
modes of action of, 440
mycotoxin, 443
neurotoxin, 440–442
phytotoxin, 442
in scarlet fever, 441
of *Shigella dysenteriae*, 442
staphylococcal, 441, 635
streptolysin O, 441
streptolysin S, 441–442
in tetanus, 441
Eye:
anatomy of, 693–695
flora in conjunctiva of, 695
infections of, 695
gonococcal conjunctivitis, 695–696
herpes corneales, 699
inclusion conjunctivitis, 696t, 698
pinkeye, 697
trachoma, 697t, 698
by viruses, 698–699
Eyepiece, 54

F

F particles, 307–308, 313
F_{ab} domain, 454–455
F_c domain, 454–455
F_d domain, 455
Facultative organisms:
anaerobes, 244
bacteria, 146t, 147
parasites, 718
Families, 32
Fats, 82
carbohydrate metabolism and, 280
Fatty acids, 82
Feedback inhibition, 288–289
Fermentation, 15
in alcoholic beverage production, 737–739
in amino acid production, 741–742
in butter production, 753–754
in buttermilk production, 754
in cheese production, 754–755
citric acid production by, 742
in clostridia, 275
germ theory of, 15–17
industrial, 737
lactic acid production by, 742
in measuring metabolism, 290–291
microbiology applied to, 8–9
of milk, 753–755
organic alcohol production by, 742t, 743
oxidation and reduction occurring in, 275–276
in pickling process, 751–753
in sauerkraut production, 751–752
in sour cream production, 754
in vinegar production, 740–741
of yeasts, 171
Ferritin-conjugated antibodies, 469t, 480–481
Fetal antigen, 712–713
Fever, 425–426
Fever blister, 576t, 593t, 594
Fibrinogen, 416
Fibrinolysin, 437
Filariasis, 723t
life cycle in, 723–724
nematode causing, 722t
prevention of, 724
transmission of, 723
Filariform larvae, 722
Filopodia, 181
Filter-paper disks, 400–401
Filtration, 370t, 379
air, 381–383
asbestos, 380
cellulose acetate membrane, 380–381
diatomaceous earth, 379–380
enzyme-coated, 382
fritted glass, 380
and germ theory, 19–20
high-efficiency particulate air, 383
liquid, 379–381
paper, 380
as sterilization procedure, 370
Fimbriae, 167, 168
5-Fluorocytosine, 404, 405t
Five-kingdom classification system, 34, 37–38
Flagella:
function of, 120
pili differentiated from, 122
of protozoa, 182, 189
shape and arrangement, 120
ultrastructure of, 120–122
Flagellates, 189, 190f
Flagellin, 122
Flash pasteurization, 375
Flatworms, 726–727
cestodes, 727, 728t
trematodes, 727, 729–732
Flaviviruses, 689, 690t
Flavobacterium:
flagella in, 121
temperature and growth of, 325t, 326
Flea-borne typhus, 650–651t, 653
Fleas, 537
in disease transmission, 538
life cycle of, 537–538
Fleming, Alexander, 26, 27f, 387
Flexibacter, 149
Flocculation test, 517
Flora, 413
of conjunctiva, 695
of gastrointestinal tract, 624–625
in mouth, 582–585
in respiratory tract, 599
of urinary tract, 661, 663
See also Normal flora
Flowing fresh water, 770–771
Fluke infections, 729t, 732t
Fluorescence microscopy, 63–64
Fluorescent antibody techniques:
direct method, 478–479
indirect method, 479–480
Fly, 535
Focal infection, 584–585
Fomites, 534
Food:
antibiotics in preservation of, 387
digestion of, 623–624
fermented, 751–755
infectious diseases spread by, 533
microbiology applied to, 8–9
microorganisms as, 755–757
preservation of, 761t
canning, 759–761
chemical, 761–762
drying, 759
spoilage by microorganisms, 757–759, 761
Food chain, 324
Food poisoning, 633–634
botulism, 634
exotoxin involved in, 439t
perfringens, 635
staphylococcal, 635
Foraminiferida, 188–189
Forespore, 134
Fork-tailed cercaria, 730
Formaldehyde, 364–365
Formed elements, 416
Forssmann antigen, 451–452
Fossils, 43–45
Fox, Sidney, 42, 43f
F-prime particle, 309
Framboise, 678
Francisella, 146t
Francisella tularensis:
interferon stimulation by, 428
in tularemia, 653
See also Tularemia
Freeze-fracture, 71–72
Frei test, 481
Freshwater habitats, 769
Fructose, 84f
Frustules, 198
Fungi, 161
aflatoxins produced by, 173
agricultural damage due to, 162
ascomycetes, 170–171
basidiomycetes, 171–172
cell mass determination of, 262
chemotherapy against, 403–405
classification of, 169–170
complement-fixation tests for, 478t
cultivation of, 168–169
as decomposers in ecosystem, 324
dermatophytes, 572–573
deuteromycetes, 172–173
differences from bacteria, 162
dimorphic, 165
distinctive mycelia in, 169
distribution of, 161
edible, 171
energy sources for, 162
fermentation in, 275
fimbriae in, 167, 168
in five-kingdom classification system, 137–138
as food, 756t
food spoilage associated with, 758t, 759
gasoline decomposition by, 350
harmful effects of, 171–176
identifying, 547
imperfecti, 172–173
infections due to:
blastomycosis, 615–616
Candida, 575
coccidioidomycosis, 614–615, 617t
cryptococcosis, 592t
dermatophytes, 572–575
histoplasmosis, 615
oral, 590–592
in plants, 543
respiratory, 614–616
ringworm, 573–575
skin, 571–575
latex agglutination tests for, 471–472
and lichens, 205–206
mechanisms of action in disease, 435t

Fungi (*continued*)
metachromatic granules in, 130
molds, 162, 163f
in mouth flora, 584, 585t
mutualism with garden-cultivating ant, 332
myxomycetes, 175–177
nitrate metabolism by, 345
in normal flora, 414t
oomycetes, 174
in penicillin production, 739–740
pH effect on growth, 245, 326
in plant diseases, 543
recombinant DNA studies on, 319
reproduction of, 165–166
salt concentration and growth of, 325–327
selective medium for, 249
in single-cell protein, 756t
skin diseases caused by, 571–575
skin tests for, 482t
specimen collection for, 549t
spores of, 165–167
structure of, 162–165
superficial, 572
surfaces of, 168
toxins of, 443
ultrastructure of, 167–168
viruses of, 236
yeasts, 162, 164f, 165
zinc action on, 363–364
zoonoses of, 531t
zygomycetes, 174–175
Fungi imperfecti, 572
Fungicide, 357t
Fungistatic, 357t
Furuncle, 564t, 569
See also Staphylococci; *Staphylococcus aureus*
Fusobacterium, 146t

G

Gaffky, Georg, 254
Gall, 726
Gamma globulin, 517–518
See also Immunoglobulins
Gamma-hemolysis, 249
Gamma-hemolytic streptococci, 569
Gas chromatography, 294
Gas gangrene, 564t, 566
exotoxin in, 439t, 441
organisms causing, 566
passive immunization against, 464
specimen collection in, 548t
transmission of, 566
See also Clostridium; Clostridium perfringens
Gas Pak system, 556
Gas vacuoles, 132
Gastrointestinal immunity, 412
Gastrointestinal tract, 622
bacterial infections of, 625–626
bacillary dysentery, 626t, 631–632
botulism, 634
brucellosis, 626t, 629
cholera, 626–629
food poisoning, 633–635
gram-negative, 627t
infant epidemic diarrhea, 633
leptospirosis, 626t, 629–630
salmonellosis, 626t, 630–631
traveler's diarrhea, 626t, 633
typhoid fever, 626t, 632
microbial ecology of, 624–625
normal flora of, 624–625
parts of, 622–624
protozoan infections of:
amoebic dysentery, 640, 641t
balantidiasis, 641–642
giardiasis, 641t, 642
viral infections of, 636
cytomegalovirus inclusion disease, 636t, 637
hepatitis, 636–640
infectious mononucleosis, 636t
picornaviruses, 636–637
Genes, 104
amplification of, 318–319
manipulation of:
potential benefits, 316
potential hazards, 316–317
techniques for, 317–319
mapping in bacteria, 313–314
Genetic code:
DNA and, 90, 300
and protein synthesis, 285–288
Genetic engineering, 7
Genetic recombination, 299, 304
Genetics:
applications of, 314–316
and biological assays, 314–315
chemistry of, 299–301
microbial, 7
percent G + C comparison among species, 315
and taxonomy, 315–316
Genitourinary immunity, 412
Genome:
in procaryotic cells, 129
viral, 212
Gentamicin, 395–396
Genus, 32
Geotrichosis, 592t
Geotrichum, 327
Germ theory:
of disease, 22–24
of fermentation, 15–17
Germ tubes, 166
German measles. *See* Rubella
Germicide, 357t
Germination, 136–137
Giardia lamblia, 642
Giardiasis, 641t, 642
Gilchrist's disease, 615–617
Gingiva, 583
Gingivitis, 588
Gliding bacteria, 146t, 149
Globulins, 452
Glomerulonephritis, acute, 667
Glossina palpalis, 692
Glucose, 84f
See also Carbohydrates
Glucoside, 84
Glutamic acid synthesis, 741
Glutaraldehyde, 364
Glycogen, 86
Glycolysis, 274–275
Glycosides, 84–85
Golgi complex, 107
Gonidia, 150
Gonorrhea:
in adult conjunctivitis, 697
causative agent of, 671
chemotherapy of, 391t
external, 671
in eye of newborns, 674, 695–697
internal, 671, 674
mechanism of disease by causative agent, 435t
ophthalmia neonatorum, 674, 695–697
organism causing, 61t
prevention of, 363, 674
silver nitrate in prophylaxis of, 363
specimen collection in, 548t
transmission of, 532, 671
vaccine for, 512–513t
See also Neisseria gonorrhoeae
Gonyaulax catenella, 203
Graft rejection, 505–506
Graft-versus-host reaction, 505
Gram, Hans Christian, 59
Gram stain, 59–62
See also Gram-negative bacteria; Gram-positive bacteria
Gram-negative bacteria, 60–61t
aerobic bacilli, 556
aerobic diplococci, 555–556
aerobic rods, 146t
anaerobic cocci, 147t
anaerobic rods, 146t
cell wall of, 125–126
chemolithotropic, 147t
chemotherapy of, 391t
classification of, 146–147t
coccal bacilli, 146t
cocci, 146t
endotoxin formation from, 437–438
enteric, 555–556
facultatively anaerobic rods, 146t
in gastrointestinal infections, 627t, 633
identification of, 555–556
lysozyme action on, 427
MacConkey agar for culturing, 250
nonfermentative aerobic, 555
in nosocomial infections, 539
phagocytin action on, 427
phototrophs, 155
properdin action on, 428
sensitivity to ionizing radiation, 379
staining characteristics of, 59
Gram-nonreactive bacteria, 59
Gram-positive bacteria, 60–61t
bacilli, 554–555
cell wall of, 125–126
chemotherapy of, 390t
classification of, 147t
cocci, 147t
identification of, 553–555
lysozyme action on, 427
mesosomes in, 128–129
non-spore forming rods, 147t
pathogenic cocci, 553–554
staining characteristics of, 59
streptokinase and invasiveness of, 437
Gram-variable bacteria, 59, 62
Grana, 110
Granulocytes, 418
Granuloma inguinale, 672t, 674
Granuloses, 227
Green algae:
ecologic importance of, 198
economic importance of, 197–198
reproduction of, 197
structure of, 197
Griseofulvin, 404, 405t
Group A streptococci, 569
Growth, 3
lag phase, 259–260
logarithmic death rate, 261
logarithmic phase, 260
measurement of, 262–267
stationary phase, 261
Guanine, 86
Guinea worm infestation, 722t
Gummas, 677

H

H chains, 454
Habitat, 325
aquatic, 328
freshwater, 769
micro, 329
microbial, 329
terrestrial, 328
Haekel, Ernst, 34
Haemagogus mosquitoes, 538t, 539
Hair, tinea infections of, 574
Haldane, B. A., 41–43
Half-life, 292
Halobacterium, 146t
Halobacterium salinarum, 325t, 326
Haloprigin, 405t
Hand, foot and mouth disease, 593t
Hanging drop technique, 57–58
Hansen, Armauer, 566
Hansen's disease. *See* Leprosy
Hansenula, 325t
Hapten, 450
Hay fever, 496
Heart:
anatomy of, 646
diseases of, 647
rheumatic fever, 647–648
subacute bacterial endocarditis, 648
Heat sterilization. *See* Sterilization, heat
Heavy chains, 454–455
Heavy metals, 360t, 363–364
Hektoen Enteric media, 254
Helminths, 718
adaptation to parasitic existence, 718
bentonite flocculation test for, 472
complement-fixation tests for, 478t
distribution of, 720
equipment of, 718

flatworms, 726–727
fleas in transmission of, 538
hosts of, 718–720
hyaluronidase and invasiveness of, 437
identifying, 547
infections of:
cestodes, 727, 728t
eosinophilia in, 720
filariasis, 723–724
hookworm, 722–725
laboratory diagnosis in, 720
mechanism of action in, 435t
nematodes, 722–726
in plants, 726
symptoms in, 720
transmission of, 538, 720
treatment of, 720
trematodes, 727, 729–732
trichinosis, 722–723t, 725, 726f
life cycle of, 719–720
skin test for, 482t
Hemagglutination, 470–471
cold, 471
in embryonated egg viral cultures, 231
pili detected by, 122
in serologic diagnosis, 469t
Hemagglutination inhibition (HI), 469t, 472
Hemoglobin, 418
Hemolysin, 476
Hemolysis tests:
antistreptolysin, 477–478
complement fixation, 475–477
Hemolytic disease of newborn, 486–487
Hemolytic streptococci, 553–554, 569
Hemophilus, 146t
opportunistic infections of, 440t
in pinkeye, 697
Hemophilus aegypticus, 697
Hemophilus ducreyi, 670–672
Hemophilus influenzae:
capsule and invasiveness of, 436
chemotherapy of, 391t
growth factors required by, 247
role in influenza, 616
Henle, Jacob, 23
Hepatitis. *See* Viral hepatitis
Hepatitis B surface antigen, 639, 640
Hepatitis virus, 638–639
danger of infection with, 371
disinfection of, 367
immune electron microscopy for, 480
prevention of infection by, 517, 639–640
See also Viral hepatitis
Hermaphroditic, 727
Herpangina, 593
Herpesviruses, 228t, 576–578
chemotherapy against, 406t
congenital infection by, 679
eye infections by, 699
fluorescent antibody technique for, 480
genital infection by, 672t, 678
latent infections of, 444
mechanism of action in disease, 435t
in oral cavity, 593t, 594
role in cancer, 707–709
skin infections of:
chickenpox, 576t, 577
herpes simplex, 576t, 577
herpes zoster, 576–578
structure of, 215
Heterocysts, 138, 157
Heterofermentative, 275
Heterophile antigens, 451–452
Heterotrophs, 147–155, 281, 282t
and bacterial cultures, 243
chemosynthetic, 285
in ecosystems, 324
photosynthetic, 284–285
protozoa as, 182
Hexachlorophene, 362
Hexuronic acids, 109
Hfr cells, 308–309, 313
High frequency of recombination, 308–309, 313
High temperature short time method, 375
High-efficiency particulate air (HEPA) filtration, 383
High-voltage electron microscopy, 72
Histocompatibility antigens, 504–505
Histoplasma capsulatum, 615
Histoplasmosis:
mechanism of disease by causative agent, 435t
in oral cavity, 592t
skin test for, 482t
specimen collection in, 549t
transmission of, 615, 617t
Hives, 496
Holozoic protozoa, 182–183
Homofermentative, 275
Hooke, Robert, 49f, 101
Hookworm, 723t, 724
Hormogonia, 138, 157
Hospital infections. *See* Nosocomial infections
Host, 9, 335
definitive, 719
different types of, 719
reservoir, 719
Host-controlled modification, 222
Host-versus-graft reaction, 505
Humus, 766
Hyaluronidase, 437
Hybrid DNA, 316
Hydrocarbon degradation, 349
Hydrogen bond, 79
Hydrogen peroxide, 362
Hydrogenomonas, 284t
Hydrophilic, 83, 104, 363
Hydrophobia. *See* Rabies
Hydrophobic, 83, 104, 363
Hydrosphere, 328
Hyperplasia, 703
Hypersensitivity, 494
allergy of infection, 502–503
Arthus reaction, 500–501
atopy, 498–500
autoimmunity, 506–507
categories of, 494–496
cell-mediated, 501–507
classic intermediate, 496
contact dermatitis, 503–504
cytotoxic, 500
delayed, 495, 501–507
factors in determining, 497
immediate, 495
immune-complex mediated, 500–501
serum sickness, 501
Shwartzman reaction, 501
tissue transplantation reactions, 504–506
Type I, 496–500
Type II, 500
Type III, 500–501
Type IV, 501–507
See also Immunity
Hyphae, 162, 163f
Hyphomicrobium, 146t, 151
Hypochlorite, 361
Hyposensitization, 499–500
Hypotrophs, 243

I

Id reaction, 574
Identification of disease agent:
acid-fast bacteria, 556–557
anaerobic bacteria, 556
approaches to, 546–548
bacteria, 547
biochemical testing in, 550–551
blood cultures in, 551–552
fungi, 547
general procedures for, 552
gram-negative bacteria, 556
gram-positive bacteria, 553–555
helminths, 547
media in, 550–551
protozoa, 547
quality control in, 557–558
specimen collection in, 548–549
IgA, 456–457, 495
IgD, 456, 495
IgE, 456, 495, 499
IgG. *See* Immunoglobulin G
IgM, 456–457, 495, 500
Ileum, 623
Immune cytolysis, 475
Immune globulins, 416, 418
See also Immunoglobulins
Immune response, 449–450
Immune serum, 516
Immune serum globulin:
for hepatitis exposure, 640
recommendation in travelers, 521t
use in passive immunization, 517–518
Immune system, 410–411
antibody formation in, 449
blood components role in, 416–419
deficiency in Chediak-Higashi syndrome, 424
inflammation in, 424–426
leukocytes in, 418–419
lymphatic system, 419–420
mechanisms in, 415
phagocytosis, 421–424
reticuloendothelial system, 420
serum globulins in, 416, 418
use in cancer treatment, 714
See also Antibodies; Immunity
Immune-complex-mediated hypersensitivity, 500–501
Immunity:
acquired, 462–465
active, 462–464
adoptive, 464–465
antibody production in, 456
artificially acquired, 464–465
and cancer, 713
cell-mediated, 458
complement in, 426–427
conditions hindering, 429–431
deficiencies in, 430t
development of, 457–461
disorders of:
anaphylaxis, 496–498
Arthus reaction, 500–501
atopy, 498–500
autoimmune diseases, 506–507
cytotoxic, 500
hypersensitivity, 494–507
primary immunodeficiencies, 493
secondary immunodeficiencies, 493–494
Shwartzman reaction, 501
and transplantation, 504–506
eyes in, 412
gastrointestinal, 412
genitourinary, 412
humoral, 458
immunoglobulin properties relating to, 454t
importance of, 492–493
innate, 462
interferon in, 426t, 428–429
leukins in, 426t, 427
lymphocytes role in, 458–460
lysozyme in, 426t, 427
mechanical barriers, 411–412
mucous membranes, 412
naturally acquired, 462–464
nonspecific, 411
passive, 462–465
phagocytin in, 426–428
properdin in, 426t, 428
skin in, 412, 561
species resistance, 411
specific, 410
spermine in, 426t, 428
states of, 462–465
thymus gland role in, 457–458
tissue antimicrobial substances in, 426
transplacental, 458, 463–464
See also Antibodies; Antigens; Immune system
Immunization:
for international travel, 521
methods of, 464
passive, 452, 487, 516–518
schedule recommended for, 515t
value of, 510–511
See also Vaccines
Immunodeficiencies, 493–494
Immunodepression, 435t
Immunodiffusion, 469t
applied to *Corynebacterium diphtheriae* culture, 310
radial, 473–474
Immunoelectron microscopy, 469t
Immunoelectrophoresis, 452, 453f
two-dimensional, 474
Immunofluorescence, 64
Immunogenicity, 449–450

Immunogens, 449
antigen determinant sites on, 450
primary response to, 456
secondary response to, 456
properties of, 449
Immunoglobulin A (IgA), 456–457, 495
Immunoglobulin D (IgD), 456, 495
Immunoglobulin E (IgE), 456, 495, 499
Immunoglobulin G (IgG), 456–457
role in hypersensitivity, 495, 500
transplacental transfer of, 458
use in passive immunization, 517–518
Immunoglobulin M (IgM), 456–457, 495, 500
Immunoglobulins, 453
in autoimmune disorders, 507
failure to produce, 493
in hypersensitivity, 495
implicated in autoimmune disease, 451t
in multiple myeloma, 493–494
normal flora and, 415
properties of, 454t
sources in man, 456–457
structure of, 454–455
subclasses of, 453–454
use in passive immunization, 517–518
See also Antibodies
Immunologic paralysis, 462
Immunologic procedures:
antisera production for, 470
blood compatibility testing, 487–488
blood typing, 484
Coombs test, 488
cross matching, 487–488
with electron microscopy, 480–481
ferritin-conjugated antibodies, 480–481
fluorescent antibody techniques, 478–480
in identifying microorganisms, 469t
immunohematology, 482–487
incorporating differential staining, 478–480
precipitin reaction, 472–475
Rh typing, 485–487
rising antibody titers in, 470
skin tests, 481–482
virus neutralization, 481
in vitro hemolysis tests, 475–478
in vivo, 481–482
See also Serology
Immunological tolerance, 506
Immunology, 5
Immunosuppression, 430t
to inhibit graft rejection, 506
methods for, 461–462
opportunistic infections due to, 440t
Immunotherapy, 499–500
Impetigo:
features of, 564t
streptococci associated with, 570
transmission of, 569
In vitro, 242
In vivo, 242
Incidental parasites, 718
Inclusion conjunctivitis, 696t, 698
Inclusions:
in bacteria, 130–132
in cells, 112
membrane-enclosed, 131–132
Incubation:
aerobic, 256
anaerobic, 256–258
capneic, 256
checking anaerobic systems, 257–258
Incubatory carrier, 529
Indicator, anaerobic, 257–258
Industrial microbiology, 737
aerobic versus anaerobic processes in, 737
alcohol production, 737–739
amino acid production, 741–742
in antibiotic production, 739–740
automation in, 746
in enzyme production, 743–744
fermentation processes, 737–743
food fermentation, 751–755
food preservation, 759–762
food spoilage, 757–759
in insecticide production, 745, 746t
steroid transformation, 744
use of microorganisms as food, 755–757
vinegar production, 740–741
vitamin production, 741t, 742
Infant epidemic diarrhea, 633
Infectious diseases, 435
acute glomerulonephritis, 667
acute pyelonephritis, 663t, 665–666
African sleeping sickness, 691–693
amoebic dysentery, 640, 641t
amoebic meningoencephalitis, 693
by animal viruses, 227, 229
anthrax, 562–564, 566
by bacteriophages, 222–226
balantidiasis, 641–642
blastomycosis, 615–617
botulism, 634
brucellosis, 626t, 629
candidiasis, 575
Chagas' disease, 693
chancroid, 670–672
chickenpox, 576t, 577
cholera, 626–629
circulatory system role in pathogenesis, 644–645
coccidioidomycosis, 614–615, 617t
common cold, 605, 606t
congenital, 677–679, 691
croup, 606
cryptococcosis, 592t
cystitis, 663t, 666
cytomegalovirus inclusion disease, 636t, 637
delayed-type skin tests of, 503
diphtheria, 601–603
of ear, 603
endemic, 527
endotoxin in, 438
epidemic, 527
epidemic typhus, 650–653
erysipelas, 570
exotoxins and, 439–440
of eye, 695–699
conjunctivitis, 697
epidemic keratoconjunctivitis, 699
inclusion conjunctivitis, 696t, 698
of female genital tract, 669–670, 678–679
filariasis, 722–724
flea-borne typhus, 650 651t, 653
food poisoning, 633–635
of fungi:
oral, 590–592
respiratory, 614–616
skin, 571–575
gas gangrene, 564t, 566
of gastrointestinal tract, 622, 625–626
amoebic dysentery, 640, 641t
balantidiasis, 641–642
botulism, 634
brucellosis, 626t, 629
cholera, 626–629
food poisoning, 633–635
giardiasis, 641t, 642
gram-negative bacterial, 627t
hepatitis, 636–640
infant epidemic diarrhea, 633
infectious mononucleosis, 636t
leptospirosis, 626t, 629–630
protozoan, 640–642
traveler's diarrhea, 626t, 633
typhoid fever, 632
viral, 636–640
giardiasis, 641t, 642
gonorrhea, 671, 672t, 674, 695–697
granuloma inguinale, 672t, 674
of hair, 574–575
of heart, 647–648
of helminths:
cestodes, 727, 728t
filariasis, 722–724
hookworm, 722–725
laboratory diagnosis of, 720
nematodes, 722–726
symptoms of, 720
treatment of, 720
trematodes, 727, 729–732
trichinosis, 722–723t, 725, 726f
hepatitis, 636–640
herpes, 576–578
congenital, 679
corneales, 699
genital, 672, 678t
histoplasmosis, 615, 617t
hookworm, 722–725
identifying agents of, 546–548
impetigo, 570–571
infant epidemic diarrhea, 633
infectious mononucleosis, 636t, 656–657
influenza, 616–617
invasiveness and, 436–437
isolation in control of, 542
kala azar, 654–655, 658t
latent, 444
leprosy, 565–568
leptospirosis, 626t, 629–630
lymphogranuloma venereum, 672t, 674
malaria, 655–656, 658t
measles, 578–579
mechanisms of pathogens causing, 435
meningitis, 684–686
microbial toxin production in, 437–443
morbidity and mortality rates of, 527–528
mumps, 594
of mucoplasma, 607–608, 610–611t
of nails, 574
natural immunity to, 462–463
of nervous system, 682
African sleeping sickness, 691–693
amoebic meningoencephalitis, 693
arthropod-borne, 689–690
aseptic meningitis, 684t, 686
brain abscess, 682–684
Chagas' disease, 693
coxsackievirus, 686–687
meningitis, 684–685
poliomyelitis, 686
protozoan, 690–693
rabies, 687
by slow viruses, 688–689
toxoplasmosis, 690–691
viral, 686–690
noncommunicability of, 527
nosocomial, 534, 539–543
opportunistic, 440t, 445
oral, 590–594
dental caries, 589
gingivitis, 588
fungal, 590–592
Ludwig's angina, 589
osteomyelitis, 586, 587t
pericoronitis, 586, 587t
periodontal, 587–588
picornaviruses, 636–637
plague, 648–651
in plants, 235, 543
pneumococcal pneumonia, 606–607, 610–611t
by *Pneumocystis carinii*, 618
poliomyelitis, 686
prevention by immunization, 510–511
See also Vaccines
protozoan:
of gastrointestinal tract, 640–642
of nervous system, 690 693
systemic, 654–658
psittacosis, 608, 610–611t
puerperal fever, 669–670
Q fever, 608, 610–611t
rabies, 687
relapsing fever, 650–652
reportable, 528, 529t
resistance to. *See* Immune system; Immunity
of respiratory tract, 599–600
blastomycosis, 615–617
coccidioidomycosis, 614–615, 617t
common cold, 605, 606t

control of, 600
croup, 606
diagnosis of, 600
diphtheria, 601–603
histoplasmosis, 615, 617t
influenza, 616–617
mycoplasma, 607–608, 610–611t
otitis media, 601t, 603
pneumococcal pneumonia, 606–607, 610–611
by *Pneumocystis carinii*, 618
psittacosis, 608, 610–611t
Q fever, 608, 610–611t
streptococcal sore throat, 601t, 604
tuberculosis, 608–613
whooping cough, 610–611t, 614
rickettsial, 154, 650–653
rickettsialpox, 650–651t, 653
ringworm, 573–575
Rocky Mountain spotted fever, 650–651t, 653
rubella, 579–580, 679
scrub typhus, 650–651t, 653
of skin, 564–566
anthrax, 562–564, 566
candidiasis, 575
chickenpox, 576t, 577
clostridial, 571
erysipelas, 570
fungal, 571–575
gas gangrene, 564t, 566
herpes simplex, 576t, 577
herpes zoster, 576–578
impetigo, 570–571
leprosy, 565–568
poxviruses, 579–580
Pseudomonas, 564–565, 568
ringworm, 573–575
staphylococcal, 564t, 568–569
streptococcal, 569–571
viral, 575–580
warts, 578
skin tests for, 481–482
slow viral, 444, 688–689
smallpox, 580
sources and reservoirs of agents of, 528–529
sporadic, 527
streptococcal sore throat, 601t, 604
subclinical, 463
syphilis, 673–678
systemic:
malaria, 655–656, 658t
plague, 648–651
protozoan, 654–658
relapsing fever, 650–652
subacute bacterial endocarditis, 648
tularemia, 650t, 653–654
typhoid fever, 650t, 654
TORCH complex, 679
toxoplasmosis, 690–691
trachoma, 697t, 698
transmission of:
by accidental inoculation, 534
in African sleeping sickness, 692
airborne, 533–534
in amoebic dysentery, 640
in anthrax, 566
by arthropods, 534–539
autoinfection, 720
in bacillary dysentery, 631–632
in balantidiasis, 642
biological, 532
in brucellosis, 629
in cholera, 628
in coccidioidomycosis, 615
by cockroaches, 539
in cytomegalovirus inclusion disease, 637
in diphtheria, 602
by direct contact, 532
dustborne, 533–534
in epidemic typhus, 652–653
in filariasis, 723–724
by fleas, 537–538
by fomites, 534
in food poisoning, 635
in gas gangrene, 566
in gonorrhea, 671
by helminths, 720
in histoplasmosis, 615
in hookworm infection, 724
in hospital, 539–543
in impetigo, 569–571
by indirect contact, 533
in infant epidemic diarrhea, 633
in infectious mononucleosis, 656
in leptospirosis, 630
by lice, 536–537
mechanical, 531–532
by mites, 535–536
by mosquitoes, 538–539
in pinworm infections, 724–725
in plague, 649
in pneumococcal pneumonia, 607
in psittacosis, 608
in rabies, 687
in rickettsial infections, 652
in rubella, 579
in salmonellosis, 631
in scarlet fever, 570
in staphylococcal infections, 569, 635
in streptococcal infections, 570, 604
in syphilis, 676
in tetanus, 571
by ticks, 535–536
in toxoplasmosis, 690–691
in trichinosis, 725
in tuberculosis, 609
in tularemia, 653–654
in typhoid fever, 632, 654
in viral hepatitis, 637–638
water contamination and, 774–775
in whooping cough, 614
traveler's diarrhea, 626t, 633
trichinosis, 722–723t, 725, 726f
trichomoniasis, 673t, 678–679
tuberculosis, 608–613
tularemia, 650t, 653–654
typhoid fever, 632, 650t, 654
typhus, 650–653
of urinary tract, 663–665
acute pyelonephritis, 663t, 665–666
anaerobic, 667
cystitis, 663t, 666
nonspecific urethritis, 663t, 666–667
vaccines for, 449, 464
venereal diseases, 669–679
viral:
of gastrointestinal tract, 636–640
of nervous system, 686–690
oral, 593–594
of skin, 575–580
viral pathogenicity in, 443–445
virulence, dosage, resistant state and, 436
warts, 578
whooping cough, 610–611t, 614
zoonoses, 529–531
Infectious hepatitis. *See* Viral hepatitis
Infectious mononucleosis, 636t, 656–657
cancer and, 708
diagnosis and treatment of, 657
Epstein-Barr virus in, 708
heterophile antigen in, 452
transmission of, 656
virus causing, 228t
Infestation, 718
Inflammation:
conditions producing, 424
exudate associated with, 425
fever in, 425–426
mechanism of, 425
pus formation in, 425
signs of, 425
Influenza, 616–617
in animals, 531t
chemotherapy of, 406t
complications of, 616
hemagglutination inhibition for, 472
immunity after, 616–617
prevention of, 617
transmission of, 531t
vaccine for, 512t
virus causing, 228t
Inoculation technique, 251–254
Inorganic, 79
Insecticide, microbial, 745, 746t
Insects in disease transmission, 536–539
Insulin synthesis with recombinant DNA, 319
Interface tests, 473–475
Interferon:
action of, 429
for common cold, 605
immune, 428–429
properties of, 429
role in immunity, 426t, 428–429
therapeutic value of, 429
Intine, 138
Invasiveness, 436
bacterial factors contributing to, 436–437
coagulase and, 436–437
hyaluronidase and, 437
presence of capsule and, 436
streptokinase and, 437
Iodine, 360
5-Iodo-2′-deoxyuridine (IDU), 405–407
Ions, 79
Iris diaphragm, 56
Irritability, 3
Isoantibodies, 451
Isoantigens, 451
Isograft, 504
Isohemagglutination, 451, 482–483
Isolation:
in bacteriological cultures, 254–256
in control of nosocomial infections, 542
reverse, 542
Isonicotinic hydrazide (INH), 396–397
Isopropyl alcohol, 359, 361
Isotope, 292
Iwanowski, I., 6

J

Janssen, Hans, 54
Janssen, Zaccharias, 54
Jaundice, 624
Jejunum, 623
Jenner, Edward, 7f, 520, 522
Joubert, Jules, 23
Juang particle, 639

K

Kala azar, 531t, 658t
in animals, 531t
life cycle of, 654
prevention of, 654–655
transmission of, 531t
Kanamycin, 395–396
Kappa particles, 312–313
Karyogamy, 196
Karyolymph, 104–105
Kelps, 202–203
Kepone, 352
Keratitis, 696–698
Kidney:
anatomy of, 661, 662f
infections of, 663t, 665–666
Killer system, 312–313
Kinetosome, 182
Kingdoms, 32
Kinins, 498
Kirby-Bauer method, 401–402
Klebsiella pneumoniae, 146t
capsule and invasiveness of, 436
opportunistic infections of, 440t
pneumonia caused by, 607, 610t
Koch, Robert, 14, 22–25, 254, 358, 502–503, 566, 608, 612
Koch phenomenon, 502–503
Koch's postulates, 23–24
Kochs-Weeks bacillus, 697
Krebs cycle, 105, 276–278

L

Lactic acid:
in fermentation process, 16

Lactic acid (*continued*)
industrial production of, 742
production by organisms, 275
Lactobacillus, 147t
fermentation in, 275
in food fermentation, 751–752
in lactic acid production, 742
in stabilization of intestinal flora, 415
Lactose, 85
Lag phase, 259–260
Lamellae, 36
Lancefield, R., 569
Landsteiner, Karl, 450, 482, 485
Large intestine, 624
Larvae, 721
filariform, 722
in nematodes, 721–722
rhabditiform, 722
in trematodes, 729
Latent viral infection, 444
Latex agglutination tests, 471–472
Lavoisier, Antoine, 19
Lecithinase, 437
Lecithins, 83
Lederberg, J., 302–303, 309
Leeuwenhoek, Anton van, 14–15, 18, 110, 116, 180
Legionnaire's disease, 154
Legumes, 344
Leishman, William, 654
Leishmania donovani, 189, 654
Leishmaniasis:
in animals, 531t
mechanism of disease by causative agent, 435t
skin test for, 482t
transmission of, 531t
Leprosy, 565t, 566
chemotherapy of, 391t
difficulty of applying Koch's postulates to, 24
early descriptions of, 566–567
mechanisms of action of causative agent, 435t
of oral cavity, 590t
organism causing, 61t
predisposing factors to, 567
prevention of, 567–568
skin test for, 482t
sources of infection, 567
transmission of, 567
Leptospira, 146t, 152t, 629–630
Leptospirosis, 626t, 629
in animals, 531t
causative agents, 152, 629–630
prevention of, 630
transmission of, 531t, 630
Leptothrix, 146t
manganese metabolism in, 352
sheath-forming ability of, 150
Leptotrichia, 146t
Leucothrix, 146t
movement of, 149
Leukemia, 705
Leukins, 426t, 427
Leukocytes, 418–419
chemotaxis of, 423
differential count of, 419
in disease states, 419
in immune system, 419
in inflammation, 425
ingestion by, 424
in phagocytosis, 421–422
Leukopenia, 419
Leukoplastids, 110
L-forms, 127
Lice:
in disease transmission, 537
diseases caused by, 536–537
life cycle of, 537
Lichens, 195, 205–206
importance of, 206
mutualism of, 331
Liebig, Justus von, 15
Lieskeella, 150
Light:
amplitude of, 51
frequency of, 52–53
refraction of, 53
wavelength of, 52–53
Light chains, 454
Light microscope, 49
components of, 54–56
compound, 54
electron microscope compared with, 67t
micrometry in, 57
specimen preparation for:
hanging-drop method, 57–58
staining, 58–63
Light reaction, 111
Limnology, 769
Limulus assay, 438
Linkage, 306
Linnaeus, Carolus, 31–33
Lipase, 743
Lipid inclusions, 131
Lipids:
in cells, 80
fats, 82
fatty acids, 82
functions of, 82
oils, 82
phospholipids, 83
steroids, 84
waxes, 82
Lister, Joseph, 14, 22, 357–358, 361
Listeria, 147t
Lithosphere, 328
Littoral zone:
of fresh water, 770
marine, 772
Liver, 624–625
Liver fluke, 729t
Loa loa, 722t
Loam, 766
Lobopodia, 181
Lockjaw. *See* Tetanus
Loeffler, Friedrich, 6, 254, 602
Loeffler medium, 250
Logarithmic death rate, 261
Logarithmic phase, 260
Lophotrichous, 120, 121f
Ludwig's angina, 589
Lumpy jaw, 60t
Lung fluke, 732t
Lungs, 599
Lupus erythematosus, 451t
Luria, S. E., 302–303
Lymphatic system, 419–421
Lymphocyte toxicity test, 505
Lymphocytes, 419–420
atypical, 656–657
B-type, 458–460
in delayed hypersensitivity, 502
in infectious mononucleosis, 656–657
role in immunity, 458–460
thymus-derived, 457–460
Lymphogranuloma venereum, 672t, 674
mechanism of disease by causative agent, 435t
organism causing, 154
skin test for, 481, 482t
Lymphokines, 502
Lymphoma, 705
Burkitt's, 708
Epstein-Barr virus role in, 708
Lyngbya, 226
Lysine synthesis, 741t
Lysogeny, 223, 310
Lysosomes, 107
anatomy of, 107
immunity and, 430t
in phagocytosis, 424
primary and secondary granules of, 424
Lysozyme, 426t
bactericidal action of, 427
in bacteriophage infections, 224, 225
effect on cell walls, 127
in filtration sterilization, 382
in tears, 412, 695
Lytic cycle, 223–225

M

M concentration, 261
MacConkey agar, 250
Macrocystis, 202
Macromolecules, 79
Macrophages, 420
B- and T-cells associated with, 458
complement synthesized by, 427
fixed, 423
in phagocytosis, 423
in tuberculosis inflammation, 612
wandering, 423
Major blood groups, 483
Malaria, 658t
historical aspects of, 655
identifying agents of, 547
life cycle of parasite causing, 191, 655–656
mechanism of disease by causative agent, 435t
mosquitoes and transmission of, 532
prevention of, 656
protozoa causing, 181
treatment of, 656
Malassezia furfur infection, 573–575
Malformins, 173
Malignant, 703
Malnutrition and opportunistic infections, 440t
Maltose, 85
Manganese metabolism, 352
Mannitol Salt agar, 250
Manometry, 291
Mansonia mosquitoes:
in filariasis, 723
life cycle of, 538–539
Mantoux test, 481, 613
Mapping genes, 313–314
Marek's disease, 708
Marine environments, 771–773
Mastigophora, 189, 190f
Measles, 578
complications of, 578
immune serum globulin after exposure to, 517
immunity after, 578
mechanism of action of causative agent, 435t
in oral cavity, 593t
prevention of, 579
vaccine for, 512t
complications of, 520
preparation of, 514
virus causing, 228t
Measles-mumps-rubella (MMR), 515
Measurement units, 49–51
Media, 242
agar plates, 252
for anaerobes, 250–251
for blood cultures, 551
broth, 252
carbon sources in, 246–247
differential, 249–250
early development of, 25–26
enriched, 249
for fungi, 168–169, 572–573
in identifying organisms, 550–551
Loeffler, 250
MacConkey agar, 250
Mannitol Salt agar, 250
mineral salts in, 247
nitrogen sources in, 246
osmotic pressure of, 248
oxygen-reduction potential of, 244
preparation of, 248
prereduced anaerobically sterilized, 251
properties of, 245
selective, 249–250
slants, 252
storage of, 251
thioglycollate, 251, 257
vitamins in, 247
water in, 247
Meiosis, 102, 196
Membrane:
cell, 103–104
nuclear, 104
plasma, 109
Membrane filter techniques, 776
Meninges, 682
Meningitis, 684
anaerobes causing, 685
aseptic, 684t, 686
mechanisms producing, 684–685
meningococcal, 684t, 685
Meningococcal meningitis, 684t, 685
See also Neisseria meningitidis
Mercury as disinfectant, 363
Merozoites, 655
Mesophiles, 244
Mesosomes, 128–129
Messenger RNA, 90, 106–107
absence in endospores, 135–136
in bacteria, 130

genetic code and, 285–288, 300
operons and, 289–290
synthesis in bacteriophage infections, 225
Metabolism, 3, 272
anabolism, 3, 246, 272
catabolism, 3, 272
control of, 288–290
measurement of, 290–294
fermentation in, 290–291
manometry in, 291–292
oxidation-reduction activity in, 292
radioisotopes in, 292–293
See also Carbohydrates, metabolism of
Metachromatic granules, 130
Metastasis, 703
Metazoan parasites, 9
Methane producing bacteria, 147t, 341
in anaerobic decomposition of wastes, 780
anaerobic respiration in, 279
evolutionary significance of, 44
Methanobacterium, 147t, 279
Methanococcus, 147t
Methanogenesis, 348–349
Methanosarcina, 147t
Methisazone, 405–407
Methyl-bromide vapor, 365
Methylococcus, 341
Methylotrophs, 155
Metric system, 50–51
Miconazole, 405t
Microaerophilic, 771
Microaerophilic organisms, 152, 243
Microbacterium, 131
Microbial infallibility, 347–348
Microbiology, 3
applied, 8–9
automation for, 746
biochemistry and, 77–78
challenges for, 11
classification in, 31–41
early development of, 14–15, 25–26
food, 8–9
germ theory in, 15–17
growth of, 26–27
impact on cancer, 703–704
industrial, 737
integrative approach to, 6–8
literature of, 10–11, 26
medical, 9
nomenclature in, 32
scientific method in, 9–10
spontaneous generation theory in, 17–21
subdivisions of, 4–8
taxonomic approach to, 4–6
veterinary, 9
Microbodies, 107
Micrococcus, 147t
glutamic acid production by, 741
radiation resistance of, 379
Microcyclus, 146t
Microfibrils, 109, 168
Microfilaria, 723
Micrometry, 51, 57
Micromonospora, 395
Microorganisms:
adaptability of, 4
antibiotics produced by, 387, 388t
cells as, 101
five-kingdom approach to classification of, 34, 37–38
in food spoilage, 757–759
growth of, 3
heat killing of, 371–377
interactions in ecosystems, 329–336
irritability in, 3
metabolism of, 3
mutations in, 4, 301–303
natural habitats of, 328–329
nomenclature of, 32
in normal flora, 414
organization of, 4
procedures used to disrupt, 119
rarity of pathogenic nature of, 434–435
reproduction of, 3
in sewage, 773–775
widespread existence of, 3
See also Algae; Bacteria; Fungi; Protozoa; Viruses
Microphages, 423
Microscope, 14
compound, 54
dark-field, 63
electron, 49, 65–73
fluorescence, 63–64
light, 49, 54–65
limitation of, 51
phase, 64–66
resolving power of, 52–53, 55–56
Microspheres, 42, 43f
Microtomy, 70–71
Microtubules, 107–108
Microvilli, 103
Middle lamella, 109
Migula, Walter, 33
Milk:
fermentation of, 753–755
infectious diseases transmitted by, 533
Miller, Stanley, 42
Minimal active concentration (MAC), 389
Minimal inhibitory concentration (MIC), 388
determination of, 400
Minimal medium, 301–302
Mites:
differentiation from ticks, 536
in disease transmission, 535–536
life cycle of, 535–536
Mitochondria:
anatomy of, 105, 106f
duplication of, 311
Mitogens, 428–429
Mitosis, 102
Mixed leukocyte reaction, 505
MMR, 515
Moist heat. *See* Sterilization, heat
Molds, 162, 163f
bread, 174–175
nitrogen assimilation by, 345t
slime, 175–177
Molecular biology, 7–8
Molecule, 78
Mollicutes, 148–149
Molluscum contagiosum:
in oral cavity, 593t
virus causing, 228t
Monera, 38
Moniliasis:
specimen collection in, 549t
vaginitis, 672t
Monoclonal gammopathy, 493–494
Monocytes, 419
in phagocytosis, 423
Monospora bicuspidata, 422
Moraxella, 146t
in eye infections, 697–698
Morbidity rates, 527–528
Mortality rates, 527–528
Mosquitoes:
Aëdes, 538–539, 723
Anopheles, 538–539, 655, 723
Culex, 538, 723
in disease transmission, 531t, 532, 538–539
in filariasis, 723–724
life cycle of, 538–539
in malaria transmission, 532, 535, 655
Mansonia, 538–539, 723
Most probable number method, 775–776
Mouth:
flora in, 582–585
structure of, 583
See also Oral infections
Mucormycosis, 592t
Mucous membrane immunity, 412
Multiple myeloma, 493
Mumps, 594
hemagglutination inhibition for, 472
naturally acquired immunity to, 462–463
in oral cavity, 593t, 594
vaccine for, 512t
virus causing, 228t, 531
Murein sacculus, 126
Mushrooms:
Amanita, 171
cultivation of, 171
life cycle of, 172
poisoning by, 171
Must, 738
Mutation, 4, 298–299
agents causing, 301
chemistry of, 300–301
indirect selection procedure to study, 302–303
in microorganisms, 301–303
misreading of genetic code due to, 300
spontaneous nature of, 302
in viruses, 40
Mutualism, 155
in algae, 195
intermicrobial, 331
microbe-animal, 332–333
microbe-plant, 331–332
rumen symbiosis, 333, 335
Mycelia, 162, 163f
and fungi cultivation, 169
Mycobacteria, 147t
acid-fast staining of, 62
isolation of, 556–557
lipid inclusions in, 131
lysogenic conversion in, 310
mesosomes in, 128
in nontubercular diseases, 608–609
petroleum decomposition by, 350
Mycobacterium avium, 128
Mycobacterium leprae:
chemotherapy of, 391t
difficulty of applying Koch's postulates to, 24
leprosy caused by, 565t, 566
See also Leprosy
Mycobacterium tuberculosis:
capneic incubation of, 256
chemotherapy of, 391t, 397–398
culture medium for, 250
fluorescence microscopy applied to, 64
formaldehyde vapor effect on, 364
glutaraldehyde effect on, 364
identification of, 557
inadequacy of phagocytosis of, 422, 424
mechanism of action in disease, 435t
opportunistic infections of, 440t
pneumonia caused by, 607
spermine action on, 428
in tuberculosis, 608–609
See also Tuberculosis
Mycology, 5
See also Fungi; Yeasts
Mycoplasma, 147–149
bacteriophage occurring in, 220f
cold agglutinins in infections of, 471
medical importance of, 148
in nonspecific urethritis, 667
Mycoplasma hominis, 667
Mycoplasma pneumoniae:
chemotherapy of, 391t
pneumonia caused by, 148, 607–608, 610–611t
Mycoses, 443
classification of, 572
"id" reaction in, 574
of oral cavity, 590–592
superficial, 571–573
systemic, 572
tinea infections, 573–575
Mycotoxins, 173, 443
in cancer, 712
Mycotoxicoses, 443
Mycoviruses, 236
Myxamoebae, 177
Myxobacteria, 137
Myxomycetes, 175–177

N

N-acetylglucosamine, 124, 125f
N-acetylmuramic acid, 124, 125f
NAD, 274
NADH, 274
NADP, 274
Naegleria gruberi, 693
Nägeli, Carl, 33
Nail infections, 574
Nanometer, 51

Necatur americanus:
in human disease, 722t
structure of, 721
Needham, John, 18–19
Neisseria, 146t
identification of, 555–556
smear used as quality control, 557
Neisseria gonorrhoeae:
in acute prostatitis, 670
capneic incubation of, 256
carbon dioxide in culture of, 243
chemotherapy of, 391t
conjunctivitis due to, 695
fermentation of, 556
in gonorrhea, 671, 674
identification of, 555–556
immunizing properties of, 513
inadequacy of phagocytosis of, 422
leukocytes in, 419
See also Gonorrhea
Neisseria meningitidis:
capneic incubation of, 256
capsule and invasiveness of, 436
fermentation of, 556
identification of, 555–556
inadequacy of phagocytosis of, 422
mechanism of action in disease, 435t
in meningitis, 685
specimen collection for, 549
vaccine for, 512t
Nematodes, 722t
infections of, 721, 722t
filariasis, 722–724
hookworm, 722–725
in plants, 726
trichinosis, 722–723t, 725, 726f
larval forms in, 721–722
life cycle of, 722–723
Neoplasm, 703
Neorickettsia, 147t
canine disease caused by, 154
Nephelometer, 263
Neritic zone, 772
Nervous system. *See* Central nervous system
Neurospora crassa:
creating mutations in, 314–315
life cycle, 170f
mercury methylation in, 352
mutation studies on, 301–302, 306
Neurotoxin, 440–442
of botulism, 634
in tetanus, 571
Neurotropic viruses, 686
Neutralization, viral, 469t, 481
Neutrophils, 419
in phagocytosis, 423
Newcastle disease virus, 231
Niche, 325
Nirenberg, Marshall, 285
Nitrates as nitrogen source, 342
Nitrobacter, 147t
energy-yielding reactions of, 284
role in nitrogen cycle, 344–345
Nitrococcus, 147t
Nitrogen cycle, 342–345
Nitrogen fixation, 156
in nitrogen cycle, 342–344
nonsymbiotic, 343–344
organisms involved in, 343–344
symbiotic, 344
Nitrosomonas:
energy-yielding reactions of, 284
role in nitrogen cycle, 344
Nocardia, 147t
chemotherapy of, 391t
identification of, 557
opportunistic infections of, 440t
petroleum decomposition by, 350
specimen collection for, 549t
survival in distilled water, 327
Nomenclature, 32
Nonimmune phagocytosis, 422
Nonspecific urethritis, 666–667
Nonsusceptibility, 411
Normal flora, 413
amphibiont sites of, 413
antibody production and, 415
benefits of, 414–415
of conjunctiva, 695
development of, 413–414
in nutrition, 415
opportunists, 413
of respiratory tract, 599
space travel and, 415
of urinary tract, 661, 663
variety of microorganisms in, 414
Nosocomial infections, 534, 539
control of:
hand washing, 541–542
institutional policies in, 542–543
isolation in, 542
medical asepsis, 540–541
surgical asepsis, 541
factors contributing to, 539
medical devices and, 540, 541t
sources of contamination in, 539
Nucleic acids, 80, 86, 88
See also DNA; RNA
Nucleocapsid, 213
Nucleoid, 35–36
Nucleolus, 101, 102f, 105
Nucleoplasm, 102, 104, 129
Nucleoside, 87
Nucleotides, 86–87
Nucleus, 104–105, 129
Numerical aperture, 56
Nutrition:
and immunity, 431t
normal flora in, 415
Nystatin, 405t

O

Objectives, 54–56
Obligate organisms, 718
anaerobes, 243–244
intracellular, 145, 152–155
viruses, 6
Oceanography, 771
Ocular, 54
Oil-immersion lens, 56
Oils, 82
Old Tuberculin, 612
Onchocerca volvulus, 722t
Oncogene hypothesis, 711–712
Oncogenic, 703
Oncogenic viruses, 227, 234
current strategies for determining, 715
DNA-containing, 707–709
oncogene hypothesis for, 711–712
protovirus hypothesis for, 712
provirus hypothesis for, 710–711
RNA-containing, 706–707
structural differences among, 706–707
One-gene, one-enzyme hypothesis, 302
One-step growth curve, 226
Oöcyst, 655
Oökinete, 655
Oomycetes, 169t, 174
plant disease due to, 174
Opalinata, 188
Oparin, A. I., 41–43
Operational taxonomic unit, 40
Operons, 286
control of metabolism and, 289–290
Ophthalmia neonatorum, 674, 695–697
Opisthorchis sinensis, 729t
Opportunistic fungi, 572
Opportunistic infections, 440t, 445
Opportunists, 413
Opsonization, 422
Optical density, 263
Optochin, 554
Oral infections:
bacterial, 590
candidiasis, 590–592
dental caries, 589
dry socket, 586
focal, 584–585
fungal, 590–592
gingivitis, 588
herpangina, 593
herpes simplex, 594
Ludwig's angina, 589
mumps, 594
osteomyelitis, 586, 587t
pericoronitis, 586, 587t
periodontal, 587–588
viral, 593–594
Orders, 32
Organelles, 102–103
functions and activities of, 112t
Organic, 79
Origin of life:
bacterial evolution in, 44
fossilized evidence for, 43–45
Oparin-Haldane concept, 41–43
Oparin's theory, 41
Origin of Species, 298
Orthromyxovirus, 228t
Osmotic pressure:
of bacteriological media, 248
effect in ecosystems, 326–327
regulation by protozoa, 183
Osmotic work, 103
Osteomyelitis in oral cavity, 586, 587t
Otitis media, 603
Ouchterlony test, 474–475
Oudin test, 473
Oxidation, 80–81
Oxidation-reduction reactions:
in ATP production, 274
in measurement of metabolism, 292
Oxidative phosphorylation, 278–279
Oxygen cycle, 346–347
Oxyuriasis, 722–725

P

Paleomicrobiology, 43–44
Pandemic, 527
Pap smear, 712
Papilloma warts, 578
Papovavirus, 228t
role in cancer, 707, 709t
Para-aminobenzoic acid (PABA), 392
Para-aminosalycylic acid (PAS), 396–397
Paragonimiasis, 729t, 732t
Paragonimus westermani, 729t
Paralytic shellfish poisoning, 203
Paramecium:
excretion by, 183
killer system of, 312–313
structure of, 184
Paramyxovirus, 228t
measles, 578–579
Parasites, 9, 335
coprozoic, 718–719
facultative, 718
incidental, 718
metazoan, 9
obligate intracellular, 145
pseudo-, 719
worms as, 717–718
See also Helminths; Protozoa
Parasitism, 335–336
obligatory, 435
Parasitology, 9
Parasporal bodies, 136
Paratyphoid fever vaccine, 512t
Parfocal, 56
Parrot fever. *See* Psittacosis
Parvovirus, 228t
Passive agglutination, 471–472
Passive immunity:
artificially acquired, 463–464
naturally acquired, 463–464
Passive immunization, 452
antimicrobial sera in, 517–518
antitoxins in, 516–517
in prevention of Rh disease, 487
usefulness of, 511
Passive transport, 103
Pasteur, Louis, 20–23, 358, 566, 688, 760
Pasteurella. See Francisella
Pasteurization:
flash, 375
in food processing, 760
in preventing milk-borne diseases, 374–376
of wine, 16
Patch test, 503
Pathogenicity, 436
Pathogens, 435
identifying, 546–548
mechanisms in causing disease, 435

opportunists differentiated from 445
Pebrine, 23
Pediococcus halophilus, 327
Pelagic zone, 772
Pellicle:
in algae, 201
in protozoa, 183–184
Penicillin:
analogs of, 393
discovery of, 26
effect on cell wall, 126–127, 393–394
hypersensitivity reaction to, 503–504
mechanism of action of, 394–395
production of, 739–740
range of activity of, 394
structure of, 393
Penicillin G, 393
Penicillinase:
plasmid effect on, 400
role in antibiotic resistance, 398
Penicillium, 172
asexual life cycle of, 163f
competition by, 330
microscopic appearance of, 173f
Penile infections, 670
Pentose, 84
Peptide bond, 80, 91
Peptococcus, 147t
Peptostreptococcus, 556
Percent G + C comparison, 315
Perfringens poisoning, 635
Pericardium, 646
Pericoronitis, 586, 587t
Periodontal disease, 587–588
Peritrichous, 120
Peroxisomes, 107
Pertussis. *See* Whooping cough
Pesticides:
accumulation in biosphere, 352
metabolism by bacteria, 351
microorganisms used as, 745, 746t
Petri dish, 25
Petroleum degradation, 349
pH, 81
bacteria cultures and, 244–245
of common substances, 245t
effect in ecosystem, 325t, 326
fungi growth and, 245
Phaeophycophyta, 202–203
Phage. *See* Bacteriophages
Phage typing, 222
Phagocytes, 420
Phagocytin, 424, 426–428
Phagocytosis, 421–422
bacterial capsule and inhibition of, 436
by basophils, 419
chemotaxis in, 423
complement enhancement of, 427
diseases associated with interference of, 435t
failure of, 424
ingestion in, 424
intracellular destruction, 424
lysosome role in, 107
macrophages in, 420, 423
microphages in, 423
neutrophils in, 419
noncellular blood components in, 422
opsonization in, 422
stages in, 423–424
surface, 422
Phagolysosome, 424
Pharynx, 597
Phase microscopy, 64–66
Phenol coefficient test, 365–366
Phenols, 360–362
Phormidium, 226
Phospholipids, 83
in cell membrane, 104
Phosphorus cycle, 345–346
Phosphorylation, 273–274
oxidative, 278–279
photosynthetic, 273
substrate, 274
Photobacterium fischeri, 332–333
Photoreactivation, 378
Photosynthesis:
in algae, 198, 201, 205
anoxygenic, 155
in autotrophic bacteria, 283
in bacteria, 130, 155, 283–285
in carbon cycle, 340
chemical reaction of, 111
dark reaction in, 111
in ecosystem, 324
in heterotrophic bacteria, 284–285
light reaction in, 111
in oxygen cycle, 347
phosphorylation by, 273
radioisotopes in study of, 293
Phototrophs, 146t, 155–157
Phragmidiothrix, 150
Phycobilisomes, 130, 157
Phycobillins, 110
Phycology, 5–6
See also Algae
Phyla, 32
Phylogenetic classification, 31
Physiology, 7
Phytoplankton, 195, 769
Phytotoxins, 442
Pickling process, 751–753
Picornaviruses, 228t
central nervous system infections by, 686–687
gastrointestinal infections by, 636–637
Piedra, 573t, 575
Pili, 122–123
immunizing properties of, 513
Pilin, 122
Pinkeye, 697
Pinocytosis, 103
Pinta, 675t, 678
Pinworms, 722–724
life cycle of, 724–725
transmission of, 724–725
Plague:
in animals, 531t
bubonic, 651
chemotherapy of, 391t
exotoxin involved in, 439t
features of, 650t
fleas in transmission of, 538
forms of, 651
historical significance of, 648–649
mechanism of disease by causative agent, 435t
organism causing, 61t
pneumonic, 651
prevention of, 651
sylvatic, 649
transmission of, 529, 531t, 649
vaccine for, 512t, 521
Plankton, 195, 198
Plant cells, 109–112
Plant viruses:
cultivation of, 234–235
infections by, 235
structure of, 234
Plants:
in five-kingdom classification system, 37, 38t
infectious diseases of, 543
nematode parasites of, 726
phytotoxins in, 442
Plaque assays, 234
Plaque purification, 234
Plaque-forming unit, 234, 264–265
Plaques:
in bacteriophage cultures, 221–222
in viral tissue cultures, 233–234
Plaquing technique, 234–235
Plasma, 416
Plasma cells, 458
Plasma membrane:
in bacterial cells, 127–128
in plant cells, 109
Plasmids:
in bacteria, 129
bacteriocins, 310–311
metabolic, 311
replication in bacteria, 310–311
resistance transfer factor, 311, 318–319
role in transfer of antibiotic resistance, 399–400
transposons, 311
Plasmodium:
diseases caused by, 191
interferon stimulation by, 428
life cycle of, 191
in malaria, 655
mosquitoes as vector for, 538
in slime molds, 175
See also Malaria
Plasmogamy, 196
Plasmolysis, 248
Plasmoptysis, 225, 248
Plasmotomy, 186
Plastids, 109
chloroplasts, 110–111
chromoplastids, 109
leukoplastids, 110
Platelets, 416
implicated in autoimmune disease, 451t
Platyhelminthes, 726–727
See also Flatworms
Plectonema, 226
Pleura, 599
Pleuropneumonia-like organisms. *See Mycoplasma*
Pneumococcal pneumonia, 610–611t
cause of, 606–607
complications of, 607
immunity after, 607
predisposing factors, 607
prevention of, 607
transmission of, 607
See also Streptococcus pneumoniae
Pneumococcus. *See Streptococcus pneumoniae*
Pneumocystis carinii, 618
Pneumonia:
bacteria causing, 607, 610–611t
pneumococcal, 606–607, 610–611t
See also Streptococcus pneumoniae
Polepieces, 68
Poliomyelitis, 686
pathogenicity of, 444
tissue culture cultivation of, 232
vaccine for, 512t
oral administration of, 518–519
preparation of, 514
virus causing, 228t, 444
Pollutants:
effect on ecosystem, 328
and immunity, 430t
Polyene antibiotics, 403–404
Polyhedroses, 227
Polymorphonuclear leukocytes, 419
Polymyxin B, 397
Polypeptides:
as antimicrobials, 397
origin of, 42
Polysaccharides, 85–86
granules, 130–131
Polysomes, 106–107
Polyunsaturated, 82
Populations, 323–324
Portals of exit, 529
Potato spindle tuber disease, 236
Pour-plate technique, 254
Poxvirus, 228t, 576t, 579–580
in cancer, 709t
PPLO. *See Mycoplasma*
Prausnitz-Küstner reaction, 499
Precipitin reactions, 469t, 472–473
double diffusion, 473
Ouchterlony test, 474–475
Oudin test, 473
radial immunodiffusion, 473–474
ring tests, 473–475
two-dimensional immunoelectrophoresis, 474
Predation in ecosystem, 330
Priestly, Joseph, 19
Primary atypical pneumonia, 608, 610–611t
See also Mycoplasma
Procaryotes, 102
budding, 151
carbon and energy supplies for, 147
cellular organization in, 34–36
chemical composition of, 139t
differentiation of, 132
eucaryotes compared with, 36t
functions of, 139t
gas vacuoles in, 132
nucleus in, 129
properties of, 139t
recombination in, 304–309
stalked, 150–151
See also Bacteria
Proglottids, 727
Properdin, 426t, 428

Prophage, 223
Propionibacterium, 147t
Prostatitis, 663t, 670
Prosthecate bacteria, 150–151
Prosthetic group, 94–95
Protease, 743
Proteinase, 437
Proteinoid, 42
Proteins, 90
  amino acids in, 90–91
  in cells, 80
  dietary sources of, 756–757
  enzymes, 93–95
  involvement in cell functions, 90
  primary structure of, 91
  secondary structure of, 91
  single-cell, 755–757
  synthesis of:
    carbohydrate metabolism and, 280–281
    feedback inhibition in, 288–289
    ribosomes in, 106–107
    steps in, 285–288
  tertiary structure of, 92
Proteus:
  antimicrobial action against, 391t, 396
  identification of, 555
  opportunistic infection by, 440t
  sulfur metabolism in, 346
  Weil-Felix test and, 471
Proteus mirabilis:
  chemotherapy of, 391t
  flagella in, 121f
Proteus vulgaris, 439t, 440t
Protista, 34, 37, 38t
Protoplasm, 102
Protoplasts, 126–127
  in culturing plant viruses, 235
Prototroph, 302
Protovirus hypothesis, 712
Protozoa, 180–181
  asexual reproduction in, 186
  beneficial effects of, 181
  budding of, 186
  chemotherapy against, 404
  cilia of, 182
  ciliata of, 187–188
  classification of, 187, 188t
  cold agglutinins in infections, 471
  complement-fixation tests for, 478t
  as consumers in ecosystem, 324
  cultivation of, 187
  cyst stage, 185
  distribution of, 181
  excretion by, 183
  feeding by, 182–183
  flagella of, 182
  functions of, 181–184
  harmful effects of, 181
  infections by:
    African sleeping sickness, 691–693
    amoebic dysentery, 640, 641t
    amoebic meningoencephalitis, 693
    balantidiasis, 641–642
    Chagas' disease, 693
    gastrointestinal, 640–642
    giardiasis, 641t, 642
    kala azar, 654–655, 658t
    malaria, 655–656, 658t
    nervous system, 690–693
    respiratory, 618
    systemic, 654–658
    toxoplasmosis, 690–691
  mastigophora, 189,190f
  mechanism of action in disease, 435t
  metachromatic granules in, 130
  movement of, 181–182
  in normal flora, 414t
  opalinata, 188
  osmoregulation by, 183
  pellicle in, 183–184
  predation by, 330
  protective structures of, 183–184
  pseudopodia of, 181
  regeneration of parts in, 187
  sarcodina, 188–189
  sexual reproduction in, 186–187
  skin test for, 482t
  sporozoa, 191
  structure of, 181–184
  suctoria, 188
  termites related to, 189
  trichocysts in, 184
  trophozoite stage, 185
  viruses and, 236
  zoonoses of, 531t
Protozoology, 6
  See also Protozoa
Providencia, 555
Provirus hypothesis, 710–711
Pseudomonas, 146t
  bacteriocin in, 310–311
  carbenicillin for, 393–394
  denitrification in, 279
  flagellum in, 121f
  gentamicin activity against, 396
  hydrocarbon degradation in, 349
  in meningitis, 685
  mercury methylation in, 351–352
  metabolic plasmids in, 311
  nitrate metabolism by, 345
  opportunistic infections by, 440t
  osmotic pressure and growth of, 325t, 327
  phytotoxins of, 442
  urinary infections after catheterization, 664
Pseudomonas aeruginosa:
  bacteriophages attacking, 221
  chemotherapy of, 391t
  DNA hybridization in, 316
  identification of, 555
  inhibition of *Candida* by, 415
  in pesticide production, 745
  skin infections of, 564–565t, 568
  use in testing detergents, 366
Pseudomonas cepacia, 325t, 327
Pseudomonas diminuta, 121f
Pseudomonas putida, 349
Pseudomycelia, 164f, 165
Pseudoparasites, 719
Pseudopodia, 181
Psittacosis, 608, 610–611t
  chemotherapy of, 391t
  control of, 608
  organism causing, 154
  skin test for, 482t
  transmission of, 608
Psychroduric, 244
Psychrophiles, 244
  temperature and growth of, 325–326
Ptomaine poisoning, 633
Puerperal sepsis, 669–670
Punnett square technique, 484–485
Purified Protein Derivative (PPD), 612
Purines, 86, 300
Pus, 425
Pyelonephritis, acute, 663t, 665–666
Pyemia, 436
Pyorrhea, 588
Pyrenoids, 197
Pyrimidines, 86, 300
Pyrogen, 426
Pyrrophycophyta, 203
Pyrivic acid and ATP synthesis, 277

Q

Q fever, 608
  chemotherapy of, 391t
  pasteurization in prevention of, 375
  ticks in, 537t
  transmission of, 652
Quaternary ammonium compounds, 360t, 363

R

Rabbit fever. *See* Tularemia
Rabies, 684t
  in animals, 530, 531t, 687
  control of, 688
  epidemiologic varieties of, 687
  passive immunization against, 464
  serologic diagnosis of, 469t
  transmission of, 530, 531t, 687
  treatment of, 687–688
  vaccine for:
    complications of, 520t
    preparation of, 513t
    recommendation in travelers, 521t
    use after rabies exposure, 688
  virus causing, 228t
Radial immunodiffusion, 473–474
Radiation sterilization:
  ionizing, 378–379
  ultraviolet, 370t, 377–378
Radioimmunoassay, 469t
Radioisotopes:
  accumulation in biosphere, 352–353
  in metabolic studies, 292–293
Rat-bite fever, 529
Rats in plague transmission, 649
Reaction of identity, 474
Reaction of nonidentity, 475
Reaction of partial identity, 475
Recombinant DNA
  potential benefits of, 316
  potential hazards of, 316–317
  restriction endonuclease in study of, 317–318
  RTF plasmids in study of, 318–319
Recombination, 299, 304
  transformation, 304–306
Rectum, 624
Red algae, 204–205
Red blood cells, 418
  in autoimmune disease, 451t
Red tide, 203, 442, 769
Redi, Francesco, 17–18
Reduction, 80–81
Reed, Walter, 6, 689
Refraction, 53
Refractive index, 53
Regeneration in protozoa, 187
Relapsing fever:
  in animals, 531t
  epidemiology of, 651–652
  features of, 650t
  organism causing, 152
  transmission of, 531t, 537
Reovirus, 228t
Reproduction, 3
  in algae, 196
  asexual, 3, 186
  regeneration, 187
  sexual, 3, 186–187
Reproductive system:
  anaerobic infections of, 669–670
  female, 667–669
  male, 668f, 669
  See also Venereal diseases
Resistance:
  to bacteriophage infection, 223
  species, 411
  See also Immunity
Resistance transfer factor (RTF). *See* Plasmids
Resolving power, 14, 52–53, 55–56
Respiratory chain, 278
Respiratory syncytial virus, 135t
Respiratory tract, 596–597
  infections of, 599–600
    bacterial, 601–604, 606–614
    control measures for, 600
    diagnosis of, 600
    fungal, 614–617
    viral, 605–606, 616–617
  normal flora of, 599
  structures of, 597–599
Restriction endonuclease, 317–318
Reticuloendothelial system, 420
Retrovirus, 228t
Reverse transcriptase, 709
Rh system, 485–486
  in hemolytic disease of the newborn, 486–487
  nomenclature in, 486
  prevention of isoimmunization in, 487
  typing in, 486
Rhabditiform larvae, 722
Rhabdovirus, 228t
Rheumatic fever, 647
Rheumatic heart disease, 647–648
  prevention of, 647
  streptolysin O effect in, 441
Rheumatoid arthritis, 451t
Rhinoviruses, 605
Rhizobium, 344
Rhizoids, 162, 175
Rhizopodia, 181

Rhizopus nigricans, 174–175
Rhodomicrobium, 146t
division cycle of, 151
Rhodophycophyta, 204–205
Rhodotorula, 325t
Riboflavin synthesis, 741t
Ribonucleic acid. *See* RNA
Ribose, 84f, 85
Ribosomal RNA, 90, 130
Ribosomes:
in bacterial cells, 130
formation in nucleolus, 105
function of, 106–107, 287–288
genetic code and, 287–288
immunizing properties of, 513
Ricketts, Howard Taylor, 652
Rickettsia, 147t
infections due to, 154, 652
epidemic typhus, 650–653
flea-borne typhus, 650–651t, 653
general clinical features of, 650–651t
rickettsialpox, 650–651t, 653
Rocky Mountain spotted fever, 650–651t, 653
scrub typhus, 650–651t, 653
transmission of, 652
trench fever, 653
interferon stimulation by, 428
mechanism of action in disease, 435t
properties of, 154
vaccines for, 511, 512t
Weil-Felix test for, 471
Rickettsia akari, 653
Rickettsia prowazekii, 652
Rickettsia rickettsii:
chemotherapy of, 391t
discovery of, 652
in Rocky Mountain spotted fever, 653
See also Rocky Mountain spotted fever
Rickettsia tsutsugamushi, 653
Rickettsia typhi, 653
Rickettsialpox, 651t, 653
mites involvement in, 536
Rickettsiella, 147t
nonpathogenicity of, 155
Rifampin, 398
Ring tests, 473–475
Ringworm:
in animals, 531t
antimycotic agents for, 405t
characteristics of, 573–575
fungi causing, 172–173
prevention of, 574
of scalp, 173f
specimen collection in, 549t
transmission of, 531t
treatment of, 573
Ripening, 754–755
Rivers, T. M., 24
Rivers' postulates, 24
RNA, 86
different kinds of, 90
interferon stimulation by, 428
messenger, 90, 106–107
oncogenic viruses containing, 706–707
in plant viruses, 234
ribosomal, 90, 130
structure of, 89f, 90
in viruses, 212–213, 218t
RNA viruses, 228t
oncogenic, 706–707
Rochalimaea, 147t
Rocky Mountain spotted fever:
in animals, 531t
chemotherapy of, 391t
features of, 650–651t
organism causing, 61t, 154
serologic diagnosis of, 469t
tick involvement in, 536t
transmission of, 531t, 653
vaccine for, 512t
Rosaniline dyes, 362
Roundworms. *See* Nematodes
Rous, Francis Peyton, 706
Rous sarcoma virus, 227
transformation assay for detecting, 234
Roux, Pierre, 602
Rubella, 576t, 579
congenital, 679
control of, 579
determining immune status toward, 469t
effect on pregnant women, 579
hemagglutination inhibition for, 472
immune serum globulin to prevent, 517
naturally acquired immunity to, 462
passive immunization against, 464
syndrome in affected infants, 579
vaccine for, 512t, 520t
Rubeola. *See* Measles
Rumen, 333, 335

S

Sabouraud medium, 168–169, 572–573
Sac fungi, 170
Saccharomyces:
in beer production, 738
fermentation by, 171
osmotic pressure and growth of, 325t
in sake production, 739
in vinegar production, 740–741
in wine production, 738
Saccharomyces carlsbergensis, 738
Saccharomyces cerevisiae, 15, 171, 738, 740–741
Saccharomyces ellipsoideus, 738
Saccharophilic yeasts, 327
Sake production, 739
Salivary glands, 583
Salk vaccine, 514
Salmonella, 146t
in antitumor therapy, 714
bacteriophages attacking, 221
in carcinogen detection test, 713
DNA hybridization in, 316
in food infection, 631
Forssmann antigen and, 451–452
identification of, 555
lysogenic conversion in, 310
mechanism of action in disease, 435t
in septicemia, 632
specimen collection for, 548t
sulfur metabolism in, 346
transduction in, 309
in typhoid fever, 654
use in testing disinfectants, 365–366
Salmonella choleraesuis, 632
Salmonella enteritidis, 714
Salmonella typhi:
chemotherapy of, 391t
and phage typing, 222
in typhoid fever, 632
Widal test for, 471
Salmonella typhimurium, 221, 316
Salmonellosis, 626t, 630–632, 654
in animals, 531t
causative agents of, 631
control of, 631
prevention of, 631
transmission of, 531t, 631
Salvarsan, 387
Sanitizer, 357t
Saprophytes, 162
Sarcina, 116, 118f, 147t
osmotic pressure and growth of, 325t, 326
Sarcina morrhuae, 325t, 326
Sarcodina, 188–189
Sarcomas, 705
Saturated, 82
Sauerkraut production, 751–752
Scabies, 536
Scanning electron microscope, 73
Scarlet fever:
exotoxin in, 439t, 441
features of, 565t, 570
predisposing factors to, 570
skin test for, 482
transmission of, 570
See also Streptococcus pyogenes
Schick test, 482, 603
Schistosomiasis, 729t, 732t
life cycle in, 730
skin test for, 482t
Schizogony, 186, 655
Schleiden, Matthew, 101–102
Schönlein, Johann, 23
Schröder, Heinrich, 19
Schulze, Franz, 19
Schwann, Theodor, 15, 19, 102
Scientific method, 9–10
Scolex, 727
Scrub typhus, 650–651t, 653
Seaweed. *See* Algae
Selective medium, 249–250
Semmelweis, I., 357–358
Sensitivity testing:
agar-overlay method, 402
of antiviral agents, 406
cylinder method, 400
drug diffusion methods, 400–402
filter-paper disk method, 400–401
Kirby-Bauer method, 401–402
minimum inhibitory concentration determination, 400
Septicemia, 436
conditions predisposing to, 440t
Serology:
cross-reactions in, 475
importance of, 468–469
for viruses, 481
See also Immunological procedures
Serratia marcescens, 146t
in antitumor therapy, 714
opportunistic infections of, 440t
Serum, 416
Serum sickness, 501
Sewage:
microorganisms in, 773–775
properties of, 773–774
treatment of:
advanced, 781–782
aerobic stabilization in, 780
anaerobic digestion in, 779–780, 782
preliminary, 778
primary, 778–779
secondary, 779–781
trickling filter in, 780–781
Sexduction, 304, 307–309
F particles, 307–308
F-prime particle, 309
Hfr cells, 308–309
Sexual reproduction, 3
Sexually transmissible diseases, 671–673
See also Venereal diseases
Shadow casting, 69
Sheathed bacteria, 146t, 150
Shellfish poisoning, 203
Shells, protozoan, 184
Shiga, Kiyoshi, 631
Shigella, 146t
in bacillary dysentery, 626t, 631
identification of, 555
mechanism of action in disease, 435t
specimen collection for, 548
Shigella dysenteriae:
chemotherapy of, 391t
exotoxin of, 439t, 442
Forssmann antigen and, 451–452
vaccine against, 512t
See also Bacillary dysentery
Shingles, 576–578
chemotherapy of, 406t
identity to virus causing chickenpox, 577
means of transmission of, 578
See also Herpesviruses
Shwartzman reaction, 501
SI system, 50
Sickle cell disease, 440t
Silver in gonorrhea prophylaxis, 363
Similarity coefficient, 40
Single-cell protein, 756–757
microorganisms used to produce, 756t
Skerljevo, 678
Skin:
bacterial infections of, 564–571
fungal infections of, 571–575
organization of, 561–562
types of lesions affecting, 562, 563t
variety of pathogens affecting, 561
viral infections of, 575–580
Skin immunity, 412
Skin test:
in antitoxin standardization, 517
for atopic states, 499
diagnostic, 481–482

Skin tests (*continued*)
  Schick, 603
  for tuberculosis, 612–613
Skin-challenge test, 517
Sleeping sickness, African. *See* African sleeping sickness
Slime layers, 123
Slime molds, 175–177
Slow virus diseases, 688–689
Small intestine, 622–624
Smallpox, 580
  eradication through immunization, 522
  naturally acquired immunity to, 462–463
  in oral cavity, 593t
Smears, 57
Smith fermentation tube, 291
Soil, 328
  formation of, 765–767
  humus in, 766
  microorganism contributions to, 765
  water cycle effect on, 767–768
  weathering in formation of, 765–766
Solid waste disposal, 783–784
Somatic (O) antigen, 438
Sour cream production, 754
Spallanzani, Lazzaro, 19
Spawn, 171
Species, 32
Species resistance, 411
Specimen collection, 548–549
  swabs in, 548
  transporting after, 549
Spectrophotometer, 263
Spermine, 426t, 428
Sphaerophorus, 556
Sphaerotilus, 146t, 150
Spheroplast, 126–127
Spines, 123
Spiral bacteria, 146t, 152
Spirillum, 118, 146t, 152
  cellulose decomposition by, 330
  flagella in, 121f
  lipid inclusions in, 131
  salt concentration and growth of, 326–327
Spirochetes:
  axial filaments of, 128
  characteristics of, 146t, 152
  movement of, 128
Spiroplasma, 147–149
Spontaneous generation, 17–21
Sporangium, 133, 175
Spores:
  in algae, 196
  auxospore, 200
  calcium in, 247
  chemical makeup of, 135–136
  cortex of, 135
  dormancy of, 134
  free, 133
  in fungi, 162, 165–166
  heat resistance of, 372, 374
  protozoan, 191
  resistance to ionizing radiation, 379
  staining of, 63
  thermal resistance of, 136
  See also Endospores
Sporocide, 357t
Sporogony, 655
Sporosarcina, 147t
Sporotrichous, 592t
Sporozoa, 191
Sporozoites, 191, 655
Sporulation, 133
  chemical substances required for, 134
  physical factors required for, 134
  stages involved in, 134–135
Spray dish, 257
Spread plate technique, 255
Staining, 57
  acid-fast, 62–63
  differential, 59
  dyes used in, 58
  electron, 70
  gram, 59–62
  simple, 58–59
  spore, 63
Stalk cells, 177
Stalked procaryotes, 150–151
Standard plate count, 777–778
Standing fresh water, 769–770
Stanley, W., 6
Staphylococcal food poisoning, 635
Staphylococci, 116, 118f, 147t
  capsule and invasiveness of, 436
  coagulase and invasiveness of, 436–437
  detergents activity against, 363
  enterotoxin presence after pasteurization, 376
  in eye infections, 698
  glutaraldehyde effect on, 364
  inadequacy of phagocytosis of, 422, 424
  infections due to, 564t, 568
    food poisoning, 635
    furuncle, 569
    impetigo, 569
    prevention of, 568–569
    transmission of, 568
  phagocytin action on, 427
  streptokinase and invasiveness of, 437
Staphylococcus aureus:
  antibiotic resistance in, 398, 399
  chemotherapy of, 390t
  culture medium for, 250
  exotoxin involved in disease, 439t, 441, 635
  food poisoning by, 635
  identification of, 553
  in kidney infections, 663t, 666
  leukocytes in, 419
  opportunistic infections of, 440t
  penicillinase production by, 398
  and phage typing, 222
  recombinant DNA studies with, 317–318
  resistance transfer factor in, 311
  role in influenza, 616
  skin infections of, 564t, 568–569
  use in testing detergents, 365–366
Staphylococcus epidermidis, 553
Starch, 85
Starter cultures, 751
  lactic, 753
Static effect, 390
Sterilization, 357t
  autoclaving, 370t, 373–375
  boiling, 374
  cold, 359
  direct flaming, 376
  ethylene oxide, 360t, 364
  filtration, 370t, 379
    air, 381–383
    liquid, 379–381
  heat:
    dry, 370t, 376–377
    mechanism of effect, 372
    moist, 373–376
    monitoring, 372–373
    in oil or silicone fluid, 377
    terminology of thermal kill in, 371–372
  heat transfer, 370t, 377
  hot-air, 376
  ionizing radiation, 378–379
  pasteurization, 374–376
  preparing materials for, 370–371
  ultraviolet radiation, 370t, 377–378
Steroids, 84
  microorganisms in transformation of, 744
Stolons, 175
Stomach, 622
Stool pathogens, 555
Streaking, 25
Streak-plate technique, 254–255
Strep throat, 601t, 604
Streptobacillus, 146t
Streptococci, 116, 118f, 147t
  differential media for, 249
  fermentation in, 275, 753
  group A, 569
  hemolytic reactions of, 249, 553–554, 569
  identification of, 553–554
  infections of, 564–565t, 569–571
    acute glomerulonephritis after, 667
    chemotherapy of, 390t
    consequences of, 571
    erysipelas, 570
    in eye, 698
    in female genital tract, 669
    impetigo, 570–571
    opportunistic, 440t
    prevention of, 604
    scarlet fever, 565t, 570
    on skin, 564–565t
    sore throat, 601t, 604
    transmission of, 570, 604
  inhibition of *Candida* by, 415
  mechanism of action in disease, 435t
  phagocytin action on, 427
  phagocytosis of, 424
  role in rheumatic fever, 647
  streptokinase and invasiveness of, 437
  streptolysins produced by, 441–442
  in tooth decay, 589
  virulence of, 569
  in water quality determination, 776–777
Streptococcus cremoris, 753
Streptococcus faecalis, 776–777
Streptococcus hemolyticus, 390t
Streptococcus mutans, 589
Streptococcus pneumoniae:
  capsule and invasiveness of, 124, 436
  carriers of, 607
  chemotherapy of, 390t
  eye infections due to, 698
  Forssmann antigen associated with, 451–452
  hyaluronidase and invasiveness of, 437
  identification of, 554
  leukocytes in, 419
  mutation to avirulent form, 304–305
  pathogenicity of, 304
  phagocytosis of, 424
  pneumonia caused by, 607
  role in influenza, 616
  vaccine for, 512
Streptococcus pyogenes:
  bacteriophage influence on exotoxin of, 439
  erythrogenic toxin of, 441
  exotoxin involved in disease, 439t
Streptococcus salivarius, 589
Streptococcus sanguis, 589
Streptodornase, 743t
Streptokinase, 437, 743t
Streptolysin O, 441
  serologic test for, 477–478
Streptolysin S, 441–442
Streptomyces, 147t
  antimicrobials produced by, 395, 398
Streptomycin:
  development of resistance to, 398
  production of, 395
  range of activity of, 396
Strickland reaction, 275
Strongyloides stercoralis, 722t
Subacute bacterial endocarditis, 648
Subacute sclerosing panencephalitis (SSPE), 688
Substage condenser, 56
Substrate, 95, 274
Sucrose, 85
Suctoria, 188
Sulfa drugs, 390, 392, 398
Sulfolobus, 325t, 326
Sulfur cycle, 346
Sulfur storage in *Thiobacillus*, 352
Suppurative otitis media, 603
Surface, bacterial, 119–127
Surface phagocytosis, 422
Surface replicas, 70
Sylvatic plague, 649
Symbiosis:
  commensalism, 335
  in ecosystem, 330–336
  mutualism, 331–335
  parasitism, 335–336
  rumen, 333, 335
Symbiotes, 147t
  nonpathogenicity of, 155
Symbiotic relationship:
  of bacterial viruses, 221
  of protozoa, 181
Syngamy in protozoa, 186
Syntropism, 330
Syphilis:
  arsenic for, 363
  arteritis in, 677
  chemotherapy of, 391t
  clinical features of, 675t

complement-fixation test for, 477, 478f
congenital, 677–678
dark-field microscopy for, 63, 676
endemic, 678
incidence of, 675
late benign, 677
of oral cavity, 590t
organism causing, 61t, 152
primary, 676
secondary, 676–677
serological diagnosis of, 469t
specimen collection in, 548t
tertiary, 677
transmission of, 532, 676
Treponema pallidum in, 675–676
See also Treponema pallidum
Système International d'Unités, 50
Systemic infections. *See* Circulatory system
Systemic lupus erythematosus, 451t, 507

T

Taenia saginata, 728t
Taenia solium, 728t
Tapeworms:
infections by, 728t
structure of, 727
Target theory, 378
Tatum, Edward, 301–302
Taxonomy, 31
genetics and, 315–316
Linnaean system, 32
microbial, 8
in microbiology, 4–6
molecular approach to, 41
numerical, 40
Teeth:
anatomy of, 583
decay of, 589
See also Oral infections
Temperate virus, 223
Temperature effect in ecosystem, 325–326
Template hypothesis, 460
Termites, protozoa related to, 189
Tetanus, 571
antitoxin preparation for, 516–517
chemotherapy of, 390t
exotoxin in, 439t, 441
features of, 565t
immunization in, 571
organism causing, 61t
passive immunization against, 464
transmission of, 571
vaccine for, 512t
Tetracyclines, 395
Tetrahymena pyriformis, 328
Thallus, 205
Thermal death point, 371
Thermal death time, 371
Thermal exhaustion, 761
Thermal kill, 371
Thermoactinomyces, 325t, 326
Thermoduric, 244
Thermophilic organisms, 244, 326
Thermoplasma, 147–149
Thin sectioning, 70–71
Thiobacillus, 147
energy-yielding reactions of, 284
pH and growth of, 325t, 326
sulfur storage by, 352
Thioglycollate medium, 257
Thiothrix, 149
Throat, 597
Thrush, 575
Thunberg tube, 292
Thylakoids, 110, 130, 157
Thymine, 86
Thymus gland:
lack of development of, 493
role in immunity, 457–458
Thyroiditis, 451t
Ticks:
differentiated from mites, 536
in disease transmission, 531t, 535–536
life cycle of, 535–536
in relapsing fever, 651–652
in Rocky Mountain spotted fever, 653
Tinea infections, 573–575
See also Ringworm
Tissue cultures:
in animal virus cultivation, 231–234
indications of viral infection in, 233–234
in plant virus cultivation, 234–235
preparation of, 233
in protozoan cultivation, 187
T-lymphocytes, 458–460
in BCG role as immunological stimulator, 714
in hypersensitivity, 495, 501–502
Togaviruses, 228t, 576t, 579, 689
Tolnaftate, 405t
TOPV, 515
TORCH complex, 679
Toxicity index, 367
Toxins, 435
conversion into toxoids, 513
in diphtheria, 602
See also Endotoxin; Exotoxin
Toxoid:
adsorbed, 513
alum precipitated, 513
aluminum-hydroxide adsorbed, 513
natural fluid, 513
plain, 513
preparation of, 513
use in immunization, 464
Toxoplasma gondii:
disease caused by, 191
in toxoplasmosis, 679, 690–691
transmission of, 690–691
Toxoplasmosis, 181, 690
in animals, 531t
congenital, 679, 691
organism causing, 181, 191
prevention of, 691
transmission of, 531t, 690–691
Trachea, 599
Trachoma, 697, 698
chemotherapy of, 391t
organism causing, 154
Transcriptase, 216
reverse, 709
Transcription, 286
Transduction, 304, 309
Transfection, 306
Transfer RNA, 90
initiator, 288
in protein synthesis, 285
Transfer techniques, 252–253
Transformation, 304–306, 319
Transformation assays, 234
Transforming principle, 304
Transfusion reaction, 483, 500
with O type blood, 483
prevention of, 487–488
Rh incompatibility causing, 485–486
Translation, 286–287
Translocation, 301
Transmission electron microscope, 65–68
Transpiration, 767
Transplantation, 504
categories of, 504
genetic control of reactions to, 504–505
graft rejection after, 505–506
opportunistic infections after, 440t
Transposons, 311
Trauma and immunity, 431t
Traveler's diarrhea, 626t, 633
Trematodes, 727, 729
infections by, 729t
life cycle of, 729–730
Trench fever, 651t, 653
organism causing, 154
Treponema, 146t, 152
Treponema carateum, 675, 678
Treponema pallidum:
appearance of, 118
chemotherapy of, 391t
in congenital syphilis, 677–678
diagnostic characteristics in syphilis, 675–676
fluorescent antibody technique for, 480
hypersensitivity to, 677, 678
mechanism of action in disease, 435t
in primary syphilis, 676
in secondary syphilis, 676–677
See also Syphilis
Treponema pertenue, 675, 678
Treponematoses, 674–675
pinta, 675t, 678
syphilis, 672–676
yaws, 675t, 678
Triatoma, 537
Trichinella spiralis, 722, 725
Trichinosis, 722t, 723t
causative agent of, 725
hosts in, 722
life cycle of, 726f
skin test for, 482t
transmission of, 725
Trichocysts, 184, 187–188
Trichome, 157
Trichomonas hominis, 667, 678, 679
Trichomoniasis, 673t, 678–679
Trichuris trichiura, 722t
Trickling filter, 780–781
Triglycerides, 82, 83f
Trivalent oral poliomyelitis vaccine (TOPV), 515
Trophozoite, 185, 655
Trypanosoma cruzi, 693
Trypanosoma gambiense, 189
See also African sleeping sickness
Trypanosoma rhodesiense, 189
Trypanosomiasis, 691–692
American, 693
in animals, 531t
cold agglutinins in, 471
life cycle of, 692
prevention of, 693
transmission of, 531t, 692
See also African sleeping sickness
Trypsin in filtration sterilization, 382
Tsetse fly, 531t, 692
Tsutsugamushi fever, 653
Tubercle bacillus. *See Mycobacterium tuberculosis*
Tuberculin test, 481, 482t, 503, 612–613
Tuberculosis, 608, 610–611t
causative agent of, 608–609
chemotherapy of, 391t, 397–398
conditions predisposing to, 440t
healing of lesions in, 612
hypersensitivity reaction in, 502–503
of oral cavity, 590t
organism causing, 61t
pathogenesis of, 609, 612
pathology of, 612
predisposing factors to, 609
prevention of, 515–516, 613
skin tests for, 481, 482t, 612–613
specimen collection in, 548t
transmission of, 533, 609
vaccine for, 512t
See also Mycobacterium tuberculosis
Tubulins, 108
Tularemia, 650t
in animals, 531t
immunity after, 654
organism causing, 61t
tick involvement in, 536t
transmission of, 531t, 653–654
vaccine for, 512–513t
Tulip break, 234, 235f
Tumor, 703
Tumor-specific antigen, 713
Tyndall, John, 21
Typhoid fever, 626t, 632, 650t
causative agent of, 632, 654
chloramphenicol for, 395
mechanism of disease by causative agent, 435t
naturally acquired immunity to, 462–463
organism causing, 61t, 154
serologic diagnosis of, 469t
transmission of, 533, 632, 654
vaccine for, 512t, 521t
Widal test for, 471
Typhus:
epidemic, 650–652
flea-borne, 538, 650–651t, 653
lice and, 537

Typhus (*continued*)
mites and, 536
murine, 650–651t, 653
scrub, 650–651t, 653
serologic diagnosis of, 469t
transmission of, 536–538
vaccine for, 512t, 521t

U

Ultraviolet radiation sterilization, 370t, 377–378
Universal donor, 483
Universal recipient, 483–484
Unsaturated, 82
Upper respiratory infections, 600, 602
antibiotics in, 605
common cold, 605, 606t
croup, 606
diphtheria, 601–603
of ear, 601t, 603
streptococcal sore throat, 601t, 604
Uracil, 86
Ureaplasma, 148–149
Ureteral infections, 666
Urethritis:
nonspecific, 663t, 666–667
specific, 671
Urey, Harold, 42
Urinary tract, 661
anatomy of, 663
infections of, 663–664
acute pyelonephritis, 663t, 665–666
anaerobic, 667
conditions predisposing to, 440t, 664
cystitis, 662t, 666
diagnosis of, 664–665
nonspecific urethritis, 663t, 666–667
routes of infection, 664
symptoms of, 665
ureteral, 666
normal flora of, 661, 663
Urticaria, 496
Use-dilution test, 366

V

Vaccines, 464
administration of, 518–519
anamnestic responses and, 456
attenuated, 513–514
autogenous, 511, 513
for cancer, 708
cholera, 629
combined, 515
complications associated with, 519–521
currently in use, 514–515
hepatitis B, 640
immunogenic substances for, 449
inactivated, 514
injection of, 518
intranasal, 519
oral, 518–519
preparation of:
bacterial, 511–513
viral, 512–514
rabies, 688
radiation sterilization in production of, 379
requirements for use, 464
rickettsial, 511, 512t
safety of live versus inactivated, 514
Salk, 514
stock, 511
toxoids, 513
value of, 510–511
Vaccinia, 580
Vacuole:
contractile, 183
food, 183
in pinocytosis, 103
in plant cells, 111–112
Vaginitis, 672t
Valence, 450
Valine production, 741t
Valley fever. *See* Coccidioidomycosis
Varicella, 576t, 577
See also Chickenpox
Vectors, 154, 235–236
Vegetables, fermented, 751–752
Veillonella, 147t
electron micrographs of, 71f
Veins, 646
Venereal diseases, 661, 670, 672–673t
chancroid, 670–672
genital herpes, 672t, 678
gonorrhea, 671, 672t, 674
granuloma inguinale, 672t, 674
lymphogranuloma venereum, 672t, 674
syphilis, 673–677
trichomoniasis, 673t, 678–679
Venezuelan equine encephalitis vaccine, 379
Vesicle in pinocytosis, 103
Vibrio, 118, 146t
Vibrio cholerae:
in cholera, 628
immune cytolysis of, 475
immunizing properties of, 513
isolation media for, 245
pH and growth of, 245, 325t, 326
Vibrio parahemolyticus, 221
Vincent's infection, 588
Vinegar production, 740–741
Viral hepatitis:
causative agents of, 637–639
features of, 636t, 637
pandemic, 527
passive immunization against, 464
transmission of, 637–638
vaccine for, 640
Virchow, Rudolf, 102
Virion, 212
Virogene, 711
Viroids, 236
Virology, 6
See also Viruses
Virucide, 357t
Virulence, 436
Viruses, 212
animal:
cultivation of, 230–234
diseases caused by, 227
properties of, 228t
replication of, 227, 229
arthropod-borne, 689–690
associated with eucaryotes, 235–236
in autoimmunity, 506
bacteriophages, 218–226
in cancer:
current strategies to determine, 715
early history of, 706
hypotheses of mechanism for, 709–712
capsid organization, 216
cell transformation by, 705–706
chemotherapy against, 405–407
classification of, 39–40, 216, 218f
comparison with other microorganisms, 214t
complement-fixation tests of, 478t
cultivation of, 264–265
cyanophages, 226–227
cytopathic effect of, 445
enveloped, 215
eye infections by, 698–699
fungal, 236
helical, 215, 216f
hemagglutination inhibition in detection of, 469t, 471, 472
immune electron microscopy for, 480
inclusions in cells infected by, 227
infections due to:
arthropod borne, 689–690
aseptic meningitis, 684t, 686
chickenpox, 576t, 577
common cold, 606t
coxsackievirus in, 686–687
cytomegalovirus inclusion disease, 636t, 637
in eye, 698–699
in gastrointestinal tract, 636
hepatitis, 636–640
herpangina, 593
herpes simplex, 576t, 577, 594
herpes zoster, 576–578
infectious mononucleosis, 636t, 656–657
influenza, 616–617
latent, 444
mumps, 594
in nervous system, 686
picornavirus in, 636–637
poliomyelitis, 686
poxviruses in, 579–580
rabies, 687
slow virus disease, 688–689
smallpox, 580
warts, 578
in insect control, 227
interferon action on, 429
latent infections of, 444
lysogenic cycle of infection, 223
lytic cycle of infection, 223–225
mechanism of action in disease, 435t
in mouth flora, 584, 585t
neurotropic, 686
neutralization of, 469t, 481
nucleic acid of, 212–213, 225
nucleocapsid in, 213
oncogenic, 221, 227, 234
oral cavity infections by, 593–594
pathogenicity of, 443–445
pathological effects of, 444
in plant diseases, 234–235, 543
proportional counting of, 266
resistance to boiling, 374
respiratory tract infections of, 605–606, 616–617
Rivers' postulates for, 24
serologic procedures for, 481
shape of, 215
skin diseases caused by, 575–580
slow, 444, 688–689
specific properties of, 212
structure of, 212–216
temperate, 223
vaccines of, 512–514
viroids, 236
virulent, 222–223
zoonoses of, 531t
Vital dye, 267
Vitamin B_{12} synthesis, 741t
Vitamins:
in bacteriological media, 247
production of, 741t, 742
synthesis by normal flora, 415
Volutin, 130
von Dusch, Theodor, 19–20
Vulvovaginitis, 674

W

Wandering macrophages, 420, 423
Warts, 578
virus causing, 228t
Wasserman test, 477
Waste treatment, 773
advanced, 781–782
aerobic stabilization in, 780
anaerobic digestion in, 779–780, 782
composting, 784
in lagoons, 782
preliminary, 778
primary, 778–779
problems with, 784
secondary, 779–781
sewage properties, 773–774
solid, 783–784
trickling filter in, 780–781
Water:
contamination by microorganisms, 774–776
diseases transmitted in, 774–775
environmental properties of, 768–769
blooms, 769
and contamination, 774–775
estuaries, 771–772
flowing fresh water, 770–771
freshwater habitats, 769–771
littoral zone, 772
marine environment, 771–773
neritic zone, 772
oxygen content and, 768–769
pelagic zone, 772

standing fresh water, 769–770
temperature and, 768
fresh, 769
flowing, 770–771
standing, 769–770
microorganisms found in, 768
nutrient contamination of, 778
quality standards for, 776–778
in sewage, 773–774
ultraviolet radiation treatment of, 378
Water activity, 759
Water cycle, 767–768
Waxes, 82
Weathering, 765
chemical, 766
mechanical, 765–766
Weil-Felix test, 469t, 471
Weil's disease. *See* Leptospirosis
Wet-mount preparation, 58
Wheal-and-flare reaction, 482, 498
Whipworm infestation, 722t
White blood cells. *See* Leukocytes
Whittaker, Robert, 37
Whooping cough, 610–611t, 614
chemotherapy of, 391t
exotoxins involved in, 439t
organism causing, 61t
prevention of, 614
transmission of, 614
vaccine for, 512t
Widal test, 469t, 471
Wine production, 738–739
Wöhler, Friedrich, 15
Worms, 717–718
See also Helminths
Wound botulism, 571
Wuchereria bancrofti, 722t, 723
Wuchereria malayi, 723–724

X

Xanthomonas:
bacteriophage attacking, 221
phytoxins of, 442
Xanthomonas oryzae, 221
Xenograft, 504
Xenopsylla, 649

Y

Yaws, 675t, 678
of oral cavity, 590t
Yeasts, 162, 164f, 165
in beer production, 738
budding, 164f, 171
counting chamber for, 267
fermentation of, 171
hydrocarbon degradation by, 349
nitrate assimilation by, 345t
nitrogen fixation by, 344t
petite colony mutant of, 311
reproduction of, 162, 165
in wine production, 738–739
Yellow fever:
in animals, 531t
mosquitoes in, 538t
transmission of, 531t, 538t
vaccine for, 513t, 521t
virus causing, 228t
Yersin, Alexander, 602, 649
Yersinia, 146t
opportunistic infections of, 440t
Yersinia pestis:
chemotherapy of, 391t
exotoxin producing disease, 439t
in plague, 648–649
See also Plague

Z

Z value, 371–372
Zernike, Fritz, 65
Ziehl-Neelson procedure, 62
Zinc as antifungal agent, 363–364
Zoogloeal masses, 781
Zoonoses, 529–531
Zooplankton, 195, 769
Zoospores, 196
Zygomycetes, 169t, 174–175